# THE ARCHIVES
OF
# INTERNAL MEDICINE




VOLUME VII

1911

CHICAGO

AMERICAN MEDICAL ASSOCIATION

PUBLISHERS

1566

# CONTENTS OF VOLUME VII

## JANUARY, 1911. NUMBER 1


PAGE

Observations on the Spirilla of Relapsing Fever. Henry A. Christian, M.D., Boston .......... 1

Diphtheria Bacillus-Carriers, with a Report of a Case Treated by Overriding the Infected Area with Staphylococcus Pyogenes Aureus. Henry Page, M.D., Manila, P. I. .......... 16

A Study of Streptococci with the Complement-Fixation and Conglutination Reactions. Homer F. Swift, M.D., and W. C. Thro, M.D., New York .......... 24

A Report of Fifty Examinations of Cerebrospinal Fluid with Special Reference to the Cell-Count. Addison Bybee, M.D., Elgin, Ill., and W. F. Lorenz, M.D., Kankakee, Ill .......... 38

Observations on Schürmann's Color Test for Syphilis. Robert Goldsborough Owen, M.D., Detroit .......... 52

Is Hemoglobinuric Fever a Manifestation of Malaria or a Disease Sui Generis? Charles F. Craig, M.D., Washington, D. C. .......... 56

A Study of the Ventilation of Sleeping-Cars. Thomas R. Crowder, M.D., Chicago .......... 85

Book Review:—Medical Education in the United States and Canada. By Abraham Flexner .......... 134


## FEBRUARY, 1911. NUMBER 2


The Diagnostic Value of the Orthodiagram in Heart Disease. J. G. Van Zwaluwenburg, M.D., and L. F. Warren, M.D., Ann Arbor, Mich. .......... 137

Studies of Malaria in Panama. II. Treatment of Blackwater Fever: Pernicious Malaria with Hemoglobinuria and Erythrolytic Hemoglobinuria. Walter Brem, M.D., Colon Hospital, Cristobal, Canal Zone .......... 153

Meralgia Paresthetica Due to Pressure of the Corset. Joseph L. Miller, M.D., Chicago .......... 182

The Energy Metabolism of Mother and Child Just Before and Just After Birth. Thorne M. Carpenter, B.S., Boston, and John R. Murlin, Ph.D., New York .......... 184

The Ameboid Activity of Megaloblasts. William Sidney Thayer, M.D., Baltimore .......... 223

The Function of the Sino-Auricular Node. Alfred E. Cohn, M.D., and Leo Kessel, M.D., New York .......... 226

Studies on the Biology of and Immunity Against the Bacillus of Leprosy with a Consideration of the Possibility of Specific Treatment and Prophylaxis. Charles W. Duval, M.D., and Fraser B. Gurd, M.D., New Orleans .......... 230

A Blood-Crisis Occurring with Primary Sarcoma of the Stomach. LeRoy H. Briggs, M.D., Oakland, Cal. .......... 246

A Study of the Technic of the Cammidge Reaction and of the Substance Giving Rise to the So-Called Typical Crystals. Joseph C. Roper, M.D., and Ralph G. Stillman, M.D., New York .......... 252

Allergy. C. E. von Pirquet, M.D., Baltimore .......... 259

*CONTENTS OF VOLUME VII*

## MARCH, 1911. NUMBER 3


PAGE

A Study of Two Cases of Adams-Stokes' Syndrome with Heart-Block. W. S. Thayer, M.D., Baltimore and F. W. Peabody, M.D., Cambridge, Mass. .......... 289

A Case of Poisoning Due to Eating Poison-Hemlock (Cicuta Maculata), with a Review of Reported Cases. Anfin Egdahl, M.D., Menomonie, Wis. .......... 348

The Opsonic Index in the Diagnosis of Mixed Infection in Pulmonary Tuberculosis. Roswell T. Pettit, Ottawa, Ill. .......... 357

Entamœba Tetragena as a Cause of Dysentery in the Philippine Islands. Charles F. Craig, M.D., Washington, D. C. .......... 362

The Acidosis Index: A Clinical Measure of the Degree of Acidosis. T. Stuart Hart, M.D., New York .......... 367

Acute Yellow Atrophy of the Liver: Report of Two Cases. Emil Novak, M.D., and E. L. Whitney, M.D., Baltimore .......... 376

Allergy. C. E. von Pirquet, M.D., Baltimore .......... 383

Book Review:—Innere Sekretion. Ihre physiologischen Grundlagen und ihre Bedeutung für die Pathologie. By Dr. Artur Biedl, Vienna .......... 437


## APRIL, 1911. NUMBER 4


Blood-Pressure in Tuberculosis. Haven Emerson, M.D., New York .......... 441

Pyrogenic Action of Salt Solutions in Rabbits. Henry F. Helmholz, M.D., Chicago .......... 468

The Retention of Alkali by the Kidney with Special Reference to Acidosis. Herman M. Adler, M.D., Hathorne, Mass., and Gerald Blake, M.D., Boston .......... 479

The Effects of Certain Internal Secretions on Malignant Tumors. G. L. Rohdenburg, M.D., F. D. Bullock, M.D., and P. J. Johnston, M.D., New York .......... 491

The Duration of Trypanosome Infections. John L. Todd, M.D., Montreal, Canada .......... 500

The Pathological Anatomy of the Human Thyroid Gland. David Marine, M.D., and C. H. Lenhart, M.D., Cleveland, Ohio .......... 506

Studies on Water-Drinking. IV. The Excretion of Chlorids Following Copious Water-Drinking Between Meals. S. A. Rulon, Jr., M.D., and P. B. Hawk, Ph.D., Urbana, Ill. .......... 536

The Use of Digipuratum in Heart-Disease. William F. Boos, M.D., L. H. Newburgh, M.D., and Henry K. Marks, M.D., Boston .......... 551

A Case of Strongyloides Intestinalis with Larvæ in the Sputum. John G. Gage, M.D., New Orleans .......... 561

Book Review:—The Elements of the Science of Nutrition. By Graham Lusk .......... 580


## MAY, 1911. NUMBER 5


Oriental Sore in Panama. S. T. Darling, M.D., Ancon, C. Z. .......... 581

The Use of Blood Charcoal as a Clearing Agent for Urine Containing Glucose. R. T. Woodyatt, M.D., Evanston, and H. F. Helmholz, M.D., Chicago .......... 598

Chlorid and Water Tolerance in Nephritis. Karl M. Vogel, M.D., New York .......... 602

PAGE

Studies on Water-Drinking. V. Intestinal Putrefaction During Copious and Moderate Water-Drinking with Meals. W. M. Hattrem and P. B. Hawk, Ph.D., Urbana, Ill ........ 610

The Determination of the Catalytic Activity of the Blood as a Clinical Diagnostic Method. M. C. Winternitz, M.D., G. R. Henry, M.D., and F. McPhedran, M.D., Baltimore ........ 624

A Study of the Internal Function of the Pancreas in Carbohydrate Metabolism. Joseph H. Pratt, M.D., and Lesley H. Spooner, M.D., Boston ........ 665

Tuberculous Retroperitoneal Adenitis Connecting by Sinus with the Duodenum. Report of a Case with Autopsy. Merrick Lincoln, M.D., Worcester, Mass. ........ 680

Synchronous Cardiac and Respiratory Rate. Report of a Case. George William Norris, M.D., Philadelphia ........ 691

The Utilization of Fats and Oils given Subcutaneously. Lloyd H. Mills, M.D., New York, with the Assistance of Ernest A. Congdon, Chemist ........ 694

## JUNE, 1911. NUMBER 6

Calcification and Ossification. H. Gideon Wells, M.D., Chicago ........ 721

Intra-Abdominal Pressures. Haven Emerson, M.D., New York ........ 754

The Effects on Blood-Pressure of Intravenous Injections of Extracts of the Various Anatomical Components of the Hypophysis. Dean Lewis, M.D., Joseph L. Miller, M.D., and S. A. Matthews, M.D., Chicago ........ 785

The Value of Trophic Bone Changes in the Diagnosis of Leprosy. A. B. Herrick, M.D., and T. W. Earhart, M.D., Ancon Hospital, Canal Zone ........ 801

An Experimental Study of the Causes Which Produce the Growth of the Mammary Gland. Robert T. Frank, M.D., and A. Unger, B.S., New York ........ 812

Index ........ 839

# THE ARCHIVES OF INTERNAL MEDICINE

## A CHANGE IN FORM

Letters of complaint regarding the bulkiness of the ARCHIVES in its former shape have prompted the Editorial Board to change the form slightly.

The change consists in a narrowing of the margins, the type page being the same in width, but containing three more lines in length. The quality of the paper is slightly improved, and is of softer finish.

We believe that in its present form the ARCHIVES will give more satisfaction, especially to those who desire to carry a copy with them.

# The Archives of Internal Medicine

Vol. VII | JANUARY, 1911 | No. 1

## OBSERVATIONS ON THE SPIRILLA OF RELAPSING FEVER *

HENRY A. CHRISTIAN, M.D.
BOSTON

The recent study of Darling[1] on the relapsing fever of Panama has called renewed attention to the probable existence of several distinct varieties of spirilla or spirochetes[2] causing types of relapsing fever. The subdivision of these organisms into varieties depends for the greater part on differences in the results obtained after animal inoculation, and as relatively only a few organisms have been so studied up to the present time, it seems desirable to record certain observations which I have been able to make on spirilla obtained from a patient admitted to my service at the Carney Hospital. These observations are far from complete. It was impossible to secure more than three monkeys at that time in the American market, and the local supply of white rats was too small for the simultaneous inoculation each day of several animals. These facts caused the paucity of observations on the monkeys and the early loss of the organism from failure of two rats to develop the infection after their inoculation. The observations made, however, will have some value in connection with those of other investigators.

### REPORT OF CASE

*History.*—The patient, P. N., married, aged 23, from whom the spirilla were obtained, was a native of Macedonia, who had just landed in Boston, and who had been a farmer in his home. He was admitted to the medical service at the Carney Hospital, Feb. 23, 1910. He had had no previous illness. Eighteen days before admission he sailed from a Mediterranean port. He became seasick almost immediately, vomited much during the entire trip and felt very weak. During the last five days of the voyage, he was reported to have had fever. He said that in his native town his wife and others had had a sickness with chills and fever,

---

* From the Medical Clinic of the Carney Hospital and the Laboratory of the Department of the Theory and Practice of Physic, Medical School, Harvard University.

1. Darling, S. T.: The Relapsing Fever of Panama, The Archives Int. Med., 1909, iv, 150.

2. The term "spirilla" will be used in this communication, since it is the term more generally used by clinicians in connection with descriptions of relapsing fever. It seems advisable to continue this usage until investigators are more fully agreed as to the proper classification and terminology for organisms of this group.

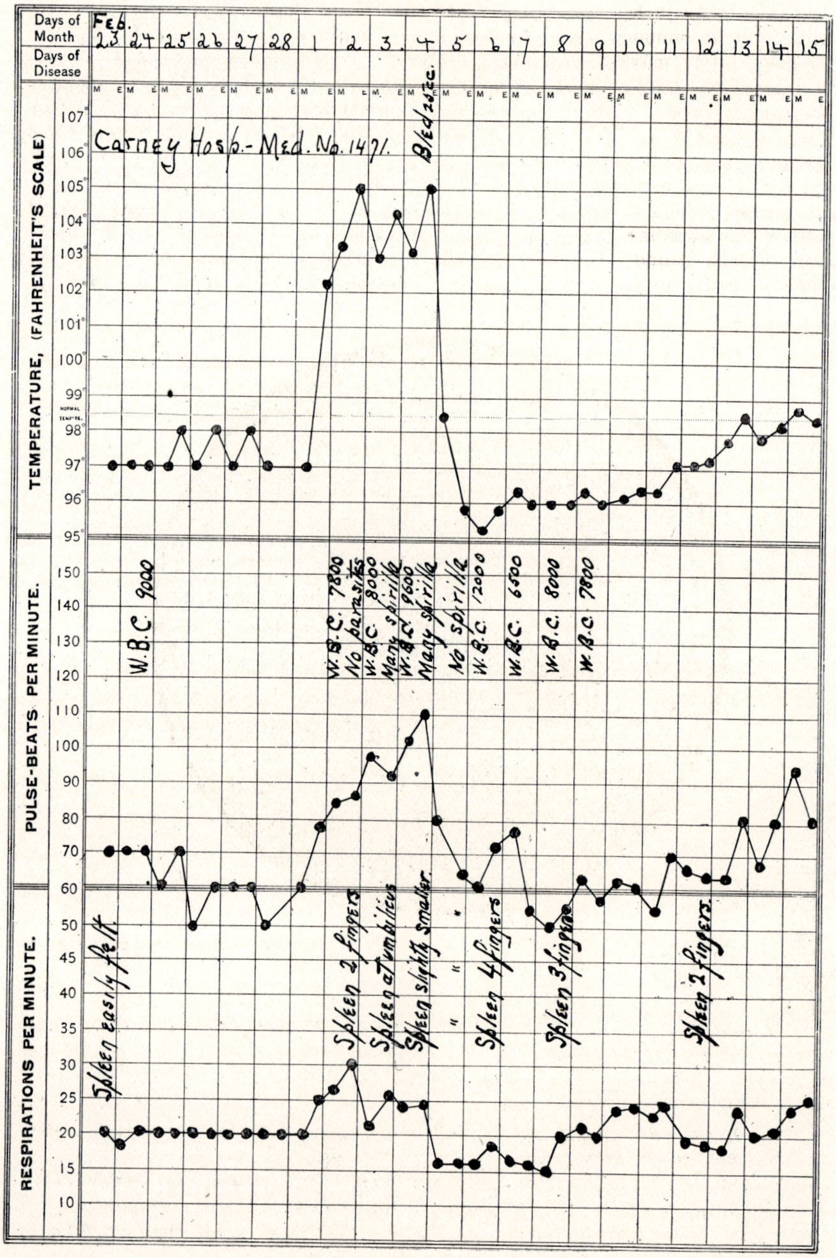


Fig. 1.—Chart of temperature, pulse and respiration of patient with relapsing fever.

but no other information as to the possible frequency of relapsing fever in his native land could be obtained.

*Physical Examination.*—A poorly developed, poorly nourished young man, lying comfortably in bed, breathing at ease. Eyes: Pupils equal, regular, react to light and accommodation; external ocular muscles appear normal. Mouth: Teeth poor, fairly marked pyorrhea alveolaris. Tongue clean, protruded in mid-line. Pharynx negative. Neck: Small, palpable glands on both sides, no rigidity or visible pulsation. Chest: Thin-walled, symmetrical, numerous scratch marks (patient had many lice, pediculi vestimentorum and pediculi capitis, on him when admitted). Heart: Upper border of percussion dulness at the third rib, right border at right sternal margin, left border 3¼ inches from mid-sternal line; heart action slow and regular; sounds distinct, no murmurs. Lungs: Good resonance throughout; a few râles and diminished breath sounds at both bases behind; breath sounds throughout rest of both lungs appeared to be normal. Abdomen: Soft, no tenderness, spasm or masses. Liver dulness from fifth rib

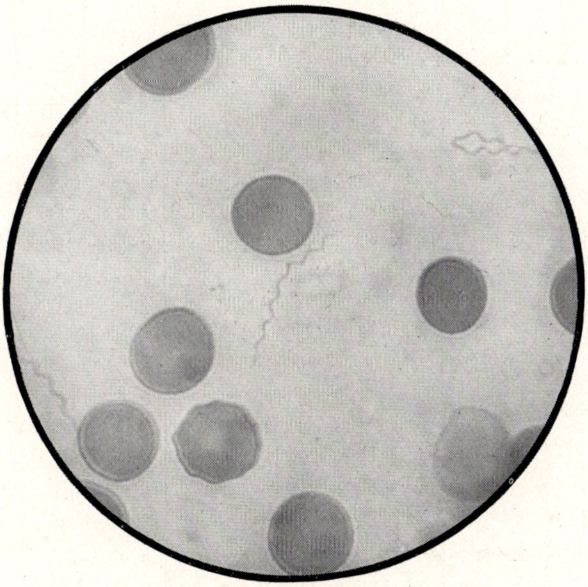

Fig. 2.—Monkey 2: Smear from peripheral circulation stained with Wright's stain, showing spirilla. Magnification, 1,500 diameters.

to costal margin, edge not felt. Spleen outline not made out, edge easily felt. Radial arteries slightly thickened. Pulses equal, regular, slow, of good volume and tension. Reflexes: Knee-jerks present, no Babinski, no Kernig, no ankle-clonus. Extremities appear normal.

*Course of Disease.*—February 27: Condition good, temperature normal, pulse slow. Patient seems very weak.

March 1: Patient had chill this afternoon while sitting up; temperature rose to 103°, pulse became rapid (Fig. 1). Lungs clear, throat normal.

March 2: This morning spleen seemed to be a little larger than previously, came about two-fingers' breadths below costal margin.

March 3: At about midnight last night the patient was complaining of pain in left upper quadrant of abdomen, which seemed distended. Spleen extended nearly to umbilicus and was tender. There was spasm over the whole of left upper quadrant. Temperature at 8 p. m., 105° F. This morning spasm had disappeared and patient appeared more comfortable. Splenic dulness from fifth interspace in mid-axilla to umbilicus. Spleen could be felt extending out to mid-line and in the left flank 6½ inches from mid-line. By percussion and palpation spleen appeared to be about 11 inches long and 9 inches wide.

March 4: Spleen seems to be a little smaller. At 8 p. m. temperature was 104° F.; at midnight it was normal. At noon to-day 25 c.c. of blood were taken from the median basilic vein, defibrinated and used for animal inoculations.

(See second paragraph following this report; also section headed "Animal Reactions.")

March 5: Temperature subnormal, patient comfortable. Spleen smaller.

March 6: Spleen extends 4 inches below costal margin in mammillary line; upper limit of percussion dulness at sixth rib. Lungs clear.

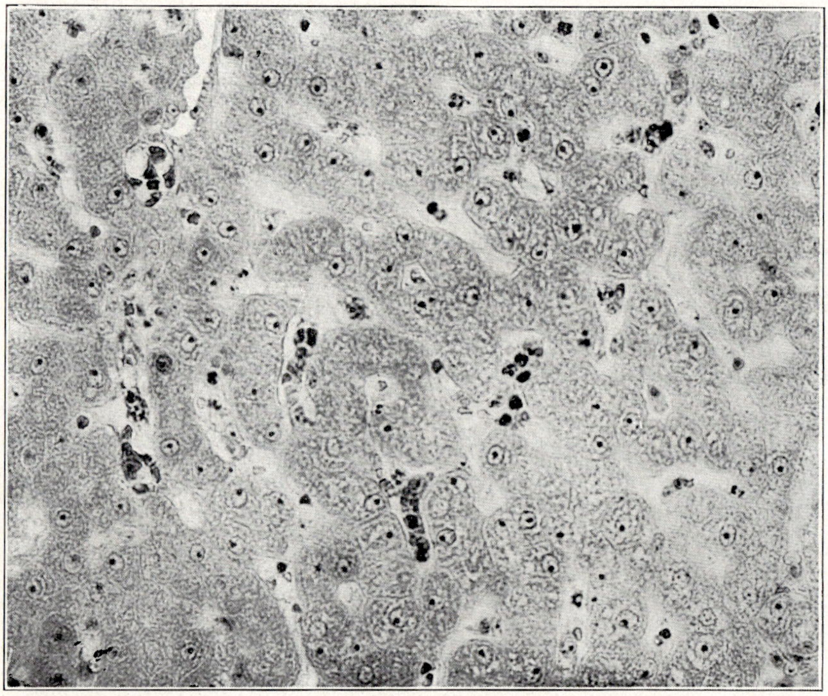

Fig. 3.—Monkey 2: Liver, showing accumulation of polynuclear leukocytes in sinusoids of the liver. Magnification, 375 diameters.

March 8: Spleen extends from ninth rib in mid-axillary line to a point 3¼ inches below costal margin in mammillary line. General condition good. Patient out of bed.

March 16: Temperature normal; no change in condition since last note.

March 30: General condition improving. Temperature remains normal. Spleen is still palpable.

April 3: No further rise in temperature since March 5. Patient discharged to-day.

*Blood Examinations.*—February 24: Hemoglobin, 90 per cent.; leukocyte count, 9,000. Smear shows no parasites.

March 2: Leukocyte count, 7,800. Smear shows no parasites.

March 3: Leukocyte count, 8,000. Smear shows spirilla.
March 4: Leukocyte count, 9,600. Smear shows spirilla.
March 5: No spirilla found.
March 6: Leukocyte count, 12,000.
March 7: Leukocyte count, 6,500.
March 8: Leukocyte count, 8,000.
March 9: Leukocyte count, 7,800.
March 20: Leukocyte count, 10,000.

The most interesting clinical feature in this case was the very rapid and very marked enlargement of the spleen, which occurred in less than twenty-four hours. The tension on the capsule of the spleen in this distention was marked enough to produce much pain, tenderness and spasm

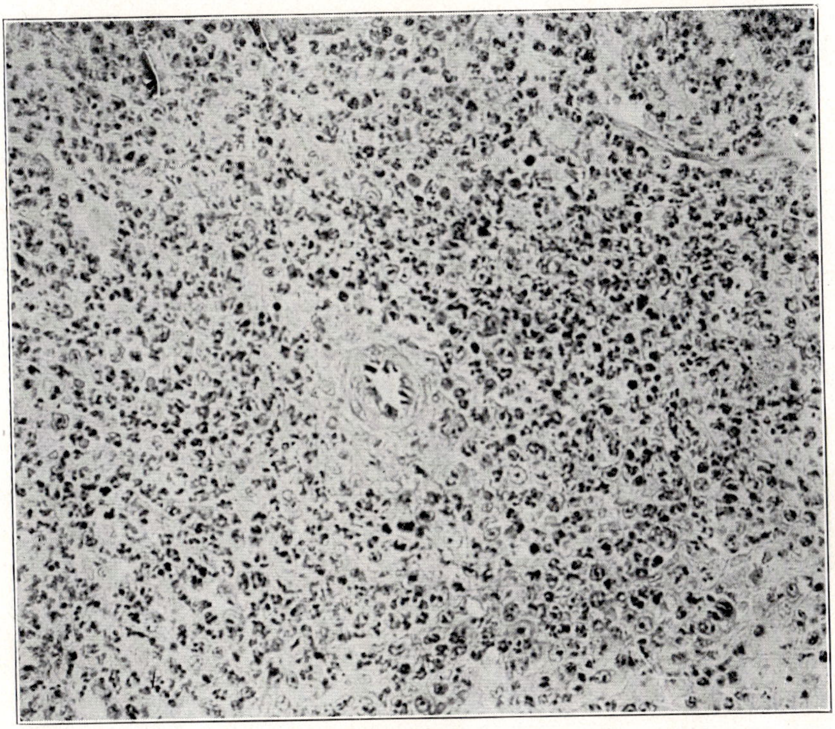

Fig. 4.—Monkey 2: Spleen, showing central portion of the Malpighian follicle, with very great infiltration with polynuclear leukocytes. Magnification, 375 diameters.

in the adjacent abdominal muscles. The suddenness of the enlargement during the night aroused fears in the house-officer in charge of the patient (Dr. Quigley) that the spleen might rupture. The spirilla were found in the circulating blood for the first time during the second day of the febrile period. They were absent the previous day; they were still present on the third day, and entirely disappeared with the fall in temperature on the fourth day after the onset of fever. During a month's subsequent observation organisms were not again found, and the patient had no recurrence of fever. From the somewhat imperfect history obtained from the patient through an interpreter, it is probable that the febrile period observed in the hospital was the second febrile period of the disease, and, as it proved, the last.

Blood obtained from the patient on the third day of the febrile paroxysm was defibrinated and inoculated into rats, rabbits, guinea-pigs and a monkey. The monkey was inoculated intraperitoneally. The rats and guinea-pigs were inoculated both intraperitoneally and subcutaneously. One rabbit was inoculated intravenously and another intraperi-

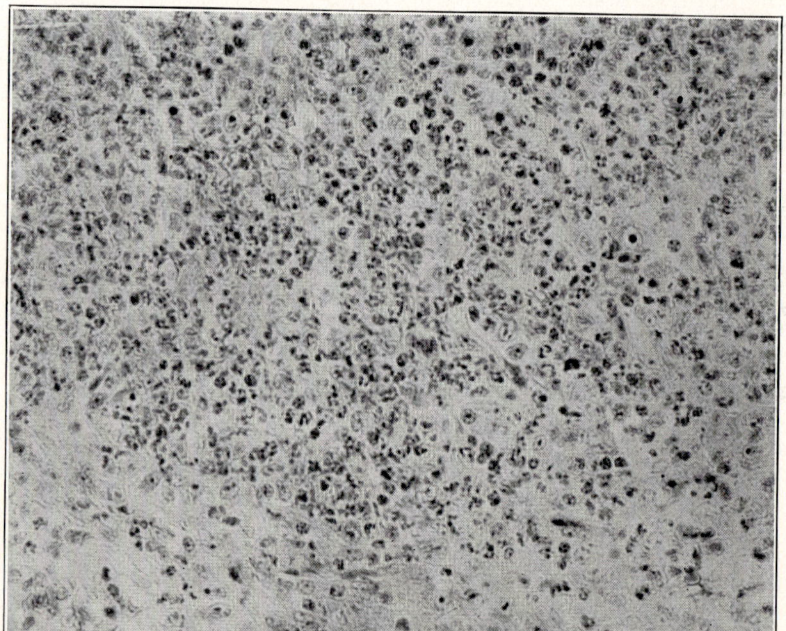

Fig. 5.—Monkey 2: Spleen, showing edge of Malpighian follicle, with marked infiltration with polynuclear leukocytes. Magnification, 375 diameters.

toneally. Each animal received from 1 to 1.5 c.c. of the blood from the patient.

### MORPHOLOGY OF THE SPIRILLA

Spirilla were numerous in the circulating blood of the patient and of the rats and monkeys which reacted positively to the inoculations. They presented the typical wavy appearance in smear preparations, and stained readily with Wright's stain. The morphology in such preparations is shown in Figure 2, a specimen from Monkey 2. Most of the spirilla in smear preparations from the patient varied in length from 16 to 22 microns. The very long forms probably represented more than one organism joined end to end. Those in smear preparations from the monkey (Monkey 2) varied in length within the same limits. The average thickness of the spirilla varied very slightly whether the forms were short or long. Blood from the human being and from the animals was studied also by means of the dark field illumination apparatus. This method of study proved very convenient as a rapid means of determining the presence or absence of spirilla in a given case. When examined in this way in fresh preparations, it was seen that the spirilla had, instead of the more wavy structure observed in the dry smears, a distinct cork-

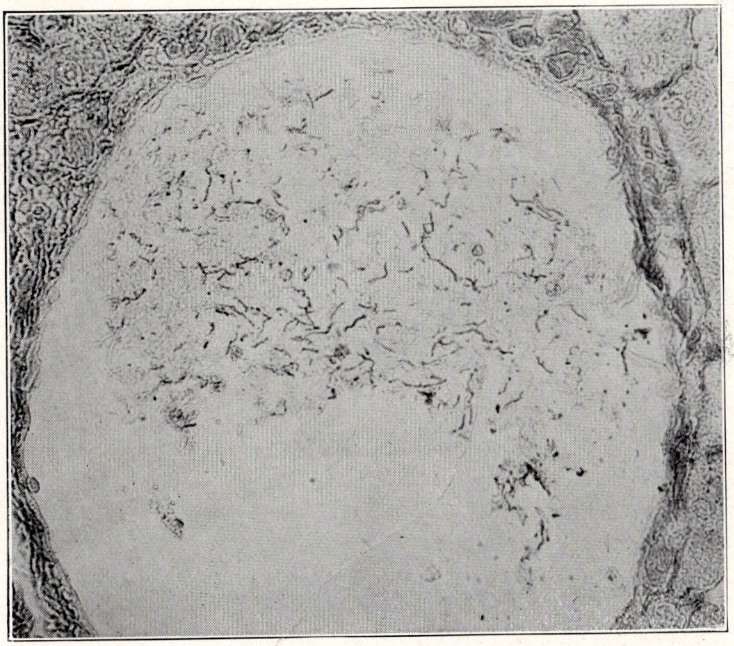

Fig. 6.—Monkey 2: Liver stained by the Levaditi method of silver impregnation, showing a vein containing spirilla. Magnification, 1,000 diameters.

screw arrangement of curves, the individual curves being very much closer together and so more numerous in the given organism than was the case when seen in smear preparations. Soon after the blood was drawn the spirilla had a very active motility, moving rapidly to and fro about the field. No effort was made to determine the range of motion, but the organisms frequently appeared and disappeared from a given field. As the activity of motion decreased, it became apparent that the organisms had a complex motion, consisting of an undulatory motion and a rotary motion. The rotary motion appeared to be sometimes in one direction, at other times in the other and while watching a given organism, sometimes the impression was made that the organism reversed its motion. This, however, could not be actually determined, and easily might have been merely an optical illusion.

Some of the blood obtained from the patient on March 4 was kept under aseptic precautions at room temperature. Twenty-four hours later the motility of the spirilla was still very great, and it seemed as if there had been probably some actual increase in the number of organisms. This, however, was more an impression than otherwise, since no means to actually count the organisms were taken. The temperature of the room during these observations was 66 F. Forty-eight hours later the same

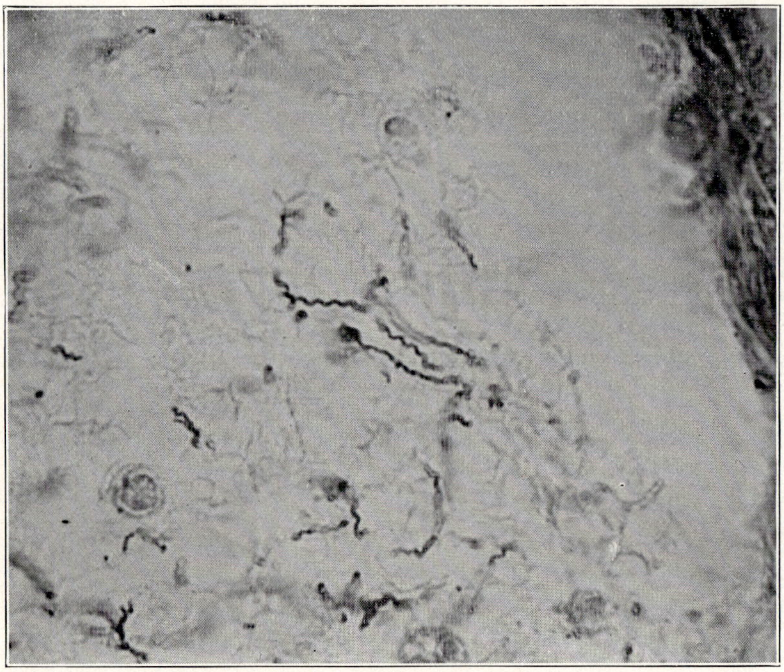

Fig. 7.—Monkey 2: Liver stained by the Levaditi method of silver impregnation, showing a vein containing spirilla. Magnification, 1,500 diameters.

organisms still showed active motility. Four days later, on March 8, there were still a moderate number of motile organisms in this same blood. No further observations were made upon this blood for a period of about two weeks, at which time living organisms no longer could be found.

ANIMAL REACTIONS

Three monkeys were utilized in studying the reaction of monkeys to the spirilla. All three of these were Macacus monkeys. Monkey 1 was inoculated intraperitoneally on March 4 (see Table 1) with blood from

TABLE 1.—INOCULATIONS OF MONKEYS WITH SPIRILLA OF RELAPSING FEVER.

*Monkey 1.*

| Date. | A.M. | P. M. | Temp. (Cent.) | Result. | Remarks. |
|---|---|---|---|---|---|
| 3/4 | .... | 1:15 | .... | ............ | Inoculated from patient. |
| 3/5 | 10:00 | .... | 39 | No spirilla. | |
| 3/6 | 11:40 | .... | 39.7 | No spirilla. | |
| 3/7 | 10:00 | .... | 39.7 | Many spirilla. | Bled (see Monkey 2). |
| 3/8 | .... | 6:15 | 41.5 | Many spirilla. | |
| 3/9 | .... | .... | ... | Blood not examined. | |
| 3/10 | 9:00 | .... | 39 | No spirilla. | Killed. |

*Monkey 2.*

| Date. | A.M. | P. M. | Temp. (Cent.) | Result. | Remarks. |
|---|---|---|---|---|---|
| 3/7 | .... | 6:15 | ... | ............ | Inoculated from Monkey 1. |
| 3/8 | .... | .... | ... | Blood not examined. | |
| 3/9 | .... | .... | ... | Blood not examined. | |
| 3/10 | 9:00 | .... | 39.5 | Few spirilla. | |
| 3/11 | 11:30 | .... | 40.2 | Many spirilla. | Killed (see Monkey 3). |

*Monkey 3.*

| Date. | A.M. | P. M. | Temp. (Cent.) | Result. | Remarks. |
|---|---|---|---|---|---|
| 3/11 | .... | 12:45 | ... | ............ | Inoculated from Monkey 2. |
| 3/12 | .... | 4:20 | 39.9 | No spirilla. | |
| 3/13 | .... | .... | ... | Blood not examined. | |
| 3/14 | .... | 4:00 | 39 | No spirilla. | |
| 3/15 | .... | 6:00 | 39 | Few spirilla. | |
| 3/16 | .... | 3:40 | .... | Many spirilla. | |
| 3/17 | 11:00 | .... | 40.7 | Many spirilla. | |
| 3/18 | 9:15 | .... | 39 | Many spirilla. | |
| 3/19 | 9:45 | .... | 39.2 | No spirilla. | |
| 3/20 | 10:45 | .... | 39.2 | No spirilla. | |
| 3/21 | 9:45 | .... | 39 | No spirilla. | |
| 3/22 | 10:45 | .... | 39.1 | No spirilla. | |
| 3/23 | 9:45 | .... | 39 | No spirilla. | |
| 3/24 | .... | 3:30 | 40 | No spirilla. | |
| 3/25 | 9:15 | .... | 39.7 | No spirilla. | |
| 3/26 | .... | 3:10 | 39.2 | No spirilla. | |
| 3/27 | 10:30 | .... | 39.2 | No spirilla. | |
| 3/28 | .... | 4:00 | 39.1 | No spirilla. | |
| 3/29 | .... | 4:15 | ... | No spirilla. | |
| 3/30 | 9:00 | .... | 39.8 | No spirilla. | |
| 3/31 | .... | 3:15 | 39.8 | No spirilla. | |
| 4/1 | .... | 2:10 | ... | No spirilla. | |
| 4/2 | 8:30 | .... | 39 | No spirilla. | |
| 4/3 | 10:00 | .... | 38.8 | No spirilla. | |
| 4/4 | .... | 3:15 | ... | No spirilla. | |
| 4/5 | .... | 2:15 | ... | No spirilla. | |
| 4/6 | .... | 5:30 | ... | No spirilla. | |
| 4/7 | 9:30 | .... | ... | No spirilla. | |
| 4/8 | .... | .... | ... | No spirilla. | |
| 4/10 | 10:30 | .... | ... | No spirilla. | |
| 4/11 | .... | 4:45 | ... | No spirilla. | |
| 4/12 | 10:30 | .... | ... | No spirilla. | |
| 4/13 | .... | 5:30 | ... | No spirilla. | |

the patient, and on March 7 numerous organisms were found. On that date, March 7, Monkey 1 was bled, and with this blood Monkey 2 was inoculated, as shown in Table 1, where the various results of the monkey inoculations are tabulated. Monkey 3 was in turn inoculated with blood from Monkey 2. From this table it is seen that infection takes place in the monkey following intraperitoneal inoculation in three to four days.

What is of particular interest is that Monkey 3, though his blood was examined during a period of twenty-six days following the last appearance of organisms in his circulating blood, failed to show them again. In other words, in the only monkey observed over a period of time following the infection, no relapse took place, and in this respect the organism studied by us seems to differ from those previously studied. Though this is but a single observation, it shows that spirilla causing relapsing fever in man may not necessarily produce a relapse in monkeys.

Table 2.—Inoculations of Rats with Spirilla of Relapsing Fever.

| Date. | A. M. | P. M. | Result. | Remarks. |
|---|---|---|---|---|
| | | | *Rats 1, 2, 3, 4 and 5.* | |
| 3/4 | .... | .... | ............ | Inoculated from patient. |
| 3/5 | .... | .... | Blood not examined. | |
| 3/6 | 10:45 | .... | No spirilla. | |
| 3/7 | .... | 4:30 | No spirilla. | |
| 3/8 | .... | 5:30 | No spirilla. | |
| | | | *Rat 1.* | |
| 3/12 | 10:00 | .... | ............ | Reinoculated from Rat 9. |
| 3/13 | 10:15 | .... | No spirilla. | |
| | | | *Rat 8.* | |
| 3/7 | .... | 6:30 | ............ | Inoculated from Monkey 1. |
| 3/8 | .... | 6:00 | No spirilla. | |
| 3/9 | .... | .... | Blood not examined. | |
| 3/10 | .... | 5:30 | No spirilla. | |
| | | | *Rats 9, 10, 11, 12, 13 and 14.* | |
| 3/11 | .... | 1:00 | ............ | Inoculated from Monkey 2. |
| 3/12 | 9:00 | .... | Many spirilla. | |
| 3/12 | .... | 4:00 | Many spirilla. | |
| 3/13 | 10:15 | .... | Many spirilla in some rats; no spirilla in some rats. | |
| | | | *Rat 15.* | |
| 3/12 | 10:00 | .... | ............ | Inoculated from Rat 9. |
| 3/12 | .... | 4:10 | No spirilla. | |
| 3/13 | 10:15 | .... | Many spirilla. | |
| | | | *Rat 16.* | |
| 3/13 | 11:45 | .... | ............ | Inoculated from Rat 15. |
| 3/14 | .... | 4:00 | No spirilla. | |
| 3/15 | 10:00 | .... | No spirilla. | |
| | | | *Rat 17* | |
| 3/15 | .... | 6:40 | ............ | Inoculated from Monkey 3. |
| 3/16 | .... | 3:30 | No spirilla. | |
| 3/17 | 10:00 | .... | No spirilla. | |
| | | | *Rat 18.* | |
| 3/15 | .... | 6:40 | ............ | Inoculated from Monkey 3. |
| 3/16 | .... | 3:40 | Many spirilla. | |
| 3/17 | 10:00 | .... | Many spirilla. | |
| | | | *Rat 19.* | |
| 3/17 | 10:00 | .... | ............ | Inoculated from Rat 18. |
| 3/18 | 8:45 | .... | Many spirilla. | |

*Rat 20.*

| Date | A.M. | P.M. | Result | Remarks |
|---|---|---|---|---|
| 3/17 | 10:00 | .... | ............ | Inoculated from Rat 18. |
| 3/18 | 8:45 | .... | No spirilla. | |
| 3/18 | .... | 5:45 | No spirilla. | |
| 3/19 | 9:45 | .... | No spirilla. | |
| 3/20 | 12:15 | .... | No spirilla. | |
| 3/20 | 10:45 | .... | No spirilla. | |

*Rat 21.*

| Date | A.M. | P.M. | Result | Remarks |
|---|---|---|---|---|
| 3/18 | 11:45 | .... | ............ | Inoculated from Rat 19. |
| 3/19 | .... | 1:30 | No spirilla. | |
| 3/19 | .... | 5:00 | No spirilla. | |
| 3/19 | .... | 11:45 | No spirilla. | |
| 3/20 | 10:45 | .... | No spirilla. | |
| 3/21 | 9:30 | .... | No spirilla. | |
| 3/22 | 10:30 | .... | No spirilla. | |

In studying the reaction of the spirilla in white rats, twenty-one rats were employed. Five rats were inoculated on March 4 with blood obtained from the patient (Table 2). These inoculations were all intraperitoneal and 1 to 1.5 c.c. of blood was used in each instance. These rats were inoculated between 1:30 and 2 p. m. on March 4. They were not examined on March 5, but were all found to be negative at 10:45 a. m. on March 6. In other words, no one of the five rats inoculated directly from the patient showed organisms in its circulating blood forty-five hours after the inoculation, nor were any organisms found on examination during two subsequent days. As was subsequently shown in this study, the spirilla usually appear in the rat in less than twenty-four hours, and in some have disappeared in less than forty-eight hours. Consequently it may have been true that rats inoculated with blood from the patient became infected, but this infection was not detected owing to failure to examine the rats early enough. On the other hand, it has been claimed by some observers that the spirilla of Obermeier are not inoculable into rats directly from man, but that it is necessary to pass them first through monkeys, after which the rat is susceptible to the organism. The only further evidence that we have on this point is an experiment at a later date, which tends to show that one of the rats inoculated directly from the patient attained immunity to the organism, for on March 12 one of these rats was reinoculated with blood from a positive rat (Rat 9) at 10 a. m., and the next day, March 13, at 10:15 a. m., his blood showed no organisms, while a control rat not previously inoculated with the patient's blood, Rat 15 (also inoculated from Rat 9) showed an infection. As is seen from the results in other rats, however, not all of our rats, even though previously untreated, were susceptible, and so no definite conclusions can be drawn from these observations. Rat 8, inoculated on March 7 with blood obtained from Monkey 1, showed no organisms after twenty-four hours, and none at a subsequent date. Six rats, however, inoculated on March 11 with blood from Monkey 2, showed organisms in their circulating blood on the next day, while twenty-four hours later some still showed the organisms and others were negative. A second generation of organisms of this strain was obtained in Rat 15, but in Rat 16 a third generation did not result. Two rats were inoculated with blood from Monkey 3. One of these rats was positive, the other negative. A second generation of this strain was obtained in Rat 19, but not in Rat 20. Here again a third generation was not obtained, as shown in the results of inoculation of Rat 21.

Of the two guinea-pigs inoculated with blood, one subcutaneously, the other intraperitoneally, from the patient on March 4, both were negative on the day, March 7, on which Monkey 1, similarly inoculated, was positive. No examination of the guinea-pigs had been made previous to March 7.

The two rabbits inoculated March 4, one intravenously, the other intraperitoneally, showed no organisms on March 6, no examination having been made on March 5. The rabbits were similarly negative on March 7, after which time no systematic examinations were made.

An attempt was made to inoculate white mice with blood obtained from the patient, but these mice, as well as control mice newly brought to the laboratory, for some reason died in from twenty-four to forty-eight hours, and so no results were obtained from these inoculations.

Darling classifies the organisms of relapsing fever into four groups:

*Group A.*—The group causing a relapsing or recurring infection in man, monkeys, white mice and white rats, including *Sp. duttoni* and the tick fever of Africa.

*Group B.*—The group causing a recurring infection in man, monkeys and white mice, but with a single paroxysm in white rats. This group comprises the relapsing fever of Panama and the two cases cited by Carlisle.[3]

*Group C.*—The group causing a recurring infection in man and monkeys, but failing to cause an infection in small rodents with blood direct from human sources, yet causing an infection in small rodents after a preliminary passage through the monkey. This group includes the relapsing fever of Europe caused by *Sp. obermeieri.*

*Group D.*—The group causing recurring infection in man and monkeys, but only transient infection in white rats and white mice. This group includes the relapsing fever of Bombay caused by *Sp. carteri.*

The patient studied by me came almost directly from Macedonia, and it is probable that the organism belongs to Group C, spirilla of Obermeier. There are, however, some slight differences as shown by rather incomplete animal inoculations. It may be that more extensive study of this group of organisms by means of animal inoculation will show additional groups or subgroups of the spirilla causing this general type of disease, clinically known as relapsing fever, and that the organism studied by me represents such a subgroup.

---

3. Carlisle, R. J.: Jour. Infect. Dis., 1909, iii, 233.

## HISTOLOGY OF THE LESION OF THE MONKEY

For study of the lesion produced by inoculation into monkeys of blood infected with the spirilla there were available two monkeys: Monkey 1, killed three days after the first appearance of spirilla in the circulating blood, and forty-two hours after they were last observed in the circulation (though it is possible that this does not represent the time elapsed between the actual disappearance and the time the animal was killed, since the blood was not examined between 6:15 p. m., March 8, and 9 a. m. March 10, at which latter time no organisms were found, and the animal was killed three hours later); and Monkey 2, killed twenty-six hours after first finding of spirilla in the circulating blood, and at a time when the blood was teeming with organisms. Monkey 2 will be described first.

Monkey 2.—This animal was killed with chloroform anesthesia at 12:30 p. m., March 11, after having been partially bled. The body cavities were free from fluid; there was moderate congestion of the intestines; the lungs and heart were normal. The spleen seemed firm; capsule was tense; numerous grayish points, 1.5 to 2 mm. in diameter, were plainly visible through the capsule, while other parts of the spleen were of a dark purplish red color. The cut surface showed grayish areas, 1.5 to 2 mm. in diameter, standing out distinctly against a red background. The cut surface was not moist and was firm. The liver, kidneys, adrenals, stomach, large and small intestine all appeared normal. Mesenteric lymph-nodes along the root of the mesentery were distinctly enlarged, pinkish gray in color, and moist. The bone-marrow was reddish gray. Brain was normal in appearance. The tissues in part were hardened in Zenker's fluid, stained with eosin and methylene blue, and with Mallory's phosphotungstic acid hematein. Of these, the heart, lung, kidney, adrenal, stomach, intestine, striated muscle, cerebrum, cerebellum and spinal cord all appeared normal. The liver showed no definite lesion of the liver cells. In the sinusoids were collected an increased number of polynuclear leukocytes, usually aggregated in distinct foci, very completely filling the sinusoids at these points (Fig. 3). In addition to polynuclear leukocytes, there were a moderate number of mononuclear cells of the endothelial type. Some of these latter were phagocytic, and contained polynuclear leukocytes as inclusions. The spleen was the only organ to show a very marked lesion. This consisted of a focal infiltration with polynuclear leukocytes. These foci varied in size from quite small ones to areas a little over 1 mm. in diameter. In these foci polynuclear leukocytes were closely packed together, almost completely replacing the other cells of the spleen. Most often the polynuclear leukocytic foci occurred in the Malpighian follicles, sometimes very largely replacing the lymphocytic cells of the follicles (Fig. 4). The smaller foci in the Malpighian follicles usually occupied a part of the peripheral portion (Fig. 5). There were also foci of leukocytes, usually smaller, scattered in the pulp. In addition to these foci of polynuclear leukocytes, the only other demonstrable lesion consisted in a proliferation of the cells, both in the pulp and the Malpighian follicles, evidenced by a considerable number of mitotic figures. No active phagocytic cells were seen in the spleen. There was present a slight amount of coarse yellow-brown pigment. The bone-marrow was cellular, fairly actively hyperplastic, as indicated by the occurrence of scattered mitotic figures. The proliferation appeared to concern the cells of the polynuclear leukocyte series more than the other bone-marrow cells, but the change was not preponderatingly a leukocytic hyperplasia. The lymph-node was slightly hyperplastic.

Part of the tissue was hardened in formaldehyd solution, and stained by the Levaditi method of silver impregnation, in order to demonstrate the spirilla. Throughout the various viscera (heart, liver, kidney, lung, gastro-intestinal tract, striated muscle, bone-marrow and brain) numerous spirilla were seen within the blood-vessels (Figs. 6 and 7), but not outside the blood-vessels in the tissue itself. In the liver, some of the spirilla contained in the sinusoids appeared to be within phagocytic cells of the endothelial type, though most of the spirilla were evidently free in the plasma. The polynuclear leukocytes did not appear to take up the spirilla. In the spleen, since some of the reticulum took a black stain with the Levaditi method, interpretation of the findings was rather more difficult. but spirilla intact enough for positive identification were very infrequent in the general splenic tissue. There were present, however, in cells numerous granules which took the silver stain, and occasionally what appeared to be definitely remains of spirilla. These appeared to be present in the phagocytic cells of the endothelial type and not in the polynuclear leukocytes. Besides these, in the foci of polynuclear leukocyte increase, there were present quite numerous fragments of spirilla. For the most part these fragments appeared to be extracellular, though some undoubtedly were contained in cells that belonged to the leukocyte series. All of these fragments were short compared with the normal spirilla.

Monkey 1.—Killed by chloroform anesthesia, 9:15 a. m., March 10. Body cavities were free from fluid. Peritoneal cavity showed a long omentum covering distinctly congested intestine in which the larger individual vessels stood out prominently. Spleen was firm, felt tense. Its cut surface showed grayish points about 1 mm. in diameter on a red background. Cut surface was rather dry, retained its shape. The general color was rather pale red, with small grayish points as described above. The lungs were pink, soft, appeared normal on the outside. On cross-section, the lungs showed scattered dark-brown to black areas about 1 to 2 mm. in diameter. The liver showed a smooth surface of a grayish red color, cut surface the same. Heart, adrenals, kidneys, and brain and spinal cord all appeared normal. The tissues in part were hardened in Zenker's fluid, and stained with eosin and methylene blue and Mallory's phosphotungstic acid hematein. Of these, as in Monkey 2, all appeared normal, with the exception of the liver and spleen. The liver showed a slight focal increase of polynuclear leukocytes and phagocytic cells in the sinusoids. This, however, was much less marked than in Monkey 2. In the spleen, the Malpighian follicles were relatively smaller and the pulp more abundant than was the case in Monkey 2. In places the pulp was distinctly poor in cells. Scattered through the spleen were small foci of infiltrating polynuclear leukocytes. These occurred principally in the peripheral portion of the Malpighian follicles and adjacent to the trabeculæ of the spleen. Scattered through the pulp there were also polynuclear leukocytes, but these were not so numerous as in Monkey 2. Mitotic figures were fairly numerous throughout the spleen. Scattered here and there was a considerable amount of rather coarse yellow-brown pigment.

Part of the tissue was hardened in formaldehyd solution, and stained by the Levaditi method of silver impregnation, in order to demonstrate the spirilla. Throughout the various viscera (heart, liver, kidney, lung, gastro-intestinal tract, bone-marrow and spinal cord) no spirilla were seen free within blood vessels and none outside the blood-vessels in the tissue itself. In the liver, a very occasional recognizable fragment of a spirillum was seen within an endothelial cell, either free in the sinusoid or still attached to the wall of the sinusoid. In the same way in the spleen a very occasional recognizable fragment of a spirillum was seen, usually within a cell of endothelial type. Apparently in these tissues the spirilla had disappeared almost completely.

SUMMARY

In the circulating blood of a patient suffering from relapsing fever spirilla were found on the second and third days of a three-day paroxysm of fever. These spirilla were inoculated successfully into monkeys and white rats. Both failed to show recurrence of the organism after the first infection. The lesion produced in monkeys consists of an accumulation of polynuclear leukocytes and endothelial cells in the sinusoids of the liver, and a focal infiltration of the spleen with polynuclear leukocytes. The spirilla appear to be removed from the circulation in the monkey by phagocytosis, to a slight extent in the liver, more actively in the spleen.

252 Marlborough Street.

# DIPHTHERIA BACILLUS-CARRIERS

## WITH A REPORT OF A CASE TREATED BY OVERRIDING THE INFECTED AREA WITH STAPHYLOCOCCUS PYOGENES AUREUS

HENRY PAGE, M.D.
MANILA, P. I.

The army medical officer and physicians associated with schools and factories are far more concerned about prophylactic measures than they are about the treatment of individual cases. It is far more important to guard an army corps or a large school or factory against an invasion of diphtheria or typhoid than it is to display great ability in treating such cases after they have arisen.

This distinction is that which separates the "sanitarian" from the "physician," a distinction that is broader than it should be, for while a sanitarian may, without prejudice to his calling, be uninterested in the cure of disease, the physician cannot neglect his sanitary functions without fatal results. In a paper entitled "Diphtheria Carriers,"[1] by Myer Solis-Cohen, read in the Section on Hygiene and Sanitary Science of the American Medical Association, Chicago, 1908, the sanitary responsibility of the physician who treats cases of infectious disease is very ably emphasized. No physician can read this article and be easy in conscience unless he makes in the future a more careful sanitary survey of his diphtheria cases than has been customary in the past.

### AGENCIES IN THE SPREAD OF DIPHTHERIA

The evidence of this work and the writings of such masters as Graham-Smith[2] tend to show that the following agencies (briefly related) are chiefly active in the spread of diphtheria and suggest that it will perhaps be better hereafter to discredit "bad odors" and "defective plumbing" until a search for the "carrier" has failed.

1. *Diphtheria Convalescents.*—Graham-Smith's[3] and Cobbett's tables show that the period of persistence of virulent bacilli in clinical cases is as follows:

1. Solis-Cohen, Myer: Diphtheria Carriers, Their Discovery and Control, Jour. Am. Med. Assn., 1909, lii, 111.
2. Graham-Smith: Bacteriology of Diphtheria, Cambridge, 1908.
3. Graham-Smith: Bacteriology of Diphtheria, Cambridge, 1908, p. 421.

| Period of persistence of bacilli in days: | No. of cases: |
|---|---|
| 1-5 | 2 |
| 6-20 | 19 |
| 21-30 | 22 |
| 31-40 | 8 |
| 41-50 | 4 |
| 51-60 | 5 |
| 61-90 | 6 |
| 91-100 | 1 |
| Above 100 | 0 |

The mean period of persistence in these cases was 31.6 days. Fisher[4] reports three cases lasting 106, 107 and 111 days, respectively.

2. *Contacts.*—Park and Beebe[5] found that in fourteen families where isolation was imperfect, 50 per cent. of contacts harbored virulent bacteria. In families where isolation was good 10 per cent. of these living in the same houses became infected. Many of these infected contacts failed to develop clinical diphtheria.

3. *Apparently Normal Persons not Known to Have Been Exposed.*—The Massachusetts Board of Health[6] states that of persons not known to have been exposed to infection 3 per cent. harbored Klebs-Loeffler bacilli; of those known to have been exposed, from 8 to 50 per cent., Park[7] examined 330 apparently healthy persons and found 9.7 per cent. who harbored bacilli. Only 2.4 per cent. of these were virulent. Holmes[8] and Fisher[4] give a much smaller percentage (about 2 per cent.) and emphasize the very important fact that very few really healthy throats harbor the bacilli. These observations simply mean that in localities where throat diseases are prevalent greater care should be used to detect carriers.

4. *Fomites.*—Park[9] isolated living Klebs-Loeffler bacilli from a tiny bit of membrane four months after its removal from the throat. Bugbee[10] reports an epidemic transmitted through a library book which had been wrapped in paper, fumigated and opened only after eleven months had elapsed. Other illustrations are unnecessary.

5. *Tonsillitis.*—Every case of tonsillitis is diphtheria until it is proved to the contrary. It is believed that the personal experience of every physician confirms this axiom.

4. Fisher, J. W.: A Diphtheria Epidemic, Its Bearing on the Question of Bacillus Carriers, Animal Carriers and the Necessity of More Strict Quarantine Regulations, Jour. Am. Med. Assn., 1909, lii, 439.
5. Park and Beebe: New York Med. Rec., xlvi, 385.
6. Report of Massachusetts Assn. Board of Health, July, 1902.
7. Park: Pathogenic Bacteria and Protozoa.
8. Holmes: New York Med. Jour., 1908, lxxxvii,
9. Park: New York Med. Rec., 1892,
10. Bugbee: Am. Med., viii, 318.

6. *Animals.*—It is a general belief that cats are often the carriers of diphtheria. Low, Dawson and Klein are among the few that have studied this subject. Cows can be infected with diphtheria and in such cases Klein[11] believes that infection of the milk often results. Fisher[4] reports an epidemic in which rats and cats as bacillus-carriers were the chief sources of infection.

This is by no means the last word on the subject of sources of infection, but it is enough to illustrate the necessity of a thorough sanitary survey of each diphtheria case. Of these sources of infection the most troublesome of all is the human carrier. For while infected rats or cats can be killed, clothing burned, the dairyman reported to the board of health and rooms disinfected, the human carrier, whether he be a diphtheria convalescent or a person who has never been sick, is the most dangerous of all sources of infection and in most cases it is impossible to control his association with others. It is with this source of infection that this paper chiefly deals.

In addition to the diphtheria convalescent carrier Watson Williams classifies human carriers into three groups, as follows:

1. Patients who have general symptoms of ill health in association with chronic tonsillitis, membranous rhinitis, otorrhea, sores, etc., which prove to be diphtheritic. There is no question but that these cases have given rise to general epidemics.

2. Persons who have no symptoms of ill health but who have one or more of the above diphtheritic lesions. The reports of Burnett,[12] Newsholme,[13] Park and Beebe, and many others, leave no room to doubt the dangerous character of these cases.

3. Persons without ill health and without local symptoms, but in whom Klebs-Loeffler bacilli have been found by culture tests: This class consists of healthy infected contacts.

Williams quotes instances in which healthy infected contacts in institutions mixed freely with non-infected persons without ill results and implies that these infected contacts are harmless until they develop local symptoms.

Graham-Smith[2] aptly remarks that even if this opinion be correct a member of this group may at any time develop a cold, and become a member of Group 2, and hence these carriers are quite as dangerous as those of Group 2. The same author also quotes many instances in which perfectly healthy contacts have transmitted the disease, and believes that careful observation could probably multiply such examples. Bugbee,[14]

11. Klein: Etiology of Diphtheria, Local Gov. Board Rep., London, 1889, xxix.
12. Burnett: Brit. Med. Jour., 1900, xxi.
13. Newsholme: Public Health Lab., Univ. of Manchester, 1904.
14. Bugbee: Am. Med., 1904, viii.

Park and Beebe,[15] White,[16] Peck,[17] and many others support Graham-Smith's opinion that perfectly healthy persons carrying diphtheria proved to be virulent by animal inoculation, can give rise to epidemics even though remaining themselves in perfect general health and without developing any local symptoms.

### DIAGNOSIS OF CARRIERS

Every author on the subject of diphtheria insists that no carrier shall be released from quarantine until at least three or four negative cultures are obtained.

Graham-Smith[2] says that infected persons must be proved bacillus-free by three successive bacteriological examinations.

Fisher[4] affirms that in institutions four successive negative cultures, including two nasal cultures, are imperative.

Ricards[18] states that 22 per cent. out of nearly 2,000 persons released on laboratory findings were found positive. These quotations indicate that a single negative finding is inconclusive, and, did space permit, it could be shown that not only should four throat cultures be taken, but a bacteriological examination should be made of all throat, nose, eye, ear, skin lesions and even lesions of the genitalia.

### VIRULENCE OF CULTURES

No one should be regarded as a carrier and subjected to quarantine until the virulence of the bacilli found has been determined. Positive culture findings in convalescents or infected contacts may be accepted as evidence of virulency (this is not true of unexposed persons). If, however, the duration of persistence exceeds two or three weeks it becomes necessary to inoculate animals with the cultures to determine virulency. According to Graham-Smith in a few instances Klebs-Loeffler bacilli in throats have apparently lost their virulence to some extent, but in the great majority they have retained their full virulence up to date of final disapearance.

Prip[19] records a case in which diphtheria bacilli, diagnosed by morphological appearances alone, lasted 669 days; Meyer, one lasting 547 days; Le Gendre and Pochon,[20] one lasting 458 days. It is manifestly impossible to insist on quarantine for such lengthy periods.

15. Park and Beebe: New York Med. Rec., 1894, xlvi.
16. White: Boston Med. and Surg. Jour., 1901, cxlv.
17. Peck: Brit. Med. Jour., 1895, i.
18. Ricards: Am. Jour. Pub. Hyg., 1906, xvi.
19. Prip: Ztschr. f. Hyg., 1906, xxxvi.
20. Le Gendre and Pochon: Rev. obst., 1895, i.

### TREATMENT OF CARRIERS

"No one antiseptic seems to affect the presence of these bacilli in carriers more than another" (Meikle[21]). I am unable to quote any positive statement in conflict with this opinion. This same author states that season, sex, age, duration of illness, amount of membrane, locality of lesions and the amount of antitoxin given do not affect the duration or persistence of the bacilli.

Wassermann[22] claims to have hastened the disappearance of the bacilli by giving tabloids made from the serum of horses immunized against several strains of living diphtheria bacilli.

Martin[23] asserts that by injecting bacillary bodies intravenously or intraperitoneally he obtained a serum that applied locally hastened the disappearance of the bacilli.

Graham-Smith[3] notes a case in which the deep crypts of the tonsils were irritated with mustard oil to produce a local inflammation; the result was not successful. Peyler[24] reports several cases in which lingering bacilli were removed by total extirpation of unhealthy tonsil and adenoid tissue.

The use of diphtheria vaccines made from the patient's culture has never been tried. I wished to try it in the case reported in this paper and it was refused. It is probably not only a dangerous procedure but promises little prospect of success.

Stitt, of the U. S. Navy, suggested the use of a 2 per cent. dilution of liquor formaldehydi in glycerin, painted on the throat, relying on the properties, as shown by Rosenau, which that drug possesses of neutralizing toxins. This failed to give any result in the case reported below.

### CARRIERS TREATED SUCCESSFULLY BY OVERRIDING WITH STAPHYLOCOCCUS PYOGENES AUREUS

For many years outbreaks of tonsillitis in which *Staphylococcus pyogenes aureus* alone was found on culture have been reported. In my practice during the past thirty days I have seen seven such cases. As in this instance, such outbreaks have often been coincident with true diphtheria cases, but no report has been made showing that diphtheria resulted from the staphylococcus infections. On the other hand I recall many cases at the children's hospital in Philadelphia in which my cultures following positive findings were returned as having only large staphylococcic growths.

---

21. Edinburgh Med. Jour., 1906, xx.
22. Wassermann: Deutsch. med. Wchnschr., 1902, xxviii.
23. Martin: Compt. rend. Soc. de biol., 1903, iv.
24. Peyler: Brit. Med. Jour., 1905.

Schiotz,[25] of Copenhagen, was much impressed with the fact that a patient with staphylococcus sore throat, installed in a diphtheria ward by error, did not contract diphtheria and also with the fact that intercurrent attacks of staphylococcus sore throat in several cases terminated positive Klebs-Loeffler findings in the case of convalescents from bacteria. Acting on the presumption that the staphylococcus was the cause of immunity on the one hand and of cure on the other he inoculated altogether six carriers with staphylococci with complete success in each instance.

W. E. Musgrave, of Manila, suggested this treatment in the case reported below and the results lead me to believe that the problem of the treatment of carriers has at last been solved by a method perfectly safe, easy to administer and promising complete success.

As to the latter it is realized that one instance doesn't make a sufficient basis for generalization, and as this is only the seventh case reported it is as yet too early for positive deductions. It is, however, not too much to state the belief that as all else has failed this measure is worthy of an extended trial.

### REPORT OF CASE

January 6: Miss B., daughter of a naval officer, had severe sore throat, fever and toxic symptoms; diagnosis, tonsillitis.

January 19: Case seen by Major D. C. Howard, M. C. U. S. A.

January 20: Cultures positive for diphtheria; 2,000 units of antitoxin given. No clinical symptoms remaining.

January 27: Two thousand units of antitoxin given. Cultures positive.

February 10: Four thousand units of antitoxin given. Cultures positive.

February 16: I assumed charge of the case.

March 1: Guinea-pig inoculated with one loopful of bouillon culture died in less than forty-eight hours. Post-mortem findings positive for diphtheria. A control pig given the same dose but protected by antitoxin still lives. Experiments made by Major Chamberlain, Medical Corps U. S. Army, president of the Army Tropical Board.

March 18: Above experiment repeated with like result.

April 2: Throat cultures every four days from January 19 have always but once proved positive. Throat sprays had no effect.

April 3: Dr. Teague of the Bureau of Science of Manila kindly continued experiments in the absence of Major Chamberlain. Inoculation as on March 1 of four pigs proved positive for diphtheria. Death occurred within thirty-nine hours; those protected by antitoxin still living. A bouillon tube was inoculated with several loops of *Staphylococcus pyogenes aureus*[27] and the patient's throat sprayed with the inoculated bouillon through an atomizer every two hours during day hours. At night no treatment given.

April 4: A culture from the throat was taken before treatment was resumed at 8 a. m. A fresh tube of staphylococcus was given patient for use in spraying throat. The throat was mopped also with an applicator, care being taken to enter the deep crypts of the tonsils.

---

25. Schiøtz, A.: Cure of Chronic Diphtheria Bacillus-Carriers, Ugesk. f. Laeger, 1909, lxxi, 1373; abstr. in Jour. Am. Med. Assn., 1910, liv, 422.

26. Slack, F. H., Arms, B. L., Wade, E. M. and Blansharck, W. S.: Diphtheria Bacillus-Carriers in the Public Schools, Jour. Am. Med. Assn., 1910, liv, 951

27. Stock virulent culture of the Philippine Bureau of Science.

April 5: Cultures from throat taken on April 4 positive, but few diphtheria bacilli were found.

April 6: Culture of April 5 negative.

April 9: Culture of the 6th, 7th and 8th negative. Examination made by the Tropical Board and Bureau of Science. Case released from quarantine.

April 10: Throat cultures inoculated into guinea-pigs by Dr. Teague showed no reaction in pigs unprotected by antitoxin other than in those protected by antitoxin.

April 11: All treatment stopped.

April 24: Numerous cultures examined by the Tropical Board and Bureau of Science all negative.

*Clinical Note.*—On March 28 Miss B. complained of paresthesias of the extremities. It had also been noted that, while there was no paralysis, her throat was very insensitive. It was feared that unless Miss B. had a good supply of antitoxin in her blood the large number of bacteria in her throat might be manufacturing enough toxin to produce serious nerve lesions. Dr. Ruediger of the Bureau of Science made the following experiments with her blood serum and found that she was almost entirely unprotected. I intended to give her weekly doses of antitoxin as a protective measure but the elimination of the bacteria by the staphylococcus made this unnecessary.

*Dr. Ruediger's Test of Patient's Serum.*—To ten times the minimum lethal dose of toxin varying quantities of patient's blood serum were added. The mixtures stood for one hour and were then injected under the skin of 250 gm. guinea-pigs. In a control series normal human serum was also inoculated with toxin.

TABLE OF TESTS OF PATIENT'S SERUM*

| Serum c.c. | Result | Serum c.c. | Result |
|---|---|---|---|
| 1. | animal lived | 1. | animal lived |
| 0.8 | animal lived | 0.8 | animal lived |
| 0.6 | animal lived | 0.6 | animal lived |
| 0.4 | animal lived | 0.4 | animal lived |
| 0.2 | animal lived | 0.2 | animal lived |
| 0.1 | animal died | 0.1 | animal died |
| 0.05 | animal died | 0.05 | animal died |
| 0.025 | animal died | | |
| 0.0125 | animal died | | |

*Ten times the minimum lethal dose was added to each dose of serum.

The results shown in the accompanying table indicate that ten times the minimum fatal dose of toxin was neutralized by 0.2 c.c. of patient's serum and also by 0.2 c.c. of normal serum, whereas in neither patient's nor in normal serum was 0.1 c.c. enough to neutralize this amount of toxin.

This test is sufficiently exact to prove that Miss B. was not manufacturing antitoxins in much, if any greater, amounts than normal persons possess.

These experiments are given in detail to emphasize a point that has received but little attention, viz: that a carrier of diphtheritic bacilli may have practically no protection in his blood serum against the toxin that must constantly be elaborated in his throat and, as this toxin is a nerve poison, steps to prevent serious nerve lesions are imperative.

In conclusion I wish to state again that Dr. Musgrave suggested the staphylococcus treatment of this case and the laboratory experiments of Major Chamberlain and Dr. Teague and Dr. Ruediger made the scientific treatment of it possible.

SUMMARY

1. A sanitary survey should be made after every diphtheria outbreak to eliminate carriers, whether they be human or animal.

2. The human carrier is the most dangerous.[26]

3. By animal inoculation a distinction should be made between the virulent and the "morphological" carrier.

4. Four negative daily cultures are necessary before quarantine is raised.

5. Treatment of carriers has heretofore proven useless. Local measures, while necessary, fail to influence the virulence or duration of the bacilli. Antitoxin has no influence on the bacillus in a carrier.

6. Pure cultures of *Staphylococcus pyogenes aureus* sprayed in throats has, in seven cases, now reported, destroyed the Klebs-Loeffler bacilli in carriers in forty-eight to seventy-two hours.

7. This method of treatment is harmless and should be used in all cases of carriers.[28]

8. This method has been found useful immediately after convalescence from an acute attack.

9. It is probable that its use during an acute attack of diphtheria would be successful.

10. As yet it is inadvisable to attempt its use in any save mild acute cases.

---

28. A doubt has been expressed as to the safety of inoculating throats with virulent *Staphylococcus pyogenes aureus*, as was done in this case. Since the above was written Musgrave of Manila reports that it has been used by the members of the Philippine Bureau of Science without any disagreeable results.

# A STUDY OF STREPTOCOCCI WITH THE COMPLEMENT-FIXATION AND CONGLUTINATION REACTIONS *

HOMER F. SWIFT, M.D., AND W. C. THRO, M.D.
NEW YORK

The study of the streptococci associated with various diseases, in which these organisms seem to play some part, has thus far led to no very definite conclusions concerning their importance in etiology. One reason for this is that the methods of study so far applied to the streptococcus are not specific enough to distinguish the various strains of the organism.

It is the object of this communication to present the results of a study of several streptococci by means of the complement-fixation, and the conglutination reaction, and incidentally, the agglutination reaction.

The extensive application of the Wassermann reaction for the diagnosis of syphilis has led to a general understanding of the principles of the fixation reaction. It is, therefore, rather surprising that it has not been used more extensively in the study of other infections.

Seven years ago Besredka[1] applied the reaction to the study of horses which had been immunized to streptococci, and found that the serum of such horses, when inoculated with streptococci, bound complement, while the serum of horses which had been immunized by means of soluble toxins produced no fixation. Both serums were protective, indicating that fixation is not always a concomitant of protective power. The various serums were, however, specific in nature, producing fixation only with the streptococcus which had been used to produce the serum tested. He, therefore, concluded that we have in the fixation phenomenon a means of differentiating streptococci. Besredka and Dopter[2] then applied the reaction to the study of scarlet fever without positive results. In both of these studies twenty-four-hour cultures of living organisms were used as antigen.

Foix and Mallein[3] later studied scarlet fever with this reaction and obtained positive results with nine different cultures of streptococci which

---

* From the Department of Pathology, the University and Bellevue Hospital Medical College, New York. Aided by a grant from the Committee on Scientific Investigation of the American Medical Association.

1. Besredka: Ann. de l'Inst. Pasteur., 1904, xviii, 363.
2. Besredka and Dopter: Ann. de l'Inst. Pasteur, 1904, xviii, 373.
3. Foix, C. and Mallein, E.: Presse méd., 1907, xv, 777.

had been isolated from the throats of scarlet fever patients. The serum of ten out of twelve patients with scarlet fever gave positive reactions, while nine controls, among which were four serums of erysipelas and one of puerperal sepsis, gave negative results.

Castex[4] studied patients with erysipelas, scarlet fever, a streptococcus abscess, puerperal sepsis, a streptococcus pleurisy and a septic arthritis, apparently using the same strain of streptococcus as antigen in all, and obtained a fixation in all except three of five cases of scarlet fever. He expresses, therefore, his belief in the unity of the streptococcus.

In all of these studies fresh living cultures were used as antigen. Investigators of the German school under Wassermann's leadership have used extracts of bacteria in place of the living organisms, and have shown that such extracts are more satisfactory.

Leuchs and Schöne[5] demonstrated clearly that the most satisfactory way of extracting typhoid bacilli was by heating to 60 C. for twenty-four hours, and then shaking at room temperature for a like period. By preparing extracts in this way Leuchs[6] shows that the various members of the colon-typhoid group can be distinguished by the fixation reaction.

In all antigens used in the fixation reaction two properties are present: first, anticomplementary; second, fixing. The anticomplementary property causes a non-specific destruction of complement; the fixing property is specific; hence the most desirable antigen is one that will give the maximum of fixation with the minimum of anticomplementary action. To the solution of this problem the present study is devoted.

Before describing our method of preparing these antigens, the method of complement-fixation as used by us will be given.

## *TECHNIC OF COMPLEMENT-FIXATION*

### REAGENTS

1. *Complement.*—Fresh guinea-pig serum in the quantity of 0.05 c.c. made up to 0.5 c.c. with normal salt solution.

2. *Immune or Normal Rabbit Serum.*—The serum was heated to 56 C. one-half hour, and used in diminishing amounts, so diluted with salt solution that 0.5 c.c. of the dilution represented the amount of serum required.

3. *Antigen.*—(See below).

4. *Red Blood-Cell Suspension.*—Defibrinated sheep's blood was washed three times with salt solution and made up to 5 per cent. suspension with saline; 0.5 c.c. of this was used in each tube.

---

4. Castex, M. R.: Presse méd., 1909, xvii, 324.
5. Leuchs, J. and Schöne, C.: Ztschr. f. Hyg., 1908, lx, 149.
6. Leuchs, J.: Berl. klin. Wchnschr., 1907, xliv, 68.

5. *Hemolysin.*—The serum of a rabbit immunized to sheep red-cells was so diluted that 0.5 c.c. of the dilution represented two hemolytic units. The hemolytic unit was determined each day.

After mixing the complement, rabbit's serum, and antigen, all the tubes were filled to 1.5 c.c. with normal salt solution, and incubation carried on in a water-bath at 37 C. for one hour. The red cells and hemolysin were then added and the incubation continued another hour, after which the tubes were placed in the refrigerator over night and the readings made the next morning. The controls are shown in the protocol.

PROTOCOL 1.—COMPLEMENT-FIXATION METHOD

| Rabbits' Serum (Inactivated). | Antigen (Bacterial Extract). | Complement, 10 % c.c. | | Sheep Cells, 5 % c.c. | Hemolysin, 2 units, c.c. | | Result. |
|---|---|---|---|---|---|---|---|
| Immune serum.......................... | With decreasing amounts | 0.5 | All | 0.5 | 0.5 | Incu- | ? |
| " " | " " " | 0.5 | tubes | 0.5 | 0.5 | bation | ? |
| " " | With constant amount... | 0.5 | filled | 0.5 | 0.5 | con- | ? |
| " " | " " " | 0.5 | to | 0.5 | 0.5 | tinued | ? |
| | Controls | | | | | | |
| Normal serum (as with immune serum) | As with immune serum... | 0.5 | 1.5 c.c. | 0.5 | 0.5 | 1 hour. | C. H. * |
| " " " | " " | 0.5 | with | 0.5 | 0.5 | Then | C. H. |
| 2 × maximum amount immune serum | .......................... | 0.5 | saline. | 0.5 | 0.5 | on | C. H. |
| 2 × maximum amount normal serum.. | .......................... | 0.5 | Incu- | 0.5 | 0.5 | ice | C. H. |
| .......................................... | 2 × maximum amount... | 0.5 | bation | 0.5 | 0.5 | over | C. H. |
| .......................................... | .......................... | 0.5 | 1 hour | 0.5 | 0.5 | night. | C. H. |
| .......................................... | .......................... | 0.5 | at | 0.5 | ... | | No H.† |
| .......................................... | .......................... | ...... | 37 de- | 0.5 | 0.5 | | No H. |
| .......................................... | .......................... | ...... | grees C. | 0.5 | ... | | No H. |

* C. H. indicates complete hemolysis.
† No H. indicates no hemolysis.

## THE PREPARATION OF ANTIGENS

Early in the study the bacteria were grown as follows: On large surfaces of plain agar were placed 1.5 c.c. sterile horse serum and 2 c.c. of a twenty-four-hour bouillon culture of streptococci, and incubation allowed for twenty-four hours. The resulting growth was removed with sterile salt solution and centrifuged, after which the supernatant fluid was taken up with a pipette and the residue again washed. The fluids of both washings were united and saved for testing. The residue (bacteria) was divided into two portions, one-half of which (E) was dried *in vacuo* over sulphuric acid. To the other half was added 60 c.c. sterile salt solution and 0.5 per cent. phenol. This mixture was well shaken, and divided into four equal portions, A, B, C and D, and treated as follows:

A.—Kept on ice.

B.—Kept twenty-four hours at 37 C. Shaken twenty-four hours at room temperature.

C.—Kept twenty-four hours at 44 C. Shaken twenty-four hours at room temperature.

D.—Kept twenty-four hours at 60 C. Shaken twenty-four hours at room temperature.

E.—Having first been dried, was ground in a mortar, after which 60 c.c. of 0.5 per cent. phenolized saline solution were added, and the mixture shaken for twenty-four hours at room temperature.

The preparations, B, C, D, and E were then centrifuged at high speed. A slight opalescence usually persisted in the supernatant fluid, which was carefully pipetted into tightly stoppered, dark brown glass bottles and kept on ice.

After all the extracts were prepared, the anticomplementary dose was determined for each, and on the following day this part of the experiment was repeated with the addition of the determination of the fixing dose with both immune and normal serum. The results of this experiment are shown in Table 1.

TABLE 1.—DETERMINATION OF ANTICOMPLEMENTARY AND FIXING POWER OF DIFFERENT FORMS OF STREPTOCOCCUS ANTIGENS

| | Amount of Rabbit Serum. c.c. | Amount of Antigen. c.c. | Antigen A. | Antigen B. | Antigen C. | Antigen D. | Antigen E. |
|---|---|---|---|---|---|---|---|
| Anticomplementary Power. | ... | 0.8 | C. I......... | Sl. I......... | V. Sl. I..... | V. Sl. I..... | V. Sl. I. |
| | ... | 0.4 | Mkd. I...... | V. Sl. I..... | C. H........ | C. H........ | C. H. |
| | ... | 0.2 | Mkd. I...... | C. H........ | C. H........ | C. H........ | C. H. |
| | ... | 0.1 | Sl. I......... | C. H........ | C. H........ | C. H........ | C. H. |
| | Immune Rabbit Serum. | | | | | | |
| Fixing Power | 0.1 | 0.2 | ............. | ............. | Mkd. I...... | Mkd. I...... | C. I. |
| | 0.1 | 0.1 | C. I......... | Sl. I......... | Sl. I......... | Sl. I......... | Part I. |
| | 0.1 | 0.05 | Mkd. I...... | V. Sl. I..... | V. Sl. I..... | C. H........ | Sl. I. |
| | 0.1 | 0.025 | Sl. I......... | C. H........ | C. H........ | C. H........ | V. Sl. I. |
| | 0.1 | 0.012 | C. H........ | C. H........ | C. H........ | C. H........ | C. H. |
| | Normal Rabbit Serum. | | | | | | |
| | 0.1 | 0.2 | ............. | C. H........ | C. H........ | C. H........ | C. H. |
| | 0.1 | 0.1 | Mkd. I...... | C. H........ | C. H........ | C. H........ | C. H. |
| | 0.1 | 0.05 | Sl. I......... | C. H........ | C. H........ | C. H........ | C. H. |
| | 0.1 | 0.025 | C. H........ | C. H........ | C. H........ | C. H........ | C. H. |
| | Ratio of fixing to anticomplementary power | | 0.5—1 / 1 | 1 / 4 | 2 / 4 | 2 / 8 | 2 / 8 |

C. I. indicates complete inhibition. Mkd. I., marked inhibition. C. H., complete hemolysis. Part I., partial inhibition. Sl. I., slight inhibition. V. Sl. I., very slight inhibition.

It will be noted that the suspension of whole bacteria gave fixation in the smallest quantity, but was also the most anticomplementary and gave fixation of complement with normal rabbit's serum; while none of the extracts gave fixation with the normal serum. The extract made from dried bacteria gave the most complete fixation in proportion to its anticomplementary action.

Similar preparations and experiments were made with a culture of *Staphylococcus aureus.* The final results are shown in Table 2.

TABLE 2.—DETERMINATION OF ANTICOMPLEMENTARY AND FIXING POWER OF DIFFERENT FORMS OF STAPHYLOCOCCUS AUREUS ANTIGENS *

| | Amount of Rabbit Serum. c.c. | Amount of Antigen. c.c. | Antigen A. | Antigen B. | Antigen C. | Antigen D. | Antigen E. |
|---|---|---|---|---|---|---|---|
| Anticomplementary Power. | ... | 0.8 | ............ | Mkd. I...... | Part I...... | Sl. I......... | C. H.† |
| | ... | 0.4 | C. I......... | C. H........ | Sl. I......... | C. H........ | C. H. |
| | ... | 0.2 | Mkd. I...... | C. M........ | C. H........ | C. H........ | C. H. |
| | ... | 0.1 | C. H........ | C. H........ | C. H........ | C. H........ | C. H. |
| | Immune Rabbit Serum. | | | | | | |
| Fixing Power | 0.1 | 0.4 | ............ | C. I......... | ............ | C. I......... | C. I. |
| | 0.1 | 0.2 | ............ | C. I......... | C. I......... | C. I......... | C. I. |
| | 0.1 | 0.1 | C. I......... | C. I......... | C. I......... | Mkd. I...... | Mkd. I. |
| | 0.1 | 0.05 | C. I......... | Mkd. I...... | Mkd. I...... | Part I...... | Part I. |
| | 0.1 | 0.025 | Mkd. I...... | Mkd. I...... | Part I...... | Sl. I......... | Sl. I. |
| | 0.1 | 0.012 | Part I...... | Sl. I......... | Part I...... | Sl. I......... | Sl. I. |
| | 0.1 | 0.006 | Sl. I......... | Sl. I......... | Sl. I......... | Sl. I......... | Sl. I. |
| | Normal Rabbit Serum. | | | | | | |
| | 0.1 | 0.4 | ............ | Mkd. I...... | Mkd. I...... | Mkd. I...... | Sl. I. |
| | 0.1 | 0.2 | ............ | Sl. I......... | Sl. I......... | Sl. I......... | C. H. |
| | 0.1 | 0.1 | V. Sl. I..... | C. H........ | C. H........ | C. H........ | C. H. |
| | 0.1 | 0.05 | C. H........ | C. H........ | C. H........ | C. H........ | C. H. |
| | Ratio of fixing to anticomplementary power | | $\frac{0.5}{2}$ | $\frac{.1}{8}$ | $\frac{1}{4}$ | $\frac{2}{8}$ | $\frac{2}{16}$ |

* Abbreviations same as in Table 1.
† 1.6 c.c. of Antigen E caused partial inhibition.

The anticomplementary action of the bacterial suspension was here also the most marked. It decreased in the heated extracts in proportion to the amount of heat applied, and was the least marked in the extract prepared from dried bacteria. The fixing power of the latter extract was also the highest compared to the anticomplementary power.

The reduction in anticomplementary power of normal serum, as the result of heating, has been noted by many in the Wassermann reaction for syphilis. We have tried the effect of drying on the anticomplementary substances in the fluid in which the bacteria were washed. It was found that this fluid was very anticomplementary, so part of it was dried in the same way as the bacteria, and afterwards made up to original volume with sterile water plus 0.5 per cent. phenol. Water was used in order to maintain the same salt tonicity. The anticomplementary power of both preparations was then determined. For the original solution this was 0.05 c.c. and for the dried substance 0.2 c.c. Thus, the anticomplementary power of the dried form was only one-fourth of that of the original fluid. To determine whether any of the fixing substances had been dissolved out of the cocci in washing, the two solutions (dried and original) were tried against an immune rabbit's serum, and found to have but little more fixing power than anticomplementary power. That the anticomplementary action of the washing fluid is due to the presence of horse serum and bouillon has been shown by the following experiment: One and a half c.c. horse serum and 2 c.c. sterile bouillon were placed on plain agar and incubated twenty-four hours, then washed off with the same amount of salt solution that had been used to wash the bacteria. The anticomplementary power of this solution was the same as that of the fluid in which the bacteria had been washed. This shows the necessity of thoroughly washing bacteria which are to be used in the fixation test. It also indicated the advisability of growing the bacteria without the addition of horse serum or an excess of bouillon. So, for the remainder of our work, bacteria were grown as follows:

The organisms grown for twenty-four hours on agar were mixed with a small amount of sterile salt solution and sprayed on plain agar in large pans with the aid of an atomizer. After incubation for twenty-four hours, the plates were flooded with 0.9 per cent. salt solution and the bacteria scraped off. A mixture was thus obtained consisting of bacteria and salt solution only. Particles of agar, if present, were removed by filtering through glass wool and the bacteria were afterwards separated by centrifuging.

By this method, the five different methods of preparation of antigen, A, B, C, D, and E, were again tried with a culture of another streptococcus, and tested as in the experiments above detailed. It was found here also that the extract E was the least anticomplementary, and that the ratio of fixing power to anticomplementary action was higher in this extract than any other.

Thus, for both streptococci and staphylococci the best method of extraction of bacteria in the preparation of an antigen for use in the fixation test, is shown to be by drying, grinding and shaking with salt solution.

This method of extraction offers several advantages:

1. The bacteria can be grown in large quantities and after drying can be kept indefinitely, and fresh extracts made as required.

2. A number of extracts from different strains of bacteria can be prepared simultaneously, so that the mechanical manipulations occupy the same length of time.

3. The extracts can be made up by weight, and hence are more comparable one with another than those made up by volume or by using the growth from a surface of media of a given size. Different strains of streptococci vary so much in their rate and abundance of growth, that it is unsatisfactory to use agar cultures of a certain size as a standard.

In the subsequent work, therefore, the organisms were grown on plain agar, well washed, and dried *in vacuo* over phenol, and kept in this dried state until used. They were then extracted as follows:

Dried bacteria were ground in normal salt solution (containing 0.5 per cent. phenol) in the proportion of 0.001 gm. to 1 c.c. The mixture was shaken at room temperature for twenty-four hours, and centrifuged to clearness. The clear solution was pipetted into dark brown, tightly stoppered bottles, and kept on ice. The extracts of the different organisms were all prepared simultaneously, so that the age of the extracts was the same.

In applying the fixation test the following organisms were used:

No. 1.—The *Diplococcus rheumaticus* of J. W. Beattie, sent to us by Dr. Ruth Tunnicliffe, of the Memorial Institute for Infectious Diseases of Chicago. In broth it occurs in pairs (which are spherical or slightly elongated), or in chains of four to eight, or in clumps of four to eight. It does not liquefy gelatin. Milk is coagulated by it at the end of seventy-two hours. Litmus agar plus lactose becomes acid, but in the same medium plus inulin the reaction is neutral. In blood-agar plates the colonies are small and green.

No. 2.—A streptococcus, isolated from a rheumatic joint, obtained from Dr. Bertha Anthony, of the Research Laboratories of New York City Board of Health. In broth it occurs as cocci in pairs and fours. Gelatin is not liquefied and milk is not coagulated by it. Litmus agar plus lactose becomes acid, but the same plus inulin remains neutral. In blood-agar plates the colonies are green, but not as large as those of Nos. 4 and 5.

No. 3.—A streptococcus, also obtained from Dr. Anthony, isolated from the blood of scarlet fever. In broth it occurs as short chains of cocci. Gelatin was not liquefied and milk was not coagulated by it. In litmus agar containing lactose the reaction was slightly acid and in the same with inulin, neutral. In blood-agar plates the colonies were not green and did not hemolyze, though originally hemolysis was noted.

No. 4.—A streptococcus, obtained from Dr. Anthony, said to have been isolated from a tonsil. In broth it grows in very long chains. In blood-agar plates the colonies are green and in this respect as well as in size they are similar to No. 5. The organism has been under cultivation longer than No. 5.

No. 5.—An organism, isolated from the blood of malignant endocarditis by the agar plate method. In twenty-four hours the colonies (0.5 mm. in diameter) appeared as greenish-black points surrounded by a clearer green zone. No hemolysis occurred. Smears showed diplococci, none of them elongated, in short chains and small clumps which were Gram-positive and without capsules. Capsules were never demonstrated with Hiss' capsule stain, although frequent trials were made during three and one-half months from cultures on blood-agar and ascitic broth. The colonies were very adherent to the agar media. In ascitic broth they occurred in twos and chains of four and six, some spherical and some lance-shaped. This organism differed from true pneumococcus in that it grew readily on plain agar and the cultures were kept alive without difficulty. Hiss' serum inulin, which was tried soon after isolation, was partly coagulated at the end of several days. Milk was coagulated and gelatin was not liquefied. In litmus agar with both lactose and inulin there was a slight acid reaction. In broth the bacteria tended to clump.

No. 6.—A strain of *Staphylococcus aureus* which liquefies gelatin and coagulates milk. In lactose litmus agar the reaction is acid while in inulin it is alkaline.

No. 7.—Pneumococcus, isolated from a pneumonic sputum. The first cultures showed cocci that suggested the morphology of *S. mucosus capsulatus*, but they finally assumed a diplococcus form, frequently lance-shaped, and always with a well-developed capsule. The cultures were kept alive with great difficulty, if blood was not used. North's media was found most satisfactory. It did not coagulate milk or liquefy gelatin. Hiss' inulin serum was coagulated to solidity in twenty-four hours, after the organism had been cultivated for several weeks on artificial media. In both lactose and inulin litmus agar, the reaction was slightly acid. In blood-agar plates the colonies were small and green.

The cultural characteristics are tabulated and contrasted in Table 3

## *IMMUNITY EXPERIMENTS*

Rabbit 1 was immunized[7] by seven injections of Streptococcus 1, and bled twelve days after the last injection. Table 5 illustrates fixation with its serum.

Rabbit 2 received three injections of Streptococcus 2 and was bled six days after the last injection. Fixation occurred as shown in Table 5.

It will be noted that, although Streptococci 1 and 2 were both from cases of rheumatism and had very similar cultural characteristics, there was a specific fixation with each serum.

Rabbit 3 had eight injections of Streptococcus 3, but showed no fixation with any streptococcus; it then had daily injections for three days with persisting negative results; then two more injections were made of organisms, heated only five minutes, with no fixation. At the final testing two days later the result was still negative.

Rabbit 4 had received nine injections of Streptococcus 4, and was bled four days after the last injection. The serum reacted as shown in Table 6.

The interesting fact is here brought out that the serum of Rabbit 4 fixes complement with Streptococcus 5 to the same degree as Streptococcus 4, but with none of the other streptococci. The growth on artificial media

7. Method of Immunization: Injections of organisms, killed by heating at 60 to 65 C. for one-half hour, were made into the ear vein of the rabbit every four days. The initial dose was 0.5 mg. (estimated) increasing to 6 mg. If the animal showed a loss of weight the injections were discontinued, and resumed when the condition of the animal improved. Although some animals died under this treatment, it was found to be accompanied by a lower mortality than other methods.

TABLE 3.—CULTURAL CHARACTERISTICS OF ORGANISMS USED IN FIXATION TESTS

| No. | Source. | Morphology. | Broth. | Plain Agar. | Blood-Agar Plates. | Gelatin. | Milk. | Hiss' Serum Inulin.* | Lactose Litmus Agar. | Inulin Litmus Agar. |
|---|---|---|---|---|---|---|---|---|---|---|
| 1 | Micr. rheumaticus, J. W. Beattie. | Small cocci, some elongated, 2s, 4s, 8s. | Faintly clouded, small amount of sediment. | Small separate colonies. | Green; very small colonies. | Not liquefied. | Coagulated. | Not coagulated. | Very acid. | Neutral. |
| 2 | Rheumatic joint. | Cocci in 2s and 4s. | Faintly clouded, small amount of sediment. | Small separate colonies. | Green colonies, larger than No. 1 but smaller than Nos. 4 and 5. | Not liquefied. | Not coagulated. | Not coagulated. | Slightly acid. | Neutral. |
| 3 | Blood; scarlet fever. | Cocci in short chains. | Faintly clouded, small amount of sediment. | Small separate colonies. | Not green; no hemolysis. (Did hemolyze at an earlier period.) | Not liquefied. | Not coagulated. | Not coagulated. | Slightly acid. | Neutral. |
| 4 | Tonsil. | Cocci, very long chains in broth. | Clouded, moderate amount of sediment. | Small separate colonies. | Green colonies like No. 5. | Not liquefied. | Partly coagulated. | Not coagulated. (Had been under cultivation a long time.) | Slightly acid. | Neutral. |
| 5 | Blood endocarditis. | Cocci and lance-shaped 2s, 4s and clumps, no capsules. | Very faintly clouded, bacteria tend to form clumps. | Small separate colonies which stick to media. | Green surrounded by pale green area. | Not liquefied. | Coagulated. | Partly coagulated at end of three days. | Slightly acid. | Slightly acid? |
| 6 | ...................... | Cocci in clumps. | Moderately clouded, moderate sediment. | Large amount of spreading yellow growth. | .................. | Liquefied. | Coagulated. | ............... | Slightly acid. | Very alkaline. |
| 7 | Sputum pneumonia. | Cocci and lance-shaped pairs and short chains; encapsulated. | Very slightly clouded. | Small flat transparent colonies; poor growth. | Green; small colonies. | Not liquefied. | Not coagulated. | Coagulated; solid at end of 24 hours. | Slightly acid. | Slightly acid. |

* Nos. 1, 2, 3 and 4 had been cultivated on artificial media a long time when this medium was tried.

TABLE 4.—FIXING POWER OF SERUM OF RABBIT 1*

| Amount Serum. c.c. | Antigen. c.c. | Strepto-coccus 1. | Strepto-coccus 2. | Strepto-coccus 3. | Strepto-coccus 4. | Strepto-coccus 5. | Staph-ylo-coccus. | Pneumo-coccus. |
|---|---|---|---|---|---|---|---|---|
| 0.1.............. | 0.1 | N. C. I. | C. H. | C. H. | C. H. | C. H. | C. H. | C. H. |
| 0.05.............. | 0.1 | N. C. I. | C. H. | C. H. | C. H. | C. H. | C. H. | C. H. |
| 0.025.............. | 0.1 | Sl. I. | C. H. | C. H. | C. H. | C. H. | C. H. | C. H. |
| 0.012.............. | 0.1 | C. H. | C. H. | C. H. | C. H. | C. H. | C. H. | C. H. |

* In this table the results of controls are omitted. Abbreviations same as in Table 1.

TABLE 5.—FIXING POWER OF SERUM OF RABBIT 2*

| Amount Serum. c.c. | Antigen. c.c. | Strepto-coccus 1. | Strepto-coccus 2. | Strepto-coccus 3. | Strepto-coccus 4. | Strepto-coccus 5. | Staph-ylo-coccus. | Pneumo-coccus. |
|---|---|---|---|---|---|---|---|---|
| 0.1.............. | 0.1 | C. H. | N. C. I. | C. H. | C. H. | C. H. | C. H. | C. H. |
| 0.05.............. | 0.1 | C. H. | Sl. I. | C. H. | C. H. | C. H. | C. H. | C. H. |
| 0.025.............. | 0.1 | C. H. | C. H | C. H. | C. H. | C. H. | ...... | ...... |

* In this table the results of controls are omitted. Abbreviations same as in Table 1.

TABLE 6.—FIXING POWER OF SERUM OF RABBIT 4*

| Amount Serum. c.c. | Antigen c.c. | Strepto-coccus 1. | Strepto-coccus 2. | Strepto-coccus 3. | Strepto-coccus 4. | Strepto-coccus 5. | Staph-ylo-coccus. | Pneumo-coccus. |
|---|---|---|---|---|---|---|---|---|
| 0.1.............. | 0.1 | C. H. | C. H. | C. H. | C. I. | C. I. | C. H. | C. H. |
| 0.05.............. | 0.1 | C. H. | C. H. | C. H. | C. I. | C. I. | C. H. | C. H. |
| 0.025.............. | 0.1 | C. H. | C. H. | C. H. | C. I. | C. I. | ...... | ...... |
| 0.012.............. | 0.1 | C. H. | C. H. | C. H. | C. I. | C. I. | ...... | ...... |
| 0.006.............. | 0.1 | C. H. | C. H. | C. H. | C. I. | C. I. | ...... | ...... |
| 0.003.............. | 0.1 | C. H. | C. H. | C. H. | C. H. | C. H. | ...... | ...... |

* In this table the results of controls are omitted. Abbreviations same as in Table 1.

TABLE 7.—FIXING POWER OF SERUM OF RABBIT 5

| Amount Serum. c.c. | Antigen. c.c. | Strepto-coccus 1. | Strepto-coccus 2. | Strepto-coccus 3. | Strepto-coccus 4. | Strepto-coccus 5. | Staph-ylo-coccus. | Pneumo-coccus. |
|---|---|---|---|---|---|---|---|---|
| 0.1.............. | 0.1 | C. H. | C. H. | C. H. | C. I. | C. I. | C. H. | C. H. |
| 0.05.............. | 0.1 | C. H. | C. H. | C. H. | C. I. | C. I. | ...... | ...... |
| 0.025.............. | 0.1 | C. H. | C. H. | C. H. | N. C. I. | C. I. | ...... | ...... |
| 0.012.............. | 0.1 | C. H. | C. H. | C. H. | C. H. | C. H. | ...... | ...... |

of Streptococci 4 and 5 are more nearly alike than any of the other organisms. Therefore, these two strains, although from widely different sources, are apparently closely related both culturally and biologically.

Rabbit 5, which had received four injections of Streptococcus 5, was bled one day after the last injection and showed no fixation. It was then given daily injections of the killed streptococci for three days and bled the following day. This serum then reacted as shown in Table 7.

This experiment confirms the view of the close relationship between Streptococci 4 and 5. Although the fixation was not as marked as in the case of Rabbit 4, the fixing limits with the two extracts are practically the same. Streptococcus 5, from a malignant endocarditis, although it closely resembles the pneumococcus in many of its cultural characteristics, must, on account of its fixation reaction, be included with the streptococci.

Rabbit 6 received twelve injections of staphylococci and the serum was tested nine days after the last injection. Nearly complete inhibition of hemolysis was noted with 0.0012 c.c. of this serum and 0.1 c.c. of the staphylococcus extract, while there was no fixation with any of the streptococci or the pneumococcus.

Rabbit 7 received four injections of pneumococci at four-day intervals, and was bled one day after the last injection. No fixation was obtained. Daily injections were then given for three days, with a like result. Then the entire growth from an agar-slant, heated only five minutes, was injected on two successive days, with still negative results. After a further interval of two days the animal was again bled; the serum gave marked inhibition in the strength of 0.1 c.c., slight inhibition with 0.05 and 0.025 c.c., but no fixation with any of the streptococci or with the staphylococcus.

Thus complement-fixing bodies were demonstrated in six out of seven animals.

The four rabbits which were treated with the green non-hemolyzing streptococci all showed the presence of antibodies which were specific, except in the case of Rabbits 4 and 5. Because of the cross-reaction between these two serums and their corresponding extracts, it is very probable that the two strains of streptococci are similar. In all the other cases the fixation was specific.

## THE CONGLUTINATION REACTION

In 1906 Bordet and Gay[8] described a colloidal substance in beef serum heated to 56 C., which has the property of causing a characteristic clumping and increased lysis of red blood-cells, when treated with a heated specific hemolytic serum and fresh alexin (complement). Bordet and Streng,[9] in later studies on this substance, gave to it the name "conglutinin." Streng[10] continued these studies with bacteria and found that a typical clumping was produced by the mixture of bacteria, fresh complement, conglutinin and a specific immune serum from which the

8. Bordet, J. and Gay, F. P.: Ann. de l'Inst. Pasteur, 1906, xx, 467.
9. Bordet, J. and Streng, O.: Centralbl. f. Bakteriol., 1909, xlix, 260.
10. Streng, O.: Centralbl. f. Bakteriol., 1909, L. 47.

agglutinins had been removed by absorption. By dialyzing the beef serum the conglutinin was shown to be present in the globulin fraction, and the reaction took place as well with bacteria, killed by heat or 0.1 per cent. liquor formaldehydi, as with live organisms.

In a study of dysentery in infants, Lucas, Fitzgerald and Schorer[11] first applied this reaction to clinical diagnosis. They found it more sensitive and specific than either the agglutination or fixation test.

In their work, cultures of the Flexner and Shiga dysentery bacilli, treated with 0.1 per cent. liquor formaldehydi were used. They conclude that in the conglutination test we have a means of diagnosis far superior to any other form.

## METHOD USED

In our studies of streptococci with the conglutination reaction, the following method was used:

The beef serum was heated to 56 C. for one-half an hour, then dialyzed in running water for twenty-four hours. By means of centrifuging, the precipitate was washed three times in sterile distilled water, after which it was made up to the original volume of the beef serum with normal salt solution to which 0.5 per cent. phenol had been added. The globulin did not completely dissolve in the salt solution, so that thorough agitation was necessary each time before using. The solution was kept on ice and the same preparation was used throughout the entire work in the amount of 0.1 c.c. in each tube.

*Bacterial Suspension.*—The bacteria were grown as for the fixation test, washed and suspended in the following solution:[12]

| | |
|---|---|
| Normal salt solution .......................... | 89.5 parts |
| Glycerin .......................................... | 10 parts |
| Phenol .............................................. | 0.5 parts |

We have adopted this solution because the glycerin prevents, to a certain extent, the spontaneous agglutination to which the streptococci are so liable. We proved that the glycerin had little deleterious influence on the conglutination reaction by actual trial with staphylococci.

All the different strains of streptococci were made up to the same density, and 0.5 c.c. of the suspension was used in each tube.

*Complement.*—Fresh guinea-pig serum was mixed with equal parts normal salt solution and 0.1 c.c. of this dilution, or 0.05 c.c. of the serum, was used in each tube.

---

11. Lucas, W. P., Fitzgerald, J. G. and Schorer, E. H.: Methods of Serum Diagnosis in Bacillary Dysentery (Infectious Diarrhea) in Infants, Jour. Am. Med. Assn., 1910, liv, 441.

12. This mixture has been used with satisfactory results for several years in the Presbyterian Hospital (New York) for the suspension of typhoid bacilli in the macroscopic agglutination test.

*Immune Serum.*—This was the same as was used in the fixation tests, diluted so that 0.5 c.c. of the dilution represented the actual amount of serum.

PROTOCOL 2.—CONGLUTINATION TEST WITH STAPHYLOCOCCUS AUREUS

| | Immune Rabbit Serum. | Complement. 50 % c.c. | Conglutinin, c.c. | Bacterial Emulsion, c.c. | Normal Saline, c.c. | Result. |
|---|---|---|---|---|---|---|
| Conglutination | 0.05 | 0.1 | 0.1 | 0.5 | ... | ++ |
| | 0.025 | 0.1 | 0.1 | 0.5 | ... | ++ |
| | 0.012 | 0.1 | 0.1 | 0.5 | ... | ++ |
| | 0.006 | 0.1 | 0.1 | 0.5 | ... | + |
| | 0.003 | 0.1 | 0.1 | 0.5 | ... | +— |
| Agglutination | 0.05 | ... | ... | 0.5 | 0.2 | — |
| | 0.025 | ... | ... | 0.5 | 0.2 | — |
| Controls | Normal Rabbit Serum. | | | | | |
| | 0.05 | 0.1 | 0.1 | 0.5 | ... | — |
| | 0.025 | 0.1 | 0.1 | 0.5 | ... | — |
| | ..... | 0.1 | 0.1 | 0.5 | 0.5 | — |
| | ..... | 0.1 | ... | 0.5 | 0.6 | — |
| | ..... | ... | 0.1 | 0.5 | 0.6 | — |
| | ..... | ... | ... | 0.5 | 0.7 | — |

++ Complete clumping and complete clearness of fluid.
+ Marked clumping and slight cloudiness of fluid.
+— Slight clumping and cloudiness of fluid.
— No clumping.
It will be noted that the agglutination reaction is a necessary control.

After the various dilutions and control tubes were filled, as shown in Protocol 2, all the tubes were made up to 1.2 c.c. with salt solution, incubated at 37 C. for two hours, and allowed to stand at room temperature over night before the readings were made. We found that the reactions were sharper after this procedure than when the dilutions were merely allowed to stand twenty-four hours without incubation, as recommended by Lucas, Fitzgerald and Schorer.

The results of this study are shown in Table 8.

The test could not be tried with the serum of Rabbit 4, because Streptococcus 4 emulsion showed spontaneous agglutination. The results with the serum from the staphylococcus rabbit are shown in Protocol 2. This serum gave conglutination only with the staphylococcus emulsion and not with emulsion of the streptococci and the pneumococcus.

In these few trials we found little more clumping in the conglutination than in the agglutination test. The agglutinins caused clumping of streptococci generally, but were not specific for any particular strain of streptococcus. With Serums 1 and 2 the conglutination persisted in higher dilutions than the agglutination, and was, with the exception of Serum 5, slightly more specific.

The distinct reaction with the staphylococcus proved that the conglutinin was active and that the glycerin did not prevent the reaction.

TABLE 8.—CONGLUTINATION AND AGGLUTINATION TESTS

| | Amount of Serum. | Strepto-coccus 1. | Strepto-coccus 2. | Strepto-coccus 3. | Strepto-coccus 4. | Strepto-coccus 5. | Staph-ylo-coccus. | Pneumo-coccus. |
|---|---|---|---|---|---|---|---|---|
| RABBIT I. Conglutination: | 0.05 | ++ | + | ++ | Spontaneous agglutination in all tubes and with normal salt solution. | — | — | — |
| | 0.025 | + | +— | +— | | — | — | — |
| | 0.012 | +— | — | — | | — | .. | .. |
| | 0.006 | +— | — | — | | — | .. | .. |
| Agglutination: | 0.05 | ++ | — | ++ | | — | — | — |
| | 0.025 | + | — | +— | | — | — | — |
| | 0.012 | — | — | — | | — | .. | .. |
| RABBIT 2. Conglutination: | 0.05 | + | ++ | — | | — | — | — |
| | 0.025 | +— | ++ | — | | — | — | — |
| | 0.012 | +— | + | — | | — | .. | .. |
| | 0.006 | — | +— | — | | — | .. | .. |
| | 0.003 | — | — | — | | — | .. | .. |
| Agglutination: | 0.05 | +— | ++ | — | | — | — | — |
| | 0.025 | — | ++ | — | | — | — | — |
| | 0.012 | — | + | — | | — | .. | .. |
| RABBIT 5. Conglutination: | 0.05 | — | ++ | + | | ++ | — | — |
| | 0.025 | — | + | +— | | + | — | — |
| | 0.012 | — | +— | — | | — | .. | .. |
| | 0.006 | — | +— | — | | — | .. | .. |
| | 0.003 | — | — | — | | — | .. | .. |
| Agglutination: | 0.05 | — | ++ | + | | ++ | .. | .. |
| | 0.025 | — | + | +— | | + | .. | .. |
| | 0.012 | — | — | — | | — | .. | .. |

## *SUMMARY*


1. The conglutination reaction in our hands has not proved of much greater value in the differentiation of various strains of streptococci than the agglutination reaction.

2. Although the conglutination and agglutination reactions are specific for streptococci, they are not specific for individual strains of streptococci. Our experiments, however, are not sufficient in number for definite conclusions on this point.

3. The best extract of streptococci for use as antigen in the complement-fixation test is that prepared by drying the washed organisms, grinding and shaking them for twenty-four hours.

4. Immune bodies, specific for different strains of streptococci, can be demonstrated by means of the complement-fixation test. It is possible that by the use of this test we have a means of studying specific streptococcus infections.


80 West Fortieth—529 West One Hundred and Sixtieth Street.

# A REPORT OF FIFTY EXAMINATIONS OF CEREBROSPINAL FLUID WITH SPECIAL REFERENCE TO THE CELL-COUNT

ADDISON BYBEE, M.D. and W. F. LORENZ, M.D.
ELGIN, ILL. KANKAKEE, ILL.

In view of the fact that the technic employed for the examination of the cerebrospinal fluid varies greatly in the hands of the individual investigator and gives in consequence such discordant results, we have endeavored to develop a technic which shall have the advantages of uniformity and reliability, together with the simplicity requisite for ordinary bedside employment.

## REVIEW OF METHODS

The methods in common use at the present time for both quantitative and qualitative estimation of the cell contents of the cerebrospinal fluid are three in number. The first, the so-called French method, developed by Widal, Sicard and Ravaut, depends on the use of the centrifuge. The second, the cell-chamber method, was first introduced by Laignel-Lavastine and subsequently modified by Fuchs and Rosenthal. The third, that of Alzheimer, requires the use of a microtome and the necessary technic for tissue staining. Each has its advantages as well as disadvantages.

The Alzheimer method is obviously too slow and cumbersome for a routine measure. As a means of determining the number of cells present, it is subject to all the criticism offered to the centrifuge method. For cell differentiation no method has yet been developed that is as satisfactory, but the process is too time-consuming and technical for a routine measure.

The obvious errors encountered in the French method were recognized soon after its introduction. They may be briefly summarized as follows: 1. The cells show a tendency to collect in clumps. 2. Many of the cells will adhere to the bottom and sides of the centrifuge tube. 3. The size of the drops delivered from the capillary pipette will vary, as will also the area covered by the drop. 4. The speed of operation of different centrifuges, and consequently the length of time necessary for complete sedimentation, varies.

In order to overcome these difficulties, various modifications have been made by different observers to obtain a better mixture. Nissl advised blowing out the sediment from the capillary pipette and allowing it again to be drawn up. Merzbacher used a bulb-ended pipette for the purpose of securing a better mixture. E. Meyer rubbed the sides and bottom of the tip of the centrifuge tube with his pipette in order to collect as many as possible of the cells. Kafka[1] has suggested the division of the droplet of sediment into two equal parts and spreading each portion over a square centimeter of surface on suitably prepared cover-slips. He further emphasized the necessity for determining the length of time required to throw down all the cells by the particular centrifuge used.

It was found to be quite impossible to recover all the cells collected at the bottom of the centrifuge tube. After the removal of the original contents, a washing from the bottom of the tube with a small amount of cell-free fluid dried on a cover-slip, fixed and stained, invariably presented a cell content varying with the degree of lymphocytosis. Furthermore, we have frequently failed to obtain any degree of uniformity of cell mixture. Often a field is observed showing a count as high as forty or more cells, while a field directly adjacent may give a count of two or three or even none. This uneven distribution of cells makes it imperative that a large number of fields be counted. An average computed from a count of ten or twenty fields would not be a fair estimation. Consequently in this investigation we have made it a rule to count at least fifty, frequently one hundred.

The standardization of the particular centrifuge by each investigator we believe to be practically impossible. The density of the cerebrospinal fluid varies from case to case, and consequently the difference in density between the cells and the fluid on which the centrifuge depends for the precipitation of the cells must also vary. If the observation by Fischer,[2] that the cell content of the cerebrospinal fluid varies greatly at different levels of the spinal column, be confirmed, as it is by our own limited investigation in this direction, it must be conceded that there can be but slight difference in the density of the fluid and that of the cells. Fischer found that a higher cell count may exist at the lower level of the first lumbar vertebræ than that which obtains at the lower border of the fourth. Consequently, in cases in which this difference in density is slight, the centrifuge cannot be expected to throw the cells down in the same limit of time as in cases in which the difference is larger.

In a series of thirty cases this point was given special attention. All cases were treated similarly, each fluid being swung one-half hour at a rate of 1,200 revolutions per minute, two specimens being treated simultaneously. In fourteen cases this time and rate of speed were ample to throw down all the cells. The remaining sixteen cases, however, did not give the desired result, as was shown by the examination of the supernatant liquor. Often the specimens treated simultaneously would show discordant results, one still presenting cells in the supernatant liquor,

---

1. Kafka, V.: Monatsch. f. Psychiat. u. Neurol, 1910, xxvii, 414.
2. Fischer, O.: Monatschr. f. Psychiat. u. Neurol., 1910, xxvii, 512.

the other a perfectly cell-free fluid. We wish to direct attention to the fact shown by the accompanying chart, that the cases giving unsatisfactory results were not always those with a high cell count. Cases 7, 23, 29 and 36 had a count of over 50 cells per cubic millimeter, yet the supernatant liquor was free from cells. On the other hand, Cases 9, 18 and 47, all having cell counts of 19 or less per cubic millimeter, still showed cells present in the fluid after centrifugation. Case 47, it will be noted, presented only 2 cells per cubic millimeter.

The shape of the centrifuge tube used is another source of error. The tubes employed in this work were of three types. The first was a sharp-pointed, gradually tapering tube, holding 15 c.c. of fluid. With this instrument we obtained results more nearly approximating those given by Rehm,[3] Kafka,[1] and others. The second tube was of the same size, but of a blunter point. This was found to give results not so evenly positive as the first type employed. Finally we had a tube made with a capillary tip, and this likewise gave results varying widely from the count obtained by the chamber method. The distortion and fracturing of cells in this method is a feature not to be ignored.

We are told by Rehm,[3] Cornell,[4] Kafka,[1] Fischer, Fuchs and Rosenthal, and other authorities who have employed the cell-chamber method, that there may be normally present in the cerebrospinal fluid from no cells to 5 cells per cubic millimeter. With this in mind it is obvious that 3 c.c. of fluid may contain 15,000 cells, so that, were the centrifuge effective and the subsequent collection without fault, this number of cells would be present in a small droplet or a measured area on the cover-slip. Consequently positive cell counts would be expected in negative cases. This, however, does not appear to occur. Indeed, negative counts, as shown in our table, occur in positive cases, and the inferences would seem obvious; either the cells are not entirely thrown down or not entirely recovered.

The cell-chamber method was first employed by Laignel-Lavastine. This investigator first centrifuged the fluid and then used the ordinary Thoma-Zeiss blood-counting slide. This procedure is obviously open to the same criticisms as the centrifuge method. Some years later Fuchs and Rosenthal devised a method much used since. In their technic they followed the suggestion of Laignel-Lavastine in the matter of the use of the counting chamber. They employed the white blood-cell pipette, with their stain, which consists of the following:

| | |
|---|---|
| Methyl violet | 0.1 |
| Glacial acetic acid | 2.0 |
| Distilled water enough to make | 50.0 |

3. Rehm, O.: In Nissl and Alzheimer's Histologische und Histopathologische Arbeiten, 1909, iii, 201.
4. Cornell, W. Burgess: Am. Jour. Insan., 1908, lxiv, 73.

This they drew up to the 0.5 mark and then drew the fluid to be examined with this stain into the diluting-chamber. These investigators have devised a special counting-chamber, which offers no advantage over the ordinary blood-counting chamber, beyond that it contains a larger quantity of fluid. In this counting-chamber the ruled space is 4 mm. square and its depth is 0.2 mm.; thus it offers 3.2 c.mm. for counting. Cornell[4] has adduced serious objections to this method, the chief being that erythrocytes will take the stain. He has suggested instead the use of polychrome methylene-blue in the same manner and employed the ordinary blood-counting chamber with Türck's ruling, counting at least three specimens. Kafka has likewise offered the same objection to the Fuchs-Rosenthal method and suggests taking 10 drops of cerebrospinal fluid in a small pointed glass, and adding thereto an equal-sized drop of a 2, 4 or 5 per cent. solution of glacial acetic acid colored with methyl violet, shaking well and counting soon after in a Elzholz chamber. He himself draws attention to the fact that on long standing the red cells take the stain.

It can be seen from the previously described objections and modifications that the Fuchs-Rosenthal method is by no means perfect. In our hands, as well as in those of the investigators quoted, the red cells were frequently more or less stained, rendering it impossible to differentiate. The suggestion of Cornell[4] to use polychrome methylene-blue gave similar results in our hands. To overcome this difficulty we experimented with many stains, all of which proved unsatisfactory for cell-chamber use in this manner, except the Fuchs-Rosenthal stain used as described under technic.

## TECHNIC

The technic used by us differs from that of Fuchs and Rosenthal in that we employ a red-cell pipette, drawing their original stain to 0.7, and wiping away the excess of stain from the point of the pipette. The stain is then drawn up into the diluting-chamber in such a manner that it evenly coats the inner wall. This can readily be accomplished by holding the point downwards and causing the incoming air to form bubbles that paint the sides evenly. If this be attempted while the pipette is in a horizontal position, the stain will be drawn into the exit and thus the pipette rendered useless.

The first 3 c.c. of fluid to escape are collected in the centrifuge tube and subsequently used for the film method. The second 2 or 3 c.c. of fluid removed are collected in a small test-tube, the tip of the red-cell pipette is then dipped in the fluid at once (since, according to Kafka,[1] fluid on standing shows a high number of degenerate cells) and the diluting-chamber filled rapidly. The pipette is then capped and thoroughly shaken for a period of five or more minutes. After twenty minutes, the pipette is again thoroughly shaken and five Thoma-Zeiss counting-chambers are filled from this pipette and permitted to stand for one-half hour. At the end of this period the entire number of cells within the square millimeter of ruled surface, as well as an equal surface outside of the ruled space of each chamber are counted. This can readily be accomplished by the use of an Ehrlich eye-piece. We then have the number of cells in an entire cubic millimeter of cerebrospinal fluid. In those fields showing a small cell content, two or more cubic millimeters of fluid have been counted to insure greater accuracy. The calculation of the number of cells in the cubic millimeter is simple, since the dilution of the fluid is only slightly more than 1/200. In our work we ignored the dilution and considered the number counted in the cubic millimeter as the actual number present. In following this technic one is constantly impressed with the regularity of numbers appearing in each counting-chamber.

The specimen taken in the centrifuge tube to which is added 3 drops of a 40 per cent. formaldehyd solution, according to the suggestion of O. Fischer,[5] is swung at a rate of 1,200 revolutions per minute for a period of one-half hour. The specimen of the supernatant liquid is then taken by means of a newly drawn pipette, which is introduced into the column of fluid so that the fluid taken is from a point at about the juncture of the middle and lower thirds. The droplet is blown out on a freshly prepared cover-slip, permitted to dry in the air, subsequently fixed and stained and a careful search made for cells.

After removing this specimen of supernatant liquid the tube is inverted and permitted to drain thoroughly. The residue is then drawn into a freshly prepared pipette. The suggestions of Nissl and E. Meyer are followed and finally the contents of the capillary pipette are marked off into equal parts. Each part is spread over a square centimeter of surface on two freshly prepared cover-slips, in this respect following the technic of Kafka.[1] After drying in the air the film is fixed by absolute methyl alcohol, washed in distilled water and stained for ten minutes in a weak Delafield's hematoxylin (5 drops to a watch crystal of distilled water). It is then washed in distilled water and permitted to remain in tap water for a few minutes. The excess of stain is removed by immersing for a few seconds in acid alcohol (one drop of dilute hydrochloric acid in 50 drops of 70 per cent. alcohol). After thoroughly washing in distilled water the film is placed in a weak aqueous eosin solution (six drops of a 0.5 per cent. eosin to a watch-crystal of distilled water) for four or five minutes. The film is washed in distilled water, dried between blotting papers, then high above a flame and mounted in cedar oil.

The film stained in this manner was used for the most part for field and differential count. A number of films were stained with Jenner's

5. Fischer, O.: Prag. med. Wchnschr., 1904.

stain for this same purpose. The field counts were made for the purpose of comparison with the cell-chamber counts, the object being to determine the relative value of these methods in the quantitative estimation of the cells present. Their comparative values is well shown in the accompanying table. It may be noted in passing that Jenner's stain was rendered useless for the films when formaldehyd had been added to the fluid. The field-counts were made, using a 1/12 oil immersion lens (Zeiss) and a 22.5 mm. eye-piece (Zeiss).

## CELL TYPES

There has been considerable effort on the part of investigators to differentiate the cells appearing in the cerebrospinal fluid, with widely varying results. Some describe only three varieties (O. Fischer[6]), while others find as many as six types, besides a group of unclassified cells. Rehm[3] finds great variations in the cell picture and classifies in a special manner. He describes, besides large and small lymphocytes, plasma cells and polymorphic elements, a cell having a large lobed nucleus showing manifold and complex shapes, four or five times the size of a small lymphocyte and having only a slight rim of protoplasm. He also finds two groups corresponding respectively to the large and small lymphocytes, but with a much greater protoplasmic body, showing branchings and drawn out processes, with nuclei which stain more lightly and are also irregular in shape. Under the name *Gitter* (or lattice cell) is described by the same author a further type. Thus this author adds four types to the many cells already described as occurring in the cerebrospinal fluid.

From the above we think it fair to infer that the shape and staining pictures as described in the literature, as well as the names applied to the individual elements, are often largely dependent on the method employed and the taste of the investigator. As before stated, the methods employed in cell differentiation are three in number. A number of investigators attempt to do this in the cell counting chamber. Others use the film after centrifugation and still others the Alzheimer method. The Alzheimer method was not used by us as a routine measure, for the reasons given above.

The cell-chamber method as employed by Fuchs and Rosenthal, and Cornell was not satisfactory for the purpose of cell differentiation. The dyes suggested by these authors and used according to their method invariably stained many of the red cells, which are almost always present to a greater or less degree. Often red cells and nucleated elements, apparently of the same type, were stained to different depths. This may have been due to the fact that the column of stain pushed into the diluting-chamber of the pipette by the oncoming cerebrospinal fluid was at

6. Fischer, O.: Jahrb. f. Psychiat. u. Neurol., 1910, xxvii.

first entirely too concentrated for the red cells to resist, and it may also account for the wide variation in the depth of staining of the nucleated elements. Although this difficulty was not encountered when we followed our method of using the Fuchs-Rosenthal stain, yet differentiation of the nuclear elements was not so readily made, nor were the six types to be spoken of later so clearly defined as in the film preparation.

The staining of films after centrifugation is widely practiced. The stains commonly used are those employed for blood work, Leishman's, Wright's, Jenner's, Nocht's and eosin hematoxylin.

Jenner's blood-stain and eosin hematoxylin, as suggested by Kafka,[1] have been used by us exclusively in the fifty-one cases shown in the accompanying table. Cases 1 to 6, and 41 to 46, inclusive, have been differentiated by means of Jenner's stain; all others by the use of eosin-hematoxylin, as described under "technic." A reference to the table will show a variation in the number of plasma cells present with the two different methods of staining, greater than it would seem fair to suppose to be due to case variation; it emphasizes the lesson that we cannot as yet compare the results obtained with different stains and different technic.

In the differentiation of the cells in this series we have frequently seen elements partaking of the characteristics of two or more of the cell groups arbitrarily decided on by us as a suitable classification. From a study of the descriptions and illustrations in the literature, we have felt that indecision in classification was by no means peculiar to us. For instance, in Stoddart's[7] "Mind and its Disorders," is an illustration by Dr. J. G. Phillips, in which he points out side by side a plasma and an endothelial cell. It is indeed difficult, if not impossible, to see any difference in these cells. One cannot be sure that the stress of centrifugation and the manipulation, both chemical and physical, used in embedding and staining has not given these cells their exceedingly slight difference in appearance. Moreover, there is little or no difference in the tinctorial reaction of these two elements, such as is supposed to occur in the two groups of cells in question.

The two cells pictured in this same illustration as endothelial cells might well be called plasma cells, descended from an endothelial parentage, as suggested by John Turner.[8] To be sure we do not find in the nuclei of these (endothelial cells) the deep red nucleolus usually figured, but they are not always seen, as Turner shows, neither are they found in the other plasma cells figured in this article. Further, the "bitten-out appearance" with the reniform and eccentric position of the nucleus, described by Turner as occurring in the plasma cells, are

7. Stoddart, W. H. B.: Mind and Its Disorders, Blakiston's Son & Co., Philadelphia, 1909, p. 208.

8. Turner, John: Rev. Neurol. and Psychiat., viii, 151.

present here. Turner[8] speaks of the resemblance of this type of plasma cell to the large endothelial cell with oval, pale-staining nucleus lining the vessels. In this same article he also describes the origin of another type of plasma cells from lymphocytes.

The disagreement and uncertainty with regard to other varieties is quite as patent. Plate 17 of Henry A. Cotton's[9] article shows a "transitional cell." It is difficult to see why Numbers 6, 7 and 8 of this illustration should be called unquestionable plasma cells, and Number 10 a questionable transitional cell. It would be easy to illustrate the diversity of opinion and uncertainty of writers by quoting from other authors, but enough has been said to demonstrate this point.

In this article six groups of cells have been recognized and designated according to the terminology most used in the literature. They are described here in the order of frequency of occurrence as revealed with the eosin-hematoxylin stain.

1. Small lymphocytes.
2. Plasma cells.
3. Polymorphonuclear elements
4. Large lymphocytes.
5. Degenerate cells.
6. Endothelial cells.

*Small Lymphocytes.*—Cells of this type are quite generally agreed on. They appear as small, round cells, varying in size from slightly less to slightly larger than a red blood-cell. They present a darkly staining nucleus with little or no protoplasm. The larger cells of this group often stain less deeply than the smaller. Cells of apparently the same class occasionally show a narrow rim of faintly pink or rose-colored protoplasm. They range in the cases here presented from 19 to 94.5 per cent. and average 61.3 per cent.

*Plasma Cells.*—These cells vary in size from a little less than a red cell to two, and rarely three times this size. The nucleus is darkly staining, but does not approach the inky blackness of the small lymphocyte. Occasionally it is violet. The nucleus, as figured in the films studied, is variously shaped. It is often round or oval, and occasionally drawn out into a finger-like body. At other times it is reniform. Sometimes it appears indistinctly lobed. It is usually eccentrically placed, but may be only slightly removed from the center of the plasma body. Such a cell is often seen with only a narrow isthmus connecting the nucleus and the cell body. This isthmus is composed of a central thread of nuclear material with a surrounding envelope of protoplasm. The protoplasm varies, sometimes taking on a deep rose-red color; at other times it stains

9. Cotton, H. C., and Ayer, J. B.: Rev. Neurol. and Psychiat., vi, 207.

much more faintly. Plasma cells range from 0 to 57 per cent. and average 24 per cent. of the cells present.

*Polymorphonuclear Cells.*—These elements present considerable variation in size, shape, and staining characteristics as to both nucleus and protoplasm. The type occurring in the infective meningitides and those that are picked up in transit by the needle, or otherwise, enter the field as blood contamination, need no description. Cells do occur, however, usually of the size of a small polymorphonuclear neutrophil, sometimes larger, sometimes much smaller, which present some difference in appearance. The larger and medium-sized cells of this group have nuclei answering the description of the nucleus of the ordinary white cell of the blood. They take the nuclear stain with but slight variation. The smaller type of this group, however, presents a nuclear appearance which is very different. On first sight the nucleus seems to be multiple. It appears as two, three, four or five black points. On more careful study minute threads of nuclear substance can be seen bridging the intervening spaces. The protoplasm of the larger cells usually is very faintly pink, whereas the smaller types stain a deeper rose-color. Kafka and O. Fischer have called attention to the fact that they sometimes show an eosinophilic protoplasm throughout their entirety, sometimes only in the center. These cells are often round and show distinct margins, while at other times they are very irregular in outline and indistinct. They are sometimes drawn out as if about to be divided by force. In such cells the nuclei show faint strands, reaching across the thin area, giving the parallel appearance of the strings of a musical instrument. It seems worthy of special attention that Case 19, with 47.5 per cent. polynuclears, and Case 35, with a polynuclear count of 33 per cent. showed the existence of a well-marked leukocytosis in the blood. These same cases did not show a marked blood contamination in the films examined. We have also observed this feature in cases not here recorded, in which there was no question of general paralysis of the insane. They range from 1 to 47.5 per cent. and average 3.4 per cent.

*Large Lymphocytes.*—These cells range in size from slightly larger than a red cell to occasionally three times this size. Their nuclei stain less deeply than those of the small lymphocyte. Occasionally they present a rim of protoplasm which stains with the nuclear dye. The staining of the protoplasm may be slightly darker than that of the nucleus, or, so nearly that of the nucleus, that only by focusing in and out with the micrometer adjustment can the protoplasm be distinguished from the nuclear substance. Large lymphocytes range in numbers from 1 to 35 per cent. and average 7.5 per cent.

*Degenerate Cells.*—These cells sometimes appear as a faint halo of nuclear stain, enclosing spaces having much the appearance of cells showing fatty degeneration. Still again, we sometimes find an element showing a strange mixture of both the acid and the basic dye, intermingled in an indefinite manner. These cells range from 0 to 3 per cent. and average 0.43 per cent.

*Endothelial Cells.*—The endothelial cells range in size from slightly less than an ordinary polymorphonuclear leukocyte to twice this dimension. The nucleus is larger than a red blood-cell. It is round or oval, may be slightly reniform, and is usually somewhat eccentrically placed. The nucleus stains somewhat paler than the large lymphocyte and sometimes presents a slightly violet tinge. The protoplasm is abundant and takes the eosin stain quite easily. Endothelial cells range from 0 to 4 per cent. and average 0.4 per cent.

### CHEMICAL EXAMINATION

A chemical examination is made on the liquid remaining in the small test-tube, after the portion has been removed for the chamber count. Sufficient time for these tests occurred while the one specimen was being centrifuged and that in the cell-chamber was given time to settle.

As a routine procedure we performed the Noguchi butyric acid test, the serum albumin test as outlined by Nissl and Cohnheim, and a test for the reducing substance, using Fehling's solution. We also made a quantitative estimation of albumin in a certain number of cases by Brandberg's method. The Noguchi butyric acid test was made as follows: In a small test-tube, 0.2 c.c. of the cerebrospinal fluid was placed. To this was added 0.5 c.c. of 10 per cent. butyric acid in distilled water. This mixture was then heated until it bubbled. While still hot, 0.2 c.c. of a 4 per cent. solution of sodium hydrate was added. The reaction depends on the appearance within twenty minutes of a definitely flocculent precipitate. Clouding or haziness of the mixture does not constitute a reaction. This test gave thirty-nine positive reactions in forty-two clinically and cytologically positive cases of general paralysis of the insane, or 92 per cent. positive findings. Two cases, Nos. 42 and 46, clinically and cytologically negative, gave a positive Noguchi reaction. Of the nine clinically and cytologically negative cases, seven gave negative Noguchi, or 77 per cent. negative findings. In the two cases with positive reactions, a previous syphilitic history cannot be excluded.

Nonne divides the albumin test into two phases, both having varying degrees of reaction, estimated by the depth of cloudiness. The first phase is the reaction obtained by the addition of heat-saturated ammonium sulphate solution to cerebrospinal fluid in equal parts. It is asserted that this semisaturation precipitates the globulins and should be permitted to stand for three minutes, when an estimation is made of the degree of reaction. Nonne states that Phase 1 occurs in all examinations of

TABLE SHOWING COMPARATIVE RESULTS OF THE CELL-CHAMBER AND CENTRIFUGE METHODS OF CELL ESTIMATION; DIFFERENTIAL COUNT AND CLINICAL REACTIONS

| | Chamber Method. | | Centrifuge Method. | | | Differential Cell Count in Percentages. | | | | | | Chemical. | | | | | | |
|---|---|---|---|---|---|---|---|---|---|---|---|---|---|---|---|---|---|---|
| Case. | Chamber Count, Per mm. | Reaction. | Field Count, Per Field. | Reaction. | Cells in Supernatant Fluid. | Small Lymphocytes. | Plasma Cells. | Polymorphonuclear Cells. | Large Lymphocytes. | Degenerated Cells. | Endothelial Cells. | Noguchi's Test. | Ser. Albumin. | ½ Sat'd. Ammonia Sulphate. | Brandberg Test. | Fehling's Test. | Clinical G. P. I. | Case. |
| 1 | 105 | P | 18.0 | P | .. | 84.0 | 9.0 | 2.0 | 5.0 | 0.0 | 0.0 | P | P | P | ...... | P | P | 1 |
| 2 | 85 | P | 35.0 | P | .. | 80.5 | 10.0 | 0.0 | 8.0 | 1.5 | 0.0 | P | P | .. | ...... | N | P | 2 |
| 3 | 136 | P | 32.0 | P | .. | 83.0 | 6.0 | 1.0 | 9.5 | 0.0 | 1.0 | P | P | .. | ...... | N | P | 3 |
| 4 | 72 | P | 7.0 | P | .. | 88.5 | 4.0 | 0.5 | 4.0 | 1.5 | 1.5 | P | P | .. | ...... | P | P | 4 |
| 5 | 75 | P | 6.0 | P | .. | 92.0 | 3.0 | 0.5 | 4.5 | 0.0 | 0.0 | P | P | .. | ...... | P | P | 5 |
| 6 | 25 | P | 4.0 | N | .. | 90.0 | 4.0 | 0.0 | 6.0 | 0.0 | 0.0 | P | P | .. | ...... | P | P | 6 |
| 7 | 73 | P | 28.0 | P | p | 63.0 | 30.5 | 2.0 | 3.5 | 1.0 | 0.0 | P | P | .. | ...... | N | P | 7 |
| 8 | 19 | P | 13.0 | P | O | 31.0 | 57.0 | 3.0 | 9.0 | 0.0 | 0.0 | P | P | .. | ...... | N | P | 8 |
| 9 | 16 | P | 5.0 | N | p | 38.5 | 53.5 | 1.0 | 7.0 | 0.0 | 0.0 | P | P | .. | ...... | N | P | 9 |
| 10 | 12 | P | 1.0 | N | O | 57.0 | 27.0 | 0.5 | 15.0 | 0.5 | 0.0 | P | P | .. | ...... | N | P | 10 |
| 11 | 42 | P | 5.0 | N | p | 77.5 | 11.5 | 1.0 | 9.5 | 0.5 | 0.0 | P | P | .. | ...... | N | P | 11 |
| 12 | 36 | P | 3.0 | N | p | 50.5 | 35.5 | 11.0 | 3.0 | 0.0 | 0.0 | P | P | .. | ...... | P | P | 12 |
| 13 | 27 | P | 2.0 | N | p | 41.5 | 46.5 | 7.5 | 3.0 | 1.5 | 0.5 | P | P | .. | ...... | N | P | 13 |
| 14 | 33 | P | 3.0 | N | O | 77.0 | 19.0 | 1.0 | 1.5 | 1.5 | 0.0 | P | P | P | 0.0033 | N | P | 14 |
| 15 | 9 | P | 1.0 | N | O | 50.5 | 40.5 | 2.0 | 5.0 | 2.0 | 0.0 | P | P | .. | 0.0033 | N | P | 15 |
| 16 | 17 | P | 1.0 | N | .. | 41.5 | 32.5 | 13.5 | 9.5 | 3.0 | 0.0 | P | N | P | 0.0033 | N | P | 16 |
| 17 | 49 | P | 2.0 | N | .. | 46.0 | 36.0 | 8.5 | 9.5 | 0.0 | 0.0 | P | P | P | ...... | N | P | 17 |
| 18 | 18 | P | 14.0 | P | p | 68.5 | 21.5 | 8.0 | 1.0 | 0.5 | 0.5 | P | P | P | 0.0033 | P | P | 18 |
| 19 | 121 | P | 7.0 | P | p | 19.0 | 28.0 | 47.5 | 4.5 | 0.0 | 1.0 | P | P | P | ...... | N | P | 19 |
| 20 | 27 | P | 2.0 | N | O | 57.5 | 22.5 | 14.5 | 5.0 | 0.0 | 0.5 | P | P | P | 0.0033 | N | P | 20 |
| 21 | 242 | P | * | .. | .. | .... | .... | .... | .... | ... | ... | P | P | P | 0.33 | .. | P | 21 |
| 22 | 162 | P | 3.0 | N | .. | 63.0 | 19.0 | 4.5 | 13.5 | 0.0 | 0.0 | P | P | P | ...... | N | P | 22 |
| 23 | 62 | P | 15.0 | P | O | 42.0 | 36.5 | 12.5 | 9.5 | 0.0 | 0.0 | P | P | P | 0.0033 | N | P | 23 |
| 24 | 14 | P | 1.0 | N | O | 48.0 | 24.0 | 14.0 | 14.0 | 0.0 | 0.0 | P | P | P | 0.0033 | N | P | 24 |
| 25 | 80 | P | 24.0 | P | p | 33.5 | 13.5 | 80.0 | 23.5 | 0.0 | 0.0 | P | P | P | 0.33 | N | P | 25 |
| 26 | 44 | P | 6.0 | P | O | 52.5 | 38.0 | 1.5 | 8.5 | 0.0 | 0.0 | P | P | P | 0.033 | N | P | 26 |
| 27 | 25 | P | 1.0 | N | p | 50.5 | 27.0 | 13.5 | 5.5 | 2.5 | 1.0 | P | P | P | 0.033 | N | P | 27 |
| 28 | 41 | P | 2.0 | N | p | 73.5 | 23.0 | 1.5 | 1.5 | 0.5 | 0.0 | P | P | P | 0.033 | N | P | 28 |
| 29 | 74 | P | 17.0 | P | O | 50.0 | 38.5 | 9.5 | 2.0 | 0.0 | 0.0 | P | P | P | ...... | N | P | 29 |
| 30 | 49 | P | 1.0 | N | .. | † | .... | .... | .... | ... | ... | P | P | P | 0.033 | N | P | 30 |

TABLE SHOWING COMPARATIVE RESULTS—CONTINUED

| Chamber Method. | | | Centrifuge Method. | | | Differential Cell Count in Percentages. | | | | | | Chemical. | | | | | | |
|---|---|---|---|---|---|---|---|---|---|---|---|---|---|---|---|---|---|---|
| Case. | Chamber Count, Per mm. | Reaction. | Field Count, Per Field. | Reaction. | Cells in Supernatant Fluid. | Small Lymphocytes. | Plasma Cells. | Polymorphonuclear Cells. | Large Lymphocytes. | Degenerated Cells. | Endothelial Cells. | Noguchi's Test. | Ser. Albumin. | ½ Sat'd. Ammonia Sulphate. | Brandberg Test. | Fehling's Test. | Clinical G. P. I. | Case. |
| 31 | 91 | P | 6.0 | P | .. | 53.0 | 37.0 | 8.0 | 2.0 | 0.0 | 0.0 | P | P | P | ...... | N | P | 31 |
| 32 | 25 | P | 1.0 | N | p | 44.0 | 42.0 | 6.0 | 6.0 | 2.0 | 0.0 | N | N | N | ...... | N | P | 32 |
| 33 | 55 | P | 2.0 | N | p | 68.5 | 23.0 | 2.0 | 6.5 | 0.0 | 0.0 | P | P | P | 0.033 | N | P | 33 |
| 34 | 23 | P | 2.0 | N | p | 44.5 | 33.5 | 15.0 | 6.5 | 0.0 | 0.5 | P | P | P | 0.033 | N | P | 34 |
| 35 | 39 | P | 2.0 | N | p | 32.0 | 17.0 | 33.0 | 14.0 | 0.0 | 4.0 | P | .. | .. | ...... | .. | P | 35 |
| 36 | 52 | P | 3.0 | N | O | 58.5 | 22.0 | 13.0 | 4.5 | 1.5 | 0.5 | P | P | P | 0.033 | P | P | 36 |
| 37 | 18 | P | 7.0 | P | O | 52.0 | 34.0 | 8.5 | 5.5 | 0.0 | 0.0 | P | P | P | 0.033 | P | P | 37 |
| 38 | 7 | P | 2.0 | N | O | 50.5 | 43.5 | 2.5 | 2.5 | 1.0 | 0.0 | P | P | P | 0.033 | N | P | 38 |
| 39 | 7 | P | 1.0 | N | O | 80.0 | 12.5 | 0.0 | 7.5 | 0.0 | 0.0 | P | P | P | 0.0033 | N | P | 39 |
| 40 | 17 | P | 2.0 | N | .. | 78.0 | 4.0 | 0.0 | 18.0 | 0.0 | 0.0 | N | P | .. | ...... | N | P | 40 |
| 41 | 5 | N | 3.0 | N | O | 89.0 | 0.0 | 0.0 | 10.0 | 0.0 | 1.0 | P | P | .. | ...... | N | P | 41 |
| 42 | 2 | N | 0.4 | N | .. | 93.0 | 3.0 | 0.0 | 4.0 | 0.0 | 0.0 | P | P | .. | ...... | P | N | 42 |
| 43 | 1 | N | 0.4 | N | .. | 90.0 | 4.0 | 1.0 | 5.0 | 0.0 | 0.0 | N | N | .. | ...... | P | N | 43 |
| 44 | 0 | N | 0.2 | N | .. | 50.0 | 9.5 | 21.5 | 12.5 | 0.0 | 6.5 | N | P | .. | ...... | P | N | 44 |
| 45 | 1 | N | 0.3 | N | .. | 86.0 | 7.0 | 0.0 | 7.0 | 0.0 | 0.0 | N | P | .. | ...... | .. | N | 45 |
| 46 | 4 | N | 2.0 | N | .. | 92.5 | 4.0 | 0.0 | 3.0 | 0.0 | 0.5 | P | P | .. | ...... | N | N | 46 |
| 47 | 2 | N | 1.0 | N | p | 30.0 | 50.0 | 7.5 | 11.0 | 0.0 | 1.5 | N | P | N | 0.0033 | N | N | 47 |
| 48 | 2 | N | 0.2 | N | O | 25.0 | 25.0 | 37.5 | 12.5 | 0.0 | 0.0 | N | N | P | 0.0033 | N | N | 48 |
| 49 | 1 | N | 0.3 | N | .. | 42.0 | 23.0 | 0.0 | 35.0 | 0.0 | 0.0 | N | N | N | 0.0033 | P | N | 49 |
| 50 | 2 | N | 0.0 | N | .. | .... | .... | .... | .... | ... | ... | N | N | P | 0.0033 | N | N | 50 |
| 51 | ... | .. | * | .. | .. | .... | .... | .... | .... | ... | ... | N | P | .. | ...... | P | P | 51 |

P, positive; N, negative; p, present.
* Blood and bile pigment present. † Blood present.

cerebrospinal fluid. The mixture of cerebrospinal fluid and ammonium sulphate is then filtered and to the filtrate is added one drop of a dilute acetic acid and the mixture boiled. This constitutes the second phase. The appearance of a cloud is a positive reaction. This cloud is said to be due to the presence of serum albumin. The degree of cloud occurring differs widely from specimen to specimen, and on this it has been suggested that a relative estimation of the quantity of serum albumin present be made. We tabulated as positive a cloudiness obtained by a half saturation of cerebrospinal fluid with a heat-saturated ammonium sulphate solution, representing the so-called serum globulin. Our serum-albumin test corresponds to the second phase as described above.

We employed the Brandberg method of quantitative estimation of albumin in the urine for the purpose of measuring the albumin in the cerebrospinal fluid. For this purpose we constructed a special two-armed small-calibered tube, which permitted the cerebrospinal fluid to flow gently on the heated nitric acid. The nitric acid was introduced by one arm of the tube, the fluid by the other, thus getting no other contact, but that at the meniscus. The readings are tabulated in our table under the heading of "Brandberg's Test." It will be seen that varying results occurred in the twenty-three clinically and cytologically positive cases in which this test was employed; twelve gave a quantitative reading of 0.0033 per cent. and nine others gave readings of 0.033 per cent., while two cases, one of which contained both bile and a large number of red cells, gave 0.33 per cent. The other was not contaminated by blood, and we are not able to offer any explanation for the high amount of albumin present. We regard this test as giving merely relative, not absolute values.

Similar variable figures are found in the literature. Rehm gives 0.03 to 0.06, or an average of 0.02 per cent. as occurring normally in the cerebrospinal fluid. Siemerling gives 0.02 to 0.1 per cent. Sahl gives 0.025 per cent. Landois gives 0.03 to 0.06 per cent.

For the purpose of quantitative estimation of the albumin present, various means have been employed. Nissl used a graduated tube from which he read the amount of precipitated albumin in percent. Rehm used Eshbach's reagent. Stephan Szecsi[10] modified Nonne and Apelt's method by employing a graduated tube, which he centrifuged and read off on his scale the amount of precipitate. From our investigations we would conclude that the quantitative estimation of albumin is of little clinical value, although it may be noted that in the four clinical and cytologically negative cases in which this estimation was performed, none showed over 0.0033 per cent. Our table does not show the parallel increase of albumin and lymphocytosis spoken of by Kutner and Rehm.

The reduction test was performed in the following manner: To 7 c.c. of a freshly prepared and heated Fehling's solution were added, one at a time, 10 drops of cerebrospinal fluid. This was heated and set aside. If after one hour a reduction precipitate occurred, a reading of positive was made. Nine of the thirty-nine clinically and cytologically positive cases in which this test was performed showed the presence of a reducing body, or 23 per cent. Four of the nine clinically and cytologically negative cases in which this reaction was performed, only 44 per cent., gave positive reaction.

10. Szecsi, Stephan: Monatschr. f. Psychiat. and Neurol., 1910, xxvii, 152.

## CONCLUSIONS

I. The French or centrifuge method for examination of the cells in the cerebrospinal fluid is not reliable for numerous reasons:

1. The cells are not always entirely thrown down, even by prolonged centrifugation.
2. It seems probable that this failure may be due to the difference in density of cells and fluid being insufficient at all times.
3. It is impossible to collect in a pipette all the cells which are thrown down.
4. The centrifugation results in clumping of the cells, which cannot be entirely overcome.
5. This method requires the use of a centrifuge and is consequently not clinical.

II. The counting-chamber method, when modified so that the red blood cells do not stain, presents none of the above objections. It requires only the ordinary blood-counting apparatus.

III. The amount of fluid necessary for the counting-chamber method is at a minimum.

IV. In our hands all clinically and cytologically positive cases of general paralysis of the insane gave a positive cell-chamber count.[11] With the French method only sixteen positive results were obtained and twenty-four negative results. In connection with this point we would call attention to the frequent statement in the literature that a single puncture is not reliable as a negative result, and that in none of our cases was more than one puncture used.

V. Differential cell counts at present give but little additional information, except in so far as they distinguish a lymphocytosis from a leukocytosis.

VI. This paper deals more especially with the cytological problems, but it is worth noting that Noguchi's butyric acid test gave thirty-eight positive results in forty clinically and cytologically positive cases of general paralysis of the insane.

Finally we wish to thank Dr. Singer for his invaluable assistance and criticism on this paper; also Dr. Norbury and our colleagues for their hearty cooperation.

---

11. Case 41 is clinically doubtful and by the chamber method gave the maximum normal limit of cells per cubic millimeter.

# OBSERVATIONS ON SCHUERMANN'S COLOR TEST FOR SYPHILIS *

ROBERT GOLDSBOROUGH OWEN, M.D.
DETROIT

Since the introduction of the serum test for syphilis by Wassermann, Neisser and Bruck, in 1906, using the method of complement fixation or deviation as evolved by Bordet and Gengou, in 1901, a large number of modifications of Wassermann's original method have been suggested, many of which have proved of distinct value in simplifying the carrying out of the test and in rendering the diagnoses made thereby more accurate. The results of the many thousands of tests which have been made have shown the remarkable value of the reaction, but the method demands considerable skill in laboratory technic and a wide experience in interpreting its results. Any method, therefore, which would place the serum diagnosis of syphilis on a plane easily reached by the man of average laboratory training with the equipment ordinarily found in a doctor's office, or at least easily secured, should first be accurately tried out by a number of observers and then, and not until then, welcomed by the profession at large.

W. Schürmann,[1] working in the Institute for Experimental Therapy at Düsseldorf, published what he considered to be a very simple color test for syphilitic serums, and reported most favorable results from the use of his method. Schürmann based his preliminary experiments on the work of Levaditi and Marie,[2] who had shown that it was possible to carry out the Wassermann test using extract of heart muscle from healthy guinea-pigs as antigen. From this work Schürmann thought that there might be something contained in the heart muscle which was represented by some of our simple chemical compounds. Working on this theory he sought for some simple substance in syphilitic blood with which a color reaction might be obtained. Reasoning further along this line, he concluded that lactic acid might be the simple element in heart muscle which played the chief rôle in the test, and found indeed that an extract containing this substance used as antigen did give a good reaction with syphilitic serums.

---

* From Research Department, Detroit Clinical Laboratory.

1. Schürmann, W.: Verlangsamung des Stoffwechsels, Deutsch. med. Wchnschr., 1909, xxxv, 616; abstr. in Jour. Am. Med. Assn., 1909, lii, 1629.

2. Levaditi and Marie: Ann. de l'Inst. Pasteur, 1907, xxi, 138.

The presence of lactic acid is readily shown by the application of Uffelmann's test (phenol and ferric chlorid reaction), and Schürmann first used this in his work, but finding that the presence of blood pigment in the serums interfered with the carrying out of the test, he hit upon the scheme of breaking up the pigment by means of perhydrol (hydrogen peroxid, Merck).

The test is carried out as follows: to 0.1 c.c. suspected serum and 3 to 4 c.c. normal salt solution is added one drop perhydrol; this is shaken well and 0.5 c.c. of the modified Uffelmann reagent (phenol 0.5, 5 per cent. solution ferric chlorid in water 0.62, distilled water 34.5 parts) is added.

Schürmann attributes the test to the action of the watery solution of the ferric chlorid, the reaction of the perhydrol and the blood serum, whether acid or alkaline. The reagent must be freshly prepared for each set of tests.

According to this observer normal serums cause only a green or greenish-blue color, the mixture remaining uniformly clear. With syphilitic serums the color is dark brown-black and the mixture becomes opaque. Syphilitic serums also give more or less foaming. The reading of the test should be made after one or two minutes. Later changes are of no significance. Perhydrol must be added before the special reagent, or negative serums will give a positive reaction.

Schürmann compared his test with the original Wassermann test in eighty-four cases. Thirty-nine cases positive to Wassermann also responded to his test. Serums from two scarlet fever cases, 1 sheep, 2 guinea-pigs and 6 rabbits all gave negative results.

A careful study of Schürmann's paper, the essential points of which I have given above, still leaves one in doubt as to just what he considers to be the factor in syphilitic serums which responds to the modified Uffelmann test. Is it lactic acid or some of its derivatives? His line of reasoning certainly points to that belief, yet the only explanation he gives is:

"Es ist der Wassergehalt des Eisenchlorids, die Reaktion des Perhydrols und des Blutserums, ob sauer oder alkalisch, sicherlich von bedeutenden Einfluss für das Gelingen der Reaktion."

From the fact that Schürmann was able to get a fixation of complement with syphilitic serums using lactic acid preparations as antigen it would seem as though he intended to imply that some sort of lactic acid antibody was present in such serum. We know, however, that in general it is impossible to obtain antibodies to such substances as acids, alkalies, bases or salts. Moreover, his use of the modified Uffelmann reagent would point to his belief in an increased lactic acid content of a syphilitic blood-serum. This lactic acid content of blood varies markedly, however.

Irisawa[3] found the content to vary greatly in different individuals, and Gaglio[4] observed that the amount present in the blood was considerably increased after meals and decreased when experimental starvation was induced.

Whatever may be the theoretical defects in Schürmann's reasoning it is the clinical application of his method as a diagnostic procedure for the differentiation of syphilitic and non-syphilitic serum to which we must take exception.

While his results were at first confirmed by Chirivino,[5] and to a certain extent by Fiorito,[6] Turchi,[7] Braunstein,[8] Clark,[9] and others, have been unable to obtain satisfactory results.

In my experiments I made use of the serum of several syphilitics and also of that of several normal persons. These bloods were tested by the Wassermann method with positive and negative results, respectively. In addition some forty specimens of blood were obtained from individuals supposedly healthy, from tuberculous subjects, from subjects of nephritis, carcinoma, exophthalmic goiter, typhoid fever and malaria. These serums were tested according to Schürmann's method, also by varying the amounts of the different reagents. Experiments were also carried out using distilled water and normal salt solution without the addition of any serum whatever. The color reaction described by Schürmann as being specific for syphilitic serum was given by all of these specimens though the color varied very slightly in some cases. Where normal salt solution or distilled water was used without the addition of any serum there was no clouding of the mixture, nor any precipitate, but the same color changes were observed. This clouding or precipitation then was evidently due to a combination of serum albumin and ferric chlorid solution. Perhydrol, plus normal salt or distilled water on the addition of the reagent gave the same color reaction. At times a green-blue tinge was observed in the negative serum, but such mixtures changed almost immediately to a dark brown. The color reaction then, is apparently due to the action of the perhydrol on the reagent, most probably a phenol oxidation process as has been suggested by Braunstein, and is given by serums from all sources regardless of their syphilitic or non-syphilitic origin.

---

3. Irisawa: Ztschr. f. physiol. Chem., 1892, viii, 349.
4. Gaglio: Arch. f. Physiol. (Du Bois), 1886, p. 400.
5. Chirivino, V.: La cromoreazione di Schürmann per la diagnosi della sifilide, Riforma med., 1910, xxvi, 194; abstr. in Jour. Am. Med. Assn., 1910, liv, 1098; Pathologica, 1910, ii, 185.
6. Fiorito: Gazz. internaz. di med., 1910, xiii, 1; Pathologica, 1910, ii, 186.
7. Turchi: Riv. di pat. nerv. e ment., 1909, xiv, 303; Pathologica, 1910, ii, 185.
8. Braunstein: Ztschr. f. klin. Med., 1909, lxviii, 345.
9. Clark: Jour. Infect. Dis., 1910, vii, 476.

CONCLUSION

1. A simple color test for syphilis would be an ideal one.

2. The method of Schürmann, however, does not provide us with such.

3. For the present at least we must rely on the proved qualities of the Wassermann or Noguchi methods.

33 High Street, East.

# IS HEMOGLOBINURIC FEVER A MANIFESTATION OF MALARIA OR A DISEASE *SUI GENERIS*?*

CHARLES F. CRAIG, M.D.
WASHINGTON, D. C.

The present condition of uncertainty regarding the etiology of hemoglobinuric fever may well be likened to that regarding the etiology of kala-azar ten years ago, and the history in this respect of the latter disease is of peculiar interest to the students of hemoglobinuric fever, because it furnishes an excellent example of how preconceived opinions influence the work of careful observers, and illustrates the fallibility of deductions regarding the etiology of any disease when influenced by such opinions.

For many years kala-azar was regarded as a persistent form of malarial infection, or a form of malarial cachexia. As late as 1896 Leonard Rogers considered it to be a fatal form of malaria, while Ronald Ross, in 1898, stated it as his belief that it was a form of malarial fever complicated by some secondary infection. Giles, after careful study, had come to the conclusion that kala-azar was due to *Ankylostoma duodenale*, and Bentley, in 1903, regarded it as a severe form of Malta fever. The discovery of the parasite now known as *Leishmania donovani* by Leishman, which was at once confirmed by Donovan, decided the etiology of kala-azar, and proved how erroneous were the theories regarding its malarial origin.

For years the study of hemoglobinuric fever has been greatly influenced by the theory that it is due to malarial infection, and much of the data which has accumulated concerning this disease has been published by believers in the malarial theory, or in the theory that it is due to quinin. While the literature contains many authentic instances which absolutely disprove both of these theories their adherents appear to have overlooked or undervalued them, and to-day the general opinion of the medical profession appears to be in favor of the theory that hemoglobinuric fever is due to malarial infection.

To one who carefully studies the literature of this disease it is evident that, in reality, its etiology is unknown; that the preconceived opinions regarding its malarial nature and its relation to quinin have greatly hindered investigation, and influenced those who have endeavored to study its etiology from an experimental standpoint; and that there is

*Read at the seventh annual meeting of the American Society of Tropical Medicine, June 11, 1910. Published by authority of the Surgeon General, U. S. Army.

every reason to believe that further research will result in proving that hemoglobinuric fever is a specific disease. The further we inquire into its etiology, pathology, and symptomatology, the more must we become convinced that the malarial nature of the condition is far from demonstrated, and that the evidence points to its being a specific disease caused by an undiscovered parasite.

Before considering in detail the theories regarding the etiology of this disease, I desire to call attention to the fact that not a few of the cases reported in the literature as hemoglobinuric fever are in reality other forms of hemoglobinuria or hematuria, having no relation to the true disease. Therefore, in the study of this condition it is most important to be sure that we are dealing with true hemoglobinuric fever rather than other conditions which sometimes very closely simulate it. Thus we must differentiate paroxysmal hemoglobinuria, hematuria, the hemoglobinuria following the administration of poisonous drugs, and the rare instances of idiosyncrasy to quinin, resulting in the production of this symptom. True hemoglobinuric fever has a definite symptomatology and is readily recognized by those living in the endemic areas, and all cases which do not agree with the clinical characteristics which have been described by many careful observers in blackwater fever regions should be regarded with suspicion. The mere fact that a patient passes a little bloody urine is very insufficient proof that he is suffering from hemoglobinuric fever, and yet the literature contains numerous reports in which this was the only symptom present, and such cases have been used to support the several theories regarding the etiology of the disease. In this contribution I have been careful to cite only those reports in which the patients described were without doubt suffering from hemoglobinuric fever.

There are three principal theories regarding the etiology of this disease; first, that it is due directly or indirectly to malarial infection; second, that it is due to quinin; and third, that it is a specific disease. Each has its enthusiastic supporters, but, as a matter of fact, not one of them rests on a firm foundation as regards absolute proof.

## *1. THE MALARIAL THEORY*

### PRESENT STATUS OF THEORY

The theory that hemoglobinuric fever is due directly or indirectly to malarial infection is very old, and is supported by many of the greatest authorities on the fevers of tropical and subtropical countries. The names of Plehm, Stephens, Bentley, Christophers, Zieman, Mannaberg, and others of equal reputation, are associated with this theory, and the following quotations from Stephens well illustrate its present position. Stephens says:[1]

1. Stephens, J. W. W.: Blackwater Fever, in Allbutt and Rolleston's A System of Medicine, London, 1907, ii, part 2, p. 295.

The etiology of blackwater fever may be summed up by saying that it is malarial in nature, *i. e.*, that it can only occur in those who are either suffering from, or have quite recently become infected with, malaria, and that the onset of the disease is induced most commonly, though not invariably, by quinin.

Again, in another contribution, he says:[2]

We may sum up the etiology of blackwater fever somewhat in this way: It is not a disease *per se*, but rather a condition of blood in which quinin, other drugs, cold, or even exertion, may produce a sudden destruction of red cells. The condition is produced only by malaria, and generally by repeated small attacks, insufficiently treated by quinin. In such cases of chronic malaria (*i. e.*, in those suffering from anemia with repeated attacks of fever and repeated doses of quinin) blackwater fever sooner or later almost certainly supervenes, at least in tropical climates. The two main factors in hemoglobinuria are, then, malaria and quinin.

Because of the objections to the malarial theory which have arisen from time to time, its adherents have modified their views, until we now have the rather amusing spectacle of a theory supported by numerous authorities, each of whom, however, explains the relation of the two diseases in a different maner. That this is true is evidenced by the following modifications of the theory which are supported by different investigators: Hemoglobinuric fever is caused by estivo-autumnal plasmodia; it is caused by a special species of malarial plasmodium; it is a peculiar form of pernicious malaria, which may be produced by any one of the species of plasmodia; it is due to malignant tertian infection accompanied by congestion of the liver; it is due to a toxin produced by the malarial plasmodia; it is due to a toxin resulting from the destruction of the red corpuscles by the plasmodia; it is due to changes in the blood caused by previous malarial infection; it is due to a condition of susceptibility to quinin brought about by malarial infection; it is due to an autolysin produced in the blood by malarial infection; it is an idiosyncrasy of certain malarial patients; and, finally, it is simply a complication of malarial fever.

The points which are usually urged in support of the malarial theory of the origin of hemoglobinuric fever are the following:

1. The occurrence of the disease only in malarial regions.

2. The presence of plasmodia in the blood, during the period immediately preceding, or during the first days of an attack.

3. The fact that most patients who develop hemoglobinuric fever have suffered previously from malaria.

4. The more frequent occurrence of the disease in localities where pernicious forms of malaria occur.

5. The fact that long residence in a malarial locality is required before the disease can develop.

6. The fact that there is an increase in the large mononuclear leukocytes similar to that occurring in malarial infection.

---

2. Stephens, J. W. W.: Blackwater Fever, in Osler's Modern Medicine, Philadelphia, 1907, i, 455.

In order to understand clearly the relation of malaria to hemoglobinuric fever, it is necessary to consider each of the points mentioned; and I believe that a careful survey of the evidence will carry the conviction that not one of them can be accepted as proving that the disease is of malarial origin, and that taken together they speak as strongly in support of the specific theory as they do of the theory under discussion.

### THE GEOGRAPHICAL DISTRIBUTION OF HEMOGLOBINURIC FEVER AND MALARIA

It is an accepted fact that hemoglobinuric fever occurs only in regions where malarial infections are endemic, but does this prove that the disease is of malarial origin? While the disease occurs only where malarial infections are endemic, there are many regions intensely infected with malaria where this disease is unknown. This fact must be admitted by every student of the disease, and is most difficult of explanation, if we accept the malarial theory. Hemoglobinuric fever is very prevalent and wide-spread in Africa, common in Sicily and Sardinia, but rare in Italy. In India the disease occurs in very limited localities, and similar regions in that country, as regards climatic and other known conditions, and as intensely infected with malaria, are free from hemoglobinuric fever. In Italy, even in the regions where the malarial fevers are most pernicious, this disease is either absent, or occurs very rarely. In fact, it may be said that Africa is the only country in which hemoglobinuric fever is generally distributed, for, in all the other countries in which it occurs, its distribution is strictly localized, while there are many countries in which pernicious forms of malaria occur, but in which blackwater fever is unknown, or occurs only in the form of imported cases. In a personal letter Dr. Prado, health officer of Trinidad, informs me that while malaria is both prevalent and severe in Trinidad and the island of Tobago, blackwater fever is common in Tobago and very rare in Trinidad, occurring only on a part of the coast-line adjacent to Tobago, and frequented by laborers from that island.

Even in the countries in which this fever occurs, there are many regions as intensely infected with malaria which are free from the disease, although only a comparatively short distance from the endemic foci. Such regions occur in our own country, in some of the southern states, and in Italy hemoglobinuric fever is limited to very restricted localities, while some of the worst malarial portions of that country have never presented a single instance of this disease. The same is true of India, of the Straits Settlements, the islands of Polynesia, the West Indies, and the countries of South America.

The almost complete absence of hemoglobinuric fever in the Philippine Islands is an excellent illustration of the fact that a most malarial country may be free from the disease. In the Philippine Census[3] for 1902, the total number of deaths from malarial fever is stated to have been 118,476, or 26.8 per cent. of all deaths, the death-rate being seventeen per thousand, and yet not a single death is recorded as being due to hemoglobinuric fever. How is it possible to explain this fact in accordance with the theory that the disease is caused by malarial infection?

Christophers and Bentley[4] believe that hemoglobinuric fever occurs only in countries where the malarial infections are intense, and that such infections, no matter what species of plasmodium causes them, may give rise to the disease. I believe that all will admit that the vast majority of intense or malignant malarial infections are caused by the estivo-autumnal plasmodia, but even in regions where the most severe estivo-autumnal infections are prevalent, hemoglobinuric fever is often absent. At Camp Stotsenburg, in the Philippines, one of the most intensely malarial regions of which we have record, where, within six months, there were more than thirty deaths from pernicious malaria among the natives in the vicinity, a case of hemoglobinuric fever has never been known to occur, and the natives informed me that they had never heard of a single instance of the passage of bloody urine during an attack of fever. If intense malarial infection is necessary for the production of hemoglobinuric fever, then in this locality one would expect to meet instances of the disease, but it is unknown. This is equally true of every other intensely malarious region in the Philippine Islands and of similar regions in many other parts of the world. Tables 1, 2 and 3 illustrate the intensity of malarial infection in some of the islands, provinces and towns of the Philippines, and prove that intensity of malarial infection has nothing to do with the production of hemoglobinuric fever.

It is evident from these tables that the Philippines are intensely infected with malaria and that the death-rate is high from that disease; but hemoglobinuric fever is practically unknown. I know from personal observation that the death-rate as given for some of these towns is not excessive, and that there are many towns in the Philippines in which malaria causes more than 50 per cent. of the death-rate.

Christophers and Bentley state that certain conditions may be present in blackwater regions which are not present in other malarial regions, but so far as climatic conditions are concerned this is not so, for in almost every country in which hemoglobinuric fever occurs the climatic conditions are the same in the blackwater regions as in others. So far as other conditions are concerned, it is enough to say that we are absolutely ignorant of what they are, and therefore they cannot be used in proving the malarial hypothesis. The fact remains that intense estivo-

3. Census of the Philippine Islands, Washington, 1905, iii, 70.

4. Christophers, S. R., and Bentley, C. A.: Blackwater Fever, Scient. Mem., Med. and San. Depts. Govt. India, Simla, 1908, N. S., No. 35.

TABLE 1.—TOTAL DEATHS AND DEATHS FROM MALARIA IN CERTAIN ISLANDS OF THE PHILIPPINES

| Island. | Total Deaths. | Deaths from Malaria. |
|---|---|---|
| Luzon | 248,831 | 60,516 |
| Cebu | 18,955 | 6,356 |
| Panay | 75,535 | 22,478 |
| Mindanao | 12,572 | 6,423 |
| Marinduque | 3,222 | 1,466 |
| Guimaras | 1,302 | 479 |
| Baliran | 1,247 | 423 |

TABLE 2.—POPULATION, TOTAL DEATHS AND DEATHS FROM MALARIA IN THE PROVINCES OF THE PHILIPPINE ISLANDS

| Province. | Population. | Total Deaths. | Deaths from Malaria. | Pr. Ct. of All Deaths. |
|---|---|---|---|---|
| Albay | 240,326 | 11,564 | 3,103 | 26.8 |
| Antigue | 134,166 | 7,411 | 3,181 | 42.9 |
| Batangas | 257,715 | 34,257 | 13,216 | 38.5 |
| Capiz | 230,721 | 15,564 | 3,254 | 20.9 |
| Cebu | 653,727 | 20,920 | 7,020 | 33.6 |
| Iloilo | 410,315 | 51,153 | 16,572 | 32.4 |
| La Laguna | 148,606 | 15,918 | 4,877 | 30.6 |
| Misamis | 175,683 | 9,038 | 4,961 | 54.9 |
| Pampanga | 223,754 | 14,383 | 3,247 | 22.6 |
| Pangasinan | 397,902 | 24,701 | 6,531 | 26.4 |
| Samar | 266,237 | 13,614 | 3,913 | 28.7 |
| Tayabas | 153,065 | 9,418 | 3,501 | 37.2 |
| Davao | 65,496 | 557 | 256 | 46. |
| Marinduque | 51,674 | 3,222 | 1,466 | 45. |
| Masbate | 43,675 | 1,881 | 811 | 43.1 |
| Nueva Vizcaya | 62,541 | 1,228 | 511 | 41.6 |
| Dapitan | 23,577 | 397 | 152 | 38.3 |
| Romblon | 52,848 | 1,422 | 531 | 37.3 |
| Surigao | 115,112 | 3,304 | 1,200 | 36.3 |
| Negros Oriental | 201,494 | 5,972 | 2,135 | 35.8 |
| Tarlao | 135,107 | 7,088 | 2,453 | 34.6 |

TABLE 3.—POPULATION, TOTAL DEATHS AND DEATHS FROM MALARIA IN PHILIPPINE TOWNS *

| Town. | Population. | Total Deaths. | Deaths from Malaria. |
|---|---|---|---|
| Angeles | 10,646 | 431 | 119 |
| Apalit | 12,206 | 771 | 208 |
| Anao-aon | 1,481 | 90 | 59 |
| Bacuag | 2,938 | 100 | 77 |
| Camiling | 25,243 | 1,288 | 513 |
| Concepcion | 12,593 | 600 | 211 |
| Gerona | 13,615 | 635 | 257 |
| Floridablanca | 7,001 | 623 | 328 |
| Jiminez | 7,187 | 1,066 | 1,019 |
| Misamis | 5,525 | 310 | 290 |
| Mabalacat | 7,009 | 201 | 126 |
| Mainit | 1,588 | 123 | 84 |
| Orequita | 15,156 | 1,650 | 1,572 |
| Palapag | 9,609 | 200 | 122 |
| Pasig | 4,830 | 296 | 110 |
| Pambujan | 6,439 | 331 | 174 |
| Porac | 8,487 | 490 | 251 |
| San Carlos | 27,166 | 1,856 | 744 |
| Tago | 3,298 | 129 | 60 |
| Taranguan | 6,184 | 549 | 234 |
| Tigao | 946 | 16 | 8 |
| Urdaneta | 20,544 | 1,378 | 498 |

* All of these tables are compiled from the Philippine Census.

autumnal infections are prevalent in nearly all tropical regions, while hemoglobinuric fever is restricted to certain countries, and in these countries, as a general rule, it occurs only in limited localities.

In regions in which hemoglobinuric fever occurs, the disease may be limited to certain very small areas, even to certain houses, and so-called "blackwater fever houses" have been reported by Daniels, Christophers and Bentley, and others. Christophers and Bentley report instances in which two or more cases of the disease have occurred in the same house, while other houses in the vicinity remained free from the infection. Because these houses were located in malarial localities, these authors believe that the disease must have been of malarial origin, but it would appear more reasonable to believe that some specific cause was present in these houses, or that the transmitting agent, perhaps a comparatively rare insect, was to be found only in the houses mentioned.

Another fact that speaks against the theory that hemoglobinuric fever is of malarial origin is that, in some of the countries where it is now prevalent, it has only recently been observed, although malarial fevers have been present for centuries. This fact must be admitted by every one who is conversant with the literature of the disease. A. Plehn[5] states that it is only recently that the disease has appeared on the west coast of Africa, where it is increasing in frequency yearly; and the same is true of India, where it is now prevalent in limited localities. The very extensive and valuable works of such men as Carter and Fayrer contain no mention of the occurrence of this disease in India in their time, and it is impossible to believe that these keen clinical observers could have overlooked a disease so striking in its symptomatology as is hemoglobinuric fever. If, then, this fever be due to malaria, how is it possible to explain its recent appearance in countries where for centuries the most intense malarial infections have existed? While it must be admitted that the disease occurs only in malarial localities, it can by no means be admitted that, therefore, the disease is of malarial nature. Many other acute infectious diseases are most commonly observed in regions infected with malaria, such as amebic dysentery, beriberi, infections with the various intestinal parasites, yellow fever, kala-azar, sleeping-sickness, and most tropical diseases, and some of them are practically limited to malarial localities, especially kala-azar, sleeping-sickness, and yellow fever; but we do not for this reason conclude that they are caused by malarial infection. The absence of hemoglobinuric fever from many intensely malarial regions and its presence in very limited localities in the regions in which it does occur, together with its recent appearance in certain countries, is very strong presumptive evidence that it is not due to

5. Plehn, A.: The Cause, Prevention and Treatment of Hemoglobinuric Fever in Warm Countries, Jour. Trop. Med. and Hyg., 1908, ii, 294.

malaria, and I believe that the unprejudiced observer must admit that the geographical distribution of this disease, far from proving its malarial origin, points directly to its specific nature.

### LENGTH OF RESIDENCE AND HEMOGLOBINURIC FEVER

It is a well-known fact that most victims of hemoglobinuric fever have resided for some time in the infected locality, and this fact is used as an argument in favor of the malarial theory, it being claimed that repeated malarial attacks are necessary for the production of this disease, and that therefore long residence in a malarial locality is essential. While it must be admitted that most cases of hemoglobinuric fever occur after the first twelve months of residence in the infected district is completed, many instances have been reported in which the symptoms appeared within less than three months after entering the infected territory, and in individuals who had never suffered from malarial infection, so far as could be ascertained; while a few cases have been reported in which the disease appeared within a few days after entering the blackwater district. I shall mention only a few of the authors who have reported instances of this kind, but the literature contains a great many such cases. Poole[6] found that, of fifty-six cases studied by him, no less than seventeen occurred in individuals who had been in the infected district less than one year. Reynolds[7] describes one instance in which the patient developed the disease within ten weeks after reaching the infected region, and others in which the disease appeared in four months, seven months, and nine months. Berenger-Feraud[8] observed one case in which the disease developed within three months, and ten in which it developed within one year; while Christophers and Bentley[4] observed one case developing within six months, and eight within one year after exposure in infected districts. Manson[9] states that instances of infection have been observed during the second and third months after arrival in infected regions, and in the last edition of his work on tropical diseases, he says (p. 235):

> There are many cases on record in which blackwater fever occurred before any kind of "malaria" had manifested itself. Plehn, Scott, Ritchie, Cardamatis, Lynch, Hearsey, Daniels and others have reported cases of blackwater fever in robust, healthy individuals, who were attacked within two or three months of their arrival in a blackwater fever country. I have frequently been told by officers in the African colonial service that the attack of blackwater fever for which they were invalided suddenly developed while they appeared to be in perfect health and without any malarial antecedents.

---

6. Poole, W.: An Analysis of Fifty-six Cases of Blackwater Fever, Jour. Trop. Med., 1899, i, 145.
7. Reynolds, G. F.: Blackwater Fever, Some Cases and Notes, Jour. Trop. Med., 1899, i, 16.
8. Berenger-Feraud: De la fièvre bileuse mélanurique des pays chauds, Paris, 1874, Ed. I.
9. Manson, Sir Patrick: Tropical Diseases, New York, 1907, Ed. 4.

F. Plehn[10] saw two patients suffering from hemoglobinuric fever which developed within four or five weeks after their arrival in Cameroon, neither of whom had suffered from malarial infection. Gross saw a patient who developed the disease within fifteen days after reaching Gaboon, and who had never had malaria. Brem[11] saw one patient who developed the disease after only two months' residence on the Isthmus of Panama; and Ziemann[12] one case occurring twenty-seven days after reaching the infected locality, and another within six weeks. Dr. Prado, in a personal communication, informs me that blackwater fever attacks new arrivals in Tobago.

It should be remembered that these patients had not resided previously in infected districts and that in most of them no history of a previous malarial infection could be obtained. It is thus evident that a long residence in the infected district is not necessary for the development of hemoglobinuric fever and that the statement of Christophers and Bentley that many months or years of exposure to the infection is required before blackwater fever can occur is unwarranted in the light of the evidence which has accumulated regarding this question.

While it is true that the disease may occur in individuals who have been exposed only a short time, it is also true that the vast majority of cases of this disease occur between the first and third years of residence, thus proving that length of residence favors the development of the disease. As the regions in which hemoglobinuric fever occur are also malarial, it follows that most of the victims of this disease have also suffered from malarial infection, but this does not prove that malaria is the etiological factor, as will be shown in the following section.

### PREVIOUS MALARIAL INFECTION AND HEMOGLOBINURIC FEVER

A history of previous malarial infection may be obtained in a large majority of cases of hemoglobinuric fever, but not in all. Many instances have been reported of the occurrence of this disease in individuals who had never suffered from malaria, and in whom no plasmodia could be found at the onset of the disease. The fact that the disease occurs most frequently in malarial localities makes it inevitable that most patients suffering from it have previously suffered from malaria, or, indeed, may be suffering from both diseases at the same time, for, from what we know of this disease, it is very rare as compared with malaria, and therefore most patients residing long enough in a locality to develop the disease have already become infected with malaria. It has been asserted by the

10. Quoted by A. Plehn, Jour. Trop. Med. and Hyg., 1908, ii, 294.

11. Brem. W. V.: Malarial Hemoglobinuria, Jour. Am. Med. Assn., 1906, xlvii, 1992.

12. Zieman, H.: Malaria, Mense's Handbuch der Tropenkrankheiten, Leipsic, 1906, iii (Halband I), 270.

most ardent advocates of the malarial theory that not a single case is on record of the occurrence of hemoglobinuric fever in a patient who had not previously had malaria, but such an assertion can be made only by one who is but very little acquainted with the literature, for numerous cases are recorded in which the disease developed in healthy individuals within two or three months after reaching infected districts and in whom there had never been any symptoms of malarial fever. That in most of these cases the disease could not have been present in a latent form is proved by the fact that many of the patients came from countries where malaria was not present, especially from England, and had not been exposed during the sea journey. Such cases have been reported by Manson,[9] Sambon,[13] Cardamatis,[14] Curry,[15] Ritchie,[16] Murri,[17] Stalkarrt,[18] Daniels,[19] and many others. The theory of Stephens and Christophers[20] that the disease is due to an unstable condition of the blood brought about by repeated malarial infection is thus disproved. It is a well-known fact that many patients suffering from hemoglobinuric fever do not present the appearance and symptoms of malarial cachexia, although, if this theory were true, it would be expected that most malarial cachectics would develop hemoglobinuric fever. It is also a well-known fact that this disease may develop during the first outbreak of malaria, and Deaderick[21] states that while hemoglobinuric fever generally occurs only after repeated malarial attacks, it may develop during the first attack. It is more than probable that such instances are in reality combined malarial and hemoglobinuric fevers.

Again, if repeated malarial attacks result in an unstable condition of the blood which causes hemoglobinuria, it is justifiable to ask why it is that such an unstable condition occurs as the result of malaria, only in restricted localities. In some of the most intensely malarial regions known a person may suffer for years from repeated attacks of malaria, and yet never develop hemoglobinuric fever, the disease being unknown in these regions. I have already called attention to the fact that climatic and all other known conditions are the same in these regions as in the

---

13. Sambon, L. W.: The Etiology and Treatment of Blackwater Fever, Jour. Trop. Med., 1899, i, 243, 262, 295.
14. Cardamatis: La fièvre bilieuse hémoglobinurique, Paris, 1902, Ed. 1.
15. Curry, Joseph J.: Blackwater (Hemoglobinuric) Fever, Jour. Am. Med. Assn., 1902, xxxviii, 1130.
16. Ritchie: Cited by Manson, Tropical Diseases, p. 235.
17. Murri: Cited by Deaderick, A Practical Study of Malaria.
18. Stalkarrt, W. H. S.: Hemoglobinuric Fever and Paludism, Brit. Med. Jour., 1899, ii, 654.
19. Daniels, C. W.: Rep. Malarial Com. Roy. Soc., London, 1901, Series 5, p. 46.
20. Stephens, J. W. W., and Christophers, S. R.: Rep. Malarial Com. Roy. Soc., London, 1901, Series 5, p. 17.
21. Deaderick, W. H.: A. Practical Study of Malaria, Philadelphia, 1910, Ed. 1.

endemic centers of hemoglobinuric fever, so that it is very difficult to explain this discrepancy on the malarial hypothesis. The advocates of this theory, however, have urged that unknown conditions may be present, but this is simply begging the question, and admitting that malaria differs in this respect from any other known disease. So far as I am aware, there is no acute infectious disease which gives rise to a striking symptom-complex in some regions, while in others this symptom-complex never occurs, although in the latter regions the disease is as intense and pernicious in character. Yet we are asked by the adherents of the malarial theory of the origin of hemoglobinuric fever to believe that malarial infection produces blackwater fever in certain districts, while in similar districts this symptom-complex never occurs, although the malarial infections are of the same type.

To one who has studied the literature, however, it is perfectly evident that repeated malarial infection is not necessary for the production of hemoglobinuric fever, as many instances of the disease have occurred in which past malarial infection could be definitely proven not to have existed. The reports of Murri, Mould, F. Plehn, and Gros, as well as others, prove that the disease may occur in persons who have never suffered from malaria, while those of F. Plehn, Goltman and Krause, and Brem, prove that it may occur during the first symptoms of a malarial infection. It is therefore justifiable to conclude that hemoglobinuric fever is not due to repeated attacks of malarial fever, and that in many instances no previous malarial infection has existed.

## THE OCCURRENCE OF MALARIAL PLASMODIA IN HEMOGLOBINURIC FEVER

The presence of malarial plasmodia in the blood of a large proportion of patients suffering from hemoglobinuric fever is considered by many authorities as proving its malarial origin; but many other conditions are frequently encountered in malarial regions in which the plasmodia may be found in the blood, but which are never considered as being due to malarial infection. The fashion of considering an organism as causative merely because it is frequently associated with a disease has generally resulted in disaster, and in the case of kala-azar, Malta fever, and sleeping-sickness, greatly delayed the discovery of the real cause.

It is but natural that, in a malarial region, patients suffering from this disease should present malarial plasmodia in their blood in many instances. The mere presence of such plasmodia, or of pigment in the tissues, does not prove that the condition is due to malarial infection, and the absence of both pigment and plasmodia in well-authenticated cases of hemoglobinuric fever proves conclusively that malaria cannot be considered as the direct cause of the disease.

As regards the frequency of the occurrence of plasmodia in the peripheral blood in hemoglobinuric fever, it may be said that it varies in different localities and with the time that the blood is examined. I have collected 273 cases in the literature, of which 109, or 40 per cent., showed malarial plasmodia in the blood. The researches of Stephens and Christophers[4, 20] and of Mannaberg[22] have shown that the number of patients presenting plasmodia in their blood varies with the time of examination, 95 per cent. of patients showing them the day before the attack; 60 to 70 per cent. showing them the day of the attack; and only 17 to 20 per cent. showing them the day after the attack. This fact has been used in contradicting the proofs of the absence of the plasmodia in cases of hemoglobinuric fever, but there are many cases on record in which the blood was examined before, during, and after the attack, and no plasmodia could be found, even puncture of the spleen being attended with a negative result. While 95 per cent. of hemoglobinuric fever patients may show plasmodia in their blood in some regions the day before an attack, it is equally true that in other blackwater regions 100 per cent. have not shown them, for it must be remembered that it is but seldom that the blood happens to be examined at this time, and that, therefore, the number of observations are very small.

From the reports of many investigators it is justifiable to state that cases of hemoglobinuric fever have occurred in which malarial plasmodia were not present, so far as could be determined, either before, during, or after the attack, while in fatal cases no evidence of malarial infection was found at autopsy. Many of these cases are reported by staunch advocates of the malarial theory and the evidence, therefore, is not affected by an unconscious personal equation.

Poole[6] found that some of his cases were negative for plasmodia either before, during, or after an attack of blackwater, although the examination was made most carefully; Barratt and Yorke[23] carefully examined twenty cases of hemoglobinuric fever, and found that nineteen of them were negative for plasmodia on the first day of the disease. They say:

> On one occasion it happened that an examination of the blood was made within two hours of the establishment of hemoglobinuria and one hour before the administration of quinin. In this case no parasites could be recognized after careful search. It can be asserted, therefore, that in this case, hemoglobinuria was not dependent on the hemolysis, in the peripheral blood, of the red cells containing the parasites.

As regards the presence of pigment or parasites in the organs of fatal cases, Barratt and Yorke say:

---

22. Mannaberg, J.: Die Malaria-Krankheiten, Nothnagel's Encyclopedia, Berlin, 1899.

23. Barratt, J. O. W., and Yorke, W.: An Investigation Into the Mechanism of the Production of Blackwater Fever, Ann. Trop. Med. and Hyg., 1909, Series T. M., iii, 152.

The presence of malarial pigment in the blood-vessels of the organs, usually the kidneys, has been described by several authors. In the three cases in which we had an opportunity of studying this point, no pigment was found in the kidneys, spleen, or liver, nor could malarial parasites be recognized in the blood-vessels of these organs.

In one of their cases the patient had never suffered from malaria to his knowledge. In sixteen of the twenty cases the onset of hemoglobinuria was preceded for several days by more or less general disturbance. Regarding this they say:

This lasted in fourteen attacks from one to seven days, and in two attacks ten and twenty-one days, respectively. The preliminary illness was regarded as malarial, but in only one case were malarial parasites found before the onset of hemoglobinuria.

This statement effectively disposes of the assertion that malarial plasmodia are always present in the peripheral blood before the onset of blackwater fever. Barratt and Yorke performed splenic puncture in six of their cases and in none of them were they able to find parasites or pigment in the material obtained; while they examined four of their patients on the first day of hemoglobinuria, giving the peripheral blood the most careful scrutiny, and did not find plasmodia in one of them.

Koch[24] described twenty-three cases of hemoglobinuric fever in which no plasmodia could be found, although some of them were fatal infections, while in four cases he found the plasmodia both before and after the attack, thus proving that their absence is not entirely due to blood destruction, as claimed by Christophers and Bentley. Koch says:

We thus perceive that the malarial plasmodia do not perish in blackwater fever attacks; that during the attack they are either entirely absent or show no remarkable increase; that, even if they are present in great numbers, no hemoglobinuria need develop. Therefore, how can one still assert that blackwater fever is caused by malarial parasites?

Mould[25] reports a case of hemoglobinuric fever which developed in a hospital; the patient, in whose blood no plasmodia could be found, never having suffered from malarial infection. Curry[15] reports two cases in which neither during the attack nor at autopsy could any evidence of present or past malarial infection be obtained, the tissues being free from pigment and parasites, and the blood likewise. In both cases the blood was examined during the first day of the attack. He describes another case in which no parasites were found, although the blood had been carefully examined for ten days preceding the attack.

Daniels[19] was unable to find plasmodia in a single one of sixteen cases which he investigated, either during or after the period of hemoglobinuria; Christophers and Bentley,[20] while agreeing that the manifestations of hemoglobinuric fever should occur only during coincident

24. Koch, R.: Blackwater Fever (Hemoglobinuria), Jour. Trop. Med., 1899, i, 333.

25. Mould, Captain: Cited by Sambon, Jour. Trop. Med., 1899, i, 243, 262, 295.

malarial infection, in their own report describe cases in which even the splenic blood did not contain parasites. Case 20 showed no parasites, though examined during the first day of the attack, and Case 26 was also negative, while the splenic blood of other patients showed a very few plasmodia. Their results dispose of the theory that the plasmodia are really very numerous in this disease, but are not discovered because they are localized in the internal organs, especially the spleen.

Newell,[26] though an ardent advocate of the malarial theory, did not find plasmodia in any of the five cases described in his book, so far as he states. Van der Scheer,[27] Hanley,[28] Thin,[29] Howard,[30] Oeconomou,[31] Le Dantec,[32] and Gauducheau,[33] all report cases in which plasmodia were not found in the blood during an attack of hemoglobinuric fever, and many of them were negative before the onset of hemoglobinuria.

Whipple[34] has recently contributed a valuable study of the pathology of hemoglobinuric fever, and believes that malaria always precedes this disease and predisposes to it, but the evidences of malarial infection in most of his cases are slight and would appear to be insufficient to prove the importance of previous malarial infection. He studied nine cases of hemoglobinuric fever at autopsy, in only two of which were plasmodia demonstrated, and compares the pathological findings with three cases of combined hemoglobinuric fever and pernicious malaria, and with five cases of pernicious malaria. He believes that the pathological findings in the hemoglobinuric fever cases "show a great similarity to those of the pernicious malaria cases and indicate that a malarial infection is an unfailing factor in all cases." In seven of the nine cases of uncomplicated hemoglobinuric fever the only evidence of malaria consisted in a small amount of pigment in the leukocytes of the spleen, kidney, and liver, and this pigment was present in such small amount in two cases that Whipple says (p. 226):

> In autopsy 1,168 and 1,169 malarial pigment is in very small amounts and is only found in the various organs after a long search. It is included in phagocytes. The second case shows a few coarse grains of malarial pigment in the cortex of the portal gland, indicating a previous malarial infection. We cannot imagine any ferment capable of rapidly dissolving the melanin which is set free by the sporulation or death of the malarial parasite. So it seems conclusive

26. Newell, C.: Blackwater Fever (Bilious Malignant Tertian Ague), London, 1909, Ed. 1.
27. Van der Scheer: Cited by Mense: Arch. f. Schiffs- u. Tropen-Hyg., 1899, iii, 80.
28. Hanley: Jour Trop. Med., 1899, i, 85.
29. Thin: Brit. Med. Jour., 1900, ii.
30. Howard: Jour. Trop. Med., 1907, x, 81.
31. Oeconomou: Cited by Cardamatis, Progrès Méd., 1902, xx, 201.
32. Le Dantec: Pathologie exotique, Paris, 1905, Ed. 1.
33. Gauducheau: Cited by Deaderick, A Practical Study of Malaria.
34. Whipple, G. H.: Blackwater Fever and Pernicious Malaria in Panama, Malaria, 1909, i, 215.

that there could have been but very few malarial parasites in the vascular system of these two patients. This would indicate that blackwater fever may follow a very slight infection of malaria, and that the severity of the attack need necessarily bear no relation to the severity of the hemoglobinuria.

It would appear that to base a belief in the causative relation of previous malarial infection to hemoglobinuric fever on the finding of a few grains of malarial pigment at autopsy in individuals residing in a malarial locality such as the Isthmus of Panama, where Whipple made his investigations, is hardly warranted, for in most patients dying of any disease in such regions, the organs would undoubtedly show a few grains of malarial pigment. If, in such a case, death were due to yellow fever, it would hardly be justifiable to assert that the malarial pigment present proved that the disease was of malarial origin. As I have stated, numerous cases of hemoglobinuric fever are on record, in which, even at autopsy, both parasites and malarial pigment were absent from the blood and tissues. Major Walter D. Webb, Medical Corps, United States Army, retired, has recently handed me the notes of two cases of hemoglobinuric fever, observed by him, in which neither on the first day of the attack, nor at autopsy, could malarial pigment or parasites be found in the blood or in scrapings from the spleen or liver. In both of these cases the onset was sudden, while the individuals were in apparent health, and in one of the cases the patient stated that he had never suffered from malarial fever. The argument that in such cases as these the malarial infection may have been latent, is negatived by the fact that at autopsy the organs presented no evidence of malarial infection, and it is impossible for one to believe that this would be so had the patients suffered from latent malaria. In one of Webb's cases no quinin had been given before the attack.

The discordant results obtained by various observers as to the occurrence of malarial plasmodia in patients suffering from hemoglobinuric fever, and the proportion of patients showing the plasmodia before or during the attack, is very largely due to the fact that malarial infection is very much more prevalent in some blackwater fever regions than it is in others, and thus a much greater proportion of the inhabitants suffer from such infection. It appears to be most illogical to maintain that, because the plasmodia are found in a certain proportion of hemoglobinuric fever patients, the disease must be caused by these parasites, in view of the absolute proof that cases of the disease occur in which neither past nor present malarial infection has occurred. A single case of hemoglobinuric fever occurring in an individual who has never suffered from malarial infection, and in whom, even at autopsy, no trace of present or past infection can be demonstrated, should be enough to convince the most skeptical that malaria is not the cause of this disease, and many such cases are on record.

THE RELATION OF THE SPECIES OF MALARIAL PLASMODIA TO HEMOGLOBINURIC FEVER

A few authorities hold that hemoglobinuric fever is due to the estivo-autumnal plasmodia, or to a specific form hitherto undifferentiated. This theory is negatived by the fact that all species of malarial plasmodia have been found in the blood of patients suffering from this disease, and that the disease occurs in individuals in whom no plasmodia can be found either before, during, or after the attack of hemoglobinuria. It is, however, an accepted fact that the estivo-autumnal plasmodia are more frequently associated with hemoglobinuric fever than are the other species, but there are many cases reported in the literature in which the other species of plasmodia were found.

According to Deaderick,[21] the tertian plasmodium has been found in cases of hemoglobinuric fever by Ziemann, Panse, Orme, Pecori, Carducci, Van der Horst, Hughes, Koch (five cases), A. Plehn (three cases), Ollwig, McElroy, Goltman and Krauss, Brem, Herrick and Curl; while, according to the same authority, the quartan plasmodium has been found associated with this disease by Vincenzi, Grocco, Kleine, Kudicke, and Otto. These observations prove that, if this disease be due to malarial infection, it may be produced by any of the species of plasmodia, and that the more frequent occurrence of the estivo-autumnal plasmodia does not prove them to be the cause of the disease, any more than the more frequent occurrence of these species of plasmodia in kala-azar patients proves them to be the cause of that disease.

As regards the presence of an undifferentiated species of malarial plasmodium, the fact that the disease occurs associated with all of the known species of plasmodia is conclusive proof that such a species is not necessary, and, in addition, all of the plasmodia associated with this disease have been very carefully studied by eminent authorities and have not been found to differ from those usually observed in malarial infection.

The theory that hemoglobinuric fever is merely one of the forms of pernicious malaria, which is held by many French and American observers, is negatived by the fact that this peculiar form of pernicious malaria occurs only in restricted localities, and that it is absent in many regions where the worst forms of pernicious malaria occur. Koch first thoroughly disproved this theory and anyone who cares to study the literature will become convinced that it is untenable in the face of the evidence that has accumulated against it.

CHANGES IN THE BLOOD IN HEMOGLOBINURIC FEVER

The blood examination in patients suffering from hemoglobinuric fever generally demonstrates an increase in the large mononuclear leukocytes, and frequently the presence of pigmented leukocytes. The increase in the large mononuclear cells has been used as a weighty argument in favor of the malarial nature of the disease, but it is perhaps the weakest of all the arguments used by the advocates of this theory. While an increase in these cells occurs in both malaria and hemoglobinuric fever, a similar increase is more or less characteristic of other acute infectious diseases, and occurs almost constantly in sleeping-sickness, kala-azar, and recurrent fever. The fact that an increase in these cells occurs in black-water fever simply suggests that the disease may be caused by a protozoon, and is really a better argument for the specific theory than for the malarial theory.

The presence of pigmented leukocytes has little value, as they occur in the vast majority of individuals residing in intensely infected malarial localities, and sometimes persist for weeks after all other traces of malarial infection have disappeared. While the presence of pigmented leukocytes indicates that at some time the patient has suffered from malarial fever, it is very slender proof of the malarial nature of hemoglobinuric fever.

### AUTOLYSIS AND THE PRODUCTION OF HEMOGLOBINURIC FEVER

Since the remarkable development of our knowledge regarding hemolytic phenomena, the theory that an autolysin is produced in the blood of certain individuals by repeated attacks of malaria, thus leading to the production of hemoglobinuria, has become a favorite one, and is held by many observers, notably Deaderick, Bignami, Cassagrandi, and Christophers and Bentley. None of the believers in this theory have been able to demonstrate conclusively the presence of an autolysin in the blood of patients suffering from hemoglobinuric fever, although every effort has been made to do so. The theory is disproved by the fact that this disease occurs in persons who have not suffered from repeated malarial attacks, and that autolysins have not been demonstrated in the blood of man either in health or disease.

Some of the theories regarding the production of this theoretical autolysin are very complicated, but they are all negatived by the recent work of several observers who have failed to find such a body in the blood of patients suffering from hemoglobinuric fever, or in that of patients suffering from other diseases. The work of Dudgeon and Wilson,[35] Moss,[36] and Barratt and Yorke,[23] is of great interest in this con-

35. Dudgeon, L. S., and Wilson, H. A. F.: On the Presence of Hemagglutinins, Hemopsonins and Hemolysins in the Blood Obtained from Infectious and Non-Infectious Diseases in Man, Quart. Jour. Med., 1910, iii, 285.

36. Moss, W. L.: Studies on Iso-agglutinins and Isohemolysins, Bull. Johns Hopkins Hosp., 1910, xxi, 63.

nection. Dudgeon and Wilson found that, while some samples of normal serum have the power of agglutinating almost all specimens of normal red corpuscles, in no case were they able to find auto-agglutination or autohemolysis in normal blood. In blood from disease they were unable to find a single instance of autohemolysis, even in twenty-one cases of pernicious anemia, in which, as they say: "of all diseases it might well be imagined that autohemolysis could be demonstrated, but a negative result was obtained in every instance."

The very thorough work of Moss demonstrates beyond question that autohemolysis does not occur in either health or disease, and it is a significant fact that he found no constant differences between the agglutinating and hemolyzing qualities of serum in health and disease, which one would expect to find did disease tend to bring about an unstable condition of the blood leading to autohemolysis. Moss did not observe auto-agglutination in any of the 213 individuals that he studied, while autohemolysis was observed but once, and of this instance he says: "In the latter case the hemolysis may have been due to extraneous causes." He found that all of the serums investigated contained an antihemolysin which protected the homologous corpuscles.

Barratt and Yorke, in their recent and conclusive experiments regarding hemolysis in hemoglobinuric fever, were not able to demonstrate an autolysin in any of twenty-one cases which they investigated, while, in the eleven cases they examined as to the presence of an isolysin, but one gave a positive result. They conclude:

From these experiments the important conclusion follows that the mechanism of production of blackwater fever stands in an altogether different category from that of paroxysmal hemoglobinuria. The presence of hemolysin or of defect of antilysis, which is present in the latter case, is absent in blackwater fever, where, therefore, search must be made for other factors.

These authors examined the blood of two oxen suffering from Texas fever, and of two dogs suffering from piroplasmosis, and were unable to find an autolysin in the blood of any of them. This fact is significant as showing the probable relationship of these infections to hemoglobinuric fever, a relationship which has been noted by many investigators.

Whipple,[34] as the result of careful experiments, also reaches the conclusion that the blood of hemoglobinuric fever patients does not contain any hemolysin.

It will thus be seen that the presence of an autolysin in the blood in hemoglobinuric fever has been disproved, and, even were such a body present, the advocates of the malarial theory would still have to explain why malarial infection produced it in some localities and never produced it in others. In other words, the presence of such a body in the blood of hemoglobinuric fever patients would point toward its specific nature rather than toward the malarial theory.

## 2. QUININ AND HEMOGLOBINURIC FEVER

The theory that hemoglobinuric fever is due to quinin will be considered but briefly, as it is not strictly included in the subject for discussion. This theory endeavors to explain the etiology of the disease by assuming that, in certain individuals, the administration of quinin is followed by hemoglobinuria, or that this results if the drug is administered to one who has suffered from repeated malarial attacks. Veratas, a Greek physician, suggested this explanation of the disease in 1858, and in 1874, Tomaselli gave it his support. The theory is believed in by many authorities, especially by Koch, whose support was accepted for a while as almost conclusive proof of its truth. As a matter of fact, many instances of hemoglobinuric fever have been reported in individuals who had never taken quinin, while the theory that the long-continued use of the drug for malarial infection may produce the disease is negatived by the fact that thousands of individuals take quinin, at intervals, for years, and never develop the disease except in regions where hemoglobinuric fever is endemic.

The occurrence of the disease in patients who have never taken quinin has been reported by A. Plehn,[5] in twenty-two cases; Cardamatis,[14] in thirty-two cases; Shropshire,[37] in twenty-five cases; Seal,[38] in six cases, and by many other observers.

My experience among the Filipinos positively disproves this theory, for of the hundreds of cases of malarial fever which I studied among these people, most of whom had suffered for years, at intervals, from malaria, the administration of quinin was not followed in a single instance by hemoglobinuria.

In the thousands of cases of malaria I have observed in soldiers of the United States Army, all of them treated with large, and frequently, heroic doses of the drug, I have observed but two cases of hemoglobinuria following its use, and in both the symptomatology was very different from that of hemoglobinuric fever. In those instances in which hemoglobinuric fever occurs among the natives of an endemic region, and many instances of this kind are on record, in hardly a single case had quinin been administered before the attack, and this must be true of the occurrence of the disease in any region where the drug is not in use by the native race.

It must be remembered that this disease occurs in malarial localities and that those suffering from the prodromal symptoms almost always take quinin, believing that they are suffering from malaria, and thus the

37. Shropshire, W.: Hemoglobinuric Fever, Its Causes and Treatment, with Especial Reference to the Use of Quinin, Jour. Am. Med. Assn., 1903, xli, 600.

38. Seal, C. E. B.: Notes on a Few Cases of Hemoglobinuria in India, Jour. Trop. Med., 1899, i, 179.

hemoglobinuria which follows is quite naturally considered as being due to the drug.

It is true that quinin does produce hemoglobinuria in some individuals, but in such instances the symptoms following each administration of the drug may occur in regions in which hemoglobinuric fever is unknown, and differ very much from the classical symptoms of hemoglobinuric fever. These cases should not be used as an argument in favor of the etiological relationship of quinin to this disease.

If quinin be the cause of this disease, it would be expected that the administration of it to patients suffering from an attack would result in an increase in the intensity of the symptoms and that death would follow in the majority of the cases. This is not so, however, for there is undisputed evidence that the mortality is very little higher when quinin is administered than when it is not. Deaderick[39] says:

> The great majority of cases recover even under the continued use of large doses of quinin.

It is also true that the severity of an attack of hemoglobinuric fever bears no relation to the size of the doses of quinin that have been administered, nor do large doses given during the attack result in a greater percentage of deaths than small ones. Shropshire[40] reports sixty-one cases treated with less than 5 grains per day, with 26.2 per cent. mortality; while in 141 cases treated with over 20 grains per day, the mortality was only 16.9 per cent. Crosse[41] states that in his experience the administration of the drug does not aggravate the attack, and that on the Niger all hemoglobinuric fever patients are treated with quinin and a large percentage recover. Moffatt[42] details six cases in which from 60 to 120 grains of quinin were given daily and all the patients recovered; while Robson[43] has given 60 grains of the drug at a single dose with good results.

Some authorities believe that quinin produces the disease only in certain individuals having an idiosyncrasy to the drug; but if this be true, we must believe that such idiosyncrasy occurs only in certain localities, for the drug is given in large doses, for long periods of time, all over the world, but hemoglobinuric fever only occurs in limited localities.

Barratt and Yorke[23] in their recent work on the mechanism of blackwater fever reach the following conclusions regarding the effect of quinin on the blood:

---

39. Deaderick, W. H.: A Practical Study of Malaria, Philadelphia, 1910, Ed. 1, p. 165.
40. Shropshire: Med. Rec., 1903, lxiii, 798.
41. Crosse: Blackwater Fever, London, 1899, Ed. 1.
42. Moffatt: Brit. Med. Jour., 1898, i, 926.
43. Robson: Brit. Med. Jour., 1898, i, 1287.

Owing to the toxicity of quinin, its concentration in the blood cannot reach an amount sufficient to allow of its direct hemolytic action on the red cells taking place during life. The red cells during blackwater fever are not hemolyzed by quinin bihydrochlorid more readily than in health.

Again, some authorities believe that hemoglobinuric fever is produced by quinin only when a person who has been taking the drug for a long time suddenly ceases to take it, and then takes a very large dose. This is disproved by the fact that this method of taking quinin is common throughout the world, while hemoglobinuric fever is restricted in its distribution; also by the fact that the disease occurs in individuals who have never taken the drug.

From this summary of the evidence against the quinin theory of the etiology of hemoglobinuric fever I believe that it is evident that quinin *per se* is not the cause of the disease. The facts that the drug is given throughout the world in large doses to individuals suffering from malarial infections, while hemoglobinuric fever occurs only in restricted localities; that many patients suffering from the disease recover under the administration of the drug; that patients who have apparently suffered from hemoglobinuria produced by quinin do not generally relapse when the drug is given; that there exists no relation between the amount of quinin given and the severity of the disease; that the disease occurs in individuals who have never taken quinin; and that the red blood-corpuscles of patients suffering from hemoglobinuric fever are as resistant to the drug as are the red cells of the normal individual, all point conclusively to the opinion that quinin cannot be regarded as the cause of hemoglobinuric fever.

## 3. *THE SPECIFIC THEORY OF THE ETIOLOGY OF HEMOGLOBINURIC FEVER*

### PRESENT STATUS OF THEORY

From the evidence which has accumulated regarding the relationship of malaria and quinin to hemoglobinuric fever, it would appear that we cannot with justice regard either as being the etiological factor in the production of the disease, and that, therefore, we must consider the etiology of this disease as still undecided. This being so, it is but natural that many authorities have endeavored to prove that hemoglobinuric fever is a distinct disease due to a specific organism, and it must be admitted, that there is much evidence which points to such a conclusion. As early as 1892, Manson,[44] in an address delivered before the Epidemiological Society of London, stated that he believed hemoglobinuric fever to be a distinct disease; but it is chiefly to Sambon that we owe the awakened

44. Manson, Sir Patrick: Tr. Epidemiol. Soc., 1892-1893, xii, 384.

interest in the specific theory of the disease. In two excellent papers[45] this author has called attention to the inadequacy of the malarial and quinin theories and collected the evidence in favor of the specific nature of the disease. At the present time this theory is steadily gaining ground, its most ardent advocates being Manson, Sambon, Rho and Blanchard, while numerous other investigators concede that only by admitting the specific nature of the disease can the contradictions inherent in the other theories be explained. Every evidence which has been urged for the malarial nature of the disease can be used as well in advocating its specific nature, and, in adidtion, there are certain positive facts which can be accounted for only by admitting that the disease is due to some hitherto undescribed parasite.

## GEOGRAPHICAL DISTRIBUTION

As I have already pointed out, the geographical distribution of this disease is a much stronger argument for its specific nature than for the malarial theory. The fact that the disease occurs only in malarial localities simply proves that the parasite causing it finds in such localities the conditions necessary for its development or transmission, and the limited distribution of the disease in even the most malarial localities speaks still more strongly for its specific nature. The geographical distribution of kala-azar is very like that of hemoglobinuric fever, so far as its limitation to certain districts is concerned, and the latter disease, so far as I know, also occurs only in malarial localities. There are other acute infectious diseases which are still more limited as regards distribution, for instance, Rocky Mountain spotted fever, which occurs only in very restricted localities in our own country, and the tsutsugamushi disease, or flood fever of Japan, which occurs only in certain small districts along the course of rivers in northern Japan. Sleeping-sickness is another disease which occurs only in malarial localities, but we do not believe, because of its geographical distribution, that it is due to malaria.

The fact that the disease occurs in patients who have never suffered from malaria or taken quinin, and in whom, even at autopsy, no trace of past or present malarial infection can be demonstrated, is positive proof that it is not due to either of these factors, and speaks in favor of its specific nature.

The occurrence in the endemic regions of hemoglobinuric fever of certain small areas, and of certain houses in which the disease is most frequently observed, points very strongly to a specific cause and probably indicates that in such places there exist certain factors which enable the disease to be transmitted. It is evident that hemoglobinuric fever is a

45. Sambon, L. W.: Blackwater Fever, Jour. Trop. Med., 1898, i, 70; The Etiology and Treatment of Blackwater Fever, Jour. Trop. Med., 1899, i, 243, 262, 295.

comparatively rare disease, even in its endemic centers, and this fact again points to its specific nature, rather than to its being due to malaria, and indicates that the cause is some parasite which requires very particular conditions either for development or for transmission.

DISPROPORTION BETWEEN NUMBER OF MALARIAL AND HEMOGLOBINURIC FEVER CASES

The numerical disproportion between the cases of hemoglobinuric fever and of malaria, in even the worst endemic regions of the former, is a strong argument in favor of the distinct nature of this disease. No one will deny that the number of cases of hemoglobinuric fever occurring in any locality when compared with the number of malarial infections is very small; while in many regions hemoglobinuric fever is unknown, although thousands of cases of malaria occur every year. In Greece, Pampoukis observed 34,937 cases of malaria, of which only 0.7 per cent. presented hemoglobinuria; Burot and Lagrand[46] observed 559 fatal cases of malaria, and only five of hemoglobinuric fever; and Stalkarrt[18] observed many cases of severe malarial infection without seeing a case of hemoglobinuria. There are many localities in which hundreds of cases of malaria occur yearly and yet hemoglobinuric fever is so rare as to be regarded as a medical curiosity. The army statistics regarding this question are of the greatest interest and value. It should be remembered that these statistics deal with soldiers recruited from every portion of our country, and include men who have served in the United States, in Cuba, Porto Rico, and the Philippines. Table 4, compiled from the Reports of the Surgeon General of the Army, shows the number of admissions to army hospitals from malaria and hemoglobinuric fever from 1903 to 1908 inclusive.

TABLE 4.—MALARIA AND HEMOGLOBINURIC FEVER IN THE UNITED STATES ARMY FROM 1903 TO 1908, INCLUSIVE

| | Admissions for — Entire Army — | | Admissions for U. S., Cuba, Hawaii, Porto Rico and Alaska | | Admissions for — Philippines — | |
|---|---|---|---|---|---|---|
| Year. | Malaria. | Hemoglobinuric Fever. | Malaria. | Hemoglobinuric Fever. | Malaria.* | Hemoglobinuric Fever. |
| 1903...... | 13,608 | 0 | 2,685 | 0 | 10,923 | 0 |
| 1904...... | 4,955 | 0 | 2,170 | 0 | 2,785 | 0 |
| 1905...... | 4,833 | 2 | 1,942 | 1 | 2,891 | 1 |
| 1906...... | 6,077 | 3 | 2,042 | 1 | 3,766 | 2 |
| 1907...... | 3,395 | 1 | 1,280 | 1 | 1,963 | 0 |
| 1908...... | 3,030 | 0 | 1,424 | 0 | 1,484 | 0 |
| Totals .. | 35,898 | 6 | 11,543 | 3 | 23,812 | 3 |

* Of the 23,812 admissions from malaria in the Philippines at least 11,000 were due to the estivo-autumnal plasmodia.

46. Burot and Lagrand: Cited by F. Plehn, Tropenhygiene, Jena, 1906, Ed. 1.

It will be seen from Table 4 that, during the six years which it covers, there were 35,898 admissions from malaria in the entire army, and only six admissions from hemoglobinuric fever, while the fact that hemoglobinuric fever does not occur among the Filipinos, although malaria is a very common and severe disease among these people, is well shown in Table 5, which gives the number of admissions from malarial fever and hemoglobinuric fever, from 1903 to 1908, inclusive, in the Philippine Scouts, an organization composed of native Filipinos from all parts of the Islands.

TABLE 5.—MALARIA AND HEMOGLOBINURIC FEVER IN THE PHILIPPINE SCOUTS FROM 1903 TO 1908, INCLUSIVE

| Year. | Admissions from Malaria. | Admissions from Hemoglobinuric Fever. |
|---|---|---|
| 1903 | 2,565 | 0 |
| 1904 | 1,691 | 0 |
| 1905 | 2,710 | 0 |
| 1906 | 1,871 | 0 |
| 1907 | 1,463 | 0 |
| 1908 | 1,205 | 0 |
| Totals | 11,505 | 0 |

From the above table it is seen that while there were 11,505 admissions from malarial fever among the Philippine Scouts during the six years mentioned, there was not a single admission from hemoglobinuric fever. If these figures are added to those for our army, exclusive of the scouts, there are 47,403 admissions from malarial fever with but six admissions from hemoglobinuric fever, or 0.00012 per cent.

In my own experience, covering over ten years' observation of the malarial fevers, during which time I have had the opportunity of studying nearly 6,000 cases of malaria in which the plasmodia were demonstrated in the blood, I have observed only two cases of hemoglobinuria, and in both of these the symptoms were not typical of true hemoglobinuric fever. All of the malarial cases were observed in Cuba or the Philippines, or in the United States in soldiers returning from service in these countries, and almost every one of them had suffered from repeated attacks of malarial fever, fully two-thirds of them from estivo-autumnal infections. In view of these facts, is it possible to believe that hemoglobinuric fever is due to malarial infection? It appears to me that this great disproportion between the number of cases of malaria and hemoglobinuric fever is very strong proof of the specific nature of the latter disease.

## OCCURRENCE IN EPIDEMICS

The occurrence of epidemics of hemoglobinuric fever is proof of its specific nature. While there are many instances of the occurrence of epidemics of malarial fever, there are no instances of epidemics of a special symptom-complex associated with this disease, and this is what hemoglobinuric fever is believed to be by the advocates of the malarial theory. Epidemics of this disease have been reported by various observers. Sambon[13] recalls the epidemic which occurred among the laborers on the Isthmus of Corinth, and the Chinese laborers on the Congo railway; and the same disease has occurred in epidmic form on the Isthmus of Panama during the French operations on the canal. According to Dr. Wenyon[47] the disease ravaged like a plague the Chinese army on the Tonquin border of Kwansi, and the same authority instances an outbreak in a prison in Sardinia, in which twenty-four out of 800 convicts suffered from the disease. According to A. Plehn,[48] hemoglobinuric fever not infrequently occurs in epidemic form in Africa, and he mentions several such instances. In this relation may be mentioned the instances already quoted, in which several individuals in the same house develop the disease, although those living in the surrounding buildings do not suffer.

The fact that hemoglobinuric fever occurs in regions where the natives are immune to malaria is an argument for the specific nature of the disease. We are informed on the authority of A. Plehn that the negro of Africa is not immune to hemoglobinuric fever; and Doering,[49] F. Plehn,[50] and others have observed cases among the negroes of that country. It is generally accepted as proved by the researches of Koch and others that the natives of certain malarial regions in Africa, after reaching adult life, are immune to malaria, and Koch did not find the plasmodia in 100 per cent. of the adult natives whom he examined. How can we reconcile these two facts, if hemoglobinuric fever be due to malarial infection? Is it not more reasonable to believe that we are dealing with a distinct disease, due to a specific parasite?

## SYMPTOMATOLOGY AND PATHOLOGY

The symptomatology of hemoglobinuric fever is distinctive and unlike that of any form of malarial fever with which we are acquainted. The lack of periodicity in the temperature curve, the presence of an enlarged and tender liver, the repeated chills, the occurrence of marked jaundice, the leukocytosis, and the hemoglobinuria, have all been instanced by Sambon[13] and other authorities, as definitely separating the disease on clinical grounds from malarial fever. The fact that, in relapses of this disease, the symptom of hemoglobinuria is always repeated proves that we are not dealing with a pernicious form of malaria, for relapses of pernicious malaria are not always accompanied by the same

47. Wenyon: Cited by Sambon, The Etiology and Treatment of Blackwater Fever, Jour. Trop. Med., 1899, i, 243, 262, 295.

48. Plehn, A.: The Cause, Prevention and Treatment of Hemoglobinuric Fever in Warm Countries, Jour. Trop. Med. and Hyg., 1908, xi, 294.

49. Doering: Cited by Deaderick, A Practical Study of Malaria.

50. Plehn, F.: Arch. f. Schiffs. u. Tropen. Hyg., 1904, iii, 336.

symptoms. While the prodromal symptoms of hemoglobinuric fever cannot be differentiated from those of malaria, the symptoms of the fully developed attack are distinctive.

The pathologic changes in hemoglobinuric fever is very strong proof of its specific nature, for the lesions are not those of pernicious malarial fever. Even the most ardent advocates of the malarial hypothesis admit that cases occur in which not even a few grains of malarial pigment can be found in the viscera, and there is no evidence of either present or past malarial infection. It is generally conceded that, unless the lesions of a disease are found at autopsy, it is not justifiable to believe the cause of death to be due to that disease, and it would appear that it is fully justifiable to disregard the malarial theory of hemoglobinuric fever because of the pathological lesions present in fatal cases. The absence of malarial pigment or parasites in the organs, or in the blood in many cases, the condition of the kidneys, which is seldom simulated in pernicious malaria, the enlarged, but unpigmented liver and spleen, are all very different from the lesions usually observed in fatal malarial infections. The enlargement of the spleen in uncomplicated cases of hemoglobinuric fever is exactly similar to that occurring in most infectious diseases, and is no proof of its malarial origin. One would think that, after the disastrous experience regarding the significance of splenic enlargement in kala-azar, it would not again be urged as an argument for the malarial etiology of any disease, but in the case of hemoglobinuric fever it is still so used. In his study of the pathology of this fever Whipple[34] gives very completely the lesions he found in nine cases of this disease, lesions which are certainly not those encountered in the vast majority of fatal cases of malarial fever. He calls attention especially to the occurrence of extensive areas of necrosis in the viscera, especially the spleen, and, while small areas of focal necrosis are sometimes found in the spleen, liver, and other organs in pernicious malaria, they are not peculiar to malarial infections, but occur also in diphtheria, streptococcus septicemia, and other acute infections in which a toxemic condition is present. The fact that they are much more pronounced in hemoglobinuric fever would appear to prove that the etiology of this disease is not that of malarial infection.

The occurrence of necrosis of the Malpighian bodies of the spleen, spoken of by Whipple, and which, according to this author, involves almost every Malpighian body in that organ, is never found in malarial infections in my experience, and alone serves to differentiate that disease from any form of such infection. It is impossible to read Whipple's excellent account of the pathology of hemoglobinuric fever without concluding that it is not due to malarial infection, for, while the two conditions have some things in common from a pathological standpoint, the pathology of other tropical infections, such as yellow fever and kala-azar, have as much in common with malaria as does this disease. The presence of a small amount of malarial pigment cannot be held as proving the etiological importance of malarial infection, for the same pigment is found in patients dying of other diseases in malarial localities, and, as has already been shown, many cases are on record in which at autopsy no pigment could be found.

### APPARENT ABSENCE OF PARASITE

One of the arguments brought forward against the specific theory of the origin of hemoglobinuric fever is the fact that, although it has been carefully searched for, no one has been able to demonstrate a parasite which could be considered as being the cause of the disease. I am sure that all will agree with me when I say that such an argument is valueless. There are a number of infections in which the cause has not as yet been demonstrated, yet one never uses this argument as valid evidence against their specific nature. Yellow fever, dengue, Rocky Mountain spotted fever and nearly all of the eruptive fevers belong in this category, and I believe that further research will show that many of these diseases are caused by a class of organisms very closely related and probably of protozoan nature.

There are many explanations for the apparent absence of a parasite from the blood and tissues in hemoglobinuric fever, among which may be mentioned a possible cyclical appearance of the parasite in the blood; the small number in the blood at any one time; the location of the parasite in some internal organ from which it rapidly disappears after the death of the patient; and the fact that the organism may be ultramicroscopical in size. The recent researches of Miyajima[52] on a piroplasma found in the blood of cattle in Japan, and of Crawley[53] on a trypanosome occurring in the blood of our own cattle, are of interest and significance in this relation. Both of these organisms occur in such small numbers in the blood of their respective hosts that they cannot be demonstrated in that fluid with the microscope, but, if the blood be added to suitable culture media, it is possible to secure the organism in pure culture. The same may be true of hemoglobinuric fever. The parasite may be present in such small numbers that a microscopic examination of the blood will not reveal it, but cultural methods might result in success. Curiously enough, I can find no record in the literature of an endeavor to make blood cultures in this disease.

---

52. Miyajima, M.: On the Cultivation of a Bovine Piroplasma, Philippine Jour. Sc. B. Med. Sc., v, 83.

53. Crawley, H.: *Trypanosoma americanum*, N. Sp., A Trypanosome which Appears in Cultures Made from the Blood of American Cattle, Bull. 119, Bureau of Animal Industry, Dept. Agri., Washington, 1909.

## *CONCLUSIONS*

That hemoglobinuric fever is not due to malaria I believe to be proved by its geographical distribution; by the fact that it occurs in individuals who have never suffered from malaria; and by the fact that, in many instances, neither before, during, or after an attack can plasmodia be demonstrated in the blood, while, even at autopsy, no trace of malaria can be found.

That the disease is not due to quinin is proved by the fact that it occurs in individuals who have never taken the drug, and that in many regions where the drug is extensively used the disease is unknown.

For the following reasons I believe that it is due to a specific organism: its geographical distribution; its numerical disproportion to malaria wherever it occurs; its occurrence in epidemics; the character of the pathological lesions; its symptomatology; the lack of conclusive evidence that it is due to malaria; and its analogy with other well-known infectious diseases.

In concluding I desire to call attention to the peculiar relation that this disease apparently bears to the hemoglobinuric fever of cattle and to piroplasma infections in general. That hemoglobinuric fever resembles Texas fever in its symptomatology has often been noted, and there is much reason to believe that it may be due to a similar parasite, for it is a significant fact that some form of piroplasma infection has been observed in almost every region in which blackwater fever is endemic. That no piroplasma has as yet been demonstrated in the blood in this disease does not count for anything, for it may be so small as to be indistinguishable by our present lenses, or it may occur in such small numbers as to necessitate its demonstration by cultural methods. All of the parasites belonging to this class are very minute and it is not at all improbable that the parasite of hemoglobinuric fever is ultramicroscopical in size, as we believe the parasites of yellow fever, dengue, and other diseases to be. Hemoglobinuric fever is probably transmitted by an insect, perhaps a larval tick, as is the case in tsutsugamushi disease, or the adult insect, as in Rocky Mountain spotted fever; but, whatever insect is ultimately proved to be the transmitting agent, we may feel sure that it will be one of comparatively rare occurrence, or that the conditions necessary for the transmission of the disease are peculiar, either in the cycle of development of the parasite in its insect host, or in the manner in which it reaches the insect. Only in some such manner can the comparative rarity of the disease in regions in which it is endemic, and its absence from others, be explained.

I would also call attention to the extremely small number of experiments which have been made on animals in research work on this disease. It is most unfortunate that the majority of investigators who have worked on the etiology of hemoglobinuric fever have been strongly biased in favor of either the malarial or quinin theories, and have not considered animal experimentation necessary in solving the problem. That such experimental methods are of the greatest value in medical research, and absolutely indispensable, if our work is to be crowned with success, has been well shown by the results which have recently been accomplished in the study of dengue, typhus fever, Rocky Mountain spotted fever, and acute poliomyelitis.

Let us attack the problem of the etiology of this disease in a similar manner and I believe that it will not be long before we shall be able to prove beyond question that hemoglobinuric fever is a disease *sui generis* and not a manifestation of malaria.

# A STUDY OF THE VENTILATION OF SLEEPING-CARS*

THOMAS R. CROWDER, M.D.
CHICAGO

Problems of ventilation confront the designers and operators of all enclosed spaces in which one or more persons are expected to live. Demands for a supply of fresh air must be recognized by those operating hospitals, theaters, offices and to a peculiar degree by those concerned in the management of public conveyances, in which the space for each occupant is necessarily restricted. For the purpose of securing a suitable exchange of air in railway cars many types of ventilators have been suggested and not a few have been given practical tests. About three years ago I was asked to report on the efficacy of one of these which had been applied to a few sleeping-cars, which has since been applied to a large number, and which seemed to be of considerable practical usefulness.

In this connection it became evident that it would be necessary to establish some basis of comparison, since it does not seem to have been estimated in exact figures to what degree natural ventilation of a railway car is effective. Inasmuch as the problem is one of lasting importance and is likely to recur, it seemed advisable to make a fundamental study of the question and to place the results within reach of those who might have occasion to make use of them.

A very simple, if somewhat tedious, means of making this investigation was long ago established by Pettenkofer.[1] It consists of estimating the vitiation of the atmosphere by determining the amount of carbon dioxid it contains, and from this computing the amount of air supplied for ventilation.

All air contains carbon dioxid as a normal constituent. The average amount in pure air is commonly stated to be 4 parts in 10,000. This is the figure arrived at by Pettenkofer and the one generally used in ventilation computations, though recent investigation has shown it to be a little too high. Harrington[2] considers the normal as but slightly in excess of three. It varies at different times and places, but the variation is confined within very narrow limits. It is somewhat higher in cities than in the open country. The average for fifteen samples, which were collected in the country districts of Illinois in 1907, was 3.6, with a maximum of 4;

---

* Presented at the thirty-eighth annual meeting of the American Public Health Association, Milwaukee, September, 1910.

1. Pettenkofer: Ueber den Luftwechsel in Wohngebäuden, Munich, 1858.

2. Harrington: Practical Hygiene, Lea Bros. & Co., Philadelphia, 1905, Ed. 3, p. 227.

for thirty-nine samples from the streets of Chicago during the same period the average was 4.06 with a maximum of 5.

The carbon dioxid in the expired breath averages more than 4 per cent. (400 in 10,000). The amount excreted hourly varies according to age, sex and the degree of bodily activity. In a mixed community of persons at rest it will average about 0.6 cubic feet per person per hour, and the variation will be a small one.

If there were no ventilation whatever the air of an ordinary railway coach, containing 4,000 cubic feet of space and occupied by twenty people, would have 34 parts of carbon dioxid per 10,000 of air at the end of one hour of occupancy; and this would continue to increase indefinitely in a direct ratio to the time, since carbon dioxid continues to be produced by the respiration of the occupants at a practically constant rate. But no car is air-tight, consequently the carbon dioxid will never reach this theoretical limit. Fresh air from the outside is constantly entering through the numerous crevices about the doors and windows, and old air is constantly leaving. The inside air is being constantly diluted.

It is plainly impossible to measure directly the amount of air flowing into a car, since it enters at many points and at constantly changing velocities. But the amount of the interchange may be readily computed from the actual amount of carbon dioxid found from time to time by applying the figures given above to a simple mathematical procedure. To illustrate this problem: Suppose a car contains twenty people and its atmosphere is found to have an average of 10 parts of carbon dioxid per 10,000. The incoming fresh air contains 4 parts of carbon dioxid per 10,000, hence the respiratory contamination of the car air is represented by only 6 parts. Twenty people produce twenty times 0.6 cubic feet, or 12 cubic feet of carbon dioxid per hour. With what amount of air must 12 cubic feet of carbon dioxid be diluted so that the air will contain 6 parts of carbon dioxid in 10,000? The simple proportion, 6 : 10,000 :: 12 : ?, gives 20,000 as the answer. Hence there must be 20,000 cubic feet of air supplied per hour, or 1,000 cubic feet for each person present, in order sufficiently to dilute the carbon dioxid produced so as to maintain its proportion at 10 parts in 10,000. The computation is better represented by the general formula:

$$A = v p \div (x - N)$$

where $v$ = the $CO_2$ produced by one person (cu. ft. per hour),
$p$ = the number of persons in the room,
$x$ = the proportion of $CO_2$ found in the air of the room,
$N$ = the proportion of $CO_2$ in the outside air (0.0004)
and $A$ = the air-supply to the room (cu. ft. per hour).

By applying the above calculation to the conditions supposed—a room containing twenty people—we find that with the carbon dioxid at 0.0009, or 9 parts per 10,000, 24,000 cubic feet of air, or 1,200 cubic feet per person, would be necessary; at 0.0008, 30,000, or 1,500 cubic feet per person; at 0.0007, 40,000, or 2,000 cubic feet per person; at 0.0006, 60,000, or 3,000 cubic feet per person; at 0.0005, 120,000, or 6,000 cubic feet per person; at 0.00045, 240,000, or 12,000 cubic feet per person; and at 0.0004 an infinite amount per room and per person.

I have attempted to represent graphically in Chart 1 the mathematical relation between the carbon dioxid in the air of a room and the hourly air-supply per person, assuming 0.0004 as the proportion of carbon dioxid in the outside air and 0.6 cubic feet as the average hourly excretion. Manifestly the curve holds good for any number of people and is independent of the size of the room, except that the larger the room the greater time must elapse before a constant condition will be reached. It

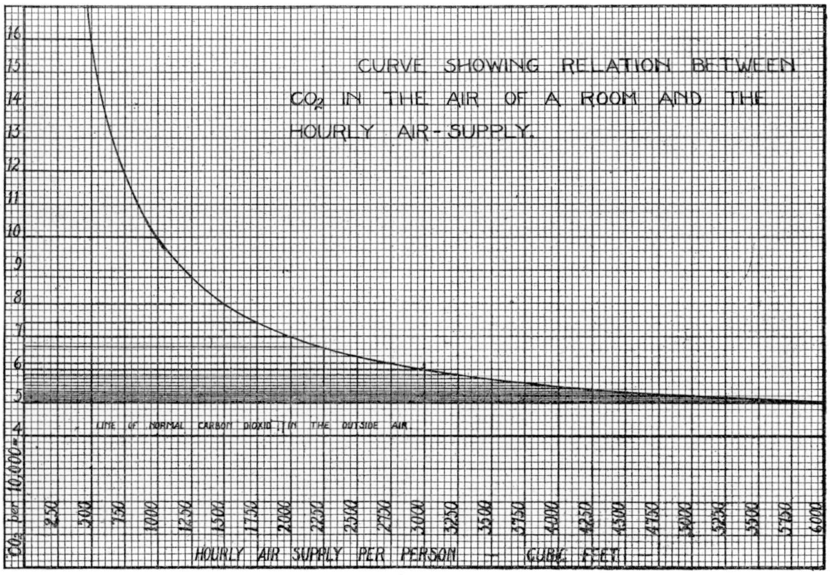


Chart 1.

is seen that the increase of carbon dioxid above the normal is in an inverse ratio to the air-supply. Six thousand cubic feet per person per hour allows an increase of 0.0001 in carbon dioxid; 3,000, an increase of 0.0002; 2,000, an increase of 0.0003; 1,500, an increase of 0.0004; 1,200, an increase of 0.0005; 1,000, an increase of 0.0006, and so on.

With any given air-supply the carbon dioxid representing respiratory contamination increases directly as the number of people present. Twenty people produce twice as much carbon dioxid as ten people, and this will cause twice the contamination of a given amount of air supplied. In Chart 2 this relation is graphically represented for various air-supplies between 10,000 and 100,000 and for any number of people up to twenty-six, the practical limit of sleeping-car occupants. The diagonal lines, representing air-supplies, simply connect the points indicating the height to which the carbon dioxid will rise when different numbers of people are in the room, the amount of air supplied being that given on the diagonal and its rate of entrance constant. This method of charting becomes valuable in certain comparisons which will be made later. It will be clear from these charts that when we are dealing with carbon dioxid which is near the normal, the slight necessary errors in determination would represent large relative errors in the calculation of air-supply. The higher the carbon dioxid the less does this latter error amount to.

The first attempt to apply Pettenkofer's methods to the air of railway cars and to place our knowledge of their ventilation upon a scientific basis seems to have been made by Wolfhügel and Lang[3] in 1875. Further investigation was carried out under the direction of the Prussian minister

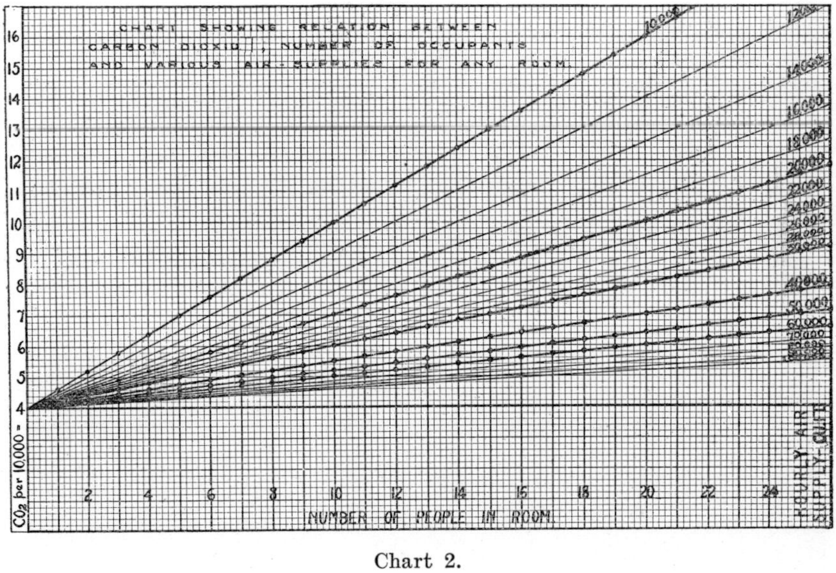


Chart 2.

of war[3] in 1887-8, in order to determine the best means of ventilating military hospital cars.

Some fifteen or twenty years ago a number of analyses of the air from passenger cars were made by Professor Nickols,[4] working under the auspices of the Board of Railroad Commissioners of the State of Massachusetts. About the same time the Pennsylvania Railroad Company[4] took up the subject and had a few tests made. In 1894 a committee of the Master Car-Builders' Association[5] made a somewhat extensive report on the subject of car ventilation, and with it submitted the results of several

3. Quoted by Brähmer-Schwechten: Eisenbahnhygiene, Gustav Fischer, Jena, 1904, p. 84.

4. Quoted by Dudley: The Passenger Car Ventilation System of the Pennsylvania Railroad Company, Pa. R. R. Co., Altoona, Pa., 1904.

5. Proc. Master Car-Builders' Assn., 1894, xxviii, p. 234.

analyses of the air from sleeping-cars, chair-cars and suburban coaches. Eight observations in sleeping-cars, with an average of 12.5 passengers, gave an average of 18 parts carbon dioxid per 10,000. The highest was 22, the lowest 11.3. Eight observations in chair-cars, with an average of 17.4 passengers, gave average carbon dioxid of 10.7 parts per 10,000; highest 15.5, lowest 7. Six observations in suburban coaches, which are stated to have been one-half to two-thirds full, averaged 13.8 carbon dioxid per 10,000; highest 21.7, lowest 6.9. No record of the conditions under which the samples were taken or of the methods employed are given. It is not stated whether the cars were moving or standing still at the time the observations were made.

In 1904 Dudley[6] reported on a part of some thirty or forty analyses made of the air of cars of the Pennsylvania Company, which were ventilated by the excellent system which he devised. He found from 10 to 18 parts of carbon dioxid per 10,000 in running cars, and 20 to 21 parts in cars standing still for twenty minutes. Fifty-two people occupied the cars, and are assumed to have produced 0.72 cubic feet of carbon dioxid each per hour; from which is estimated 26,000 to 62,000 cubic feet of air-supply per hour for the moving and 22,000 to 23,000 for the still cars.

More recently the air of cars running in the New York Subway, but more particularly of the subway itself, has been thoroughly studied experimentally by Soper.[7] Similar studies have been carried out in Paris by Lucien-Groux[8] and others. But these cars have little in common with the railway coach.

Numerous reports are to be found upon particular types of ventilators and ventilation systems as applied to railway cars. An excellent and extensive report of this order was made by a committee of the Master Car-Builders' Association,[9] in 1908, in which the various systems in general use were reviewed in detail. But unless I have missed important literature on this subject, the information concerning the actual conditions of the air in railway cars is very meager. It is adequate on the application of ventilating devices, but there is no series of analyses extensive enough on which to base any comprehensive opinion as to the deficiencies of natural ventilation to be overcome, or as to the adequacy of the devices applied in keeping the air of the breathing-zone freed from the products of respiration.

---

6. Dudley: The Passenger Car Ventilation System of the Pennsylvania Railroad, Pa. R. R. Co., Altoona, Pa., 1904.
7. Soper: The Air and Ventilation of Subways, Wiley & Sons, New York, 1908.
8. Lucien-Groux: Hygiène des métropolitaines souterraines, Deuxième Congrès internationale d'Assainissement et de la Salubrité des habitations, Genève, 1906.
9. Proc. Master Car-Builders' Assn., 1908, xlii, 338.

The ventilating device[10] upon which this report is based is designed to remove air by exhaustion from the upper portion of the car, and its operation is dependent on train motion. It was easily determined that it does exhaust air in this way. A long series of anemometer readings, made chiefly by Mr. C. S. Knapp, have shown that each such exhaust ventilator will remove an average of about 15,000 cubic feet of air per hour at a forty-mile train speed, and proportionately more or less for faster or slower speeds. While there is considerable variation under apparently similar conditions, the outward flow is a constant one. One ventilator is placed over each alternate section of a sleeping-car; thus there are six in the sleeping-compartment of the ordinary twelve-section car and eight to a sixteen-section car, while two are applied to the smoking-room and one to a stateroom. Toilet and dressing-rooms are also equipped with one each in recent practice. It is readily seen that a very large volume of air leaves the car each hour through these openings; it must enter somewhere. The question was, does it enter at such places and take such courses as to cause a free dilution of the air at the breathing level in the occupied car? There seems no adequate way to answer this question except by determining the carbon dioxid in such air, from which the amount of dilution may be computed as already indicated. It was desirable also to make determinations in cars not having the exhaust ventilators, but depending upon natural ventilation, for purposes of comparison.

The results of such determinations, while applying particularly to the specific ventilator in use, are to be considered rather as a test of the type—ventilation by exhaustion—as applied to railway cars, and may apply equally to any exhaust ventilator placed in the same location, provided only that the one used actually accomplishes its purpose of removing air in large volume and with constancy.

## METHODS

Determinations of carbon dioxid were made by the Petterson-Palmquist[11] apparatus, with a pipette of 20 c.c. capacity. This instrument furnishes a direct volumetric reading of carbon dioxid and should be sensitive to one part in 20,000 of air when carefully used. The accuracy of the method has been amply proven by Teich[12] and others.

10. The ventilator referred to, known as the Garland Ventilator, is fully described, with drawings and photographs, in the Railway Age, 1906, xli, 847. It is also well illustrated in the Railway Age-Gazette, 1910, xlviii, 1757.

11. Bericht der deutschen chemischen Gesellschaft, 1887, xx, 2129. A good description of the apparatus and its use is found in Hempel's Gas Analysis, translation by Dennis, Macmillan, 1902, p. 363.

12. Teich: Die Methode von Petterson und Palmquist zur Bestimmung der Kohlensäure in der Luft, Arch. f. Hyg., 1893, xix, 38.

About a thousand c.c. of the air to be examined was pumped into a large rubber cautery bulb, arranged with a cut-off, and was then emptied into a two-ounce bottle through a delivery tube leading to the bottom. The bottles were fitted with well-ground glass stoppers, lightly coated with petrolatum, and were immediately sealed after filling with the samples, by pressing the stopper tight and turning it around until no air channels were visible in the petrolatum. Foster and Haldane[13] have shown that when such a container is clean and dry and properly sealed no appreciable change takes place in the air within a fortnight, a fact which I have been able to verify amply. A single example will illustrate: Three bottles were filled with air known to contain 39 parts of carbon dioxid per 10,000 and duplicate analyses were made from these bottles after varying periods with the following results:

1st bottle, 3 days after filling, 39.5 and 38.5
2nd bottle, 6 days after filling, 38.5 and 39.0
3rd bottle, 11 days after filling, 39.0 and 38.5

If the bottles are liable to be subjected to much shaking about, a heavy rubber band should be passed over the ends to keep the stopper in place, and each one should be carefully inspected before proceeding to analysis. The bottles were prepared by thoroughly cleansing, washing in dilute sulphuric acid and distilled water and then drying. This process was repeated after each using.

If an average sample of the air was desired, the bulb was filled while walking up and down the middle portion of the car; if of a single place the bulb was filled in place or the air simply pumped through the bottle by means of a small hand bellows. For taking air from an occupied berth a woven tube about 14 inches in length and possessing enough stiffness to stand alone was passed its full length between the curtains into the berth, and air was withdrawn through this into the bottle. The delivery of air was into the bottom of the bottle, the old air being drawn off from the top by suction. Experiment showed that withdrawing through the bottle ten or twelve times the volume of air originally in the container always furnished a fair sample of the air to be tested. The point from which the berth air was taken lies approximately twelve inches behind the middle of the curtain. Comparative determinations from different points in the same berth have shown that this represents a fair sample of the berth air.

The samples of air collected in this manner were opened under a saturated solution of pure sodium chlorid, which had been saturated with carbon dioxid in order to remove any trace of free alkali and exposed to the air. The mouth of the bottle was closed by the finger-tip; it was then

13. Foster and Haldane: The Examination of Mine Air, C. Griffin & Co., London, 1905, p. 98.

removed from the solution and the finger replaced by a rubber stopper, through which a similar solution was immediately let into the bottle from a siphon. This forces the air out through a second very narrow rubber tube about 10 inches in length; and when the whole of the original air contained in this tube is displaced it may be connected to the pipette of the instrument and the air let in for analysis. There is no doubt a trifling interchange of gases between the outside air and that contained in the sampling bottle during the insertion of the rubber stopper; but with the equalized pressure brought about by opening the container under salt solution the change is so slight as to be undetectable and therefore negligible. Saturated salt solution is so slightly absorbent for carbon dioxid that no appreciable error is occasioned by the short time of exposure involved in this procedure. In order to test this, samples highly contaminated with carbon dioxid were collected in the rubber balloons used for collecting samples from cars, bottles were filled in the ordinary way and the air remaining in the balloon analyzed directly. Subsequent duplicate analyses were made from the bottles with the following comparative results, expressed in parts of carbon dioxid per 10,000 of air:

1. From balloon, 23.5; from bottle, 22.5 and 23.5
2. From balloon, 79.5; from bottle, 80.0 and 79.5
3. From balloon, 22.5; from bottle, 22.5 and 22.0
4. From balloon, 104.5; from bottle, 104.0 and 105.0

When water, instead of salt solution, is used for this purpose a considerable variation sometimes results.

When the air samples were taken from the cars a record was entered opposite the identifying numbers assigned to them, in which was recorded the date, line, time of day, time of occupancy, name of the car, its distance in car lengths from the locomotive, approximate speed, the place taken, the outside and inside temperature, the direction of the wind, number of passengers, whether doors, windows or decks were open, or whether the exhaust ventilators were used, the kind of lighting; and remarks were added as to the comfort, apparent ventilation, etc. Samples were collected chiefly in the course of ordinary travel, and, in general, no attempt was made to control any of the arrangements, the purpose being to study actual and general conditions as they exist normally.

All of the observations were made during the cooler months of the year, and nearly all when the outside temperature was low. This varied from below zero to 65 F., being in the majority of instances below 40 F.

The larger proportion of observations were made during the night after passengers had retired, and practically every hour of the night is represented by different parts of the work. This was necessary in order to study the chief feature of the sleeping-car, namely, the occupied berth. A group of samples from a single car is called a "series," and these series are consecutively numbered in the original records. In some of the earlier numbers more than one car was included, consequently in the tables which follow the series number is sometimes repeated.

Nearly 3,000 carbon dioxid determinations were made for all purposes in connection with this work; about 2,000 of these were of the air from over 200 sleeping-cars. A considerable number were made of the air of day coaches, suburban cars, street-cars, stores, restaurants, offices and the open air for comparative purposes, and others for the purpose of establishing certain facts experimentally.

## *RESULTS*

Before proceeding to an analysis of the findings it is necessary to know the amount of carbon dioxid in the air surrounding trains in order to have some basis for computing air-supplies to cars. The locomotive emits an enormous total volume of this gas, which, it is easily conceived, might play a considerable part in the amount of carbon dioxid found in the air of the cars. According to Leissner[14] the air surrounding trains contains from 18 to 22.8 parts carbon dioxid per 10,000. My results are at variance with this. Forty-six determinations averaged 4.04; the highest was 10, the lowest 3. A few showing 5 and over were made from the rear platform of trains running in a straight head wind, where the suction effect of the advancing body has a tendency to draw in the overhanging gases. One sample showing 10 and one showing 7.5 were taken in closed vestibules, which generally show no internal contamination. It is a matter of ready observation that any lateral wind carries all the smoke from a locomotive stack well out of the path of the following train. Presumably this is true of the invisible gases as well as the visible carbon. When the wind is straight ahead or directly with the train, the smoke and steam are, as a rule, carried high enough by their propulsion from the stack and their heated condition to allow the train to pass under with a clear interval, the heavier particles only, such as the small cinders, falling in its path. Of course, the smoke and condensed steam do not diffuse as do the invisible gases; but with these is mixed a quantity of sulphur dioxid, for which the sense of smell is very delicate. My observation has been, in the examination of tunnel air, that where flue gases have contaminated the air with 15 to 20 parts of carbon dioxid in 10,000, sulphur dioxid is readily detected. It occasionally happens that sufficient gas is carried into a train running in the open to render sulphur dioxid noticeable. It seems that my determinations of carbon dioxid in the air surrounding trains have not dealt with the conditions that could bring this about. Consequently I conclude that this is a relative rarity, and that 4 in 10,000 is a proper average to deal with in considering the air outside of moving

14. Cited by Brähmer-Schwechten: Eisenbahnhygiene, Gustav-Fischer, Jena, 1904, p. 85.

trains. Further evidence of the correctness of this conclusion will be found later; it is especially well shown by the conditions represented in Chart 5. Undoubtedly trains may run for a long distance and be surrounded by only the pure air of the open country, containing not more than 3.5 parts of carbon dioxid per 10,000. It must be realized that conditions may change almost momentarily.

It was not found feasible to make use of all the items recorded at the time of collecting the samples in the analysis of the findings. The distance of a car from the engine appears to bear no definite relation to the

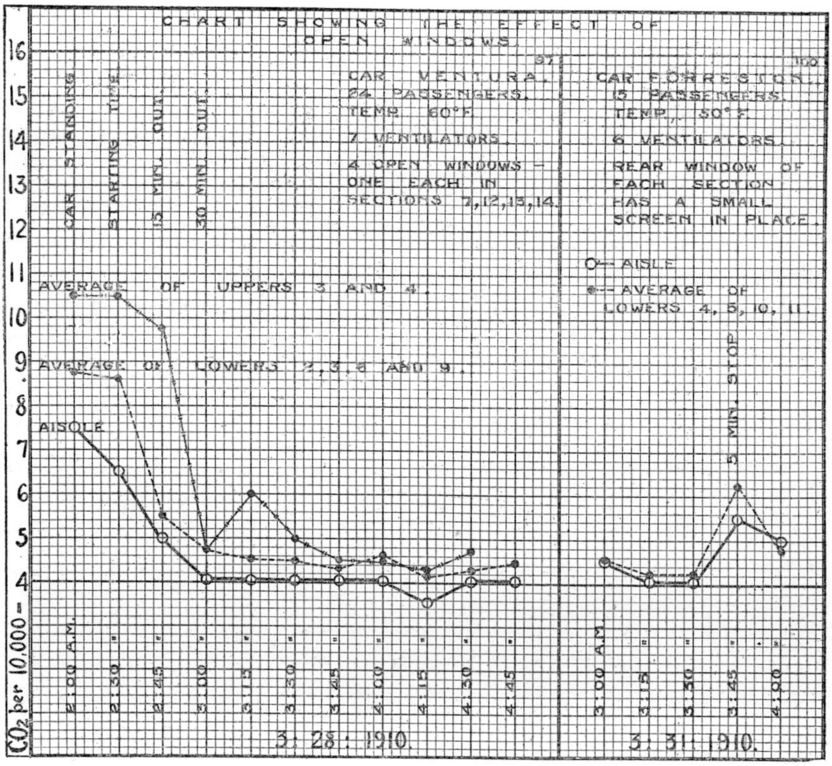


Chart 3.

amount of carbon dioxid in its atmosphere; the direction and force of the wind is so difficult to follow, especially at night, that it must generally be neglected; a car nearly always contains more carbon dioxid before starting than after it is in motion, so the length of time of its service becomes negligible; the products of illuminating gas combustion are carried out directly through the roof of the car and play no part in the air contamination; a low outside temperature is compensated for by more internal heat and seems to make no constant difference in the air-supply; the actual train speed is of less importance than the relative, that is, the rate and angle at which it cuts the wind.

It was soon observed that a few open windows in a moving train admit such a volume of the surrounding air as to render the respiratory contamination almost undetectable. The results of examination in two such cars are presented in Chart 3.

Four windows were open the full height in the car represented in the left part of the chart, though none of these were in sections where berth samples were collected. In the right-hand car one window of each section was raised about five inches with a screen in place.

The figures in the lower part of the chart indicate the time at which samples of the air were collected. Each berth examined was occupied by one person. In the right portion of this chart will be noticed the effect of a short stop, during which the carbon dioxid invariably rises; and this rise is nearly always detectable in a very few minutes. It goes down rapidly when the car is again in motion. The effect of starting is more apparent in the left portion of the chart, where the maximum conditions had been reached during a long period of standing still.

As already stated, the relative error in computations of air-supply based on findings of carbon dioxid which lie very near the normal is so great as to render the results unreliable, unless we could know the exact amount in the outside air at the particular time and place and the exact amount produced within the car or room under consideration. For parts of the series represented in this chart the computation would indicate an infinite number of cubic feet per hour—a manifest impossibility. It is obvious, however, that the air-supply must have been very large—probably over 200,000 cubic feet hourly—and its diffusion good; and that ventilation as a problem in furnishing an adequate amount of fresh air entirely disappears. This is a fact which may be easily verified by directly measuring the rate of flow of air through such an open window. I have measured up to 50,000 cubic feet per hour entering through a single side window raised only six inches.

So we may dismiss the car with open windows from further consideration, and with it the whole subject of summer ventilation, in so far as the term "ventilation" refers to supplying air and not to keeping the car cool, and turn to the car running in cold weather and with windows closed.

As already intimated, two main types of ventilation will be dealt with: the so-called natural ventilation of cars which are not equipped with any special ventilating devices, and ventilation by exhaustion with the device referred to in a previous section. All examinations were made at the ordinary breathing level unless otherwise stated. The computations of air-supply, or of ventilation efficiency, refer then to the air dilution in this breathing-zone, and to the main compartment of the car.

## NATURAL VENTILATION

The most ordinary condition for the natural ventilation of cars in cool weather is to have the doors and windows closed and a certain proportion of the small windows at the top of the car open. These small windows are herein referred to as "decks" or "deck sash," in order to avoid confusion of the term "window," which will always refer to those along the sides of the car, and of the term "ventilator," which will refer to the exhaust ventilator above mentioned.

In Table 1 are recorded 153 determinations of carbon dioxid under the above conditions, grouped and averaged for the forty-four cars included in the list. The maximum and minimum carbon dioxid observed in each car is given, together with the number of observations in which the carbon dioxid was above and below certain figures. From the average carbon dioxid and the average number of passengers is computed the hourly air-supply for each car, according to the formula given above. This we may call the ventilation equivalent. It does not necessarily equal the actual air-supply. It is the amount of fresh air with which the total amount of carbon dioxid produced by these people within an hour must be diluted in order that the proportion of carbon dioxid may be equal to the average found. The rate at which the air enters is not constant; but the rate of production of carbon dioxid is constant, and its average dilution is the nearest approximation to the average rate of air-supply. Both the maximum and minimum computations should be looked on as having only a relative value, because we cannot safely assume that the outside air always had just 0.0004 of carbon dioxid. It may be higher, and probably was higher for Cars 2 and 34 of Table 1, or it may be a trifle lower, as might be suspected for Car 32. Neither is great accuracy to be expected in computations based on four or five passengers to a car. The error in this relation is, however, generally on the safe side, as I have been able to prove experimentally where the air-supply could be measured with accuracy and the number of occupants changed. Nor is a single observation sufficient on which to base definite conclusions as to the average ventilation of a car.

It will be seen from Table 1 that there is a wide variation in the air-supply necessary to satisfy the findings under physical conditions which are apparently nearly identical. This will be noted in other tables and no doubt represents, to a large extent, actual variations, the cause of which is often difficult or impossible to determine; it may be represented in part by errors of observation.

The averages representing number of passengers and carbon dioxid in the last line are of the totals of all of the 153 observations included in Table 1, and from these figures is again computed an hourly air-supply necessary to satisfy these general averages. Inasmuch as some of these

TABLE 1.—DETERMINATIONS OF CARBON DIOXID IN CARS WITHOUT VENTILATORS, WITH OPEN DECKS, AND WITH DOORS AND WINDOWS CLOSED

| Cars. | Series. | Average Number of People in Car While Taking Samples. | $CO_2$ Per 10,000 of Air. No. of Determinations. | Average. | Extremes. Min. | Extremes. Max. | No. Over Twelve. | No. Over Ten. | No. Over Eight. | No. Under Six. | Approximate Hourly Air Supply Necessary to Maintain Average $CO_2$ | Proportion of Decks Open. |
|---|---|---|---|---|---|---|---|---|---|---|---|---|
| 1 | 4 | 12.00 | 3 | 7.66 | 5.5 | 9.0 | 0 | 0 | 2 | 1 | 19,700 | ¼ |
| 2 | 17 | 5.00 | ? | 6.75 | 6.5 | 7.0 | 0 | 0 | 0 | 0 | 10,900 | ¼ |
| 3 | 17 | 14.00 | 8 | 6.56 | 4.5 | 8.5 | 0 | 0 | 1 | 4 | 32,800 | ¼ |
| 4 | 27 | 24.00 | 1 | 11.00 | 11.0 | 11.0 | 0 | 1 | 1 | 0 | 20,600 | ¼ |
| 5 | 45 | 22.00 | 4 | 8.88 | 8.5 | 9.5 | 0 | 0 | 4 | 0 | 27,000 | ¼ |
| 6 | 46 | 24.00 | 6 | 8.58 | 8.0 | 10.0 | 0 | 0 | 4 | 0 | 31,400 | ¼ |
| 7 | 49 | 20.00 | 5 | 6.80 | 6.0 | 7.5 | 0 | 0 | 0 | 0 | 42,900 | ¼ |
| 8 | 89 | 17.00 | 4 | 7.75 | 6.5 | 9.0 | 0 | 0 | 1 | 0 | 27,200 | ¼ |
| 9 | 92 | 13.00 | 4 | 5.63 | 5.5 | 6.0 | 0 | 0 | 0 | 3 | 47,900 | ¼ |
| 10 | 93 | 16.00 | 4 | 6.75 | 6.0 | 7.5 | 0 | 0 | 0 | 0 | 34,900 | ¼ |
| 11 | 94 | 13.00 | 4 | 8.00 | 7.5 | 8.5 | 0 | 0 | 1 | 0 | 19,500 | ¼ |
| 12 | 95 | 14.00 | 10 | 7.70 | 7.5 | 8.5 | 0 | 0 | 1 | 0 | 23,300 | ¼ |
| 13 | 4 | 10.75 | 4 | 6.25 | 5.5 | 7.0 | 0 | 0 | 0 | 1 | 28,700 | ½ |
| 14 | 5 | 8.00 | 2 | 6.75 | 6.0 | 7.5 | 0 | 0 | 0 | 0 | 17,500 | ½ |
| 15 | 7 | 8.50 | 8 | 6.31 | 3.5 | 10.0 | 0 | 0 | 1 | 4 | 22,100 | ½ |
| 16 | 8 | 12.00 | 3 | 6.60 | 4.0 | 8.0 | 0 | 0 | 0 | 1 | 27,700 | ½ |
| 17 | 9 | 20.00 | 2 | 9.25 | 8.5 | 10.0 | 0 | 0 | 2 | 0 | 22,900 | ½ |
| 18 | 10 | 9.00 | 3 | 8.66 | 6.5 | 10.0 | 0 | 0 | 2 | 0 | 11,600 | ½ |
| 19 | 12 | 15.00 | 6 | 5.83 | 5.0 | 7.5 | 0 | 0 | 0 | 3 | 49,200 | ½ |
| 20 | 20 | 15.00 | 2 | 7.50 | 7.0 | 8.0 | 0 | 0 | 0 | 0 | 25,700 | ½ |
| 21 | 22 | 13.00 | 6 | 6.17 | 5.0 | 7.0 | 0 | 0 | 0 | 1 | 36,900 | ½ |
| 22 | 24 | 16.00 | 2 | 5.25 | 4.5 | 6.0 | 0 | 0 | 0 | 1 | 76,800 | ½ |
| 23 | 6 | 13.33 | 3 | 5.00 | 4.5 | 5.5 | 0 | 0 | 0 | 3 | 89,000 | ½ |
| 24 | 1 | 24.00 | 1 | 12.00 | 12.0 | 12.0 | 0 | 1 | 1 | 0 | 18,000 | ½ |
| 25 | 62 | 13.00 | 4 | 7.38 | 6.0 | 8.0 | 0 | 0 | 0 | 0 | 23,100 | ½ |
| 26 | 84 | 17.00 | 4 | 6.38 | 6.0 | 6.5 | 0 | 0 | 0 | 0 | 42,900 | ½ |
| 27 | 85 | 12.25 | 4 | 8.25 | 8.0 | 9.0 | 0 | 0 | 1 | 0 | 13,300 | ½ |
| 28 | 86 | 17.00 | 4 | 8.00 | 6.5 | 9.5 | 0 | 0 | 2 | 0 | 25,500 | ½ |
| 29 | 87 | 19.00 | 4 | 7.13 | 6.5 | 8.0 | 0 | 0 | 0 | 0 | 36,400 | ½ |
| 30 | 90 | 16.00 | 4 | 7.00 | 7.0 | 7.0 | 0 | 0 | 0 | 0 | 32,000 | ½ |
| 31 | 5 | 10.00 | 3 | 5.66 | 5.0 | 6.0 | 0 | 0 | 0 | 0 | 36,100 | All |
| 32 | 6 | 13.25 | 4 | 4.75 | 4.5 | 6.0 | 0 | 0 | 0 | 3 | 106,000 | All |
| 33 | 8 | 12.00 | 1 | 7.00 | 7.0 | 7.0 | 0 | 0 | 0 | 0 | 24,000 | All |
| 34 | 9 | 4.00 | 2 | 6.50 | 5.5 | 7.5 | 0 | 0 | 0 | 1 | 9,600 | All |
| 35 | 10 | 9.00 | 1 | 6.50 | 6.5 | 6.5 | 0 | 0 | 0 | 0 | 21,600 | All |
| 36 | 21 | 8.00 | 2 | 5.50 | 5.5 | 5.5 | 0 | 0 | 0 | 2 | 32,000 | All |
| 37 | 27 | 18.00 | 5 | 6.90 | 6.0 | 7.5 | 0 | 0 | 0 | 0 | 37,200 | All |
| 38 | 1 | 16.00 | 2 | 7.00 | 6.0 | 8.0 | 0 | 0 | 0 | 0 | 32,000 | All |
| 39 | 1 | 10.00 | 2 | 7.50 | 6.5 | 9.0 | 0 | 0 | 1 | 0 | 16,000 | All |
| 40 | 1 | 20.00 | 1 | 9.00 | 9.0 | 9.0 | 0 | 0 | 1 | 0 | 24,000 | All |
| 41 | 3 | 20.00 | 2 | 12.00 | 11.0 | 13.0 | 1 | 2 | 2 | 0 | 15,000 | All |
| 42 | 1 | 24.00 | 1 | 8.00 | 8.0 | 8.0 | 0 | 0 | 0 | 0 | 36,000 | All |
| 43 | 82 | 17.00 | 4 | 6.63 | 6.0 | 7.0 | 0 | 0 | 0 | 0 | 38,800 | All |
| 44 | 83 | 22.50 | 4 | 8.13 | 7.0 | 8.5 | 0 | 0 | 3 | 0 | 32,700 | All |
| Totals—Av. | | 15.05 | 153 | 7.19 | 3.5 | 13.0 | 1 | 4 | 31 | 29 | 28,300 | |

series do not fairly represent car averages, but only individual and temporary conditions, and sometimes strictly local conditions within the car, the plan is considered better than to average the car averages. The change would be but a slight one, however, in this case; and the two methods have been found to give results very close together in nearly all groups considered.

For the 153 observations the average carbon dioxid is 7.19 per 10,000. The maximum is 13, the minimum 3.5. The average number of passengers for the 153 observations is 15.05. A car carrying this number of people would require 28,300 cubic feet of fresh air hourly to maintain the carbon dioxid at 7.19 parts per 10,000. In other words, there would necessarily be an air-supply of 1,880 cubic feet per person hourly.

TABLE 2.—DETERMINATIONS OF CARBON DIOXID IN CARS WITHOUT VENTILATORS WHEN THE DECKS ARE OPEN AND ONE OR BOTH END DOORS INTO VESTIBULES ARE OPEN. WINDOWS CLOSED

| Cars. | Series. | Average Number of People in Car While Taking Samples. | $CO_2$ Per 10,000 of Air. No. of Determinations. | Average. | Extremes. Min. | Max. | No. Over Twelve. | No. Over Ten. | No. Over Eight. | No. Under Six. | Approximate Hourly Air Supply Necessary to Maintain Average $CO_2$. | Proportion of Deck Sash Open. | Doors Open.* |
|---|---|---|---|---|---|---|---|---|---|---|---|---|---|
| 1 | 17 | 14.00 | 4 | 5.00 | 4.0 | 5.5 | 0 | 0 | 0 | 4 | 84,000 | ¼ | F. |
| 2 | 5 | 9.75 | 4 | 5.75 | 5.0 | 7.0 | 0 | 0 | 0 | 2 | 33,400 | ½ | F. |
| 3 | 8 | 12.00 | 3 | 7.33 | 7.0 | 8.0 | 0 | 0 | 0 | 0 | 21,600 | ½ | F. |
| 4 | 9 | 16.00 | 3 | 4.50 | 3.5 | 6.0 | 0 | 0 | 0 | 2 | 192,000 | ½ | F. |
| 5 | 9 | 13.00 | 3 | 7.16 | 6.5 | 8.5 | 0 | 0 | 1 | 0 | 24,700 | ½ | F. |
| 6 | 23 | 5.00 | 9 | 5.26 | 3.5 | 8.0 | 0 | 0 | 0 | 7 | 23,800 | ½ | F. |
| 7 | 6 | 13.00 | 2 | 5.25 | 4.5 | 6.0 | 0 | 0 | 0 | 1 | 62,400 | ½ | F. R. |
| 8 | 9 | 6.00 | 1 | 5.50 | 5.5 | 5.5 | 0 | 0 | 0 | 1 | 24,000 | ½ | F. |
| 9 | 3 | 4.60 | 5 | 3.60 | 3.5 | 4.0 | 0 | 0 | 0 | 4 | ....... | ½ | F. R. |
| 10 | 5 | 12.00 | 1 | 5.50 | 5.5 | 5.5 | 0 | 0 | 0 | 1 | 48,000 | All | F. |
| 11 | 6 | 10.00 | 2 | 6.00 | 5.0 | 7.0 | 0 | 0 | 0 | 1 | 30,000 | All | F. |
| 12 | 21 | 5.50 | 2 | 4.75 | 4.5 | 5.0 | 0 | 0 | 0 | 2 | 44,000 | All | F. |
| 13 | 6 | 10.00 | 2 | 4.75 | 4.5 | 5.0 | 0 | 0 | 0 | 2 | 80,000 | All | F. R. |
| 14 | 10 | 10.00 | 1 | 5.50 | 5.5 | 5.5 | 0 | 0 | 0 | 1 | 40,000 | All | R. |
| 15 | 10 | 11.50 | 4 | 6.25 | 5.5 | 7.0 | 0 | 0 | 0 | 1 | 31,000 | All | F. R.† |
| Totals—Av. | | 9.50 | 46 | 5.40 | 3.5 | 8.5 | 0 | 0 | 1 | 29 | 40,700 | | |

* F., forward door open; R., rear door open.
† In car 15 the end doors were closed but their drop sashes, about 14 inches high, were open.

The carbon dioxid is less than 6 per 10,000 in 18.9 per cent. of the observations; it is 8 or less in 79.7 per cent., while it is over 8, 10 and 12 in 20.3 per cent., 2.6 per cent. and 0.65 per cent., respectively. Consequently the ventilation efficiency was in these cases equivalent to more than 3,000 cubic feet per person hourly in 18.9 per cent., 1,500 cubic feet or more in 79.7 per cent.; while it was less than 1,000 cubic feet in 2.6 per cent., and less than 750 in only 0.65 per cent.; 3,000, 1,500, 1,000 and 750 being the air-supplies per person per hour necessary to maintain the carbon dioxid at 6, 8, 10 and 12, respectively (Chart 1).

Adding to the open decks by opening one or both end doors to the vestibule (the outside vestibule doors remaining closed) would be expected to cause a greater air-supply. Such is the case, as shown by the forty-six observations recorded in Table 2. The general remarks made above apply equally to this table.

The maximum carbon dioxid is seen to be 8.5 against 13 in Table 1, while 64.35 per cent. of the determinations are below 6. The average carbon dioxid being 5.40 per 10,000 and the average number of passengers 9.50, there would be required 40,700 cubic feet of air hourly to meet the conditions. In Cars 3, 5 and 6 the computed air-supply is far below the average; in Car 4 it is far above, while in Car 9 it may be called infinite, since there is no detectable increase of the carbon dioxid. It sometimes happens that an end door is open and practically no air enters through it; on the other hand, an enormous volume may enter; and occasionally air may leave the body of the car through such an open door. These are facts which may be verified by noting the direction and force of the air currents as they pass. Air does not necessarily sweep through cars with doors open to the vestibules, though on the average the air supplied to the breathing-zone in the body of the car is considerably increased. There seems to be no constancy as to which door acts best in the capacity of ventilator. Sometimes the forward and sometimes the rear is most efficient.

TABLE 3.—DETERMINATIONS OF CARBON DIOXID IN CARS WITHOUT VENTILATORS AND HAVING ALL DECKS, DOORS AND WINDOWS CLOSED

| Cars. | Series. | Average Number of People in Car While Taking Samples. | $CO_2$ Per 10,000 of Air. | | | | | | | | Approximate Hourly Air Supply Necessary to Maintain Average $CO_2$. |
|---|---|---|---|---|---|---|---|---|---|---|---|
| | | | No. of Determinations. | Average. | Extremes. Min. | Extremes. Max. | No. Over Twelve. | No. Over Ten. | No. Over Eight. | No. Under Six. | |
| 1 | 10 | 16.00 | 2 | 12.50 | 10.0 | 15.0 | 1 | 1 | 2 | 0 | 11,300 |
| 2 | 14 | 6.00 | 2 | 6.25 | 5.5 | 7.0 | 0 | 0 | 0 | 1 | 16,000 |
| 3 | 17 | 14.00 | 2 | 7.50 | 7.0 | 8.0 | 0 | 0 | 0 | 0 | 24,000 |
| 4 | 18 | 15.00 | 3 | 7.33 | 7.0 | 8.0 | 0 | 0 | 0 | 0 | 27,500 |
| 5 | 50 | 18.00 | 1 | 10.00 | 10.0 | 10.0 | 0 | 0 | 1 | 0 | 18,000 |
| 6 | 1 | 15.00 | 1 | 5.50 | 5.5 | 5.5 | 0 | 0 | 0 | 1 | 60,000 |
| 7 | 16 | 10.00 | 1 | 10.00 | 10.0 | 10.0 | 0 | 0 | 1 | 0 | 10,000 |
| Totals—Av. | | 13.33 | 12 | 8.33 | 5.5 | 15.0 | 1 | 1 | 4 | 2 | 18,500 |

Only twelve observations were made where both doors and all the deck sash were closed. These are recorded in Table 3. Whatever amount of the outside air enters the car under these conditions must find its way in through natural crevices and is driven in and out by the pressure of the wind and the suction effects produced by the motion of the train.

As would be expected under these conditions, the average carbon dioxid is greater than in either of the preceding groups and the computed air-supply is smaller. The maximum carbon dioxid has advanced to 15, while the average is 8.33. Eight and three-tenths per cent. are above 12 and 33.3 per cent. are above 8, while only 16.6 per cent. are below 6. With the average of 8.33 parts of carbon dioxid per 10,000 and 13.33 passengers 18,500 cubic feet of air per hour would be required.

There were only two observations made when all the decks were closed and one end door to the vestibule was open—the rear door in each instance. The number of passengers averaged 9.5 and the carbon dioxid averaged 5.75, which would indicate a ventilation efficiency equivalent to 32,500 cubic feet of air per hour. The number of observations is too small to have any considerable value.

The comparative efficiency of natural ventilation in the four groups of conditions stands: 18,500 cubic feet of air hourly for the fully closed car; 28,300 when from one-fourth to all the decks are open; 32,500 when decks are closed and one door open; and 40,700 where end doors are open in addition to open decks. It is, of course, possible that a larger number of observations would materially change these figures, but it is not probable that their relation to each other would be greatly altered.

## VENTILATION BY EXHAUST VENTILATORS

It has been stated that one ventilator of the type described is fitted above each alternate section of sleeping-cars and that each ventilator will remove an average of 15,000 cubic feet of air per hour at a forty-mile train speed. No special intakes are provided for this air. It goes out; it must come in. But it might come in at such places and take such courses as to play no part in aerating the breathing-zone of the car—might be short-circuited, so to speak. The results of the carbon dioxid determinations of air at the breathing level shows that to a certain extent this must happen, since the air supplied to the breathing-zone, as computed from carbon dioxid determinations, is considerably less than the amount which leaves through the ventilators, as determined by actual measurement. But in spite of this the air-supply is much increased and is better regulated than in cars not so equipped.

In Table 4 are recorded 294 determinations in 67 cars which were fitted with these ventilators and in which all doors and windows were closed.

In Table 4 the first twenty-five series represent daylight or early evening; the remainder represent all hours of the night from about 10:30 p. m. to early morning. The two groups are averaged for comparison, and the final average includes both groups. None of the night determinations are of air taken from behind the curtains of berths; they are from the air of the center aisle.

As in the previous tables, there is here also a considerable variation in the computed air-supplies, though the tendency is to much more pronounced uniformity. The maximum carbon dioxid is 10 parts per 10,000 of air, the minimum 4.5 parts. The average carbon dioxid is 6.20 per

10,000 and the average number of passengers 14.88. There would be required 40,600 cubic feet of air hourly to satisfy these conditions. Of the 294 determinations of carbon dioxid only 4.4 per cent. are over 8 per 10,000 while 46.9 per cent. are below 6 and 95.6 per cent. are as low as 8. Hence the ventilation efficiency is equivalent to at least 1,500 cubic feet per person hourly 95.6 per cent. of the time and is 3,000 cubic feet or more 46.9 per cent. of the time, while it is never less than 1,000 cubic feet.

It will be noticed that the averages of the totals in this table represent essentially the same average ventilation as for those in Table 2, where to a proportion of open decks is added an open door. Probably its proper comparison would be made with the conditions of Table 1, when it is seen that there is a distinct advantage in favor of the cars equipped with exhaust ventilators over those ventilated by the decks, and that this advantage represents an average addition in the air-supply to the breathing-level of about 12,000 cubic feet of air per hour.

TABLE 4.—DETERMINATIONS OF CARBON DIOXID IN CARS EQUIPPED WITH EXHAUST VENTILATORS: ALL DOORS AND WINDOWS CLOSED

| Cars. | Series. | Average Number of People in Car While Taking Samples. | $CO_2$ Per 10,000 of Air. | | | | | | | | Approximate Hourly Air Supply Necessary to maintain Average $CO_2$. |
|---|---|---|---|---|---|---|---|---|---|---|---|
| | | | No. of Determinations. | Average. | Extremes. Min. | Extremes. Max. | No. Over Twelve. | No. Over Ten. | No. Over Eight. | No. Under Six. | |
| | | | | | DAY | | | | | | |
| 1 | 2 | 18.00 | 4 | 7.21 | 5.0 | 10.0 | 0 | 0 | 1 | 1 | 34,600 |
| 2 | 6 | 10.00 | 2 | 6.50 | 5.0 | 8.0 | 0 | 0 | 0 | 1 | 24,000 |
| 3 | 11 | 6.00 | 3 | 5.33 | 4.5 | 6.0 | 0 | 0 | 0 | 2 | 27,100 |
| 4 | 11 | 18.00 | 5 | 6.80 | 5.5 | 8.0 | 0 | 0 | 0 | 1 | 38,600 |
| 5 | 13 | 8.00 | 2 | 5.25 | 5.0 | 5.5 | 0 | 0 | 0 | 2 | 38,400 |
| 6 | 18 | 10.00 | 2 | 5.50 | 4.5 | 6.5 | 0 | 0 | 0 | 1 | 40,000 |
| 7 | 19 | 8.00 | 4 | 5.75 | 5.0 | 6.5 | 0 | 0 | 0 | 2 | 27,400 |
| 8 | 22 | 19.00 | 2 | 7.25 | 7.0 | 7.5 | 0 | 0 | 0 | 0 | 35,100 |
| 9 | 25 | 12.00 | 1 | 5.50 | 5.5 | 5.5 | 0 | 0 | 0 | 1 | 48,000 |
| 10 | 26 | 10.66 | 3 | 5.50 | 4.5 | 7.0 | 0 | 0 | 0 | 2 | 42,600 |
| 11 | 28 | 15.00 | 3 | 7.83 | 7.0 | 8.5 | 0 | 0 | 1 | 0 | 23,500 |
| 12 | 30 | 10.00 | 20 | 5.70 | 4.5 | 8.0 | 0 | 0 | 0 | 12 | 35,300 |
| 13 | 31 | 14.00 | 5 | 6.70 | 6.0 | 8.0 | 0 | 0 | 0 | 0 | 31,100 |
| 14 | 32 | 10.00 | 5 | 5.10 | 5.0 | 5.5 | 0 | 0 | 0 | 5 | 54,500 |
| 15 | 34 | 18.00 | 2 | 7.00 | 7.0 | 7.0 | 0 | 0 | 0 | 0 | 36,000 |
| 16 | 38 | 16.00 | 4 | 7.37 | 6.0 | 8.0 | 0 | 0 | 0 | 0 | 28,500 |
| 17 | 38 | 12.00 | 4 | 5.62 | 5.0 | 6.0 | 0 | 0 | 0 | 2 | 44,400 |
| 18 | 39 | 13.17 | 6 | 5.67 | 5.0 | 7.0 | 0 | 0 | 0 | 5 | 47,200 |
| 19 | 40 | 13.17 | 6 | 5.42 | 5.0 | 6.5 | 0 | 0 | 0 | 5 | 55,600 |
| 20 | 42 | 13.75 | 8 | 5.19 | 5.0 | 5.5 | 0 | 0 | 0 | 8 | 66,400 |
| 21 | 43 | 15.00 | 3 | 6.17 | 6.0 | 6.5 | 0 | 0 | 0 | 0 | 41,500 |
| 22 | 44 | 11.00 | 3 | 6.00 | 5.0 | 7.0 | 0 | 0 | 0 | 1 | 33,000 |
| 23 | 51 | 17.17 | 6 | 6.58 | 6.0 | 7.5 | 0 | 0 | 0 | 0 | 40,000 |
| 24 | 52 | 12.00 | 6 | 5.83 | 5.0 | 6.5 | 0 | 0 | 0 | 3 | 39,300 |
| 25 | 102 | 16.17 | 6 | 6.17 | 5.0 | 8.0 | 0 | 0 | 0 | 0 | 44,700 |
| Daytime Totals—Av. | | 12.88 | 115 | 6.01 | 4.5 | 10.0 | 0 | 0 | 2 | 54 | 38,400 |

TABLE 4.—CONTINUED

NIGHT

| | | | | | | | | | | | |
|---|---|---|---|---|---|---|---|---|---|---|---|
| 26 | 12 | 11.00 | 2 | 6.25 | 5.0 | 7.5 | 0 | 0 | 0 | 1 | 29,300 |
| 27 | 13 | 12.00 | 2 | 6.25 | 6.0 | 6.5 | 0 | 0 | 0 | 0 | 32,000 |
| 28 | 19 | 8.00 | 3 | 5.66 | 5.5 | 6.0 | 0 | 0 | 0 | 2 | 28,900 |
| 29 | 28 | 13.00 | 3 | 7.33 | 6.0 | 10.0 | 0 | 0 | 1 | 0 | 23,400 |
| 30 | 31 | 14.00 | 4 | 6.88 | 6.0 | 8.0 | 0 | 0 | 0 | 0 | 29,200 |
| 31 | 33 | 14.00 | 3 | 6.83 | 5.5 | 8.5 | 0 | 0 | 1 | 1 | 29,700 |
| 32 | 35 | 9.40 | 5 | 5.80 | 5.5 | 6.5 | 0 | 0 | 0 | 3 | 31,300 |
| 33 | 36 | 17.25 | 4 | 6.25 | 5.5 | 7.5 | 0 | 0 | 0 | 2 | 36,000 |
| 34 | 37 | 16.00 | 4 | 5.50 | 5.0 | 6.5 | 0 | 0 | 0 | 3 | 64,000 |
| 35 | 41 | 17.00 | 5 | 4.90 | 4.5 | 5.5 | 0 | 0 | 0 | 5 | 113,300 |
| 36 | 48 | 18.00 | 2 | 6.25 | 6.0 | 6.5 | 0 | 0 | 0 | 0 | 48,000 |
| 37 | 54 | 17.00 | 6 | 6.33 | 5.5 | 7.0 | 0 | 0 | 0 | 1 | 44,000 |
| 38 | 56 | 23.00 | 5 | 6.60 | 5.5 | 8.0 | 0 | 0 | 0 | 1 | 53,100 |
| 39 | 59 | 18.00 | 5 | 7.60 | 7.0 | 8.0 | 0 | 0 | 0 | 0 | 30,800 |
| 40 | 60 | 16.00 | 5 | 5.80 | 5.0 | 6.0 | 0 | 0 | 0 | 3 | 50,000 |
| 41 | 61 | 18.00 | 5 | 6.20 | 5.5 | 7.5 | 0 | 0 | 0 | 2 | 49,100 |
| 42 | 63 | 23.00 | 4 | 8.50 | 7.5 | 10.0 | 0 | 0 | 2 | 0 | 30,700 |
| 43 | 64 | 18.00 | 4 | 6.25 | 5.5 | 7.0 | 0 | 0 | 0 | 1 | 48,000 |
| 44 | 65 | 14.00 | 4 | 5.25 | 5.0 | 6.0 | 0 | 0 | 0 | 3 | 67,200 |
| 45 | 66 | 13.00 | 4 | 5.25 | 5.0 | 6.0 | 0 | 0 | 0 | 3 | 62,400 |
| 46 | 67 | 20.00 | 4 | 6.13 | 5.5 | 6.5 | 0 | 0 | 0 | 1 | 56,200 |
| 47 | 68 | 16.00 | 4 | 6.38 | 6.0 | 7.0 | 0 | 0 | 0 | 0 | 40,300 |
| 48 | 69 | 15.00 | 4 | 6.25 | 5.5 | 7.0 | 0 | 0 | 0 | 1 | 40,000 |
| 49 | 70 | 17.00 | 4 | 8.88 | 8.0 | 10.0 | 0 | 0 | 3 | 0 | 20,900 |
| 50 | 71 | 14.00 | 4 | 7.50 | 6.0 | 8.0 | 0 | 0 | 0 | 0 | 24,000 |
| 51 | 72 | 13.00 | 4 | 6.25 | 6.0 | 6.5 | 0 | 0 | [illegible] | 0 | 31,700 |
| 52 | 73 | 15.00 | 4 | 7.63 | 6.5 | 9.0 | 0 | 0 | 1 | 0 | 25,000 |
| 53 | 74 | 16.00 | 4 | 7.50 | 6.5 | 9.0 | 0 | 0 | 1 | 0 | 27,400 |
| 54 | 75 | 25.00 | 4 | 6.75 | 5.5 | 8.0 | 0 | 0 | 0 | 1 | 54,600 |
| 55 | 76 | 22.00 | 4 | 7.25 | 5.0 | 9.5 | 0 | 0 | 2 | 2 | 40,600 |
| 56 | 77 | 14.00 | 4 | 6.13 | 5.5 | 7.0 | 0 | 0 | 0 | 1 | 39,400 |
| 57 | 78 | 15.00 | 4 | 5.00 | 5.0 | 5.0 | 0 | 0 | 0 | 4 | 90,000 |
| 58 | 79 | 14.00 | 4 | 5.38 | 5.0 | 5.5 | 0 | 0 | 0 | 4 | 61,900 |
| 59 | 80 | 18.00 | 4 | 5.38 | 5.0 | 6.5 | 0 | 0 | 0 | 3 | 78,300 |
| 60 | 81 | 14.00 | 4 | 5.63 | 5.0 | 6.5 | 0 | 0 | 0 | 2 | 51,600 |
| 61 | 88 | 17.00 | 4 | 5.50 | 5.0 | 6.5 | 0 | 0 | 0 | 3 | 68,000 |
| 62 | 91 | 14.00 | 4 | 5.61 | 5.0 | 6.5 | 0 | 0 | 0 | 3 | 51,600 |
| 63 | 96 | 14.00 | 12 | 5.33 | 4.5 | 6.5 | 0 | 0 | 0 | 8 | 63,200 |
| 64 | 98 | 14.00 | 4 | 5.25 | 5.0 | 6.0 | 0 | 0 | 0 | 3 | 67,200 |
| 65 | 99 | 19.00 | 10 | 5.40 | 4.5 | 7.0 | 0 | 0 | 0 | 8 | 81,400 |
| 66 | 103 | 13.00 | 4 | 5.75 | 5.0 | 6.5 | 0 | 0 | 0 | 2 | 44,600 |
| 67 | 104 | 17.00 | 2 | 5.75 | 5.5 | 6.0 | 0 | 0 | 0 | 1 | 58,300 |
| Night time Totals—Av. | | 16.04 | 179 | 6.33 | 4.5 | 10.0 | 0 | 0 | 11 | 84 | 41,300 |
| Totals—Av. | | 14.88 | 294 | 6.20 | 4.5 | 10.0 | 0 | 0 | 13 | 138 | 40,600 |

Forty-eight observations in twelve cars equipped with ventilators and having one or both doors open to the vestibules are recorded in Table 5.

With an average of 14.48 passengers the carbon dioxid varies from 3.5 to 9, and averages 5.50. It is over 8 but once and is 29 times under 6 (60.4 per cent.). While the totals and average carbon dioxid are very close to those of Table 2 (where natural ventilation is carried on through open decks and doors), the number of passengers is greater and the equivalent air-supply is 57,900 cubic feet per hour against 40,700, showing again a distinct advantage in favor of the cars equipped with exhaust ventilators. A larger proportion of all doors was open in these cars than in those of Table 2.

We may bring together all these different conditions for comparison of the air-supply by using the form presented in Chart 2. This comparison will be made clear by Chart 4. The carbon dioxid found, when plotted at the place representing the number of passengers present, will always reach some diagonal which has a definite value in terms of air-supply.

TABLE 5.—DETERMINATIONS OF CARBON DIOXID IN CARS EQUIPPED WITH EXHAUST VENTILATORS AND HAVING ONE OR BOTH END DOORS TO VESTIBULE OPEN

| Cars. | Series. | Average No. of People in Car While Taking Samples. | $CO_2$ Per 10,000 of Air. | | | | | | | | Approximate Hourly Air Supply Necessary to Maintain Average $CO_2$ | Doors Open.* |
|---|---|---|---|---|---|---|---|---|---|---|---|---|
| | | | Number of Determinations. | Average. | Extremes. | | No. Over 12. | No. Over 10. | No. Over 8. | No. Under 6. | | |
| | | | | | Min. | Max. | | | | | | |
| 1 | 2a | 10.00 | 3 | 5.00 | 3.5 | 6.5 | 0 | 0 | 0 | 2 | 60,000 | F. R. |
| 2 | 2b | 12.00 | 3 | 6.50 | 6.0 | 7.0 | 0 | 0 | 0 | 0 | 28,800 | F. R. |
| 3 | 2c | 18.00 | 3 | 5.50 | 3.5 | 7.0 | 0 | 0 | 0 | 1 | 72,000 | F. R. |
| 4 | 2d | 15.00 | 6 | 7.16 | 6.0 | 9.0 | 0 | 0 | 1 | 0 | 28,500 | F. R. |
| 5 | 3 | 5.00 | 4 | 4.25 | 3.5 | 4.5 | 0 | 0 | 0 | 4 | 120,000 | F. R. |
| 6 | 18 | 10.00 | 1 | 4.50 | 4.5 | 4.5 | 0 | 0 | 0 | 1 | 120,000 | R.† |
| 7 | 22 | 12.00 | 3 | 5.50 | 4.5 | 6.5 | 0 | 0 | 0 | 2 | 48,000 | F. |
| 8 | 25 | 14.60 | 5 | 5.10 | 4.5 | 5.5 | 0 | 0 | 0 | 5 | 79,600 | F. R. |
| 9 | 26 | 19.88 | 9 | 5.22 | 4.0 | 7.5 | 0 | 0 | 0 | 6 | 97,800 | F. R. |
| 10 | 27 | 17.00 | 1 | 6.50 | 6.5 | 6.5 | 0 | 0 | 0 | 0 | 40,800 | F. R. |
| 11 | 57 | 13.00 | 5 | 5.20 | 4.5 | 6.5 | 0 | 0 | 0 | 4 | 65,000 | F. R. |
| 12 | 58 | 17.00 | 5 | 5.40 | 5.0 | 6.0 | 0 | 0 | 0 | 4 | 72,800 | F. R. |
| Totals—Av | | 14.48 | 48 | 5.50 | 3.5 | 9.0 | 0 | 0 | 1 | 29 | 57,900 | |

* F., forward door open. R., rear door open.

† Car 6 was the last car in the train, consequently the rear door led to an open and not to a closed vestibule, as did the others.

Chart 4 shows clearly that the air-supply to sleeping-cars, as computed from these 555 carbon dioxid determinations, is for all but that of the completely closed car depending upon natural ventilation, a large one relative to the number of passengers, and would not allow the average carbon dioxid to go above ten in any but this one condition unless the cars were crowded beyond their natural capacity. Such overcrowding in sleeping-cars is prevented by the assignment of space and refusing further applicants when this is all taken. It very rarely happens that sleeping-cars carry more than twenty-five passengers. Such a case did not come under my observation in the collection of these 555 and many other samples of the air.

It should be understood that all of the above observations apply to the main compartment of the standard sleeping-car in motion; and in setting down the number of passengers only those persons were counted who were actually in this compartment, and who had been there for a period of at least ten minutes at the time the samples of air were being collected. The smoking-room, the drawing-room, and other small rooms constitute separate problems.

In order to test the consistency of the results obtained, and to find if the carbon dioxid actually does go up in proportion to the number of passengers, these 555 observations were divided into four groups, accord-

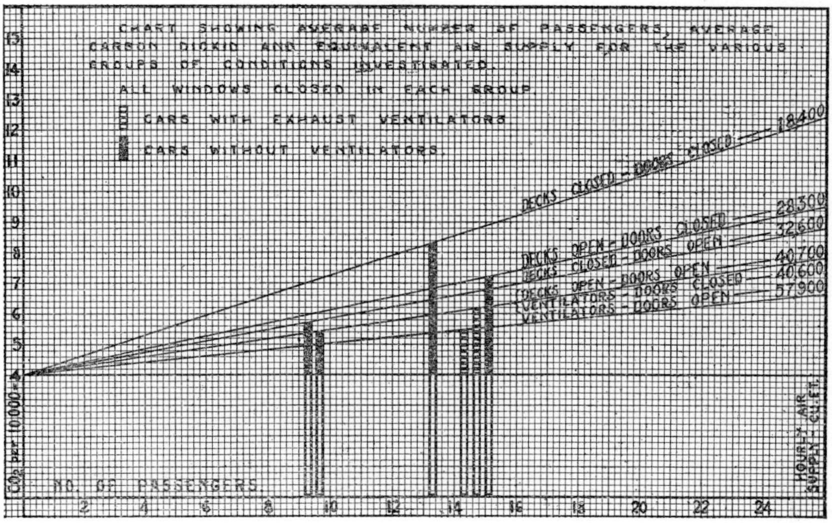


Chart 4.

ing to whether the number of passengers was below 10, between 10 and 15, between 15 and 20, or above 20. The averages of carbon dioxid and

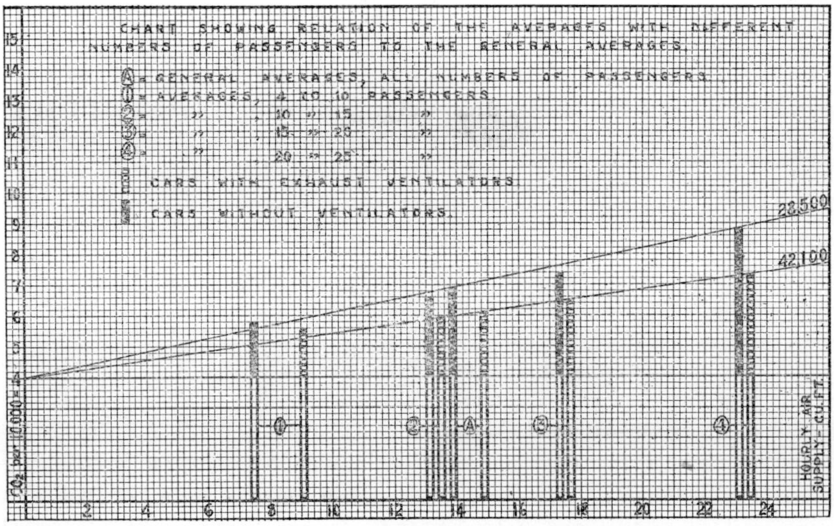


Chart 5.

number of passengers were determined for all observations falling in each of these groups for each of the two classes of cars under consideration and are shown in Chart 5 along with the general averages for each class.

For the cars depending upon natural ventilation the general averages of passengers and carbon dioxid for all observations are 13.70 and 6.88, respectively, and the equivalent hourly air-supply 28,500 cubic feet. Averaging all observations in cars when there were—

Less than 10 passengers: 7.48 and 5.91, respectively; equivalent air-supply = 23,500 cu. ft. per hour.

Between 10 and 15 passengers: 13.29 and 6.62, respectively; equivalent air-supply = 30,500 cu. ft. per hour.

Between 15 and 20 passengers: 17.57 and 7.38, respectively; equivalent air-supply = 31,200 cu. ft. per hour.

More than 20 passengers: 23.18 and 8.85, respectively; equivalent air-supply = 28,700 cu. ft. per hour.

For cars equipped with exhaust ventilators the general averages of passengers and carbon dioxid for all observations are 14.82 and 6.11, respectively, and the equivalent hourly air-supply 42,100 cubic feet. Averaging all observation in these cars when there were—

Less than 10 passengers: 9.10 and 5.58, respectively; equivalent air-supply = 34,600 cu. ft. per hour.

Between 10 and 15 passengers: 13.51 and 5.95, respectively; equivalent air-supply = 41,600 cu. ft. per hour.

Between 15 and 20 passengers: 17.65 and 6.46, respectively; equivalent air-supply = 43,000 cu. ft. per hour.

More than 20 passengers: 23.24 and 7.24 respectively; equivalent air-supply = 43,000 cu. ft. per hour.

From the figures alone it is seen that the carbon dioxid increases with increase in the number of passengers. The consistency with which the figures hold to the general statement that the excess of carbon dioxid over the normal increases directly as the number of occupants can be read from Chart 5. The dark bars indicate this increase and are placed as nearly as possible at the point on the horizontal representing the average numbers in each of the passenger groups given above. The diagonal lines, representing air-supply, are computed from the general averages of all observations in each class of cars. It will be seen that the carbon dioxid in all of the groups except where the passengers are less than 10 falls very close to these diagonals. When the number is below 10 I cannot look on the results of analyses as of great value because of the unequal distribution. In all the latter part of the work no samples were taken under these conditions; and those that were taken represent chiefly samples taken in single places in the car, and not average samples taken while walking up and down the aisle.

Chart 5 also furnishes a striking confirmation of the correctness of my previous conclusion that the average amount of carbon dioxid in the air surrounding trains is very near to 4 parts in 10,000.

A further method of determining the ventilation of the cars equipped with exhaust ventilators was applied as follows: When trains pass through tunnels the cars receive a considerable amount of engine gas.

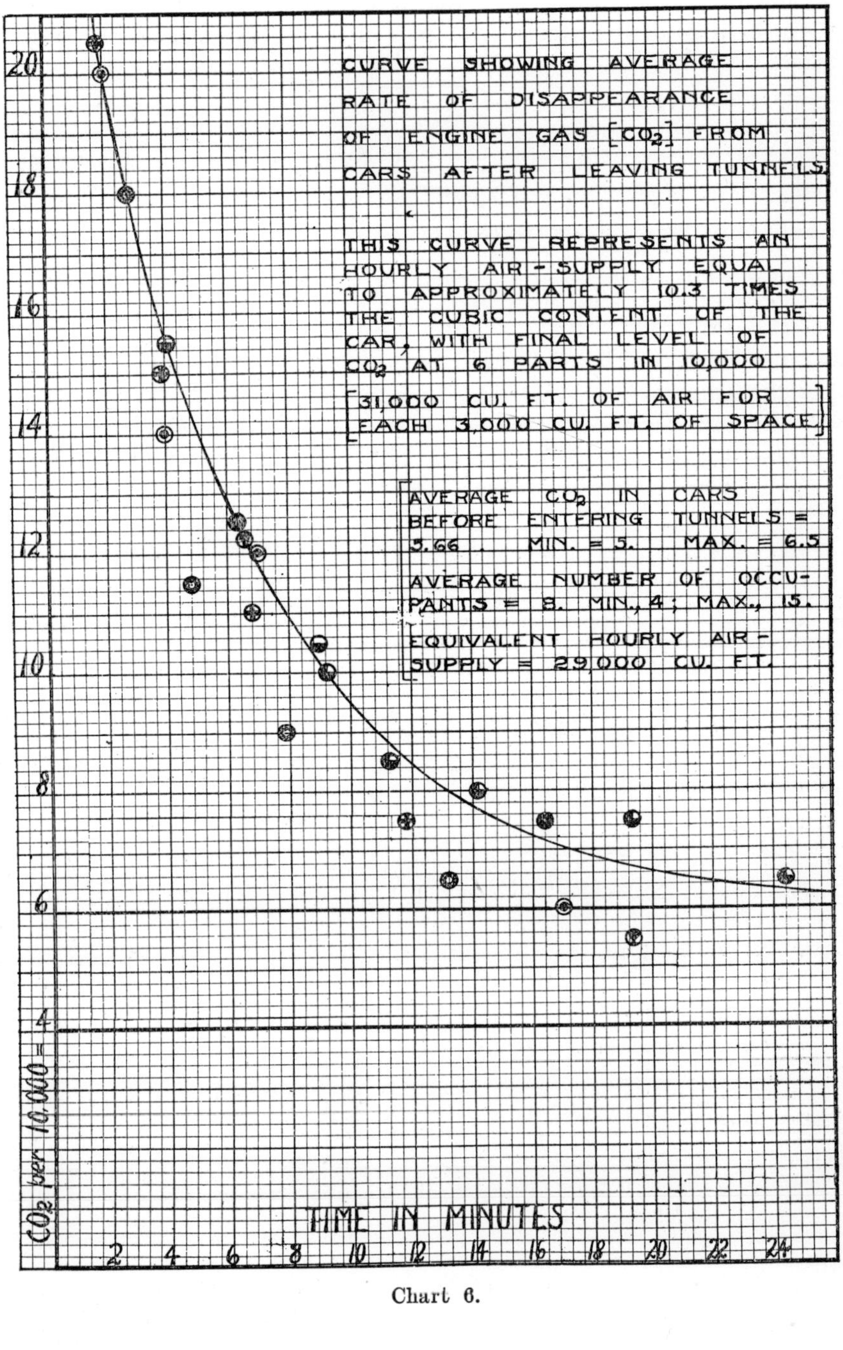

CURVE SHOWING AVERAGE RATE OF DISAPPEARANCE OF ENGINE GAS [$CO_2$] FROM CARS AFTER LEAVING TUNNELS.
THIS CURVE REPRESENTS AN HOURLY AIR-SUPPLY EQUAL TO APPROXIMATELY 10.3 TIMES THE CUBIC CONTENT OF THE CAR, WITH FINAL LEVEL OF $CO_2$ AT 6 PARTS IN 10,000
[31,000 CU. FT. OF AIR FOR EACH 3,000 CU. FT. OF SPACE]
AVERAGE $CO_2$ IN CARS BEFORE ENTERING TUNNELS = 5.66. MIN. = 5. MAX. = 6.5
AVERAGE NUMBER OF OCCUPANTS = 8. MIN., 4; MAX., 15.
EQUIVALENT HOURLY AIR-SUPPLY = 29,000 CU. FT.
$CO_2$ per 10,000
TIME IN MINUTES
20
18
16
14
12
10
8
6
4
2
4
6
8
10
12
14
16
18
20
22
24


Chart 6.

We may compute the fresh air supplied to these cars by observing the rate of disappearance of this gas (carbon dioxid) after leaving the tunnel. In Chart 6 are shown series of determinations under these conditions for six cars. Each form of figure represents the succeeding determinations of a single series.

There is considerable irregularity; but it will be seen from the explanation in the chart itself that the basic conditions also varied, and that the final level to which the carbon dioxid was approaching was different for different cars. The ideal conditions for such tests would be an empty car where the final carbon dioxid would be the same as in the outside air (0.0004). It is nevertheless clear that the disappearance of the gas is rapid and may be fairly represented by the curve drawn. This curve represents a relative decrease of 50 per cent. of the excess in four minutes, and is equivalent to sufficient air each hour to equal 10.3 times the cubic contents of the car. There are 3,000 to 4,000 cubic feet in the body of a sleeping-car; this curve would therefore represent a rate of air-supply from about 31,000 to about 41,000 cubic feet per hour.[15] It will also be noted that the observations made fall rather under than over the curve and represent a more rapid rather than a less rapid disappearance of the carbon dioxid, consequently a greater air-supply than the curve itself, thus confirming in a striking manner the computations of air-supply above recorded.

THE BERTH

When taking samples of air from the berths in the manner already described, it was the rule to take, as near simultaneously as possible, an average sample from the aisle for comparison. Samples from each place were generally repeated at fifteen minute intervals, until twenty or more had been collected in the car. Two lower berths on each side of the car were generally selected, availability determining the choice, and one or two uppers when possible. Table 6 gives the details recorded in foregoing tables, together with the temperatures, the relation between the carbon dioxid of the berths and aisles, and the equivalent air-supply per berth, for 321 analyses from lower berths and 41 from upper berths in cars not having exhaust ventilators.

---

15. The computation of air-supply in the above problem is made from the following equation:

$$A = \frac{C}{t} \log_e \frac{x_1 - N}{x_2 - N}$$

Where $C$ = the contents of the car (cubic feet)
$t$ = time in minutes
$x_1$ and $x_2$ = proportion of carbon dioxid in air of car at any two times, $t$ minutes apart
$N$ = proportion of carbon dioxid in outside air (0.0004), or the level to which it is approaching in an occupied car (assumed to be 0.0006 in this case)
and $A$ = the air-supply (cubic feet per minute).

The air-supply per berth is computed as that necessary to maintain the carbon dioxid at the average level for a small enclosure occupied by one person. All berths included in this table had a single adult occupant.

**TABLE 6.—SIMULTANEOUS DETERMINATIONS OF CARBON DIOXID IN BERTHS AND AISLES OF CARS WITHOUT VENTILATORS: ALL DOORS AND WINDOWS CLOSED**

| Cars. | Date. | Outside Temp. °F. | Series. | Average No. of people in car while taking samples. | $CO_2$ Per 10,000 of Air: Aisle. Average. | Aisle. Extremes. Min. | Aisle. Extremes. Max. | Berths. No. of Determinations for Berths. | Berths. Average. | Berths. Extremes. Min. | Berths. Extremes. Max. | No. Over 12. | No. Over 10. | No. Over 8. | No. Over 6. | Berths < Aisle. | Berths > Aisle. | Hourly Air Supply Per Berth Necessary to Maintain Average $CO_2$. | Proportion of Decks Open. |
|---|---|---|---|---|---|---|---|---|---|---|---|---|---|---|---|---|---|---|---|
| | | | | | | | | | **LOWER BERTHS** | | | | | | | | | | |
| 1 | 2/ 2/07 | 0 | 14 | 6.00 | 6.25 | 5.5 | 7.0 | 6 | 7.83 | 7.5 | 9.0 | 0 | 0 | 1 | 0 | 0 | 6 | 1.566 | 0 |
| 2 | 4/13/07 | 28 | 20 | 15.00 | 7.50 | 7.0 | 8.0 | 8 | 9.38 | 8.0 | 12.0 | 0 | 2 | 6 | 0 | 0 | 8 | 1,115 | ½ |
| 3 | 4/27/07 | 52 | 21 | 6.85 | 5.25 | 4.5 | 5.5 | 14 | 6.71 | 5.5 | 8.5 | 0 | 0 | 1 | 3 | 1 | 10 | 2,210 | All |
| 4 | 10/26/07 | 40 | 24 | 16.00 | 5.25 | 4.5 | 6.0 | 6 | 8.17 | 5.0 | 11.0 | 0 | 1 | 3 | 1 | 0 | 6 | 1,438 | ½ |
| 5 | 12/23/09 | 20 | 45 | 22.00 | 8.87 | 8.5 | 9.5 | 16 | 9.78 | 6.5 | 13.5 | 1 | 6 | 13 | 0 | 5 | 9 | 1,038 | ¼ |
| 6 | 12/25/09 | 24 | 46 | 24.00 | 8.58 | 8.0 | 10.0 | 24 | 9.13 | 6.5 | 11.5 | 0 | 5 | 18 | 0 | 6 | 14 | 1,170 | ¼ |
| 7 | 12/28/09 | 20 | 49 | 20.00 | 6.80 | 6.0 | 7.5 | 19 | 7.58 | 6.5 | 9.5 | 0 | 0 | 3 | 0 | 1 | 14 | 1,676 | ¼ |
| 8 | 12/29/09 | 6 | 50 | 18.00 | 10.00 | 10.0 | 10.0 | 6 | 9.25 | 8.0 | 10.5 | 0 | 3 | 4 | 0 | 3 | 3 | 1,143 | 0 |
| 9 | 2/16/10 | 10 | 62 | 13.00 | 7.38 | 6.0 | 8.0 | 16 | 8.88 | 7.0 | 10.5 | 0 | 2 | 12 | 0 | 2 | 12 | 1,229 | ½ |
| 10 | 3/10/10 | 30 | 82 | 17.00 | 6.63 | 6.0 | 7.0 | 16 | 6.41 | 5.0 | 7.5 | 0 | 0 | 0 | 3 | 8 | 3 | 2,473 | All |
| 11 | 3/10/10 | 30 | 83 | 22.50 | 8.13 | 7.0 | 8.5 | 16 | 9.00 | 7.0 | 12.0 | 0 | 2 | 11 | 0 | 1 | 12 | 1,200 | All |
| 12 | 3/11/10 | 30 | 84 | 17.00 | 6.38 | 6.0 | 6.5 | 16 | 9.13 | 6.0 | 18.0 | 1 | 1 | 5 | 0 | 2 | 9 | 1,170 | ½ |
| 13 | 3/14/10 | 22 | 85 | 12.25 | 8.25 | 8.0 | 9.0 | 16 | 8.88 | 7.5 | 11.0 | 0 | 3 | 11 | 0 | 3 | 10 | 1,229 | ½ |
| 14 | 3/15/10 | 22 | 86 | 17.00 | 8.00 | 6.5 | 9.5 | 16 | 8.09 | 6.5 | 10.0 | 0 | 0 | 6 | 0 | 5 | 8 | 1,467 | ½ |
| 15 | 3/15/10 | 22 | 87 | 19.00 | 7.13 | 6.5 | 8.0 | 16 | 7.97 | 7.0 | 9.5 | 0 | 0 | 4 | 0 | 1 | 12 | 1,511 | ½ |
| 16 | 3/15/10 | 32 | 89 | 17.00 | 7.75 | 6.5 | 9.5 | 16 | 8.78 | 7.0 | 11.0 | 0 | 3 | 12 | 0 | 3 | 12 | 1,255 | ¼ |
| 17 | 3/16/10 | 32 | 90 | 16.00 | 7.00 | 7.0 | 7.0 | 16 | 7.91 | 7.0 | 11.0 | 0 | 1 | 4 | 0 | 0 | 11 | 1,534 | ½ |
| 18 | 3/16/10 | 32 | 92 | 13.00 | 5.63 | 5.5 | 6.0 | 16 | 6.72 | 5.5 | 8.0 | 0 | 0 | 0 | 1 | 0 | 14 | 2,205 | ¼ |
| 19 | 3/17/10 | 36 | 93 | 16.00 | 6.75 | 6.0 | 7.5 | 16 | 7.38 | 6.0 | 10.0 | 0 | 0 | 3 | 0 | 2 | 11 | 1,775 | ¼ |
| 20 | 3/17/10 | 36 | 94 | 13.00 | 8.00 | 7.5 | 8.5 | 16 | 9.38 | 7.0 | 11.5 | 0 | 4 | 12 | 0 | 1 | 12 | 1,115 | ¼ |
| 21 | 3/21/10 | 40 | 95 | 14.00 | 7.70 | 7.5 | 8.5 | 30 | 8.49 | 6.0 | 14.5 | 2 | 4 | 14 | 0 | 11 | 17 | 1,336 | ¼ |
| Totals—Average | | | | 16.41 | 7.32 | 4.5 | 10.0 | 321 | 8.32 | 5.0 | 18.0 | 4 | 37 | 143 | 8 | 55 | 203 | 1,389 | |
| | | | | | | | | | **UPPER BERTHS** | | | | | | | | | | |
| 1 | 10/12/06 | .. | 1A | 24.00 | ...... | ...... | ...... | 1 | 9.50 | 9.5 | 9.5 | 0 | 0 | 1 | 0 | 0 | 0 | 1,091 | All |
| 2 | 10/14/06 | .. | 1B | 24.00 | 13.00 | 13.0 | 13.0 | 1 | 12.00 | 12.0 | 12.0 | 0 | 1 | 1 | 0 | 1 | 0 | 750 | ½ |
| 3 | 11/ 5/06 | 52 | 2 | 20.00 | 11.00 | 11.0 | 11.0 | 1 | 7.00 | 7.0 | 7.0 | 0 | 0 | 0 | 0 | 1 | 0 | 2,000 | All |
| 4 | 11/17/06 | 32 | 6 | 17.00 | ...... | ...... | ...... | 1 | 4.50 | 4.5 | 4.5 | 0 | 0 | 0 | 1 | 0 | 0 | 12,000 | All |
| 5 | 1/19/07 | 50 | 10 | 16.00 | 10.00 | 10.0 | 10.0 | 1 | 10.50 | 10.5 | 10.5 | 0 | 1 | 1 | 0 | 0 | 1 | 923 | 0 |
| 6 | 1/20/07 | 24 | 14 | 20.00 | 10.50 | 10.5 | 10.5 | 2 | 15.75 | 13.0 | 18.5 | 2 | 2 | 2 | 0 | 0 | 2 | 511 | 0 |
| 7 | 12/23/09 | 20 | 45 | 22.00 | 9.00 | 8.5 | 9.5 | 6 | 11.42 | 9.0 | 14.0 | 2 | 3 | 6 | 0 | 0 | 4 | 809 | ¼ |
| 8 | 12/25/09 | 24 | 46 | 24.00 | 8.58 | 8.0 | 10.0 | 12 | 8.66 | 7.5 | 10.5 | 0 | 1 | 8 | 0 | 3 | 5 | 1,287 | ¼ |
| 9 | 12/28/09 | 20 | 49 | 20.00 | 6.80 | 6.0 | 7.5 | 5 | 7.50 | 6.5 | 8.5 | 0 | 0 | 1 | 0 | 0 | 3 | 1,714 | ¼ |
| 10 | 3/15/10 | 22 | 86 | 17.00 | 8.00 | 6.5 | 9.5 | 4 | 8.00 | 7.0 | 9.0 | 0 | 0 | 1 | 0 | 2 | 2 | 1,500 | ½ |
| 11 | 3/17/10 | 36 | 93 | 16.00 | 6.75 | 6.0 | 7.5 | 7 | 8.36 | 7.5 | 9.5 | 0 | 0 | 4 | 0 | 0 | 7 | 1,376 | ¼ |
| Totals—Average.. | | | | 20.51 | 8.37 | 6.0 | 13.0 | 41 | 9.17 | 4.5 | 18.5 | 4 | 8 | 25 | 1 | 7 | 24 | 1,161 | ........ |

*Lower Berths.*—By consulting the figures for the lower berths it will be seen that the average of the carbon dioxid for the berths is higher than for the aisles in all but two instances—Car 8, where only one aisle determination was made, and Car 10, where the average is from four determinations. The average difference is one part of carbon dioxid per 10,000 of air. The highest for the aisle is 10, for the berths 18; lowest, 4.5 and 5, respectively. In 17.1 per cent. of the berths the carbon dioxid was lower than in the aisle at the same time; in 63.2 per cent. it was higher than in the aisle, and in 19.6 per cent. they were equal.

The average carbon dioxid for all berths is 8.32 and the average ventilation is equivalent to 1,389 cubic feet of air per hour per berth. The lowest average carbon dioxid for the berths of any car is 6.41 (Car 10), the highest is 9.78 (Car 5); inversely, the largest equivalent air-supply is 2,473 cubic feet per hour (Car 10), and the smallest is 1,038 cubic feet per hour (Car 5). Of the 321 determinations of carbon dioxid 1.2 per cent. are above 12 per 10,000; 11.2 per cent. are above 10; 44.5 per cent. are above 8; only 2.5 per cent. are below 6, and 55.5 per cent. are 8 or under. Hence, 55.5 per cent. of the determinations indicate that at the moment the samples were taken the air of the berth was diluted with fresh air to an extent that would necessitate ventilation of that berth with 1,500 or more cubic feet of air hourly; it was less than 1,500 feet per hour in 45.5 per cent., less than 1,000 cubic feet in 11.2 per cent., and less than 750 cubic feet in only 1.2 per cent. of the examinations.

*Upper Berths.*—If a considerable number of the upper berths are occupied the car is necessarily well filled. The higher number of passengers would logically account for a higher carbon dioxid in the body of the car (average 20.51 passengers and 8.37 carbon dioxid against 16.41 passengers and 7.32 carbon dioxid in the table for lower berths). With open decks it would be expected to find better ventilation in the upper part of the car. The figures for Car 4 indicate how this may occur. On the other hand, when the decks are closed the opposite may be the case (see Cars 5 and 6).

Of the 41 determinations of carbon dioxid 9.8 per cent. are above 12; 19.5 per cent. above 10; 61 per cent. above 8; 2.4 below 6; and only 39 per cent. are 8 or under. These figures indicate that the ventilation of these berths was equivalent to 1,500 cubic feet or more of air hourly in 39 per cent., less than 1,500 cubic feet hourly in 61 per cent., less than 1,000 cubic feet in 19.5 per cent., and less than 750 cubic feet in 9.8 per cent., while the average ventilation is equivalent to 1,161 cubic feet per berth per hour.

Of 39 times that the comparison can be made the air of the berths contains less carbon dioxid than the aisle at the same time in 17.9 per cent.; it contains more in 61.5 per cent., and they are equal in 20.5 per cent.

*Comparison of Lower and Upper Berths in Same Car.*—I am able to compare the carbon dioxid, consequently the ventilation, of the lower and the upper berths in five cars from this table, namely Series 45, 46, 49, 86 and 93, which correspond to Cars 5, 6, 7, 14 and 19 in the first part of the table and 7, 8, 9, 10 and 11 in the second part. Samples were taken from the lower and upper berths simultaneously. Table 7 will make the comparison clear.

TABLE 7.—COMPARISON OF LOWER AND UPPER BERTHS IN CARS WITHOUT VENTILATORS

| Cars. | Series. | Average $CO_2$ per 10,000. | | Equivalent hourly air supply per berth, cu. ft. | | Proportion of Decks Open. |
|---|---|---|---|---|---|---|
| | | Lowers | Uppers | Lowers | Uppers | |
| 1 | 45 | 9.78 | 11.41 | 1,038 | 809 | ¼ |
| 2 | 46 | 9.13 | 8.66 | 1,170 | 1,287 | ¼ |
| 3 | 49 | 7.58 | 7.50 | 1,676 | 1,714 | ¼ |
| 4 | 86 | 8.09 | 8.00 | 1.467 | 1,500 | ½ |
| 5 | 93 | 7.38 | 8 36 | 1,775 | 1,376 | ¼ |
| Totals—Av.... | | 8 43 | 8.85 | 1,354 | 1,237 | |

In two cars (1 and 5) there is less carbon dioxid in the air of the lower berths than in the uppers; consequently, the ventilation of these lowers is better than of the uppers. In the remaining three cars (2, 3 and 4) the carbon dioxid is lower in the uppers; consequently, the ventilation of the upper berths is more efficient than for the lower berths in the same cars. There was a total of 91 determinations for the lower berths of these cars, against 34 for the upper berths. The average of these totals gives slightly less carbon dioxid for the lowers than for the uppers; consequently, there was a slightly better average ventilation of the lowers under the conditions represented than of the uppers.

Simultaneous determinations were made for the lower and upper berth of the same section thirty-four times in these cars. The upper had more carbon dioxid than the lower 20 times (58.8 per cent.) less 8 times (23.5 per cent.), and they were equal 6 times (17.7 per cent.). The relative ventilation is, of course, inversely as the carbon dioxid.

Table 8 records the details of 690 carbon dioxid determinations of the air of lower berths and 53 of the air of upper berths in cars equipped with exhaust ventilators. The tabulation and computation is similar to that of Table 6.

*Lower Berths.*—In all but three of the forty-two cars (17, 31 and 37) the average carbon dioxid of the lower berths is higher than the average for the aisle. The average difference for all observations is 0.63 parts per 10,000 of air. The highest for the aisle is 10, the lowest 4.5; for the berths the highest is 13.5 and the lowest 4.5. In 20.4 per cent. of the berths the carbon dioxid is lower than the aisle at the same time; in 63.8 per cent. it is higher than the aisle, and in 15.8 per cent. they are equal.

The average carbon dioxid per berth is 6.96 per 10,000; the average ventilation is equivalent to 2,027 cubic feet per hour. The lowest average carbon dioxid for the berths of any car is 5.38 (Car 37), the highest is

TABLE 8.—SIMULTANEOUS DETERMINATIONS OF CARBON DIOXID IN BERTHS AND AISLES OF CARS EQUIPPED WITH EXHAUST VENTILATORS AND HAVING ALL DOORS AND WINDOWS CLOSED

| Cars. | Date. | Outside Temp. °F. | Series. | Average No. of People in the Car While Taking Samples. | $CO_2$ Per 10,000 of Air. Aisle. Average. | Aisle. Extremes. Min. | Aisle. Extremes. Max. | Berths. No. of Determinations for Berths. | Berths. Average. | Berths. Extremes. Min. | Berths. Extremes. Max. | No. Over 12. | No. Over 10. | No. Over 8. | No. Under 6. | Berths < Aisle. | Berths > Aisle. | Hourly Air Supply Per Berth Necessary to Maintain Average $CO_2$. |
|---|---|---|---|---|---|---|---|---|---|---|---|---|---|---|---|---|---|---|
| | | | | | | | | LOWER BERTHS | | | | | | | | | | |
| 1 | 1/23/07 | 24 | 12 | 11.00 | 6.25 | 5.0 | 7.5 | 4 | 8.00 | 7.0 | 10.0 | 0 | 0 | 1 | 0 | 2 | 2 | 1,500 |
| 2 | 1/24/07 | 26 | 13 | 12.00 | 6.25 | 6.0 | 6.5 | 6 | 6.75 | 5.5 | 8.0 | 0 | 0 | 0 | 1 | 2 | 4 | 2,183 |
| 3 | 4/ 5/07 | 36 | 19 | 8.00 | 5.66 | 5.5 | 6.0 | 18 | 7.97 | 6.0 | 13.5 | 1 | 1 | 9 | 0 | 0 | 18 | 1,511 |
| 4 | 1/ 5/08 | 30 | 28 | 13.00 | 7.33 | 6.0 | 10.0 | 9 | 8.00 | 7.0 | 10.0 | 0 | 0 | 3 | 0 | 2 | 4 | 1,500 |
| 5 | 2/ 6/09 | 34 | 31 | 14.00 | 6.88 | 6.0 | 8.0 | 8 | 7.67 | 5.5 | 9.0 | 0 | 0 | 4 | 0 | 1 | 6 | 1,623 |
| 6 | 2/13/09 | 36 | 33 | 14.00 | 6.83 | 5 5 | 8.5 | 12 | 8.00 | 6.0 | 11.0 | 0 | 1 | 5 | 0 | 3 | 8 | 1,500 |
| 7 | 11/27/09 | 55 | 35 | 9.40 | 5.80 | 5.5 | 6.5 | 20 | 6.73 | 4.5 | 10.0 | 0 | 0 | 3 | 5 | 5 | 15 | 2,198 |
| 8 | 12/15/09 | 10 | 36 | 17.25 | 6.25 | 5.5 | 7.5 | 12 | 6.25 | 4.5 | 10.5 | 0 | 1 | 2 | 7 | 8 | 4 | 2,666 |
| 9 | 12/16/09 | 20 | 37 | 16.00 | 5.50 | 5.0 | 6.5 | 9 | 7.94 | 5.0 | 11.0 | 0 | 2 | 5 | 1 | 0 | 8 | 1,523 |
| 10 | 12/20/09 | 18 | 41 | 17.00 | 4.90 | 4.5 | 5.5 | 20 | 5.98 | 5.0 | 9.0 | 0 | 0 | 1 | 11 | 0 | 16 | 3,030 |
| 11 | 12/26/09 | 20 | 48 | 18.00 | 6.25 | 6.0 | 6.5 | 4 | 6.88 | 6.0 | 8.5 | 0 | 0 | 1 | 0 | 0 | 2 | 2,083 |
| 12 | 1/ 3/10 | 26 | 54 | 17.00 | 6.33 | 5.5 | 7.0 | 36 | 6.58 | 5.0 | 8.5 | 0 | 0 | 5 | 3 | 12 | 20 | 2,325 |
| 13 | 1/ 6/10 | 30 | 56 | 23.00 | 6.60 | 5.5 | 8.0 | 20 | 7.55 | 5.5 | 11.5 | 0 | 1 | 6 | 1 | 5 | 14 | 1,690 |
| 14 | 1/10/10 | 18 | 59 | 18.00 | 7.60 | 7.0 | 8.0 | 20 | 8.65 | 7.5 | 10.0 | 0 | 0 | 16 | 0 | 0 | 16 | 1,290 |
| 15 | 1/20/10 | 30 | 60 | 16.00 | 5.80 | 5.0 | 6.0 | 20 | 6.40 | 5.0 | 8.0 | 0 | 0 | 0 | 6 | 3 | 14 | 2,500 |
| 16 | 1/23/10 | 28 | 61 | 18.00 | 6.20 | 5.5 | 7.5 | 20 | 6.90 | 5.0 | 10.0 | 0 | 0 | 3 | 4 | 6 | 11 | 2,069 |
| 17 | 2/17/10 | -2 | 63 | 23.00 | 8.50 | 7.5 | 10.0 | 16 | 8.19 | 6.0 | 12.0 | 0 | 2 | 6 | 0 | 10 | 5 | 1,432 |
| 18 | 2/17/10 | -2 | 64 | 18.00 | 6.25 | 5.5 | 7.0 | 16 | 6.84 | 6.0 | 8.0 | 0 | 0 | 0 | 0 | 4 | 10 | 2,113 |
| 19 | 2/17/10 | 10 | 65 | 14.00 | 5.25 | 5.0 | 6.0 | 16 | 5.81 | 5.0 | 7.0 | 0 | 0 | 0 | 8 | 1 | 9 | 3,315 |
| 20 | 2/20/10 | 30 | 66 | 13.00 | 5.25 | 5.0 | 6.0 | 16 | 5.97 | 4.5 | 10.0 | 0 | 0 | 2 | 13 | 3 | 7 | 3,046 |
| 21 | 2/20/10 | 30 | 67 | 20.00 | 6.13 | 5.5 | 6.5 | 16 | 7.72 | 5.5 | 8.5 | 0 | 0 | 4 | 1 | 0 | 14 | 1,613 |
| 22 | 2/21/10 | 18 | 68 | 16.00 | 6.38 | 6.0 | 7.0 | 16 | 7.69 | 6.5 | 9.0 | 0 | 0 | 6 | 0 | 1 | 13 | 1,623 |
| 23 | 2/21/10 | 18 | 69 | 15.00 | 6.25 | 5.5 | 7.0 | 16 | 6.84 | 5.0 | 9.0 | 0 | 0 | 2 | 4 | 5 | 10 | 2,113 |
| 24 | 2/23/10 | 0 | 70 | 17.00 | 8.88 | 8.0 | 10.0 | 16 | 9.34 | 7.0 | 12.0 | 0 | 5 | 13 | 0 | 4 | 9 | 1,123 |
| 25 | 2/23/10 | 0 | 71 | 14.00 | 7.50 | 6.0 | 8.0 | 16 | 8.19 | 6.5 | 10.0 | 0 | 0 | 8 | 0 | 3 | 9 | 1,432 |
| 26 | 2/24/10 | 18 | 72 | 13.00 | 6.25 | 6.0 | 6.5 | 16 | 7.50 | 6.0 | 8.5 | 0 | 0 | 2 | 0 | 0 | 14 | 1,714 |
| 27 | 2/27/10 | 26 | 73 | 15.00 | 7.63 | 6.5 | 9.0 | 16 | 9.16 | 7.5 | 12.0 | 0 | 4 | 10 | 0 | 0 | 15 | 1,163 |
| 28 | 2/27/10 | 26 | 74 | 16.00 | 7.50 | 6.5 | 9.0 | 16 | 8.91 | 7.0 | 11.0 | 0 | 3 | 11 | 0 | 0 | 14 | 1,222 |
| 29 | 3/ 1/10 | 30 | 75 | 25.00 | 6.75 | 5.5 | 8.0 | 4 | 7.38 | 6.0 | 8.5 | 0 | 0 | 1 | 0 | 0 | 4 | 1,775 |
| 30 | 3/ 2/10 | 52 | 76 | 22.00 | 7.25 | 5.0 | 9.5 | 16 | 7.47 | 5.5 | 10.5 | 0 | 1 | 4 | 1 | 7 | 8 | 1,749 |
| 31 | 3/ 4/10 | 50 | 77 | 14.00 | 6.13 | 5.5 | 7.0 | 16 | 6.09 | 5.0 | 8.5 | 0 | 0 | 1 | 6 | 6 | 5 | 2,871 |
| 32 | 3/ 6/10 | 40 | 78 | 15.00 | 5.00 | 5.0 | 5.0 | 16 | 6.19 | 5.0 | 7.5 | 0 | 0 | 0 | 6 | 0 | 11 | 2,739 |
| 33 | 3/ 6/10 | 40 | 79 | 14.00 | 5.38 | 5.0 | 5.5 | 16 | 6.47 | 5.0 | 8.0 | 0 | 0 | 0 | 1 | 1 | 15 | 2,429 |
| 34 | 3/ 7/10 | 28 | 80 | 18.00 | 5.38 | 5.0 | 6.5 | 16 | 6.69 | 5.0 | 9.5 | 0 | 0 | 2 | 4 | 1 | 14 | 2,230 |
| 35 | 3/ 8/10 | 34 | 81 | 14.00 | 5.63 | 5.0 | 6.5 | 16 | 6.72 | 4.5 | 10.5 | 0 | 1 | 3 | 6 | 3 | 10 | 2,205 |
| 36 | 3/15/10 | 32 | 88 | 17.00 | 5.50 | 5.0 | 6.5 | 16 | 6.64 | 5.0 | 9.5 | 0 | 0 | 4 | 7 | 2 | 9 | 2,273 |
| 37 | 3/16/10 | 32 | 91 | 14.00 | 5.63 | 5.0 | 6.5 | 16 | 5.38 | 4.5 | 8.0 | 0 | 0 | 0 | 12 | 9 | 4 | 4,348 |
| 38 | 3/24/10 | 60 | 96 | 14.00 | 5.33 | 4.5 | 6.5 | 48 | 5.51 | 4.5 | 8.0 | 0 | 0 | 0 | 36 | 19 | 17 | 3,973 |
| 39 | 3/30/10 | 66 | 98 | 14.00 | 5.25 | 5.0 | 6.0 | 16 | 6.50 | 4.5 | 10.0 | 0 | 0 | 3 | 5 | 4 | 12 | 2,400 |
| 40 | 3/30/10 | 50 | 99 | 19.00 | 5.40 | 4.5 | 7.0 | 40 | 6.36 | 5.0 | 10.0 | 0 | 0 | 3 | 11 | 3 | 28 | 2,541 |
| 41 | 4/ 5/10 | 60 | 103 | 13.00 | 5.75 | 5.0 | 6.5 | 16 | 6.25 | 4.5 | 10.5 | 0 | 1 | 1 | 6 | 4 | 8 | 2,667 |
| 42 | 4/ 6/10 | 46 | 104 | 17.00 | 5.75 | 5.5 | 6.0 | 8 | 6.13 | 5.0 | 7.5 | 0 | 0 | 0 | 2 | 2 | 4 | 2,812 |
| Totals—Average....... | | | | 15.72 | 6.33 | 4.5 | 10.0 | 690 | 6.96 | 4.5 | 13.5 | 1 | 23 | 150 | 169 | 141 | 440 | 2,027 |
| | | | | | | | | UPPER BERTHS | | | | | | | | | | |
| 1 | 1/10/10 | 18 | 59 | 18.00 | 7.60 | 7.0 | 8.0 | 5 | 8.70 | 8.0 | 9.5 | 0 | 0 | 4 | 0 | 0 | 5 | 1,277 |
| 2 | 3/ 2/10 | 52 | 76 | 22.00 | 7.25 | 5.0 | 9.5 | 4 | 9.63 | 8.5 | 10.5 | 0 | 1 | 4 | 0 | 0 | 4 | 1,065 |
| 3 | 3/24/10 | 60 | 96 | 14.00 | 5.33 | 4.5 | 6.5 | 24 | 5.75 | 4.5 | 7.5 | 0 | 0 | 0 | 15 | 3 | 12 | 3,428 |
| 4 | 3/30/10 | 50 | 99 | 19.00 | 5.40 | 4.5 | 7.0 | 16 | 6.62 | 5.0 | 9.0 | 0 | 0 | 1 | 2 | 0 | 16 | 2,290 |
| 5 | 4/ 6/10 | 46 | 104 | 17.00 | 5.75 | 5.5 | 6.0 | 4 | 7.25 | 6.5 | 8.0 | 0 | 0 | 0 | 0 | 0 | 4 | 1,846 |
| Totals—Average....... | | | | 16.72 | 5.95 | 4.5 | 9.5 | 53 | 6.70 | 4.5 | 10.5 | 0 | 1 | 9 | 17 | 3 | 41 | 2,222 |
| Lowers in these same cars: Totals—Average..... | | | | | | | | 132 | 6.51 | 4.5 | 10.5 | 0 | 1 | 23 | 50 | 31 | 73 | 2,391 |

9.34 (Car 24); the largest equivalent air-supply is 4,348 cubic feet per hour (Car 37), and the smallest 1,123 cubic feet per hour (Car 24). Of the 690 determinations of carbon dioxid only one, 0.14 per cent. is above 12 parts per 10,000; 3.3 per cent. are above 10; 21.7 per cent. are above 8; 24.5 per cent. are below 6, and 78.3 per cent. are 8 or under. Consequently the ventilation is equivalent to more than 3,000 cubic feet of air per berth hourly in 24.5 per cent. of the berths examined; it is 1,500 or more in 78.3 per cent., and less than 1,500 cubic feet in 21.7 per cent.; it is less than 1,000 cubic feet per hour in 3.3 per cent. and less than 750 cubic feet but once in 690 determinations. In this case 631 cubic feet is indicated.

*Upper Berths.*—Of the 53 determinations of carbon dioxid the highest is 10.5, the lowest 4.5. There is but one over 10 (2 per cent.); 17 per cent. are over 8; 32 per cent. are below 6, and 83 per cent. are 8 or under. The ventilation is therefore equivalent to more than 3,000 cubic feet per hour in 32 per cent.; it is 1,500 cubic feet or more in 83 per cent.; 1,000 cubic feet or more in 98 per cent., and less than 1,000 in 2 per cent., while the average ventilation is equivalent to 2,222 cubic feet per hour. The berth is higher than the aisle at the same time in 94.3 per cent. and lower in 5.7 per cent.

*Lower Berths and Upper Berths in Same Car.*—I am able to compare the lower berths with the upper berths in five cars, as shown in Table 9. Samples were taken from the lower and the upper berths simultaneously.

TABLE 9.—COMPARISON OF LOWER AND UPPER BERTHS IN CARS EQUIPPED WITH EXHAUST VENTILATORS

| Cars. | Series. | Average $CO_2$ per 10,000. | | Equivalent hourly air supply per berth, cubic feet. | |
|---|---|---|---|---|---|
| | | Lowers. | Uppers. | Lowers. | Uppers. |
| 1 | 59 | 8.65 | 8.70 | 1,290 | 1,277 |
| 2 | 76 | 7.47 | 9.63 | 1,749 | 1,065 |
| 3 | 96 | 5.51 | 5.75 | 3,937 | 3,428 |
| 4 | 99 | 6.36 | 6.62 | 2,541 | 2,290 |
| 5 | 104 | 6.13 | 7.25 | 2,812 | 1,846 |
| Totals—Average.......... | | 6.51 | 6.70 | 2,391 | 2,222 |

In all of these cars there is a lower average carbon dioxid in the air of the lower berths than in the air of the upper berths; the lower berths in these cars are therefore better ventilated than the upper berths. The averages of the totals (132 lower and 53 upper berths) and the corresponding ventilation equivalent show that this difference is very small.

Simultaneous observations of the lower and upper in the same section were made forty times. The upper had more carbon dioxid than the lower 22 times (55 per cent.), less 9 times (22.5 per cent.), and they were equal 9 times (22.5 per cent.). The greatest difference was 2 parts carbon dioxid per 10,000. It seems clear that the average ventilation of the lower berth in this type of car is on the average slightly better than the upper, but the difference is so small as to be of no practical consequence.

In a general way it is found that the average of the berths and of the aisle follow each other consistently. Both vary from time to time in a way that can be only theoretically explained, and an individual berth may show great irregularity. Chart 7 shows the variations through two of the longer series (Series 96 and 99, Cars 38 and 40 for lowers and 1 and 2 for uppers in Table 8), and will serve to render clear the manner of making up the details of the tables. The determinations made at 12:45 a. m. in the car Oswego were from samples collected just after a five-minute stop. The effect of such a stop is almost invariably shown by a similar rise of the carbon dioxid. The averages for the series represented in left part of Chart 7 are among the lowest observed.

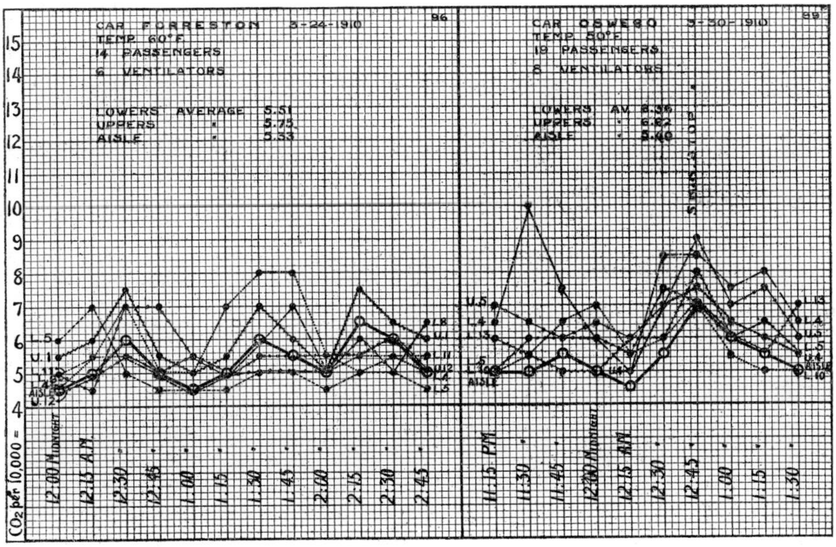


Chart 7.

In a few instances samples were taken simultaneously in two cars of the same train, both being equipped with exhaust ventilators. Such a condition is represented in Chart 8 (Series 78 and 79, Cars 32 and 33 of Table 8), where it is seen that the average carbon dioxid for both berths and aisles of the two cars show only a fractional difference.

If we bring into comparison the conditions of the two classes of cars, those without and those with the exhaust ventilators, a decided advantage is seen to lie with the latter in the study of berth conditions, as was before noted in the study of air from the car body. This comparison is graphically represented for the general averages of the lower berths and the aisles in Chart 9, and an equivalent for the upper berths of all the cars represented in Tables 6 and 8 is computed from the ratios between lower and upper berths established from the comparisons made in Tables 7 and 9.

It was possible in only two instances to make direct observations of the comparative ventilation in these two classes of cars under identical conditions by taking samples of the air simultaneously from the two on the same train. The results are shown in Chart 10.

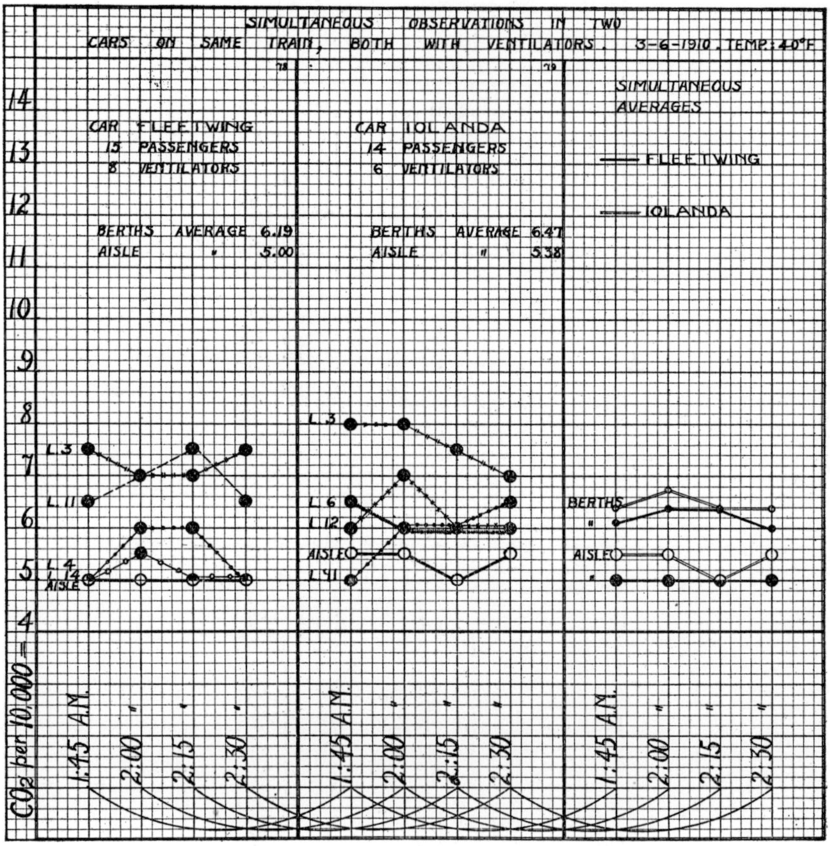


Chart 8.

On the left are represented Series 89 (Car 16, Table 6) and 88 (Car 36, Table 8); on the right are represented Series 92 (Car 18, Table 6) and 91 (Car 37, Table 8). It will be noticed that the averages lie a considerable distance apart and represent a greater air-supply to the cars with exhaust ventilators in both instances.

All of the observations recorded above refer to berths which were occupied by one person only. It sometimes happens that two people occupy a single berth. Determinations of the carbon dioxid have been made in thirty-five such instances in seven cars equipped with exhaust ventilators. The average carbon dioxid of these berths is 9.91 per 10,000.

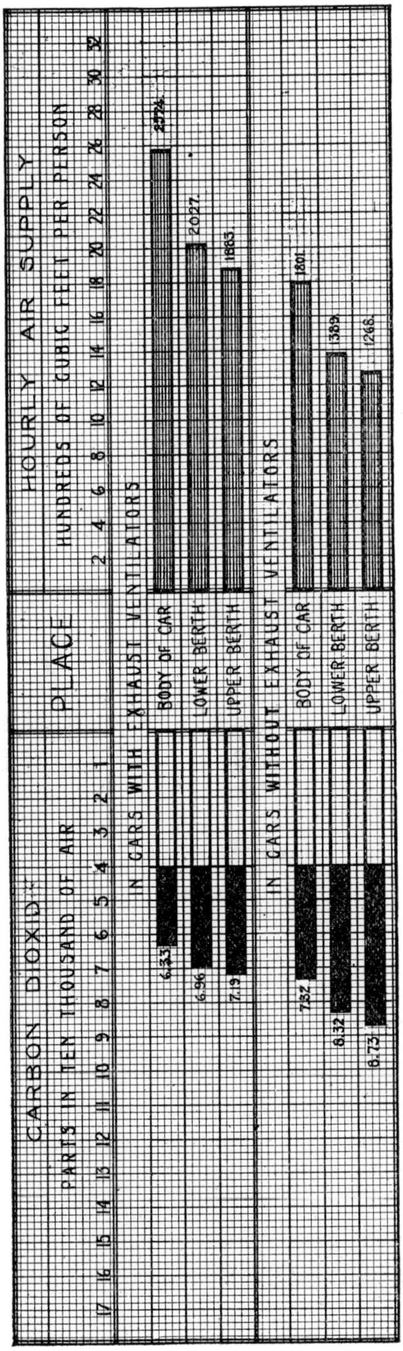
CARBON DIOXID
PARTS IN TEN THOUSAND OF AIR
17 16 15 14 13 12 11 10 9 8 7 6 5 4 3 2 1
PLACE
HOURLY AIR SUPPLY
HUNDREDS OF CUBIC FEET PER PERSON
2 4 6 8 10 12 14 16 18 20 22 24 26 28 30 32
IN CARS WITH EXHAUST VENTILATORS
BODY OF CAR
LOWER BERTH
UPPER BERTH
6.33
6.96
7.19
2574
2027
1863
IN CARS WITHOUT EXHAUST VENTILATORS
BODY OF CAR
LOWER BERTH
UPPER BERTH
7.32
8.32
8.73
1801
1389
1268

Chart 9.

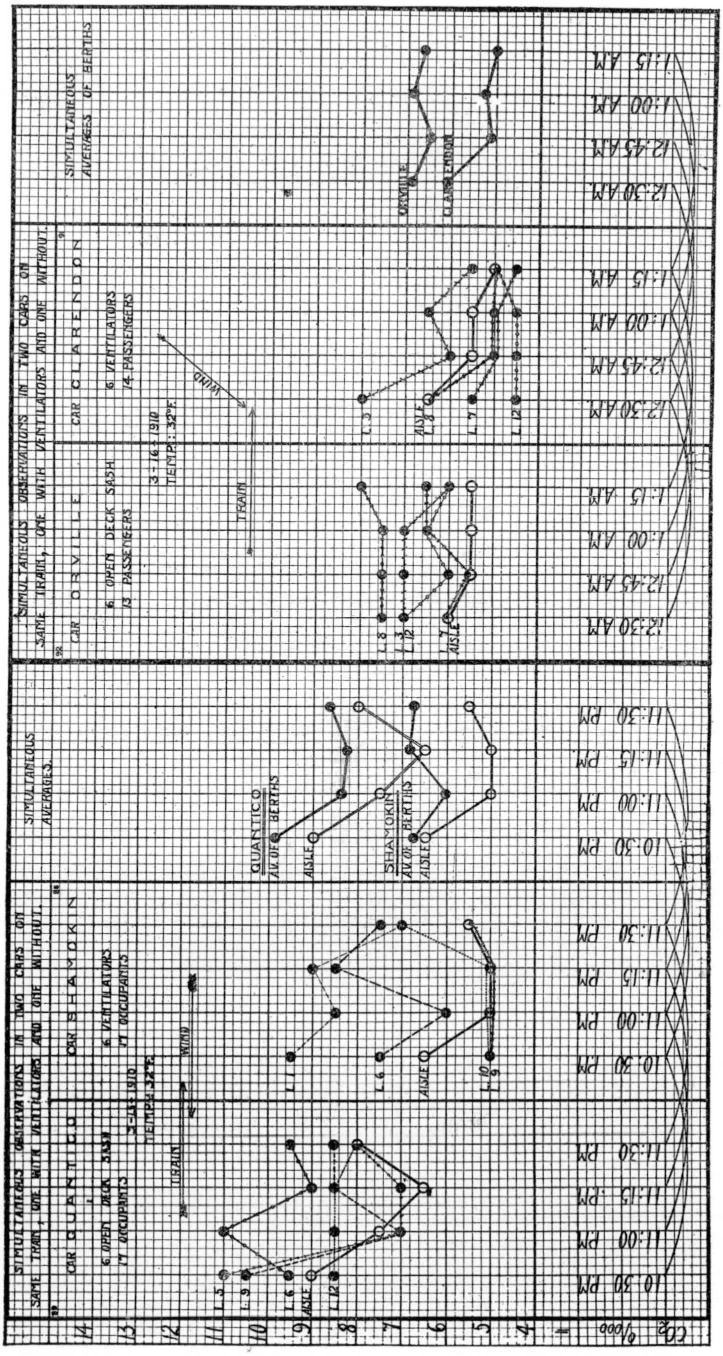
SIMULTANEOUS OBSERVATIONS IN TWO CARS ON SAME TRAIN, ONE WITH VENTILATORS AND ONE WITHOUT.
CAR QUANTICO
6 OPEN DECK SASH
17 OCCUPANTS
3-15-1910
TEMP. 32°F.
TRAIN
WIND
CAR SHAMOKIN
6 VENTILATORS
17 OCCUPANTS
SIMULTANEOUS AVERAGES.
QUANTICO
AV. OF BERTHS
AISLE
SHAMOKIN
AV. OF BERTHS
AISLE
SIMULTANEOUS OBSERVATIONS IN TWO CARS ON SAME TRAIN, ONE WITH VENTILATORS AND ONE WITHOUT.
CAR ORVILLE
6 OPEN DECK SASH
13 PASSENGERS
3-16-1910
TEMP.: 32°F.
TRAIN
WIND
CAR CLARENDON
6 VENTILATORS
14 PASSENGERS
SIMULTANEOUS AVERAGES OF BERTHS
ORVILLE
CLARENDON
CO2 %/000

Chart 10.

The maximum is 14, the minimum 6.5. Since the excess of carbon dioxid over the normal increases directly as the number of occupants it should be twice as great for two persons as for one, the air-supply remaining the same. The excess is here 5.91; half of it is 2.96; adding this

TABLE 10.—COMPARISON OF BERTHS WITH ONE OCCUPANT AND BERTHS WITH TWO OCCUPANTS

| Cars. | Series. | Berths having two occupants. | | Berths having one occupant. | |
|---|---|---|---|---|---|
| | | $CO_2$ per 10,000. | Equivalent Hourly Air-Supply per Berth, Cubic Feet. | $CO_2$ per 10,000. | Equivalent Hourly Air-Supply per Berth, Cubic Feet. |
| 1 | 48 | 11.25—(7.63)* | 1,653 | 6.88 | 2,083 |
| 2 | 29 | 10.50—(7.25) | 1,846 | 9.08 | 1,181 |
| 3 | 54 | 9.50—(6.75) | 2,183 | 6.58 | 2,325 |
| 4 | 59 | 12.10—(8.05) | 1,481 | 8.65 | 1,290 |
| 5 | 64 | 8.50—(6.25) | 2,667 | 6.84 | 2,113 |
| 6 | 73 | 11.75—(7.88) | 1,546 | 9.16 | 1,163 |
| 7 | 75 | 8.75—(6.38) | 2,521 | 7.38 | 1,775 |
| Totals—Average. | | 9.91—(6.96) | 2,027 | 7.36 | 1,785 |

* In parenthesis are given the figures representing one-half of the excess carbon dioxid plus 4. This would represent the carbon dioxid which should be found had the berth had one occupant and had the air-supply been the same. It is directly comparable with the figures in the carbon dioxid column for berths having one occupant.

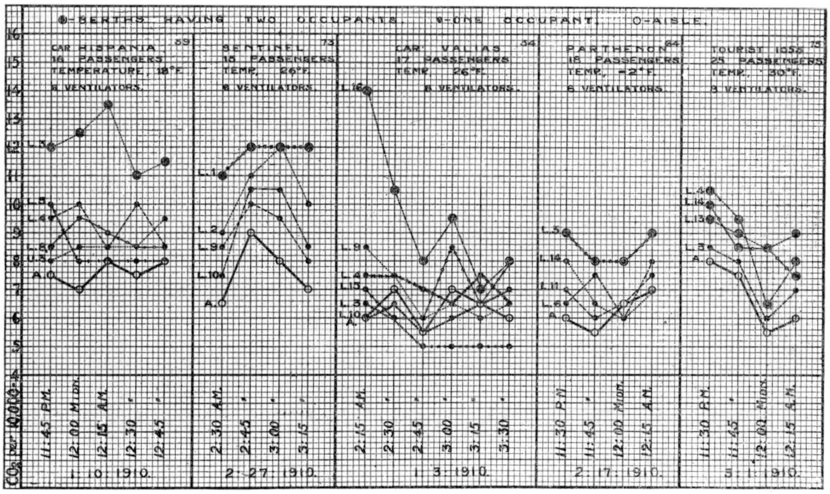


Chart 11.

half to the normal, 4, gives 6.96 which should have been the carbon dioxid in these berths with the same ventilation and only one occupant. This is, by a coincidence, just equal to the observed general average for all lower berths occupied by one person in the same class of cars; and the effective ventilation of the berths is therefore at the same rate, namely, equivalent to 2,027 cubic feet of air per hour. This equality does not hold good when we compare berths with one and with two occupants in the same cars only; but the discrepancies are not greater than might be found by comparing any two berths of the same car. Table 10 makes the comparison in detail; and the greater number of observations made when berths were occupied by two persons are shown in Chart 11.

### THE BERTH CURTAIN AND DIFFUSION

Popular opinion ascribes better ventilation to the upper than to the lower berth in a sleeping-car. The reason generally given in support of this opinion is that the berth curtain entirely covers the lower and only partly the upper. It is supposed that the curtain hinders the progress of air-currents. The findings already given show that the air contamination is not very different on the two sides of the curtain, but it may be contended that this is a matter of equalization by the diffusion of gases, and that the circulation of fresh air is chiefly through the body of the car. In order to gain some information concerning the conditions that would obtain if the closed berth had to lose its carbon dioxid by diffusion through the curtain, a series of experiments was conducted with the purpose of determining the rate of diffusion under similar conditions.

A box made of one-inch lumber, containing 6 cubic feet of space and having one open side of 4.15 square feet, was sealed by stripping all crevices. A standard berth curtain was stretched closely over the open side, which was vertically placed, thus representing a miniature berth. Carbon dioxid artificially produced was then introduced into this box, mixed by blowing in air, and time allowed for equal distribution to take place. The box was set in a closed room where every attempt was made to avoid draughts. Samples of the air from the box were then analyzed at five-minute intervals until the carbon dioxid had nearly all disappeared. As a matter of physics this is no doubt very crude experimentation; but the results have enough uniformity to indicate that a general law applies. In Chart 12 are shown the results of twelve series of analyses, the same symbol representing successive determinations in a single series; and the curve is constructed to the average rate of decrease.

Expressed according to the generally accepted theory of gas diffusion, the progress of carbon dioxid and air into each other through such a partition and under the conditions given is at the average velocity of 0.125 of a lineal foot per minute.[16] The volume of carbon dioxid which

16. The computation of this value is completed from the equation:

$$R = \frac{C}{St} \log \frac{x_1 - N}{x_2 - N}$$

Where $C$ = the contents of the box in cubic feet,
$S$ = the surface of the curtain in square feet,
$t$ = time in minutes,
$x_1$ and $x_2$ = the proportion of carbon dioxid in the box at any two successive periods $t$ minutes apart,
$N$ = the proportion of carbon dioxid in the outside air (air of the room),
and $R$ = the rate per minute (coefficient of diffusion, foot-minutes).

will so diffuse during any minute through each square foot of curtain surface is represented by the product of this rate times the concentration of the carbon dioxid in the box at the beginning of that minute over and above that in the air outside. In order readily to conceive an equivalent

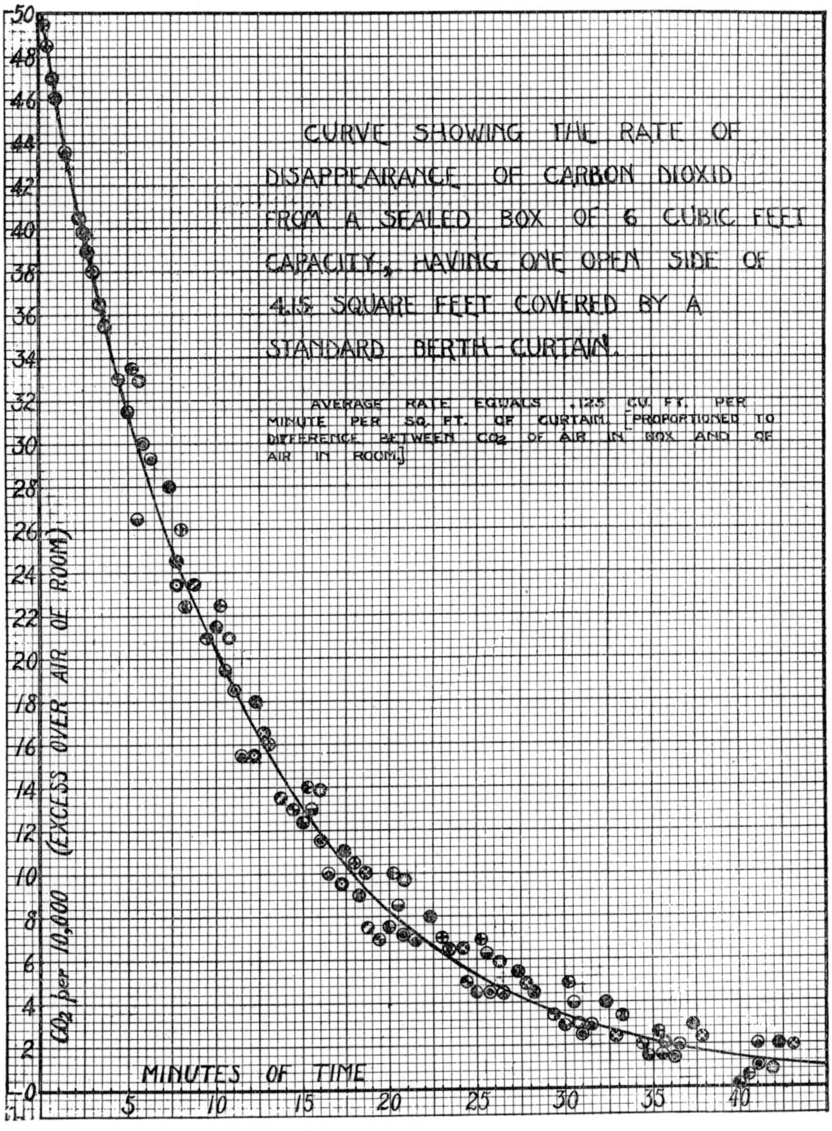


Chart 12.

of what takes place it may be supposed that through each square foot of curtain surface essentially 0.125 cubic feet of the gas mixture in the box passes out during each minute, and that an equal volume of the outside air enters to take its place; but the motion is one of molecules and not of movement in masses. This is about one-half the rate given for diffusion between air and carbon dioxid when no partition intervenes.[17]

By using boxes having different relations between the open surface and the cubic contents practically the same result for the value of $R$ was obtained. The twelve series represented by the chart represent points for taking the samples lying 4, 8, 12 and 16 inches back of the curtain, and show no essential differences. Assuming that the above established rate of interchange is essentially correct for the conditions represented by a berth, we may compute to what height the carbon dioxid of a berth would rise provided there were no air supplied and the carbon dioxid produced (0.6 cubic foot hourly or 0.01 per minute by one occupant) had to find its way out by diffusion through the curtain. The cubic contents of the lower berth are approximately 62 cubic feet and the curtain covering it approximately 18.8 square feet. Without going into the computations, which are long, these figures and the value $R = 0.125$ indicate that the carbon dioxid in the air of a berth with one occupant would be about 8 per 10,000 above that in the air of the aisle after five minutes' occupancy, 20 at the end of fifteen minutes, 30 at the end of half an hour, 39 at the end of an hour, and would reach and maintain a final difference of 42.5. This proportion would be maintained by the entrance into the berth of about 135 cubic feet of air per hour. From which it appears that diffusion of this sort has practically nothing to do with the problem in hand and that the berth must receive essentially the amount of ventilation previously determined. In other words, the berth does not act as a closed compartment, but is essentially a part of the general space of the car body, and is subject to the effects of air-supply and air-currents through and around the curtain very much as it would be were the curtain entirely absent.

### THE SMOKING-ROOM

Thirteen observations were made in crowded smoking-rooms of cars without ventilators. The occupants were from 4 to 7, the carbon dioxid from 10.5 to 20.5 per 10,000. The average carbon dioxid, 14.88, with the average occupants, 5.85, would be maintained by an air-supply of 3,225 cubic feet per hour for the room.

Eleven observations in smoking-rooms of cars equipped with exhaust ventilators had 4 to 8 occupants, and carbon dioxid from 7 to 16.5 per 10,000. The averages were 6.1 occupants and 11.41 carbon dioxid; the equivalent air-supply would be 4,940 cubic feet.

No account is taken in this connection of the carbon dioxid produced by the burning of tobacco and matches.

17. Winkelmann: Handbuch der Physik, J. A. Barth, Leipsic, 1908, Ed. 2, i, 1420.

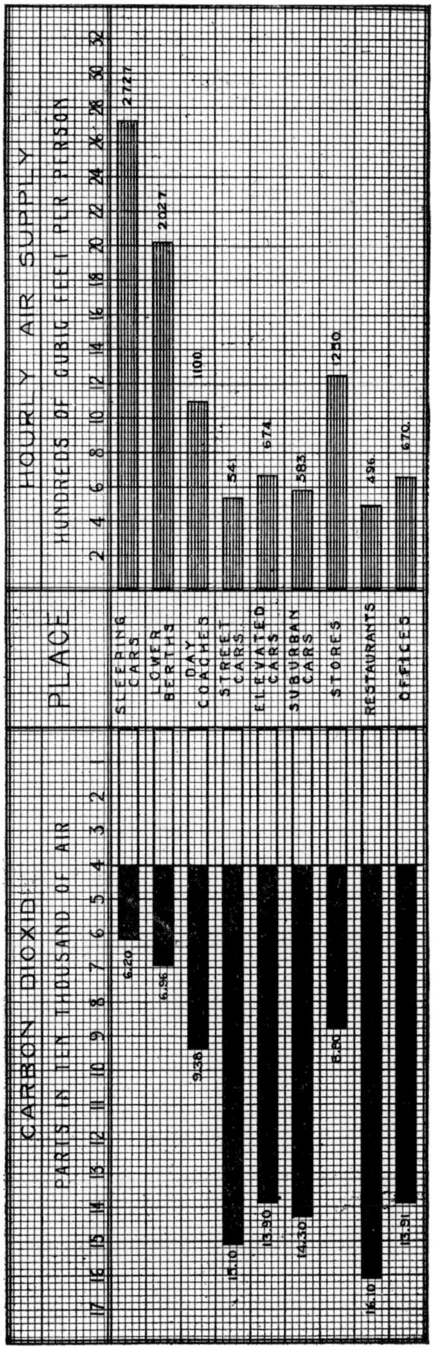
CARBON DIOXID
PARTS IN TEN THOUSAND OF AIR
PLACE
HOURLY AIR SUPPLY
HUNDREDS OF CUBIC FEET PER PERSON
SLEEPING CARS
LOWER BERTHS
DAY COACHES
STREET CARS
ELEVATED CARS
SUBURBAN CARS
STORES
RESTAURANTS
OFFICES
6.20
6.96
9.38
15.10
13.90
14.30
8.80
16.10
13.91
2727
2027
1100
541
674
583
1250
496
670

Chart 13.

DAY COACHES AND OTHER CARS

Forty-three observations were made in day coaches. The number of passengers averaged 32.63 and the carbon dioxid 9.38; the equivalent ventilation would be 36,300 cubic feet per hour. These cars were dependent upon so-called natural ventilation. The result corresponds closely to the general average for the sleeping-car, the difference in air-supply being about proportionate to the difference in size—the full length of the day coach being open to occupancy.

Determinations of carbon dioxid were made from the air of various places occupied by an unknown number of people for purposes of comparison of the contamination. These included street-cars, elevated cars, suburban steam-cars, stores, offices and restaurants. They were all made during the cooler months of the year and under various conditions. The cars were from half full to crowded, restaurants were taken at the lunch hour and the offices were well filled. The average and maximum carbon dioxid and the hourly air-supplies per person necessary to maintain the various averages, as well as those for the body and the lower birth of sleeping-cars equipped with exhaust ventilators—now standard construction—are shown in Table 11 and the general comparisons are graphically represented in Chart 13.

TABLE 11.

| Place. | No. of Observations. | $CO_2$ per 10,000. | | Equivalent hourly air supply per person, cu. ft. |
|---|---|---|---|---|
| | | Average. | Maximum. | |
| Sleeping Cars (Body) | 294 | 6.20 | 10.0 | 2,727 |
| Sleeping Cars (Berths) | 690 | 6.96 | 13.5 | 2,027 |
| Day Coaches | 43 | 9.38 | 21.0 | 1,100 |
| Street Cars | 45 | 15.10 | 29.0 | 541 |
| Elevated Cars | 17 | 13.90 | 26.5 | 674 |
| Suburban Coaches | 47 | 14.30 | 38.0 | 583 |
| Stores | 23 | 8.80 | 10.0 | 1,250 |
| Restaurants | 51 | 16.10 | 26.0 | 496 |
| Offices | 26 | 13.91 | 19.0 | 670 |

THE STILL CAR

About 200 samples of air from still cars have been analyzed. It is usual to find that the carbon dioxid rapidly increases when a train stops running. This increase reaches its maximum only after a considerable time, and the final height is variable, depending largely on the force of the outside wind. A strong wind will drive much air into the car, a light one proportionately less. Among these 200 observations the carbon dioxid passed 20 per 10,000 but twice—20.5 and 21.5, both in lower berths. It is usual to find the maximum around 15 in cars that are occupied at stations awaiting very late departures. A very good example of what may happen in a car kept closed when there is almost no wind blowing is seen in Chart 14. This car was halted by an obstructing wreck, and there was

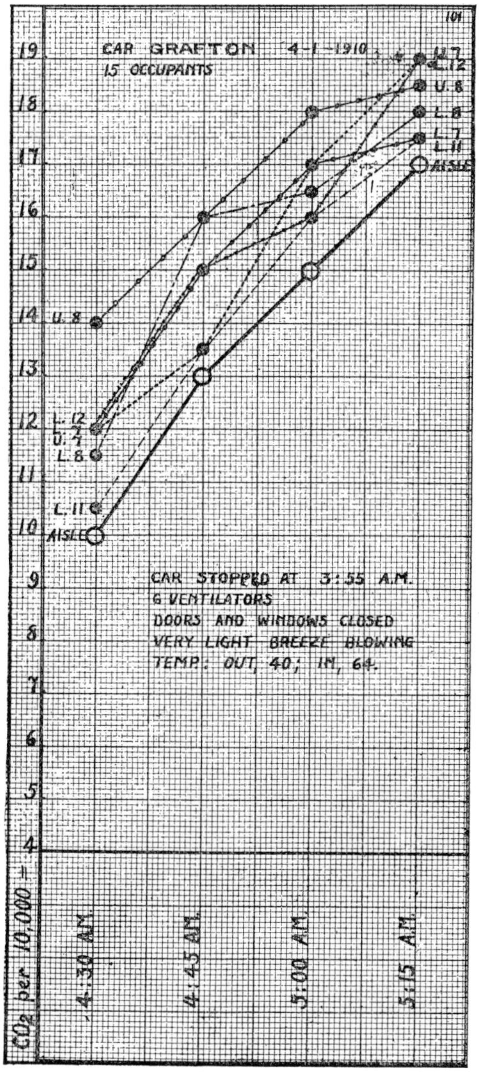


Chart 14.

not even the opening of a door while it was standing. It represents the highest average contamination, at 5:15 a. m., of any car yet examined; and had the sampling been carried forward from this time it would probably show that the increase had nearly reached its maximum.

The effect of starting the train is invariably to bring down the carbon dioxid rapidly. After thirty minutes it has reached as low a point as it can be expected to maintain. Chart 15 will illustrate the condition better than any description. A light breeze only was blowing when the observations were made.

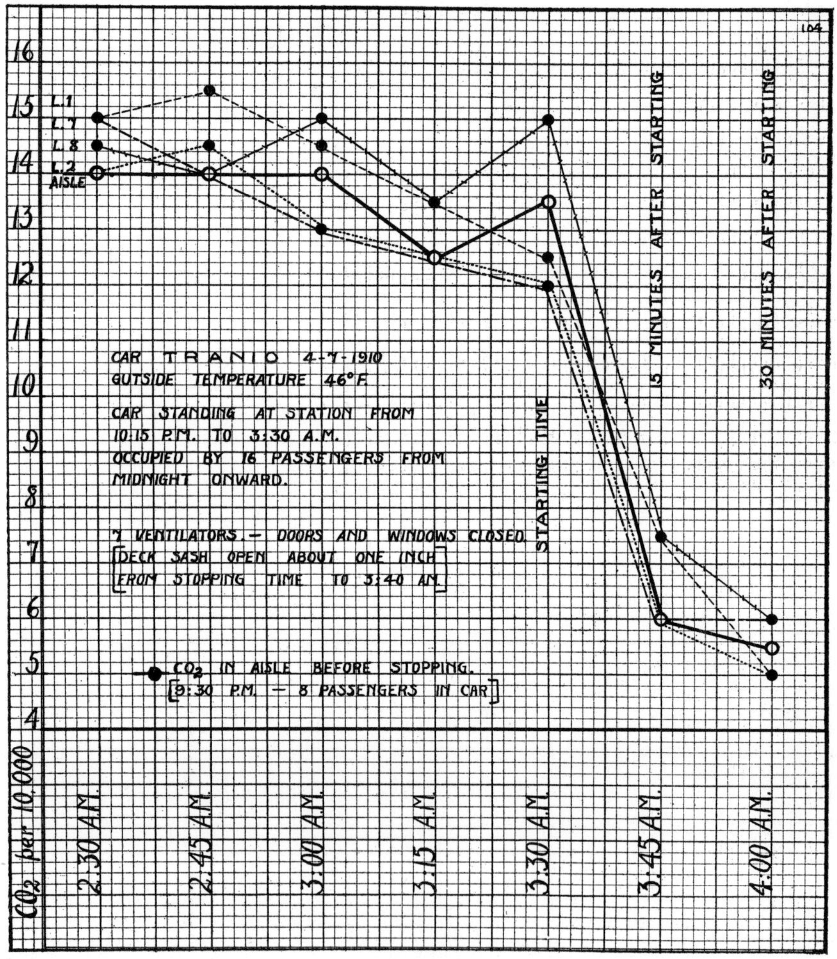


Chart 15

THE ENTRANCE AND DISTRIBUTION OF AIR

It has been shown that an average of over 40,000 cubic feet of air per hour enters the breathing-zone of sleeping-cars equipped with the type of exhaust ventilator herein considered. It has been further shown that approximately twice this much air leaves from the upper portion of the car through the six or eight ventilators used. In the absence of specific intakes it is difficult to determine exactly in what manner this air finds an entrance.

Sleeping-cars are snugly built; the crevices are small; but no crevice is too small to admit air, provided a little pressure is behind it. A row of windows covers each side of the car, another row of small ones extends along each side at the deck level, and each end has a door. There is a sum total of approximately 500 lineal feet of crevices at their edges. If they average one-fiftieth of an inch in width and admitted air at half the rate of the train speed, the 40,000 cubic feet would be more than accounted for. Some of these crevices are much larger than one-fiftieth of an inch, some are probably smaller. It is not unusual to find air entering certain areas of open windows at a rate equal to one-half the train speed, or even more. The crevices may act in the same way; the passage of air through such invisible openings is a much more important means of ventilation than might be thought. Pettenkofer[18] showed that when all visible chinks were closed in a room the rate of ventilation was decreased only 28 per cent. as compared with the rate when the doors were closed in the ordinary way. Putnam[18] showed that air entered a room through a register almost as rapidly when every means was taken to make it air-tight as when the doors stood open. There is no difficulty with the draught of an open fireplace when the room is closed, though each pound of coal consumed causes some 2,600 cubic feet[19] of air to pass up the flue.

Samples of air were taken simultaneously from various locations in sleeping-cars with exhaust ventilators and the carbon dioxid determined, in an attempt to find where the contamination is greatest. So long as the samples are taken well within the body of the car they show nearly uniform results for different levels and different locations; hence the general mixing of the air must be good. The carbon dioxid is, on the average, a little lower close to the floor than higher up. This is consistent with the upward trend of the flow to the ventilator exits. There is essentially no difference between the breathing-zone and the bell-cord level. There is a slight difference between samples taken at the breathing-level and near the ventilator exits, the latter being lower; but the difference is not so great as would be indicated by the difference in the dilution of the lower air and the amount leaving the car through these exits.[20]

The one way in which strikingly different comparative results are brought out is by collecting samples from within a few inches of the tops or bottoms of the windows and from the body of the car. Thirty-three such comparisons were made. Twenty-three times the air taken

18. Quoted by Macfie: Air and Health, E. P. Dutton & Co., New York, 1909, p. 202.

19. Notter and Firth: Quoted by Macfie, Air and Health, p. 207.

20. One must be careful in collecting samples at these exits not to breathe directly into the air being collected. The first samples collected were rendered useless by failure to observe this precaution.

from near the window crevices in this way showed no increase in carbon dioxid over the normal, while the interior had from 5 to 8 parts of carbon dioxid per 10,000. In these twenty-three instances it seems clear that fresh air was entering here at a sufficient rate to drive back all contaminated air for a distance of several inches. It is often possible to feel a draught on the hand placed near to such a crevice, especially if the outside air is cold. Now the least perceptible draught is about two miles per hour. If air is moving at this rate in the several inches lying inside a crevice it must be passing through the crevice itself at a much higher speed. Seven times the carbon dioxid by the windows was 4.5, when the car body showed 5 to 7. Twice it was 5, when the car body was 5.5 and 7. Once it was 6 when the car body was 8. In none of the thirty-three was it equal in contamination to the general air of the car.

Samples were taken from the inner ends of the passageways which lead to the end doors twenty-eight times. Seven times this air showed no contamination; the car body showed 5 to 8 parts carbon dioxid per 10,000. The other samples showed 4.5 to 8. Six times the air from the passage was higher than the average from the car. In one car four successive observations from the rear passage way showed no contamination, while the forward passageway always showed a contamination equal to or greater than the average for the body. It seems clear in this case that there was a continuous flow of air from the rear door inward—and probably an outward flow from the forward end of the car. Both doors were closed.

## *HYGIENIC INTERPRETATION*

It has been attempted to determine the ventilation of sleeping-cars in terms of air-supply, using carbon dioxid as the only available basis of computation. In order to pass judgment on the findings recorded, it is necessary to know the hygienic significance of respiratory contamination of the atmosphere, and, if possible, to establish the cause of discomfort which may arise, supposedly as the result of an insufficient air-supply.

According to the older theories the sensations of discomfort arising in enclosed spaces had their origin either in an excess of carbon dioxid or an insufficiency of oxygen. Pettenkofer cast the first serious doubt on the correctness of these theories. By the work of Hermans[21] it was proved that air containing 15 per cent. of oxygen may contain 2 per cent. to 4 per cent. of carbon dioxid and not be harmful. On removing the carbon dioxid there was no great discomfort even when the oxygen was reduced to 10 per cent. The air of certain breweries examined by Lehmann[22] contained 1.5 per cent. to 2.5 per cent. of carbon dioxid, and men

21. Hermans: Ausschaltung organischer Substanzen durch den Menschen, Arch. f. Hyg., 1883, i, 1.

22. Lehmann: Untersuchung über die langdauernde Wirkung mittlerer Kohlensäuredosen auf den Menschen, Arch. f. Hyg., 1899, xxxiv, 335.

worked continuously in this for years without any ill effects. It occasionally rose to 6 per cent. and even 10 per cent., and might then produce temporary intoxication. On the testimony of numerous experimenters it has come to be generally accepted that an atmosphere containing pure carbon dioxid below 3 per cent. and oxygen as high as 15 per cent. has no toxic effect and produces no distressing symptoms. It is very rare for the carbon dioxid produced by respiration to contaminate the air of any room, even with the poorest ventilation, to the extent of more than 50 parts in 10,000, or one-half of one per cent. It is not in accordance with the evidence to ascribe to this amount of carbon dioxid alone any harmful influence.

In relation to the subject of ventilation it has been very generally accepted that carbon dioxid in such amount as is likely to be found in inhabited rooms, even up to 50 parts in 10,000, is in itself entirely harmless, but that when this is due to respiration certain poisonous organic bodies are also present of which the carbon dioxid is an accurate index. The allowable amount of carbon dioxid as respiratory impurity has been variously placed at from 2 to 10 parts, or a total of 6 to 14 parts, in 10,000 of air, the limit being placed at that degree of contamination at which the sense of smell begins to give the first indication of closeness to one entering the room from without. It has always been recognized that high standards of personal cleanliness would allow this limit to go higher than when such standards are low, that those within do not perceive any odor as readily as one entering, and that the contamination at which discomfort develops is liable to great variation. As a result of their work Haldane and Osborn[23] recommended a limit of 12 volumes per 10,000 by day, and 20 volumes by night when gas or oil is used for lighting. It has been very generally stated that about 10 volumes in 10,000 allows a fair margin of safety.

Though poisonous bodies in the expired air had been earlier mentioned, they were first claimed to have been demonstrated by Brown-Séquard and D'Arsonval,[24] in 1888 and 1889. They injected the condensation fluid of the expired breath into rabbits and produced death. In a second group of experiments they arranged a series of cages in which rabbits were placed so that each succeeding cage received the vitiated air from the one before it. In the end cage rabbits died; but if the air received into this cage were passed through sulphuric acid the rabbits remained alive. From these experiments it was concluded that the expired air contained poison-

23. Haldane and Osborn: First Report of the Departmental Committee appointed to inquire into the ventilation of factories and workshops, London, 1902, p. 5. Quoted by Soper, The Air and Ventilation of Subways, Wiley and Sons, New York, 1908, p. 44.

24. Brown-Séquard and D'Arsonval: Compt. Rend. de l'Acad. de Paris, 1888, cvi, 106, 165; 1889, cviii, 267, 1295.

ous gases, which were considered to be of the nature of volatile ptomains or leukomains, and were looked on as exceedingly toxic. A vast amount of research was inspired by the work of Brown-Séquard and D'Arsonval, and among the many workers who attempted to confirm their results Merkel[25] stands almost the only important sponsor for the correctness of their conclusions; and with some changes in technic he was unable to get uniform results. Though as late as 1894 Brown-Séquard and D'Arsonval[26] reassert the correctness of their earlier results and insist on the existence of such poisons, most of the later investigations go to show that no such poisons exist; and errors both of technic and conclusion have been pointed out to account for the results which they obtained.

Dastre and Loya[27] exposed one dog to the expired air of others and saw no effect after six hours. They concluded from experiments that the condensation from the breath is no more toxic than distilled water, which conclusion was confirmed by Von Hoffmann-Wellenhof,[28] Lehman and Jessen,[29] Haldane and Smith,[30] Billings, Weir Mitchell and Bergey,[31] and others.

The cage experiments of Brown-Séquard and D'Arsonval were repeated by Haldane and Smith, Beu,[32] Rauer,[33] Lübbert and Peters,[34] Billings, Weir Mitchell and Bergey, Formanek,[35] and others, with the conclusion that no poison exists in the expired air, and that the animals of the last cage die only when the carbon dioxid reaches 10 per cent. to 12 per cent., with proportionate reduction of oxygen—conditions which produce death by suffocation. There have been found traces of ammonia in the breath and traces of hydrochloric acid. These have their origin in decaying teeth and particles of food or effete discharges. They exist in such small

25. Merkel: Neue Untersuchungen über die Giftigkeit der Expirationsluft, Arch. f. Hyg., 1892, xv, 1.

26. Brown-Séquard and D'Arsonval: Arch. de phys. norm. et path., 1895, xvi, 113.

27. Dastre and Loya: Recherches sur la toxicité de l'air expiré, Compt. rend. Soc. de biol., 1888, v, 91.

28. Von Hoffmann-Wellenhof: Enthält die Expirationsluft gesunder Menschen ein flüchtiges Gift, Wien. klin. Wchnschr., 1888, i, 753.

29. Lehman and Jessen: Ueber die Giftigkeit der Expirationsluft, Arch. f. Hyg., 1890, x, 367.

30. Haldane and Smith: The Physiological Effects of Air Vitiated by Respiration, Jour. Path. and Bacteriol, 1892-3, i, 168, 318.

31. Billings, Mitchell and Bergey: The Composition of Expired Air and Its Effects on Animal Life, Ann. Rep. Board of Regents, Smithsonian Inst., 1895, General Appendix, p. 389.

32. Beu: Untersuchung über Giftigkeit der Expirationsluft, Ztschr. f. Hyg., 1893, xiv, 64.

33. Rauer: Untersuchung über die Giftigkeit der Expirationsluft, Ztschr. f. Hyg., 1893, xv, 57.

34. Lübbert and Peters: Abst. in Hyg. Rundschau, 1894, iv, 1118.

35. Formanek: Ueber die Giftigkeit des Ausathmungsluft, Arch. f. Hyg., 1900, xxxviii, 1. (An excellent review of the literature.)

quantities as to have no practical bearing on the question, in the opinion of those best qualified to judge.

The researches mentioned were practically all on animals, and this may account for their conclusions not having found such general acceptance as would induce their practical application to problems of ventilation. It is common practice still for hygienists to insist that ventilation of rooms is necessary because the air becomes poisoned with gaseous excretions and that the carbon dioxid of the air is the measure of danger; and this in spite of the fact that practically all significant evidence is to the effect that no such poisonous excretions exist. The assumption seems to find its support in the fact that certain susceptible individuals suffer from oppression, malaise, headache, nausea, vomiting and even collapse under certain conditions in crowded rooms. If not due to a poison, to what then are these phenomena due?

Hermans[21] long ago suggested, since he could not find sufficient chemical changes in the air to disturb the health, that the influence is very likely a thermal one. Indeed, the symptoms are not very different from those clearly recognized as heat exhaustion, nor from those experienced in the open air on certain hot and humid days. Heat and aqueous vapor must increase enormously in ill-ventilated places with many occupants, and thus prevent the usual dissipation of body heat to the surrounding air.

In order to bring the problem into direct relation to the ventilation of rooms for human habitation, and to get nearer the cause of the disturbances often observed in closed spaces, a series of experiments were carried out about five years ago in the Institute of Hygiene in Breslau by Heymann,[36] Paul[37] and Erclentz.[38] These experiments were carried out under the direction of Flügge,[39] who has admirably summarized and interpreted the results.

Paul placed healthy individuals in a cabinet of 3 cubic meters' capacity where they were kept for a variable time up to four hours, and until the carbon dioxid had risen to 100 or 150 parts in 10,000—an accumulation of gaseous excretion practically never developed under ordinary conditions. In these experiments no symptoms of illness or discomfort developed so long as the temperature and moisture were kept low. Tests of the psychic fatigue of these individuals by means of the esthesiometer

36. Heymann: Ueber den Einfluss wieder eingeathmeter Expirationsluft auf die Kohlensäure-Abgabe, Ztsch. f. Hyg., 1905, xlix, 388.

37. Paul: Die Wirkung der Luft bewohnter Räume, Ztschr. f. Hyg., 1905, xlix, 405.

38. Erclentz: Das Verhalten Kranker gegenüber verunreinigter Wohnungsluft, Ztschr. f. Hyg., 1905, xlix, 433.

39. Flügge: Ueber Lüftverunreinigung, Wärmestauung und Lüftung in geschlossenen Räumen, Ztschr. f. Hyg., 1905, xlix, 363.

and ergograph, or by means of computations, gave negative results throughout, under similar conditions of temperature and moisture. Tests in a crowded school room were similarly negative. Erclentz made the same observations on diseased persons. Those suffering from emphysema, heart diseases, kidney diseases, etc., with the exception of a few peculiarly susceptible anemic and scrofulous school children, bore the highly contaminated air for hours without any evidence of bodily or mental depression.

The results were very different, however, when the temperature and moisture of the air of the cabinet were allowed to increase. At 80 F with moderate humidity, or at from 70 to 73.5 with high humidity, practically all persons began to show depression, headache, dizziness or a tendency to nausea. The susceptibility was not alike for all. School children reacted slightly and emphysematics slightly, while those with heart troubles were most susceptible. By means of certain objective signs of heat stagnation—the surface temperature of the forehead, and the temperature and moisture of the clothed parts of the body—it was determined that subjective symptoms appeared only when the surface temperature reached a certain height. This was for healthy people 93 F. to 95 F. on the forehead; for the more susceptible diseased 89.5 to 91.5; and with the moisture of the skin increased by 20 or 30 per cent. Under these conditions the normal dissipation of body heat is interfered with, and it is under these conditions that symptoms appear which are in every way similar to those developed in overfilled and "stuffy" rooms.

Now when these people in the cabinet suffering from such symptoms, were allowed to breathe the fresh outside air through a tube, such air being raised to the temperature and relative humidity of that within, it gave them no relief whatever; nor did the internal air produce any symptoms when breathed through a tube by one outside the cabinet. But the symptoms of discomfort and illness experienced by the person within could be almost immediately relieved either by drying the air of the cabinet, or by cooling it, or by putting it in rapid motion by means of a fan, without any chemical change being made in the air. Now what is the effect of any or all of these measures? Simply by purely mechanical means to enable the body to throw off its heat more rapidly; and thereby all symptoms disappear. Heat stagnation is the cause of the discomfort, and this is caused by the physical condition of the atmosphere quite independently of the degree of respiratory contamination or of any changes in its chemical composition.

From the long series of experiments, carried out with great care as to all the details of observation and control, it is concluded that all of the symptoms arising in the so-called vitiated atmosphere of crowded rooms are dependent on heat stagnation in the body, and that the thermic conditions of the atmosphere, its moisture and its stillness are responsible for the effects. To change any one of these elements is to change the rapidity of the loss of heat. If the change is such as to increase this loss comfort is restored. It is also considered proved beyond any reasonable doubt, by their own as well as by previous research, that there is no gaseous excretion into the surrounding air, either from the breath or from other sources, deserving of the name of poison. Angelici,[40] working independently at about the same time, concurs in these opinions; and Reichenbach and Heymann[41] later determined that objective evidence of heat stagnation in the body always precedes the development of subjective symptoms of discomfort under natural conditions, in the same way that it does under the artificial conditions of the cabinet.

The evidence presented by these investigators is such as to be convincing. It seems to be established beyond any reasonable doubt that discomfort is not due to any change in the chemical composition of the air but to physical changes only; and that to maintain a normal heat interchange between the body and the air is to avoid the development of those symptoms which are commonly attributed to poor ventilation. A certain amount of fresh air must be supplied, of course, but the most vital element of the ventilation problem becomes that of regulating the temperature of the air. The question of how to ventilate a railway car is therefore chiefly a question of how to regulate its heat.

It has happened that a few of the cars considered in this work have been uncomfortable, have been called "close" or "stuffy." The temperature of these cars has invariably been high. There has sometimes been an unpleasant odor. This cannot be ventilated away so long as its source remains. A high temperature renders such odors more noticeable. The most marked offensiveness I have ever noticed was in a day coach where the air was of such a degree of chemical purity as to indicate ideal ventilation by any standard that has ever been proposed. The car was hot and had many filthy people in it. With perfect comfort have been sometimes associated the highest chemical impurity. Such was the case in the car represented in Chart 14. It seems probable, furthermore, that one main cause of the complaint of poor ventilation in the sleeping-car berth is purely psychic. We are used to sleeping-rooms with walls and ceilings far from us. In the berth they are very close. Their very nearness is oppressive. It seems as if there cannot be enough air in this small space to supply our wants. The sensation is often quite independent of the amount of air supplied and even of the temperature.

40. Angelici: Quoted by Reichenbach and Heymann, Ztschr. f. Hyg., 1907, lvii, 23.

41. Reichenbach and Heymann: Untersuchungen über die Wirkungen klimatischer Factoren auf den Menschen, Ztschr. f. Hyg., 1907, lvii, 23.

Even under the older applied principles of ventilation, the air-supply of sleeping-cars, as determined in this study, is ample under nearly all conditions. The average carbon dioxid in the air of running cars falls well within the limits of contamination permitted by the earlier investigators, and it is relatively rare that the individual observations show more than 10 parts in 10,000. In the light of the newer conceptions, which have as yet been applied in practice only to a very limited extent, this air-supply is ample under all conditions observed. No danger to health is to be apprehended under the conditions ordinarily obtaining even in still cars. They are occupied only for short periods as a rule and are not uncomfortable if kept cool. It would seem that the results obtained by the type of exhaust ventilator investigated in this study, which is now a part of the standard equipment of Pullman cars, are entirely adequate to meet the demands of hygiene, and that those difficulties and discomforts which do sometimes arise are due to other causes than lack of a sufficient amount of fresh air or to excessive vitiation. It is extremely unlikely that increasing the air-supply, which now amounts to from six to ten or more times the cubic content of the car each hour, and must maintain considerable motion of the atmosphere, would aid in any other way than by making overheating more difficult to bring about. Overheating is the paramount evil. It is the thing to be chiefly guarded against in the attempt to maintain comfort and good hygiene. It is not feasible to cool the naturally overheated air in summer, or to dry it when excessively humid. Fan motors and open windows are the available means by which the difficulties arising in hot weather may be most readily overcome. Carry away the body heat as rapidly as possible by a strong current of air. Though the avoidance of overheating in winter would seem to be an easy thing, its accurate control to meet the rapidly changing conditions under which cars may be operated is a matter of great difficulty. Experience has shown that it is necessary to have in sleeping-cars at least twice as much radiating surface as is demanded in common practice for heating the same space in houses; this in order to warm the large volume of air received and discharged so that it will maintain comfort to inactive passengers. To decrease this surface would be to fail to maintain a sufficiently high temperature on occasion. A system is needed capable of being quickly and effectively controlled to meet rapidly changing conditions. Such a system is now being experimented with in which there are multiple units of radiating surface, each with a separate control. The results so far indicate that from this a more uniformly comfortable condition can be maintained.

Let it not be understood that any protest is here urged against the benefits of fresh air and of outdoor life. It is undoubted that crowded rooms can call forth evil consequences from the excess of heat and moisture in their atmosphere, and that foul-smelling air may be, for those susceptible to it, productive of temporary disturbances of considerable importance, though these are reflex rather than toxic in character. Flügge, in reviewing and interpreting the facts established by his co-workers, urges that life in the open should be more and more resorted to; but he would have the motive correctly understood: not that the chemical condition of inside air is harmful, but that it is the overheating of rooms that causes disturbances of health: that one should go into the open, not because one may there breathe chemically purer air, but because its almost constant motion carries away the body heat and causes a beneficial stimulation of the skin; and reflexly brings about a heightened cell activity that aids in the development of sturdy health. The chemistry of air and "crowd-poisons" have little or no part to play in the explanation of outdoor benefits or of indoor discomforts. These are both dependent upon physical conditions; and their explanation rests with the physics of heat interchange between the body and its surrounding medium.

2 Adams Street.

# BOOK REVIEW

Medical Education in the United States and Canada. A Report to the Carnegie Foundation for the Advancement of Teaching. By Abraham Flexner. With an Introduction by Henry S. Pritchett, President of the Foundation. Bulletin No. 4. Paper. Pp. 346. 576 Fifth Avenue, New York, 1910.

In this report Mr. Flexner presents a comprehensive statement, based on a thorough investigation of the conditions pertaining to medical teaching in the United States and Canada. The report is extremely timely and will do much to bring about that readjusting of our medical schools for which a number of agencies are now working. General interest in the subject has been stimulated in recent years, especially by the excellent work of the Council on Medical Education of the American Medical Association. The medical public should, therefore, be in a position at this time to accept the advanced position indicated in the constructive criticism of this report. The effort is apparent throughout to give full credit for everything that is praiseworthy in each institution. At the same time the various questions are met with directness and candor, and shortcomings are frankly and clearly pointed out. Without the comprehensive statement of facts which this report places before us many would not be able to appreciate the deplorable conditions permeating our system of medical teaching—conditions which have developed largely as the result of what we have to acknowledge as an American idea, the proprietary school of medicine. The disgraceful situation existing in many cheap diploma mills, called medical schools merely by courtesy, in which Chicago appears to take the lead, has not before been brought so clearly and definitely to the attention of the public. It is indeed refreshing and encouraging to have the situation in these institutions of quackery discussed frankly by an outsider who can have no bias or interest to serve other than the improvement of present conditions.

The report is on the whole constructive, and will no doubt serve to crystallize as well as to popularize certain ideals toward which medical education in this country is certainly tending. Foremost is the idea that the medical school must be a department of a real university and dominated by the same ideals of investigation and teaching which characterize any real university department. An immediate result which we can hope for from this report is the abandonment, at least in our better institutions, of the practice of voting into the university a proprietary medical school and dubbing it the medical department of the university, whereas in reality the medical school retains in every detail the ideals of the proprietary school and is in no sense a university department of medicine.

Another idea developed at length in this report which is fundamental in the problem of our medical schools is their relation to the hospital. The report makes quite clear the fact that the hospital is in reality a laboratory in clinical medicine and as such to be efficient it must be owned and controlled by the medical school. "One sort of laboratory may as well be borrowed as another. The university professor of physics can teach his subject in borrowed quarters quite as well as the university professor of clinical medicine. . . . The student can never be part of the organization in a hospital in which he is present on sufferance" (p. 99).

The few pages which were deemed sufficient to devote to the postgraduate school in this report contain in conclusion the statement that "advanced instruction along these lines (the specialties) will not thrive in isolation. It will be but the upper story of a university department of medicine." The smatterings of elementary instruction now constituting the teaching in these postgraduate schools will not be necessary when once the undergraduate schools are doing their work properly. Graduate work in medicine, as in any field, is a function of the university for it embodies the idea of investigation and the discussion of unsolved problems.

# The Archives of Internal Medicine

VOL. VII | FEBRUARY, 1911 | No. 2

## THE DIAGNOSTIC VALUE OF THE ORTHODIAGRAM IN HEART DISEASE*

J. G. VAN ZWALUWENBURG, M.D.

AND

L. F. WARREN, M.D.

ANN ARBOR, MICH.

The orthodiagram has been a disappointment to those clinicians who had hoped to find an accurate estimation of the size of the heart of use in diagnosis. Particularly in the field of cardiac neurosis and early myocarditis, in which the ordinary diagnostic methods fail to show any enlargement, evidence of a slight enlargement might be expected to have diagnostic or prognostic import.

The roentgenogram does not give us such evidence because of the magnification of the cardiac shadow by the divergent rays and because of the lack of definition at the margin, since the heart is in active motion while the exposure is being made. The orthodiagram, however, gives perfectly definite images of a moving organ, allows of the observation of any anomaly of motion, and depends only on the skill of the operator in the interpretation of the images viewed. In addition it leaves a permanent record of that interpretation in the actual dimensions of the organs observed.

Of the various dimensions of the heart shadow which have been proposed, the following have been most commonly adopted:

1. The right-median (M.R.) or greatest perpendicular distance from the right border to the median line (*k-l*).
2. The left-median (M.L.) or similar measurement to the left (*m-n*).
3. The total transverse (T.T.) or sum of M.R. and M.L.
4. The long diameter (L.) measured from the auriculovenous junction to the apex (*a-d*).
5. The area of the completed heart shadow. A dimension less frequently used is the transverse (trans), measured from the left auriculoventricular junction to the auriculohepatic angle (*b-c*).

M. R. and M. L. are the orthodiagraphic equivalents of the measurements obtained in routine percussion of the deep cardiac dulness, and as such have a distinct value as a check on the examiner's technic. But, because they are always measured in the horizontal direction without reference to the obliquity of the long axis of the heart, their numerical

* From the Department of Internal Medicine, University of Michigan.

value depends directly on the angle of obliquity, approaching the long diameter with a transverse position, and the transverse diameter with a vertical position of that organ. The sum of the two, therefore, bears no fixed relation to the size of the heart and any conclusions drawn from a comparison of such values must be inaccurate. The transverse diameter is also an inaccurate criterion, because its right lower extremity is not a fixed point, but depends on the position of the heart with reference to the diaphragm.

The orthodiagram of the heart is never a closed figure (Fig. 3). The outline cannot be followed through the shadows of the sternum and the

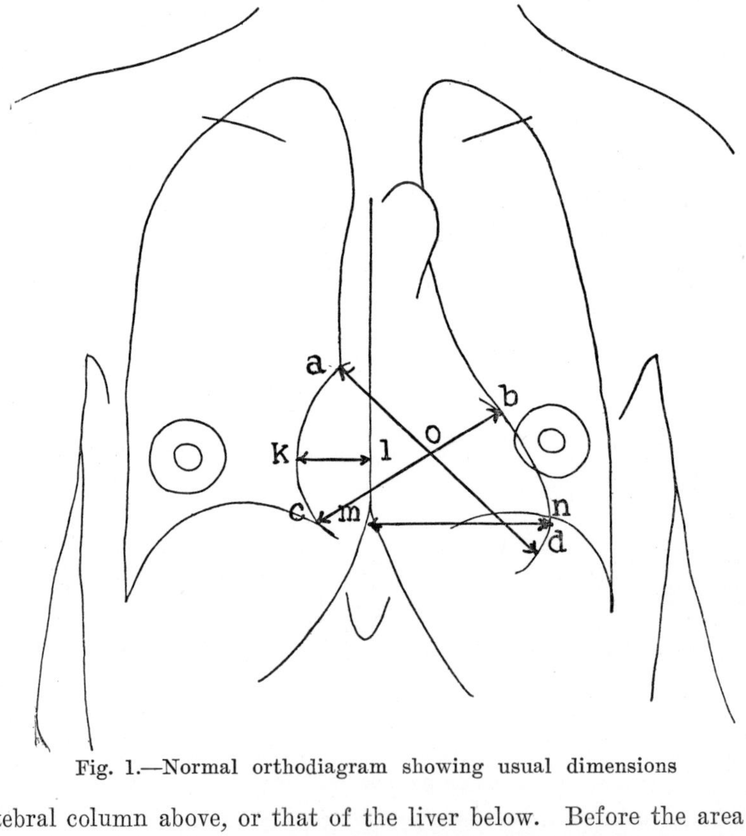


Fig. 1.—Normal orthodiagram showing usual dimensions

vertebral column above, or that of the liver below. Before the area can be determined the figure must be completed. This is usually done in free-hand, in broad curves to suit the notions of the observer. The upper border usually shows only a short defect and the probable position of the line bridging it is fairly well defined. The lower border is often so deeply sunk in the liver shadow that it is absurd to attempt to supply it. In normal hearts this lower border is a fairly straight line, but pathologically it may become considerably curved. Therefore the completed heart outline represents only the examiner's opinion of its size and shape.

The estimation of the area so enclosed is best accomplished by the use of the planimeter, an instrument used by engineers for measuring irregular areas. Its scientific accuracy is limited only by the exactness with which the circumference can be followed by a needle-point. By the kindness of Professor J. A. Moyer, of the engineering department, we are able to measure all our diagrams by this means.

One may assume that the heart shadow approximates an ellipse and apply the formula for the area of this surface, namely, 3.1416/4 times the product of the long axis and the short axis. By drawing the longest diameter (*p-q*) of the completed figure, then constructing a short diam-

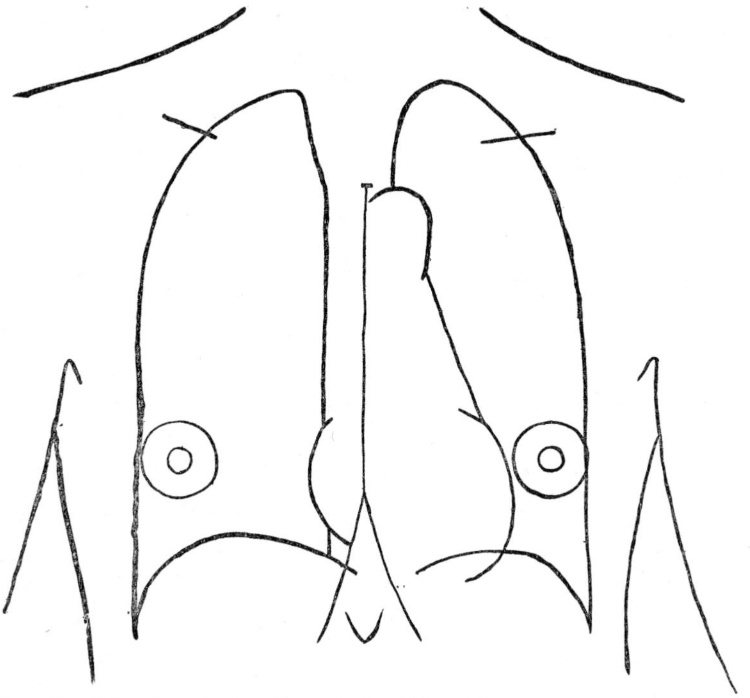

Fig. 2.—Splanchnoptosis, Case 126, M.R. 2.7 cm.; M.L. 7.8 cm.; long diameter 11.5 cm.; area 81 sq. cm.; index .830. Right auricular shadow does not meet the diaphragm shadow. Vertical position.

eter (*r-s*) normal to and bisecting this line, and using these values in the above formula, results are obtained which vary but little from the planimeter values (Fig. 4). This longest diameter (*p-q*) is not the same as the "long diameter" (*a-d*) above described. The latter is drawn from the auriculovenous angle and is frequently considerably shorter than a line drawn from some other point on the right border. To make the approximation closer, this line should be drawn as near the center of inertia of the figure as possible, although, actually, it often lies a short distance above it. The average error of the method in our series is in the neighborhood of 3 or 4 per cent. and the highest was 8 per cent. in a heart of very irregular shape.

Claytor[1] has proposed a method of approximation based on a similar calculation using the long and the transverse diameters. In a series of normal diagrams he found 70 per cent. of the product of these dimensions closely approximated the area. The two diameters intersect at such an angle that the transverse diameter always exceeds in length a perpendicular to the long diameter, thereby reducing the necessary constant factor from 0.7854 to 0.7000. The difference in length depends, however,

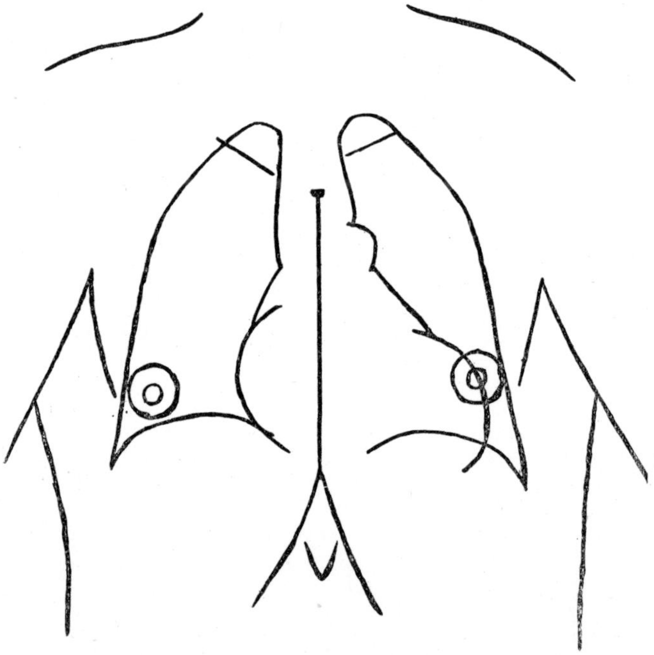

Fig. 3.—Aortic regurgitation well compensated. Snub-nosed heart. Case 58, M.R. 4.5 cm.; M.L. 9.4 cm.; long diameter 14.8 cm.; area 115 sq. cm.; index .378.

on the obliquity of this angle, which in pathological hearts is subject to wide variation, resulting in a considerable error in the majority of cases.

Before slight enlargements of the heart or changes in its position can be recognized, a standard or norm must be established. Series of measurements of normal hearts have been published by Dietlen,[2] Groedel[3, 4]

1. Claytor and Merrill: Am. Jour. Med. Sc., 1909, cxxxviii, 549.
2. Dietlen: Deutsch. Arch. f. klin. Med., 1906, lxxxviii, 55.
3. Groedel, F. M.: Die Orthoroentgenographie, Munich, 1908.
4. Groedel, F. M.: Roentgen Diagnostik, Lehmann's medizinische Atlanten, vii, Munich, 1909.

Claytor, and others. The tables of Dietlen[2] were chosen for use in the University Hospital, because the number of cases reported and the number of observations on each case are larger than in any of the others. It includes the measurements of 187 male and 74 female adults, classified according to age, weight, stature, etc. In his opinion, the dimensions follow weights rather more closely than any other one factor, and the table for adult males classified by weights was accordingly selected for a standard and is shown in Table 1.

TABLE 1.—TABLE OF DIMENSIONS OF 187 NORMAL HEARTS, AFTER DIETLEN

| | | | Ttl. Trs. Diam. (mm.) | | | Long. Diam. (mm.) | | | Area (Sq. cm.) | | |
|---|---|---|---|---|---|---|---|---|---|---|---|
| Class. | Kilos. | Pounds. | Max. | Aver. | Min. | Max. | Av. | Min. | Max. | Av. | Min. |
| I | 40-44 | 88-97 | 123 | 113 | 106 | 135 | 121 | 114 | 104 | 92 | 78 |
| II | 45-49 | 100-108 | 122 | 114 | 110 | 141 | 129 | 126 | 112 | 102 | 98 |
| III | 50-54 | 111-120 | 138 | 124 | 107 | 150 | 135 | 120 | 124 | 104 | 84 |
| IV | 55-59 | 120-132 | 147 | 129 | 114 | 151 | 140 | 128 | 128 | 112 | 101 |
| V | 60-64 | 133-134 | 146 | 131 | 104 | 159 | 141 | 127 | 138 | 114 | 91 |
| VI | 65-69 | 145-146 | 145 | 132 | 123 | 152 | 145 | 134 | 133 | 118 | 102 |
| VII | 70-74 | 157-165 | 149 | 134 | 122 | 162 | 148 | 135 | 149 | 122 | 106 |
| VIII | 75-79 | 166-175 | 150 | 145 | 131 | 161 | 155 | 136 | 139 | 131 | 120 |
| IX | 80-84 | 176-184 | 153 | 145 | 139 | 156 | 153 | 150 | 134 | 133 | 124 |

The use of this table has been found unsatisfactory. The average values appear to be too large for our cases in every class, from light weight to heavy weight. The position of the patient may be to blame for some of this, since Dietlen used only the dorsal position, while many of our orthodiagrams were taken in the erect position. A factor which is probably more important is the sort of material he used, much of it being drawn from soldiers from a neighboring military post, men who are kept in training by systematic and strenuous physical exercises, and may be expected to show hearts unusually large for their weight. Possibly also racial characteristics of build and the proportion of thorax to abdomen materially alter the obliquity of the heart's axis, and so the proportions.

Both Groedel and Claytor find somewhat smaller values on diagrams taken in the vertical position, but their series are rather too small to allow of conclusions.

A more serious obstacle to the estimation of hypertrophy is the wide variation of individual cases from the "average normal," as shown by the maximum values in any class. Naturally the greater the number compiled under any one class, the greater the liability of finding one very large and one very small heart. So we see the greatest variation in Class V, which includes thirty-four individuals, or fifteen more than the next largest class. Here the total transverse diameter reaches a maximum of 14.6 cm. with a minimum of 10.4 cm., a difference of 4.2 cm., a variation of 32 per cent. on the average of 13.1 cm. On the area the maximum reaches 138 sq. cm., with a minimum of 81 sq. cm., a difference of 47 sq. cm., or 41.2 per cent. on the average of 114 sq. cm.

The "normal average" can be of comparatively little use in the question of a pathological increase in the heart size. A given heart must be judged against the maximum which is normal for that class. Judged by these standards, we find that some hearts which are undoubtedly hypertrophied as the result of valvular disease or nephritis, do not exceed the maxima, nor is it possible to demonstrate enlargement in hearts which from a clinical point of view are manifestly insufficient. We need a more definitely established normal, with a critical study of any and all cases approaching the maxima, and excluding all cases that are clinically open to the suspicion of abnormality of any sort. From our observations it is not at all impossible that the large class of neurasthenics may have large hearts and it would seem advisable to exclude such from the list. Extremely shallow and extremely deep thoraces may also be excluded, on the ground that the depth of the mediastinal space may influence the

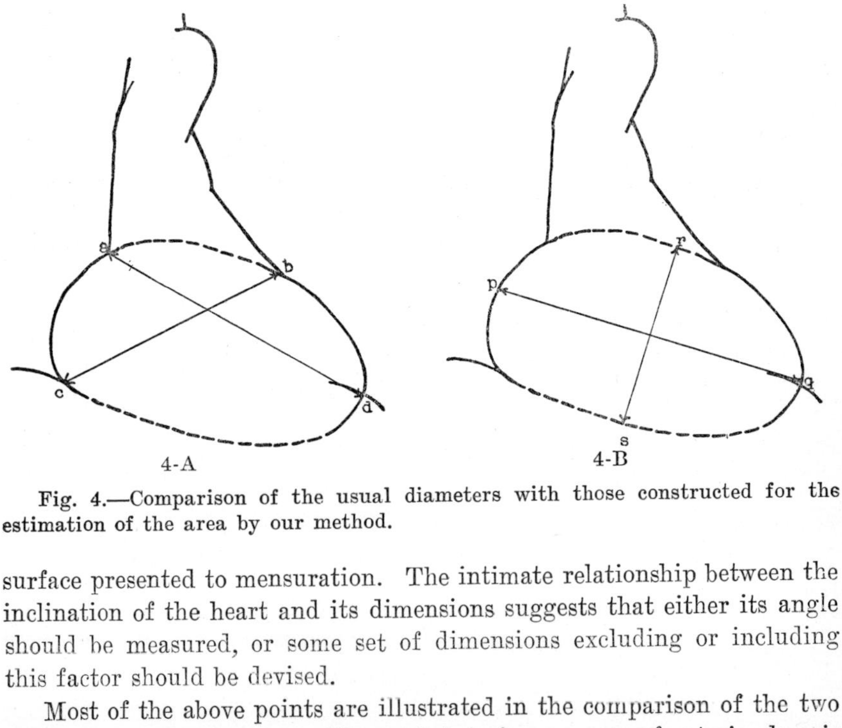


**Fig. 4.—Comparison of the usual diameters with those constructed for the estimation of the area by our method.**

surface presented to mensuration. The intimate relationship between the inclination of the heart and its dimensions suggests that either its angle should be measured, or some set of dimensions excluding or including this factor should be devised.

Most of the above points are illustrated in the comparison of the two hearts shown in Figure 5. Figure 5-A is from a case of arteriosclerosis with anginoid symptoms. Its dimensions are: M. R., 4.2 cm.; M. L., 10.4 cm.; T. T., 14.6 cm.; long diameter, 14.8 cm.; area, by planimeter, 100 sq. cm. The averages given by Dietlen for men of his weight are as follows; T. T., 13.4 cm.; long diameter, 14.8 cm.; area, 122 sq. cm. Figure 5-B is from a young adult having a mitral regurgitation following scarlet fever in his eighth year. Except for a chronic bronchitis, the patient has no symptoms at present. The dimensions are as follows: M. R., 4.2 cm.; M. L., 9.7 cm.; T. T., 13.9 cm.; long diameter, 14.7 cm.; area, by planimeter, 121 sq. cm. Dietlen's values for his class are T. T., 14.5 cm.; long diameter, 15.5 cm.; area, 131 sq. cm., with a minimum of 120 sq. cm. Here is a heart which is certainly hypertrophied from a clinical point of view, yet all its linear dimensions are smaller than that of a heart which has an area 20 per cent. smaller. Moreover, its area exceeds Dietlen's minimum dimensions by only 1 sq. cm., while it lies 10 sq. cm. below the normal average and 18 sq. cm. below the normal maximum (see Class VIII of Table 1).

Groedel[5] asserts that valuable information may be obtained by the careful analysis of the component arcs of the two heart borders, thereby judging of the relative hypertrophy or dilatation of the anatomical sub-

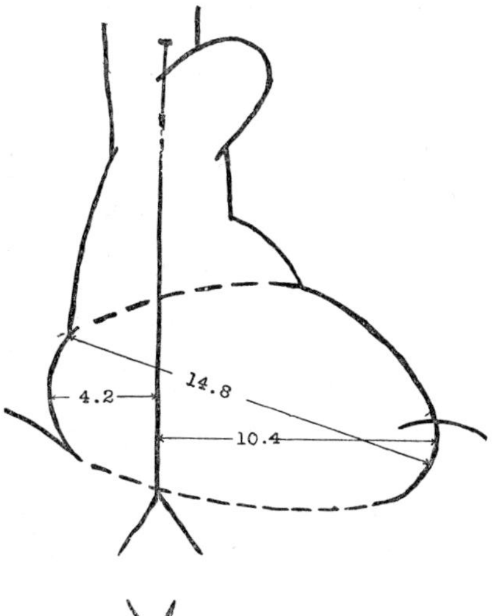


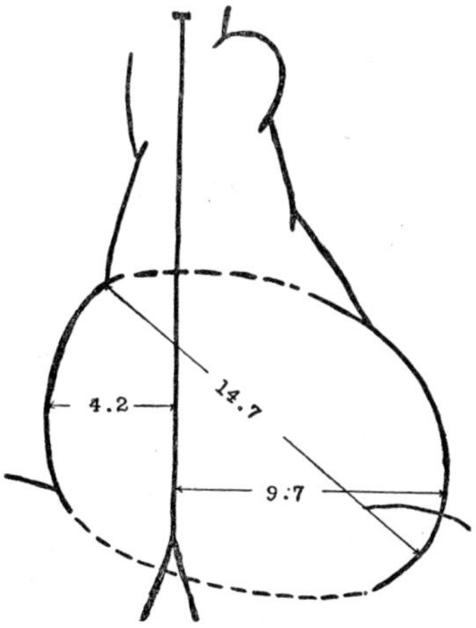


Fig. 5.—Showing the unreliability of the conventional linear dimensions. The smaller diagram has equal and larger dimensions than the larger one to the right. The latter is hypertrophied from an old mitral regurgitation.

divisions represented by these arcs. This principle is accepted by nearly all orthodiagraphists at the present time. Several characteristic shadows are recognized, of which the most typical are the "round heart" (Fig. 6), of mitral disease and the "snub-nosed" heart or "shoe-shaped" heart of aortic disease. Neither of these is pathognomonic of their respective lesions, but each materially assists in the diagnosis of doubtful cases. The altered shape is often the only evidence of the relative severity of two combined lesions, or the only suggestion of the secondary character

5. Groedel, F. M.: Deutsch. Arch. f. klin. Med., 1908, xciii, 79.

of the one or the other. It may be noted from the examples given how closely the heart of nephritis approaches that of aortic regurgitation in many cases (see Figures 3, 10 and 11).

It was felt that a numerical expression of the shape of the heart silhouette would be of assistance in the study of such combined lesions and of cardiac changes which were not secondary to valvular disease. For this purpose, there are only four available fixed landmarks on the circumference of the heart shadow (Fig. 1), namely, the right auriculovenous junction (*a*), the auriculohepatic angle (*c*), the upper extremity of the left ventricular border (*b*), and the apex of the heart (*d*). With good illumination these landmarks may be fixed in the majority of cases, especially in the erect position, which is the position chosen in our work. In this position the diaphragm rests at a lower level and the apex

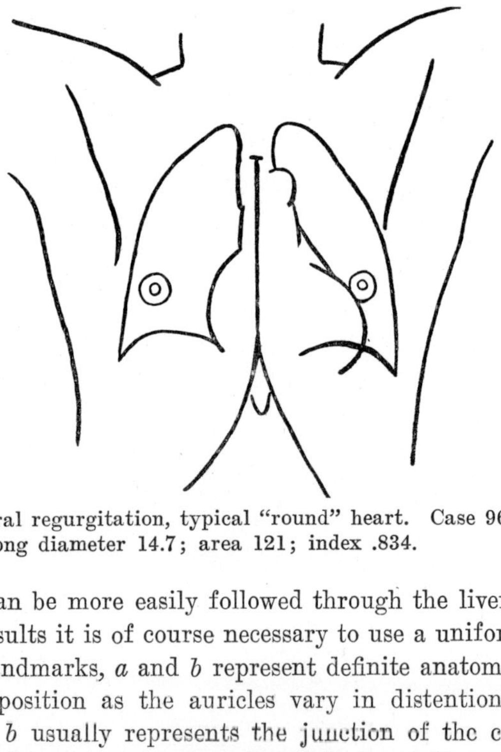

Fig. 6.—Mitral regurgitation, typical "round" heart. Case 96. M.R. 4.2 cm.; M.L. 9.7 cm.; long diameter 14.7; area 121; index .834.

of the heart can be more easily followed through the liver shadow. For comparable results it is of course necessary to use a uniform technic.

Of these landmarks, *a* and *b* represent definite anatomical points and will vary in position as the auricles vary in distention and size. In normal cases, *b* usually represents the junction of the conus arteriosus and the ventricle, but in enlarged hearts the left auricle frequently presents, and it then represents the junction of its shadow with that of the ventricle. Point *c* varies with a number of conditions, such as the degree of dilatation of the right auricle, changes in the obliquity of the cardiac axis, lengthening of the arch of the aorta, elevation of the diaphragm from abdominal distention or its depression in emphysema, splanchnoptosis, and so forth. The apex (*d*) is the most important of the four, because on its position depends the value of the long diameter and the area. It is also the most difficult to fix exactly. It represents the thinnest part of the heart; its motion has the widest excursion; and it lies depressed beneath the diaphragm shadow in the shadow of the left lobe of the liver. It is perhaps the least reliable of all.

By joining *a* and *d* we have the ordinary long diameter. The line *b-c* represents the transverse diameter as measured by Moritz. These two lines intersect at an oblique angle at 0, the obliquity depending on both the shape and the position of the heart.

The line *b-c* does not accurately represent the auriculoventricular septum either in position or in direction, but it may be assumed that the two areas into which the heart shadow is so divided are roughly representative of the auricular and ventricular areas, and, if the two segments are

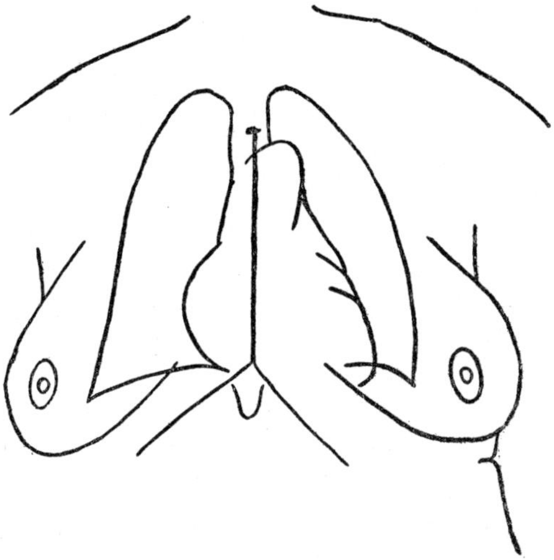

Fig. 7.—Mitral stenosis, showing prominence of left auricular shadow, with low position of the l. auriculoventricular junction. Case 97. M.R. 5.2 cm.; M.L. 9.0 cm.; long diameter 15.1 cm.; area 119; index 1.030.

similar with a common base and the obliquity of the axis equal, the areas will be in proportion to the fractional diameters *a-o* and *o-d*, and the ratio $a : o :: o : d$ will roughly represent the surface relations of the auricles and ventricles. Since distention of the auricles is a marked feature in a mitral lesion, the ratio should be larger than normal with mitral disease, and, since hypertrophy and dilatation of the ventricle bear a similar relation to an aortic lesion, it should be smaller in this condition.

Although the assumptions of the previous paragraph are scarcely justified by the conditions, it so happens that most of the errors tend to exaggerate the difference in ratio in the two classes of cases and we believe that the tables shown justify the acceptance of this ratio as an index of the heart form on empirical grounds alone. We have selected from the 170 orthodiagrams available all those which are technically satisfactory, which show definite enlargement and which have an adequate clinical diagnosis.

Our series of normal orthodiagrams is too small to allow of deductions. The indices of the few cases we have observed range between 0.534 and 0.704, but it is probable that the ratio is less fixed in normal than in pathological cases, because the greater mobility of the heart results in variations in the point *c*.

Our results have been tabulated according to conditions, the uncomplicated cases being separated from those showing such complications as might have some bearing on the shape of the heart, and the latter complications are noted in the last column.

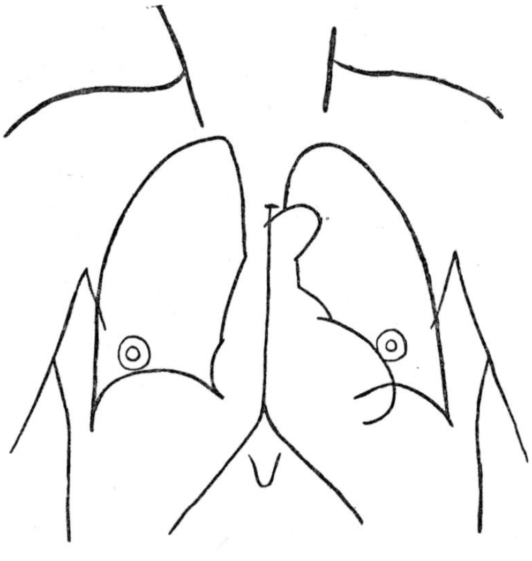

Fig. 8.—Arteriosclerosis. Prominent arch and transverse position. Case 99, M.R. 4.2 cm.; M.L. 10.4 cm.; long diameter 14.8 cm.; area 100; index .386.

It will be seen that all cases of mitral stenosis show an index in excess of .880, even in the presence of a complicating mitral regurgitation and irrespective of the degree of enlargement. This high value is due in part to the low position of the point *b*, because of the enormous enlargement of the left auricular shadow. This form of heart shadow is very striking and is almost pathognomonic of mitral stenosis.

The clinically uncomplicated mitral regurgitants range from 0.657 to 0.834 (Fig. 6). The two cases complicating nephritis have a value of 0.815 and 0.822, respectively; three cases combined with mitral stenosis exceed 1,000 while one case of mitral regurgitation and aortic regurgitation shows a value of 0.420, placing it more nearly with the latter condition.

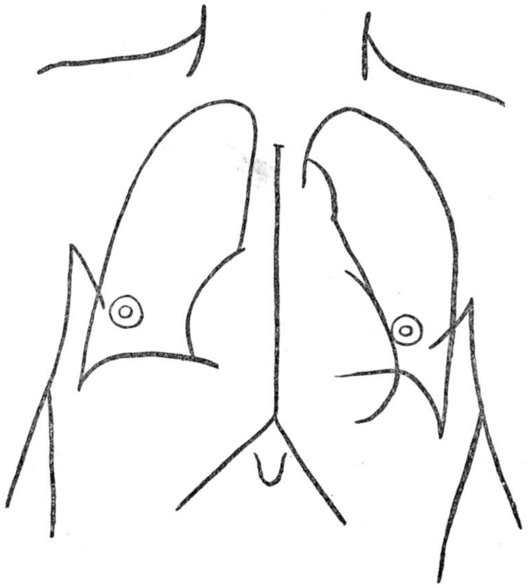

Fig. 9.—Chronic parenchymatous nephritis, mitral regurgitation, typical round heart, both following scarlet fever. Case 100. M.R. 6.8 cm.; M.L. 9.5 cm.; long diameter 16.8 cm.; area 172 sq. cm.; index .711.

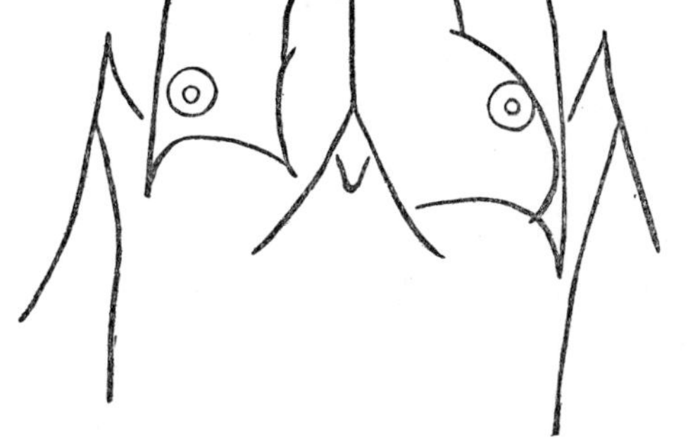

Fig. 10.—Chronic interstitial nephritis, signs of aortic regurgitation. Snub-nosed heart. Case 95. M.R. 4.4 cm.; M.L. 12.2 cm.; long diameter 17.7 cm.; area 177 sq. cm.; index .479.

Only one case of uncomplicated aortic regurgitation came under our observation and gave an index of 0.378 (Fig. 3). Of the cases showing higher than 0.400, one was complicated with pernicious anemia, and the other three showed well-marked mitral murmurs, probably as a result of dilatation. Two of the latter are also classified under the nephritics and show the largest areas in our series.

The class of arteriosclerotics is so poorly defined that only the most marked cases are noted. The index ranges between 0.282 and 0.393, with one exception (No. 84), which showed a perpetually irregular pulse, and

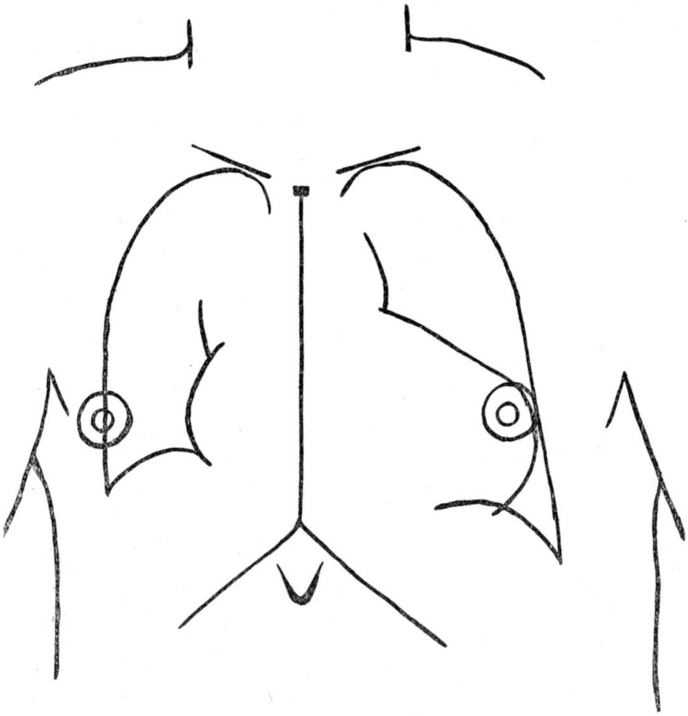

Fig. 11.—Chronic interstitial nephritis. Cardiac failure. Case 59. M.R. 6.1 cm.; M.L. 13.3 cm.; long diameter 19.3 cm.; area 186 sq. cm.; index .280.

this is held to account for the value of 0.492. The explanation of the low value in these cases is probably the low and transverse position of the heart (Fig. 8), due to the lengthening of the arch of the aorta. The result is to bring the point *c* higher up on the right auricle. The closely related group of angina pectoris shows similar relations.

Under the head of "myocarditis" have been grouped all the cases of cardiac failure without obvious lesions. Because of the difficulty of diagnosis, the number was limited to these five cases, although this probably represents only a small fraction of the total number. Two showed the permanent type of irregularity and two others are classified with the nephritics. The lowest value was found in the latter complication with relatively little insufficiency of the heart.

The group of nephritics shows a wide range in index as well as in area. We are not in a position to offer any interpretation of this variability. In a general way we find the cases with cardiac complaints at the lower end of the scale and those complaining of headaches, loss of vision, gastric complaints, etc., near the upper end.

The athletes were taken from long-distance runners and range well above the average, lying between 0.731 and 0.912. Casual inspection of

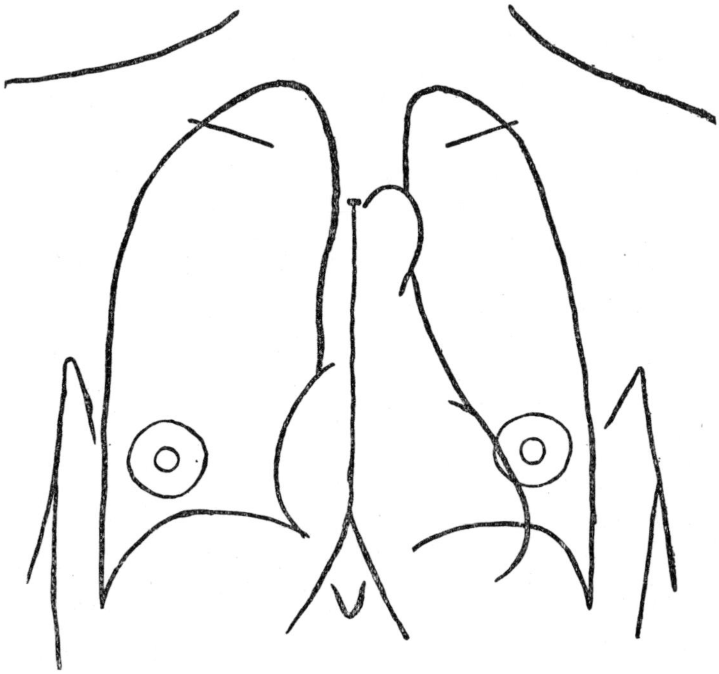

Fig. 12.—Athletic heart. Two-mile runner. Case 142. M.R. 5.3 cm.; M.L. 8.5 cm.; long diameter 14.5 cm.; area 98 sq. cm.; index .735.

the orthodiagram shows a pyriform shadow with a long and wide right auricular border on a comparatively transverse heart. The areas of these figures are all well within the maxima given by Dietlen.

As representatives of the heart form described as the pendulous heart, we have listed five cases of splanchnoptosis (Fig. 2). These hearts are all small, falling near or below the minima for their class. They are characterized by a very low position of the point *c*. Indeed, the auricular border may meet the vertebral shadow above the diaphragm so that the heart appears to be freely suspended above the diaphragm. In such case *c*, as defined above, does not exist and the meeting of the right border with the vertebral border must be taken as the lower extremity of the transverse diameter. The index accordingly ranges above 0.816. We believe that this high value may be taken as demonstrating that the thoracic viscera partake of the general relaxation and ptosis found in this remarkable condition.

Although our series of sixty cases is too small to allow of any but the broadest generalizations, we believe that we are justified in the conclusion that an abnormal index is an early evidence of the increase in size of one or more chambers of the heart and may occur before such

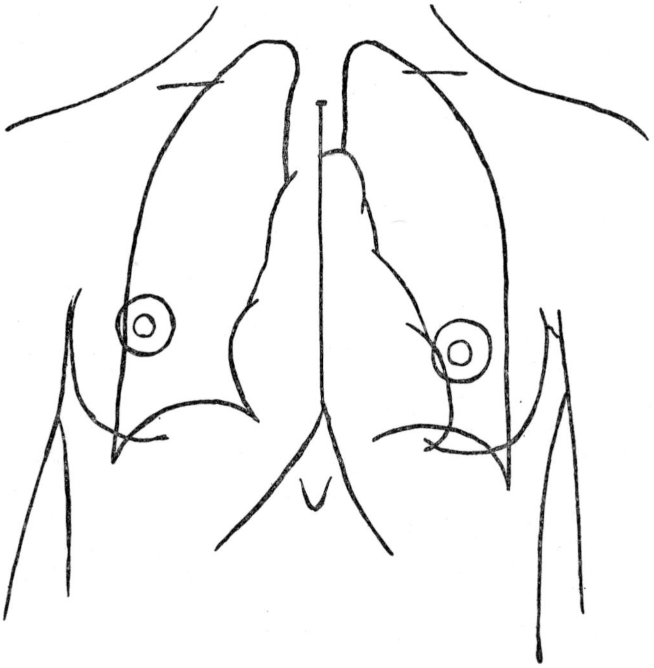

Fig. 13.—Diagram of a case showing a presystolic roll at the apex and a diastolic blow in the third left interspace. Pulse quick but not collapsing. The orthodiagram shows the form and index of mitral stenosis as against aortic regurgitation with an Austin Flint murmur. The latter lesion is either absent or must be insignificant. Case 170. M.R. 5.3 cm.; M.L. 7.2 cm.; long diameter 13.6 cm.; area 96 sq. cm.; index 1,000.

increase can be demonstrated by other means; that a decrease in the index results from left ventricular hypertrophy and dilatation, and an increase indicates a dilatation of the auricles with or without hypertrophy of the right ventricle. In combinations of these two antagonistic factors the index will depend on the predominance of the one or the other (Fig. 13). The wide variation shown in valvular diseases should make the index valuable in the diagnosis of doubtful or combined lesions, and it is hoped that the smaller fluctuations found associated with renal conditions may sometime be of diagnostic and prognostic value.

TABLE 2.—TABLES OF DIMENSIONS OF 60 ORTHODIAGRAMS CLASSIFIED ACCORDING TO DISEASES

| | | | | | | | | | Areas. | | | |
|---|---|---|---|---|---|---|---|---|---|---|---|---|
| Case. | Index. | Sex. | Age. | Weight. | M.R. | M.L. | Trans. | Long. | Planimeter. | Claytor's Est. | Author's Approx. | Complications |
| **Mitral Stenosis Uncomplicated** | | | | | | | | | | | | |
| 21 | 990 | F. | .. | 150 | 53 | 95 | 120 | 159 | 136 | 135 | 128 | |
| 139 | 1000 | F. | 48 | 145 | 45 | 82 | 111 | 128 | 81 | 99 | 77 | |
| 97 | 1030 | F. | 53 | 180 | 52 | 90 | 125 | 151 | 119 | 132 | 114 | |
| **Mitral Stenosis—Complicated** | | | | | | | | | | | | |
| 170 | 1000 | F. | 28 | 128 | 53 | 72 | 110 | 136 | ... | 105 | 96 | Mitral regurg. |
| 145 | 1040 | F. | .. | ... | 53 | 82 | 117 | 137 | 108 | 112 | 107 | Mitral regurg. |
| 60 | 1110 | F. | 22 | 130 | 46 | 96 | 105 | 150 | 113 | 111 | 110 | Mitral regurg. |
| 46 | 685 | M. | 60 | 125 | 68 | 90 | 130 | 173 | 141 | 157 | 133 | Perm. irreg'ty. |
| **Mitral Regurgitation—Uncomplicated** | | | | | | | | | | | | |
| 120 | 657 | F. | .. | 158 | 72 | 110 | 161 | 183 | 171 | 206 | 158 | |
| 47 | 690 | M. | 17 | 120 | 53 | 78 | 113 | 143 | 124 | 113 | 123 | |
| 57 | 706 | F. | 16 | 118 | 38 | 86 | 115 | 132 | 91 | 107 | 89 | |
| 55 | 714 | M. | 28 | 125 | 50 | 98 | 115 | 130 | 103 | 105 | 107 | |
| 31 | 781 | F. | 20 | 128 | 46 | 74 | 106 | 130 | 86 | 97 | 84 | |
| 96 | 834 | M. | 26 | 170 | 42 | 97 | 122 | 147 | 121 | 127 | 122 | |
| **Mitral Regurgitation—Complicated** | | | | | | | | | | | | |
| 49 | 420 | M. | 53 | 118 | 66 | 115 | 143 | 183 | 160 | 183 | 167 | Aortic regurg. |
| 76 | 815 | F. | 53 | 106 | 30 | 95 | 109 | 135 | 108 | 103 | 110 | Nephritis. |
| 100 | 822 | M. | 22 | 185 | 68 | 95 | 148 | 168 | 172 | 174 | 169 | Nephritis. |
| 26 | 936 | F. | 17 | 90 | 38 | 77 | 98 | 127 | 82 | 86 | 84 | Splanch'tosis. |
| 170 | 1000 | F. | 28 | 128 | 53 | 72 | 110 | 136 | ... | 105 | 96 | Mitral stenosis. |
| 145 | 1040 | F. | .. | ... | 53 | 82 | 117 | 137 | 108 | 112 | 107 | Mitral stenosis. |
| 60 | 1110 | F. | 22 | 130 | 46 | 96 | 105 | 150 | 113 | 111 | 110 | Mitral stenosis. |
| **Aortic Regurgitation** | | | | | | | | | | | | |
| 58 | 378 | M. | 26 | 127 | 45 | 94 | 108 | 148 | 115 | 112 | 112 | |
| **Aortic Regurgitation—with Complications** | | | | | | | | | | | | |
| 87 | 319 | M. | 62 | 136 | 33 | 117 | 113 | 152 | 107 | 121 | 104 | Arterioscl'sis. |
| 88 | 355 | M. | 52 | 136 | 61 | 132 | 161 | 205 | 211 | 231 | 208 | Nephritis. |
| 49 | 420 | M. | 53 | 118 | 66 | 115 | 143 | 183 | 160 | 183 | 167 | Mitral regurg. |
| 11 | 448 | M. | 61 | 126 | 50 | 107 | 112 | 177 | ... | ... | ... | Pernic. anemia. |
| 78 | 466 | M. | 48 | 140 | 56 | 124 | 136 | 175 | [150?] | 166 | ... | Nephritis. |
| 95 | 479 | M. | .. | 154 | 44 | 122 | 133 | 177 | 177 | 164 | 170 | |
| **Arteriosclerosis** | | | | | | | | | | | | |
| 80 | 282 | M. | 60 | 150 | 47 | 87 | 104 | 141 | 105 | 102 | 102 | |
| 143 | 336 | M. | 55 | 138 | 34 | 84 | 100 | 119 | 91 | 85 | 94 | |
| 118 | 393 | M. | 52 | 156 | 45 | 67 | 105 | 131 | 83 | 96 | 83 | |
| **Arteriosclerosis—Complicated** | | | | | | | | | | | | |
| 87 | 319 | M. | 62 | 136 | 33 | 117 | 113 | 152 | 107 | 121 | 104 | Aortic regurg. |
| 99 | 386 | M. | 62 | 138 | 42 | 104 | 110 | 148 | 100 | 114 | 101 | Nephr. angina. |
| 84 | 492 | M. | 71 | ... | 36 | 96 | 98 | 144 | 100 | 99 | 101 | P.I.P. |

| Case. | Index. | Sex. | Age. | Weight. | M.R. | M.L. | Trans. | Long. | Areas. Planimeter. | Areas. Claytor's Est. | Areas. Author's Approx. | Complications. |
|---|---|---|---|---|---|---|---|---|---|---|---|---|
| **Nephritis—Uncomplicated** | | | | | | | | | | | | |
| 59 | 280 | M. | 61 | 177 | 61 | 133 | 132 | 193 | 186 | 177 | 181 | |
| 77 | 304 | M. | .. | ... | 40 | 110 | 118 | 160 | 118 | 131 | 116 | |
| 68 | 445 | M. | 49 | 188 | 58 | 121 | 128 | 188 | ... | ... | ... | |
| 74 | 454 | M. | .. | ... | 40 | 120 | 110 | 193 | 136 | 148 | 144 | |
| 43 | 482 | M. | 56 | 126 | 40 | 118 | 108 | 165 | 114 | 126 | 109 | |
| 61 | 564 | M. | .. | ... | 38 | 93 | 116 | 133 | 101 | 108 | 101 | |
| 37 | 564 | M. | 57 | 125 | 58 | 69 | 109 | 136 | 92 | 103 | 88 | |
| 168 | 610 | M. | 53 | 103 | 40 | 108 | 129 | 161 | ... | 140 | 139 | |
| 158 | 728 | M. | 48 | 114 | 43 | 88 | 112 | 142 | 101 | 112 | 100 | |
| 154 | 755 | M. | 36 | 152 | 40 | 111 | 120 | 156 | 108 | 131 | 101 | |
| 85 | 793 | M. | 51 | 160 | 40 | 83 | 105 | 130 | 90 | 95 | 86 | |
| **Nephritis—Complicated** | | | | | | | | | | | | |
| 88 | 355 | M. | 52 | 136 | 61 | 132 | 161 | 205 | 211 | 231 | 208 | Aortic regurg. |
| 99 | 386 | M. | 62 | 138 | 42 | 104 | 110 | 148 | 100 | 114 | 101 | Arterioscl'sis. |
| 78 | 466 | M. | 48 | 140 | 56 | 124 | 136 | 175 | ... | ... | ... | Aortic regurg. |
| 95 | 479 | M. | .. | 154 | 44 | 122 | 133 | 177 | 177 | 164 | 170 | Aortic regurg. |
| 69 | 539 | M. | .. | ... | 40 | 120 | 119 | 180 | 163 | 150 | 167 | Myoc. insuf. |
| 67 | 561 | M. | 45 | 136 | 49 | 93 | 109 | 142 | 98 | 109 | 93 | Anemia. |
| 42 | 625 | F. | 54 | 134 | 50 | 103 | 120 | 156 | 123 | 131 | 123 | P.I.P. |
| 41 | 625 | M. | 64 | 129 | 48 | 134 | 145 | 184 | 164 | 187 | 167 | P.I.P. |
| 167 | 750 | M. | 50 | 120 | 43 | 113 | 127 | 162 | ... | 144 | 138 | Myoc. insuf. |
| 76 | 815 | F. | 53 | 106 | 30 | 95 | 109 | 135 | 108 | 103 | 110 | Mitral regurg. |
| 100 | 711 | M. | 22 | 185 | 68 | 95 | 148 | 168 | 172 | 174 | 160 | Mitral regurg. |
| **Angina Pectoris** | | | | | | | | | | | | |
| 94 | 450 | M. | 51 | 148 | 54 | 78 | 109 | 143 | 117 | 109 | 119 | |
| 79 | 495 | M. | .. | ... | 60 | 99 | 128 | 164 | 139 | 146 | 138 | |
| **Angina—Complicated** | | | | | | | | | | | | |
| 99 | 386 | M. | 62 | 138 | 42 | 104 | 110 | 148 | 100 | 114 | 101 | Nephritis. |
| **Myocardial Insufficiency** | | | | | | | | | | | | |
| 62 | 925 | M. | .. | ... | 51 | 137 | 145 | 187 | 163 | 190 | 160 | |
| **Myocardial Insufficiency with Complications** | | | | | | | | | | | | |
| 69 | 539 | M. | .. | ... | 40 | 120 | 119 | 180 | 173 | 150 | 167 | Nephritis. |
| 12 | 688 | M. | 67 | 170 | 48 | 103 | 124 | 152 | ... | ... | ... | P.I.P. |
| 167 | 750 | M. | 50 | 120 | 43 | 113 | 127 | 162 | ... | 144 | 138 | Nephritis. |
| 73 | 862 | M. | 32 | 152 | 56 | 106 | 111 | 176 | 162 | 163 | 166 | P.I.P. |
| **Athletes—Track Team** | | | | | | | | | | | | |
| 39 | 731 | F. | 24 | 108 | 34 | 84 | 103 | 142 | 100 | 101 | 103 | |
| 142 | 735 | M. | 23 | 158 | 53 | 85 | 117 | 145 | 98 | 119 | 92 | |
| 141 | 736 | M. | 28 | 123 | 42 | 95 | 113 | 137 | 96 | 109 | 92 | |
| 169 | 739 | M. | 22 | 155 | 50 | 84 | 122 | 135 | ... | 115 | 109 | |
| 156 | 768 | M. | 25 | 145 | 48 | 91 | 111 | 144 | 103 | 113 | 100 | |
| 149 | 781 | M. | 20 | 142 | 57 | 130 | 147 | 145 | 114 | 113 | 113 | |
| 157 | 825 | M. | 22 | 155 | 45 | 95 | 115 | 146 | 101 | 118 | 96 | |
| 140 | 841 | M. | 21 | 127 | 36 | 61 | 91 | 117 | 66 | 74 | 71 | |
| 146 | 912 | M. | 20 | 132 | 48 | 79 | 118 | 131 | 98 | 109 | 95 | |
| **Splanchnoptosis—Uncomplicated** | | | | | | | | | | | | |
| 115 | 816 | F. | 32 | 112 | 30 | 62 | 87 | 110 | 63 | 67 | 65 | |
| 126 | 830 | M. | 36 | 136 | 27 | 78 | 98 | 115 | 81 | 79 | 79 | |
| 2 | 1035 | F. | .. | 94 | 47 | 64 | 94 | 112 | 68 | 74 | 72 | |
| **Splanchnoptosis—with Complications** | | | | | | | | | | | | |
| 23 | 920 | F. | 17 | 102 | 27 | 79 | 83 | 122 | 79 | 71 | 84 | Chlorosis. |
| 26 | 936 | F. | 17 | 90 | 38 | 77 | 98 | 127 | 82 | 86 | 84 | Mitral regurg. |

# STUDIES OF MALARIA IN PANAMA. II. TREATMENT OF BLACKWATER FEVER

## PERNICIOUS MALARIA WITH HEMOGLOBINURIA AND ERYTHROLYTIC HEMOGLOBINURIA*

WALTER BREM, M.D.
COLON HOSPITAL, CRISTOBAL, CANAL ZONE

"Blackwater fever" is a term commonly used to designate fever with hemoglobinuria, associated more or less definitely with malaria. It embraces, I believe, two types of hemoglobinuria, which should be clearly differentiated for purposes of treatment and of study. The first type is associated with enormous numbers of malarial organisms, and, like the hemoglobinuria of piroplasmosis, its intensity is in direct relation to the severity of the infection. The mechanism of its production is, I am led to believe, the immediate destruction of erythrocytes by segmenting parasites, and differs from the mechanism of the second type, which is due, it is generally conceded, to the solution of erythrocytes by an unknown hemolysin (erythrolysis). I venture to propose, therefore, that the terms "blackwater fever," "malarial hemoglobinuria," "hemoglobinuric fever," etc., be abandoned as leading to confusion and possibly to grave errors in treatment, and that the two types of hemoglobinuria be described under a differential nomenclature.

*Type 1.*—Pernicious malarial fever with hemoglobinuria. The etiology is known and it is better that the condition or symptom of hemoglobinuria should not receive a more prominent place in the diagnosis.

*Type 2.*—Erythrolytic hemoglobinuria. Our knowledge of the etiology of this type is incomplete, and until an etiologic terminology can be rationally applied it would seem best to use one based on the mechanism of production, and on the most prominent feature of the symptom-complex.

If I may be permitted to do so, I shall employ this nomenclature.

### *PERNICIOUS MALARIAL FEVER WITH HEMOGLOBINURIA*

A typical example of this type is presented in the case reports (Case 1, Chart 1). The hemoglobinuria was anticipated from the examination of blood about thirty-four hours before it appeared; 15.6 per cent. of red blood corpuscles in the peripheral blood were infected; the urine had the characteristic appearance of "blackwater."

---

* Read at the seventh annual meeting of the American Society of Tropical Medicine, St. Louis, June 11, 1910.

Since my attention was drawn to the separation of this type of hemoglobinuria, eight patients with pernicious malaria have been admitted to the hospital, and in the urine of all we were able to demonstrate the presence of hemoglobin; in the last six the blood examination led us to suspect its imminence, and to foresee approximately the time of its onset.

The hemoglobinuria varies in degree from traces of hemoglobin in the sediment discernible only by special tests to the intensity of "blackwater." Two of the eight patients mentioned voided typical "blackwater" urine;

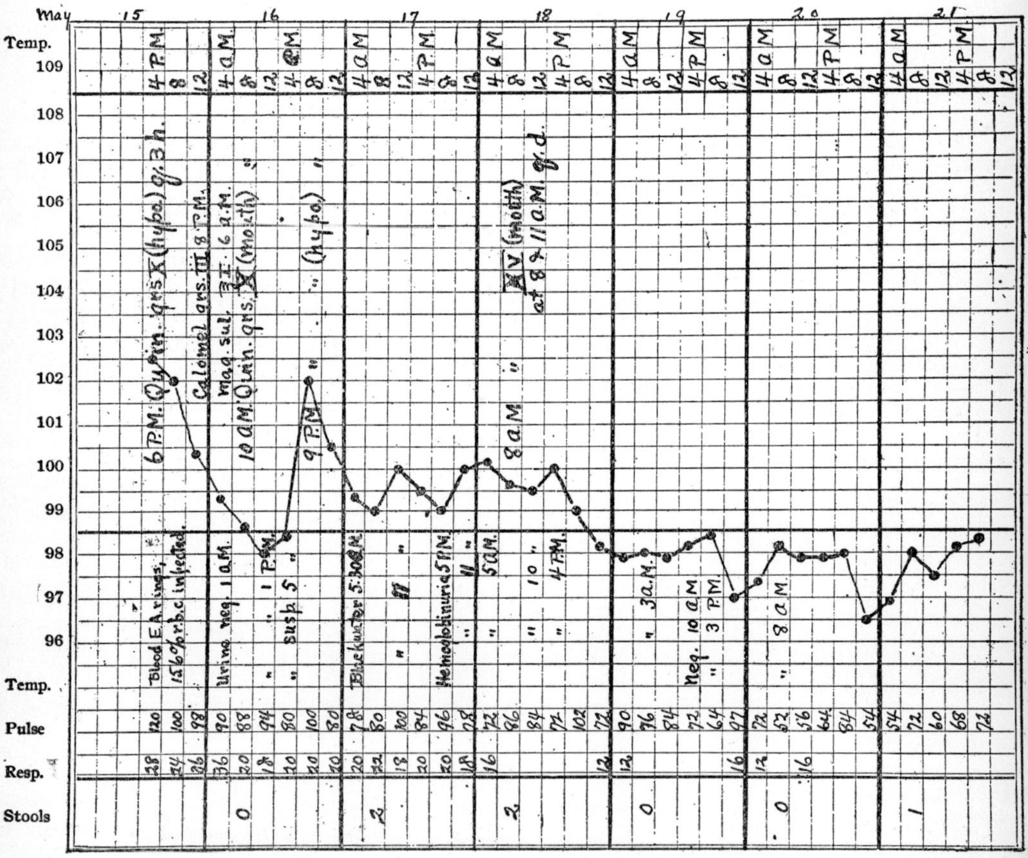


Chart 1.—Showing conditions in Case 1.—Pernicious malarial fever with hemoglobinuria.

three voided urine recognizable by the eye as probably hemoglobinous; one passed reddish-brown urine with a suggestive grayish-brown sediment; the other two, urine that, to the eye, gave no suggestion of hemoglobin, which was demonstrable only in the sediment. The guaiac and turpentine test for hemoglobin was employed. Controls were made by testing the urine of hundreds of patients with mild or moderate malarial infections, and uniformly negative results were obtained. I feel confident, therefore, in saying that a positive reaction of the urine to the guaiac and turpentine test means the presence of hemoglobin.[1] Only a definite blue color was considered as indicating a positive reaction.

It is my belief at present that future examinations will demonstrate hemoglobinuria at some time during the course of every pernicious malarial infection. In some of the cases an examination of each specimen voided must be made, the urine must be sedimented, preferably in a conical glass, and the sediment used in the test for hemoglobin. If this belief proves to be well founded, the mortality of this type will be the mortality of pernicious malarial fever. Of my eight patients, one died from the malarial infection, the capillaries of his brain being stuffed with parasites; another died, after his malarial infection was controlled, from a subsequent infection with an organism (isolated at autopsy from the spleen) apparently belonging to the typhoid-colon group, but possessing atypical fermenting properties (no malarial parasites were found in smears from the spleen, bone-marrow and brain); the other six made rapid recoveries. I have been able to recall four other cases and to find records of two more. One of the four was a fatal case seen in Baltimore in Osler's wards in the Johns Hopkins Hospital and mentioned by me in a former report.[2] Five of these six patients died. This mortality is very high, because the diagnosis was made from the gross appearance of the urine, and hemoglobinous urine of blackwater intensity occurs only in the most severe infections. Among twenty deaths that I have seen associated with blackwater, five of them, or 25 per cent., were due to pernicious malarial infections. It would seem, therefore, that a considerable percentage of deaths, heretofore reported as due to blackwater fever, were really due to pernicious malarial fever with hemoglobinuria, which fact has an important bearing on comparative mortality statistics under differ-

---

1. The following modification of the guaiac-turpentine test has been developed in the clinical laboratory of Colon Hospital for the examination of urine: Place 3 to 5 c.c. of urine containing sediment in a test-tube, add a few drops of glacial acetic acid; after a moment add 1 to 2 c.c. of ether and agitate gently, then a pinch of powdered guaiac resin, and lastly 10 to 20 drops of old turpentine. A pale blue to a blue-black color indicates a positive reaction, which may take a few moments to develop. If the ether does not separate well, a few drops of alcohol will facilitate the separation. The blue color may be brought out and the test rendered more delicate in doubtful cases by the following procedure: To the ether-turpentine mixture add chloroform drop by drop until all of the resultant mixture, except a thin layer, has been sunk to the bottom. To the thin layer remaining at the top, add carefully two or three drops of alcohol, then a few drops more of old turpentine. If inadvertently all of the ether-turpentine mixture has been sunk by adding too much chloroform, the alcohol and turpentine may be added as before and then a few drops of the sunken mixture recovered with a small pipette and added to the top layer.

2. Brem, W.: Malarial Hemoglobinuria, Jour. Am. Med. Assn., 1906, xlvii, 1896, 1992.

ent systems of treatment. Among twelve cases of blackwater fever in Panama, reported by Whipple,[3] in a pathologic study, three appear to have been of this type, and Whipple separates them from the ordinary type by designating them as "pernicious malaria and blackwater fever." Whipple made the important observation that the pathology of these cases, and, also, of pernicious malaria without apparent hemoglobimuria does not differ esssentially from that of "blackwater fever." Whipple did not observe evidence of hemoglobinuria in five other cases of pernicious malaria reported in the same study. But the detection of a mild

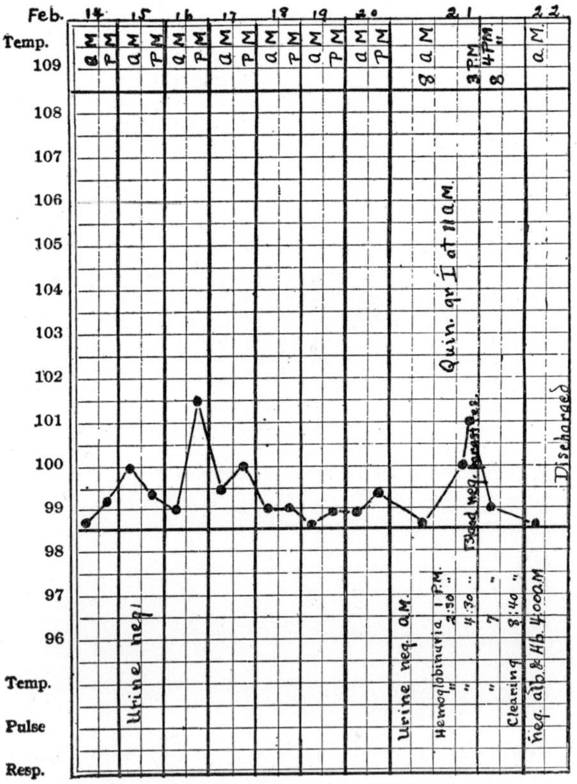


Chart 2.—No. 23,831. Patient, Frenchman, who had been on Isthmus six years, was admitted to Ancon hospital, Feb. 14, 1907. The patient had had several previous attacks of fever, "blackwater" being precipitated by quinin. The spleen was about 6 cm. below costal margin. The patient consented to take 1 grain of quinin as an experiment; blackwater followed in two hours. (Case from the clinic of Dr. A. B. Herrick, who kindly permits me to use it.)

grade of hemoglobinuria by a microscopic examination of kidneys would be a difficult or impossible task, and, as Whipple points out, the differ-

3. Whipple, G. H.: Blackwater Fever and Pernicious Malaria in Panama, Malaria, Leipsic, 1909, i, 4, 215.

ence in the pathology is one of degree and not of kind. Moreover, the hemoglobinuria of pernicious malarial fever seems to be in proportion to the absolute number of parasites, and in treated cases these are always decimated by quinin in the general circulation, while death is usually produced by those blocking the capillaries of the brain. This is well illustrated by one of Whipple's cases (No. 1431). As a rule, then, when treated patients come to autopsy, the hemoglobinuria has almost or entirely disappeared.

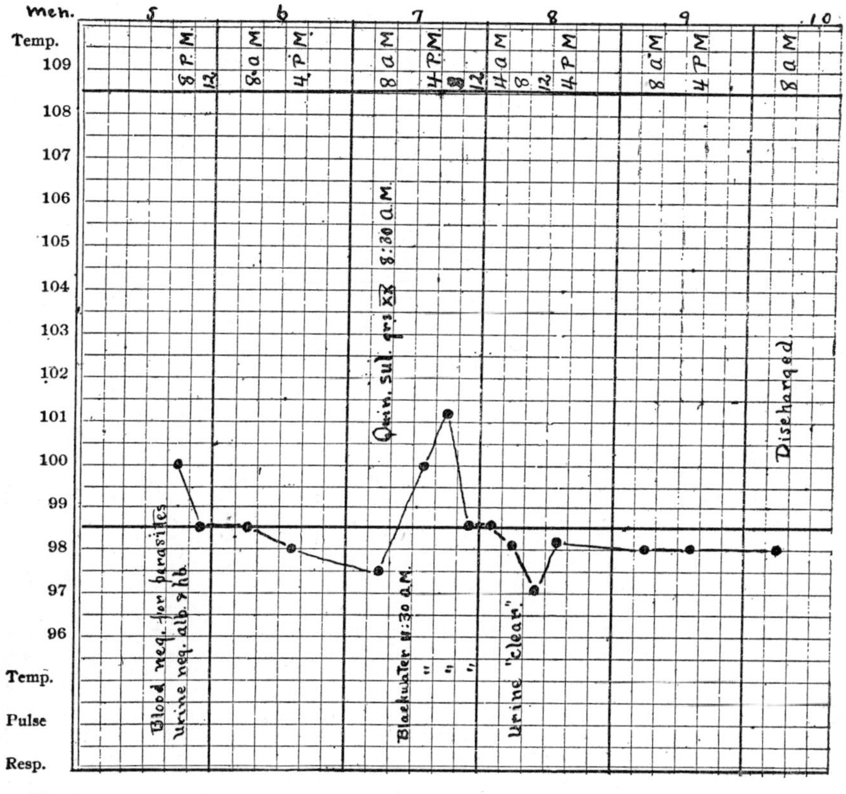


Chart 3.—No. 10,077. Patient, colored man from Antigua, W. I., who had been on the Isthmus five months, was admitted to Colon hospital, March 5, 1908. The patient passed "bloody urine" after taking quinin three weeks before admission. On the day before admission he felt sick and took 15 or 20 grains of quinin, after which he passed "bloody urine" again. After admission the urine was negative for albumin and hemoglobin. Quinin was withheld until the third day at 8:30 a. m., when 20 grains was given. "Blackwater" appeared at the third urination, two hours after quinin, and hemoglobinuria persisted until the next morning.

The differentiation of pernicious malarial fever with hemoglobinuria from erythrolytic hemoglobinuria rests chiefly on blood examinations. But occasionally parasites may not be numerous in the peripheral blood while they may be swarming in the internal organs. In such a case, cerebral symptoms (delirium, stupor or coma), which are rare in erythrolytic hemoglobinuria, may lead one to a correct diagnosis. The importance of the differentiation from the standpoint of treatment is obvious, for whatever may be one's belief regarding the treatment of erythrolytic hemoglobinuria, there can be no question but that in the pernicious malarial type the infection overshadows the hemoglobinuric condition, and that quinin in large doses must be introduced promptly into the blood-stream. If the patient is not vomiting and the attack seems only

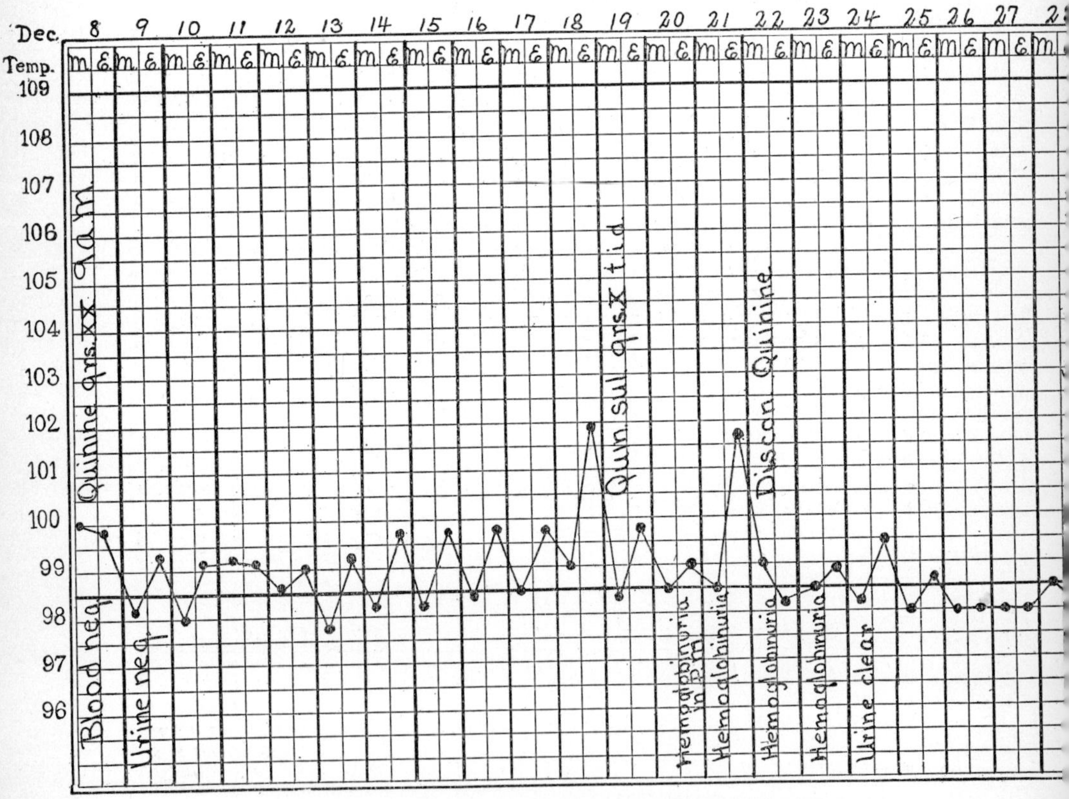


Chart 4.—No. 8,711. Patient, colored man from Jamaica, who had been in Panama two and a half years, was admitted to Colon hospital, Dec. 8, 1907. The patient had chill with blackwater Nov. 19, 1907, about nineteen days before admission. Hemoglobinuria did not follow one dose of quinin given on admission. After ten days quinin grs. x, t. i. d. was ordered, and hemoglobinuria developed the next day; it subsided when quinin was discontinued. The patient's brother was in the hospital at the same time with hemoglobinuria (Chart 15).

moderately severe, 10 grains of quinin in solution by mouth every three or four hours may be sufficient, the absorption being determined by tests for the drug in the urine. If vomiting supervenes, quinin must be given by intramuscular injection or intravenously. In the severer infections an intravenous injection of 15 or 20 grains should be given at once and repeated every eight hours, for four doses. Between these doses 15 or 20 grains should be given by mouth or, if necessary, by intramuscular injections. It should be one's object to destroy the parasites

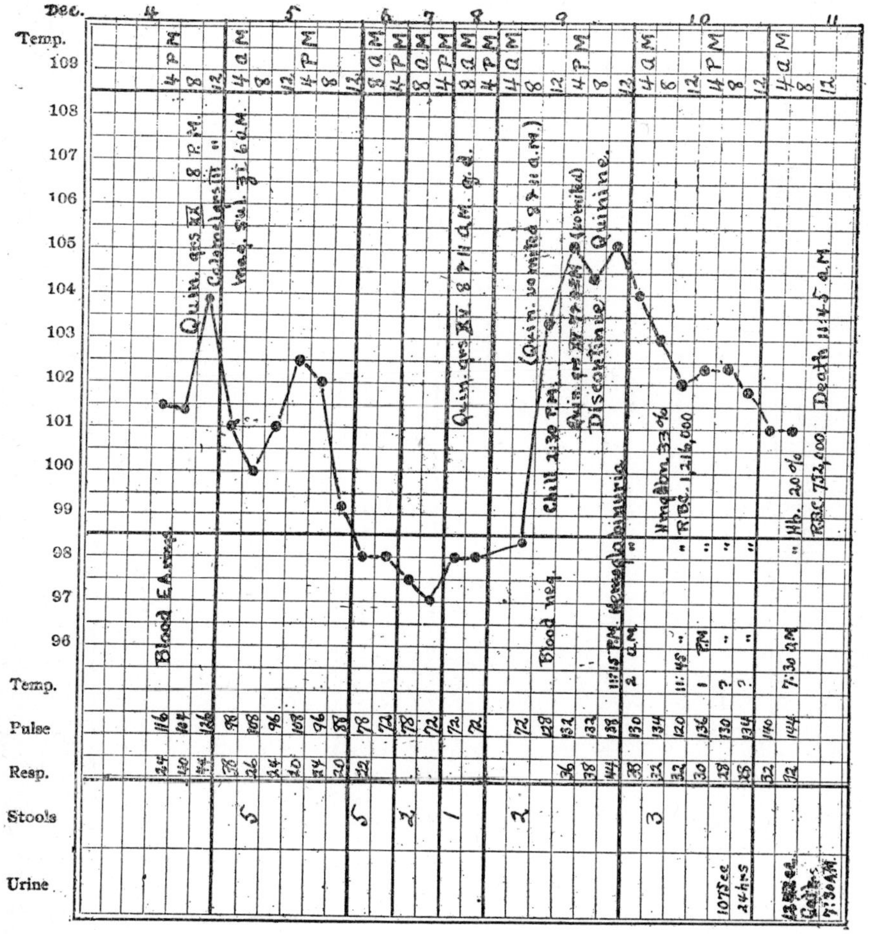


Chart 5.—No. 16,520. Patient, white, American, aged 21, from Fort Dodge, Iowa, who had been on the Isthmus four months, was admitted to Colon hospital, Dec. 4, 1908. The patient had had no previous malaria, had been sick three days and had taken quinin before admission. Quinin was ordered and 20 grains given on admission, but omitted by mistake afterward. The temperature dropped to normal and patient improved rapidly. On the third day of normal temperature the omission of quinin was discovered and it was re-ordered. On the following day a violent chill occurred, the temperature rose to 105, and hemoglobinuria followed. Quinin was discontinued, but the course was rapidly downward, urination was free, but blood destruction was extreme, and death took place forty-eight hours after the temperature began to rise.

in the intracorpuscular stage of the cycle, and thus to prevent them from reaching maturity. It seems certain that a large proportion of them can be killed in this stage, and the evidence is good that many infected corpuscles can be saved. (Case 1, hemoglobin and r. b. c. records).

### *ERYTHROLYTIC HEMOGLOBINURIA*

This type of hemoglobinuria is of course the common one and the one under special discussion in this paper. The material for my study has been collected from the records of Ancon Hospital from 1904 to

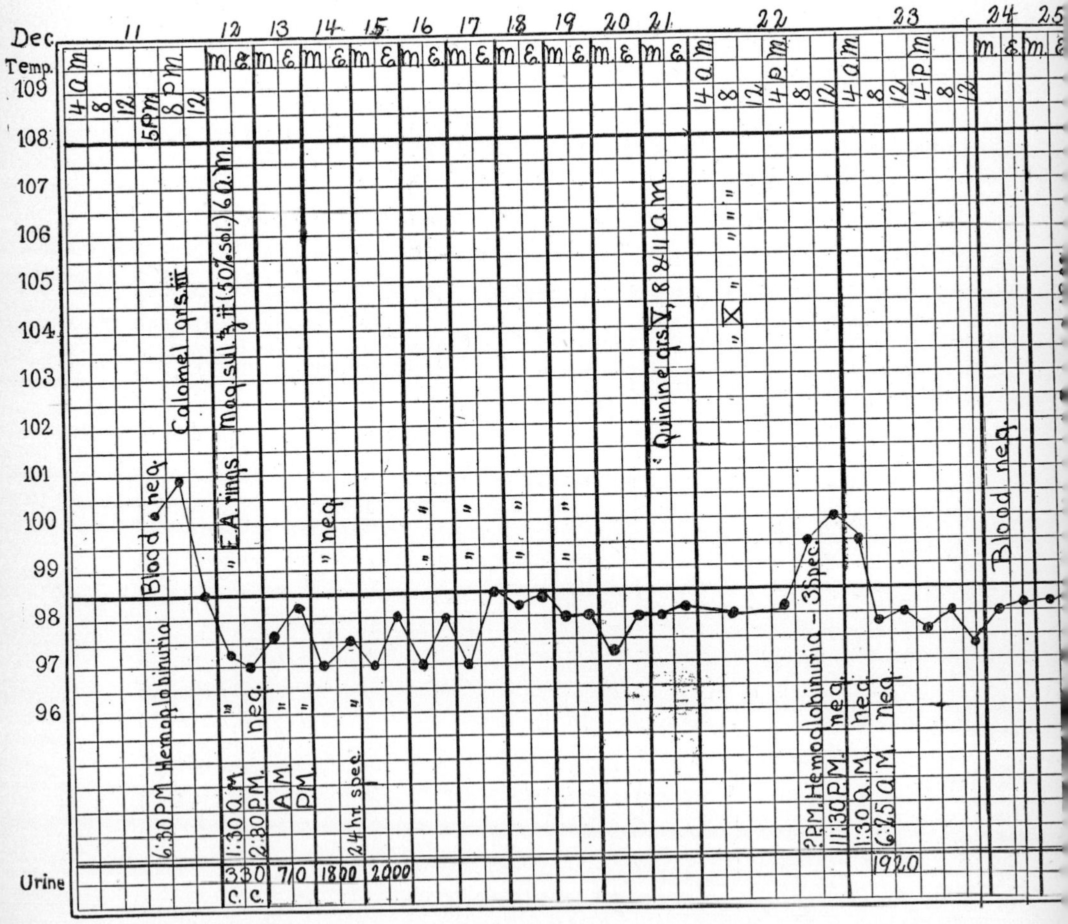


Chart 6.—No. 16,605. Patient, white, Austrian, who had been on the Isthmus one year, was admitted to Colon hospital, Dec. 11, 1908. The patient had had three previous attacks of "blackwater," had been sick two days, and had taken a quinin tablet every day for past ten days. On the morning of Dec. 11 the patient took 15 grains of quinin and at 4 p. m. noticed "blackwater." There was hemoglobinuria on admission. Estivo-autumnal (E. A.) parasites were found on second day. Quinin, grains x, were given on December 21 and grains xx on December 22. A transient hemoglobinuria followed.

April, 1910, 162 cases, and Colon Hospital from November, 1907, to May, 1910, fifty-nine cases—a total of 221 cases. For certain reasons all of the records of Colon Hospital prior to November, 1907, and many of the records of Ancon Hospital were not accepted and the cases excluded. There were eighteen recurrences in the hospitals among the 221 cases, and these have been considered separate attacks, since it sometimes happened that an initial attack was treated by one method while the recurrence was treated by another. The recurrences were considered separate attacks only when a period of not less than two days of hemoglobin-free urine intervened between attacks. There were, then, 239 attacks of blackwater represented by the 221 cases. These 221 cases include twenty cases previously reported by Gorgas,[4] which in turn included fourteen cases reported by me.[2] They include, also, Herrick's nine cases referred to in my report.[5]

The 221 cases have been divided into two series, the first of which includes cases directly or indirectly under my care, the second all other cases.

*Series 1.*—My cases, seventy-three patients, eighty-four attacks. (Hemoglobinuria verified in almost every attack by the demonstration of hemin crystals or by the guaiac and turpentine test.)

*Series 2.*—Other cases, 148 patients, 155 attacks. (Hemoglobinuria often verified by above tests and diagnosis often made from appearance of urine with a heavy transient albuminuria.)

### GENERAL TREATMENT

The most important general measure is the introduction of fluids by mouth, by rectum, subcutaneously or intravenously. The passage of a large quantity of urine is of the utmost importance, for the gravity of the prognosis increases with a decreased urinary output, and the majority of patients who die have suppression of urine. Sweat baths and the various diuretics may be tried, but I think that little is to be expected from them, and there is always a possibility of drug irritation of the affected kidneys. In a large number of the cases of Series 2, however, Basham's mixture was used as a routine procedure, and there appears to have been no injury done by it, although no good either. The bowels should be opened with calomel (3 to 5 grains is sufficient) followed by a saline cathartic; or, if vomiting prevents, enemas may be used.

The diet should consist of nourishing liquids, and during convalescence the patient's appetite may be the guide.

---

4. Gorgas, W. C.: Malaria in the Tropics, Jour. Am. Med. Assn., 1906, xlvi, 1417.
5. In order that no confusion may arise in future leading to repeated reports for mortality statistics of the same cases, a list of the hospital numbers of the cases included in this report is appended.

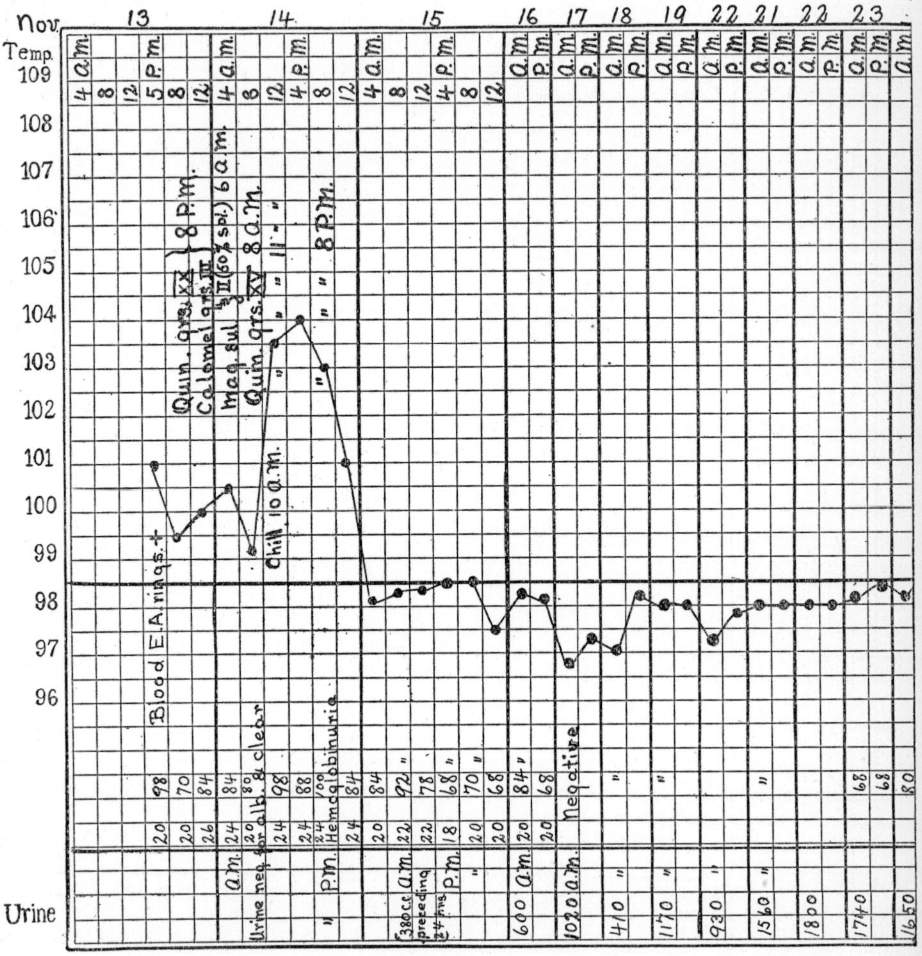


Chart 7.—No. 16,141. Patient, white, Spaniard, who had been in Panama nineteen months, was admitted to Colon Hospital July 25, 1909. The patient had had six previous attacks of malaria, and had been sick one day with present illness. Both attacks of hemoglobinuria in the hospital were apparently precipitated by quinin. Estivo-autumnal parasites were found on six separate examinations. Quinin was discontinued when hemoglobinuria developed, but when death approached quinin was ordered to be given by intramuscular injection. Autopsy was made fifteen hours after death. No parasites were found in smears from the brain, spleen, bone-marrow and liver.

For vomiting and restlessness morphin in repeated small doses given hypodermically is harmless and by far the most useful and satisfactory remedy. Crushed ice, also, may be useful.

Strychnin is the most satisfactory stimulant in cardiac or respiratory depression.

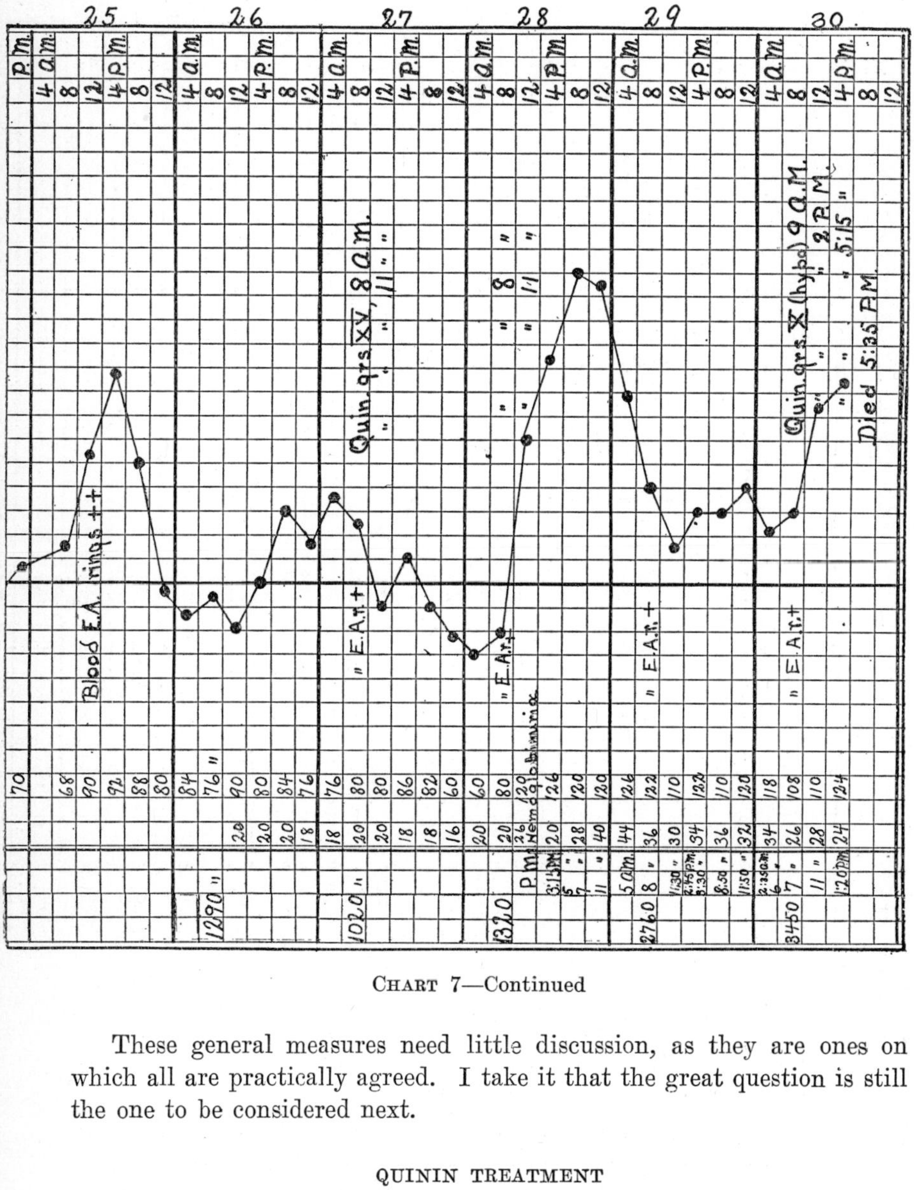

CHART 7—Continued

These general measures need little discussion, as they are ones on which all are practically agreed. I take it that the great question is still the one to be considered next.

## QUININ TREATMENT

### *Relation of Quinin to Etiology.*

Before one discusses whether or not it is wise to use quinin in the treatment of erythrolytic hemoglobinuria, it is meet that one's confession of faith be made regarding the relation that quinin bears to the onset of the disease. In Charts 2 to 11 inclusive, evidence that seems to be conclusive is presented in favor of the view that in certain cases, whatever may be the predisposing condition, quinin is the exciting cause. On the other hand, the recurrences in Charts 11, 12 and 13 furnish evidence that in other cases the onset may be in no way connected with the drug. The negative quinin history in the case represented by Chart 14 seems to be reliable. I have previously reported another attack occurring in an intelligent American who denied having taken quinin before the passage of blackwater.[2] The onset of many other attacks in this series was apparently associated with quinin (Chart 16), and in many the his-

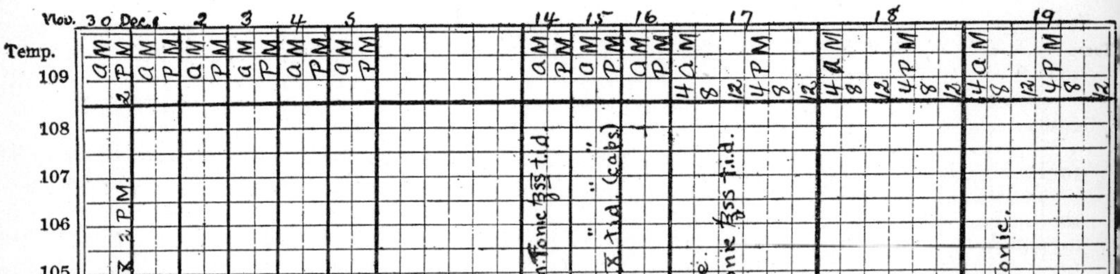


Chart 8.—No. 50,017. Patient, white, Spaniard, who had been on the Isthmus four and one-half months, was admitted to Ancon Hospital Nov. 30, 1908. The patient had been sick and passing "blackwater" five days before admission; had been jaundiced four days. "Blackwater" was present on admission. Recurrence followed iron and quinin tonic, which contained 15 grains of quinin in one ounce.

tory was indefinite or not solicited. The charts referred to represent the attacks most strikingly illustrating the truth in the views that quinin is and is not the exciting cause. That the number of striking instances of attacks precipitated by quinin is greater than the number arising without it is due, partly at least, to the fact that evidence in favor of the latter view is more difficult to obtain. More or less fever usually precedes the onset of blackwater, and residents practically always take quinin on the slightest suggestion of fever. It follows, then, that nearly all patients who have hemoglobinuria in Panama have taken quinin before the onset, but it would be absurd to conclude that quinin precipitated the condition in every case or even in the majority of cases.

To sum up, I am sure that a few attacks of erythrolytic hemoglobinuria are precipitated by quinin, and also that a few develop without

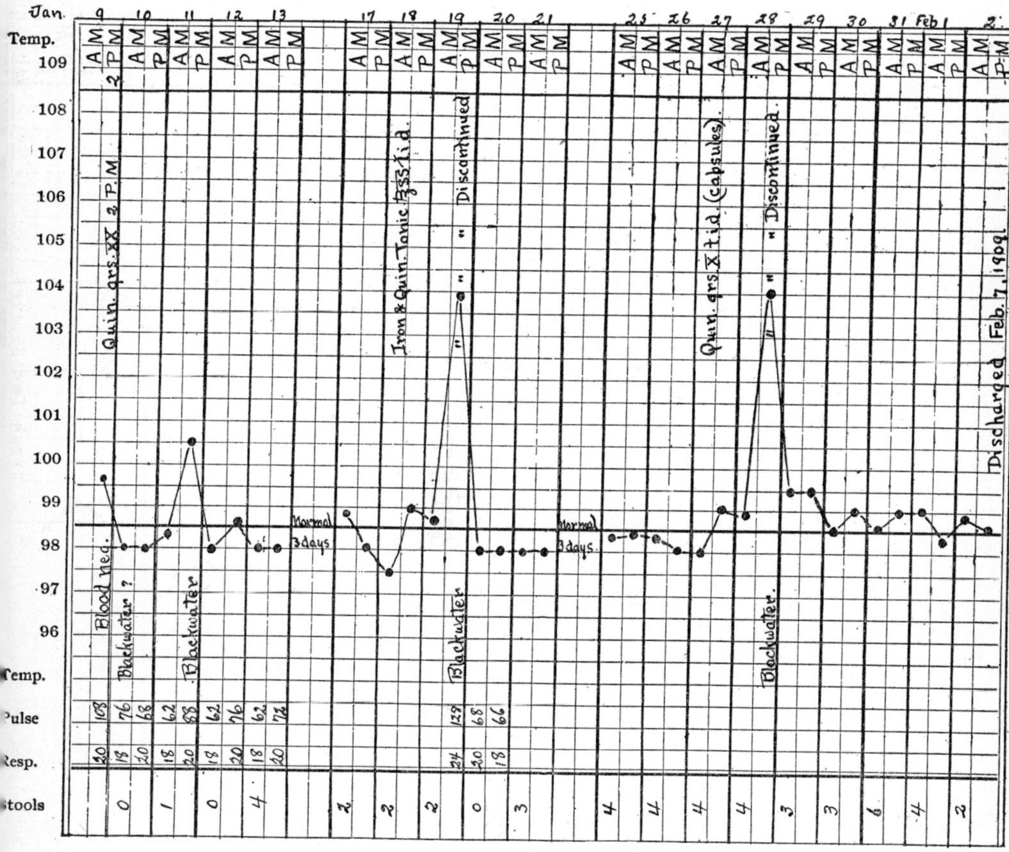


Chart 9.—No. 52,291. Patient, white, Jamaican, who had been on the Isthmus two years, was admitted to Ancon Hospital, Jan. 9, 1909. The patient had had "blackwater" on one previous admission to hospital. He had been sick three days and passed "blackwater" on day before second admission. Presence or absence of "blackwater" on admission was not stated in record. Iron and quinin tonic, 15 grains quinin to one ounce was given, and "blackwater" followed.

quinin, and good evidence is afforded that such is the case. I believe that a considerable number of the attacks that remain are precipitated by quinin and that a larger number are not connected with the drug, but I cannot present evidence in proof.

Our knowledge, so far, of the part that quinin plays in the etiology of erythrolytic hemoglobinuria does not aid us greatly, therefore, in settling the question of its use in the treatment. Attacks that are precipitated by quinin (such as those represented by Charts 2 to 11) of course should not be treated with quinin. But these attacks cannot be definitely separated from others except in occasional recurrences that take place

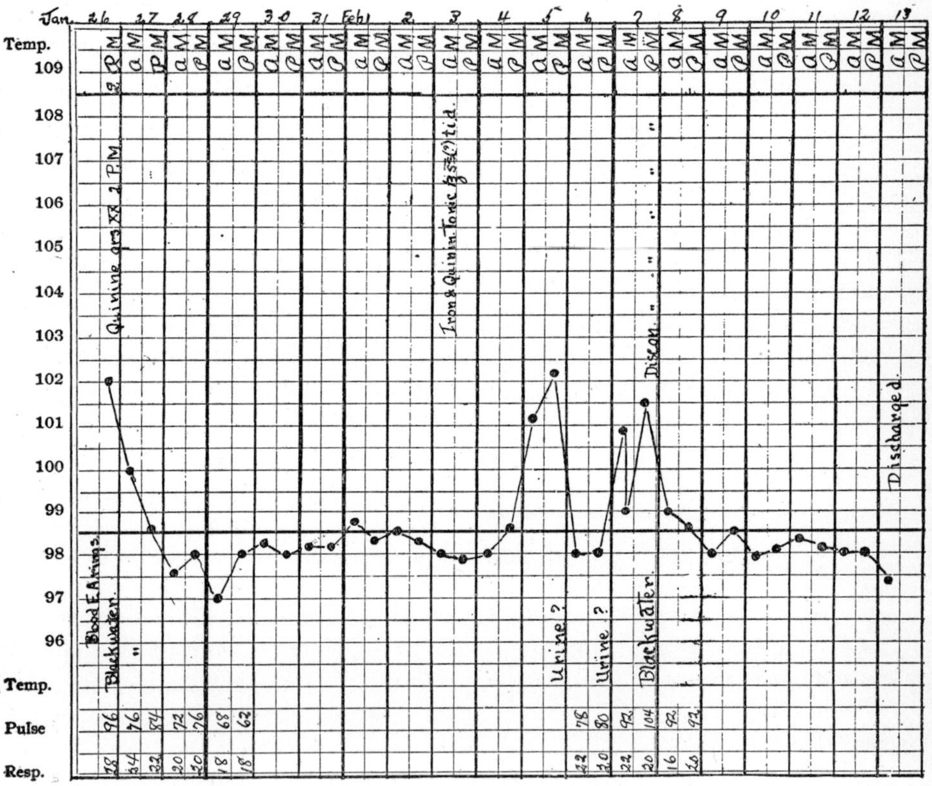


Chart 10.—No. 53,409 (Ancon). Patient, white, Italian, who had been on the Isthmus twenty-four months, was admitted to Ancon Hospital, Jan. 26, 1909. The patient had been previously admitted to hospital because of "blackwater"; had left hospital only nine days before second admission. He had been sick five days. The night before admission he passed "blackwater." Character of urine February 5 and 6 was not recorded, and the dose of iron and quinin tonic was not stated in record, probably half an ounce three times a day or quinin 7½ grains t. i. d.

while the patient is under observation and which follow promptly the administration of quinin after a period of apyrexia and hemoglobin-free urine.

One must turn to statistical studies and his own personal observations for guidance in a matter about which there is so much genuine difference of opinion.

*Statistical Study*

Deaderick's compilation of statistics in his recent book[6] practically settles the matter in favor of treatment without quinin. The summary is as follows:

| | Cases. | Deaths. | Mortality. |
|---|---|---|---|
| Treated with quinin................ | 1821 | 472 | 25.9 % |
| Treated without quinin.............. | 1006 | 112 | 11.1 % |
| Treatment mixed or not recorded..... | 3210 | 684 | 21.3 % |

Deaderick thinks that "this number of cases probably eliminates all errors and should be convincing," in which opinion he is probably correct. My own statistics tend to confirm the above compilation, but the result is not nearly so striking. The difference may be partly a matter of interpretation, for I have found it not always an easy matter to classify a given case, and I have separated no class as having received mixed treatment, for the following reason. During the latter part of 1907 and the first eight months of 1908 we were treating all cases of blackwater fever with quinin in large quantities, usually by intramuscular injections. The treatment was never curtailed in severe cases, and all of the attacks could be placed frankly among those treated with quinin. In September, 1908, we began to treat a series of cases without quinin, and a certain number of them were of course severe and proceeded towards a fatal termination. It sometimes happened that the ward physician in immediate charge of such a case felt that nothing was being done for the patient, and the natural desire was that an attempt be made to do something, the courage required to watch the battle without interference failed, and the patient received quinin (Chart 7). It would certainly be misleading to take these fatal cases out of the class treated without quinin, for the mortality of this class would thereby be artificially lowered. I cannot but believe that this has happened to some extent in the statistics that Deaderick has done such able work in collecting. As for the mortality of the class treated with quinin, it is certain that in it have been placed all those cases of pernicious malaria in which hemoglobinuria was recognizable as "blackwater," and that these cases, belonging to the severest type of the disease, have very much increased the mortality of the class. After all is said, however, the difference is so great that one would be, perhaps, ultracritical not to accept the general indication of the statistics in favor of withholding quinin in erythrolytic hemoglobinuria.

An attempt has been made in analyzing the cases of this report to avoid errors like those indicated above, and the cases have been placed

6. Deaderick: Practical Study of Malaria, W. B. Saunders Co., Philadelphia, 1909, p. 299.

in the class to which they belonged when the course was downward and the prognosis became grave. This was sometimes a difficult question to decide, but in the main I think that the result is trustworthy.

Table 1.—Result of Treatment With and Without Quinin

SERIES I: WRITER'S CASES, SEVENTY-THREE PATIENTS, EIGHTY-FOUR ATTACKS

| Treated with quinin— | Attacks. | Deaths. | Mortality. |
|---|---|---|---|
| Whites | 31 | 4 | 12.9 % |
| Blacks | 10 | 4 | 40. % |
| Total | 41 | 8 | 19.5 % |
| Treated without quinin— | | | |
| Whites | 28 | 5 | 17.8 % |
| Blacks | 15 | 2 | 13.3 % |
| Total | 43 | 7 | 16.3 % |

SERIES II: OTHER CASES, ONE HUNDRED FORTY-EIGHT PATIENTS, ONE HUNDRED FIFTY-FIVE ATTACKS

| Treated with quinin— | Attacks. | Deaths. | Mortality. |
|---|---|---|---|
| Whites | 36 | 5 | 13.9 % |
| Blacks | 18 | 5 | 27.8 % |
| Total | 54 | 10 | 18.5 % |
| Treated without quinin— | | | |
| Whites | 83 | 12 | 14.5 % |
| Blacks | 18 | 3 | 16.6 % |
| Total | 101 | 15 | 14.8 % |

SERIES I AND II: TWO HUNDRED TWENTY-ONE PATIENTS, TWO HUNDRED THIRTY-NINE ATTACKS

| Treated with quinin— | Attacks. | Deaths. | Mortality. |
|---|---|---|---|
| Whites | 67 | 9 | 13.4 % |
| Blacks | 28 | 9 | 32.1 % |
| Total | 95 | 18 | 18.9 % |
| Treated without quinin— | | | |
| Whites | 111 | 17 | 15.3 % |
| Blacks | 33 | 5 | 15.2 % |
| Total | 144 | 22 | 15.3 % |

The mortality of the white patients of each series and of the combined series shows a difference, under the two methods of treatment, so small that one death credited to the group of quinin-treated cases would even up the percentages. This difference is within the limits of error in classification. The mortality of colored patients treated without quinin is almost exactly equal to that of white[7] patients, while of those treated with quinin more than double the percentage died. As far as the statistics go, therefore, they appear to indicate that in regard to life it makes little difference whether or not white patients receive quinin, while from colored patients it should be withheld.

## *Personal Observations*

In a former communication[2] I concluded that quinin was strongly indicated in "malarial hemoglobinuria," that it should be given in large doses, and that properly given it appeared to be almost a specific. I beg

7. The kidneys of blacks appear to be much more susceptible to injurious influences than the kidneys of whites.

leave here to abandon that view, which I consider now to be erroneous. In spite of the fact that my mortality statistics present only qualified support of the antiquinin view, observation of a fair number of cases treated by both methods has convinced me that quinin does no good in any case of erythrolytic hemoglobinuria, and that in many it is emphatically injurious. With it the patients usually suffer more, the disease is more frequently severe, and in many instances the fever and the passage of blackwater are prolonged in a manner that one rarely sees when quinin is withheld (Chart 16). Weight is added to this view by the cases cited in which quinin certainly precipitated the attack, and by the less striking evidence that there are numbers of other instances in which the drug was probably responsible for the onset. In a number of cases, also, hemoglobinuria persisted while quinin was being given, but promptly ceased when it was withheld (Chart 15).

TABLE 2.—RESULT OF TREATMENT WITH AND WITHOUT QUININ IN BOTH THE PRESENCE AND ABSENCE OF MALARIAL PARASITES

| | PARASITES PRESENT | | | | | | PARASITES ABSENT | | | | | |
|---|---|---|---|---|---|---|---|---|---|---|---|---|
| | Quinin+ | | | Quinin— | | | Quinin+ | | | Quinin— | | |
| | No. attacks. | No. deaths.. | Mortality per cent.. | No. attacks. | No. deaths.. | Mortality per cent.. | No. attacks. | No. deaths.. | Mortality per cent.. | No. attacks. | No. deaths.. | Mortality per cent.. |
| Whites (Series 1)..... | 7 | 1 | 14.3 | 15 | 3 | 20 | 24 | 3 | 12.5 | 13 | 2 | 15.4 |
| Whites (Series 2)..... | 18 | 4 | 22.2 | 31 | 4 | 12.9 | 18 | 1 | 5.6 | 52 | 8 | 15.4 |
| Total (Series 1 and 2).. | 25 | 5 | 20.0 | 46 | 7 | 15.2 | 42 | 4 | 9.5 | 65 | 10 | 15.4 |
| Blacks (Series 1)..... | 3 | 1 | 33.3 | 7 | 1 | 14.3 | 7 | 3 | 42.9 | 8 | 1 | 12.5 |
| Blacks (Series 2)..... | 9 | 1 | 11.1 | 3 | 1 | 33.3 | 9 | 4 | 44.4 | 15 | 2 | 13.3 |
| Total (Series 1 and 2).. | 12 | 2 | 16.7 | 10 | 2 | 20.0 | 16 | 7 | 43.7 | 23 | 3 | 13.0 |
| Whites and blacks (Series 1)........... | 10 | 2 | 20.0 | 22 | 4 | 18.2 | 31 | 6 | 19.4 | 21 | 3 | 14.3 |
| Whites and blacks (Series 2)........... | 27 | 5 | 18.5 | 34 | 5 | 14.7 | 27 | 5 | 18.5 | 67 | 10 | 14.9 |
| Total (Series 1 and 2).. | 37 | 7 | 19.0 | 56 | 9 | 16.1 | 58 | 11 | 19.0 | 88 | 13 | 14.8 |

### *Relation of Malarial Parasites to Quinin Therapy*

Writers on blackwater fever have usually divided the cases into two groups according to the presence or absence of malarial parasites in the peripheral blood, and have recommended that quinin be employed in treating the first group and withheld from the second. Deaderick[8] and Stephens[9] are exceptions to this rule. It is Deaderick's opinion that "the only conditions in which quinin is indicated are, first, where the parasites show no tendency to disappear after forty-eight hours from onset; second, in the infrequent cases of intermittent hemoglobinuria where the outbreak corresponds with parasitic sporulation." Stephens goes a little

8. Deaderick: Practical Study of Malaria, p. 383.
9. Stephens: Osler's Modern Medicine, i, 458.

further and says, "if parasites still persist with a continuance of the fever then the question must be carefully weighed...If it can be avoided we should say it is better to abstain." Deaderick was unable to divide the cases of which he collected reports into groups according to the presence or absence of parasites. The attacks of the present report, however, can be grouped in such a manner and they bear on this point.

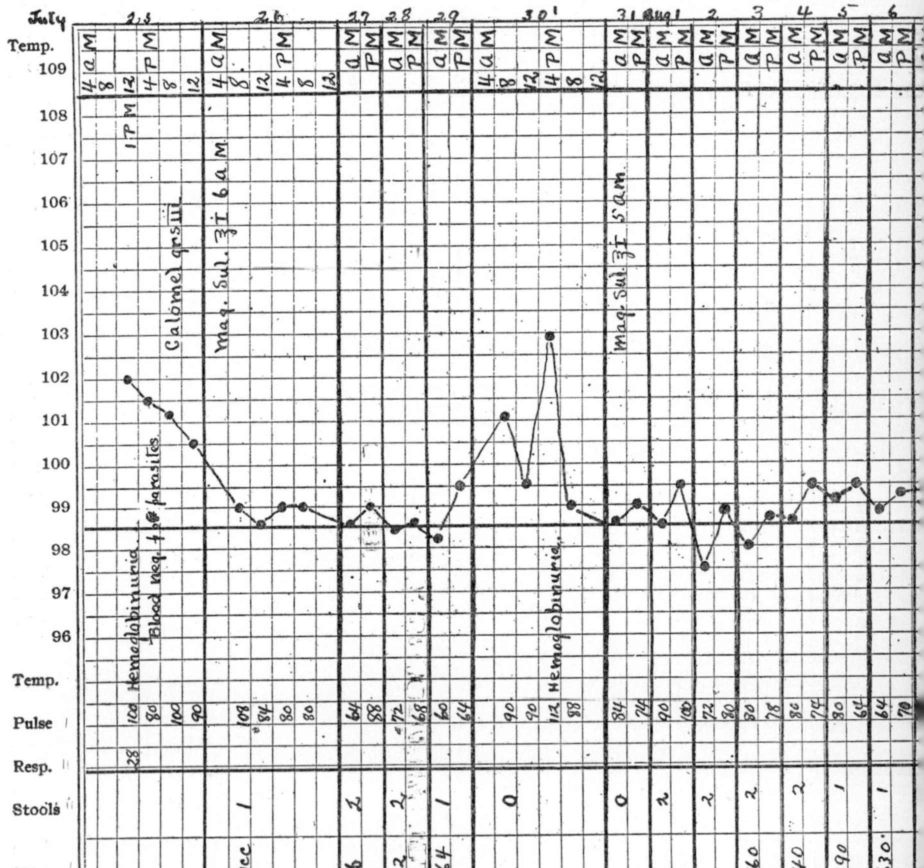


Chart 11.—No. 19,162. Patient, white, Spaniard, who had been on the Isthmus nineteen months, was admitted to Colon Hospital July 25, 1909. The patient had had malaria eight times previously, and before admission had been sick three days; had taken quinin and on the second day had passed "blackwater." He had been taking 9 grains of quinin daily before onset of the present illness. There were two recurrences; one arose spontaneously and one after taking quinin.

The whites of the "parasites present" group show a considerably higher mortality with quinin treatment than without it; the whites of the "parasites absent" group show a higher mortality without quinin than with it. The mortality among the blacks occurs somewhat more according to expectation. The mortality of the combined whites and blacks of both groups is slightly smaller in the attacks treated without quinin. Therefore the presence or absence of malarial parasites appears to make no difference in the mortality. Nor have I been able to detect any difference in the clinical courses of members of the two groups.

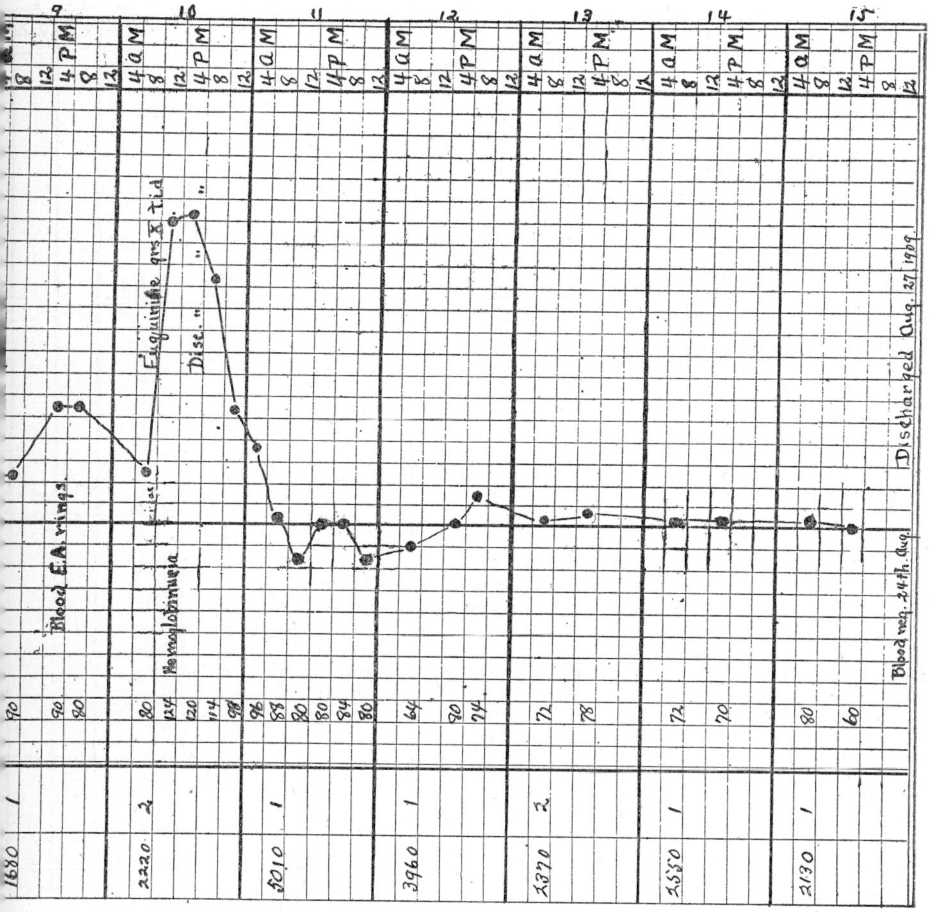


CHART 11—Continued

It is my opinion, therefore, that Deaderick and Stephens are quite right, as far as they go, in advising the withholding of quinin in most cases of blackwater fever, even if parasites be present in the blood. I should go a little further, however, and say that quinin should never be given during the passage of blackwater in cases belonging frankly to the erythrolytic type of hemoglobinuria. If parasites persist in or return to the peripheral blood during convalescence, as frequently happens, or if a malarial type of fever recurs, quinin may be given with caution, beginning with small doses and gradually increasing. It may be fatal to begin at once with large doses of quinin (See Chart 7).

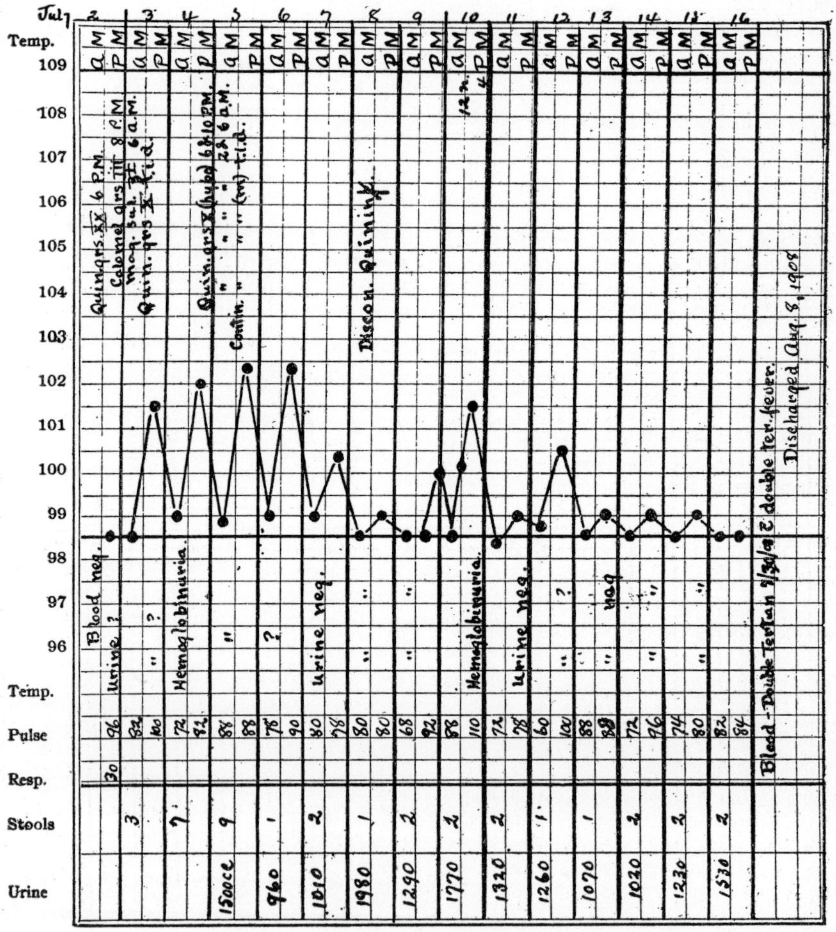


Chart 12.—No. 12,145. Patient, white, Spaniard, who had been on the Isthmus six months, was admitted to Colon Hospital July 2, 1908. The patient had had no previous malaria (?)—the present being the first time in hospital—and had never passed black urine. The patient had been sick four days and had taken quinin in solution twice daily since onset. The urine was "highly colored," but not black. It is not certain from the record whether or not the patient had "blackwater" on admission. It apparently developed on the third day in the hospital. There was a recurrence three or four days after hemoglobinuria had ceased and two days after quinin had been discontinued. The double tertian infection possibly occurred in the ward. Quinin was given, 10 grains, t. i. d., and "blackwater" did not develop.

## *Serum Therapy*

It would scarcely be proper to close without referring to the work of Christophers and Bentley[10] and their suggestion that a serum therapy, such as that used in paroxysmal hemoglobinuria, is possibly in sight. Their work on iso-agglutinins and isohemolysins and their conclusions[11]

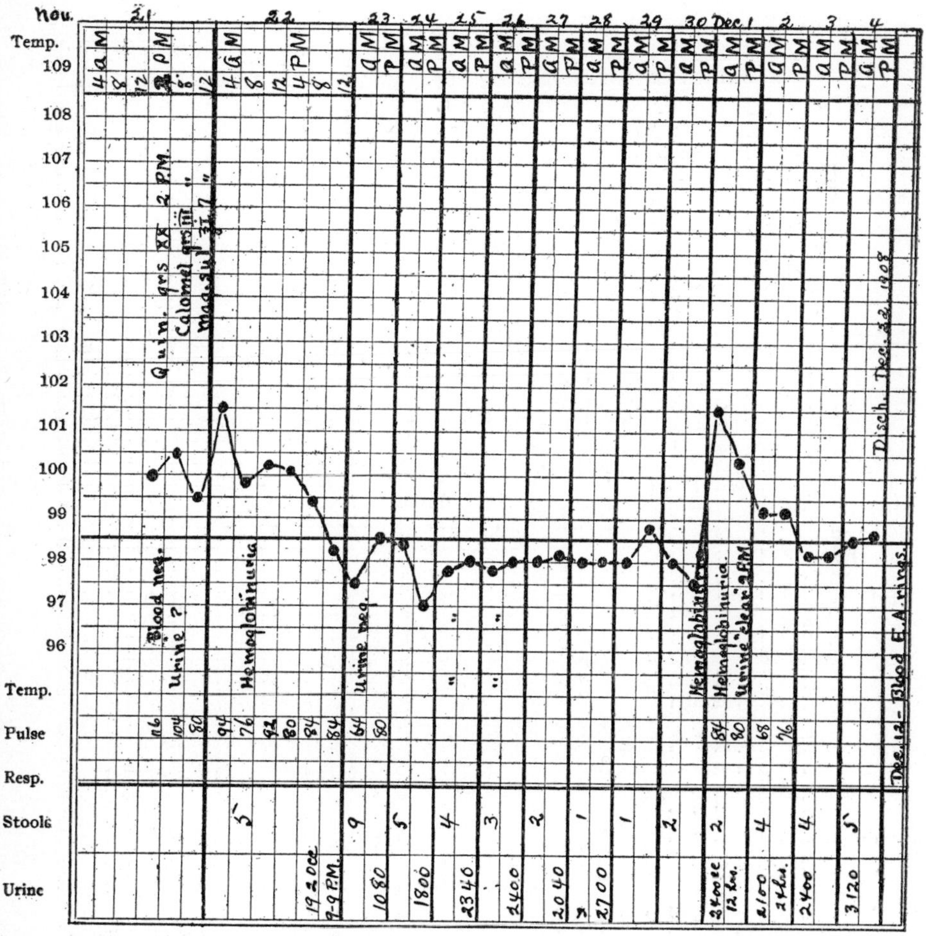

Chart 13.—No. 49,539. Patient, white, Portuguese, who had been on the Isthmus fifteen months and in hospital four times, was admitted to Ancon Hospital Nov. 21, 1908. The patient had been sick three days, passing "blackwater" two days. There was spontaneous recurrence of hemoglobinuria. Fever recurred on Dec. 12 and estivo-autumnal organisms were found. The patient was given 30 grains of quinin daily without recurrence of "blackwater."

10. Christophers and Bentley: Blackwater Fever, Scient. Mem. Gov. India. (new series), 1908, No. 35, pp. 181, 182.

11. Christophers and Bentley: Blackwater Fever, Scient. Mem. Gov. India. (new series), 1908, No. 35, pp. 154-179.

are interesting, but in the light of Moss'[12] recent extensive and excellent studies of normal and pathologic bloods, it seems probable that they misinterpreted their results, attributing to the influence of malaria merely normal variations of serums and corpuscles. When their monograph came into my hands, I attempted to repeat some of their work,

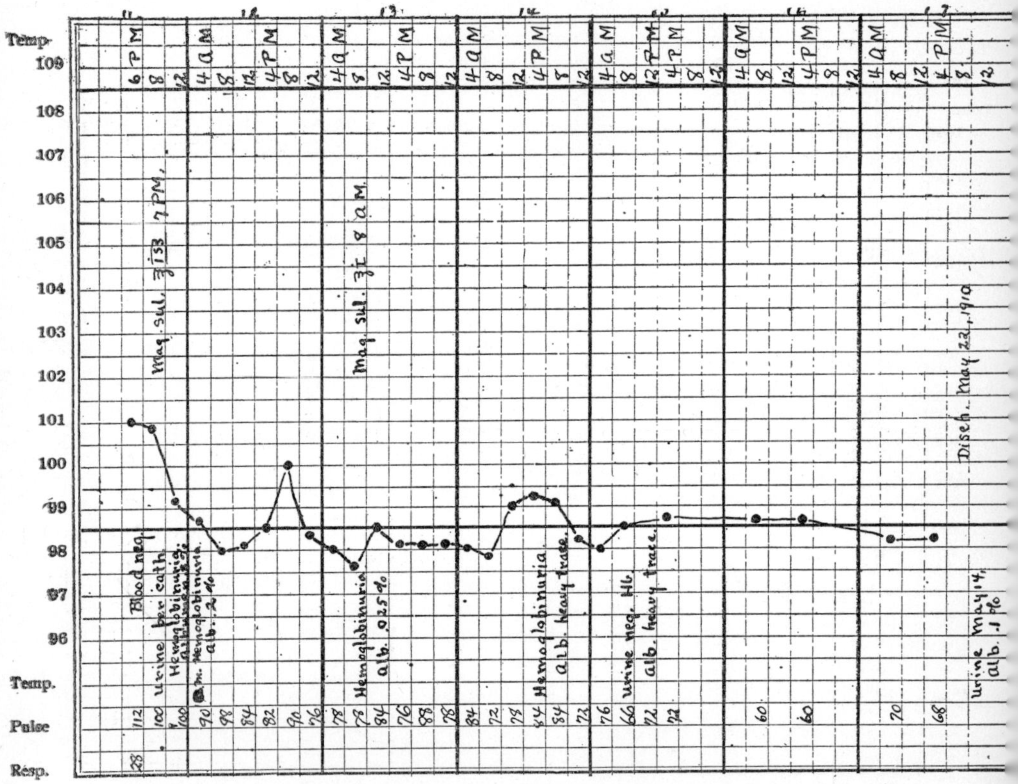


Chart 14.—No. 23,174. Patient, colored woman, Jamaican, who had been on the Isthmus two years, was admitted to Colon Hospital, April 11, 1910. The patient had had several light attacks of fever in Jamaica, but no "ague," and took no quinin, and one prolonged attack of fever three months after coming to Isthmus. She then took medicine, but did not think it was quinin. She has had a little fever now and then during past eight months, but took no quinin. The patient was eight months pregnant; first baby. In the present illness of two days convulsions occurred before admission and a severe one shortly afterward. The patient was semicomatose, passed very little urine. She had taken no quinin. There was no uterine hemorrhage. Urine per catheter showed hemoglobinuria, albumin 0.8 per cent. (Esbach). Recovery was good. Patient did not abort. On May 4 the patient developed toxemia and labor was induced under stovaine anesthesia. Good recovery and child lived. Urine on May 14 showed albumin 0.1 per cent., hyaline and hyalogranular casts.

---

12. Moss, M. L.: Isoagglutinins and Isohemolysins, Bull. Johns Hopkins Hosp., 1910, xxi, 63.

but in the beginning I met results which were incapable of explanation by their hypotheses, and which were explained only when Moss' paper appeared. Moss was able to classify all human bloods into four groups according to the agglutinating reactions of serums and corpsucles. With this classification as a working basis, we shall be able now to approach the study of the blood in erythrolytic hemoglobinuria with a degree of comprehension hitherto not possessed.

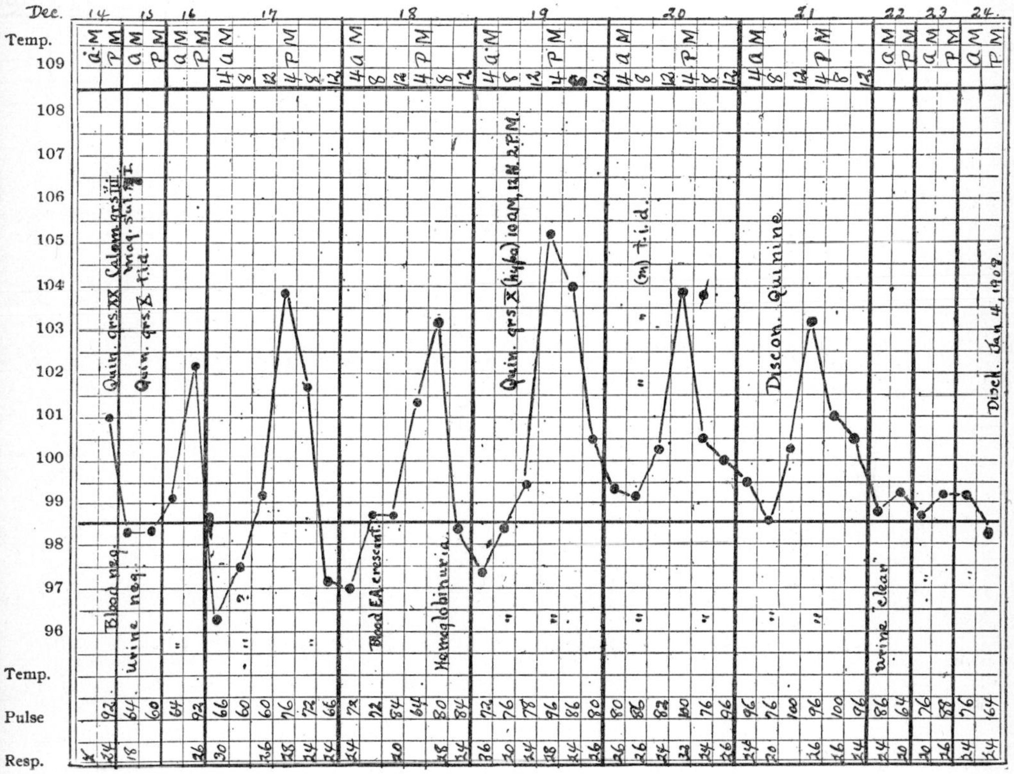


Chart 15.—No. 8,877. Patient, colored man, Jamaican, who had been on the Isthmus three years, was admitted to Colon Hospital Dec. 14, 1907. The patient had "blackwater" fever in Jamaica, 1903; no quinin had been given previous to onset; patient treated with quinin and "blackwater" lasted six days. "Blackwater" fever again occurred on the Isthmus, March, 1907, but the patient did not remember whether or not he took quinin before onset; he was then treated with quinin by intramuscular injection, and "blackwater" continued five days. On present admission no "blackwater," which was apparently precipitated by quinin and continued until quinin was discontinued. Patient's brother was in hospital at same time with "blackwater," apparently precipitated by quinin (Chart 4).

## *SUMMARY*

1. Blackwater fever is a term that includes two types of hemoglobinuria more or less definitely associated with malaria. It is important

that the two types be separated for study and treatment. The indications for treatment are diametrically opposed. The two types probably differ in the mechanism of their production and their clinical phenomena are different.

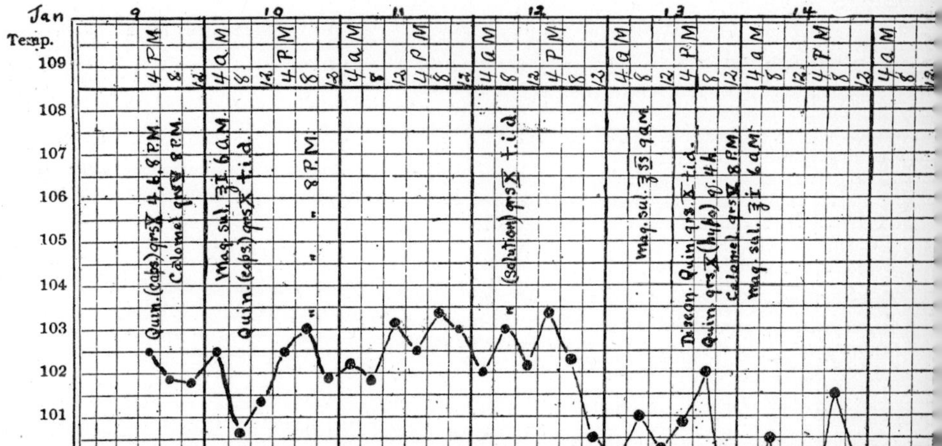


Chart 16.—No. 9,322. Patient, white, Australian, who had been on the Isthmus over three years, was admitted to Colon Hospital, Jan. 9, 1908. The patient had had fever three times previously. "Blackwater" fever occurred three years ago on the Isthmus. Onset occurred Jan. 7, 1908, with chill and fever; January 8, chill fever and "blackwater." Quinin history was not recorded. There was no "blackwater" on admission, but continued fever, possibly "post-hemoglobinuric." Quinin in solution was given on January 12 and hemoglobinuria developed that night. The patient was treated vigorously with quinin. Prolonged, severe course followed. The hemoglobin fell to 30 per cent. January 18. Widal test was negative January 18 and 22.

2. Type 1.—Hemoglobinuria associated with pernicious malarial infections. The hemoglobinuria is probably brought about by immediate destruction of erythrocytes by enormous numbers of sporulating parasites, and the time of its appearance can generally be foretold with a

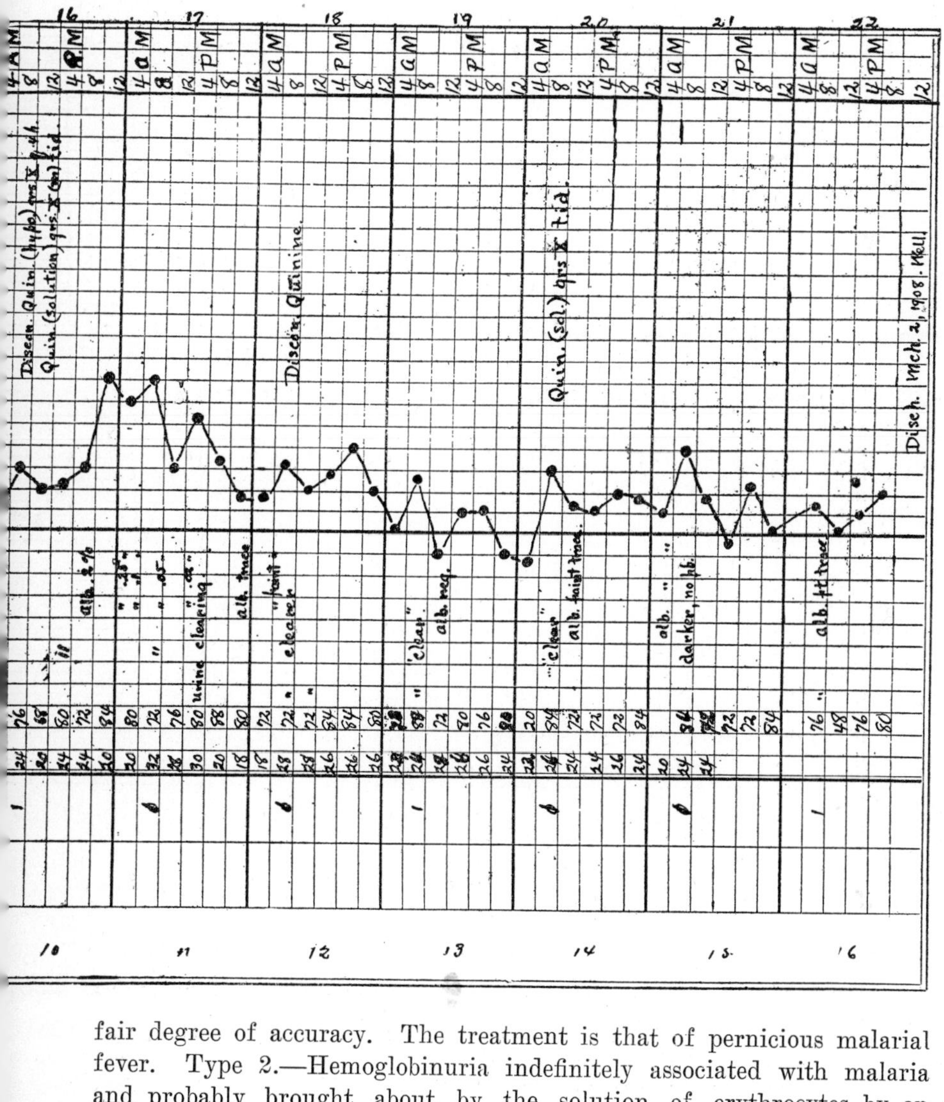


fair degree of accuracy. The treatment is that of pernicious malarial fever. Type 2.—Hemoglobinuria indefinitely associated with malaria and probably brought about by the solution of erythrocytes by an unknown hemolysin.

3. It is proposed that the terms "blackwater fever," "malarial hemoglobinuria," "hemoglobinuric fever," etc., be abandoned and that the two types of hemoglobinuria hitherto embraced by them be known as follows:

*Type 1.*—Pernicious malarial fever with hemoglobinuria.
*Type 2.*—Erythrolytic hemoglobinuria.

4. A number of attacks of erythrolytic hemoglobinuria in this series of cases were precipitated by quinin, a large number of attacks were apparently precipitated by quinin, and a few recurrent attacks developed in the wards when no quinin had been given.

5. Statistical studies of 239 attacks of erythrolytic hemoglobinuria, supplemented by personal observation indicate that quinin should never be given during hemoglobinuria.

6. The presence of malarial parasites in the blood of patients with erythrolytic hemoglobinuria has no effect on the mortality or on the clinical phenomena, and affords no indication for treatment during hemoglobinuria. When parasites persist or reappear during convalescence or when fever persists or recurs after the cessation of hemoglobinuria, quinin should be given guardedly. The dose should be small at first and gradually increased, if hemoglobinuria is not precipitated.

## REPORT OF CASES[13]

CASE 1 (Chart 1).—Pernicious malarial fever with hemoglobinuria, No. 23,811.

BLOOD EXAMINATIONS

| Time. | Hemoglobin (Sahli hemom.). | R. B. C. per c.mm. | Color index | Number R. B. C. counted. | Number infected. | Percentage infected. |
|---|---|---|---|---|---|---|
| 15— p. m. | .. | ........ | .. | 500 | 78 | 15.6 |
| 16— 9:00 a. m. | .. | ........ | .. | 500 | 47 | 9.4 |
| 16—10:00 a. m. | 85 | ........ | .. | .... | .. | .... |
| 16—11:30 a. m. | .. | ........ | .. | 500 | 27 | 5.4 |
| 16— 4:00 p. m. | .. | ........ | .. | 500 | 23 | 4.6 |
| 16— 4:30 p. m. | 85 | 4,760,000 | .89 | .... | .. | .... |
| 16— 7:00 p. m. | .. | ........ | .. | 500 | 18 | 3.6 |
| 16—12:00 m. | .. | ........ | .. | 500 | 9 | 1.8 |
| 17— 4:00 a. m. | .. | ........ | .. | 3,500 (approx.) 20 fields* | 16 | .46 |
| 17— 8:30 a. m. | .. | ........ | .. | 4,500 (approx.) 25 fields | 6 | .13 |
| 17— 9:30 a. m. | 93 | 5,192,000 | .9 | .... | .. | .... |
| 17— 4:00 p. m. | .. | ........ | .. | 5,000 (approx.) 25 fields | 5 | .1 |
| 18— 8:00 a. m. | 93 | 4,872,000 | .95 | 50 fields | 0 | 0 |
| 18— 3:00 p. m. | .. | ........ | .. | 50 fields | 0 | 0 |
| 19—10:00 a. m. | .. | ........ | .. | 50 fields | 0 | 0 |
| 19— 4:00 p. m. | 91 | ........ | .. | .... | .. | .... |
| 20— 1:30 p. m. | 84 | 5,008,000† | .84 | .... | .. | .... |
| 25—10:00 a. m. | 81 | ........ | .. | .... | .. | .... |

13. Only Case 1 is discussed in detail. Synopses of the other cases (2-16) appear as legends under the respective charts.

* B. and L. objective 1/12 and ocular 1. Actual counts of the corpuscles in a number of fields in which the corpuscles were more and less thickly spread varied from 175 to 250 per field. The estimates were made from these standards, taking into consideration the thickness of the smear.

† 8:30 a. m.

| | | | | | | | |
|---|---|---|---|---|---|---|---|
| 16— 1:20 a. m. | Brownish-red | 1,028 | Acid | Heavy trace (boiling) | Negative .......... | Mucous cloud... | A few hyaline and hyalo-granular casts; no r. b. c. |
| 16— 1:30 p. m. | Brownish-yellow | 1,033 | Acid | Faint trace ...... | Negative .......... | None.......... | A few hyaline and hyalo-granular casts; no r. b. c. |
| 16— 4:40 p. m. | Brownish-yellow | 1,030 | Acid | Trace ............ | Suspicious ......... | Pus Shred...... | A few hyaline and hyalo-granular casts; no r. b. c. + pus cells |
| 17— 5:30 a. m. | Blackwater, dark, cloudy, smoky, brownish-red by transmitted light | 1,028 | Alk. | Will not settle in Esbach tube; 25 per cent. wet | Intense reaction..... | Heavy, grayish-brown | Brown amorphous detritus; numerous hyalo-granular casts, covered with brown material; no r. b. c. |
| 17—11:00 a. m. | Blackwater, yellowish-red, less intense | 1,025 | Acid | Heavy trace...... | Supernatant urine; 1-100 dil. is robin-blue; sediment is blue-black (1-100) | Heavy, greenish brown | Brown amorphous detritus; numerous hyalo-granular casts, covered with brown material; no r. b. c. |
| 17— 5:15 p. m. | Suggests black water, brownish-red, less intense | 1,023 | Acid | Heavy trace...... | Mixed urine; 1-10 dil. is violet-blue | Heavy, greenish brown (less) | Brown amorphous detritus; numerous hyalo-granular casts, covered with brown material; no r. b. c. (fewer casts) |
| 17—10:40 p. m. | Yellowish-red, not like blackwater | .... | .... | Trace ............ | Supernatant urine; 1-10 is violet-blue | Mucous cloud... | Brown amorphous detritus; numerous hyalo-granular casts, covered with brown material; no r. b. c. (few casts) |
| 18— 4:45 a. m. | Yellowish-red, not like blackwater | .... | .... | Trace ............ | Undiluted urine is violet-blue | Mucous cloud... | Brown amorphous detritus; numerous hyalo-granular casts, covered with brown material; no r. b. c. (few casts) |
| 18—10:20 a. m. | Yellowish-red, not like blackwater | .... | Acid | Faint trace ...... | Undiluted urine is violet-blue | Mucous cloud... | Brown amorphous detritus; numerous hyalo-granular casts, covered with brown material; no r. b. c. (few casts) |
| 18— 4:30 p. m. | Yellowish-red, not like blackwater | .... | Acid | Very faint........ | Supernatant urine is negative; sediment is violet-blue | Very slight..... | Very few hyaline and hyalo-granular casts; no r. b. c. |
| 19— 3:10 a. m. | ........... | 1,023 | .... | Very faint........ | Supernatant urine is negative; sediment is violet-blue | Very slight..... | |
| 19—10:20 a. m. | ........... | 1,022 | .... | Negative ......... | Negative .......... | Very slight..... | |
| 19— 3:00 p. m. | ........... | .... | .... | Negative ......... | Negative | | |
| 20— 8:00 a. m. | ........... | .... | .... | Negative ......... | Negative | | |

*Patient.*—Colored man, Martiniquan, aged 30, laborer, admitted May 15, 1910, 4 p. m.

*History.*—The patient had been on the Isthmus thirty-one months, had had seven previous attacks of fever in Panama, and many in Martinique. During fever attacks he had never noticed that urine was black or red. He said that he had been sick three days with fever, vomiting and headache, and had not taken quinin before admission.

*Examination.*—The patient was very restless on admission, tossing from side to side in bed and complaining of great pain in his head. His mind seemed fairly clear. Examination of heart, lungs and abdomen was negative; the spleen was not palpable. The blood was found to contain enormous numbers of small ring forms of estivo-autumnal malarial parasites. The imminence of hemoglobinuria was suspected and every specimen of urine was ordered to be sent when voided to the laboratory.

*Course of Illness.*—On the following day, May 16, the patient was quiet, but seemed very ill and extremely prostrated. Leukocytes numbered 7,100. At 8 p. m. his temperature rose abruptly from normal to 102 F. There was no chill, but vomiting occurred. The next urine voided, at 5:30 a. m. May 17, had the characteristic appearance of "blackwater." The patient did not pass into coma, or even lose consciousness, but he appeared to be extremely ill and profoundly depressed. The sclerotics became slightly jaundiced, but the spleen never became palpable or enlarged to percussion. Hemoglobin could be detected in the urine in traces until 3:10 a. m., May 19. Improvement was rapid from May 18 onward.

## DISCUSSION OF THE CASE

Blackwater was prognosticated from an examination of the blood. More than 15 per cent. of the red corpuscles in the peripheral blood were infected. The number infected in the internal organs was probably much larger. In spite of the enormous infection, hemoglobin estimations and erythrocyte counts indicated but slight blood destruction, and the results were in striking contrast to the blood-picture in erythrolytic hemoglobinuria, in which, even in mild cases, blood destruction, as indicated by the same methods, is terrific. (Other cases have confirmed the blood findings given above.) The increase of hemoglobin and erythrocytes on May 17 was probably due to concentration of blood from loss of fluid by vomiting and urination. It seems quite certain that quinin in this case not only killed parasites in the intracorpuscular stage, but also prevented the destruction of many infected corpsucles. The parasites themselves showed evidence of the influence of quinin by their vacuolated and often bizarre appearance. The urine did not differ from the ordinary "blackwater" urine.

In conclusion, I wish to thank Colonel Gorgas for permitting me the use of the above material, and for consenting to the publication of the paper.

Hospital Numbers of Cases Included in Above Report

Ancon Hospital Cases, 162

| | | | | | |
|---|---|---|---|---|---|
| 98 | 12,506 | 23,573 | 49,146 | 53,646 | 58,252 |
| 400 | 653 | 719 | 303 | 681 | 413 |
| 535 | 13,445 | 831 | 317 | 696 | 637 |
| 542 | 459 | 25,282 | 419 | 806 | 59,622 |
| 1,401 | 463 | 304 | 446 | 54,016 | 664 |
| 1,469 | 879 | 362 | 539 | 202 | 776 |
| 2,065 | 14,369 | 575 | 50,017 | 292 | 61,930 |
| 2,721 | 15,093 | 26,308 | 980 | 341 | 63,139 |
| 3,060 | 938 | 31,457 | 51,364 | 394 | 274 |
| 4,263 | 945 | 32,205 | 607 | 500 | 364 |
| 4,266 | 16,525 | 34,115 | 753 | 956 | 564 |
| 4,515 | 979 | 125 | 758 | 55,111 | 696 |
| 6,418 | 17,018 | ..... | 969 | 104 | 64,680 |
| 6,970 | 18,109 | 36,162 | 971 | 189 | 65,036 |
| 7,110 | 363 | 249 | 52,192 | 218 | 66,592 |
| 8,408 | 489 | 534 | 206 | 348 | 828 |
| 8,823 | 981 | 38,349 | 291 | 468 | 966 |
| 9,004 | 19,329 | 711 | 386 | 56,137 | 976 |
| 9,372 | 20,304 | 735 | 454 | 550 | 68,273 |
| 9,925 | 158 | 47,423 | 479 | 717 | 703 |
| 10,107 | 222 | 525 | 496 | 729 | 757 |
| 10,163 | 231 | 605 | 53,031 | 969 | 759 |
| 10,474 | 433 | 637 | 52 | 57,473 | 703 |
| 11,627 | 21,975 | 781 | 55 | 617 | 873 |
| 11,991 | 22,428 | 788 | 139 | 731 | 69,290 |
| 12,271 | 762 | 48,075 | 409 | 58,065 | 516 |
| | | | | | 71,243 |
| 12,383 | 23,320 | 384 | 479 | 157 | 72,431 |

Colon Hospital Cases, 59

| | | | | | |
|---|---|---|---|---|---|
| 8,711 | 9,971 | 12,645 | 15,347 | 16,655 | 17,837 |
| 8,877 | 10,021 | 875 | 372 | 687 | 978 |
| 9,036 | 77 | 13,069 | 735 | 758 | 18,199 |
| 130 | 126 | 81 | 742 | 879 | 19,162 |
| 300 | 344 | 102 | 16,141 | 957 | 20,231 |
| 322 | 590 | 449 | 295 | 17,307 | 21,301 |
| 370 | 964 | 817 | 402 | 471 | 425 |
| 516 | 967 | 965 | 520 | 488 | 645 |
| 842 | 12,055 | 14,272 | 602 | 548 | 23,174 |
| 950 | 145 | 15,213 | 605 | 734 | ..... |

# MERALGIA PARESTHETICA DUE TO PRESSURE OF THE CORSET

JOSEPH L. MILLER, M.D.
CHICAGO

Meralgia paresthetica, described independently in 1895 by Bernhardt and Roth, although an unusual, can scarcely be considered a rare condition, inasmuch as Musser and Sailer have reported ten cases personally observed. The peculiar disturbance of the external cutaneous femoral nerve characterized by paresthesia, or more or less severe pain when the individual is in the erect position, has been ascribed to various causes. Bernhardt considered a toxic neuritis as the most important factor, as he and others have reported cases following the acute infections, especially typhoid. Others have considered pure mechanical factors as the more important; the peculiar curve of the nerve and its relation to the surrounding structure render it especially liable to compression when the thigh is extended. Roth has called attention to the following points along the course of the nerve where trauma of this character may occur: first just after the exit of the nerve where it passes beneath the psoas muscle; second where it curves around below the anterior superior spine, and finally the fibrous canal in the fascia lata. Among the mechanical factors responsible there have been mentioned pregnant uterus, pelvic tumors, varices, tight bands, direct trauma, flat-foot. Pressure on the nerve by the lower edge of Poupart's ligament was found in one case and the symptom disappeared after partial section of the ligament. Hereditary influences may play a rôle.

The pain is described as burning in character but as a rule not intense. More annoying is the paresthesia and the hypersensitiveness of the skin over the affected area, so that the slightest pressure of the clothing is annoying. Souques reports a case in which the pain was so intense that during a paroxysm it was necessary to use morphin.

The only unusual features in the case to be reported is the etiology and intensity of the pain.

*Patient.*—Miss K., aged 23, had good family history; she was employed at office work, requiring her to remain standing most of the day. She had had no recent acute illnesses. About two years ago patient first noticed a peculiar sense of numbness, when standing or walking, extending over the upper and outer side of the right thigh. A few weeks later she suffered from occasional attacks of burning or stabbing pain in the same region. The attacks of pain increased in frequency and severity until she was compelled to discontinue her work, as standing would excite such an attack, the pain promptly disappearing on sitting or lying down. Twice the patient had sudden attacks of excruciating pain, falling to the floor, unable to move the limb; during this time the slightest irritation over the affected area would cause her to scream. These attacks lasted about a half hour, and were always followed by a period of extreme hyperesthesia over the upper part of the thigh. One of these attacks came on while standing to have a dress fitted, the other while leaning over a wash-bowl, cleaning her teeth.

*Examination.*—A circumscribed area of tenderness was located below and slightly outward from the anterior superior spine of the ilium; surrounding this was an ill-defined area of hyperesthesia; no analgesia, anesthesia or thermalgesia. During one of the attacks of acute pain the area of hyperalgesia could be very easily mapped out. It was triangular in outline, the upper border forming the base, about 5 cm. above the iliac bone and extending from the crest of the ilium to 5 cm. medianward from the anterior superior spine. The apex of the triangle was located at the junction of the lower and middle third of the thigh. A general examination of the patient did not reveal anything else abnormal.

In examining to determine if pressure of the clothing could be responsible for the trouble, it was noted that the lower edge of the corset hooked over the anterior superior spine, pressing into the thigh so that when standing erect it was with difficulty that the finger could be introduced between the corset and the thigh. Following instructions, the patient cut out a portion of the corset over this region. Within a few days the relief was marked, and after the lapse of ten days the attacks of pain entirely disappeared, only slight numbness remaining. She returned to her work and reported three months later that, except for slight numbness, she considered herself cured. It was suggested that she purchase a new corset of the same style as that previously worn. After wearing this a few days, the pain again recurred, and the patient of her own accord cut out a piece of the corset as before, the pain promptly disappeared and now after the lapse of five months complains only of slight numbness.

150 Michigan Avenue.

# THE ENERGY METABOLISM OF MOTHER AND CHILD JUST BEFORE AND JUST AFTER BIRTH *

THORNE M. CARPENTER, B.S., AND JOHN R. MURLIN, PH.D.†
BOSTON NEW YORK

## INTRODUCTION

The first attempt to estimate the energy production of the mammalian fetus was that of Pflüger[1] forty-two years ago. Pflüger expressed the opinion, largely on *a priori* grounds, that the gaseous exchange of the fetus as compared with that of the mother must be insignificant in amount. This idea was apparently supported by the work of Cohnstein and Zuntz[2] on the embryo sheep, but was strongly contested by Wiener[3] and others, and within the past ten years has been refuted definitely.[4]

It is mainly to the physiological institutes of Copenhagen and Budapest headed by Bohr and Tangl, respectively, that we are indebted for the newer conception that the gaseous exchange, and therefore the energy production, of the animal embryo is greater per unit of weight than that of the adult organism. Rubner,[5] however, has drawn attention to the fact that the mammalian embryo has no appreciable weight as compared with the mother until near the middle of the gestation period, and several workers[6] using the Zuntz method have failed to find any increase in the oxygen consumption per unit of weight in pregnant as contrasted with non-pregnant women; or if such an increase appeared at all, it became evident only comparatively late in the gestation period. This has been confirmed with respect to the total energy production, as computed from the output of nitrogen and carbon, by one of us in a series of experiments on a pregnant dog.[7] The only exception to the rule is a single case

---

* From the Nutrition Laboratory of the Carnegie Institution of Washington, Boston.

* The hospital expenses for this research were partly covered by a grant from the Rockefeller Institute for Medical Research, New York City.

† Writer.

1. Pflüger: Arch. f. d. ges. Physiol., 1868, i, 61.
2. Cohnstein and Zuntz: Arch. f. d. ges. Physiol., 1884, xxxiv, 173.
3. Wiener: Arch. f. Gynäk., 1884, xxiii, 183.
4. For a complete review of the literature bearing on the metabolism of development see Grafe: Biochem. Centralbl., 1907, vi, 441; and Murlin: Am. Jour. Physiol., 1910, xxvi, 134.
5. Rubner: Arch. f. Hyg., 1908, lxvi, 185.
6. Magnus-Levy: Ztschr. f. Geburtsh. u. Gynäk., 1904, lii, 116. L. Zuntz and Franz Müller. See discussion to Magnus-Levy's address above and articles by Zuntz in Ergebn. d. Physiol., 1908, vii, 430; and Arch f. Gynäk., 1910, xc, 452.
7. Murlin: Am. Jour. Physiol., 1910, xxvi, 134.

reported by Magnus Levy,[6] in which he observed both an absolute and a relative increase in oxygen absorption as early as the third month of gestation. So far as our information at present goes, it appears, then, that the energy production and consequently the energy requirement of the pregnant organism, while certainly increased in the absolute sense by a certain small amount from the very beginning of gestation, does not undergo any significant rise until near the middle of the gestation period. From this time on the experiments cited above show that the total energy production increases steadily to the end of pregnancy.

Thus far no experiments on human subjects have sought to determine what change, if any, in the energy metabolism of mother and child may take place at birth. Does the change from intra-uterine to extra-uterine life mark a turning-point in the metabolic processes of the child? And how do the demands on the mother's metabolism of the late pregnancy compare with those of the early nursing period? In the paper cited above on the metabolism in the pregnant dog the energy production at the culmination of the pregnancy was compared in two different pregnancies with that of the same animal in sexual rest and the conclusions were reached that the extra metabolism of the pregnant organism just before parturition is proportional to the weight of the new-born, and is just about equal to the theoretical requirement of the new-born alone, under the conditions of muscular rest and ordinary room temperature. The latter conclusion means that, neglecting the muscular activities of mother and offspring, the curve representing the energy production of both combined would suffer no deflection at birth. The subject is of sufficient importance from both the theoretical and the practical standpoints to make its application to the human mother and child a matter of considerable interest. With this object in view the following observations on parturient women were made during the summer of 1909 by means of a respiration calorimeter.

### *THE SUBJECTS AND GENERAL PLAN OF THE EXPERIMENTS*

Through the courtesy of Dr. Charles M. Green, chief of the obstetrical service of the McLean Lying-In Hospital, permission was granted us to make use of the application lists of that institution for the selection of suitable subjects and through his suggestion the task of their selection was entrusted to Dr. John T. Williams, of Boston. The success which has attended the laboratory observations has been due in no small degree to the judicious care with which the selections were made. While nothing connected with the routine to which the patients were subjected entailed any particular hardship, their willingness to observe directions to the strictest letter was essential to a satisfactory outcome of the determinations. Through the kindly interest of Dr. E. P. Joslin the patients were admitted to a small ward set apart for them in the New England Deacon-

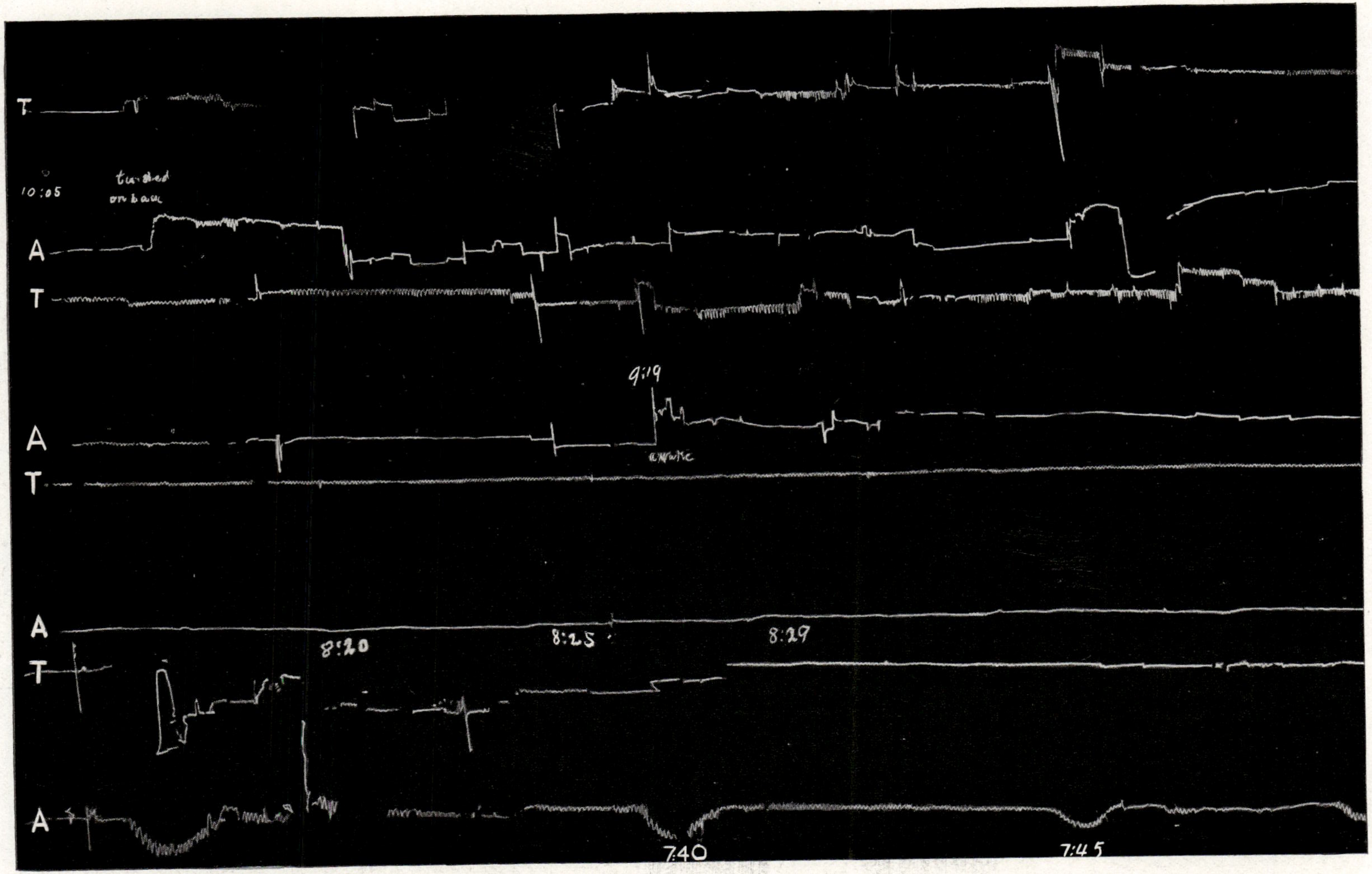


Fig. 1.—Pneumographic tracings obtained while the patient was in the calorimeter hidden from view, to show degree of composure of the [illegible] Movements of the uterus were observed at 7:40, 7:45, 7:50, etc. The woman

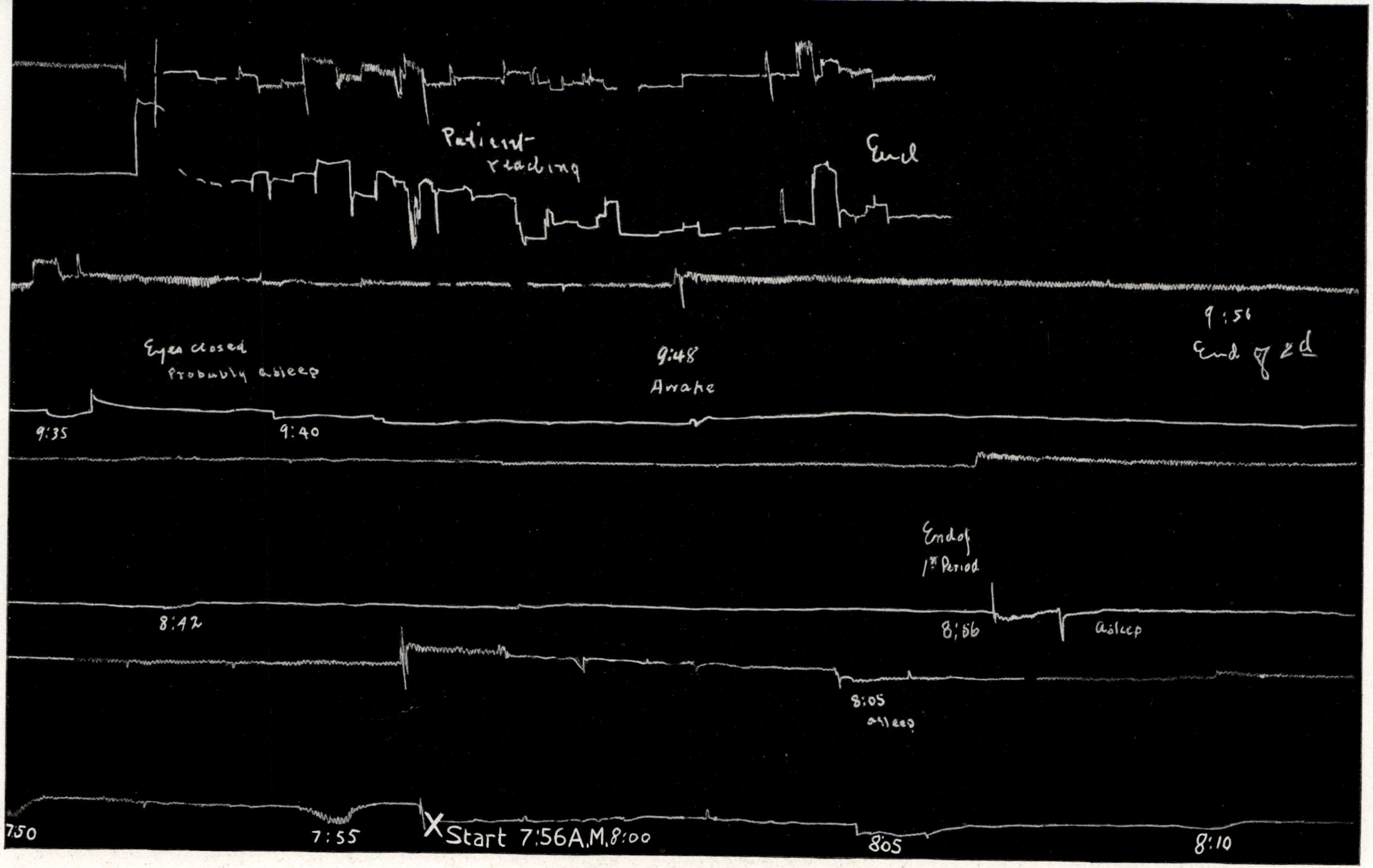


FIGURE 1—Continued

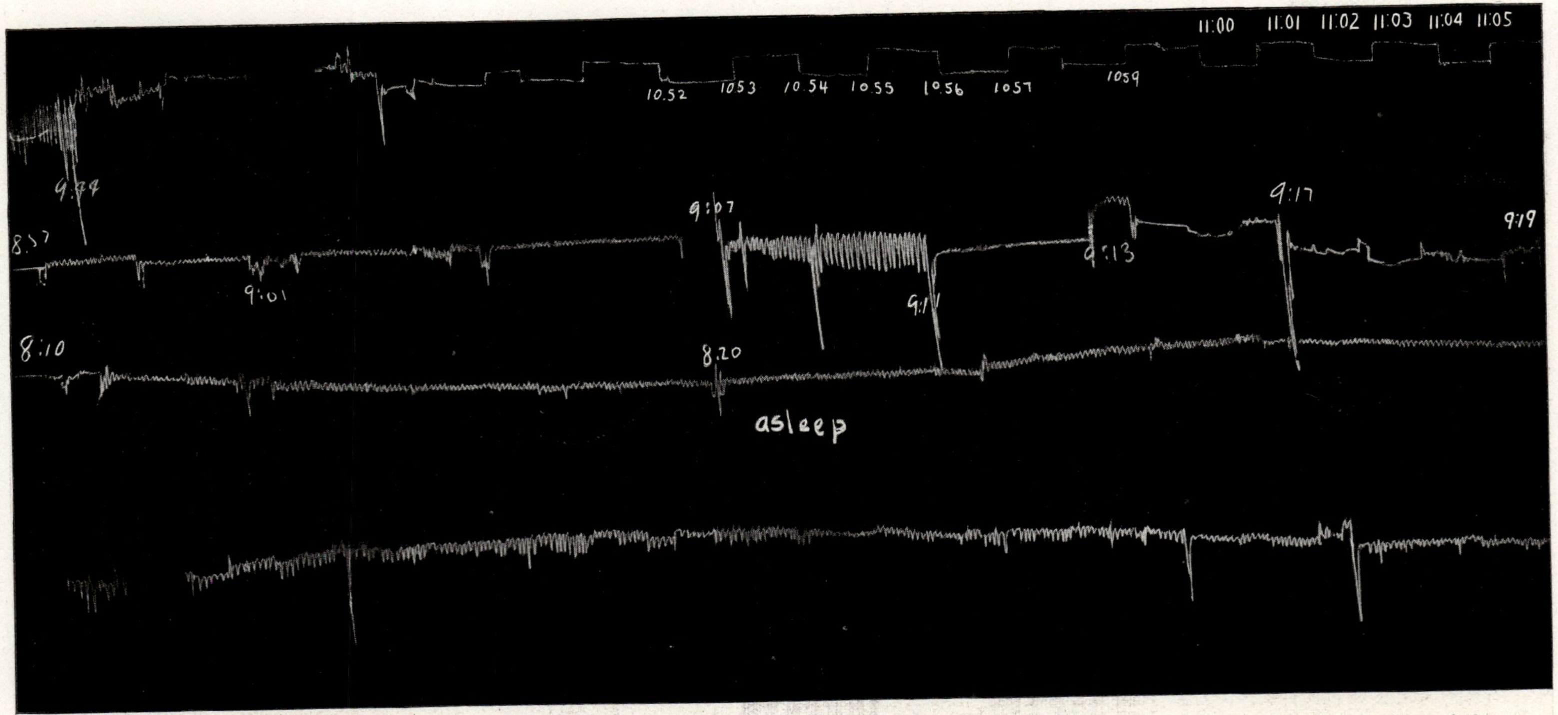


Fig. 2.—Tracing obtained from a single pneumograph about the thorax of the patient, Mrs. E. W., on May 23. The long excursions of the writing point downward were due to long breaths. Note difference while the patient was asleep. The block-like tracings on the upper line were due to differences in the positions of the patient's arms while reading opposite pages of a book.

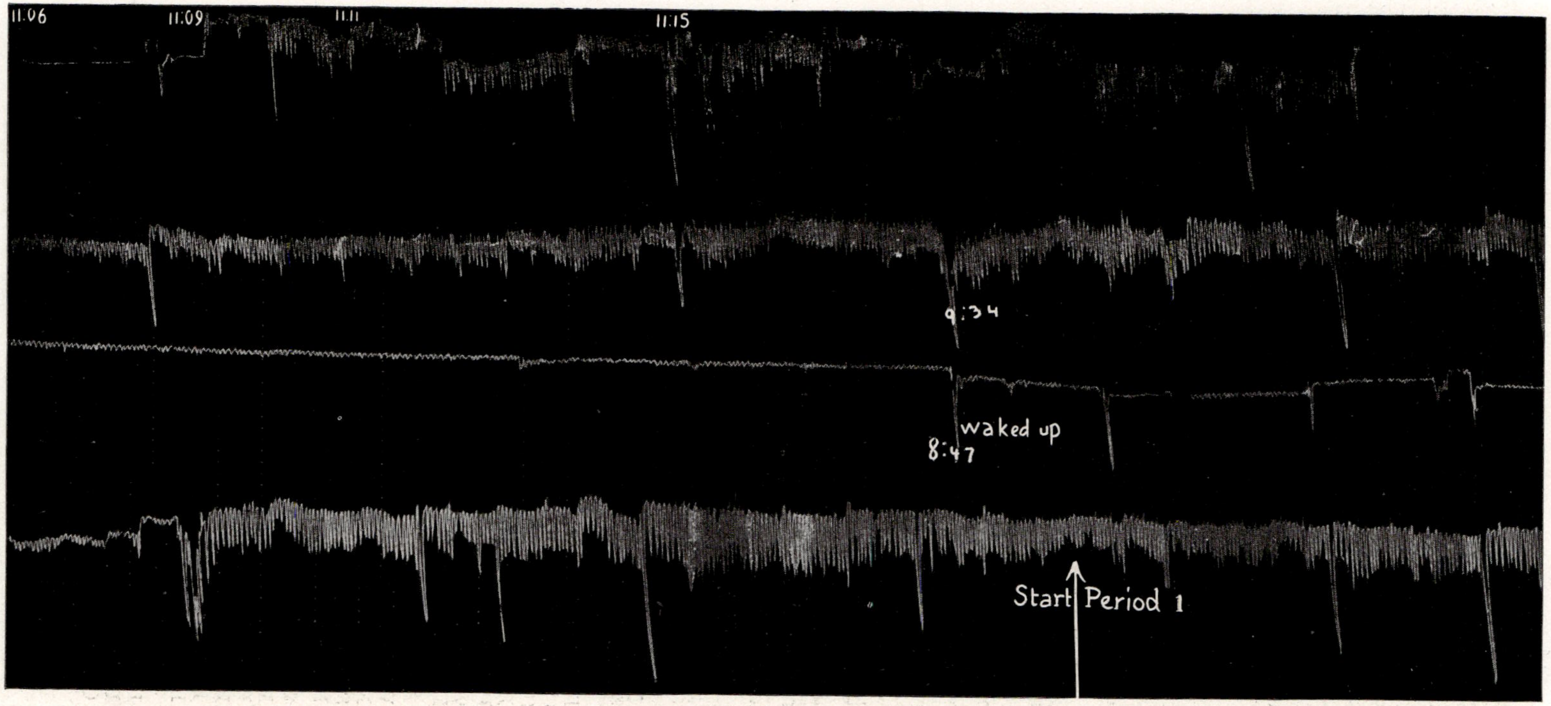


FIGURE 2—Continued

ness Hospital, situated only a short distance from the laboratory, where, through the active cooperation of Miss Zilla MacLauchlin, the head nurse, they received most excellent attention and were under the constant care of Dr. Williams. To all these persons, each of whom played an essential part in the success of these experiments, we wish to express our earnest thanks.

The observations began from one to four weeks previous to parturition and extended throughout the puerperium. Our plan contemplated observations as close up to parturition and as soon thereafter as they could be made without danger to the patient. With the first and third cases (named in order of their delivery) the patient was in the calorimeter on the day immediately preceding that of parturition. With the first and second cases the mother and child were brought to the laboratory in an ambulance on the second day following parturition, and with the third on the fourth day following, the mothers on these days being carefully kept in a horizontal position throughout. Altogether nine separate experiments—three before and six after parturition—were made with Case 1 and ten separate experiments—five before and five after—with both Cases 2 and 3.

At the hospital the patients were kept on a strictly regulated diet containing approximately a known amount of nitrogen and potential energy, and lived under the most hygienic conditions possible. Samples of the daily diet for Patients 3 and 1 are shown herewith. The first is a creatin-free diet.

SAMPLES OF DAILY DIET

*Breakfast Hour, 10:20 a. m.*

| Mrs. D. A., June 3 | Amount Prescribed gm. | Amount Eaten gm. |
|---|---|---|
| Rolled oats | 160 | 160 |
| Cream, double strength, 45% fat | 50 | 50 |
| Sugar, granulated | 24 | 24 |
| Bread, toasted | 37 | 37 |
| Butter | 13 | 13 |
| Coffee | 1 cup | 1 cup |
| Eggs | 2 | 2 |
| *Lunch Hour, 2 p. m.* | | |
| Whole milk | 280 | 280 |
| Bread | 74 | 74 |
| Sliced banana | 100 | 100 |
| Butter | 13 | 13 |
| *Dinner Hour, 6:30 p. m.* | | |
| Milk | 280 | 280 |
| Rice, stewed and steamed | 135 | 180 |
| Bread, white | 37 | 37 |
| Butter | 13 | 13 |
| Lettuce, with 1 tablespoonful of olive oil in French dressing | | all |
| Ice-cream | 60 | 60 |
| Plain sponge cake | 30 | 30 |
| Coffee, cream (25) and sugar (12) | 1 cup | 1 cup |

Total N., 8.942; total cal., 2,400 = 34 cal. per kg.
(estimated) (estimated)

*Breakfast Hour, 9 a. m.*

| Mrs. A. B., May 23 | Amount Prescribed gm. | Amount Eaten gm. |
|---|---|---|
| Rolled wheat | 120 | 120 |
| Cream, double strength, 45% fat | 50 | 50 |
| Sugar, granulated | 24 | 15 |
| Bread, toasted | 37 | 37 |
| Butter | 7 | 7 |
| Eggs | 2 | 2 |
| *Lunch Hour, 2 p. m.* | | |
| Whole milk | 280 | 280 |
| Bread | 37 | 37 |
| Sliced orange and banana | 100 | 100 |
| Cream, (what remained from breakfast) | ... | ... |
| Sugar, (what remained from breakfast) | ... | ... |
| Butter | 7 | 7 |
| *Dinner Hour, 6:30 p. m.* | | |
| Roast breast of veal, cut free of fat | 60 | 60 |
| Rice, stewed and steamed | 135 | 135 |
| Bread, whole wheat | 37 | 37 |
| Butter | 7 | 7 |
| Lettuce, with 1 tablespoonful of olive oil in French dressing | | all |
| Ice-cream | 30 | 30 |
| Plain sponge cake | 30 | 30 |
| Coffee, cream (25) and sugar (12) | 1 cup | 1 cup |

Total N., 7.396; total cal., 1,650 = 26 cal. per kg.
(estimated) (estimated)

The prescribed amounts of the articles chosen by the patient were weighed out immediately before the meal in the diet kitchen of the hospital and the amounts left on the service plates were again weighed immediately after the meal and deducted. All excreta were collected quantitatively in twenty-four-hour amounts and were carefully preserved for analyses later. The urines will form the subject of a separate paper to be published soon.

On experiment days, which we shall designate henceforth as "calorimeter days," the routine was planned so as to reduce to a minimum the effect of variations in the diet on the metabolic processes. The last meal the day before was given before 7 p. m. The patient came to the laboratory before breakfast, or after taking only a little black coffee, and entered the calorimeter usually about 7 a. m., at least twelve hours after the last meal. Numerous observations in this laboratory have shown that by this procedure the effect of *small* variations in the diet on the respiratory quotient is negligible. Of course no attempt was made to have the patient eat the same absolute amounts of protein, carbohydrate and fat every day. In fact, for two days immediately after parturition the regulation milk and broth diets were given. With these exceptions, however, the diets for each case were as nearly uniform from day to day both as to quality and quantity as the condition of the appetite would permit.

Further comments on the effect of the diet will be found in the section where the results for the respiratory exchange are discussed.

Arriving at the laboratory, the subject, accompanied always by a nurse, was taken to a small room adjoining the calorimeter room where she was prepared for her sojourn in the calorimeter by emptying the bladder, so that the urine for the calorimeter period could be saved, and by being weighed whenever this was possible without discomfort to the patient. She was then placed on a small portable bed covered by an air mattress, and the instruments for recording the pulse, respiration and temperature were adjusted to her body. The patient was clothed for the calorimeter only in her underclothing and a thin wrapper, and was covered on the bed by a doubly-folded blanket. Care was taken to have these conditions always the same for a given patient. When all was in readiness the patient, lying on the bed, was carried into the calorimeter room and the bed was pushed into the calorimeter.

The calorimeter used was the one recently described by Benedict and Carpenter[8] as the "bed calorimeter." This calorimeter admits of the entrance of the subject only in the horizontal position, which made it especially suitable for the parturient patient. All the accessory apparatus, as well as the calorimeter itself, are described in the publication cited above, so that reference will be made here only to such features of their construction as are necessary to make clear the principles involved. It should be stated, however, that after a preliminary trial made with each subject the day before she was used for the first observation recorded, and made for the express purpose of reassuring her as to the nature of the experience she was to undergo, there was no apparent apprehension or hesitation on the part of any one of them. As noted in the description referred to above, it is possible for the subject in this calorimeter to look out of the laboratory window and to read by the light of a small tungsten lamp. It was our custom to have the nurse who accompanied the subject sit immediately outside the window of the calorimeter in plain view of the subject, whence she could communicate to the latter the time of day or could observe whether she appeared to be in any distress. That none of the patients, while they were bed-ridden or before, found the calorimeter oppressive or uncomfortable in any sense, speaks well for its adaptability to subjects of this class. An examination of the pulse-records for the calorimeter periods, given in the tables beyond, will show also that there was at no time any undue psychical disturbance.

---

8. Benedict and Carpenter: Respiration Calorimeters for Studying the Respiratory Exchange and Energy Transformations of Man, Carnegie Institution of Washington, Publication No. 123, 1910.

CONTROL OF THE PATIENT WHILE IN THE CALORIMETER

Since the amount of energy produced in the body above the minimal maintenance requirement is, in general, determined by the three factors of food, muscular activity, and temperature, it is essential, in comparing the energy production for the different physiological conditions which we are here studying, that the condition of the patient with regard to the outside factors be as nearly constant as possible. We have already mentioned the precautions taken to make the food factor as constant as possible. The factor of muscular activity is the one which most affects the metabolism and is at the same time the most difficult to control. While in general it was understood by the patient that she was to lie as still as possible, it was necessary for us to know with certainty to what extent this rule was complied with. With the exception of her face and head a patient in this calorimeter is practically invisible from the outside. A satisfactory control was obtained, however, by means of the pneumograph. As noted by Benedict and Carpenter[9] the Ellis pneumograph if properly adjusted will record not only the movements of respiration but even slight extrinsic movements of the limbs, head, etc., and its record, obtained by air-tight transmission through the wall of the calorimeter, on a small kymograph placed on a table just outside, furnishes a very good index of the degree of general muscular rest. With our patients the pneumograph was placed about the lower thorax, and when fitted closely enough it always recorded such motions as turning from back to side and side to back, movements of limbs, and even of the head. Part of the time before parturition two of these pneumographs were used, one just below the breasts and the other about the umbilicus, or the point of greatest distention of the abdomen, and simultaneous records were kept on the same kymograph. The writing-point of the lower pneumograph on one occasion showed variations which were unmistakably due to movements of the uterus. As may be seen from Figure 1, these movements, obtained the day preceding parturition, occurred regularly every five minutes for about half an hour and then were lost. On another occasion the thoracic pneumograph showed peculiar block-like variations which by careful observation through the window of the calorimeter proved to be due to the movements of turning the pages of a book which the patient was reading (Fig. 2). The tracings exhibiting these two peculiar movements as well as others are reproduced for the purpose of showing how complete was our knowledge of the condition of the patient with respect to muscular activity. In Tables 1, 2 and 3 the number of extrinsic movements, counted from these records, is given for each experiment together with such additional remarks on the composure of the mother alone or mother and child, as seemed necessary. The number of respirations per minute

9. Benedict and Carpenter: Respiration Calorimeters, p. 95.

were counted with a stop-watch from the movements of the writing-point on the kymograph.

Since we hoped to keep the child asleep throughout the experiments with both mother and child, provision was made for recording movements of the mother only. In the main the end justified this expectation.

The importance of the pulse as an index of the degree of internal muscular activity, especially in fasting, has also been emphasized by Benedict.[10] It was deemed advisable to make use of such information as could be gained in this way with these patients. Accordingly a Bowles stethoscope was fitted to the naked chest wall of the patient before she entered the calorimeter and its tube was afterward attached to the ear-pieces outside by an air-tight connection passing through the wall. After several trials it was found that owing to the fulness of the breasts the best location for the stethoscope on the chest wall of the parturient patient was high up above the left breast near the clavicle. Here the heart could be distinctly heard, unless, on turning, the patient caused the stethoscope to slip from its position, in which case the failure to hear the beat was communicated by the nurse to the patient, who was usually able to replace the instrument with only a slight movement. The pulse was counted in this way every ten minutes. Incidentally also the stethoscope on the mother's chest enabled the observer to hear the baby when it cried. Fortunately this happened but twice in the whole series of experiments and it was not therefore a seriously disturbing factor.

As a further means of control of the patient, recourse could always be had to the telephone if it was thought desirable to caution her against moving at a particular time; but in these experiments, owing to their relatively short duration, and to the cheerful willingness of the patient to observe directions, its use was seldom found necessary.

The influence of variations in temperature, either directly or indirectly, on the metabolism of the subject was eliminated entirely by keeping the temperature of the air inside the calorimeter uniform from day to day within 1° C. In fact the direct heat measurements made by this calorimeter are based on the ideal of a perfectly uniform air temperature (about 20° C.) throughout the course of any given experiment, although small variations do not invalidate them in any sense, since means of correction are always at hand. The attempt was made to start the experiment each day at the same temperature. The control of the temperature of both room and calorimeter is such as to enable this to be accomplished with great exactness even when there are extreme variations of the outside temperature.

In general, we feel every confidence in saying that the conditions of each patient as regards the several factors of food, muscular activity and

10. Benedict: Influence of Inanition on Metabolism, Carnegie Institution of Washington, 1907, p. 488.

temperature to which she was exposed, were as nearly constant as possible, and that therefore the differences in metabolism observed, with certain exceptions which will be noted, may safely be taken as being due to the different physiological conditions which it is here sought to compare.

METHODS OF DETERMINATION

*A. The Respiratory Exchange.*—The respiration calorimeter as used in this laboratory has a closed circuit system of ventilation; i. e., the same residual air is circulated round and round through the chamber and through the absorption system by a blower, while oxygen is admitted automatically as required, and the respiratory products are removed as they are formed, by the absorbers. Carbon dioxid is absorbed by potash lime, and water vapor by sulphuric acid. The gross amounts of these substances given off by the patient are obtained by the gain in weight of the separate absorbers, but it is necessary to make a correction by determining whether the carbon dioxid and water content of the air residual in the apparatus has changed during the course of an experiment. This is accomplished by making analyses in triplicate of ten-liter samples of air for carbon dioxid and water both at the beginning and at the end of an experiment period. The same is true of the oxygen absorbed by the patient. The gross amount is obtained by the loss in weight of the oxygen cylinder during a period and a correction—it may be an addition or it may be a subtraction—is made by determining the change, if any, in the oxygen content of the residual air. This is effected by calculating the change in volume of the entire air due to fluctuations of the temperature and barometric pressure and subtracting from the residual volume found the volume of nitrogen (assuming it to be eight-tenths of the whole at the start of the experiment) and the volumes of carbon dioxid and water vapor taken out in the residual analyses for these substances already referred to. The accuracy of this method depends on the total volume of the calorimeter, the smaller the total volume the greater being the accuracy. The calorimeter used in these experiments is the smallest which has ever been constructed for experiments on adult human subjects, its total capacity being only about 880 liters. The accuracy of the oxygen determinations therefore is as great as can be obtained at present.[11]

*B. Water Vapor.*—The water vapor absorbed by the sulphuric acid was always determined; but with this calorimeter, and especially in the short periods used for these patients, it is of importance only as a means

11. A criticism of the oxygen determination (which at best is a very difficult matter) with all the sources of error involved, will be found in the description of the new calorimeters. Benedict and Carpenter: Respiration Calorimeters, p. 89.

of estimating the heat carried away from the calorimeter by vaporization.[12]

*C. The Heat Production as Measured.*—The heat lost from the subject's body is measured in part by the amount of heat absorbed[13] by a current of water circulated through the calorimeter and in part by the amount of water vaporized[14] in the calorimeter.

The sum of these two may not, however, be the exact amount of heat produced by the subject. Either more or less heat may have been generated in the body than was given up to the calorimeter. In the former case the patient's own body temperature would rise; in the latter case it would fall. Whether there has been any such difference can be learned, if the exact temperature of the body at the beginning and at the end of the period can be known; for the amount of heat stored or the extra amount lost from the body in the period can be calculated by multiplying the body weight by the rise or fall in temperature and by the specific heat of the human body (0.83).

The method of registering the body temperature of these patients was that first employed by Benedict and Snell[15] and by Benedict alone,[16] namely, by means of an electrical resistance thermometer inserted 10 or 12 centimeters into the rectum and connected through a Wheatstone bridge with a d'Arsonval galvanometer, the exact temperature at any time being known from the position of the slide necessary to give a zero deflection. The thermometer was sensitive to 0.01° C. and enabled us therefore to know the temperature of the body with great accuracy.[17]

The energy production, as given in the accompanying tables under the heading "direct," denotes the amount of heat eliminated and measured directly, plus or minus the change in body heat retained, as calculated from the rectal temperature. Control tests to make sure the calorimeter

---

12. Benedict and Carpenter: Respiration Calorimeters, p. 44.

13. It is assumed that with a subject lying under a cover of certain thickness the heat lost from the subject's body will pass through the cover to the heat-absorbers at a uniform rate, allowance of sufficient time being made to permit the subject to warm up the bed before measurements actually begin. In these experiments the determinations never began within less than one-half hour after the patient entered the calorimeter.

14. Whether this water comes from the subject's lungs or from the skin is a matter of indifference for this purpose.

15. Benedict and Snell: Arch. f. d. ges. Physiol., 1901, lxxxviii, 492; 1902, xc, 33.

16. Benedict: Am. Jour. Physiol., 1904, xi, 145.

17. Whether variations of the temperature in the rectum accurately represent variations of the temperature of the entire body mass cannot be known until a complete topographical study of the temperature of the human body has been made. Experiments in this direction have been planned and are now being carried out in this laboratory. Meantime the assumption that such is the case is the best means we have of estimating the fluctuations in the amount of heat retained by the body.

was working satisfactorily were made several times during the course of these experiments.

Since the weight of the new-born child is only 5 or 6 per cent. of that of the mother, it was not deemed necessary to complicate the connections with the calorimeter further by using a separate thermometer for the child. That is to say, for anything that we know the temperature of the child's body in any given period might have been falling while the temperature of the mother's body was rising and *vice versa.* The error involved would be small, however, unless the variation of the child's temperature was extreme, and this would have been revealed by the routine examination at the hospital. In only one case was there any report of a temperature for the child above normal and this was not on a calorimeter day.

The rectal thermometer was the only feature of the apparatus to which the subjects of these experiments offered any objection and this was not serious. The objection was rather to the idea than to the sensations experienced. The patient was always questioned at the termination of the calorimeter period whether she had been comfortable and in no case was the discomfort from the thermometer sufficient to account for any restlessness observed.

*D. The Heat Production as Calculated.*—As an additional source of information regarding the energy transformations in the parturient patient we have made use of the method of Zuntz and Schumburg in calculating the heat production per hour from the known quantities of nitrogen in the urine and the quantities of carbon dioxid and oxygen exchanged in the respiration. This method is based on the following constants:

1. N in urine $\times$ 2.56 = grams C from combustion of protein in respiration.
2. Total C of respiration — C of protein = C of C-H and fat in respiration.
3. N in urine $\times$ 8.45 = grams $O_2$ necessary for combustion of protein.
4. Total $O_2$ absorbed — $O_2$ of protein = $O_2$ for combustion of C-H and fat.

The number of grams of carbon from carbohydrate and from fat are then found by the following equations:

Let x be C of fat and y be C of carbohydrate in the respiration. Then

$$x + y = \text{C of fat and C-H.}$$

$$3.751\,x + 2.651\,y = O_2 \text{ required for combustion of fat and C-H.}$$

Finally the N of urine $\times$ 26 = cal. from protein,
C of fat $\times$ 12.3 = cal. from fat,
C of C-H $\times$ 9.5 = cal. from C-H.
Sum=Total cal. produced.

The figures obtained by this method of calculation are presented in the accompanying tables under the heading "Indirect."

We are well aware that the use of this method in these particular cases is open to the objection that the constant N $\times$ 2.56 may not apply to

TABLE 1.—CASE 1, MRS. A. B. (PRIMIPARA), LABORATORY RECORD

| Time of Experiments. | | Physical Condition of the Mother. | | | | Respiratory Exchange. | | | Energy Production, Calories per hour. | | | | |
|---|---|---|---|---|---|---|---|---|---|---|---|---|---|
| Day. | Periods. A. M. | Pulse, av. per min. | Resp., av. per min. | Body temp., av. °C. | No. of extraneous movements per hour. | $CO_2$ gm. per hour. | $O_2$ gm. per hour. | R. Q. | a—Direct meas. | b—Indirect | $\frac{a+b}{2}$ | Per kg. | Remarks. |
| 5/20 ...... | 8:11-10:11 | 67 | 17.5 | ? | 32 | 21.6 | 17.9 | .88 | ? | 60.6 | ? | ... | |
| 5/22 ...... | 8:20-10:50 | 59 | 18.5 | 36.7 | 19 | 21.4 | 19.0 | .82 | 61.3 | 62.6 | 61.9 | 0.96 | |
| 5/25 ...... | 7:56- 8:56<br>8:56- 9:56<br>9:56-10:56 | 62 | 17.5 | 36.8 | 19 | 21.0 | 18.3 | .84 | 58.8 | 60.7 | 59.7 | 0.95 | Patient slept 46 min. 1st period. Patient slept 23 min. 2d period. Patient restless 3d period. |
| 5/26 ...... | Parturition. | Child born at 1:45 p. m. Weight, 3.3 kg. | | | | | | | | | | | |
| 5/28 ...... | 8:32- 9:32<br>9:32-10:32 | 62 | 20 | 37.6 | 13 | 21.2 | 20.6 | .75 | 70.4 | 67.2 | 68.8 | 1.18 | Mother and child together in calorimeter; mother very quiet, child slept entire time. |
| 5/31 ...... | 8:30- 9:28<br>9:28-10:30 | 90 | 21 | 37.9 | 24 | 21.2 | 19.6 | .78 | 62.9* | 64.9 | 63.9 | 1.13 | Mother quiet, child slept most of time. |
| 6/ 7 ...... | 8:14- 9:14<br>9:14-10:14 | 82 | 19 | 36.6 | 16 | 19.3 | 17.2 | .82 | 53.5 | 56.0 | 54.7 | 1.03 | Mother quiet, child slept entime time. |
| 6/ 9 ...... | 8:12- 9:12<br>9:12-10:12 | 75 | 19 | 36.6 | 25 | 19.5 | 16.7 | .85 | 56.5 | 56.5 | 56.5 | 1.06 | Mother quiet, child slept entire time. |
| 6/10 ...... | 8:06- 9:06<br>9:06-10:06<br>10:06-11:06 | 72 | 18.5 | 36.4 | 19 | 17.8 | 15.3 | .85 | 53.5 | 54.3 | 53.9 | 1.06 | Mother alone, very quiet, slept part of time. |
| 6/12 ...... | 8:23- 9:23<br>9:23-10:23<br>10:23-11:23 | 78 | 20 | 36.8 | 25 | 19.9 | 18.2 | .79 | 62.6 | 61.4 | 62.0 | 1.14 | Mother and child; mother quiet, child slept all except few minutes at end. |

* First period only.

the urine of pregnancy, particularly in the later stages, when nitrogen is being retained in large quantity, or to the urine of the puerperium when nitrogen is being lost from the body in considerable quantity. In the absence of positive knowledge on these points we justify the use of the constant on the belief that the error produced by variations in the composition of such urines from that of normal urines would, at most, be small and therefore negligible.[18]

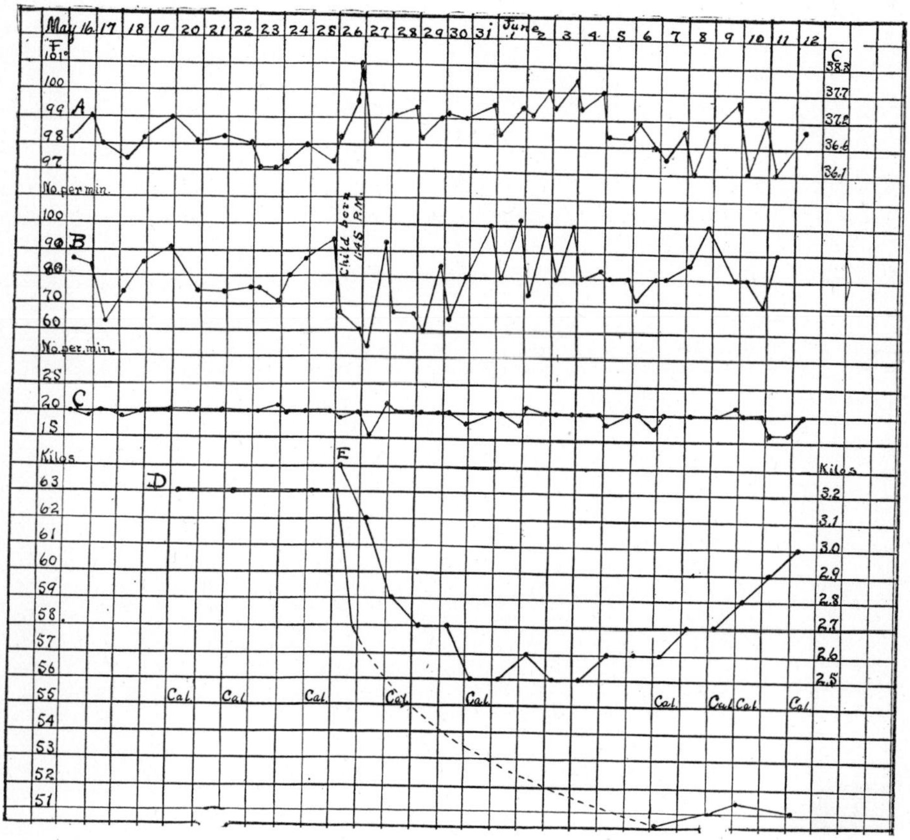


Fig. 3.—Clinical record, Case 1, Mrs. A. B., primipara. Cal., calorimeter days; A, temperature curve; B, pulse; C, respiration; D, mother's weight; E, child's weight.

## *DISCUSSION OF RESULTS*

The results of all our laboratory determinations are presented in parallel with the clinical records of the cases in the tables and charts (Figs. 3, 4 and 5).

---

18. Our analyses of these urines, while not complete at the time this is written, confirm this belief.

TABLE 2.—CASE 2, MRS. E. W. (MULTIPARA), LABORATORY RECORD

| Time of Experiments. | | Physical Condition of the Mother. | | | | Respiratory Exchange. | | | Energy Production, Calories per hour. | | | | |
|---|---|---|---|---|---|---|---|---|---|---|---|---|---|
| Day. | Periods. A. M. | Pulse, av. per min. | Resp., av. per min. | Body temp., av. °C. | No. of extraneous movements per hour. | $CO_2$ gm. per hour. | $O_2$ gm. per hour. | R. Q. | *a*—Direct meas. | *b*—Indirect | $\frac{a+b}{2}$ | Per kg. | Remarks. |
| 5/21 ...... | 8:24-10:24 | 73 | 16 | 36.5 | 64 | 22.4 | 19.9 | .82 | 63.1 | 66.7 | 64.9 | 1.11 | Patient rather restless. |
| 5/23 ...... | 7:56- 9:11<br>9:11-10:26 | 82 | 16 | 36.6 | 40 | 22.5 | 20.1 | .82 | 60.0 | 67.7 | 63.8 | 1.09 | Patient slept 15 min. |
| 5/24 ...... | 8:04- 9:04<br>9:04-10:04<br>10:04-11:04 | 85 | 17 | 36.6 | 28 | 22.2 | 19.3 | .84 | 60.5 | 64.8 | 62.6 | 1.08 | Slept 15 min. 1st period. |
| 5/26 ...... | 7:51- 8:51<br>8:51- 9:51 | 89 | 16.5 | 36.8 | 27 | 22.1 | 18.4 | .87 | 62.4 | 62.6 | 62.5 | 1.09 | Patient read book most of time; slight nausea. |
| 5/30 ...... | 8:28- 9:28<br>9:28-10:28 | 81 | 16.5 | 36.9 | 32 | 22.3 | 20.3 | .81 | 72.1 | 67.8* | 69.9 | 1.20 | Complained of severe headache. |
| 6/12 ...... | Parturition. Child born at 2 a. m. Weight, 3.6 kg. | | | | | | | | | | | | |
| 6/14 ...... | 8:28- 9:28<br>9:28-10:28 | 71 | 17 | 36.8 | 38 | 23.6 | 23.3 | .74 | 70.1 | 76.2 | 73.1 | 1.36 | Mother and child together. Child cried most of the time. Mother nursed child in calorimeter. |
| 6/16 ...... | 8:34- 9:34<br>9:34-10:34 | 67 | 16 | 36.7 | 32 | 18.5 | 17.3 | .78 | 58.3 | 56.8 | 57.5 | 1.16 | Mother alone; restless 2d period. |
| 6/17 ...... | 8:37- 9:37<br>9:37-10:37 | 66 | 17 | 36.7 | 39 | 20.5 | 18.9 | .79 | 67.9 | 63.2 | 65.6 | 1.26 | Mother and child. Child cried short time, then slept. |
| 6/23 ...... | 8:24- 9:24<br>9:24-10:24 | 59 | 17 | 36.9 | 43 | 20.8 | 19.0 | .80 | 75.3 | 63.0 | 69.2 | 1.35 | Mother quiet; child slept entire time. |
| 6/24 ...... | 8:10- 9:10<br>9:10-10:10 | 56 | 16 | 37.0 | 22 | 18.1 | 17.0 | .77 | 65.8 | 57.5 | 61.6 | 1.29 | Mother alone; quiet entire time. |

* First period only.

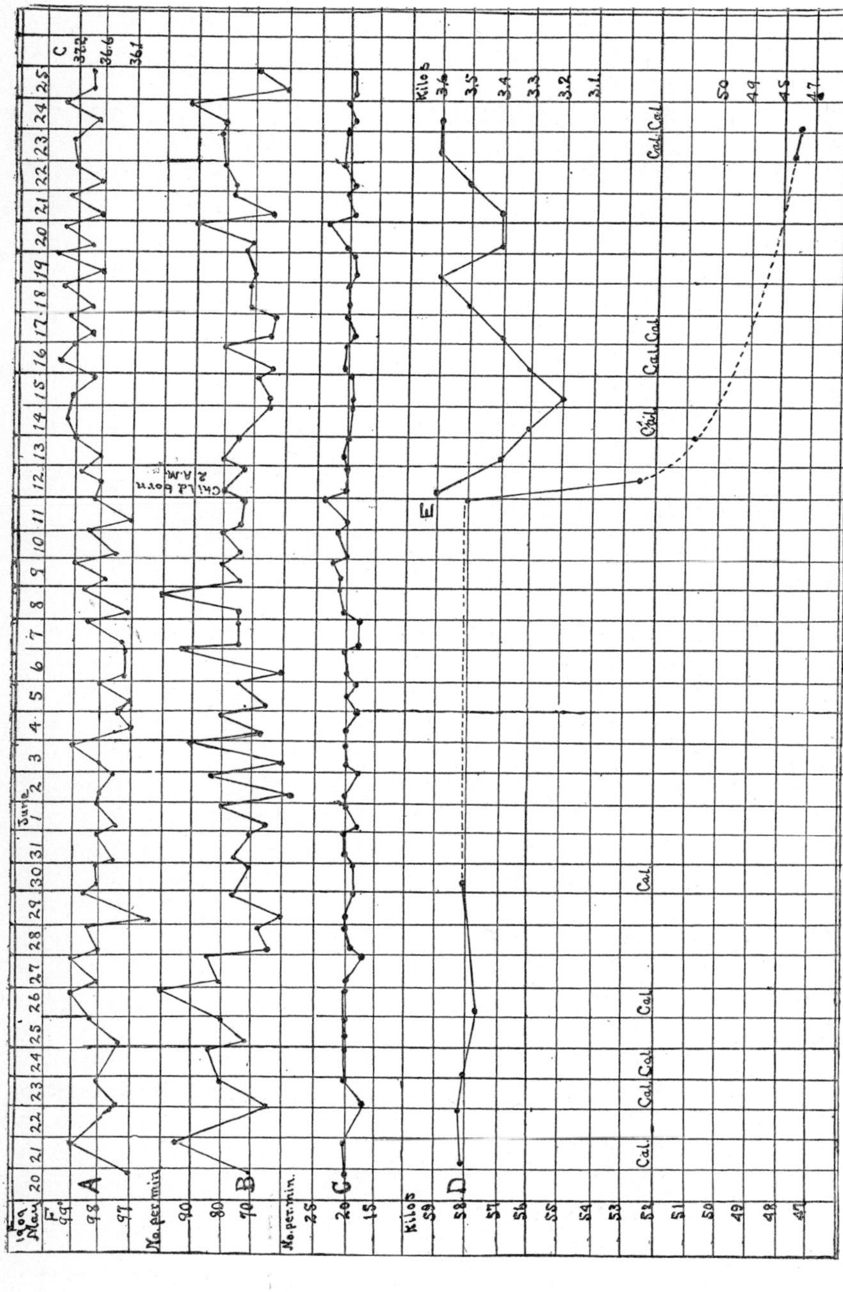

Fig. 4.—Clinical record, Case 2, Mrs. E. W., multipara. Cal., calorimeter days; A, temperature curve; B, pulse; C, respiration; D, mother's weight; E, child's weight.

TABLE 3.—CASE 3, MRS. D. A. (PRIMIPARA), LABORATORY RECORD

| Time of Experiments. | | Physical Condition of the Mother. | | | | Respiratory Exchange. | | | Energy Production, Calories per hour. | | | | |
|---|---|---|---|---|---|---|---|---|---|---|---|---|---|
| Day. | Periods. A. M. | Pulse, av. per min. | Resp., av. per min. | Body temp., av. °C. | No. of extraneous movements per hour. | $CO_2$ gm. per hour. | $O_2$ gm. per hour. | R. Q. | a—Direct. meas. | b—Indirect. | $\frac{a+b}{2}$ | Per kg. | Remarks. |
| 5/29 ...... | 8:04- 9:04<br>9:04-10:04 | 78 | 21 | 36.8 | 40 | 24.9 | 20.7 | .87 | 73.3 | 70.5 | 71.9 | 1.03 | Patient slept few minutes. |
| 6/ 1 ...... | 8:02- 9:02<br>9:02-10:02 | 76 | 20 | 36.8 | 44 | 24.9 | 20.6 | .88 | 71.4 | 70.5 | 70.9 | 1.01 | Patient slept ½ hr. 1st period; restless 2d period; backache. |
| 6/ 5 ...... | 8:18- 9:18<br>9:18-10:18 | .. | 20 | 36.4 | 18 | 23.1 | 20.2 | .83 | 66.6 | 67.7. | 67.1 | 0.95 | Very quiet throughout; no backache. |
| 6/19 ...... | 8:13- 9:11<br>9:11-10:11<br>10:11-11:11 | 66 | 18.5 | 36.5 | 24 | 23.2 | 19.4 | .87 | 72.6 | 65.6 | 69.1 | 1.01 | Patient quiet, but complained of backache. |
| 6/21 ...... | 8:17- 9:17<br>9:17-10:17 | 68 | 19 | 36.7 | 38 | 23.6 | 20.6 | .83 | 78.2 | 69.4 | 73.8 | 1.08 | Patient a little restless. |
| 6/22 ...... | Parturition. | Child born at 3 p. m. | | | Weight, 3.4 kg. | | | | | | | | |
| 6/26 ...... | 8:35- 9:35<br>9:35-10:35 | 86 | 17 | 37.1 | 26 | 23.6 | 22.3 | .77 | 76.7 | 72.1 | 74.4 | 1.19 | Mother and child together; mother quiet; child slept all but 2 or 3 min. |
| 6/30 ...... | 8:28- 9:28<br>9:28-10:28 | 89 | 19 | 37.3 | 35 | 23.4 | 20.6 | .83 | 71.6 | 68.8 | 70.2 | 1.12 | Mother and child; mother quiet; child slept entire time. |
| 7/ 1 ...... | 8:17- 9:17<br>9:17-10:17 | 82 | 17 | 37.4 | 20 | 20.5 | 18.7 | .79 | 69.7 | 62.2 | 65.9 | 1.09 | Mother alone; very quiet 1st period; little restless 2d period. |
| 7/ 3 ...... | 8:28- 9:28<br>9:28-10:28 | 79 | 18 | 37.3 | 12 | 22.3 | 19.4 | .83 | 64.3 | 65.1 | 64.7 | 1.02 | Mother and child; mother very quiet; child slept entire time |
| 7/ 4 ...... | 8:24- 9:24<br>9:24-10:24 | 77 | 20 | 37.2 | 19 | 18.9 | 16.0 | .86 | 55.8 | 54.0 | 54.9 | 0.90 | Mother alone; very quiet. |

The general curves for temperature, pulse and respiration in the clinical record show that the cases ran perfectly normal courses. The temperature, even immediately after delivery never rose to 101° F. except in Case 1 on the evening of the day of parturition. The temperature which, according to Williams,[19] is arbitrarily taken as the upper limit for the normal puerperium is 100.4° F. or 38° C., any rise above this being regarded as pathological. Applying this test we had but one pathological day (possibly two) in Case 1 and none at all with either of the other cases.

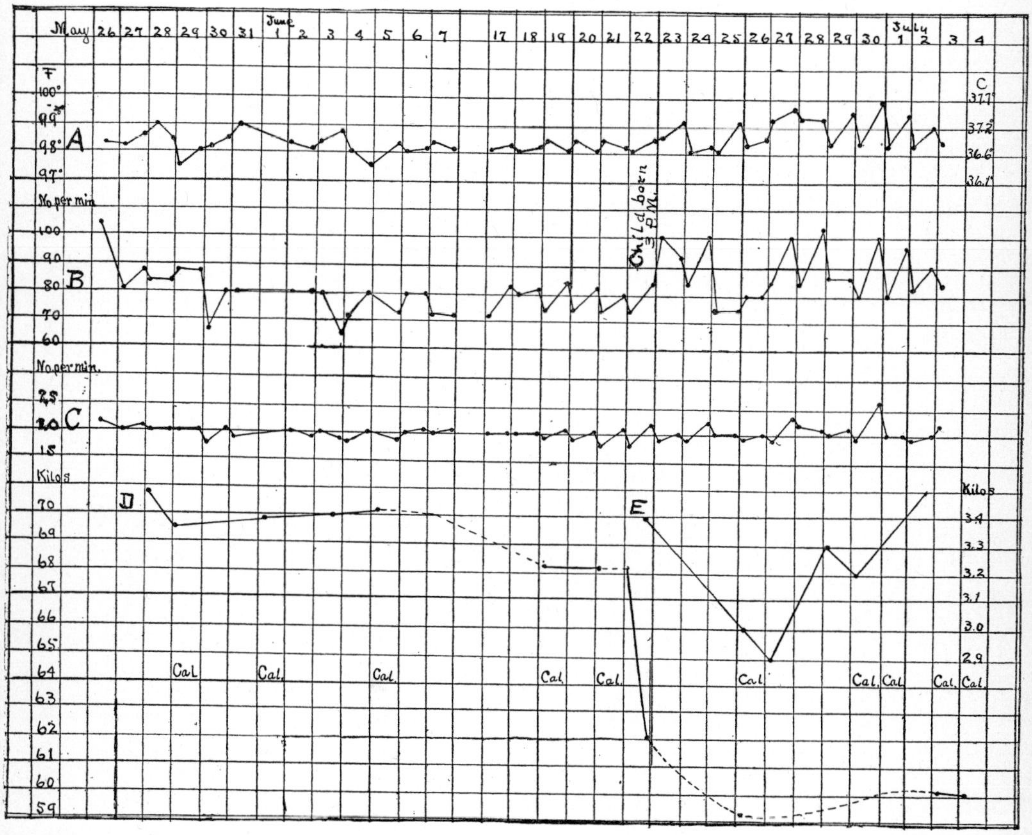


Fig. 5.—Clinical record, Case 3, Mrs. D. A., primipara. Cal., calorimeter day; A, temperature curve; B, pulse; C, respiration; D, mother's weight; E, child's weight.

The pulse in Case 2 was perhaps a little less regular than usual before parturition, but this was probably due to the nervous temperament of the patient and especially to the fact that she was in a rather badly

19. Williams: Text-Book of Obstetrics, 1908, p. 336.

run-down condition when she entered the hospital. For several days immediately preceding parturition, however, her pulse and in fact her whole clinical record is perfectly regular. It is possible that the high evening pulse and temperature of May 21 and May 26 in this case were due in some degree to the mild excitement of the laboratory experience during the morning hours, but this seems hardly probable in view of the fact that a pulse equally high was recorded on June 6 and 8, and a temperature equally high on June 3 and 9 when the patient had not been to the laboratory. On no other day can we find the slightest indication of any influence on the clinical record caused by the laboratory experience or by the journey to and fro either when the patient walked or when she was conveyed in an ambulance.

The curves representing the body weights of the mothers call for a word of explanation. Weighings in all cases were made at the laboratory just before the patient entered the calorimeter, no account being taken of fluctuations between calorimeter days. Between days when the weight is positively known the curve is represented by a continuous line. Because it was deemed necessary to keep the mother in a horizontal position immediately after delivery and because the laboratory was not provided with a scales having a platform large enough to support the ambulance stretcher, or calorimeter bed, we are obliged to interpolate the weights within the first eight or ten days of the puerperium. This has been done by making due allowance for the weight of afterbirth, which was obtained in two of the cases, and of the average weight of liquor amnii as given by Gassner[20] in 154 cases, by consulting the curves representing loss of weight in the puerperium as given by Gassner,[20] by Baumm[21] and by Heil,[22] and finally by referring to the dietary records which were strictly kept throughout. These portions of the curves are shown in broken line. While this interpolation of weights is not entirely satisfactory, we believe that no very considerable error is thereby introduced. It should be added that in most instances in the special tables which follow, the per-kilogram data are based on the known weights.

Special results of the investigation are set forth by means of the summaries contained in Tables 4, 5, 6 and 7. By way of comment on the detailed laboratory records which accompany the charts we would direct attention to the following:

## GENERAL RESULTS

1. *Pulse and Metabolism.*—The records seem to show that in patients of this class the pulse alone cannot be taken as an index of the intensity of the metabolic processes, either in the same patient or as between differ-

20. Gassner: Monatschr. f. Geburtsk., 1862, xix, 31.
21. Baumm: München. med. Wchnschr., 1887, Nos. 10 and 11.
22. Heil: Arch. f. Gynaek., 1896, li, 18.

ent patients. This was not unexpected in view of the fact that the energy of the heart is measured not by the frequency alone but by the frequency multiplied by the volume output for each beat. A simultaneous record of the pulse-pressure, if it could have been obtained with the patient in the calorimeter, would doubtless have furnished a sufficiently accurate measure of the volume output for this purpose. We did, as a matter of fact, take the blood-pressure of the patients with an Erlanger sphygmomanometer on many of the calorimeter days both before and after the calorimeter period, with this very point in view; but because of the slight disturbance to the patient incident to putting her in and taking her out of the calorimeter, we could not, without consuming more time than could be spared for the purpose, secure results which we could be sure would obtain in the calorimeter at the time the heat was being measured.

2. *Respiration.*—The respiration rate shows nothing unusual. In Case 1 it is slightly higher after parturition than before; in Case 2 about the same; and in Case 3 slightly lower. These results agree with those of L. Zuntz[23] in showing no essential change in the rate due to pregnancy. There is no indication that the number of respiratory movements bears any fixed relation to the intensity of the metabolism. We have no data on the depth of respiration.

3. *Body Temperature.*—In Case 1 the slightly febrile condition immediately after parturition may have been a determining cause of the higher heat production. In Case 2 this may have been the case previous to delivery, for example, on May 30, and on the days after parturition when the mother was alone in the calorimeter; but on the days when the baby accompanied her this factor is entirely obscured by the factor of muscular activity occasioned by the crying of the baby. In fact, this case is the only one in which the postpartum metabolism was higher than the prepartum (see summary beyond) and yet the body temperature after parturition was not distinctly higher than before. In Case 3 again where the temperature was higher after parturition the heat output was not greater than before. It is not impossible that we have in Cases 1 and 3 two distinct types of fever—the first a physiological fever caused by an increase in the heat production and the second a toxic fever caused by interference with heat loss, but showing no increased heat production.

4. *Extraneous Movements and Metabolism.*—There is a noticeable parallelism between the number of bodily movements, i. e., restlessness of the patient, and the heat production in all the cases, a circumstance which stamps this as the most important extraneous factor which we had to contend with. The variations in this respect are not so extreme as the numbers alone might indicate, for the movements were not all of the same character, sometimes being merely long breaths, at other times grosser

23. Zuntz, L.: Arch. f. Gynaek., 1910, xc, 452.

movements like turning over from side to back. The fact, however, that the metabolism does follow these fluctuations in what one may call the composure of the patient makes interpretation of any progressive difference within the last month of pregnancy or within the puerperium somewhat difficult, although, as we shall see presently, it does not invalidate the comparison of the prepartum metabolism with the postpartum, which is our chief concern. Thus without this record of movements one might be inclined to say that the metabolism per kilogram of weight in Cases 2 and 3 fell off as they approached parturition only to rise immediately before, and to refer these differences to changes in the rate of embryonic growth or at least to uterine conditions, but with the knowledge of the relative composure of the patient, the decline noted probably becomes a question of diminishing psychic effect of the calorimeter, and the rise (Case 3) just before parturition is probably secondary to restlessness induced by uterine conditions. We do not feel justified, therefore, in saying that our experiments show any progressive change in the metabolic processes due to progress of the pregnancy or to the involution processes after parturition, except as such change may be attributable to secondary causes. The experiments were limited to too short a period both before and after parturition, or were too few in number, for such a purpose.

5. *Respiratory Exchange.*—What has just been said with regard to progressive changes in total energy production, will apply also to the respiratory exchange. There is no clear evidence of a progressive change in either the carbon dioxid elimination or the oxygen absorption which is referable to progressive changes going on in the uterus.

Changes in the respiratory quotient can be accounted for in almost every case by fluctuations in the diet. Case 1 shows a falling off in the respiratory quotient as parturition is approached, while Case 2 shows in the first four days on which experiments were conducted a gradual rise in the quotient. In the former the change is due to a more restricted diet which was begun on May 21, and in the latter the change was due, probably, to improvement in the patient's appetite and in her general physical condition.

The low quotient observed in all cases immediately after parturition is due to the milk-and-broth diet on which the patients were kept at this time. That such a diet falls far short of supplying the actual energy requirement at this time can readily be shown by calculation and is emphasized by this low quotient, which is practically that of starvation. This dietetic procedure may be justifiable from the clinical standpoint, but it certainly is not from the standpoint of energy requirement. It may well be recommended to attempt supplying the full requirement of energy by fortifying the milk with lactose or other easily digested form of carbohydrate.[24] As soon as the patient returned to the diet prescribed before parturition the quotient rose, and within a week or ten days had returned to about the same level as before parturition.

The general level of the respiratory quotient is somewhat lower throughout for Case 2 than for Cases 1 and 3, a difference which we are inclined to refer to the poorly nourished condition in which this woman was received at the hospital. Both the other patients were in much better general condition, and continued so throughout.

In this connection it is of interest to compare the oxygen absorption per kilogram of weight at corresponding stages in the different patients. Thus, on the eighteenth day (June 24) before parturition in Case 2, the oxygen absorption was 0.33 gm., while on the seventeenth day (June 5) in Case 3, the absorption was only 0.28 gm., the quotient on these two days being 0.84 and 0.83, respectively. This difference is due, we believe, partly to the nutritive condition and partly also to the difference in body form. Patient 2 was tall and rather slender in build; Patient 3 was no taller, but weighed about 12 kilograms more—that is, she was comparatively fat. The effect of body fat in diminishing the heat production per kilogram of body weight is a well-known phenomenon. Again, on the first day before parturition in Case 1, the oxygen absorption per kilogram was 0.29 gm.; in Case 3 it was 0.3—or almost exactly the same. Both patients were primiparæ and were approximately of the same general build. The respiratory quotient on these two days was 0.84 and 0.83 respectively.

6. *Energy Production.*—It will be observed that the energy production directly measured and that calculated agree fairly well on most of the experiment days. This is notably true, with few exceptions, of Cases 1 and 3. The agreement is not so good in Case 2, due possibly to irregularity in the quantity of nitrogen excreted by the kidneys in the calorimeter periods. One method shows variations about as great as the other. Taking the mean of the two we have a figure which probably represents more accurately than either one alone the total energy production per hour at the different stages of the experiments. Where the physical conditions of the patients were the same, or approximately so, previous to parturition, the metabolism per kilogram of body weight, by taking the mean of direct and indirect measurements, agrees very well from day to day, e. g., Case 1, May 22 and 25; Case 2, May 24 and 26; Case 3, June 1 and 19. Naturally it was much more difficult to secure physical conditions for both mother and child which would be the same on different days of the experiment, yet where this chanced to be approximately true,

---

24. See Shaffer, P. A., and Coleman, W.: Protein Metabolism in Typhoid Fever. The Archives Int. Med., 1910, iv, 538; also Murlin: The Nutritive Value of Gelatin. II. The Influence of Carbohydrate, etc., Am. Jour. Physiol., 1907, xx, 234.

as in Case 1, June 7 and 9, and Case 3, June 26 and 30, the agreement again is fairly good, better than it would have been by taking the direct measurements alone. In each case the metabolism per kilogram was highest for mother and child immediately after parturition. In Case 1, this was due to the febrile condition of the mother; in Case 2, in part at least, to the restlessness of the child, and consequently of the mother; in Case 3, the cause is not so clear, but it may have been the nervousness of the patient so soon after parturition. (See also "Comparison of the Metabolism of Mother and Child Before and After Birth.")

## SPECIAL RESULTS

### I. COMPARISON OF THE METABOLISM OF PREGNANT AND NON-PREGNANT WOMEN

We have already seen from *a priori* considerations as well as from the few experiments which have been reported that there is no significant increase in the metabolism of the pregnant organism, even in the absolute sense, until near the middle of the gestation period, and that the single experiment of Magnus-Levy is the only one on record so far in which an increase per kilogram of weight has been reported before the middle of pregnancy. We were fortunate enough to receive the recent paper of L. Zuntz[23] in time to find that, so far as the respiratory metabolism alone is concerned, this general conclusion is confirmed by the complete report of his experiments. Zuntz reports three cases on two of which he made observations by means of the Zuntz-Geppert method throughout the gestation period and on the third a few observations in the sixth month only. He compares the results with figures previously obtained from the same subjects in sexual rest. The first two increased considerably in weight during the gestation period, quite independently of the product of conception, so that the amount of oxygen absorbed, when expressed per kilogram of body weight, was even less in the ninth month (Case C) than it had been in sexual rest, or was so little greater (Case B) that Zuntz believed the difference was entirely due to the increased labor of respiration. In the third case, however, the weight was less in the sixth month than it had been previous to conception, the oxygen absorption being as a consequence significantly larger per unit of weight in the pregnant condition. On the basis of this experiment and that of Magnus-Levy, Zuntz concluded that at the end of pregnancy the respiratory metabolism normally would be considerably higher than in sexual rest and that this is not altogether due to increased labor of respiration.

This paper has been purposely delayed for the sake of obtaining results on the metabolism of non-pregnant women for comparison with those obtained in this investigation. Such determinations have recently been made in this laboratory on seven different women ranging in age from 18 to 55 years, and in weight from 37 to 66 kilograms. We have also been fortunate enough to induce the subject of our Case 1 to return to the laboratory, just one year from the date of her confinement, for three one-hour determinations. The results for this woman show certain discrepancies with those obtained from her a year previously, due possibly to differences in her physical condition at the time of the experiment. For this reason the results are included only in the average for the normal woman (Table 4).

TABLE 4.—COMPARISON OF THE ENERGY METABOLISM IN PREGNANT AND NON-PREGNANT WOMEN, COMPILED FROM ALL SOURCES KNOWN TO-DAY

| | Pregnant (ninth month). | | | | Non-pregnant. | | | | |
|---|---|---|---|---|---|---|---|---|---|
| Subjects. | Weight kg. | $O_2$ abs. c.c. per kg. and min. | R. Q. | Heat production cal. per kg. and min. | Weight kg. | $O_2$ abs. c.c. per kg. and min. | R. Q. | Heat production cal. per kg. and min. | Remarks. |
| s-Levy's case (1896-97) | 115 | 3.3 | ... | .... | 108 | 2.9 | ... | .... | |
| tz' Case A (1905) | 50 | 3.9 | .79 | .... | 50.9 | 3.47 | .85 | .... | Sixth month of pregnancy. |
| tz' Case B (1904-5) | 58 | 3.7 | .87 | .... | 48.6 | 3.5 | .84 | .... | |
| tz' Case C (1903-4) | 67 | 3.4 | .84 | .... | 54.7 | 3.75 | .81 | .... | Mean of all four cases to this point 3.4 c.c. $O_2$. |
| s' Case 1 (1909) | 63 | 3.4 | .85 | 0.96 | 51.4 | 3.46 | .85 | 1.06 | 1st, 4th and 6th days prepartum; 15th day postpartum. |
| s' Case 2 (1909) | 58 | 3.9 | .83 | 1.11 | 48.5 | 4.12 | .78 | 1.23 | Mean of 13, 17, 19, 20 and 22d days prepartum; 4th and 11th days postpartum. |
| s' Case 3 (1909) | 69.1 | 3.4 | .85 | 1.02 | 60.1 | 3.34 | .83 | 1.00 | Mean of 1st, 3d, 17th, 21st and 24th days prepartum; 9th and 12th days postpartum. |
| Mean. of 1, 2 and 3 | | | | | 3.65 | ... | 1.10 | | |
| e of eight normal women, laboratory (1910) | .. | ... | ... | .... | 37-66 | 3.48 | .88 | 0.99 | This average includes Case 1 for May 24, 1910. |
| e of all cases | .. | 3.57 | .84 | 1.03 | .... | 3.49 | .88 | 1.02 | |

It is surprising how close is the agreement between the results obtained with the respiration calorimeter and those obtained by the Zuntz-Geppert method. Zuntz' Case C agrees perfectly as far as $O_2$ absorption is concerned, with our Cases 1 and 3. The agreement between his Case B and our Case 2 is not so close as seems at first sight, for it is certain that his subject was much fatter than ours, and the quotient is higher. The mean oxygen absorption per kilogram and minute in the non-pregnant woman before conception is 3.45 c.c. (for first four cases in the table, 3.4 c.c.; for the eight normal women recently experimented on in this laboratory, 3.48 c.c.) but the mean for our three cases taken during the puerperium is 3.65 c.c., an increase of 5.8 per cent.[25] This higher average, however, is entirely due to the high figure given by Case 2, which exhibits a much lower respiratory quotient, a result probably attributable to the food factor. Neglecting this case we can say that the oxygen absorption per kilogram and minute is the same in the puerperium as in complete sexual rest. The mean result for all non-pregnant subjects is 3.49 c.c. For the pregnant woman the result is 3.57 c.c.—3.5 per cent. more than the amount obtained for all the cases taken in complete sexual rest and 2.2 per cent. less than the average for the puerperium.

As for the heat production per kilogram and hour, the only data available are from our own cases. The mean result for the pregnant woman is almost exactly the same as the average for all the non-pregnant subjects summarized in the table—1.03 calories for the former, 1.02 calories for the latter. For the woman in complete sexual rest, however, the mean result for the eight cases is 0.99 calories per kilogram and hour, i. e., about 4 per cent. less than for the pregnant woman. The agreement between the oxygen difference and the total energy difference is very satisfactory indeed. The *conclusion which we may draw with entire confidence is,* that *the energy metabolism, expressed per kilogram and hour, of the pregnant woman in the last month of her pregnancy, is but little larger (4 per cent.)*[26] *than for a woman in complete sexual rest.*

While we have no data as to the depth of respiration or as to the increased labor of respiration in pregnancy, we are inclined to think that so slight a difference might be attributable entirely to such a cause, instead of only partly so, as L. Zuntz believes. In fact, according to Zuntz' own estimate of the increased labor of respiration in his Case B the difference in oxygen absorption between the pregnant and the non-pregnant condition is exactly accounted for in this way. This conclusion would mean, very clearly, that the metabolism of the fetus, together with all the accessory structures, is the same as so much maternal tissue. If the metabolism of the fetus itself were slightly higher in the human being, as it seems, from Bohr's[27] experiments, to be in the guinea-pig, this factor would be counterbalanced by the fact that the liquor amnii (and possibly the membranes) takes no part in the metabolism (see, however, the discussion of the metabolism per unit area of surface).

On the other hand the heat production in the puerperium is distinctly higher than that for complete sexual rest or for the pregnant condition—

25. Magnus-Levy (Ztschr. f. klin. Med. 1897, xxxiii, 258) gives results on the respiratory exchange of twelve normal women ranging in weight from 31 to 76.5 kg., and in age from 18 to 40. The average amount of $O_2$ absorbed was 4.1 c.c. (Zuntz method).

26. If Rubner's law of skin area is strictly true for subjects of this class the difference is really about 10 per cent. (see end of Section IV, Metabolism per Unit Area of Body Surface).

27. Bohr: Skandin. Arch. f. Physiol., 1900, x, 413.

the average for our three cases being 1.10 calories per kilogram and hour, or 11 per cent. higher than the average for the former and 7 per cent. higher than the average for the latter. The three cases actually agree in this better than appears from the summary in Table 4. By reference to Table 3 it may be seen that Case 3 showed a heat production of 1.09 calories per kilogram and hour on the ninth day and that the low figure given in Table 4 is due to the unusually low result obtained on July 4, the last day of the series, when the patient was extraordinarily quiet.

What is the explanation of this higher energy production of the puerperient mother? That it was not fever is apparent from the very accurate temperature measurements made by the rectal thermometer. It is quite conceivable that the processes of involution, which were not yet entirely complete at the time our observations were made, set free decomposition products which stimulate the general heat production in a manner analogous to the stimulation of the mammary glands by fetal products. If so, the processes by which heat is lost from the body (evaporation of water, radiation and conduction) must be equally stimulated, for there is no accumulation of heat. A state of hyperactivity of the sweat-glands, especially during the early days of the puerperium, is a phenomenon well known to obstetricians and it is possible that this activity is a primary cause of the increased heat production—a cooling of the body surface generally resulting in a reflex stimulation of the heat-producing tissues. We believe, however, that the most important factors are the activity of the mammary glands and the specific dynamic action[28] of the foodstuffs burning—especially the increased protein combustion[29] due to involution of the uterus. All of our patients were nursing their babies and at the time of the experiments the breasts were overfull of milk, though there was, so far as we know, no irritation from this condition. The lower respiratory quotient found in the puerperium which, as we have seen, is to be ascribed to the restricted diet very commonly imposed immediately after delivery, is a sign that the patient has used up her store of glycogen during labor and is thrown back on her reserve of fat, and on the protein resorbed from the uterus, for her supply of energy. The dynamic action of the latter would considerably increase the heat production.[30]

## II. COMPARISON OF THE METABOLISM OF MOTHER AND CHILD BEFORE AND AFTER BIRTH

A comparison between the prepartum and postpartum metabolism of mother and child is shown in Table 5. Taking the mean of all experiment days both before and after birth, we find that the temperature of

28. Consult Lusk: Science of Nutrition, Philadelphia, 1909, p. 156.
29. Cf. Murlin: Am. Jour. Physiol., 1910, xxvii, 177.
30. Cf. Rubner: Energie-Gesetze,, p. 370.

the mother's body (and, we might add, the other physical conditions as well) shows but little change. The greatest difference occurred in Case 3, where the temperature remained about half a degree higher up to the time the experiments terminated (eleventh day) than it was before parturition. This, however, it will be noted, did not increase the total metabolism.

The carbon dioxid output in each case is higher before parturition than after; the oxygen, on the contrary, is slightly higher after parturition than before, differences which, of course, are reflected in the lower quotient following parturition. The energy production expressed in absolute figures in both Cases 1 and 3, is almost the same before and after

TABLE 5.—ENERGY METABOLISM OF MOTHER AND CHILD TOGETHER BEFORE AND AFTER PARTURITION

| Case. Mean of all days before and after delivery. | Average body temp °C | Respiratory Exchange. $CO_2$ gm. per hour. | $O_2$ gm. per hour. | R. Q. | Energy Production, Calories per hour. *a*—Direct. | *b*—Indirect. | $\frac{a+b}{2}$ | % difference. | per kg. | % difference. |
|---|---|---|---|---|---|---|---|---|---|---|
| Case 1— 1st, 4th and 6th before delivery | 36.75 | 21.3 | 18.4 | .85 | 60.0 | 61.3 | 60.7 | .... | 0.96 | .... |
| 2d, 5th, 12th, 14th and 17th after delivery | 36.9 | 20.2 | 18.5 | .80 | 61.2 | 61.2 | 61.2 | + .87 | 1.11 | +15.6 |
| Case 2— 13th, 17th, 19th, 20th and 22d before delivery | 36.68 | 22.3 | 19.6 | .83 | 63.6 | 65.9 | 64.7 | .... | 1.11 | .... |
| 2d, 5th and 11th after delivery | 36.8 | 21.7 | 20.4 | .78 | 71.1 | 67.5 | 69.3 | +7.1 | 1.32 | +18.9 |
| Case 3— 1st, 3d, 17th, 21st and 24th before delivery | 36.64 | 23.9 | 20.2 | .86 | 72.2 | 68.7 | 70.6 | .... | 1.02 | .... |
| 4th, 8th and 11th after delivery | 37.23 | 23.1 | 20.3 | .81 | 70.8 | 68.6 | 69.7 | — .9 | 1.11 | + 8.8 |

parturition. In Case 2 there is an increase of about 7 per cent. in the postpartum metabolism over the prepartum. It is gratifying to note that this general result would not be materially changed in either case if the figures as obtained by direct measurement, or those obtained by calculation were used alone instead of the mean of the two. The slight increase in Case 2 can perhaps be accounted for by the crying of the baby on two out of the three postpartum days. We feel justified therefore in drawing the conclusion, that *the postpartum metabolism of mother and child is not greater in absolute amount than the prepartum metabolism.* In other words, the extra metabolism of pregnancy at its culmination, due in part to the activity of the accessory maternal structures as well as to the fetus, is just compensated by an extra metabolism set up after the child begins an independent existence. Ruling out the factor of muscular activity in mother and offspring, therefore, as we have succeeded in doing in Cases 1 and 3, the curve of total energy metabolism in mother and child suffers no deflection at birth. This conclusion is the same as that drawn by one of us from experiments on the pregnant dog.[31]

Calculated per kilogram of total weight of mother and child, the post-partum metabolism shows an increase of from 9 to 19 per cent. over the prepartum. That is, while the absolute amount of energy produced by mother and child is just the same after birth as before, each average kilogram of mother-and-child material is producing more energy after birth. To understand this we must bear in mind two facts:

1. The total weight after birth is considerably less than before and a part of the material whose weight is to be deducted (liquor amnii, blood, membranes, placenta, etc.) did not participate at all in the metabolism and the remainder of it probably did not participate so actively as mother and fetus proper. The metabolism before birth is diluted or toned down, so to speak, by a certain weight of inanimate and relatively inert material.

2. We have seen in the previous section that in spite of this fact the metabolism per unit of weight of the mother alone in the puerperium is but 11 per cent. at most more than that of a woman just before parturition. Hence, it follows that the greater energy production per unit of weight after birth is due in considerable part to the more active metabolism of the new-born child. It is a remarkable fact that the compensation mentioned above should be so perfect that the increase in energy production in the child when it passes from the warm environment of its mother's uterus to that of the outside world (in bed beside its mother) plus the increase in the mother's own metabolism, should be so nearly equal to the energy required by the fetus and the accessory parts which supported it *in utero*.

Just how much the child's metabolism increases at the time of birth we have as yet no certain means of knowing. That it is considerable —that the change represents indeed a turning-point, in the quantitative sense, in the metabolism of the child—is evident, by analogy at least, from Bohr's[27] results on the guinea-pig, where the metabolism of the embryo was found to be only 10 per cent. greater per unit of weight than that of the mother, and from the results which will be given in the next section. The demands on the digestive system of the mother, however, are not greater. She is called on to supply the same amount of energy in potential form to herself and child immediately after parturition that she did to herself and child immediately before.

31. Murlin: Am. Jour. Physiol., 1910, xxvi, 134.

## III. ENERGY METABOLISM OF THE NEW-BORN CHILD

It was not our intention at the outset to attempt determinations of the metabolism of the child, but as the experiments progressed we saw the possibility of obtaining this by difference. The bed calorimeter is not calculated to measure a total quantity of heat as small as that produced by a new-born child with a high percentage of accuracy; but it is calculated to measure the quantity produced by adults with an accuracy much greater (that is, with an error much less) than the metabolism of the infant alone would amount to. If, therefore, we obtain the metabolism of

TABLE 6.—ENERGY METABOLISM OF NEW-BORN CHILD

| Case. | Av. weight kg. | Body temperature of mother. | Respiratory Exchange. $CO_2$ gm. per hour. | $O_2$ gm. per hour. | R. Q. | Energy Production, Calories per hour. *a*—Direct. | *b*—Indirect. | $\frac{a+b}{2}$ | Per kg. | Remarks. |
|---|---|---|---|---|---|---|---|---|---|---|
| Case 1— Mother and child; mean of 5 days after parturition...... | ... | 36.9 | 20.2 | 18.5 | .80 | 61.2 | 61.2 | 61.2 | 1.11 | |
| Mother alone; 15th day after parturition .............. | ... | 36.4 | 17.8 | 15.3 | .85 | 53.5 | 54.3 | 53.9 | 1.05 | |
| Child by difference........... | 2.7 | .... | 2.4 | 3.2 | .56 | 7.7 | 6.9 | 7.3 | 2.70 | =2.57 times that mother (1.05) |
| Case 2— Mother and child; mean of 3 days after parturition...... | ... | 36.8 | 21.7 | 20.4 | .78 | 71.1 | 67.5 | 69.3 | 1.32 | |
| Mother alone; mean of 4th and 11th days after parturition.. | ... | 36.8 | 18.3 | 17.2 | .78 | 62.0 | 57.2 | 59.3 | 1.21 | |
| Child by difference........... | 3.4 | .... | 3.4 | 3.2 | .77 | 9.1 | 10.3 | 9.7 | 2.88 | 2.34 times tha mother (1.21 |
| Case 3— Mother and child; mean of 3 days after parturition...... | ... | 37.2 | 23.1 | 20.8 | .81 | 70.8 | 68.7 | 69.7 | 1.09 | |
| Mother alone; mean of 9th and 12th days after parturition.. | ... | 37.3 | 19.7 | 17.4 | .83 | 62.7 | 58.1 | 60.4 | 1.00 | |
| Child by difference........... | 3.2 | .... | 3.4 | 3.2 | .73 | 8.1 | 10.6 | 9.3 | 2.90 | 2.9 times tha mother. |
| Mean of 1, 2 and 3 (child).... | ... | .... | 3.1 | 3.3 | .68 | 8.3 | 9.3 | 8.8 | 2.82 | 2.6 times tha mother. |

the mother and child with a satisfactory degree of accuracy and that of the mother alone with the same accuracy the difference, or the metabolism of the child, ought to be at least fairly accurate, provided the conditions of the different determinations are comparable. Acting on this thought we made one determination in Case 1 on the mother alone on a day immediately adjoining that of a determination on mother and child, and two such determinations in both the other cases. Without attempting to select the days which would be most nearly comparable, we have taken the mean of all in each case (Table 6) in the belief that the conditions throughout were as nearly constant as it would ever be possible to get them. It should be understood that the results here obtained represent the metabolism of a child while sleeping only (Cases 1 and 3) or at least comparatively quiet and sleeping most of the time (Case 2) and while kept warm in bed beside the mother. It should be added also that in every determination with mother and child, the child had been allowed to nurse immediately before the experiment.[32]

The respiratory quotient, it will be observed, is comparatively low in each case, and in Case 1 is probably too low to be trustworthy. Quotients as low as this have been reported for new-born infants by Scherer[33] and by Babák,[34] but one feels very loath to believe that these results can be reliable unless it can be shown that some oxygen-rich substance is being formed for storage out of some oxygen-poor substance by utilizing oxygen absorbed from the lungs.

The average respiratory quotient obtained by both Scherer and Babák for a child exposed to ordinary room temperature is about 0.7, with which our own results in the latter two cases agree very well. These are the only determinations on infants as young as ours which we have been able to find in the literature. Recent determinations on infants above 4 months of age made by Schlossmann, Oppenheimer and Murschhauser[35] make the quotient as high as 0.9.

The heat production, expressed per kilogram and hour, of our three infants agree very well with that obtained by Babák in the experiments above mentioned on infants from one hour to eight days old with a compensating calorimeter of the d'Arsonval type, and by Rubner and Heubner[36] on an infant nine weeks old with the Voit-Pettenkoffer apparatus. Babák's results vary between 2.42 calories per kilogram and hour at 24° C. and 3.83 calories at 12.1° with an average of 3.15 calories for the seven experiments. Rubner and Heubner found 2.93 calories.

Perhaps the most interesting thing about our determinations of the metabolism of the infant is the opportunity we had for a direct comparison with the metabolism of the mother under conditions which would influence the energy production to about the same extent. While the mother had had no breakfast, the child had just been fed; but while the mother was awake, the child was asleep (with the exception of two days

32. The urine of the child was not collected. Such error as this produces would make the indirect measurement too high: see method, D. "The Heat Production as Calculated," under "Methods of Determination."

33. Scherer: Jahrb. f. Kinderh., 1896, xliii, 471.

34. Babák: Arch. f. d. ges. Physiol., 1902, lxxxix, 154.

35. Schlossmann, Oppenheimer and Murschhauser: Biochem. Ztschr., 1908, xiv, 385.

36. Rubner and Heubner: Ztschr. f. Biol., 1898, xxxvi, 1.

in Case 2, as already noted). The differences would therefore tend to equalize each other.

*The first infant showed a metabolism per kilogram and hour two and a half times that of its mother, the second two and three-tenths, and the third two and nine-tenths—an average for the three of a little over two and a half.*

## IV. METABOLISM PER UNIT AREA OF BODY SURFACE

We have already seen that the metabolism of the pregnant woman, expressed per unit of weight is about 4 per cent. greater than that of the non-pregnant woman. It becomes of special interest now in view of the generally recognized importance of Rubner's law of skin area to consider what influence the change in shape of the woman's body may have had in producing this higher metabolism. Has the abdominal distention and other hypertrophy characteristic of the last month of pregnancy brought about a greater exposure of skin surface in proportion to weight, and, if so, how may it be conceived to affect the rate of heat loss and consequently of heat production? To any one familiar with Rubner's law it is evident at once that the higher metabolism per unit of weight in a person of greater weight must mean either a change in the relationship of surface to weight or an increase in the metabolism per unit of surface, because with the formula $S = K\sqrt[3]{W^2}$, the larger the weight becomes the smaller (proportionally) becomes the surface. This will be readily understood by comparing the energy production of the mother before and after delivery as calculated from the above formula (employing Rubner's factor 12.3 as the constant) with that of women in complete sexual rest.

Table 7 shows that the energy production per square meter of surface and hour is higher for the pregnant woman in each case than it is for the eight normal women (last line of table). The increase is 3.9 per cent. for Case 1, 15.8 per cent. for Case 2 and 12.2 per cent. for Case 3; or 10.6 per cent. as the average for the three. The percentage increase per unit of surface, in other words, is apparently greater than the percentage increase per unit of weight. We say "apparently" because in reality if the metabolism per unit of surface were the same in two individuals differing as much in weight as these two groups of individuals did (about 20 per cent.) the difference per kilogram would be at least 6 per cent. in favor of the smaller individual, which, added to the increase of 4 per cent. in favor of the larger individual which we found, makes the percentage increase per unit of weight actually the same as that per unit of surface. This, however, is a mere coincidence. For the metabolism per unit of surface ought to be the same, according to Rubner's law, which seems to be fairly well established. Is the increase then per unit of surface due to a change in the relation of surface to weight (i. e., does the formula need to be modified for pregnant women), or to a specific difference?

Anticipating this problem, we made some measurements on two of the patients both before and after delivery, with the idea of estimating the difference in skin area due to pregnancy. These measurements apply to the abdomen only and assume that the extent of the abdominal wall near the close of the puerperium would be essentially the same as that of a woman in complete sexual rest. The shape of the abdomen in the non-pregnant woman we considered as roughly that of a cylinder, and the shape in the last few weeks of pregnancy with the patient on her back, as she would be most likely to lie in the calorimeter, to be roughly that of one-half of a sphere added to one-half of a cylinder. To

TABLE 7.—METABOLISM OF MOTHER (BEFORE AND AFTER PARTURITION) AND OF CHILD PER SQUARE METER OF SURFACE *

| | Weight kg. | Skin area sq. m. | $CO_2$ gm. per hour. | $O_2$ absorbed gm. per hour. | Heat production calories per hr. | $CO_2$ thermal quotient. | $O^2$ thermal quotient. |
|---|---|---|---|---|---|---|---|
| Case 1— | | | | | | | |
| Mother before parturition..... | 63 | 1.94 | 11.0 | 9.5 | 31.4 | 35.0 | 30.2 |
| Mother after parturition..... | 51.4 | 1.70 | 10.5 | 9.0 | 31.7 | 33.1 | 28.4 |
| Child ...................... | 2.7 | 0.24 | 10.0 | 12.9 | 30.5 | .... | .... |
| Case 2— | | | | | | | |
| Mother before parturition..... | 58 | 1.84 | 12.1 | 10.6 | 35.1 | 34.4 | 30.2 |
| Mother after parturition....... | 48.5 | 1.64 | 11.1 | 10.5 | 36.2 | 30.6 | 29.0 |
| Child ...................... | 3.4 | 0.28 | 12.2 | 11.5 | 34.9 | .... | .... |
| Case 3— | | | | | | | |
| Mother before parturition..... | 69.1 | 2.07 | 11.5 | 9.8 | 34.0 | 33.8 | 28.8 |
| Mother after parturition..... | 60.1 | 1.89 | 10.4 | 9.1 | 31.9† | 32.6 | 28.5 |
| Child ...................... | 3.2 | 0.28 | 13.6 | 13.1 | 33.2 | .... | .... |
| Average of eight normal women (1910) .................. | 37-66 | .... | 11.0 | 9.1 | 30.3 | 36.3 | 30.0 |

* Formula $12.3\sqrt[3]{(W)^2}$

† Taking ninth day only after parturition this figure would be 34.7.

make sure that we did not underestimate the increase we calculated the skin area, indeed, as if two-thirds of a sphere were added to two-thirds of the cylinder. Thus on July 3, with Case 3 we found the length of the abdominal cylinder from pubis to ensiform process to be 75 cm., and the circumference of the cylinder at the umbilicus to be 36 cm.—a total skin area for this part of the body therefore of 0.27 sq. M. On June 3, about three weeks before delivery this same woman measured from pubis to ensiform 42 cm. and around the body at the umbilicus 98 cm. Calculating the area of a sphere with circumference of 98 cm. by the formula $4 \pi r^2$, taking two-thirds of that amount and adding to two-thirds of the area of the cylinder we get 0.383 sq. M. as the area of the abdomen of the pregnant woman, an increase therefore over the area ten days after delivery of 0.113 sq. M. This method is confessedly crude, but it gives a figure for the increase in skin area of the pregnant woman, which is at least large enough and is probably much too large. Nevertheless this amount is not so large as is obtained by calculating the surface from the weight on the two dates given above and taking the difference. On July 3, the weight was 60 kg. and by the formula $12.3 \sqrt[3]{W^2}$ the surface at this time would have been 1.885 sq. M. On June 3 the weight was 70 kg. and the surface by the same formula would be 2.089 sq. M. This makes the difference in surface 0.204 sq. M. It is clear, therefore, that the same formula would not apply to the pregnant women. Reversing the process and estimating what factor would be necessary to give an increase in surface of 0.113 sq. M. for a weight of 70 kg. over that of 60 kg., we find that the factor 12.3 would need to be changed to 11.8. Applying the same method to Case 2 we found that in order to give the increase of skin area which could be demonstrated by regarding the pregnant abdomen as two-thirds of a sphere added to two-thirds of a cylinder, the factor 12.3 in the formula would need to be changed to 11.4. This woman, it may be remembered, was very slender and was also a multipara, while Patient 3 was the fattest of the three patients and was a primipara. Hence these figures may be taken as representing sufficient range for the deviation from Rubner's factor of 12.3 which would be necessary to express the relationship of skin area to weight produced by the distention of the abdomen, although the deviation itself may not be large enough. This estimate is sufficiently liberal also, we think, to cover the enlarged mammary glands and any other increase in surface such as that due to hypertrophy of the pelvis generally. We may fairly conclude then that the relation of body surface to body weight in the pregnant woman presents a considerable departure from that of the normal adult—that, in fact, the amount of surface in proportion to weight is relatively less than that of a normal adult. It is a singular fact and one probably not without its significance that the factor necessary to express the relationship of surface to weight in the pregnant woman should approach that found by Meeh[37] for infants.

It is evident, however, that this change in relationship cannot account for the higher metabolism per unit of weight; for a smaller surface would mean a diminished heat loss and a corresponding decrease in heat production. This forces the conclusion, therefore, that a higher metabolism in the pregnant woman is a specific one. The heat production in some part of the body is higher and the heat loss is consequently greater

---

37. Meeh: Ztschr. f. Biol., 1879, xv, 425.

per square meter surface than it is in the average normal woman. For illustration, employing the factor 11.8 and calculating the heat production per square meter surface for Case 1, we get 32.5 calories instead of 31.4 as given in the table. This would make the lowest of our results for the pregnant woman over 7 per cent. greater per unit of surface than for the average of the eight normal women. We cannot commit ourselves to this conclusion quite without reserve, for the reason that the individual variation among the normal women, as well as among the pregnant women, is more than 7 per cent. It is possible that this same woman (Case 1) under identically the same outward circumstances would have produced in sexual rest as much energy per unit of surface as she did in pregnancy. The evidence, as far as it goes, taking averages in both sets of observations, however, supports the general conclusion stated above. If this conclusion should be confirmed by other observations it would be necessary to suppose that the energy production in the child just before it is born is enough greater to more than offset the dead weight of liquor amnii, etc., which take no part in the metabolism, or else that the extra heat loss is due to the greater vascularity of the organs contained in the abdomen, to the thinness of the abdominal wall—the extra good conduction, in short, from uterus to the outside world. It is scarcely conceivable that any other part of the body can play any important rôle in the greater loss. But several points in this connection must wait for further data.

The metabolism after delivery when calculated per unit of surface is likewise, of course, higher than that of the woman in sexual rest. In Case 1 it is 4.6 per cent.; in Case 2, 19.1 per cent.; in Case 3, 5.2 per cent. (or employing the figure 34.7 given in the note at the bottom of the table, 14.5 per cent.). The average is 9.6 per cent. at least or 12.7 per cent. at most. The difference on the basis of weight was 11 per cent.

Calculated per unit of surface and per unit of weight the increase appears to be about the same. This again is a mere coincidence, for the average weight of the puerperient woman was 53 kg. while that of the women in sexual rest was only 50 kg., a difference which, as just seen, would accentuate the higher metabolism per unit of surface in the puerperium. Reasoning similar to that employed for the pregnant woman would lead us to the conclusion that this higher metabolism is a specific one, for it is scarcely possible that the skin surface is 9 per cent. greater than that of the normal woman.

An interesting side-light on the metabolism of the newly delivered and nursing woman is obtained from the thermal quotients.

## THERMAL QUOTIENTS

Inspection of Table 7 shows that the amount of carbon dioxid eliminated per unit of surface is higher for two of the pregnant women than it is for normal women and for the other it is just the same. On the other hand, for two of the puerperient women the amount of carbon dioxid is lower than for normal women and for the other it is the same. The column for the oxygen absorption shows that the amount for pregnant women is uniformly higher than for normal women, while for the puerperient women it is the same in two cases and higher in the other.

These comparisons have little meaning unless considered in relation to the heat production. In the last columns of this same table are shown the carbon dioxid and the oxygen thermal quotients—that is, the number of grams of carbon dioxid given off and of oxygen absorbed in the production of every 100 calories of energy.[38] Here it is seen that the oxygen absorption for two of the pregnant women is quite normal while for the third it is somewhat lower. For the puerperient women the oxygen absorption is distinctly lower than normal in all of the cases. If these figures are borne out in the future we shall be led to the belief that heat is being produced in the latter condition by some other process than that of oxidation.

The carbon dioxid thermal quotient is below that of the normal women for all cases, both in the pregnant condition and after delivery. This is readily explained by the higher respiratory quotient in the normal women (see Table 4), which in turn is to be explained by the presence of more carbohydrate in the diet. Similarly the lower carbon dioxid thermal quotient for the newly delivered woman is due to the difference in foodstuffs burning.

## V. METABOLISM PER UNIT AREA OF SURFACE IN THE CHILD

We do not feel disposed to draw sweeping conclusions as to the bearing of our determinations on the metabolism per unit of surface of the child as compared with that of the adult woman. As is well known, the experiments of Sondén and Tigerstedt[39] and those of Magnus-Levy and Falk[40] seem to show a higher metabolism per unit of surface in children than in adults, while the experiments of Rubner and Heubner,[36, 41] and especially the more recent experiments of Schlossmann[42] and his co-workers on infants, tend to confirm the idea that the metabolism of the young is not specifically higher except in so far as the surface is greater.

Our experiments show a heat production per square meter of surface a little higher for the child than for a woman in sexual rest in Cases 2

38. Cf. Benedict: The Influence of Inanition on Metabolism, p. 504.

39. Sondén and Tigerstedt: Skandin. Arch. f. Physiol., 1895, vi, 53.

40. Magnus-Levy and Falk: Arch. f. Anat. u. Physiol., Supplement Bd., 1899, 344.

41. Rubner and Heubner: Ztschr. f. exper. Path. u. Therap., 1905, i, 1.

42. Schlossmann, Oppenheimer and Murschhauser: Biochem. Ztschr., 1908, xiv, 385. Schlossmann and Murschhauser, Ibid., 1909, xviii, 499.

and 3 and about the same in Case 1. On the other hand, as compared with its own nursing mother the heat production is lower in two of the cases and higher in one. Any error in this latter comparison due to differences in conditions, such as the fact that the mother was awake while the child slept, would tend to be equalized by the fact that the child had just been fed while the mother was on empty stomach, that the result for the child is confessedly a little higher because of the omission of the urine in the calculation, and finally by the fact that we have used the same constant (12.3) in computing the surface of the child as for the mother, while one ought perhaps to use a constant somewhat lower. To what extent the greater warming of the child by the mother than of the mother by the child would influence the results we do not attempt to say. We wish it borne in mind that our results on the child alone are not only indirect but largely incidental to the main purpose of the experiments. We can merely say that there is no evidence from them that the metabolism of the infant beside its nursing mother in bed is higher per unit of surface than is that of the mother in the same bed alone, although there is evidence that it is higher than that of a woman in complete sexual rest. To make the comparison complete we should have had the child alone in the same bed, but that was impossible on account of the size of the calorimeter.

## *SUMMARY*

1. In agreement with the results of one of us on the dog, we find that the curve of total energy production of mother and child suffers no deflection at birth. The extra metabolism of the pregnant woman at the culmination of pregnancy, due in part to the accessory structures as well as to the fetus, is just equalled by the extra metabolism set up in the newborn child by exposure of its body to the outside world, and in the mother by activity of the mammary glands, etc.

2. The energy metabolism, expressed per unit of weight, of the pregnant woman is about 7 per cent. less than that of the same woman newly delivered, and about 4 per cent. more than that of women in complete sexual rest. Expressed per unit of surface ($12.3\sqrt[3]{W^2}$) the energy metabolism of the pregnant woman is specifically higher than that of women in complete sexual rest, probably because of a higher metabolism in the uterus and because of more rapid conduction of heat through the abdominal wall. In the newly delivered and nursing mother the metabolism is likewise higher per unit of surface than that of either the pregnant or normal woman. This is probably due in part to the activity of the mammary glands and in part to the dynamic action of protein liberated by the involution processes.

3. The energy metabolism of the new-born child expressed per unit of weight and found by subtracting the metabolism of mother alone from that of mother and child together, is two and a half times that of the mother. Expressed per unit of surface (same formula) the energy metabolism of the new-born child is not greater than that of the nursing mother, but is higher than that of a woman in complete sexual rest.

In conclusion we wish to express our sincere thanks to Dr. F. G. Benedict, director of this laboratory, for placing at our disposal a considerable part of the laboratory staff for this work, and for many helpful suggestions during its progress.

# THE AMEBOID ACTIVITY OF MEGALOBLASTS

WILLIAM SYDNEY THAYER, M.D.
BALTIMORE

In the study of the blood and blood-forming organs so much attention has been given to methods of fixation and staining that the careful examination of the fresh specimen or tissue is too often neglected. Certain biological characteristics of the cells, such, for instance, as ameboid activity, may easily be overlooked.

In the study of the blood of a case of Addisonian anemia of a chronic course, I have observed characteristic ameboid movements in a megaloblast. Phylogenetically, it is not remarkable that a megaloblast should possess the powers of ameboid activity; indeed, one might expect that this should be so. Inasmuch, however, as the present observation is apparently the first of this nature, it would appear to be worthy of record.

*History.*—R., aged 39, a patient of Dr. G. A. Hartman, consulted me on Sept. 27, 1905. His family, personal history and habits were excellent. Two years previously he had had several "spells" of faintness which occurred about a week apart. These were associated with a slight feeling of confusion. He never actually fell, the attacks lasting but a minute. Shortly after this, his ankles and legs began to swell. He became more and more short of breath after exertion. There were periods of diarrhea; no blood in the stools. Somewhat over two months before consulting me he had been obliged to give up work on account of great weakness and diarrhea.

*Physical Examination.*—The patient was a rather sparely nourished man, with marked yellowish pallor of the face, lips and mucous membranes; conjunctivæ were subicteric; slight arcus senilis. Pulse in the recumbent posture 28 to the quarter. There was nothing remarkable on examination of the lungs or the heart, except a soft systolic murmur heard all over the cardiac area in the recumbent posture, which almost disappeared at the apex in the erect posture. The abdomen was a little full. Hepatic flatness began at the sixth rib above, border palpable 2 to 3 cm. below the costal margin in the mammillary line. In the median line, by percussion, it extended to a point about 5 cm. above the umbilicus. The spleen was palpable; knee-jerks active; deep reflexes in the arms very lively. On the left side there was a distinct ankle-clonus. Sensation appeared to be good in the legs, both of which were bandaged because of edema.

Blood: Fresh specimen showed a very marked poikilocytosis; numerous very large elements; color of the individual corpuscles apparently good. Leukocytes were scanty, the proportion of whites to reds being apparently rather high.

| | |
|---|---|
| Red blood cells | 1,464,000 |
| White blood cells | 4,000 |
| Hemoglobin | 30 to 35 per cent. |

A differential count of the leukocytes showed:

| | Per Cent. |
|---|---|
| Polymorphonuclears | 71.9 |
| Small mononuclears | 17.3 |
| Large mononuclears | 4.8 |
| Eosinophils | 3.0 |
| Myelocytes | 1.6 |

During the differential count one megaloblast and three normoblasts were seen.

Oct. 10, 1905: Examination of Stool: A large liquid stool, with a few small formed particles, yellowish-brown in color. Microscopically, much granular detritus; numerous muscle cells and vegetable cells; few triple phosphate and many Charcot-Leyden crystals; very large number of cercomonads; no eggs of parasites.

Rest and arsenic in increasing doses were prescribed. The patient remained at home under the care of his physician, Dr. Hartman, and improved slowly.

Jan. 7, 1906: Red blood cells, 1,692,000; white blood cells, 4,500; hemoglobin was 55 per cent. No eosinophils were found; there was an increased percentage of small mononuclears.

Feb. 18, 1906: Red blood cells, 2,394,000; white blood cells, 4,000; hemoglobin amounted to 58 per cent.

May 16, 1906: Red blood cells, 2,584,000; white blood cells, 6,500; hemoglobin amounted to 65 per cent.

Nov. 15, 1906: The patient has been steadily improving. Color looks much better. Has gained twelve pounds in weight. Hemoglobin 80 to 90 per cent. by Tallquist.

The patient was not seen again for a year and a half. He consulted me again on May 30, 1908. Since the winter, he had been failing. A morning diarrhea had set in during the winter which had exhausted him greatly, obliging him to give up work. There had been a slight purpuric eruption on his legs; three weeks previously, nose-bleed. There was marked pallor, slightly subicteric; pulse of rather low pressure, rapid at the beginning of examination; slight protodiastolic gallop at the apex; a soft systolic murmur all over the cardiac area. The abdomen was a little full; liver about one and one-half fingers' breadths below the costal margin, soft and smooth. The spleen was readily palpable and, on quiet breathing, visible about two fingers' breadths below the costal margin. Knee-jerks were active.

Blood: On examination of a fresh specimen, the following note was made: "Corpuscles on the average very large; great difference in size; marked poikilocytosis. Leukocytes, scanty. One megaloblast seen in the fresh specimen.

"Under observation, this megaloblast shows typical ameboid movements. Small round pseudopodia are projected into which the colored protoplasm flows in much the same manner seen with the ordinary intestinal amebas. Slight changes in shape occur at times in the nucleus. The movements of the cell are marked, strikingly like those in leukocytes, and entirely unlike the gradual changes of shape sometimes seen in red blood corpuscles in the fresh specimen. The pseudopodia that are projected are exactly like those seen in the movements of a polymorphonuclear leukocyte; that is, on the edge of the cell there appear sometimes very small round buds, several at a time, which coalesce and form larger processes. The absolute homogeneity of the protoplasm does not allow one to observe the rolling motion so clearly as in the case of *Amœba coli* or a leukocyte containing granules. At times, however, the movement is really rather active as shown in the few drawings that I have made. The change is so distinct that in the course of five minutes the whole picture is different."

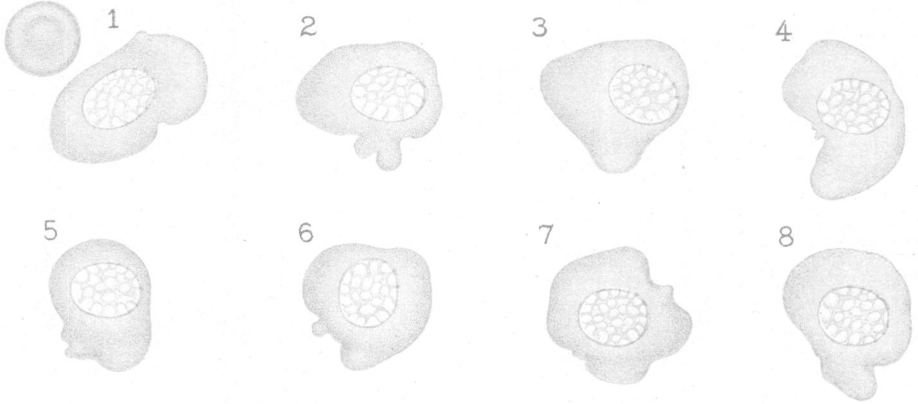


Megaloblasts in a case of Addisonian anemia showing true ameboid movements. The outline drawn by the author from the fresh specimen represents eight successive phases of the movement of the cell. The original drawings were elaborated in detail and colored by Mr. Herrman Becker under the supervision of the author from a similar megaloblast selected from the bone-marrow of a new-born infant.

On the left and above is seen a normal red blood corpuscle. Figs. 1 to 8, Ameboid movements of the megaloblasts.

The accompanying illustration shows six successive phases of this cell which I drew from the fresh specimen. The picture was so remarkable that I demonstrated the specimen to my neighbor, Dr. Hamman. By the time Dr. Hamman had arrived, the movements had become very sluggish, but the projection of one pseudopod, into which the protoplasm gradually flowed, was clearly observed. Red blood cells, 1,488,000; hemoglobin, Tallquist, 30 per cent.

The patient was not seen again for over a year. On Nov. 1, 1909, however, he consulted me again, stating that he had picked up during the summer of 1908, but in the spring of 1909, had begun to fail again, recovering remarkably, however, under atoxyl. The general appearance of the patient was very much better. He was still a little pale and looked rather thin, but the great pallor which he had shown before had almost entirely disappeared.

The fresh blood showed a remarkable change in appearance. The corpuscles were rather deeply colored, and, on the average, of rather large size. There was little poikilocytosis, but occasional pear-shaped and saucepan-shaped cells were observable. The leukocytes were obviously diminished. No nucleated reds were seen in the fresh specimen. There were occasional microcytes. Red blood cells, 3,600,000; hemoglobin, 87 per cent.

The patient was seen again on Aug. 24, 1910. He was rather pale, but on the whole in fairly good condition. The physical examination showed nothing remarkable. The liver and spleen were of about the same size as on the last note. Red blood cells numbered 2,207,000; white blood cells, 3,350; hemoglobin was 62 per cent. The fresh specimen showed considerable difference in the size of the corpuscles; there was a number of microcytes, but macrocytes were especially numerous; there was considerable poikilocytosis; leukocytes were very scanty. Vital staining by Vaughan's and Widal's methods showed very few corpuscles with intracellular staining. Little polychromatophilia. The corpuscles showing vital staining were certainly fewer than 1 to 100. Differential count of the leukocytes showed: lymphocytes, 38.6 per cent.; large lymphocytes, 0.6 per cent.; large mononuclears, 2.8 per cent.; eosinophils, 0.4 per cent.; unclassified, 1.2 per cent. There were no myelocytes, basophils or nucleated reds seen in counting 250 white corpuscles. The reds were of good color. There was well-marked anisocytosis and poikilocytosis. The resistance of the red blood corpuscles to solutions of sodium chlorid showed the onset of hemolysis at 0.325 per cent.; complete hemolysis at 0.275 per cent.

## SUMMARY

In a typical instance of Addisonian anemia, ameboid movements were observed in a characteristic megaloblast. These movements were altogether analogous to those seen in polymorphonuclear leukocytes.

In the early stage of development represented by the megaloblast, the red blood corpuscle is then, probably, a cell with powers of active progression.

In conclusion, it may be well to urge the more frequent study of the behavior of the various elements of the blood and blood-forming tissues, wherever they may be obtained sufficiently early, in the fresh state under conditions as nearly approaching the normal as may be.

# THE FUNCTION OF THE SINO-AURICULAR NODE *

ALFRED E. COHN, M.D., AND LEO KESSEL, M.D.
NEW YORK

Since the time Keith and Flack[1] (April, 1907) described and Koch[2] substantiated the presence and site of the sino-auricular node in the mammalian heart no experiments dealing with the physiology of this node have been attempted.[3] The earlier experiments which busied themselves with this subject were those of Langendorff and Lehmann[4] in 1906, Erlanger and Blackman[5] in 1907, and Hering[6] in 1907 and 1909. We desire to give a brief report of some experiments that have been carried on during the course of the past winter.

It will be remembered that the so-called sino-auricular node has its location at the point where the superior vena cava enters the right auricle and is found just to the right of the right extremity of the right auricular appendix, and near its upper border. It is a structure of small size, roughly from 10 to 15 mm. long, 1 to 3 centimeters according to Koch[2] and about one-third as wide. It lies directly under the pericardium. It is easily differentiated from the surrounding auricular muscle, with which it freely communicates, and resembles closely the now familiar structure of the auriculoventricular node. Its relation to a moderately large vessel and its close proximity to nerve structures has been dwelt on elsewhere

---

* From the Pathological Laboratory of the College of Physicians and Surgeons, Columbia University.

1. Keith and Flack: The Form and Nature of the Muscular Connections between the Primary Divisions of the Vertebrate Heart. Jour. Anat. and Physiol., 1907, xli, 172.

2. Koch, W.: Ueber die Struktur des oberen Cavatrichters und seine Beziehungen zum Pulsus irregularis perpetuus. Deutsch. med. Wchnschr., 1909, No. 10; Weitere Mitteilungen über den Sinus-Knoten des Herzens. Verhandl. Deutsch. path. Gesellsch., 1909, p. 85.

3. Hering's discussion of stimulus production (München. med. Wchnschr., 1909, lvi, 845) gives neither curves nor the facts of technic or results, and details no experiments.

4. Langendorff, O., and Lehmann, C.: Der Versuch von Stannius am Warmbluterherzen, Arch. f. d. ges. Physiol. (Pflüger's), 1906, cxii, 352.

5. Erlanger, J., and Blackman, J. R.: A Study of Relative Rhythmicity and Conductivity in Various Regions of the Auricles of the Mammalian Heart. Am. Jour. Physiol., 1907, xix, 124.

6. Hering, H. E.: Ueber die Automatie des Säugethierherzens. Arch. f. d. ges. Physiol. (Pflüger's), 1907, cxvi, 143; Ueber den normalen Ausgangspunkt der Herztätigkeit und seine Aenderung unter pathologischen Umständen, München. med. Wchnschr., 1909, lvi, 845.

(Koch, Keith and Mackenzie[7]). The connections between the sino-auricular and the auriculoventricular node which Thorel[8] claims to have seen have been emphatically denied by Keith and Mackenzie,[7] Koch, Aschoff,[9] and Mönckeberg.[10] One of us has examined carefully several human, dog, monkey and rat hearts, without being able to observe this connection.

Langendorff and Lehmann were inspired to do experiments at the site of the entrance of the superior vena cava, at a time when a differentiated nodal structure was unknown, by the cooling and warming experiments which H. Adam[11] had performed and in which prompt response in rate of the heart to changes of temperature had been observed. Adam had found that the only portion he could so influence was that between the entrances of the superior and the inferior vena cava, especially that nearer the latter. Langendorff and Lehmann, working with excised rabbits' hearts perfused with Locke's solution, cut away with scissors portions of the right auricle. Exactly which portions they excised is not mentioned, though it was their intention to excise the sinus. The result of their experiments was, briefly, that after excision the heart ceased to beat for variable lengths of time, after which only the ventricles again took up their activity, but at a very much slower rate. The auricles never beat again. The stoppage was averted when the fluid employed in the perfusion contained defibrinated blood.

Erlanger and Blackman[5] took up the work where Langendorff and Lehmann left it. They worked with perfused rabbits' hearts. Their technic made the excision of definite amounts of tissue impossible; and they state (p. 133) that the amount varied in different experiments. It may be that just these differences, as we hope our experiments may show, caused the differences in the results at which they arrived. Unlike Langendorff and Lehmann, they performed experiments in which the auricles did not go into asystole, but continued to contract after operative interference. In this particular our experiments agree. Furthermore, they found that several of these hearts did not stop after the excision, either

7. Keith, Arthur, and Mackenzie, Ivy: Recent Researches on the Anatomy of the Heart. Lancet, London, 1910, i, 101-103.

8. Thorel, Charles: Nachweis von sogenannten Reitungsfasern an der Vorhofkavagrenze, München. med. Wchnschr., 1900, 890; Vorläufige Mitteilung über eine besondere Muskelverbindung zwischen der Cava superior und dem Hisschen Bundel; München. med. Wchnschr., 1909, lvi, 2159; Ueber den Aufbau des Sinusknotens und seine Verbindung mit der Cava superior und den Wenckebachschen Bundeln; München. med. Wchnschr., 1910, lvii, 183.

9. Aschoff, L.: Die Herzstörungen in ihrer Beziehung zu den spezifischen Muskelsystemen des Herzens, Centralbl. f. allg. Path. u. path. Anat., 1910, xxi, 434.

10. Mönckeberg, J. G.: Beiträge zur normalen und pathologischen Anatomie des Herzens, Centralbl. f. allg. Path. u. path. Anat., 1910, p. 437.

11. Adam, H.: Experimentelle Untersuchungen über den Ausgangspunkt der automatischen Herzreize beim Warmbluter, Arch. f. d. ges. Physiol. (Pflüger's), 1906, iii, 607.

because other portions not affected by the insult were equally rhythmical or because the pace-maker, the dominating area, may have resided in some other portion. We trust that this problem may be resolved by investigating microscopically the portions excised in the experiments. They found variations in the correlation of auricle to ventricle, just as will appear in the experiments here to be reported.

Hering,[6] on the evidence gained from inspecting the dying heart, thinks that the last portion to die is that at the entrance of the superior vena cava, sometimes the portion about the inferior vena cava, and that in any case, the right auricular appendix is never involved in stimulus production. He has been able to cut away the region of the venæ cavæ at their entrances and beyond and yet has found the right auricle continue to beat with regularity, though he does not give the rate after the operation (p. 145). He is of the opinion that not all supraventricular portions are capable of automatism and certainly not the left auricle, but he gives no exact site for this activity. However, he mentions the fact that a small incision in the region of the superior vena cava which separated the sinus from the right auricle at a small place only, caused auricular asystole. We have been unable to make a similar incision. It will be seen that definite statements, both as to the site of production of the normal stimuli and experimental evidence for localizing such a site, are wanting.

The experiments we wish briefly to report here were done on the excised hearts of small dogs, which had been perfused with Locke's solution. The plan differed from the other series of experiments, in that, first, an attempt was made to excise only the known node-bearing area, and, second, to show that even multiple incisions did not influence the rate (except to accelerate it), while a final incision which cut away the window that had been made on three sides, did in ten of sixteen experiments successfully cause the stoppage of the entire heart. In two the stoppage is not noted in the protocol, though the rates fell from 114 to 81.9 in one, and from 121.5 to 63 in another. In three others the node is probably not excised, and in a fourth final incision was not made. The experiments gave a fairly uniform result and are reported here without detail. Curves and histological examinations of the excised portions are subsequently to be published.

After the heart had been suspended the experiment was not undertaken until it was seen to be beating regularly and in coordination. Suspension curves of the left auricle and right ventricle were written. Then incisions 1, 2, 3 (figured in the diagram) were made, and additional pieces of curve written. Finally incision 4 completed the excision of the sinus-bearing area. After incisions 1, 2, 3, the hearts beat for the most part at an accelerated speed, varying from 6.75 and 8.4 contractions in two, to between 21 and 50 in others. After incision 4, the hearts stopped beating entirely for periods varying from 7 to 92 seconds. Then the rate gradually, but rather rapidly, quickened and remained at an approximately fixed speed, always much slower than before the incisions, for the remainder of the experiment. It happened only once that the auricle ceased permanently to contract after the excision of the node-bearing area. In some experiments, the auricular systole preceded the ventricular, in others the reverse took place, in still others they beat simultaneously. We cannot conclude from our experiments that a definite anatomical site takes up the pace-making function for the entire heart as a substitute for the sino-auricular node after the sino-auricular node is excised. If various portions of the heart possess this automatic power, as Keith[1] and

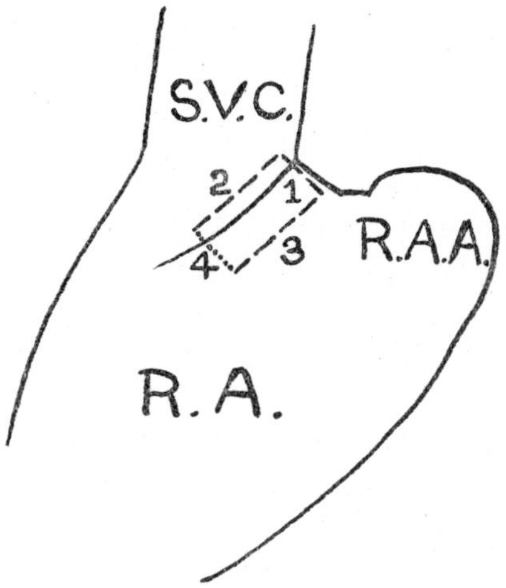


Diagram of incisions: S. V. C., superior vena cava; R. A., right auricle; R. A. A., right appendix auriculæ; 1, 2, 3, 4, incisions.

Erlanger[5] thought, sometimes one and sometimes another steps in for the usual dominating area, which, if we may conclude from the uniformly slower rate after its excision, resides normally in the sino-auricular node.

The conclusion is not justified from our experiments that simple incisions cause a stoppage of the whole heart (as Hering states), and the phenomena subsequently noted. We have shown that excision is necessary to produce this result. We are led to conclude, therefore, from our experiments that, as has long been supposed, and as former experiments have seemed to indicate, normal impulse formation takes place and normal rate is produced in the sino-auricular node.

Received for publication, Aug. 12, 1910.

# STUDIES ON THE BIOLOGY OF AND IMMUNITY AGAINST THE BACILLUS OF LEPROSY

## WITH A CONSIDERATION OF THE POSSIBILITY OF SPECIFIC TREATMENT AND PROPHYLAXIS *

CHARLES W. DUVAL, M.D., AND FRASER B. GURD, M.D.
NEW ORLEANS

Since an earlier communication[1] on the cultivation of *Bacillus lepræ* and the experimental production of leprosy by one of us (Duval) considerable light has been thrown on further study into the biology of the organism, especially with regard to its pathogenicity and viability, properties little understood prior to the cultivation of the bacillus. In the present paper we propose to give briefly our researches in this particular phase of the subject together with the results of our studies in immunity.

Soon after the cultivation of the specific organism the possibility of a serum therapy for the treatment of leprosy presented itself, and with this in view we set about to study the blood of lepers in the hope that something might accrue which would aid in subsequent work on the artificial production of an immune serum. Before beginning the work along this line it was thought advisable first to determine whether in cases of human leprosy specific antibodies are present, and if so, to find out as far as possible their nature and the mechanism of production.

### PATHOGENICITY

Heretofore our attempts to infect or produce lesions in animals other than the Japanese dancing mouse have been unsuccessful; but of late we have succeeded in producing the lesion in white mice and monkeys, not only with the infested tissue from human leprosy, but with cultures. One strain of *B. lepræ* in particular readily gives rise to fatal infection in the white mouse. The success with this strain has led us to test again the infectibility for the white mouse of four strains isolated more than a year ago. To our surprise, one of these (Culture II), with which we failed in former experiments to infect the white mouse, now proves infectious after more than fourteen months under cultivation, producing multiple lesions following intraperitoneal injection. The failure before

---

*From the Laboratories of Pathology, Tulane University, New Orleans.

1. Duval, C. W.: The Cultivation of the Leprosy Bacillus and the Experimental Production of Leprosy in the Japanese Dancing Mouse, Jour. Exper. Med., 1910, xii, 649.

to infect this species must be attributed to some error, for it cannot be conceived that a culture would alter in this particular feature under conditions of artificial cultivation. One is led to infer, however, from the present behavior of the culture, that the infectivity of some strains of *B. lepræ,* at least, are not appreciably altered by a year's sojourn outside of the animal body. It may be stated that not all strains are capable of infecting either dancing or white mice.

Thus far the experimental work would indicate that there is a considerable range in infectibility for cultures with respect to these animals; and the same is true for the bacilli used directly from the human tissues. An illustration of this variation has been observed in a rather remarkable stem that was recently isolated from the necrotic tissues of an acute case of human leprosy which had developed numerous soft subcutaneous leprous masses and had had repeated attacks of leprous fever. The initial growth resulted directly from bits of the transferred necrotic material on tryptophan agar. The acid-fast bacilli in the necrotic tissue were in enormous numbers and uncontaminated by other organisms as was subsequently proved by cultural tests.

A series of animals including four each of rats and white and Japanese dancing mice were inoculated, some subcutaneously and others intraperitoneally, with small quantities of the grumous material (0.5 c.c. emulsified in 1 c.c. of normal saline solution). The two white mice which received intraperitoneal injection died fourteen days after the inoculation. At autopsy both showed a general infection of the peritoneum with a pure growth of *B. lepræ,* while the mesentery, omentum, visceral and parietal peritoneum contained numerous minute, firm grayish white nodules that on microscopic section proved to be typical leprous lesions. The most surprising feature was the occurrence of a slightly turbid semigelatinous peritoneal exudate which microscopically consisted almost entirely of large mononucleated cells (macrophages). Great numbers of these cells were filled with acid-fast bacilli, and scarcely any were found that did not contain a few. A pure culture of *B. lepræ* was recovered from the exudate on a variety of special media, including tryptophan and glycerinated blood-agar.

The ability of *B. lepræ* to cause a fatal infection in so short a period, and to induce the production of a peritoneal exudate is a new rôle for the organism in our experience with the eight stems now under cultivation. At first we were inclined to believe that death in the case of these animals had resulted from the liberation of large quantities of toxins introduced with the necrotic material and augmented by the liberation of more toxic bodies due to lytic action on the injected bacilli. This hypothesis, however, is hardly tenable if we consider the length of time that elapsed between the inoculation and death of the animal (fourteen days), and the fact that the bacilli had increased in number within the peritoneum and were cultivated from the exudate.

The rats which received injections of the necrotic material have not as yet developed any signs of infection; nor have the Japanese dancing mice which were injected subcutaneously evinced any evidence of the disease. In two of the Japanese mice, however, which were sacrificed four weeks after the inoculation, small 1-mm. leprous nodules were found in the spleen, liver and inguinal lymph-nodes. Unfortunately, no Japanese mice were inoculated intraperitoneally with the bacilli of the necrotic tissue.

Another series of white and dancing mice were injected in a similar manner with the artificial culture obtained from this case, four standard loops of a heavy homogeneous suspension of bacilli being used. All the animals which received intraperitoneal injection became infected, the white mice dying one in three weeks and the other in twenty-eight days. At autopsy a semigelatinous exudate partially filled the peritoneum. In the Japanese mice, though numerous minute lesions studded the peritoneum, there was no evidence of exudate.

With regard to dancing mice, though lesions almost invariably develop after intraperitoneal injections of *B. lepræ,* none of the animals die as a result, although some of them have now been under observation for more than eight months. The mice that have been sacrificed, however, present small macroscopic lesions in various organs of the body. In some instances, the mice killed five months afterward have shown no demonstrable lesions; presumably in these animals the bacilli were destroyed and the lesions in consequence healed. This assumption is based on the fact that all dancing mice killed four to ten weeks after inoculation have shown small well-defined leprous lesions. Experimentation with these animals has proved that no intermediate host is necessary in the transmission of the disease. Attempts to infect rats, rabbits and guinea-pigs have so far given negative results.

The culture which produces fatal infection in white mice is now being used in the attempt to infect larger animals, more especially the *Macacus rhesus* monkey. In one animal of this species which has received at weekly intervals large subcutaneous doses of the bacilli have developed at the various points of inoculation firm subcutaneous nodules many of which have increased in size. The blood of this animal shows specific agglutinins and amboceptors in the presence of the culture antigen.

With the exception of two cultures (one isolated in December, 1909, and the other in October, 1910) *B. lepræ,* in our experience, has failed to give rise to a fatal infection in any of the laboratory animals employed. Many of the animals show multiple lesions after from four to eight weeks, but the lesions are small and tend to retrogress after a period of several months.

The experimental lesions of leprosy are histologically identical with those in the human tissue. Although to the naked eye they appear as tubercles, they are more minute and circumscribed than the lesions of tuberculosis and do not caseate. It cannot be said, however, that they are indistinguishable from early miliary tubercles, but one accustomed to seeing the experimental leprous tubercle has very little trouble in recognizing even macroscopic differences and on microscopic examination any previously existing doubt is at once dispelled.

Though at present we are not prepared to discuss *in extenso* the toxic body of *B. lepræ* it may be stated that experiments show apparently the presence of a soluble toxin. Four hundred million leprosy bacilli treated with 2 c.c. of a 5 per cent. glycerin solution and centrifugalized yield an extract which gives a well-marked cutaneous reaction in doses of 0.4 c.c. at the end of twenty-four hours.

## VIABILITY

The question of the viability of *B. lepræ* outside of the animal body is of the greatest practical importance from the standpoint of sanitation and preventive medicine. The fact that *B. lepræ* cultures will remain alive and virulent for months under the most unfavorable conditions would explain much heretofore not understood about the transmission of the disease.

The bacilli can be readily cultivated from bits of infested leprous tissue which have been kept in salt solution at room temperature for more than eight months. Again, they live and retain their virulence in culture associated with other bacteria for more than a year when precaution is taken to avoid against drying of the medium. Fresh growth can also be obtained from cultures which are more than a year old, whether kept at 10 C., 32 C. or 37 C. Even in material overgrown with saprophytic bacteria, the lepra bacilli remain viable for months and will multiply when separated from these and transferred to a suitable medium. There is no evidence to show that the ordinary pyogenic or saprophytic bacteria interfere with the longevity of *B. lepræ;* as a matter of fact, the organism seems to live and flourish best in symbiosis. Where the contaminator is a non-spore-bearer it is an easy task to rid it from the culture by heating at 60 C. for one hour. In order to obtain a pure growth of *B. lepræ* from a culture contaminated with saprophytic spore-bearers, the mixture may be injected intraperitoneally into a mouse, the animal killed in ten days to two weeks, and the acid-fast bacillus recovered from the peritoneum.

The leprosy bacilli will multiply slowly in transplanted bits of tissue kept at 25 C. We have found that the temperature conditions in which the bacillus will multiply range between 25 C. to 39 C., the optimum being about 32 C. In a previous paper it was stated that with the four strains then under cultivation growth would not occur at 37 C. We wish to correct this statement, as recent work with cultures shows that multiplication does occur at body temperature, though the best growth is obtained at from 32 to 35 C.

In our experience cultures will withstand higher degrees of temperature and for a longer period of time than any of the better-known acid-fast bacilli, growth resulting after heating the bacilli for thirty minutes at 70 C. or at 65 C. for one hour. Heating at these temperatures apparently does not alter the infectivity of the bacilli for mice. Whether the organism's resistance to high temperature is due to its fatty envelope, as in the case of the tubercle bacillus, or to spores, is still undetermined. We do not doubt that the fatty substance in and about the organism protects it to a certain extent against moderate degrees of heat, but this in itself would not explain the resistance shown by some cultures. These higher resistant cultures possess "clear spaces" and deeply staining bodies within the bacilli, which in many respects are morphologically similar to the ordinary bacterial spore. That certain cultures of *B. lepræ,* more especially those containing these "clear spaces," resist higher temperatures than cultures that do not contain them, has been repeatedly demonstrated by us. The true nature of these bodies is, however, still problematic and work is now in progress to determine whether or not *B. lepræ* under certain conditions forms spores.

## CULTIVATION

The initial growth of *B. lepræ* from the human tissue on an artificial medium is in all cases obtained with considerable difficulty. The bacilli outside of the animal body multiply more slowly in the initial transplants than do bovine tubercle bacilli, and it is necessary to transfer large quantities of the macerated tissue to the culture medium unless amino-acids are used in order to insure growth, which at best is feeble and not visible macroscopically before several weeks. Again, transplantation of large numbers of bacilli from the tissues is necessary, because not one-third of the planted bacilli will multiply. The rods do not differ in size and shape from the parent organisms and grow in dense clusters, which are broken up with great difficulty. In some instances, multiplication can be accelerated by rubbing up the bits of transplanted tissue after the first week or ten days, which frequently is the occasion for prompt appearance of growth within another few days, as it seems to stimulate to further development certain lepra bacilli, perhaps the more saprophytic forms in and around the tissue bits. Once the bacilli are accustomed to the new environment, however, there is no difficulty in increasing the rapidity of growth by frequent subculturing. In two of our older cultures the transfers now multiply with great rapidity and reach the maximum growth in three days.

Once *B. lepræ* has started to grow rapidly, special media such as tryptophan, cystein, etc., are not essential. The culture now does well on any neutral or slightly alkaline medium of human or rabbit blood-agar and glycerinated serum-agars.

Attempts have been made to cultivate the lepra bacilli from nasal secretions in cases in which large numbers of them are found in the serous discharge, and even though they may be contaminated with other bacteria, growth has resulted in two out of five cases in which we have attempted it. The contaminating bacteria, provided there are no spore-bearing varieties present, may be first eliminated by suspending some of the infested secretion in saline solution and heating the suspension at 60 C. for thirty minutes. It is much more difficult to obtain cultures of *B. lepræ* from nasal discharges than from the tissues, because in the latter, bits of tissue are unavoidably carried over in the transplants, which serve as pabulum for the culture until growth is well started. The same, of course, holds true for other acid-fast species, more especially the tubercle bacillus, whose initial cultivation in many respects is attended with the same difficulties as that of the lepra bacillus.

In a previous paper[1] on the cultivation of *B. lepræ* it was stated that the morphology of the bacillus under artificial growth conditions corresponded closely with that of the organism found in the tissues. This in the main is true, but as two of the original four strains studied have recently undergone a marked change in size, shape and manner of arrangement, we feel that much is yet to be said on the variation in morphology for artificially grown lepra bacilli.

The organisms, when freshly isolated from the animal tissues, are slightly curved and distinctly beaded, a feature that is constant for all early cultures, no matter on what medium they are grown. In some of the older cultures, however, those many generations removed from the parent stem, the bacilli undergo a decided change in size, shape and manner of their arrangement. Not only is the growth more rapid, which naturally would be expected, but the arrangement of the bacilli is diplobacillary, the individual organisms resembling in size the young forms of bovine tubercle bacilli. The difference is so marked that on morphological appearance alone it is quite easy to determine cultures of recent isolation from those that are many generations removed from the animal body. In the first dozen or so subplants from the parent stem the bacilli invariably grow in felt-like masses of slightly curved, slender, beaded rods, while in cultures which are many generations removed they grow diffusely over the medium and occur in pairs of short, ovoid, plump rods. This diplobacillary arrangement of egg-shaped rods is a characteristic feature for the older cultures. In the examination of stained microscopic preparations it is difficult to find single bacilli or clusters of more than two pairs. If such a preparation is stained by any of the ordinary anilin dyes it would be hard indeed to distinguish the organism from *Diplococcus lanceolatus*.

Though this transformation indicates that a given lepra culture is rapidly growing and has become accustomed to a saprophytic existence it is no criterion that the organism has lost its virulence. The same number of bacilli produce lesions in animals as quickly as they did when recently isolated. It is noteworthy in this connection that the bacilli passed through the animal body again become long slender "beaded" rods without a suggestion of pairing, and their recovery from the animal on artificial medium is accompanied with the same difficulty as in the case of the human tissue, growing at first slowly and only on special media.

The staining reaction of the diplo-forms with respect to acid-fastness remains unaltered; in fact they retain more tenaciously the carbol-fuchsin dye than formerly, since they take the stain more intensely and resist for a longer period the decolorizing agents. This form of *B. lepræ* multiplies rapidly on a variety of media, good growth occurring in forty-eight hours after incubation at 32 C. or 37 C. The culture gives the luxuriant growth common to other bacteria that divide as rapidly, and reaches its maximum growth in three days. These older, actively growing cultures still retain their virulence for white and dancing mice.

In some cultures, especially where growth has attained its maximum, many of the diplo-forms of *B. lepræ* undergo still another change in morphology. Occasionally in a given culture a great number of the bacilli will show as spindle-shaped rods with swollen centers. This central bulging often appears as an oval clear space with the chromatin densely massed at both poles. These cultures, when heated at 70 C. for thirty minutes, are still capable of reproduction. In two of our older cultures this central bulging with the formation of egg-shaped central bodies has repeatedly occurred. Just what factors determine sporulation (assuming that these spaces represent spores) we have not been able to determine, but from analogy, the same factors that influence spore-formation in well-known bacteria do not seem to apply to *B. lepræ,* as not all cultures under unfavorable conditions of food, temperature, etc., form "clear spaces." Spore-formation with *B. lepræ* might account for successful cultivation after heating at 60 C. but, as in the case of tubercle bacilli, the fatty envelope always has to be taken into account, which in itself may sufficiently protect the organism against moderate degrees of heat.

In the cultures that change in morphology the transformation is easily followed. From the granular substance within the bacilli that are lightly stained and distinctly beaded, ovoid masses develop. The chromatin of the parent bacilli seems to undergo amitotic division into two equal parts, which lie end to end in the long diameter of the organism.

These chromatin masses become more and more definite in outline until two well-formed, deeply staining oval bodies appear in the parent cell. The old cell membrane then undergoes metamorphosis, freeing the pair of oval bodies as a diplobacillus. All forms, from small irregular masses of chromatin to perfect diploid bodies, can be seen in a single field of a preparation of *B. lepræ*. There is no mistaking the manner of reproduction of the bacilli during this period of transformation. As soon as the culture has lost all its long beaded forms, however, reproduction then occurs by simple fission. In stained preparations from cultures undergoing this transformation the contrast in density of coloring between the old slender beaded rods and the new oval forms is very striking; the new forms always take the carbol-fuchsin stain more deeply and in consequence decolorize with more difficulty.

Under some conditions, more especially when the organisms are grown in an acid medium or when they are associated with a too profuse growth of symbiotic bacteria, the diplobacillary forms undergo still another change in which one organism in a pair will swell up to twice the size of its fellow and become distinctly spindle-shaped; or both organisms of a pair will simultaneously show the same alteration, forming lancets that are pointed at the distal and flattened at the proximal ends, giving rise to the appearance of certain forms of pseudo-diphtheria bacilli (*B. hofmani*). These so-called "involution forms" will take place in forty-eight hours when conditions are unfavorable. In old cultures in which growth has ceased, however, they may be kept for months without showing any change in the size and shape of the bacilli. The question of how the administration of different amino-acids, as well as the direct and indirect supply of oxygen influence the growth of parasitic organisms is being studied by one of us (Duval) in collaboration with Dr. Gustav Mann.

## IMMUNITY

Following the cultivation of *B. lepræ* our attention was naturally drawn to the possibility of producing an active artificial immunity which might be made use of in the treatment of the disease. In this respect our efforts have been directed along two distinct lines: patients suffering from the disease were inoculated with suspensions containing leprosy bacilli and their toxins; and animals have been inoculated with larger doses of culture in the hope of producing in their serums immune bodies which might be used in the passive immunization of human subjects. In addition an effort has been made to identify the presence of such bodies in the blood from patients suffering from the disease. By means of these qualitative and quantitative tests it was hoped that some circumstantial evidence, at least, might be adduced which would suggest the probable outcome of efforts in serum or vaccine therapy.

In our first examination four bodies were looked for, namely, specific amboceptors, agglutinins and opsonins against the leprosy bacillus and variations in the complement content from the normal and in patients suffering from the disease at its different stages and types. At present we are prepared to report on the complement and amboceptor content in twenty-eight serums from lepers of different types. It has been determined that the complement content does not differ from that in normal individuals to any demonstrable extent, nor does the stage or type of the disease produce any alteration in the quantity of this body present. A paper is now in process of preparation by one of us which will discuss, *in extenso,* the variations of complement in different diseases, both acute and chronic and in normal individuals; therefore, space will not be taken up here with the discussion of the methods employed nor with a more precise statement of the variations found.

We consider that since complement is present in leprous patients in normal quantities it will probably be of the utmost importance in the treatment of the disease by serum therapy if it is found possible to produce a serum in animals which will contain a high amboceptor content against the *Bacillus lepræ.*

In testing for the specificity as well as the quantity of the amboceptor two antigens were utilized: first, a suspension in saline solution of cultures of the organism grown on tryptophan medium; and secondly the so-called syphilitic antigen consisting of acetone-insoluble lipoids extracted from the human heart by alcohol and ether was employed. Of the twenty-eight serums fifteen were from cases of tubercular types of the disease, seven from anesthetic and six from the so-called mixed type. Although most of the cases showed well-marked and unmistakable evidence of the activity of the disease, few could be classified as advanced and in certain others which will be referred to later there had existed a doubt in the clinician's mind as to the actual presence of the disease in the individuals during the past few years. As is seen from Table 1, the serum from this last group of cases failed to show the presence of specific antibodies. We wish to note here that it was not until the attention of the clinician was drawn to the absence of specific antibodies in those cases that we were informed that the patients were considered free from active disease. In determining the presence of specific antibodies active serum was used, and in reading the results those cases marked (+ +) represent serums in which at least three quantities of complement are bound. In those marked weakly positive (— +) at least two, and in those marked doubtful (— ±) only one quantity is fixed. Before proceeding to a discussion of the results obtained and their significance as interpreted by us, Table 1 will be considered.

TABLE 1.—RESULTS OF COMPLEMENT FIXATION TESTS WITH LEPROUS SERUMS

| | Leprosy Antigen. | | Lipoid Antigen. | |
|---|---|---|---|---|
| 1. Tubercular early | — | + | + | + |
| 2. Anesthetic | — | ± | — | — |
| 3. Anesthetic | — | + | + | + |
| 4. Tubercular | + | + | + | + |
| 5. Mixed | — | + | — | + |
| 6. Mixed | — | + | — | — |
| 7. Tubercular | — | — | — | — |
| 8. Tubercular | + | + | + | + |
| 9. Tubercular | + | + | + | + |
| 10. Mixed | — | + | — | + |
| 11. Mixed | — | + | + | + |
| 12. Tubercular | + | + | + | + |
| 13. Anesthetic | — | + | — | — |
| 14. Anesthetic | — | ± | + | + |
| 15. Tubercular | + | + | + | + |
| 16. Tubercular | + | + | + | + |
| 17. Tubercular | + | + | + | + |
| 18. Mixed | — | + | + | + |
| 19. Tubercular | + | + | + | + |
| 20. Tubercular | — | + | — | + |
| 21. Mixed | — | + | + | + |
| 22. Tubercular | + | + | + | + |
| 23. Tubercular | + | + | + | + |
| 24. Tubercular | + | + | + | + |
| 25. Tubercular | + | + | + | + |
| 26. Tubercular | + | + | + | + |
| 27. Anesthetic | — | — | — | — |

In this table several interesting points are noted; in the first place all but three cases show bodies capable of combining with and fixing complement in the presence of leprosy bacilli and in thirteen cases this binding power is well marked. Of the serums giving a complete reaction with the bacilli, all give a similar reaction in the presence of phosphate containing lipoid substances; and all giving negative results with the organisms are also negative with the phosphatids as an antigen. When the second part of the table is examined, seventeen cases are seen to possess a marked binding power, and eight give negative results. In all instances cases showing no complement-binding power in the presence of the lipoids have been found to possess either little or none when the bacillary emulsion was employed.

To control the reactions with the leprous serums similar reactions were carried out with the blood from patients other than lepers, and at first a most astonishing result was obtained, the significance of which was not at first understood. As controls, serums collected for diagnosis by the Wassermann reaction were utilized, and it was found that a large number of these gave positive results with the bacillary suspension. It was found in the first ten serums tested that six gave a marked binding and two a weak reaction, only two failing to fix any complement whatever. This result was unlooked for, and seemed to upset any inferences whicn might have been drawn from the results of reactions with serums from leprous individuals. It is further noted, however, that of those cases fixing complement in the presence of leprosy bacilli all give a marked Wassermann reaction and are undoubtedly syphilitic cases, while one, a tabetic, gave a weak Wassermann reaction.

Table 2.—Results of Complement Fixation in Serums from Cases Other than Leprous

| | Leprosy. | | Lipoids. | |
|---|---|---|---|---|
| 1. Syphilis | + | + | + | + |
| 2. Syphilis | + | + | + | + |
| 3. Non-luetic | — | — | — | — |
| 4. Tabetic | — | + | — | + |
| 5. Syphilis | + | + | + | + |
| 6. Syphilis | — | + | + | + |
| 7. Normal | — | — | — | — |
| 8. Syphilis | + | + | + | + |
| 9. Syphilis | + | + | + | + |
| 10. Syphilis | + | + | + | + |
| 15. Syphilis | + | + | + | + |
| 16. Syphilis | — | + | ∓ | + |
| 17. Syphilis | + | + | + | + |
| 18. Syphilis | — | + | + | + |
| 19. Syphilis | + | + | + | + |
| 20. Syphilis (treatment) | — | + | + | + |
| 21. Non-luetic | — | — | — | — |
| 22. Normal | — | — | — | — |
| 23. Syphilis | + | + | + | + |
| 24. Syphilis | + | + | + | + |
| 25. Non-luetic | — | — | — | — |
| 26. Primary | — | + | — | — |
| 27. Syphilis | — | ∓ | — | ∓ |
| 28. Syphilis treated | — | + | ∓ | + |
| 29. Normal | — | — | — | — |
| 30. Normal | — | — | — | — |

Of the three leprous patients failing to give any reaction with either antigen, two (Numbers 13 and 27) are individuals whose history shows that the disease has been present for twenty or twenty-five years and in whom for many years past no progression of the disease has been noted. Both are free from macular or tuberculous lesions and are detained in the home chiefly because the ravages of the disease during the active stage have resulted in so great a deformity that it would be impossible for the patients to go about among society without being subject to criticism. The other patient (No. 7) is a young man in whom all evidence of leprosy has disappeared but who is dying from a severe tuberculous infection. Of the cases giving the weakest reaction all show very little if any evidence of active disease.

Repeated tests prove amply that the suspension of leprosy bacilli used possessed neither anticomplementary powers nor hemolytic properties. There remains, therefore, but one apparent explanation of the phenomenon of cross-reaction between syphilitic and leprous patients with both lipoid bodies and the leprosy bacilli as antigen. Whatever may be the cause of the phenomenon producing antibodies against phosphatids in the blood of syphilitic patients, it is apparent that it is easy to explain the presence of antibodies against fatty materials in leprous patients, since it is generally accepted that a fatty or waxy substance forms an important constituent of the leprosy bacillus.

In order, therefore, to prove the presence or absence of specific amboceptors in leprous serums against the other substances in the bacilli, two methods of experimentation were utilized. First, it was endeavored to bind by means of an excess of lipoid body and complement the antibodies against the fatty substances, and then by adding a further content of complement and leprosy bacilli, to bind, if possible, more complement by means of the specific amboceptor against the constituents or toxins of the bacilli other than the fatty substances. In the second series of experiments we attempted to demonstrate the presence of such antibodies by an examination of various serums, especially those in which a small amount of lipoid body was present, carrying out two series of reactions simultaneously in the presence of varying amounts of complement. Up to the present we have been unable to demonstrate by either of these methods specific bodies in leprous serums capable of fixing complement in the presence of products of the bacilli other than the lipoid substances.

In attempting to identify specific agglutinins against the *Bacillus lepræ,* we have found that serums from certain patients at least will agglutinate thoroughly broken-up suspensions of the bacilli in dilutions of 1 to 50 in two hours. Serum from normal individuals has failed to agglutinate bacilli in dilutions of 1 to 10. We have not found cases from which the serum would agglutinate in dilution of 1 to 100 or more.

So far, we are only in a position to report regarding the immune bodies developed in one experimental animal; namely, a monkey (*Macacus rhesus*), which was injected at intervals with living leprosy bacilli. Up to the time of examination four doses of a suspension of from 20 to 100 million live lepra bacilli had been injected into the subcutaneous tissue over the chest and in the groin. Following each inoculation a swelling had appeared about the point of inoculation within two or three days which gradually increased in size. The reactions performed on his blood at the end of one month showed that the serum agglutinated the bacilli in dilutions of 1 to 50, whereas the serum from the normal monkey showed not the slightest tendency toward agglutination. In determining the amboceptor in the monkey's serum it has been found that it binds complement in the presence of phosphatids, even in small quantities, so that further tests are necessary to determine the presence of amboceptors in the serum of this animal.

On October 22, twelve patients were inoculated with a suspension of leprosy bacilli containing eight million organisms to the cubic centimeter. The vaccine was prepared by preliminary heating at 70 C. for ten minutes and subsequently the finely divided bacilli were treated in a 2 per cent. phenol solution for forty-eight hours. The material was then diluted to six times its volume and used in this manner.

The human cases in which we used the inoculations consisted of moderately advanced tubercular or mixed types together with one long-standing anesthetic case. On the occasion of the first inoculation, doses varying from 0.1 to 0.25 c.c. were used, being given either into the true skin or into the subcutaneous tissue. Following the first administration four patients, each of whom had received 0.2 c.c., reacted locally as evidenced by a small zone of redness about the point of inoculation.

On the second dose (October 29) the quantity injected was increased to from 0.25 c.c. to 4 c.c. without the development of a reaction in any case. Four treatments have so far been given, the dose having been arbitrarily placed at four million bacilli. We cannot, at present, report on any definite progress in the clinical condition of any of these patients, but it may at least be said that no harmful results have ensued.

### SUMMARY AND DISCUSSION

*B. lepræ* may be cultivated on a variety of artificial media, and are capable of living and retaining their infectibility for months under adverse conditions outside of the animal body. The bacilli can also be cultivated from contaminated leprous tissue and from the nasal discharge that has been kept at room temperature for more than a year. Remarkable as it may seem, it is nevertheless the case that contaminating micro-organisms have no appreciable effect on the viability and infectivity of some strains of lepra bacilli.

Pure cultures of *B. lepræ* can be obtained directly from the infested leprous tissue on a variety of special media including tryptophan and glycerinated blood-agar without first growing them in the presence of amebas and their symbiotics. From two cases of leprosy we have cultivated in pure growth the specific organism directly from the tissues on Novy-McNeal rabbit blood-agar to which 1 per cent. glycerin had been added. As a rule, multiplication of *B. lepræ* on artificial medium takes place slowly, but once the growth has started it can be readily accelerated by frequent transplantation.

At the present writing we have succeeded in cultivating *B. lepræ* from the cutaneous nodules in eight cases of leprosy, two cases of nasal discharge, and from the experimental lesion in a number of monkeys and white and Japanese dancing mice. That the cultures are leprosy bacilli, and not some other acid-fast species, has been definitely proved by cultural and animal tests.

The experimental study on the virulence and viability of leprosy bacilli shows the necessity of early diagnosis and the need of strict segregation of certain types of the disease. The length of time *B. lepræ* will live and retain its infectiousness outside the body indicates plainly the risk to a community in allowing leper patients at large, in particular those who have open lesions. Especially dangerous from the standpoint of source of infection are the patients discharging the bacilli in the secretions from the nasal mucous membrane. These patients are a constant menace to those with whom they associate because of the possibility of indirect transmission of the bacilli that are unconsciously deposited on articles about the household where the leper resides.

The mere fact that the organism lives for so long a time outside of the animal body may explain why the disease continually reappears in households that have harbored a leper. The bacilli escaping from the infected individual, who for months may not be aware of his malady, are a constant menace to others of the household or to subsequent tenants, even though it be years after the direct source of infection has been removed. The animal experiments do not tend to support the view that leprosy may reside for years in the human body before manifesting any outward signs of the disease.

Direct inoculation from man to man may occur, but it is the exception. On the other hand, in the light of our present knowledge the indirect evidence of transmission is by far the more significant. We believe that this is the most likely condition that renders transmission of the disease possible. It is recognized that other conditions, such as virulence of the bacilli, suitable port of entrance and susceptibility, play an important part, as they do in all infectious diseases. Our investigations also confirm the belief that the mucous membrane of the nasal pharynx is the port through which the bacilli gain entrance to the body, as well as the chief source from which infection spreads.

The results of animal experimentations demonstrate the fact that direct communication of the disease may take place from individual to individual without the presence of the bed-bug or other parasites as intermediate hosts.

On two occasions we have succeeded in infecting mice by rubbing cultures into the nares after gentle scarification of the mucous membrane. These experiments support the view that the chief portal of entrance for *B. lepræ* to the human body is by way of the nasopharynx. There is also evidence to show from animal experiments that the bacilli may gain entrance to the human body through breaks in the skin without giving rise to lesions at the entrance site.

In the examination of blood from patients suffering from leprosy the serum has been shown to contain specific antibodies of different kinds against certain constituents of the *B. lepræ*. In addition to the presence of specific bodies, we have demonstrated that complement is present in normal quantities. Agglutinins are present, though not in very large amounts. The opsonic content is probably affected at different stages of the disease, but with reference to the activity of this body our researches have so far not proved conclusive.

Specific amboceptors are undoubtedly present in comparatively large quantities. In confirmation of the results of others we have found that not only specific bodies are present in the blood of leprous patients binding complement with leprosy bacilli, but also substances capable of fixing this body in the presence of phosphatids prepared by the extraction of human heart muscle. Not only has this phenomenon been constantly present, but it has been demonstrated that the complement-binding power is as great in the presence of the lipoids as in the presence of the bacilli themselves. Thus serums fixing nine units of complement when treated with a suspension of *B. lepræ* are likewise found to be capable of fixing a similar quantity when the lecithin antigen is employed; in the same way serums fixing two units with one antigen have fixed two units with the other. That the reaction is quantitatively as well as qualitatively specific is shown by the fact that with few exceptions, even the delicate reaction depending on the fixation of only one complement unit, it has been equal with both materials as antigen.

On the other hand we have been unsuccessful in demonstrating the presence in leprous serums of specific amboceptors other than those combining with the lipoid bodies. Again, we have found that not only is the complement-binding power in the presence of the two antigens a characteristic of leprous cases but it is also found in the serum from luetic individuals. Apparently, then, the constituents of the leprosy bacillus against which the most active antibody is produced is the lipoid material.

Furthermore, we have been successful in extracting from the bacilli by means of ether and alcohol fatty substances in comparatively large quantities, the greater portion of which is insoluble in acetone. This acetone-insoluble content has by analysis been found to contain phosphorus, proving that it belongs to the phosphatid group of fats. Since chemically the fatty material in the bacilli is closely related to the lecithins as extracted from the human heart, and the amboceptor content of the serum of both leprous and luetic cases is quantitatively as well as qualitatively the same whether the artificially prepared lipoids or the bacilli themselves are used, we consider that it is justifiable to assume that these two lipoids can differ but slightly from one another. Furthermore, in view of the fact that the serum of leprous individuals contains chiefly antibodies against the fatty content of the bacterium, and since specific immune bodies are usually produced in a manner in which they will be most useful to the host, we think it reasonable to infer that it is the fatty constituent of the bacillus which offers the greatest protection to the bacilli against the action of the individual's resistant forces.

The idea that the fatty material in the bodies of both tubercle and leprosy bacilli is a powerful protection against the body fluids and cells is by no means new. In fact, in the treatment of leprosy both tuberculin and nastin have been employed in the hope of increasing the resistance of the individual against this protective covering on the bacillus. The absence of satisfactory results following the employment of both these materials can be explained in two ways. First, the fatty constituents of both these preparations differ to a greater extent from that present in the leprosy bacillus than do the phosphatids prepared from cardiac muscle; and secondly, along with the fatty material injected a larger or smaller quantity of toxic bodies other than the lipoids is inoculated, rendering the use of large doses impossible.

We have been sufficiently impressed by the apparent importance of the specific bodies against the phosphatid fat in the immunization against the *B. lepræ* to have undertaken animal experimentation in the hope of preparing a serum of sufficient antilipoid potency to be of service in the passive immunization of human cases. Leprous patients are also being subjected to injections of emulsions of the fats to determine the possibility of the production of a more marked active immunity than that produced normally by these cases.

Although we consider that our researches suggest the prime importance of this phase of the immunity leading to the destruction of the bacillus, we believe that this method may probably be supplemented by the production of either a passive or active immunity against the toxins and protein constituents of the bacillus. We have proved the presence of soluble toxins and may assume apparently the presence of endotoxin and toxalbumin, against all of which it should be our aim to develop specific bodies if the greatest advantage in the treatment of the disease is to be achieved. To this end we are continuing the vaccine treatment of cases and are proceeding with the attempt to produce an active immunity in animals.

# A BLOOD-CRISIS OCCURRING WITH PRIMARY SARCOMA OF THE STOMACH *

LE ROY H. BRIGGS, M.D.
OAKLAND, CAL.

The coincidence of two such interesting features as these in the same patient is unusual enough to warrant the case being reported somewhat in detail.

*Patient.*—An engineer, aged 39, was seen on Feb. 26, 1910. The family history and the patient's past and personal history were negative. The habits of the patient were good.

*Present Complaint.*—Some eight months before, the patient noticed a belching of gas, sour or bitter, usually after meals. There was never any localized pain or any pain with reference to food, but rather a general abdominal distress "due to gas" relieved by belching or by pressure and massage over the epigastrium. The bowels had been obstinately constipated, requiring enemas to move them. The appetite had been good, but food causes distress on account of the belching and eructation following. Weakness had been progressive, and for the last month the patient had been almost constantly in bed. His weight, normally about 185, was now 130. Five months before examination he was under a physician's care, and with "dietary and silver nitrate treatment" gained considerable weight. Vomiting had occurred but twice; four months before admission, after a dietary indiscretion the patient immediately expelled the ingested food, and again, several days prior to entrance, he vomited dark, finely granular, semiliquid material. There had been no difficulty with swallowing and no regurgitation of food. There was no jaundice. Lately there had been some tenderness over the epigastrium.

*Examination* (on admission).—The patient was a man of large frame, markedly emaciated and anemic. Head and face were negative; likewise the chest, save for a well-marked systolic murmur over the pulmonary area, and one of less intensity over the apex, neither transmitted. Pulse 80, regular, full volume, with pressure of 95 mm. of Hg, and arteries not sclerotic. The abdomen as a whole was sunken, but there was a slight bulging visible on the left side, just below the costal margin; no rigidity. A hard tender mass, corresponding to the bulging, extended to within 5 cm. of the mid-line, and to 5 cm. above the umbilical level. The upper and posterior borders of the spleen could be made out in their normal positions, but owing to tenderness it was impossible to say whether the mass was continuous with the spleen or not. The liver was enlarged downward about two finger-breadths below the costal margin, and was smooth and slightly tender. The kidneys were not palpable. The genitalia were normal. On inflating the colon, there was no change in the mass, and the tympany extended to, but not beyond, it. Rectal examination was negative. There was no edema. No nodules could be felt on any bone. The deep and superficial reflexes were all normal.

Urine and Feces: The urine was clear, 1.015-20, acid, no sugar nor albumin, with a trace of indican. Microscopically, an occasional leukocyte and spermatozoon, but no casts. A Cammidge reaction was not done. The stools were

---

* From the medical service of the Samuel Merritt Hospital.

examined three times, with always the same findings: dark-colored (tarry) solid stool, very slight odor, no mucus, pus or fresh blood. Occult blood, very strongly positive. No ova or parasites. Staining by Gram showed no Boas-Oppler bacilli.

The Elsberg carcinoma reaction (the injection of washed human red blood cells under the skin) was negative.

Owing to the extremely poor condition of the patient, the stomach-tube was not passed, nor was inflation done.

Blood: The pathology of the blood presented probably the most interesting phase of the present case, and the findings are here given in full. The counting was done as carefully as possible, at the same hour, with the same pipettes and chamber, and by the same observer. In estimating the hemoglobin the Dare instrument was used, the lowest reading of which is 10 per cent. In no instance was the percentage above that, and often below. However, the readings were all recorded as 10 per cent. on account of the uncertainty of a lower degree. The personal factor was eliminated here by having several different individuals make the readings each time. For the differentials, between 1,500 and 2,000 cells were counted in every case, affording a fair basis for the calculation of the nucleated red cells. Wright's and Hasting's stains were used. The red cells showed marked central pallor, were as a rule of normal size and shape and with comparatively little poikilocytosis and anisocytosis. Polychromatophilia and basophilic degenerations were common, particularly in the earlier counts, becoming less marked later as the nucleated reds increased. Platelets seemed about normal. Regarding the classification of the nucleated reds: Cells classed as megaloblasts were those in which the nucleus was at least the usual size of a red cell, 7 to 8 microns, and the cell body itself considerably larger. Normoblasts were those the same size as the normal cell and with a densely staining, sharply outlined nucleus; intermediate forms, those a trifle larger than the normoblasts, with the nucleus staining less densely and either fragmented, lobulated or undergoing mitosis, and the cell protoplasm in practically all, showing basophilic or polychromatophilic degenerations. This class would therefore include the immature nucleated red cells of Howell.

BLOOD EXAMINATIONS

| Date. | Red cells, per c. mm. | Hb. per cent. | Whites, per c. mm. | Polys., per cent. | L. M., per cent. | Lymp., per cent. | Eo., per cent. | My., per cent. | Nuc. Reds, per c. mm. | Nor., per cent. | Int., per cent. | Meg., per cent. |
|---|---|---|---|---|---|---|---|---|---|---|---|---|
| 2/28...... | 1,304,000 | 10 | 10,400 | 84.0 | 5.0 | 11.0 | 0 | 0 | 0 | .... | .... | 0 |
| 3/ 5...... | 1,108,000 | 10 | 10,600 | 85.2 | 4.6 | 10.0 | 0.2 | 0 | 158 | .... | .... | 0 |
| 3/ 8...... | 1,008,000 | 10 | 10,600 | 83.0 | 4.0 | 13.0 | 0 | 0 | 925 | 60 | 40 | 0 |
| 3/10...... | 974,000 | 10 | 10,200 | 86.0 | 3.5 | 10.3 | 0.2 | 0 | 1,350 | 69.5 | 30.0 | 0.5 |
| 3/12...... | 1,220,000 | 10 | 16,300 | 88.5 | 3.8 | 7.5 | 0.2 | 0 | 1,695 | 68 | 31 | 1 |
| 3/13...... | 1,120,000 | 10 | 14,100 | 90.9 | 1.6 | 7.3 | 0 | 0.2 | 1,850 | 58.5 | 40.5 | 1 |
| 3/15...... | 1,131,000 | 10 | 17,400 | 90.8 | 1.8 | 7.2 | 0.1 | 0.1 | 1,914 | 72 | 27.5 | 0.5 |
| 3/17...... | 1,028,000 | 10 | 20,200 | 93.0 | 1.4 | 5.2 | 0 | 0.4 | 3,456 | 64.2 | 34.3 | 1.5 |
| 3/19...... | 1,172,000 | 10 | 15,400 | 94.0 | 1.5 | 4.1 | 0 | 0.4 | 1,198 | 74.5 | 25.5 | 0 |
| 3/21...... | 1,181,000 | 10 | 12,200 | 92.3 | 1.2 | 6.3 | 0 | 0.2 | 793 | 78 | 22 | 0 |

*Course of Disease.*—The case progressed steadily downward. The temperature for the first week ran an irregular course, at times rising to 102, but after that it remained normal, with a pulse-rate of about 100, until the end. Emaciation and weakness were progressive, but practically no pain was complained of. The mass increased rapidly, causing marked bulging of the entire upper left quadrant of the abdomen; on palpation a few days before death its limits were the midline and the umbilical line. There was no vomiting or jaundice. Bowel movements were obtained only by enemas. No nodules developed on any of the bones. No therapy of any sort was attempted. Death occurred March 22, twenty-four days after entrance to hospital.

*Diagnosis.*—The case was considered one of neoplasm in the alimentary tract, the only question being as to the location. Owing to the lack of stomach symptoms, the constipation and the position of the mass, especially with reference to the inflated colon, a tentative diagnosis of neoplasm of the splenic flexure of the colon was made.

*Autopsy.*—Thoracic cavity: No fluid or adhesions. Pericardium contained about 20 c.c. of clear fluid. Heart showed a slight dilatation and the muscle was flabby, soft and pale. Lungs and pleuræ were normal.

Abdominal cavity: This contained free gas of fecal odor. The stomach, transverse colon, spleen, left kidney, pancreas, omentum and numerous enlarged lymph-glands were bound together in a dense mass and the whole attached to the diaphragm and lateral abdominal wall on the left side. With the exception of the kidney the individual organs could not be separated out. A perforation the size of a dollar had occurred on the anterior wall of the stomach, probably within forty-eight hours, but had been covered by liver, omentum and a thick, white exudate. There were no evidences of peritonitis in the lower abdominal cavity.

The stomach was enlarged, 14 by 23 cm., but both openings were clear. The anterior and posterior surfaces at the fundus were the seat of a wide-spread malignant infiltration. This extended with a fairly clear edge of demarcation, to a point 9 cm. above the greater curvature, and from the cardiac end 16 cm. toward the pyloric end. At least one-half of the greater curvature was involved, but none of the lesser. The walls in this area were 2 to 4 cm. in thickness, fairly soft, and the mucous membrane shaggy and necrotic. Beyond the lesion they were of normal thickness and appearance. The anterior wall was extremely necrotic, tearing with the slightest manipulation, while the posterior was much more dense in structure. There were numerous glands, varying from the size of a pea to that of a cherry, along both curvatures, in the omentum, mesocolon and mesentery. Almost the entire transverse colon was involved in the fibrous tissue about the stomach and at a point 8 cm. from the splenic flexure the lumen was constricted to 1 cm. in diameter by adhesions and the presence of a particularly enlarged gland in the mesocolon. Just proximal to this point, for about 10 cm. back, the colon was markedly dilated. There was no involvement of the wall itself.

The liver showed slight uniform enlargement. A portion of the left lobe, overlying the stomach perforation was covered with a flaky exudate and was necrotic on the surface. On section the liver tissue was pale, but otherwise normal. There were no metastases. The gall-bladder was normal.

The spleen was enlarged (13 by 6 by 5 cm.), soft, its anterior surface necrotic and covered with exudate. The pulp was normal. No metastases. The pancreas was densely bound to the posterior wall of the stomach and a portion of the tail was involved in the growth. The kidneys were normal. The bone-marrow of the ribs and sternum was apparently unchanged, but unfortunately it was not examined histologically. There were no metastases on any of the vertebræ.

Tissue taken from the advancing edge of the neoplasm, including part of the unattacked wall, showed that the growth was undoubtedly a sarcoma of the round-cell type. Advance took place in the muscular layers, the fibers of which were first invaded, then disintegrated and finally entirely replaced. At the edge, which was quite sharply defined, intact mucous membrane and submucosa covered the growth for some distance back, even over portions where the other layers were entirely gone. Further back these layers were invaded and later replaced by the sarcomatous cells, so that not a vestige of the original structure remained. (See illustration.) The cells themselves were approximately round and their diameter averaged a trifle less than twice that of a red-blood cell. The nucleus, oval or round, occupied the major portion of the cell and in the resting stage the reticulum was of fairly coarse mesh. Cells in all steps of mitotic division were present, although far outnumbered by those in the resting stage. Intracellular substance was scanty.

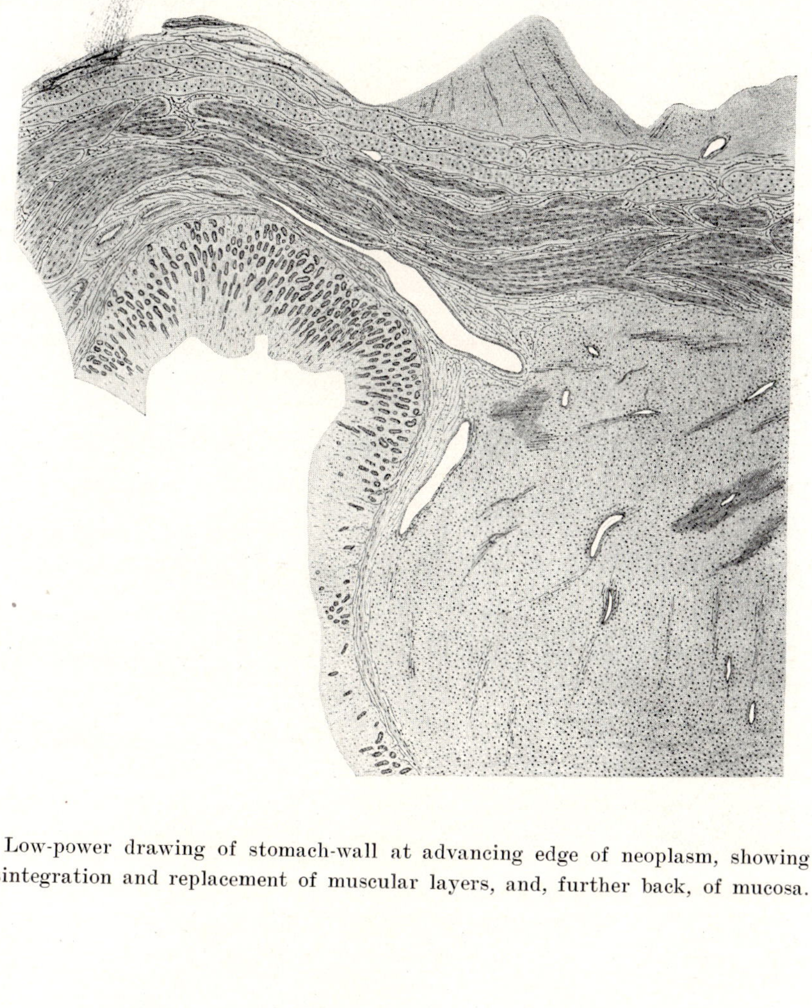

Low-power drawing of stomach-wall at advancing edge of neoplasm, showing disintegration and replacement of muscular layers, and, further back, of mucosa.

We thus have a case that presents two interesting sides pathologically: a primary sarcoma of the stomach; and a most extreme secondary anemia, during the course of which there was a distinct rise and fall of the red blood cells, the so-called "blood-crisis." In addition the individual clinical features merit a passing word. The paucity of gastric symptoms, the Gram-negative stools, the position of the mass, and the obstinate constipation, all combined to point to the colon as the seat of the growth, rather than to the stomach; yet at autopsy there was found the most widespread malignant involvement of the latter, with a mere mechanical obstruction of the former.

Primary sarcoma of the stomach is considered uncommon enough to justify the reporting of observed cases, and in consequence the literature is yearly becoming more extensive. No attempt is made here at a detailed review since several have appeared within the year. Clendening,[1] in a recent article, reviews seventy-three cases, including two of his own, and sets the frequency as next to that of carcinoma. About the same time Ziesche and Davidsohn[2] report three cases from the Breslau clinic, and give a most comprehensive analysis of 146 additional, gathered from a search of all literature. Since then three others have been reported, one by Dickinson[3] and two by Lofaro.[4] It would appear, therefore, that about 150 cases in all, of primary sarcoma of the stomach have been put on record up to the present time.

The term "blood-crisis" was coined by Von Noorden[5] to signify the temporary presence in the blood during a severe anemia, of numbers of nucleated red cells, which increase to a certain maximum and then diminish again, sometimes within a few days. At times followed by a rise in the red cell content, Von Noorden thought them to be a sign of an active blood regeneration, especially as they are accompanied by a leukocytosis.

Whatever may be the cause of the crisis, it by no means always bespeaks a good prognosis, and in pernicious anemia may be a terminal event in the disease, although marked improvement occasionally does occur. It would seem that crises in which the adult nucleated forms, the normoblasts, predominate, are followed by a rise in the red cell count, while those in which the younger forms and megaloblasts are present to any extent are not. It is in the idiopathic pernicious anemias that crises are most frequently found (19 per cent. of the Johns Hopkins series[6]). Here nucleated reds are almost always present, and for the definition

---

1. Clendening: Am. Jour. Med. Sc., 1909, cxxxviii, 191.
2. Ziesche and Davidsohn: Mitt. a. d. Grenzgeb. d. Med. u. Chir., 1909, xx, 377.
3. Dickinson, G. K.: Gastric Sarcoma, Jour. Am. Med. Assn., 1909, liii, 117.
4. Lofaro: Arch. gén. de chir., 1909, iii, 771.
5. Von Noorden: Charité-Ann., 1891, xvi, 217.
6. Emerson: Clinical Diagnosis, ed. 2, p. 568.

of a crisis an arbitrary line has been set at more than fifty nucleated reds per 1,000 leukocytes.[6] In some secondary anemias, particularly the post-hemorrhagic, crises, as stated by all writers, do occur, yet reports of this interesting phenomenon are strikingly rare, a search of the literature revealing but three. This may be due to the fact that the condition was not deemed sufficiently noteworthy to report, or if reported, was indexed under the disease causing the anemia.

Emerson[7] reports two cases in which crises occurred during the course of typhoid fever.

In his first case, that of a male negro aged 27, on the twenty-first day of illness the blood count was: reds, 3,752,000; hemoglobin, 55 per cent.; whites, 4,200. Within the next twenty-four hours an intestinal hemorrhage of about 500 c.c. occurred, with a drop in the temperature to subnormal. On the twenty-fourth day the crisis commenced, the count being: reds, 2,104,000; hemoglobin, 30 per cent.; whites, 16,000, of which 0.2 per cent. were myelocytes; and 64 nucleated reds per c.mm. The leukocytes and nucleated reds rose rapidly to 33,300 of the former, and 26,000 of the latter on the twenty-seventh day, the percentage of myelocytes at that time being 6.46. The next day there were but 1,006,000 red cells per c.mm., and on the thirtieth, the day of death, the whites were 10,000, and the nucleated reds 900. The necropsy showed the usual findings of typhoid fever, and examination of the bone-marrow gave *Bacillus typhosus* in pure culture, with histologically, wide-spread areas of necrosis. During the rise of the crisis, from 20 to 40 per cent. of the nucleated reds were megaloblasts and intermediate forms, and it is significant in this regard to notice the failure of the attempt of the marrow to cope with the rapidly developing anemia. This would bear out the observation that a megaloblastic crisis occurs where a patient is losing ground and is an evidence of the insufficiency of the marrow to regenerate the blood.

His second patient was a man aged 47, with hematemesis and melena from a bleeding esophageal varix, probably secondary to hepatic cirrhosis, admitted to hospital with an infection by *Bacillus typhosus* as proved by blood cultures. On admission the count was: reds, 1,300,000; hemoglobin, 25 per cent.; whites, 71,500, of which 8.8 per cent. were myelocytes. There were 3,500 nucleated reds per c.mm. with about 10 per cent. megaloblasts and intermediate forms. Two days later the nucleated reds numbered 90,000. Death occurred on the following day, no autopsy being permitted.

In both these cases there was a severe secondary anemia, partially due to hemorrhage, a pronounced leukocytosis with a decided increase in the number of myelocytes, and sharp blood-crises in which the megaloblasts

7. Emerson: Bull. Johns Hopkins Hosp., 1907, xviii, 412.

and intermediate forms predominated. In neither did any improvement in the blood occur, although in the second case death supervened at the heighth of the crisis.

Kerr and Spriggs[8] report a crisis in the case of a man of 30 with amyloid disease of the kidney following syphilis, complicated by hemorrhages from the kidneys and bowels. On entrance the count was: reds, 1,100,000; hemoglobin, 29 per cent.; whites, 13,600, of which 1.1 per cent. were myelocytes; and nucleated reds, 20,672 per c.mm. These were classified according to the shape of the nucleus as single, double and polynucleated. If we can assume that by the double and polynucleated forms are meant the immature intermediate varieties, these were present to the extent of 29 per cent. Three weeks later the count was: reds, 3,950,000; hemoglobin, 58 per cent.; whites, 17,700; no myelocytes, and only two nucleated reds seen in making the differential count. The general condition improved considerably for a time, but death occurred within a month. In this case there was a temporary improvement in the anemia.

The blood-crisis in the present case is a small although a typical one. The hypocythemia and low index, exceptional as it is, may be explained on the basis of the combined factors of a constant occult hemorrhage, and the toxins of an extremely malignant growth. Thus, a diminution of the red count to 1,000,000 or under does not necessarily rule against a malignancy. Also, it may be that the occurrence of a blood-crisis during a severe secondary anemia is a more frequent feature than the records would indicate, and it is partly in the hope that this particular point be observed in other cases that this report is offered.

In conclusion I wish to express my indebtedness to Professor Alonzo E. Taylor, late of the University of California, for his kindness in examining and passing upon sections of the tissue, and also to his assistant, William T. Jane, for his trouble in preparing them and to Mr. Richard W. Harvey for the drawing.

Central Bank Building.

8. Kerr and Spriggs: Lancet, London, 1909, clxxvi, 378.

# A STUDY OF THE TECHNIC OF THE CAMMIDGE REACTION AND OF THE SUBSTANCE GIVING RISE TO THE SO-CALLED TYPICAL CRYSTALS *

JOSEPH C. ROPER, M.D., AND RALPH G. STILLMAN, M.D.
NEW YORK

P. J. Cammidge[1] discusses in detail the "chemical pathology" of the pancreas, describing three methods, classed as A, B and C, for the examination of the urine in cases of suspected pancreatic disease. The A and B reactions were discarded because, when positive, they result in precipitates which "consist of two parts, one a phenylhydrazin compound of glycuronic acid, and the other the osazone of a sugar." To overcome this and other difficulties, the "improved" or "C" reaction was introduced, "in which the presence or absence of pancreatitis is indicated by the examination of a single specimen."

The technic of the "C" reaction is as follows:

The urine is freed from albumin (by heat and acetic acid) and from sugar (by fermentation) and filtered several times through the same paper. Forty c.c. of this clear filtrate are boiled for ten minutes with 2 c.c. strong hydrochloric acid (specific gravity 1.16) in a small flask with a funnel condenser. This is cooled and diluted up to 40 c.c. with cold water. Then 8 gm. lead carbonate are added slowly, the liquid allowed to stand for a few minutes, cooled again in running water and filtered until perfectly clear. The filtrate is then shaken well with 8 gm. powdered tribasic lead acetate, and filtered as clear as possible, the filtrate being repeated several times if necessary. It is then shaken well with 4 gm. powdered sodium sulphate, heated to boiling point, cooled in running water and filtered carefully. Ten c.c. of this perfectly clear transparent filtrate are diluted to 17 c.c with distilled water and added to 2 gm. sodium acetate, 0.8 gm. phenylhydrazin hydrochlorid, and 1 c.c. 50 per cent. acetic acid. This is boiled for ten minutes in a small flask with a funnel condenser, filtered while hot through paper moistened with hot water and the filtrate diluted to 15 c.c. with hot water if necessary. The crystals separate in a few hours in a characteristic reaction, but it may be necessary to leave the preparation over night before a deposit occurs.

---

* From the Department of Clinical Pathology of the New York Hospital.

1. Cammidge, P. J.: The Pancreas: Its Surgery and Pathology, 1907, p. 206 *et seq.*

"The 'improved method' or 'C reaction' is based upon the different behavior of glycuronic acid and the sugars in acid solutions, to tribasic lead acetate, the former being precipitated and the latter remaining in solution." "The result is an absolute one, and is therefore independent of the personal bias of the investigator."

The results obtained with the Cammidge reaction by different investigators, are not so absolute as one might be led to expect from the above statements. Roth[2] obtained unsatisfactory results in thirty-two cases, and regards it as of little value in the diagnosis of pancreatic disease. Petroff[3] concludes that it is not pathognomonic, is influenced by diseases of the duodenum, and that the precipitate is rarely an osazone of glycuronic acid but is usually an osazone of inverted saccharose. Also that the reaction is a test of the assimilation of beet sugar, and that no facts

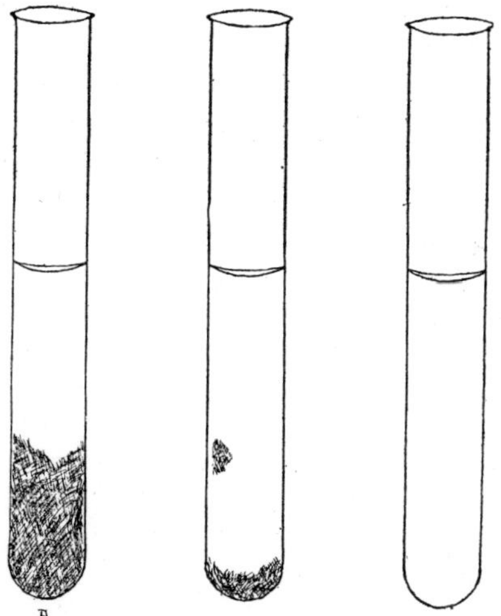


Quantity of typical Cammidge crystals obtained from 10 c.c. diluted to 40 c.c.: A, after boiling urine with HCl and neutralizing with sodium carbonate; B, after completion of Cammidge reaction; C, after completion of mortar technic.

have been adduced[2] to show that pentose is the cause of the positive reaction.

Ochsner[4] thinks that further development of the test is necessary. Kreinitz'[5] results were in accord with the findings at operation in 80 per cent. of the cases, although he had positive reactions in diseases of the intestinal tract, biliary tract, diabetes and carcinoma of organs other

2. Roth: Ztschr. f. klin. Med., 1909, lxvii, 222.
3. Petroff, N. Y.: Russk. Vrach, 1909, viii, 1498, 1536.
4. Ochsner: Surg. Gynec. and Obst., 1908, vii, 621.
5. Kreinitz: Arch. f. Verdaungskr., 1909, xv, 53.

than the pancreas. Deaver[6] is inclined to regard it as "a fairly constant sign of pancreatic disease rather than of great value in the differential diagnosis."

Goodman[7] admits difficulties but is enthusiastic in its favor. Spiese and Goodman,[8] as the result of experimental work on dogs, found it constant in hemorrhagic pancreatitis, mechanical injuries of the gland, as crushing and partial or total extirpation—inconstant in subacute pancreatitis. They are uncertain of the nature of the phenylhydrazin compound, but think (on what grounds is not plain) that the reaction is indicative of altered carbohydrate metabolism, due to disturbance of the internal secretion of the pancreas. Smolenski,[9] investigating the *Mutter-Substanz,* concluded that, in the case under observation, the crystals were due to the presence of saccharose. Schumm and Hegler[10] conclude that many positive reactions are nothing else than positive grape-sugar tests, and that the result is influenced more or less by accidental occurrences. Swan and Gilbride[11] think it a mistake to interpret every positive reaction as indicative of organic disease of the pancreas.

The varying results obtained by us in the early part of our work in the examination of cases led us to agree, with Schumm and Hegler, that these results were influenced by accidental occurrences. Attempts to control these accidents led to a slight modification of the technic. This modification consisted in rubbing up in a mortar with their appropriate filtrates, the lead acetate and sodium sulphate, instead of mixing them in a beaker by shaking. This procedure insured thorough mixing and gave perfectly clear filtrates and uniformly negative results in cases which, by the original method, might be positive one day and negative the next. Having made, with this technic, 125 negative examinations on thirty cases, we naturally concluded that the reaction, when positive, was due to some substance normally present in the urine, split off by boiling with hydrochloric acid and incompletely removed by the lead acetate, and that the substance was probably glycuronic acid.

Regarding the typical crystals, Cammidge says: "By collecting large quantities of urine from well-marked cases of pancreatitis, we were able to investigate the character of this (the 'sugar' giving rise to the typical crystals) and found that it gave the reactions of a pentose. We have been unable to discover any evidence of the presence of a pentose in the untreated urine from any of our cases, so that it is probable that the pentose giving rise to the characteristic 'pancreatic reaction' was formed

6. Deaver, John B.: Chronic Pancreatitis, Jour. Am. Med. Assn., 1908, li, 374.
7. Goodman: Ann. Surg., 1909, xlix, 183.
8. Spiese and Goodman: Am. Jour. Med. Sc., 1909, cxxxviii, 108.
9. Smolenski: Ztschr. f. physiol. Chem., 1909, lx, 119.
10. Schumm, O., and Hegler, C.: München. med. Wchnschr., 1909, lvi, 2054.
11. Swan and Gilbride: New York Med. Jour., 1910, xci, 781, 852.

by hydrolysis from some antecedent substance in the urine, during the process of heating it with the dilute acid."

We cannot agree with this opinion. Working with the urine from a case of essential pentosuria, we found that small amounts of pentose were destroyed or removed in the course of the Cammidge reaction. This specimen gave positive reactions for pentose, and crystals with a typical melting-point were obtained from it by the ordinary procedure. At the conclusion of the Cammidge reaction, on the other hand, no crystals could be obtained. If, however, the precipitation with lead acetate were omitted, atypical crystals, which were probably a mixture of pentose and glycuronic acid, were formed.

Cammidge's contention, that the improved or "C" reaction removed the glycuronic acid, is not supported by facts. A. Jolles[12] has called attention to the impossibility of precipitating all the glycuronic acid with lead acetate when the former is present in excess. Even when present in small amounts, it will not, in every instance, be completely precipitated by the ordinary Cammidge procedure. When present in large amounts it can be positively identified in the filtrates obtained after precipitation with lead acetate and sodium sulphate, even when the precaution is taken of carefully mixing the reagents in the mortar.

For the demonstration of this last fact we used specimens of urine from two patients who were taking from 20 to 40 grains of chloral a day. Chloral, as is well known, increases the amount of conjugate glycuronates in the urine. For the positive identification of glycuronic acid, the urine is boiled with an acid to split up the conjoined glycuronates, and after neutralization, is boiled a short time with parabromphenylhydrazin hydrochlorid. This gives a compound with a characteristic melting-point. The employment of this parabromphenylhydrazin hydrochlorid is necessary because glycuronic acid, by virtue of its carboxyl and aldehyd groups, forms with phenylhydrazin hydrochlorid a hydrozone, an osazone, a hydrazid, a hydrazin salt, a hydrazone hydrazid, an osazone hydrazid and intermediate condensation products.[13] Most of the phenylhydrazin compounds with glycuronic acid are mixtures of these substances:

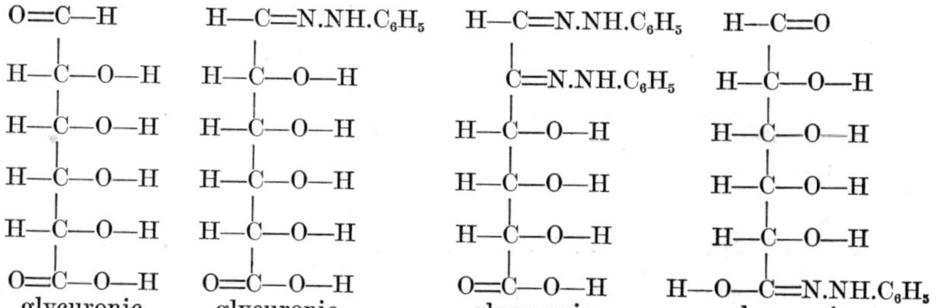

glycuronic acid — glycuronic acid hydrazone — glycuronic acid osazone — glycuronic acid hydrazid

12. Jolles, A.: Zentralbl. f. inn. Med., 1909, xxx, 1097.
13. Mayer, P.: Ztschr. f. physiol. Chem., 1900, xxix, 59.

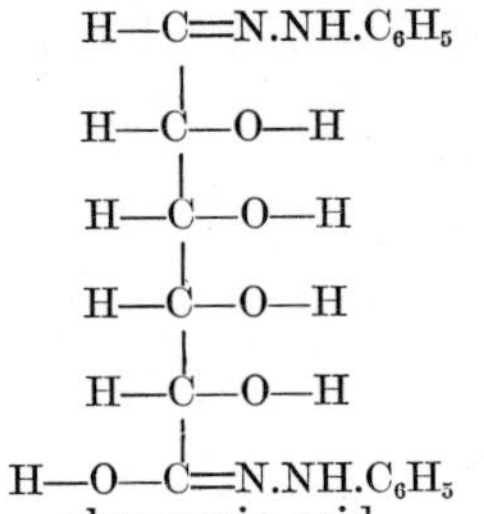

glycuronic acid
hydrazone hydrazid

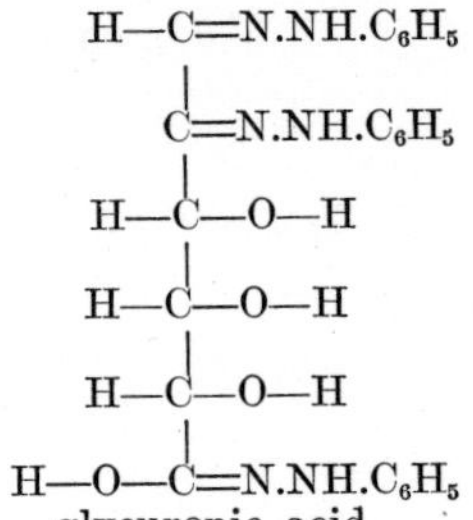

glycuronic acid
osazone hydrazid

This fact explains the different melting-points obtained by other workers and ourselves in attempts to identify the Cammidge crystals. These different melting points were 114-115 C., 160-173 C., 180-185 C. and 200-204 C.

P. Mayer[13] has shown that one molecule of glycuronic acid combines with one molecule of phenylhydrazin to form a compound which, when crude, melts at 199-205 C., when recrystallized, at 210-217 C.; that one molecule of glycuronic acid combines with two, three, or four molecules of phenylhydrazin to form a compound which melts at 159-164 C. These two compounds have melting-points identical with those of glucosazone and pentosazone, respectively. Thierfelder obtained a compound containing one molecule of glycuronic acid and two and one-half molecules of phenylhydrazin, which melted at 114 C.

Mayer and Neuberg,[14] however, have demonstrated that combinations of parabromphenylhydrazin hydrochlorid with glycuronic acid have a specific melting point of 235-240 C. This compound can be obtained only when the urine contains large amounts of glycuronic acid.

Using 40 c.c. of the urines mentioned above (from patients taking chloral) we were able to isolate compounds of glycuronic acid and parabromphenylhydrazin hydrochlorid with the characteristic melting point, 235-240 C., from the filtrates obtained at each step of the Cammidge reaction. Obtaining this characteristic compound from 10 c.c. of the filtrate resulting after boiling with acid and neutralizing, showed that glycuronic acid was present in large amount in the original specimen. Obtaining this same compound from 10 c.c. of the filtrate resulting from the precipitation with lead acetate showed that this procedure had not removed all the glycuronic acid. Obtaining it also from 10 c.c. of the filtrate resulting after the treatment of the lead acetate filtrate with sodium sulphate, demonstrated that glycuronic acid was present at the completion of the reaction. Parallel tests of the above filtrates with ordinary phenylhydrazin hydrochlorid gave typical Cammidge crystals with melting points between 114 and 204 C.

---

14. Mayer and Neuberg: Ztschr. f. physiol. Chem., 1900, xxix, 257.

When 40 c.c. of the urines containing large amounts of glycuronic acid were used, a negative result could not be obtained with the modified or mortar technic. By employing 10 c.c. diluted to 40 c.c., however, a negative result was obtained by the mortar technic while the regulation Cammidge procedure still showed a deposit of typical crystals. The illustration shows the volume of the precipitate of typical Cammidge crystals obtained from 10 c.c. of this urine: A, after boiling and neutralizing; B, after completion of the reaction by the Cammidge; and C, by the mortar technic.

In specimens which do not contain enough glycuronic acid to permit of the demonstration of the specific melting point of its parabromphenylhydrazin compound, recourse must be had to other reactions. We employed the orcein test and the naphtoresorcin test of Tollens.[15] In specimens giving typical crystals by the C technic, these tests were positive in the filtrates obtained after treatment with sodium sulphate, and negative in the corresponding filtrate obtained in parallel tests by the mortar technic, the latter giving no typical crystals.

The number of examinations on which this article is based is 175, on forty cases representing all types of disease. Before adopting the mortar technic, the result of the test was frequently at variance with the findings at autopsy or operation. Since adopting this modification, with its uniformly negative or readily explained results, we have been able to demonstrate marked pancreatic lesions in two "negative" cases at autopsy. The specimens giving a positive reaction when 40 c.c. were employed (due, as we have demonstrated, to glycuronic acid) were not from pancreatic cases but from patients with high arterial tension, usually with associated constipation, who were taking large doses of chloral.

An excess of glycuronic acid in the urine cannot be accepted as indicating disease of the pancreas. Glycuronic acid is an intermediate product of carbohydrate metabolism. It is normally present in the urine, as shown by Mayer and Neuberg,[14] while Tollens and Stern[16] have found that the average output in health amounts to 0.025 gm. per 100 c.c. in the twenty-four-hour urine. It is excreted in combination with indoxyl, skatoxyl and phenol, and will vary as these substances vary. The administration of camphor, salicylates or chloral markedly increases its elimination, in which case it may amount to 1.4 gm. in the twenty-four hours. It is apparently saved from destruction by combination with these substances. Of its origin little is known. In a starving dog, administration of chloral or camphor leads to the elimination of the corresponding glycuronate, suggesting the possibility of its formation in the body.

---

15. Tollens, C.: München. med. Wchnschr., 1909, lvi, 652.

16. Tollens and Stern: Ztschr. f. physiol. Chem. (Hoppe-Seyler's), 1910, lxiv, 39.

We could not satisfy ourselves that any substance other than glycuronic acid was responsible for the reaction. The elaborate technic suggested would be unnecessary and indeed unsuitable for the demonstration of small amounts of glucose or pentose. That saccharose, as such, was not present in any of our cases seemed apparent from the absence of the characteristic changes in rotation.

## CONCLUSIONS

The "C" reaction proposed by Cammidge, for the demonstration of a characteristic substance in the urine of patients suffering from diseases of the pancreas, does not rest on a sound scientific basis, as not all the glycuronic acid is removed in every instance by the technic of this reaction. The formation of the typical crystals is due to the presence of glycuronic acid. As this substance is present in the urine of persons in normal health, and is increased in amount in many conditions in no way associated with disease of the pancreas, the demonstration of these so-called typical crystals can have no diagnostic value.

255 West Eighty-Fourth Street—120 West Fifty-Fifth Street.

# ALLERGY

C. E. VON PIRQUET, M.D.
BALTIMORE

A person who has once had measles, smallpox or whooping-cough does not, as a rule, have the infection a second time. We call this immunity. On the other hand, there are infectious diseases, such as pneumonia and erysipelas, which leave behind a greater sensibility, which we call predisposition.

For half a century the medical world has worked on the mechanism of these phenomena. The great discoveries made in this field have been the result of our knowledge of the pathogenic micro-organism, together with that of the morphological elements and the soluble constituents of the blood and other organs. It is not surprising that the greatest attention has been paid to microscopic observations and animal experimentation, while the study of the clinical phenomena has been comparatively neglected.

## *THE CLINICAL OBSERVATION OF THE MECHANISM OF IMMUNITY*

The question we put ourselves is: what occurs if we try to reinfect an immune individual? Suppose we choose as a point of reinfection the skin, and study with the naked eye the course of events at the point of reinfection. Here it is of no consequence to us whether the micro-organism is destroyed outside the cells or taken up by the leukocytes. Neither the macrophages nor the side-chains need concern us.

Cowpox inoculation affords us the best opportunity for our study. The disease called forth by vaccination with cowpox is just as real a disease as smallpox, but less severe. Let us first inoculate an individual who has been inoculated two years previously with a drop of lymph. This individual is to all appearances "immune." On the other hand, let us inoculate a person who has not yet gone through this process, and note the results carefully. Will there be no manifestations in the immune individual? Not at all; if we return in twenty-four hours, we shall find in the immune an infected scratch, a very small, but elevated, inflamed and itching reddening, whereas the newly vaccinated person shows only a little scab, without any sign of inflammation.

Is the person, therefore, hypersensitive, who has been inoculated previously? If we wait a few days conditions will change. The papule on the person previously inoculated will turn brown and grow smaller in size; a little blister on the other hand will develop under the scab on the one inoculated for the first time. This will grow larger and will be surrounded by a large red area and then turn into a pustule. We now perceive that the newly inoculated person is the more sensitive, for he has pain, fever and considerable local inflammation, while the one formerly inoculated does not show any signs of infection.

We shall understand the value of this "early reaction" of the immune, if we consider how a real reinfection occurs in smallpox. Let us suppose that, instead of the infection with attenuated cowpox, a virulent smallpox germ had been deposited in the throats of both individuals: the vaccinated would have had a slight redness around the spot within twenty-four hours, while the unvaccinated person would have gone through the whole severity of a smallpox fever and exanthem. The fact, however, which I wish to emphasize here is that both persons, after the infection with cowpox, react, the one sooner, the other later, one with a papule, the other with a pustule, one hardly noticeable, the other with considerable symptoms. The "immune" person does not become insensible to inoculation, but the time, quality and quantity of his reaction is changed.

Therefore, we might rightly use the word "allergy": from *ergeia,* reactivity, and *allos,* "altered," a changed reactivity as a clinical conception without being prejudiced by the bacteriological, pathological or biological findings. As the oldest observation of allergy—even though not under this name and not conceived in the same way as to-day—one may cite the knowledge of the modification of the form of smallpox by means of a previous vaccination. During the great smallpox epidemics, from 1813 to 1830, very many, who had been vaccinated in childhood, became ill with an eruption resembling smallpox, though in a milder form, and disappearing more rapidly. This was contrary to the early expectations of Jenner. It was termed "varioloid" by Thomson, in 1820. Wolfert, Dornblueth and Harder then showed that one inoculation of vaccinia was not a sufficient protection against smallpox for a lifetime, that a revaccination was necessary, and that the clinical manifestations of this revaccination are as different from that of the first vaccination as varioloid is from variola.

In 1839 Magendie made an observation which represents a quite different and apparently useless kind of allergy; he saw that rabbits which had been injected with egg albumin died after a repetition of the injection.

In 1882 Pohl Pincus made a histological study of first and repeated cowpox vaccination, and found that the reactive inflammation appears early after the repeated inoculation. He reached the conclusion that the vaccine micro-organism secretes a toxin, which, at its first entry into the human organism, is capable of paralyzing the reactive powers of the human body.

Arloing, in 1888, was led to an apparently contrary opinion, finding that repeated injections of micro-organisms have fatal results.

In 1891, Courmont studied this question with the tubercle bacillus. The Lyons school repeated the observations with staphylococci and streptococci, *Bacillus pyocyaneus* and other bacteria.

The study of bacterial toxins furnished new evidences in this direction and the results are described here as hypersensibility and paradoxical reaction. In 1895, Brieger reported the case of a goat highly immunized against tetanus, whose blood and milk contained great quantities of antitoxin, but in spite of this the animal was subject to tetanus. Knorr (1895) studied more closely this unexpected effect, which had made itself felt chiefly as a practical difficulty in immunizing animals against tetanus toxin. Von Behring and Kitashima found a similar case with diphtheria in an immune horse (1901). They determined quantitatively the hypersensibility of guinea-pigs, and showed that the animals died of a typical diphtheritic intoxication after they had been inoculated with an amount of toxin containing only 1/800 of the minimal deadly dose. That this was not brought about by cumulative effect of the toxin in the sense of a mere addition of separate doses of the poison is shown by the fact that by the addition of all the toxic doses, only 1/400 of the minimal deadly dose was obtained (cit. after Otto). Von Behring conceived the hypersensibility as purely histogenetic; the explanations of Kretz, in the sense of Ehrlich, are very closely allied to his conception. He regards the side-chains anchored to the cells as a cause of this paradoxical phenomenon.

The French physiologist, Richet, found (1902) that the poison of the actinia on a second injection after an interval of several days goes into action much more intensely and acutely than the first time; if the animal survives, however, it conquers the disease in a shorter time than after a first injection. He states that two different substances are contained in this poison, one concerned in establishing an immunity, the other in calling forth a hypersensitiveness, but thus far the separate existence of both these hypothetical substances has not been proved. The conception of anaphylaxis, which has been sharply separated here for the first time from immunity, has been maintained. On the instigation of Richet, Arthus undertook similar experiments with horse-serum in animals (1903). It was found that a first injection of an apparently harmless substance changed the organism in such a manner that a repeated injection now acted on it as a violent poison.

Independent of these authors, observations at the bedside called my attention to phenomena standing in a certain relationship to those just cited. In 1902 a child at Escherich's clinic received a second injection of horse-serum. The first injection had been followed by clinical symptoms on the tenth day, but after the second injection they appeared in the course of the same day. On the basis of this observation I reached the conclusion that the prevailing theory with regard to the time of incubation could not be correct. I proposed a theory that the disease-producing organism calls forth symptoms only when it has been changed by antibodies; the time if incubation is the time necessary for the formation of these antibodies. I was confirmed in this opinion by the statements of von Dungern, pointing out that a rabbit forms precipitins more quickly after a second injection of alien serum.

In an effort to treat all infectious diseases from the same point of view, I looked for analogies and found one in the early appearance of reactions in cases of revaccination. In association with B. Schick, I made all the diseases which seemed to correspond to these views the subject of investigation, and we cited vaccination, smallpox, measles, recurrens, injection of serum, streptococci, tuberculin and mallein. In a comprehensive study of serum disease we pointed out the difference between accelerated and immediate reactivity. We called attention to the diagnostic value of the latter; that is, we showed that it enables us to decide whether the organism had been previously infected. Our idea was that substances of the character of an antibody digest the foreign substances, and that the products of digestion act as poisons.

These views remained unnoticed for several years, and until to-day the main point of the theory, the difference in the time of reaction, has not been understood by many scientists.

In 1904 Detre-Deutsch wished to explain the question why a luetic man cannot acquire a primary infection of syphilis a second time, although he still shows symptoms of the disease, and is, therefore, not insensitive to syphilis. To this end he made reinjections of tuberculosis in guinea-pigs, and emphasized the difference in phenomena between the first and second superinfection. His explanation of the immediate effect of the latter is the same as that held by Koch on the result of tuberculin injections (*Additionstheorie*).

In 1904 Wolff-Eisner wrote a general treatise "Ueber Grundgesetze der Immunität," starting from the pure idea of hypersensibility in the sense of Pfeiffer's antitoxin theory. He studied microscopically the lysis of blood-corpuscles of doves and of human spermatozoa after first and second injection in the peritoneal cavity of a guinea-pig, and stated at the same time that the animals died regularly after repeated injections. He explained the phenomenon by the hypothesis that poisonous bodies, endotoxins, contained within the cells pass out after the solution of their shells. This solution is accomplished by means of lysins formed as a result of the first injection.

Since that time several authors, more or less independently, have noticed hypersensibility as an important phenomena, and studied it (Löwenstein, Friedemann and Isaac, Saeli, Batelli, De Waele). Theobald Smith, of Boston, found that guinea-pigs which are used for standardizing the strength of diphtheria antitoxin often die after a second injection of serum. Otto studied these phenomena more closely, and since then has published several important works in this connection. The best work has been contributed by Rosenau and Anderson, who started out from the investigation of the sudden death which was attributed to the use of antidiphtheritic serum. These authors demonstrated by a great number of experiments the action of horse-serum and other substances in guinea-pigs. Most of the experimental work has been done on that animal, by Vaughan and Wheeler, Lewis, Gay and Southard and others, to whose experiments I shall have to refer in the special part, as well as to those of Kraus, Doerr and Russ, Sleeswijk, Besredka and others who have made very valuable contributions during the last years.

My plan is to take all the morbid entities in which symptoms of allergy are to be found one after another, and then to collect those facts which all of them have in common. I begin with those groups which are carefully worked out, and later go on to those in which only one or the other symptom allows an analogy.

## *SERUM DISEASE*

### HORSE-SERUM IN MAN

The first injection of horse-serum which we use as a carrier of antitoxin in diphtheria, tetanus, scarlet fever and epidemic meningitis has not only an antitoxic influence, but often causes symptoms of its own, which consist in urticaria, fever, edema and pains in the joints. They are due to the horse-serum, for they show themselves also after injection of the serum of healthy horses not previously treated with diphtheria or other toxins (Bokay, Johannessen).

These symptoms to which Schick and I have given the name of "serum disease" occur only occasionally immediately after the injection. There is nearly always an incubation time of eight to twelve days up to the outbreak of the symptoms. On a repetition of the injection a different behavior is noted.

E. E., injection of 200 c.c. scarlatina serum of Moser. On the evening of the seventh day a severe serum disease set in, which consisted in a swelling of the regionary lymph-glands, fever up to 40.5, edema and rash, the latter first consisting of urticaria; later on it had the character of erythema multiforme (Marfan's *érythème marginé aberrant*). Thirty-eight days later fifteen children received immunizing doses of 1 c.c. antidiphtheritic serum, among them E. E., who showed after eight hours, fever and a swelling of the skin of the lower arm on the point of injection. The next morning a diffuse red, painful swelling up to the middle of the upper arm was noticed, and in the afternoon a general rash of urticaria character. The fever lasted thirty-six hours, then the swelling decreased gradually On the sixth day after this injection, again a general rash.

We shall study in these cases the properties of allergy against horse-serum in man.

1. *Allergy According to Time.*—The symptoms after the first injection of E. E. appeared on the seventh day; after reinjection, after eight hours.

2. *Quantitative Allergy.*—Of the fifteen children who were injected at the same time with E. E., 10 had not received the serum previously. Only one of them showed a very slight swelling at the same time that E. E. showed his severe symptoms. Between the sixth and eighth day, slight general symptoms were noticed in four of them.

The severe reaction which E. E. showed was, therefore, not due to a property of the horse-serum which was used in this second injection, but was due to a subjective disposition. He was extremely hypersensitive, and this hypersensitiveness was an acquired one, for he had not reacted in that way after the first injection.

3. *Qualitative Allergy.*—After the first injection there were no local reactions on the point of injection, but general symptoms, such as fever, urticaria and hydrops. The second injection provoked an intense redness and swelling at the point of inoculation. In other cases the reinjection is followed by general phenomena of short duration, which are sometimes accompanied by collapse. This collapse is never seen in serum disease occurring after a normal incubation time.

Goodall remarked in his paper of 1907, that as early as 1898 he had mentioned three cases in which the injection of antitoxin was immediately followed by fever and other symptoms. In all three cases a previous first injection had produced serum disease in the second week after the injection. The third case is extremely typical: Within a quarter of an hour after the reinjection, the child became very ill, showed an urticaria-like rash, stiffness for half an hour, cyanosis, rapid and weak pulse. At that time Goodall did not draw conclusions from these cases, but simply recorded them.

The most important feature of allergy is certainly the immediate reaction. In addition to the cases noted by von Pirquet and Schick, Lehndorff, Lemaire, Goodall, Currie, Netter and Debre give the figures shown in Table 1 for the day on which the serum disease appeared after injection.

TABLE 1.—TIME OF APPEARANCE OF SERUM DISEASE

| Day of appearance of serum disease | 1-2 | 3 | 4 | 5 | 6 | 7 | 8 | 9 | 10 | 11 | 12 | 13 | 14 | 15 | 16 | 17-20 |
|---|---|---|---|---|---|---|---|---|---|---|---|---|---|---|---|---|
| First injection | 3 | 1 | 5 | 2 | 11 | 21 | 35 | 32 | 23 | 17 | 18 | 10 | 12 | 9 | 8 | 7 |
| Reinjection | 89 | 6 | 9 | 14 | 20 | 24 | 7 | 2 | 1 | .. | .. | .. | .. | .. | .. | .... |

We see from this table that after the first injection, serum disease appears seldom before the sixth day, mostly on the eighth and ninth day, but frequently later. In reinjected children, however, we find that the symptoms usually appear as an "immediate reaction" within twenty-four hours. The first and second day in the table are taken together, because clinically they are difficult to distinguish, as the hour of injection is not often noted in histories. A second maximum of the onset of the disease is shown on the sixth and seventh day; this is about two days earlier than the maximum in patients injected for the first time. Von Pirquet and Schick call this therefore "accelerated reaction."

The accelerated reaction is clinically similar to the normal type of reaction. It consists of fever, urticaria, etc., without a special involvement at the point of inoculation, but it disappears more rapidly. It has in common the quantitative allergy with the immediate reaction. If the same amount of serum is given, reactions occur more frequently than in children injected the first time. It is not to be understood that after each injection or reinjection all these symptoms occur. They are seen only in part of the cases, but if present, follow the given rules of time, quantity and quality.

As a whole, serum disease occurs the more frequently, the larger the amounts of serum administered.

TABLE 2.—FREQUENCY OF SERUM REACTIONS WITH DIFFERENT QUANTITIES OF SERUM *

| Total Amount of Serum in c.c. | Cases Showing Reaction. | Cases Observed 10 Days and More Showing No Reaction. | Total Cases. | Per Cent. Showing Reaction. |
|---|---|---|---|---|
| 1- 9 | 9 | 73 | 83 | 10.9 |
| 10- 19 | 52 | 137 | 189 | 27.5 |
| 20- 29 | 40 | 100 | 140 | 28.5 |
| 30- 49 | 47 | 73 | 120 | 39.0 |
| 50- 79 | 46 | 138 | 92 | 50.0 |
| 80-280 | 42 | 111 | 69 | 61.0 |

* After Weaver, George H.: Serum Disease, THE ARCHIVES INTERNAL MEDICINE, 1909, iii, 485.

Very often, the first injection is not followed by marked symptoms, but after the reinjection we find an early or accelerated reaction. Explicit statistics on these facts are given by Goodall and Currie.

Both forms—"immediate" and "accelerated" reaction—may follow one another as in the example of E. E. This double reaction is especially common when there is a certain interval of time between the first and second administration of serum. In the cases of von Pirquet and Schick and of Lehndorff, grouped according to interval of time, it is found, as shown in Table 3.

Allergy in the form of accelerated reaction lasts for years. As the first serum disease is seen only after an incubation time, so also the allergic condition does not occur immediately after the first injection, but only after a certain period. If the second injection is made within the first ten days after the first injection, it does not provoke a local edema or other immediate symptoms. This incubation time of allergy has nearly the same duration as the normal incubation time of serum disease, or as the period required for the active formation of antibodies against serum. We shall return later to the inferences to be drawn from this analogy.

TABLE 3.—DOUBLE REACTION

| Interval Between First and Second Injection. | Reaction: Only "Immediate." | Double. | Only "Accelerated." | Sum. |
|---|---|---|---|---|
| Ten days to one month | 21 | 3 | .. | 24 |
| One month to six months | 21 | 7 | 5 | 33 |
| More than six months | 2 | 2 | 30 | 34 |

Von Pirquet and Schick found that the shortest interval between the injections giving rise to an allergic reaction was twelve days; Lehndorff found ten days; Marfan and Lemaire and Currie cite three more cases with so short an interval as ten days.

## REACTION OF MAN AGAINST OTHER SERUMS

The action of horse-serum is the only one which has been thoroughly investigated in man, because for therapeutic purposes horse-serum is used nearly exclusively. Several other serums seem to act in the same way as horse-serum does. Thus Dellera cites a case in which ten days after the transfusion of lamb's blood, a general urticaria occurred. Similar symptoms have also been seen after an injection of rabbit-serum. We see, however, in man a primary action of the serums of some animals, without incubation time. This primary action is probably due to thermolabile bodies, according to the findings of Doerr, which will be discussed in the next chapter. The serums of pigs and of cattle seem to have a primary action.

Bier, who tried to influence malignant tumors by the injection of pig's blood, observed fever and local reaction on the following days. Schlossmann and Salge saw in nurslings, after injections of only 0.1 c.c. cattle-serum, intense actions within the first twenty-four hours. The question whether this action of cattle-serum is analogous to symptoms sometimes seen in nurslings after the first feedings with cow's milk, has been discussed by Hamburger, Moro and Schlossmann, but definite conclusions have not been reached as yet.

## SERUM DISEASE IN ANIMALS

The experiments might be increased manifold if we should undertake to test the serum of each species on all of the other species, as Nuttall did in studying the precipitin reaction. Thus far numerous experiments of this kind have been conducted and their results may be divided into three groups:

*Group 1.*—Primary toxic action of the foreign serum at the first injection. Uhlenhuth found that serum of cattle, sheep and pigs kill the guinea-pig in doses of 6, 11 and 12 c.c. per kilogram. Of eel serum only 0.02 c.c. per kilogram is sufficient according to Mosso.

H. Pfeiffer showed that after a subcutaneous injection of guinea-pigs with the serum of cattle, doves, pigs and man, a local necrosis is found; at the same time these serums dissolve the red corpuscles of the test animals. Pfeiffer states that this necrotizing substance is destroyed by heating to 56, and he claims to have made an antitoxic serum against it. The latter point has been denied by Uhlenhuth and Haendel. They explain the immunization found by Pfeiffer by deviation of complement.

The primary toxic action of eel-serum has been studied thoroughly by Doerr and Raubitscheck. They found that it was destroyed by heating to 60 C., but that another action of the serum was left which produced an allergic condition toward a second injection, so that the property of eel-serum heated to 60 corresponds to that of horse-serum. The primary toxic substance gives rise to an antitoxin, the second substance to an anaphylactic antibody.

The slight primary toxicity of cattle-serum is also due to a thermolabile body. After heating it (Doerr and Russ, Olaf Thomsen), only the second thermostabile body is left.

To exclude this primary action in experiments of allergy or anaphylaxis, one ought always to use serums heated to 56. The work of Pick and Yamanouchi and Heilner on anaphylaxis is not free from objection because they used large quantities of fresh serum in which the thermolabile body may have caused part of the symptoms.

*Group 2.*—Action like that produced by horse-serum in man; serum disease after a certain incubation time. Thus we see that horse-serum in cattle, according to Beclère, Chambon and Menard, causes rashes of an urticarial or measles-like character, and pains in the joints after an incubation time of four days.

*Group 3.*—No certain action after the first injection, but an immediate and severe reaction after a reinjection made after an interval of at least eight days. To this group belong the symptoms which were studied very thoroughly after an injection of horse-serum in rabbits and guinea-pigs.

## HORSE-SERUM IN RABBITS

The first injection of horse-serum causes no definite symptoms, even if very large doses (10 per cent. of the body weight) are given.

The only data which may be explained as symptoms similar to a first serum sickness are given by Lemaire, who states that nearly all rabbits show a loss of weight in the second week after the first injection. It might be that the diminution of complement which Ehrlich and Morgenroth and Moreschi found ten to twelve days after the injection are to be considered in the same light.

The event occurring after reinjection are quite different. Arthus first noted these symptoms, and they are called, therefore, "phenomenon of Arthus." After a subcutaneous reinjection, a local edema occurs which reaches its maximum after twenty-four hours. On repeated injections, more severe changes of the skin are seen, even gangrene. In intravenous injections, very severe general symptoms occur, leading often to death.

Arthus cites the following instance: A rabbit which had been previously treated three times, receives 2 c.c. horse-serum in the auricular vein; after one minute the animal begins to sneeze, becomes anxious and restless, lies on its abdomen, the respiration becomes frequent, loose passages of the bowels occur, then the rabbit turns on its side, throws its head back, moves its extremities, then becomes quiet and the breathing ceases. After a short pause, it breathes again a few times, and finally dies about four minutes after the injection.

Arthus did not consider the interval of time between the injections as very significant, but the repetition of the injections. Von Pirquet and Schick showed that the previous treatment with one injection is sufficient, and that time is the principal factor in the development of allergy. In a series of experiments they showed that even the second injection produces an infiltration, if given after an interval of ten days.

Recently rabbits have often been used to produce an anaphylactic antibody. The results of these experiments will be considered in the next section, as these antibodies have been demonstrated chiefly in guinea-pigs. Friedemann notes that passive anaphylaxis in rabbits is best seen if one injects horse-serum and antibody simultaneously in given proportions with a comparatively small amount of horse-serum. The work of Heilner on rabbits differs so much in its method from the work of other authors, that it is difficult to classify its results. He injected more than 10 per cent. of the body weight and investigated the nitrogen excretion in the urine, without obtaining any very clear results.

## HORSE-SERUM IN GUINEA-PIGS

The difference between the normal and the allergic animal betrays itself in the guinea-pig even more sharply than in the rabbit. Here most severe symptoms and death occur not only after intravenous, but also after subcutaneous injections. Theobald Smith observed that many guinea-pigs which had been used to test diphtheria antitoxin (by injections of a mixture of toxin and antitoxin) died if injected later on with normal horse-serum.

He reported in 1906 in a discussion of a paper of Rosenau's, that he had become interested in the phenomena as long ago as 1902, but without going into an analysis of it. In this discussion he gave a report of about 117 experiments. Of eighteen animals which had been treated previously with mixtures of toxins and antitoxins, thirteen had shown symptoms on reinjections; ten of them died. It was not clear, however, why, of fifty-eight animals not previously treated, nine died also after the same injection of normal horse-serum.

Ehrlich proposed the name of "phenomenon of Theobald Smith" for this form of hypersensitiveness. These observations incited Otto to make a thorough investigation of this subject. Otto injected subcutaneously with 6 c.c. of normal horse-serum, 22 animals, which had been used one to three months before for antitoxin tests. All showed severe symptoms; a few minutes after the injection, the animals became restless, then fell over with symptoms of a severe dyspnea. The respiration became very frequent, the heart's action weak, and half of the animals died about thirty or sixty minutes after the injection in convulsions; the other half slowly revived, and soon became quite normal again. These animals were not in the least hypersensitive against serum of rabbits, goats and cattle. Otto showed later on that diphtheritic toxin alone caused no hypersensitiveness. Simultaneously with Otto, Rosenau and Anderson began their studies, to which I shall have to refer later on very frequently.

The incubation time, after which the allergy can be tested, depends somewhat on the locality of the first injection. Rosenau and Anderson found that the animals which were treated by a cerebral injection of 0.01 c.c. became sensitive after the eighth day, whereas a subcutaneous injection of the same amount created sensitiveness only after two more days. The amount of the first injection has, according to Rosenau and Anderson, no influence on the length of the incubation time, whereas Otto, Lewis, Vaughan and Wheeler, Gay and Southard, believe that after larger doses the sensitiveness occurs later. At the first injection very small doses are sufficient to produce allergy ("sensitizing dose"). According to Rosenau and Anderson, 1 mg. gives allergy with certainty, and in some cases 0.001 mg. (1 micromilligram) was sufficient. For the second injection a somewhat larger amount is necessary to produce symptoms of disease ("toxic dose"), but still 0.1 c.c. is enough to kill a sensitive animal, whereas in a first injection 10 c.c. are borne without any symptoms.

The symptoms after a reinjection of guinea-pigs, the "anaphylactic shock," are by most authors looked on as of central origin, but it is not to be forgotten that the local symptoms are cut off by the rapid death, the event on which general attention has been concentrated. Lewis has taken an interest in those animals which survived the anaphylactic shock. These, after a recovery from the first symptoms, look quite healthy for some hours; then they appear weak, tired, have watery eyes, and after twenty-four hours one finds an intense local redness (after subcutaneous injection), which may extend over the whole thorax and abdomen. Later on an ulcer of long duration may develop. If the animals die in this state, hemorrhagic necroses in the spleen, as well as changes in the blood and other organs, are found.

### CATTLE-SERUM IN GUINEA-PIGS

In the last year Doerr and Russ have reexamined the data published by Otto, Rosenau, Anderson and others, using cattle-serum instead of horse-serum. The possibility that the animals used for the experiments may be descendents of animals which had been used for standardizing diphtheria antitoxin introduces a disadvantage in the work with horse-serum, inasmuch as the results may be influenced to some degree by this relationship. This objection does not hold for cattle-serum, if it is applied after heating to 56, thereby depriving it of its primary action. Doerr and Russ give the first injection subcutaneously over the xyphoid process on the breast. The reinjection, which I call farther on the test, is given intravenously in the right jugular vein.

These authors make the test in the following way: the skin is scraped on the neck parallel to the jugular vein; the vein is laid free, and on both sides clamps are applied. The point of the syringe is then introduced into the vein and the central clamp removed. After a slow injection of the serum the central clamp is again applied, the vein is ligated, and the skin closed with clamps.

The time of incubation for the fully developed allergy is eight to nine days, when for the first injection 0.01 c.c. and for reinjection 0.2 c.c. are used.

All animals tested nine to fourteen days after the first injection died. Of those tested after seven to eight days, only half died. Five or six days after the first injection only slight symptoms of an anaphylactic character were to be observed in the test. In intravenous tests made thirteen days after the first injection, the minimal fatal dose was found to be 0.04 c.c., while 0.01 produced distinct symptoms. The surely sensitizing dose leading to death on reinjection of 0.2 c.c. was 1 mg. One one-thousandth mg. did not sensitize at all, and 0.1 and 0.01 mg. not in all cases. With these minimal amounts the incubation time of allergy is lengthened: After a first injection of 1 mg., the test made after eight days produced a deadly shock, whereas after a sensitizing dose of 0.1 mg., a deadly test was found only after nineteen days, and after a first injection of 0.01 mg. only after twenty-five days. The smallest toxic dose is therefore a thousand times greater than the smallest sensitizing dose. This is a fact which is of great importance in explaining several questions which have been raised as to the difference between the sensitizing and toxic property of the serum.

## SYMPTOMS OF LESSENED SUSCEPTIBILITY—"ANERGY"—"ANTIANAPHYLAXIS"

Whereas Arthus and Wolff-Eisner thought that the sensitiveness increased in intensity with each added injection, von Pirquet and Schick show in several instances that in man a diminution of the degree of sensitiveness can occur. Furthermore, in serum disease hypersensitiveness and immunity cannot be absolutely distinguished. Rosenau and Anderson found that after daily injections of horse-serum, an immunity was produced in guinea-pigs. Otto was the first who directly described the phenomenon which is now known as antianaphylaxis; that is, if a guinea-pig survives the acute shock and is injected again a short time afterward, it shows no more general symptoms. Whereas Besredka and Steinhart considered this state as a definite and lasting immunity, or even as a return to the normal state, Otto and Gay and Southard found that it is only a passing one and lasts longer the larger the doses which have been used in the reinjections. I call this clinical phenomenon of lessening of reactivity "anergy" (lack of reactivity), in contrast to the term "allergy." I apply this name quite generally to the absence of clinical manifestation of reaction; an instance of this anergy is the phenomenon in question, which was called antianaphylaxis by Nicolle (1907), who found that repeated injections during incubation time were not only innocuous, but even immunizing. Besredka called this action of horse-serum *propriété vaccinante,* and tried to prove that it was due to a body different from the sensitizing and the toxic. We shall see later on that it is now absolutely proved that all these actions are produced by the same body.

Rosenau and Anderson tried to lessen the hypersusceptibility by other substances than the allergen (the horse-serum) itself. They used injections of pancreatin, sodium oxalate, pepsin, peptone, sulphate and oxalate of calcium twenty-four hours before the reinjection of horse-serum, but the action of the latter was not lessened. Kraus and Biedl found in dogs that peptone injected previously prevented the allergic reaction. Gay and Southard lessened the effect of the shock by injecting 10 c.c. physiological salt solution in the peritoneum ten minutes before the horse-serum.

It is immaterial whether the "antianaphylactic" injection is given into the brain, in the peritoneum, or subcutaneously (Rosenau and Anderson). If the animals survive the shock at all, which is most probable after a subcutaneous injection, they do not show any general symptoms after a second test made twenty-four hours later.

*Effect of Anesthesia on the Anaphylactic Shock.*—Besredka made the remark that the anaphylactic phenomenon could be avoided completely if the animals were etherized before the second injection. Banghof and Famulener found the same effect after intramuscular injection of chloral hydrate. According to Rosenau and Anderson, this action of anesthesia is only an apparent one. Symptoms which would not lead to death are only masked by the anesthetic. The animals do not show the states of excitement and paralysis, whereas fatal doses are not at all influenced in their action by the narcosis. Kraus and Biedl came to similar conclusions, using dogs in their experiments. They found that the characteristic lowering of the blood-pressure was not prevented by the narcosis.

## THE TOXIC SUBSTANCE

This leads us to the question as to what substances in the serum are the causes of the allergic phenomena. Here we must distinguish (*a*) the sensitizing substance, for which I proposed the name "allergens;" in analogy to Detre's expression "antigens"; (*b*) a substance which acts as a poison after the reinjection (toxic substance); and (*c*) the substance which acts protectively and causes the phenomenon of antianaphylaxis or anergy. It is *a priori* probable that *a, b* and *c* are identical, if one considers not only the symptoms in guinea-pigs, but also the serum disease in man. In the latter instance we have the great advantage that we know the symptoms following a first injection. Although there is some difference between these symptoms and those of a second injection (no edema at the point of injection, no collapse), they have a great clinical similarity with regard to the fever, and especially to the urticarial-like rashes.

Rosenau and Anderson took the trouble to prove the identity between *a* and *b* in guinea-pigs, examining separately the physical and chemical properties of the sensitizing and the toxic substances.

They found that these properties of the horse-serum are not altered by heating to 60 C. for six hours, but are both destroyed by heating to 100 C. for a quarter of an hour. They are not destroyed by drying, by standing for several years, by the addition of different chemical substances (butyric acid, permanganate of potash, formaldehyd, alcohol, hydrogen peroxid, or by diastase, pancreatin, invertin, pepsin, or by atropin, strychnin, caffein, or finally by chloroform, trikresol, or by *x*-rays).

Gay and Southard tried to solve this question in another way. They showed that the serum of allergic guinea-pigs sensitizes other fresh guinea-pigs; it contains therefore the sensitizing substance. Then they tried whether the same serum acts in a toxic way on other already allergic guinea-pigs. This not being the case, they came to the conclusion that the toxic and the sensitizing qualities were different. A thorough study of this question has lately been made by Doerr and Russ, who confirm absolutely the findings of Rosenau and Anderson. They state (1) that the sensitizing, toxic and antianaphylactic properties of the serum act quite identically on being heated. All these properties are destroyed when the serum was exposed to a temperature between 70 and 80 C. for an hour.

Besredka claimed to have separated the two substances by heating. The toxic substance, he says, is partially destroyed at 56 C., and completely at 100 C., whereas he had "the impression that the sensitizing property is even a more intense one if the serum was heated above 100." Kraus confirmed Besredka's statements. The findings of Besredka and Kraus are probably due to the fact that drops of serum, which are left on the upper part of the test-tube, do not get heated as well as the serum at the bottom of the tube. On pouring out the substance from the test-tube, these drops mix with the heated part. Such a minimal amount is enough to act as a sensitizer, but too small to produce toxic effects (Doerr and Russ).

Wells thinks that heating does not directly destroy the anaphylactic substances, but inhibits their action only in making insoluble the albuminous substances in which the active bodies are contained. Rosenau and Anderson confirmed this hypothesis: they heated dry horse-serum and dissolved it afterward. In this way heating to 130 or 170 C. had no influence on the sensitizing property, or on the toxicity of the serum.

Doerr and Russ say (2) that in fractional precipitation with ammonium sulphate, the sensitizing and toxic properties are both contained in the globulin fraction of the serum. The albumin fraction is ineffective.

These results contradict the opposing views of Gay and Adler, who claimed to have found a difference between these substances by fractional precipitation. Sleeswijk dialyzed the serum against water. The sensitizing property was retained, while the toxic was diminished. But he explains these results by the dilution of the serum. It must be remembered that about a thousand times more serum is required to elicit the toxic effect than to produce the hypersensitiveness.

### SPECIFITY OF SERUM ALLERGY

If an animal be treated with a given allergen, its organism acquires an allergic condition directed only against the allergen used. Using a somewhat different substance for reinjection, the allergic reaction does not appear. Arthus stated that horse-serum produces hypersensitiveness only to horse-serum, cow's milk to cow's milk, so that animals treated with the one do not react to a later injection of the other. Von Pirquet and Schick pointed out the difference existing in this direction between horse and pig-serum. These conditions have been studied extensively by Rosenau and Anderson. Guinea-pigs prepared with horse-serum do not react against other albuminous bodies, such as egg albumin or milk, and on the contrary, guinea-pigs which are prepared with these substances do not react when tested with horse-serum. Just as in the case of the precipitin reaction, the specificity to the blood serum is not absolute. Animals treated with the serum of one species will react not only on a reinjection with the serum used previously, but with that of a number of an allied species, although less intensely. The reinjection with the serum of a number of a remote species is not followed by any symptoms.

In contradiction to the statements of Gay and Southard that the anaphylactic reaction is not strictly specific, Rosenau and Anderson have lately demonstrated again sharp differences between egg albumin, horse-serum and cow's milk. Uhlenhuth has proved that the precipitin reaction called forth by injections of organ extracts like those of liver, lungs, spleen, etc., is not specific for the organs used, but for all the organ extracts as well as the serum of the species. Thus, for instance, the liver of a dog does not produce a precipitin for the liver of the horse, but for every organ of the dog. There seems to be only one exception, that is the lens of the eye. The extract of lenses forms a precipitin which does not react with other organs of the species from which the lens is taken, but with the extract of lenses of any other species. In analogy, Kraus, Doerr and Sohma found, that the anaphylactic reaction of the lens extract is not specific for the species but for the lens organ.

Bornstein fed rabbits with lenses of cattle. He found that most of the animals died after continued daily feeding with this substance for several weeks. The relation of these experiments to anaphylaxis is not clear.

Ranzi tried to use the anaphylactic reaction for the differential diagnosis of malignant tumors, but it was shown that these tumors again produced no specificity depending on their kind, but depending only on the species of animals from which they were taken.

Levaditi and Laijchmann proposed the question whether the sensitizing substance is absorbed by the stroma of cells, and found that this is the case with red blood corpuscles, somewhat less with white corpuscles and brain cells. Very interesting experiments in this direction have been made lately by Sleeswijk.

Gay and Southard have found that the injection of the serum of animals anaphylactic against horse-serum, produces again anaphylaxis when injected into a second generation. As I think that this latter is to be considered rather as an active anaphylaxis due to sensitizing with a very small amount of horse-serum circulating in the allergic animals, I have not mentioned these results in the chapter on passive anaphylaxis. If it were a passive anaphylaxis, it ought to appear at least the next day and not only after a fortnight. This view is confirmed by further experiments of Gay and Southard, that such an injection had no effect when made with the serum of the second generation. The amount of sensitizing substance in the second generation is apparently too small to cause hypersensitiveness again. It might have been expected that a passive anaphylaxis would be transmissible also from a second generation.

The same criticism must be applied to the views of Pick and Yamanouchi, who think that the serum of allergic animals acquires a new property of allergy different from the allergen of the horse-serum. There is no reason for such a hypothesis, since the result can be explained very well on a simpler supposition.

Not all albuminous bodies are capable of acting as allergens. Peptone acts only very weakly, and further products of digestion such as leucin and tyrosin not at all. I shall have to return to these facts in the last chapter. Rosenau and Anderson propose to use the anaphylactic properties as a method of distinguishing higher and lower albuminous substances.

## TRANSMISSION OF ALLERGY BY SERUM OF ALLERGIC ANIMALS—PASSIVE ANAPHYLAXIS

Von Pirquet and Schick differentiated an immediate from an accelerated reaction. The former depends on the presence of antibodies not identical with the precipitins, but formed in a similar way. These antibodies, when brought in contact with the allergens of the horse serum in the organism, produce a toxic substance as the result of some unknown biochemical reaction. Von Pirquet and Schick designated these bodies *antikörperartige Reactionsproducte* or antibodies of vital reaction. Later on I proposed the name of ergins for the same substances. By this I understood bodies which are concerned in the production of the altered reactivity of the organism. The term has a purely clinical meaning, and I do not connect with it any definite chemical or biological character. In the case of serum allergy, it has lately been demonstrated by Friedemann, Friedberger, Doerr and Russ, that the antibody in question, the ergin responsible for this part of the phenomenon, is identical with the precipitins. In other processes certainly the altered reactivity depends on other kinds of antibodies. On the basis of the experiments of Babes and Preisich on tuberculosis, von Pirquet and Schick gained the idea that the allergy must be transmissible with the serum of the allergic animal. Their experiments with regard to the transmission of serum allergy did not lead to sharply defined results. In these experiments horse-serum was injected following an injection of the supposed antibody (ergin) or horse-serum combined with this antibody. But when rabbits were injected first with horse-serum and one day later with the serum of an allergic rabbit, an edema occurred on the point of injection. Nicolle, however, in 1906, obtained local edema if he injected first a large quantity of the serum of an allergic rabbit, and twenty-four hours later horse-serum. Otto was the first who produced an anaphylactic shock in animals, such as guinea-pigs, into which he had injected serum of an allergic guinea-pig twenty-four hours previously. He was also the first to study more closely the antibody question. He did not consider the antibody identical with the precipitin, or with the amboceptors, which cause a deviation of complement. The antibody did not suffer by heating to 55 C. and its action was not altered by addition of complement.

According to Rosenau and Anderson, the anaphylactic antibody in guinea-pigs can best be demonstrated by the following experiment: A guinea-pig receives a subcutaneous injection of 0.01 c.c. of horse-serum, and is bled fourteen days afterwards. Ten c.c. of this serum after defibrination and centrifugalization are injected subcutaneously into a new guinea-pig. After forty-eight hours, the latter gets 6 c.c. of horse-serum subcutaneously, or 0.22 c.c. in the brain. Death does not occur frequently, but symptoms of an anaphylactic shock are generally observed.

The anaphylactic antibody appears in the serum at the time when the sensitiveness begins (Rosenau and Anderson). The anaphylactic antibody displays its action not only in animals of the same species, but also in animals of another species. According to Doerr and Russ, this is best seen when rabbits are treated systematically with the foreign serum, and when the serum of these rabbits is then injected in guinea-pigs. These authors worked out a quantitative test of the antibody, and proposed to take as a unit a serum of which 1 gm., injected into the peritoneal cavity of a guinea-pig, makes the latter so sensitive that 0.2 antigen, injected intravenously twenty-four hours later, kills rapidly.

When a mixture of the antibody and the allergen is injected, no immediate symptoms are seen; therefore it is probably necessary for the antibody to unite first with the cells of the organism. In order to display the effect of the antigen, it is then necessary that this union be broken by a disintegration of the cells. When the anaphylactic antibody is injected intravenously, this disintegration takes about four hours; when intraperitoneally, twelve to twenty-four hours.

### TRANSMISSION OF ALLERGY TO THE OFFSPRING

Anderson has shown that the offspring of allergic guinea-pigs present a positive anaphylactic test if treated within the first ten days of life. This allergy depends only on the mother; an allergic state of the father has no influence (Anderson). The offspring of mothers who are in an antianaphylactic state, or in a state of "anergy," are not anergic, but anaphylactic (Gay and Southard). Lewis observed a clinical difference in the anaphylaxis of the offspring when compared with that of grown-up animals. They never show slight symptoms after the test, but either death or nothing at all. This state of passive allergy in the offspring lasts about two months (Otto).

### ACTIVE ALLERGY OF NEWLY BORN ANIMALS

Schlossmann and Moll found that serum disease after injection of diphtheritic serum in nurslings is remarkably rare. Therefore, Moll made a study of the antibody formation in very young animals. Whereas grown-up rabbits always form precipitins, rabbits from four to eight weeks of age hardly ever produce them. Similar findings were made by Schkarin. Moll found furthermore that immune globulins and agglutinins are scarcely formed during this early period of life. In agreement with these findings he was unable to produce a state of anaphylaxis at this time of life with repeated injections of albumin. These results are of great importance, inasmuch as they may throw light on the occurrence of the first symptoms of lues, as well as on the tuberculous infection during the first months of life (Rietschel).

Studying the changes of the blood in connection with the serum disease and serum allergy, Hamburger and Moro were the first (1903) who found that man forms precipitins after the injection of horse-serum. Precipitin was present after the appearance of serum rashes; therefore they suggested a connection between serum exanthema and precipitin formation, without looking on the precipitation itself as a cause of the rash. Francioni, Marfan and Lemaire pleaded for this direct connection, whereas Rosenau and Anderson, Otto and Arthus were not in favor of it. Von Pirquet and Schick found in men no determinable relationship between the appearance of precipitin and serum disease, and in rabbits between precipitin formation and immediate reactivity. They reached, therefore, the conclusion that the production of the substance concerned in bringing about the clinical phenomena—the antibody of the vital reaction—may run parallel with the formation of precipitin, but that the antibody is not identical with the precipitin. Lemaire, in serum disease of man, found precipitin in only about half of the cases. As a rule it appeared one to five days after the beginning of serum symptoms. The most important analogy between allergy and precipitin formation is that the appearance of both is accelerated after reinjection. For the precipitin this has been found by von Dungern and confirmed by Hamburger and von Pirquet and by Lemaire. Rabbits always form precipitin after subcutaneous injection of horse-serum. It appears between the eighth and fourteenth day, or on an average after ten days; after reinjection it appears within three to ten days, or, on an average, in five days.

The relation of precipitin and serum allergy has already been very often discussed. Within the last year much light has been thrown on this relationship. Friedberger, in May, 1909, advanced the theory that all anaphylactic phenomena could be explained by precipitation. Friedemann, in June, 1909, came to similar conclusions in comparing serum allergy with hypersensitiveness against blood. Finally, Doerr and Russ, in July, 1909, brought very strong proofs of the identity of the anaphylactic antibody with the precipitin. In quantitative investigations they found that the amount of the anaphylactic antibody in the serum of rabbits was always parallel to its precipitin content. The most conclusive experiment seems to be that where the serum of a rabbit previously treated with sheep-serum was used, this serum was highly charged with precipitin against sheep-serum. This immune serum was tested with a series of serum of different species, both *in vivo* and *in vitro*. *In vitro* the precipitin reaction was observed. *In vivo* the experiments were arranged so that a guinea-pig was first injected with the immune serum, and after twenty-four hours it received one of the serums to be tested. The severity of the anaphylactic symptoms, as well as the amount of serum necessary to produce these symptoms, depended solely on the source of the serum used for the second injection; that is, on the biological relationship of the serum donors. The power of a given serum to produce anaphylactic symptoms corresponded absolutely with the intensity of the precipitin reaction it gave with the immune serum. A further proof of the identity of allergen with the precipitable substance is the following:

A washed precipitate which therefore contains only precipitin and that part of the other serum which has been precipitated, that is the precipitable substance, has a toxic action. It contains, therefore, allergen. The presence of the allergen in the precipitate can be explained only on the assumption that it is identical with the precipitable substance.

Furthermore, animals which do not form precipitins, like white mice, are equally incapable of forming the anaphylactic antibody.

One phase of our problem has not as yet received a satisfactory explanation. It is not understood why there does not exist a parallelism between active hypersensitiveness and the appearance of antibody in the serum.

## PATHOLOGICAL FINDINGS

Gay and Southard described typical macroscopical and microscopical lesions in animals which died in the acute anaphylactic shock. They found principally hemorrhages: regularly in the mucous membrane of the stomach (thirty-two times in forty-one cases); more rarely in other organs. Miller (with Rosenau and Anderson) found these hemorrhages in only 25 per cent. of the cases. He denies the importance of fatty degeneration of the endothelia of the vessels, which Gay and Southard emphasize. According to Rosenau and Anderson, the dilatation of the small veins and capillaries, which is found more regularly in hemorrhages, is not pathognomonic, since they occur in other acute toxic cases and conditions of shock.

### CONDITION OF THE LEUKOCYTES

I shall not take into consideration the acute changes which are found in the first hour after a first injection (Hamburger and von Reuss). I consider here those changes which are synchronous with the normal time of serum disease. They were studied by von Pirquet and Schick, and more closely by Bienenfeld. After a slight leukocytosis during the incubation time, mostly between the seventh and ninth days, a leukopenia sets in, which comes to a minimum between the tenth and nineteenth days, and then slowly disappears. This leukopenia is characterized by a decrease in the number of neutrophil granulated polymorphonuclear leukocytes. A large number of transitional forms and large mononuclear cells at the end of the leukopenia, suggest a destruction of leukocytes (Bienenfeld). Lazar found in rabbits a similar leukopenia after an incubation time of several days. Concomitant with an accelerated reaction in men, a very sharp fall of the number of leukocytes was found by von Pirquet and Schick.

### CONDITION OF THE COMPLEMENT

Francioni states that a lack of complement is found in serum disease. This corresponds to the findings of Ehrlich and Morgenroth and Moreschi, who, after the first injections of rabbits with serum, found the complement diminished between the eighth and tenth days. Sleewijk made an exact examination of the alexin content after the anaphylactic shock. He found a very intense but rapidly disappearing decrease of the alexin. Thirty minutes after the injection, the amount of alexin fell to a minimum one; after two hours, however, it is again normal.

### OTHER PHENOMENA

Sleeswijk also proved an intense injury to the red blood corpuscles during the anaphylactic shock; Kraus and Biedl, intense decrease of the blood-pressure and of the coagulation time of the blood. Of this I shall speak later on. Pfeiffer described as an anaphylactic symptom the lowering of the body temperature, which is also mentioned in Vaughan's works. This phenomenon seems to appear only under certain conditions.

### SYMPTOMS AFTER THE INCORPORATION OF OTHER ALBUMINOUS BODIES

The toxin of actinias, which Richet used in the first systematic studies of anaphylaxis, has some relation with blood-serum and belongs probably to the eel-serum group. It acts as a primary poison on dogs in amounts of 1.2 gm. per kilogram, but death occurs only after four to nine days.

After the reinjection, animals die in a far shorter time, say two hours, and after a small amount. Richet states that the anaphylaxis appears only after several days. By extraction he got two bodies: the thalassin and the congestin, the latter being very much more toxic primarily. He thought that it also acted in a manner contrary (anaphylactic) to the action of the first component, to which he attributed a prophylactic influence.

The result of Weichardt and Wolff-Eisner, who tried to obtain Pfeiffer's phenomenon after injection of different cellular material, belong to this group. Wolff-Eisner injected rabbits with the spleen and glands of cattle, and stated that the second or later injection had a fatal effect.

### BLOOD-CORPUSCLES

The therapeutic transfusions of blood in the seventeenth and eighteenth centuries were sometimes followed by urticaria, a phenomenon which must be considered in conjunction with normal serum disease of man.

As early as 1895 Flexner stated that animals often died after several injections of blood. Wolff-Eisner, in 1904, investigated the lysis of blood-corpuscles in the peritoneal cavity of guinea-pigs.

After the first injection the erythrocytes remained quite unchanged from three to four hours. After twelve to eighteen hours polynuclear exudation appeared containing some macrocytes and a small number of phagocytes. This exudate increases slowly, and after sixty-four hours all macrocytes are filled with blood-corpuscles. Hardly any extracellular lysis occurs. If the injection is repeated after five days, the phagocytes begin to appear after an hour and a half, and there is besides an extracellular lysis. If a third injection is performed after ten days, hemolysis begins within fifteen minutes and ends within three hours before the appearance of phagocytes in larger numbers.

Friedemann lately tried the injection of washed blood-corpuscles of cattle in rabbits, and finds that an anaphylactic shock occurs if a second injection is made after the appearance of hemolysins in the serum of the rabbits. Antianaphylaxis could not be produced, but a passive anaphylaxis can easily be demonstrated. It is seen best on a simultaneous injection of blood-corpuscles and antiserum in certain quantitative proportions. The antibody is thermostabile and probably identical with the hemolysin itself.

I have mentioned previously that Rosenau and Anderson tested a great many albuminous bodies, and found that hemoglobin, egg albumin, and extract of peas act analogously to serum. The effect of injections of milk was studied by Arthus, Rosenau and Anderson.

Recently Besredka investigated all anaphylactic phenomena observed after the injection of milk. He used boiled milk, 1 c.c. intraperitoneally as a sensitizing, and 0.25 c.c. injected in the cerebral cavity as an anaphylactic dose. He obtained very curious results with regard to the antianaphylactic substance. He contends that it is conserved after heating to 135 C., when both the other properties, the sensitizing and the toxic, have been destroyed. And this antianaphylactic condition could be produced by giving the milk per rectum, and even per os.

## ALBUMIN OF BACTERIA

The early experiments of Arloing and Courmont and especially of Rist, working with diphtheria bacilli, must be mentioned. Rosenau and Anderson tried the action of extracts of colon bacteria, yeast, etc. and tubercle bacilli. The sensitiveness appears after ten to fourteen days. Vaughan and his pupils also worked in this direction but from a different point of view. By extracting bacteria and albumin, they obtained two substances, one of which showed an immediate toxic action while the other acted only as a sensitizer. Kraus and Doerr tried to use the anaphylactic reaction for an exact differentiation of bacteria. The paradoxical phenomenon and the work contributed by Behring and Knorr with diphtheria and tetanus toxin have already been cited.

Axamit found that after the injection of yeast, rabbits are allergic even after six days; the anaphylactic state is of only short duration and disappears after three to four weeks. The time elapsing before the appearance of the anaphylaxis and the duration of the latter seem to be very short, when we compare these data with those obtained by Rosenau and Anderson, moreover keeping in mind our knowledge about similar processes.

## URTICARIA

We return from our excursion into the field of animal experimentation to human pathology. There is a disease having a great clinical similarity with serum disease, that is, the urticaria which occurs after eating certain kinds of food or after coming into contact with substances against which a so-called idiosyncrasy exists in an individual. Wolff-Eisner was the first who claimed that these processes were to be considered as hypersensitiveness against albumin, and were to be brought into analogy with the animal experiments. We see here the highest susceptibility to minimal amounts of substances innocuous for normal man. Until now the difficulty existed that the analogy between these phenomena and the experiments with serum was incomplete, inasmuch as it was not known whether this sensitiveness was inherited or acquired. In order to construct an analogy, it has to be supposed that the first introduction of the substance under consideration should not cause any toxic symptoms, and the allergy against a second introduction should betray itself only when after the first introduction sufficient time has elapsed corresponding to that required for the formation time of antibody.

*Satinwood Dermatitis.*—This supposition has been realized thus far in one form of idiosyncrasy, the satinwood dermatitis. Wechselmann gives the history of a carpenter who felt an itching in his lower arms eight days after beginning to work on satinwood. Fourteen days after the first work, suddenly severe pains in the lower arm set in with an erysipelas-like reddening and swelling of the lower arm and of the face and neck, with spots of moist eczema. Two other workmen became ill ten to fourteen days after their first contact with satinwood. As the work had been continued daily, it is not quite clear whether the symptoms are to be considered as analogous to those of normal serum disease, caused by first contact, or as an anaphylactic reaction caused by the last incorporation. The latter explanation is more probable, because from that time minimal amounts of satinwood acted immediately. Wechselmann made the test by rubbing the cheek with the dust of satinwood. Two hours afterward a reddening appeared; after two more hours, moist dermatitis. The hypersensitiveness against primroses also appears after an incubation time of ten to seventeen days (Hirth, Priza and Nestler, cited by Wechselmann).

*Idiosyncrasy Against Egg Albumin.*—In this an incubation time after the first incorporation has not yet been proved, but here we have exact descriptions of the immediate reaction. Landmann gave to a man, who knew his great idiosyncrasy against egg albumin, a very small amount of it, about the size of a pea, on the point of the tongue. After fifteen seconds the man felt a burning, then appeared a swelling of the tongue and an intense edema of the palate and the throat; later on saliva began to flow, the eyes became watery, and there was a burning in the Eustachian tubes and vomiting. Fifty minutes after the test, the first loose movement took place. Within some hours the patients' bowels moved twelve times, an intense weakness made itself manifest but gradual recovery set in after eight hours; the attack then was completely over. Landmann tried also the application on the skin. After ten minutes he saw a urticaria-like erythema. In this patient, then a man of 35, a bad result had been noted when he was a year old, after taking soup and egg. In his ninth year the influence of egg albumin on his skin had been noted first.

Here we see reactions of skin and mucous membrane occuring after very much smaller doses than those producing the serum disease in animals. Similar small amounts we find sufficient to produce reactions in hay fever and in tuberculosis.

*Buckwheat Poisoning (Phagopyrismus).*—In this H. L. Smith was able to show a typical cutaneous reaction with buckwheat flour. The patient was a man aged 45. The first attack was noted at the age of 9 years, when after eating buckwheat cakes, he suffered with a severe urticaria and nausea. Since that time his sensitiveness to buckwheat reached such a degree that he could detect the adulteration of pepper and other spices with buckwheat by his reaction. On W. S. Thayer's advice, the patient was vaccinated with buckwheat. At the same time a vaccination with wheat flour was made, and three non-susceptible persons were vaccinated with both kinds of flour. In this manner the specificity of the patient's reaction to buckwheat flour was shown.

Within fifteen minutes after the vaccination, the patient complained of a tired feeling in his chest and of nausea. He began to cough,, asthmatic sounds were heard, and there was a rapid pulse which soon became intermittent. A suffusion of the conjunctiva was also noticed, together with an erythema mostly on the upper part of the body, intense pruritus, a slight swelling of the face, hands and fingers, giddiness, restlessness, and unsteadiness of gait. At the point of vaccination there was a urticarial wheal the size and shape of a half-dollar piece.

The most important problem awaiting its solution with regard to the urticaria is the determination of the incubation time of the first attack, and furthermore the elucidation of the different allergic phenomena coupled with subsequent attacks. In this connection the observations recorded by Bruck are of great interest. A man reacted with an urticaria, each time after eating pork, betraying in this manner an idiosyncrasy against this meat. Bruck was able to demonstrate the presence of an anaphylactic antibody to pig-serum in the patient's blood during such an attack. The blood of the patient was obtained by puncture of a vein, allowed to coagulate and 10 c.c. of the serum were injected subcutaneously in guinea-pigs. Twenty-four hours later 5 c.c. pig-serum heated to 56 C. were injected. The animals showed a typical shock. Other guinea-pigs first treated with normal human serum did not react.

*Insect-Poisoning.*—It is a well-known fact that the reaction of different individuals to the sting of bees and wasps varies within very wide limits. We here have a range between immunity and all degrees of hypersensibility, The reaction to the bites of fleas and mosquitoes shows the same width of scope. No efforts have been made, thus far, to make these every-day observations the subject of exact investigations, and to consider these phenomena in analogy with the known allergic reactions.

*Eclampsia.*—Rosenau and Anderson advanced the theory that the toxemias of pregnancy might be due to hypersensitiveness against soluble protein substances deriving their origin from the fetus or the placenta. Weichardt in 1901 had already tried to explain these toxemias on the basis of "cytolytic antibodies." Rosenau and Anderson found that guinea-pigs could be sensitized by extracts of placenta of their own species when the placenta was autolyzed. The theory of Rosenau and Anderson would gain much in strength if it could be shown that the injection of placental elements in the skin of eclamptic women gives rise to a local reaction, or that the serum of the patients yields a precipitate when brought in contact with placental extracts.

## HAY-FEVER

Individuals subject to hay-fever show a uniform series of symptoms at certain definite seasons, either in early summer or in autumn. These symptoms are a reddening and swelling and watering of the eyes, sneezing, a sore feeling of the throat and larynx, and asthmatic troubles. Elliotson in 1831 was the first to show that the cause of this disease was to be sought in certain kinds of pollen, and his observations were confirmed by Blackley and Dunbar. In this connection it is of special interest that we are able to produce this disease at will and at any time, even in winter, by exposing individuals subject to hay-fever to a small amount of pollen, while normal individuals do not react in the least under the same conditions. We owe the study of this reaction as a phenomenon of hypersusceptibility to Wolff-Eisner, whose monograph I have followed mainly in the presentation of this subject.

The pollen test is usually made in the following manner: One centigram of pollen is taken up in 5 c.c. physiological salt solution. Two drops of this solution are applied to the conjunctiva. Normal individuals feel at the most a slight itching; subjects of hay-fever react with its typical symptoms. A few seconds after the instillation, an itching is felt in the eye, particularly on the plica. After the lapse of a few minutes, the conjunctiva becomes injected and this injection rapidly advances to a chemosis. The nasal mucous membrane swells, the patient begins to sneeze and finally asthmatic symptoms supervene. The analogy of this reaction to serum disease and to hypersensitiveness to tuberculin is strengthened by the important fact that the administration of pollen through other channels leads also to inflammatory symptoms. Dunbar experimented with subcutaneous injections.

One minute after the injection the patient became giddy; fifteen minutes later he began to sneeze; and after two minutes a cough, reminding one of whooping-cough, started. This cough lasted very long. At the same time a discharge from the nose was noted, with a swelling of the nasal passages. The conjunctiva became chemotic, the face swollen and cyanotic. The mucous membrane of the larynx participated in the inflammation, accompanied by an inspiratory stridor. On the point of injection hives made their appearance. The symptoms lasted nearly twenty-four hours. The injection in normal individuals was not followed by ill results.

The conjunctival reaction is elicited on an average after an instillation with a 1 per cent. solution of pollen (Wolff-Eisner), but in a subject of high sensitiveness even 1/40 of a milligram is sufficient to produce symptoms (Luebbert).

## VACCINIA AND SMALLPOX

Of all infectious diseases, cowpox is best fitted for exact clinical and experimental studies. The first vaccination in healthy children shows an extremely constant symptom-complex. Some minutes after the vaccination, a traumatic reaction, in the form of a very slight redness, appears, which lasts for about one day, and leaves a small scab surrounded with normal skin. On the third or fourth day a small red papule appears, which indicates the beginning of the specific reaction. Between the fourth and the sixth days, the middle portion of the papule becomes more elevated ("papilla" formation), the outer part becomes flat, and forms a small red circle then the "aula" around the papilla. From now on, the papilla increases in size quite regularly, about 1 mm. a day, and the solid papule is transformed into a blister. The aula remains of the same width, and is protruded only by the extension of the papilla.

Between the eighth and the eleventh days the aula increases to a large, slightly elevated inflammatory plaque, the "area." The papilla ceases to grow and becomes yellow. Between the eleventh and the fifteenth days the area reaches its highest development and then disappears slowly, whereas the papilla dries and a large scab falls off, leaving a scar. During the time of the area formation general symptoms appear in association with this local reddening. The special features are fever and leukopenia. On revaccination, characteristic changes of reactivity are seen. If daily vaccinations be made for a fortnight, the allergy evinces itself most distinctly. Here it becomes necessary to regard separately the growth of the papilla and the formation of the area. The papillæ of the later vaccination appear in order corresponding to the day of inoculation, and are not much influenced by one another. The development of the area behaves quite differently. The most striking feature of it is that this inflammation appears on all the vaccination points simultaneously. Although the vaccinations were made on successive days, the area develops around all the vaccination points at the same time, that is, at the time when its development is due on the first vaccination points. From now on the papillæ also of the later vaccinations stop growing as does the papilla of the first vaccination. In those vaccinations which have been made from this time on, the state of papilla formation is no longer reached. Another type of reaction occurs, "early reaction." In this reaction a papula is formed, reaching its maximal development in twenty-four hours and from then on gradually disappearing. Whenever the vaccination is repeated later this formation of a papula takes place. If, however, several months or years have elapsed after a first vaccination, on repeating it, this type of very early reaction is replaced by another. Here the reaction occurs somewhat later, within the second day, reaching its maximum on the third or fourth day ("torpid early reaction"). The longer the interval of time between the first and second vaccination, the more frequently more intense reactions are seen going on, perhaps, to the formation of papilla and area. Nevertheless these reactions still show some difference from a first vaccination, inasmuch as the area develops sooner and therefore the growth of the papilla is interrupted at an earlier stage ("accelerated reaction"). The area generally does not reach the size of that of a first vaccination; only exceptionally it shows very large dimensions (hyperergical accelerated reaction). As in serum disease, the change in the reactivity, that is, the allergy, expresses itself in the intensity of the reaction, or quantitatively, in the kind of lesions produced, or qualitatively and in its time relations.

*Comparison of Time.*—Comparing the time at which the individual reacts on revaccination with that of a first vaccination, there are the "early," and the "accelerated" reaction.

*Qualitative Comparison.*—After a first vaccination, the reaction progresses to the differentiation of papilla and area, the "early" reaction stops with the formation of a papula.

*Quantitative Comparison.*—Comparing the sum total of the events of a first vaccination with those of revaccination, there exists a hypersensitiveness the first time vaccinated, with the extensive local inflammation, fever and other general symptoms. The revaccinated overcomes the whole process with a very slight local reaction a few millimeters in size; but observing the reaction on the day following the vaccination, it appears that the revaccinated is hypersensitive because at this time the first vaccinated does not show any reaction, while the revaccinated responds with a local inflammatory process. This hypersensitiveness becomes very prominent when it is increased as follows: Repeating the vaccination very frequently on the skin of my lower arm, I finally became hypersensitive to such a degree that within twelve hours a papule of 9 mm. in diameter developed, a size which after a first vaccination is not reached before the seventh day.

*Hyperergic Early Reaction.*—This type of early reaction concerns an absolutely local condition, and here no such influence is noted as that which a first vaccination has on subsequent vaccinations. Each point of vaccination runs an independent course of its own. The size of the early reaction depends quantitatively on the amount of vaccinia used. With fresh undiluted lymph, early reactions to 30 mm. in diameter were obtained with formation of vesicles. With successive dilutions of the lymph, the size of the reactions decreases, and with a concentration of 1 to 500 the threshold limit is reached. The results obtained on first vaccination are quite different. Here the amount of vaccine does not influence the size of the reaction. Using a large amount of vaccine, the area appears earlier, as had been pointed out by Nourney, a fact which I confirmed by exact experiments. Diluting the lymph, the appearance of the area could be postponed three days, while the diameter of the local lesions was not influenced. There exists a peculiar, thus far unexplained, phenomenon. If an individual is vaccinated for the first time simultaneously with undiluted and diluted lymph, the reactions of the vaccinations made with diluted lymph develop just as fast as those made with undiluted lymph and progress exactly like them. The latter must, therefore, have a stimulating effect on the former.

The allergy in smallpox is completely analogous with that in vaccinia. Here also a typical early reaction appears in frequent revariolation (experiences of John Mudge); we see the accelerated reaction in the so-called "local pustule formation." A new element without analogue in vaccinia is the "varioloid" exanthema, an allergic modification of the smallpox exanthema. The hemorrhagic variola met with in healthy adults having been vaccinated in their early youth, I consider as an analogon to the hyperergic reaction in vaccinia.

*Subcutaneous Injections of Vaccine.*—Knoepfelmacher gave an analysis of the symptoms after subcutaneous injections of vaccine, according to my findings in cutaneous inoculation. After the first injection of an individual, an infiltration and an erythema on the point of injection is noticed between the tenth and the fourteenth days; the erythema (corresponding to the area) disappears after some days. The infiltration (corresponding to the papilla) is slowly absorbed. On daily successive injections of lymph in a first vaccinated child, all reactions appear simultaneously with the reaction of the first injection point. Later injections react within twenty-four hours.

This early reaction is much more marked after an injection than after a cutaneous inoculation, and its extent is dependent on the amount of lymph injected. After an injection of 0.1 gm. of lymph, intense reddening and swelling appear, giving place, with smaller doses down to about 0.01 mg., to a slighter reaction. Such a reaction is also found after an injection of inactive lymph, whether it has been heated up to 70 C., or deprived of its virulence by the action of blood-serum of vaccinated persons. A heated lymph does not give well-defined local symptoms when used in an individual not previously vaccinated. At the same time, however, it establishes an allergy, although not so marked as in vaccination or inoculation with virulent lymph. Cutaneous inoculations made after an injection of heated lymph are followed by an "accelerated reaction." Only exceptionally the allergy is so intense that a cutaneous reinoculation is without effect, and a subcutaneous one leads to an "early reaction."

## GLANDERS

The injection of extracts of the *Bacillus mallei* in animals sick with glanders, produces characteristic local and general symptoms. Helmann and Kalning were the first who realized the diagnostic value of this reaction. High doses of mallein influence also animals free of glanders, but in sick animals a very small dose is sufficient to cause fever. There are to be distinguished:

1. *Temperature Reaction.*—Six to twelve hours after the injection of mallein, a steep ascent of temperature sets in. Besides the fever, and

somewhat corresponding to its height, there are general symptoms of weakness, and anorexia.

*2. Local Reaction.*—After six to ten hours, the subcutaneous tissue shows a swelling sharply defined and hard. On the second day the heat and pain diminish, while the swelling extends to the sides, and the greater part becomes softer and in from three to eight days disappears, leaving no trace.

Wladimiroff in 1905 had expressed the opinion that this edema was specific and a sign of some immunity. "We must consider this enormous accumulation of fluid, found around the inoculated toxin, as a specific means of defence, of which only the infected organism is capable. The result of several of our experiments confirms this idea, for it was found that this fluid neutralizes the toxic action of mallein."

*3. Cutaneous Reaction.*—Vallée, repeating my experiments on animals, extended his investigations with mallein to horses afflicted with glanders. He describes an intense papule formation, setting in eight hours after the vaccination. Later a papilla develops which disappears more quickly than a tuberculin reaction. The cutaneous test with mallein in man is also followed by an intense local reaction. Martel observed it on himself fourteen years after having passed through an attack of glanders. Controls made on healthy persons showed negative results.

*4. Percutaneous Reaction.*—Schnuerer rubbed the shaved skin with a rough cloth and afterwards with mallein. A diffuse and hot swelling appears.

*5. The Conjunctival Reaction.*—This, according to Schnuerer, is very marked. An abundant discharge of pus, an intense swelling of the conjunctiva and the eyelids appears within twelve hours and reaches its maximum in twenty-four hours. Schnuerer recommends to begin the examination with a conjunctival test. When positive, the horses are to be killed. Those reacting negatively are submitted to further tests: subcutaneous injection and agglutination. De Blieck came to similar results. He has further proved that the incorporation of mallein does not cause an allergy in healthy animals, and that horses with glanders do not react with tuberculin.

## ACTINOMYCOSIS

Corresponding to the close clinical connection between actinomycosis and tuberculosis, it is to be expected that cutaneous and subcutaneous application of extracts of actinomyces will bring forth allergic reactions, and that these may be used for diagnostic purposes. Up to the present time we know only of experiments on rabbits, which prove that the symptoms of sickness appear after an incubation time, and that the reinfection produces immediate reaction (Nakayama and Verliac).

### LEPRA

De Beurman and Gougerot made experiments with leprolin of Rost, an extract of lepra bacilli analogous to tuberculin. Its action in leprosy is similar to that of tuberculin in tuberculosis—fever and focal reactions. These authors could not produce cutaneous and conjunctival reaction, probably because the extract was too weak. Leprolin and tuberculin are related; their action does not seem to be strictly specific, so leprolin causes fever in tuberculous people and *vice versa.* It has been known for a long time (Joseph Kaposi) that focal reactions can be produced by tuberculin in leprosy. According to Klingmueller, the histological findings are not identical with those in tuberculous foci.

### SYPHILIS

The course of syphilis indicates that this disease will prove a very interesting field for the study of allergic phenomena. Thus the primary lesion appears after an incubation time of two to three weeks; in the secondary state it manifests itself in periodical waves of different general symptoms; the primary, secondary and tertiary lesions show a qualitative difference. At present, besides the theoretical studies of Detre, the findings of Finger and Landsteiner are the only exact data at our disposal. They state that after a second infection of monkeys with syphilis, the incubation time is abbreviated, and further, that contrary to the general opinion, syphilitics are not immune in every state against repeated infection, but react with local specific phenomena. In tertiary syphilis the reaction after an injection of syphilitic material is sometimes a definite local erythema which reminds us very much of allergic phenomena in serum disease and tuberculosis. Finger and Landsteiner obtained these signs of an immediate allergic reaction after injection of syphilitic tissue which, of course, contained besides a small number of micro-organisms of syphilis, a far greater amount of body fluid which not only diminishes the concentration of the virus, but probably neutralizes it to a certain extent. I personally feel quite sure that it will be possible to make the diagnosis of syphilis by means of cutaneous and subcutaneous inoculation as soon as the syphilis virus can be obtained in pure cultures. This will be necessary in order to prepare extracts like the tuberculin, containing the virus without admixture and in sufficiently concentrated form. Meirowsky tried cutaneous reactions with extracts and filtrates of his cultures of *Spirochæta pallida,* but did not reach definite results. I do not consider this negative result as a final one, particularly because he was unable to produce syphilis in animals with his preparations.

(*To be continued*)

The Archives of Internal Medicine

Vol. VII | MARCH, 1911 | No. 3

# A STUDY OF TWO CASES OF ADAMS-STOKES' SYNDROME WITH HEART-BLOCK

W. S. THAYER, M.D., AND F. W. PEABODY, M.D.
BALTIMORE CAMBRIDGE, MASS.

Despite the numerous observations of recent years on the subject of auriculoventricular dissociation there is much that remains unexplained. Two cases of heart-block, which came under our observation during the past year, have presented features of such unusual interest as to justify special consideration.

## CASE 1

*Adams-Stokes' syndrome; partial and complete auriculoventricular dissociation without essential lengthening of the a-c time; striking relief of certain phases of partial block of atropin; recovery.*

A man, aged 53, consulted one of us on Nov. 28, 1908. His father died at 65 of angina pectoris. In other respects there was nothing of note in the family history. He had been a man of excellent habits, was in active business and had always been well and strong. As a young man he had what was probably typhoid fever. He was married and had had two children. There was no history of venereal disease. He did not drink, but had been a rather heavy smoker (pipe and cigarettes) and had been in the habit of taking very active physical exercise (bicycle riding). For the last two years he had been rather more easily tired than previously. This had not, however, interfered with his work.

*Present Illness.*—Nine days before consulting me he awoke in the morning with a feeling of nausea. Shortly afterward he heard some one call, "Did you fall?" and found that he was on the floor. He realized that he must have fainted. On the following morning, while in the bathroom he again lost consciousness and fell to the floor. Dr. Earnshaw,[1] who was summoned immediately, found that his pulse was exceedingly slow and irregular. The patient was put to bed. The pulse remained slow and irregular. Attempts to move or rise were followed by slight, general convulsive seizures, of which the patient was quite unconscious. Several of these occurred during the day. These were accompanied by sensations of impending death, as if, as the patient expressed it, he "was just going off;" they began with a sinking feeling, as if "something were going." There were frequent attacks of vomiting throughout the day, and the sensations of flushing and sinking lasted for two days. There was at no time any pain. The urine showed a slight trace of albumin. Since that time he has felt a little weak, but reasonably well.

*Physical Examination* (W. S. T.)—This showed a healthy-looking man, of good color. The pupils were equal, responding quickly to light and accommodation. The pulse was 66, the radial just palpable, slightly more so on the left than on the right, probably a little thickened. The rhythm was regular, although, while feeling the pulse off and on for about two minutes, one intermission which,

1. An excellent account of the features of this remarkable case observed by Dr. Earnshaw may be found in Am. Jour. Med. Sc., 1910, 503.

at the time, was regarded as an extrasystole, was felt. The pulse showed the normal respiratory variations; it was accelerated by deep inspiration, slower at the beginning of expiration. Pressure (Janeway): maximum, about 150; minimum, apparently between 110 and 120.

Thorax: Symmetrical; costal angle, about 90. Heart: Point of maximum impulse not visible or distinctly palpable when patient was in the dorsal decubitus. On percussion the dulness extended to a point in the fifth space just outside the mammillary line, about 11 cm. from the median line, to the right, 3.7 cm. from the median line. The first sound was heard loudest at about the point of outermost dulness. The first sound began fairly sharply, and was continued into a blowing systolic murmur of moderate intensity which, however, was lost before the midaxilla. The murmur was a little louder in the aortic area than elsewhere, and the aortic second sound was a little sharper than the pulmonic second. The same systolic souffle was heard rather louder in the xiphisternal notch. In the erect posture the murmur was not audible in the back, and was heard with diminished intensity at the apex, but remained of about the same intensity at the base. Lungs: Resonance and respiration everywhere clear. Abdomen: Natural. Liver: Not distinctly felt, the dulness extending about a finger's breadth below the costal margin in the mammillary line and, in the median line, a little below the xiphoid.

Cardiographic and sphymographic tracings were taken on the same day. They showed the pulse to be regular, at the rate of 63 to the minute. The jugular tracing (Tracing 1) showed a well-marked *a* wave, followed by *c* and *v* waves. The *a-c* time averaged 0.18 second.

*Course of Disease.*—The patient was advised to lead a careful life and to avoid excitement or overexertion. He remained perfectly well up to the last week in December, when there was a recurrence of attacks similar to those from which he had previously suffered. From Dec. 27, 1908, until May 15, 1909, the patient has been under constant observation in Bryn Mawr under the care of Dr. Earnshaw, or under our care at the Johns Hopkins Hospital.

During this time there have been three periods in which he has had attacks of bradycardia, often associated with syncopal attacks or convulsions. In the intervals between these periods the pulse has been for the most part regular and of a normal rate, and the general condition has been in the main satisfactory.

The first recurrence of attacks lasted from December 27 until January 16; these attacks were more severe than those which occurred during the later periods. During sixteen days there were two hundred and three hours in which there was distinct evidence of partial or complete heart-block. The longest individual attack lasted continuously for ninety-six hours. During the second period, which lasted from March 15 to March 29, there were seventeen hours of heart-block on six of the fifteen days. During the third period, from April 11 to 19, there were sixteen hours of block on five of the nine days. A fourth period, lasting from June until August, occurred while the patient was under the care of Dr. Earnshaw of Bryn Mawr, Pa. These have been described by Dr. Earnshaw.[1] Since August the patient remained in good health until the latter part of February, 1910, when, while walking on the street in Philadelphia, he suddenly fell to the ground. There was a momentary loss of consciousness. By the time his physician saw him his pulse was regular and of normal rate. In May the patient again suddenly lost consciousness and for nearly a week the pulse was very slow and irregular and numerous syncopal and convulsive attacks occurred. Since then he has been apparently well.

## GENERAL CHARACTER OF THE ATTACKS

The general characteristics of the attacks were similar. They always began with a sudden fall in the rate of the pulse, often to about 30 beats to the minute. The onset was usually without apparent cause. Sometimes, however, it seemed to follow overexertion or exhaustion. During the attacks the heart's action was usually very irregular, the rate ranging from 10 to 49. Occasionally, during a short attack, the rate was regular at about 30 or 35, but usually there were several beats at more or less regular intervals, shorter or longer, followed by complete cessation of the ventricular contractions, lasting from a few seconds up to as much as twenty-five seconds. Toward the end of the longer pauses the patient often fell into a slight, momentary, partial or general convulsion.

The onset of these attacks was rather characteristic. With the longer pauses in the ventricular contractions the pallor of the lips increased the pupils dilated, the eyes rolled slightly upward, and the face, hands and legs showed clonic twitchings which sometimes became general. This was followed usually by a flush which coincided with the return of the patient's radial pulse. The convulsion ceased and the patient broke into a rather profuse perspiration. At the end of each long pause there occurred usually one or two very forcible heart-beats, followed by a series of much more rapid beats. During these attacks the auricular pulsation was easily visible in the veins of the neck. The rate was usually 100 or above, once as high as 130. The respiration was slow, often as slow as eight or ten to the minute. During the long intermissions in ventricular contractions, there were periods of apnea as long as thirty-five seconds.

The onset of the attack was always noticed by the patient, who complained of "weak, sinking feelings" at the beginning of a pause in ventricular contractions, and always experienced a feeling of well-being when the ventricular contractions returned. Except occasional sensations of blurring or yellow spots before the eyes, subjective symptoms were, for the most part, absent. There was never a distinct aura. During the attacks there was frequent vomiting, and all paroxysms were marked by sweating, which came in successive outbursts with the resumption of pulsations of the ventricles after long pauses. The output of the urine was generally decreased.

There was, almost invariably, a tendency to constipation and flatulence. The end of the attacks came almost always suddenly and without warning, but occasionally the pulse-rate gradually increased up to about 60 or 70.

At the end of each of the three long periods of bradycardia the patient was much exhausted, and from each attack the convalescence was slow. During the convalescence the pulse-rate of the patient usually ranged from 60 to 80, and was regular, except for occasional intermissions. The intermissions were noticed usually between two and three in the morning, and were rarely associated with subjective discomfort; but his nurse, Miss Dewey, who watched him with unusual care, often reported that, for a series of eight or ten beats, there appeared to be a distinct weakening in

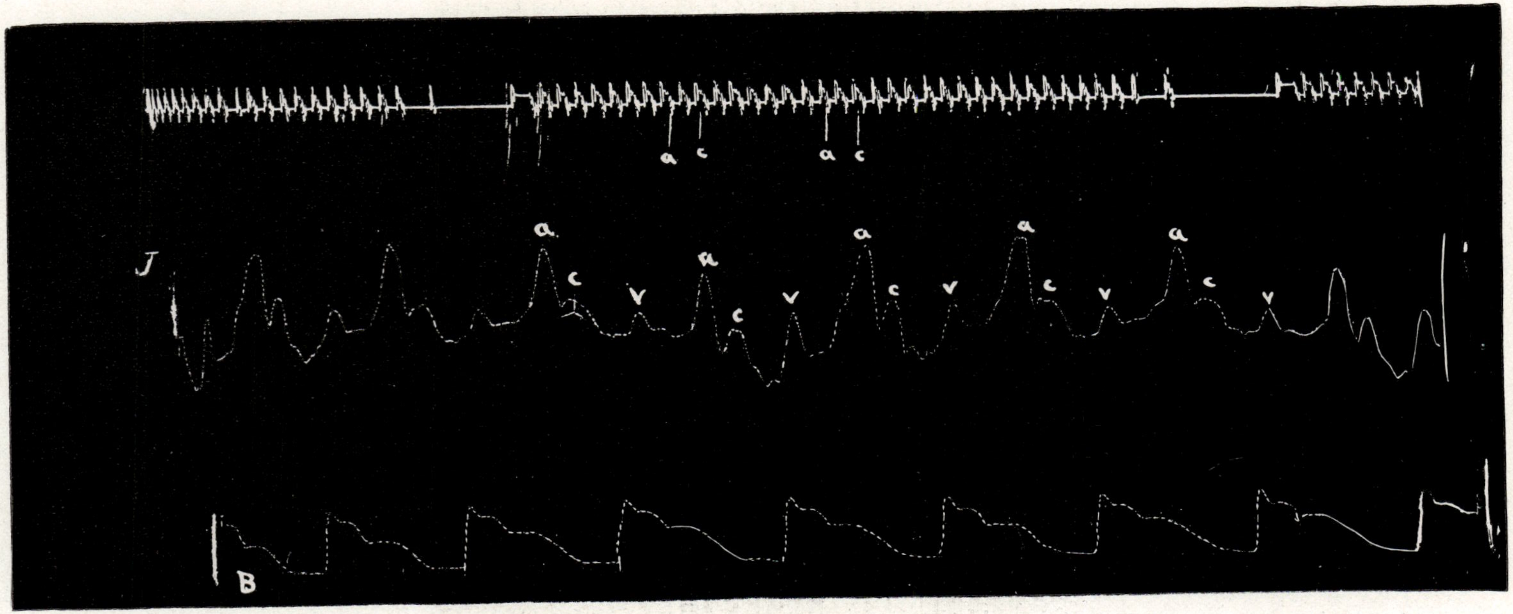


Tracing 1.—Case 1; Nov. 28, 1908. Right jugular and brachial. Normal rhythm; *a-c* time under 0.2 second.

the force of the pulse, and sometimes an apparent intermission. On several occasions one of us (F. W. P.) saw the patient during the night and was able to observe these periods during which the pulse seemed to become peculiarly small, but we were never able to obtain records which permitted us to determine the exact character of the occasional intermission described by the nurse.

### CLINICAL NOTES ON SPECIFIC ATTACKS

The patient was seen by one of us (W. S. T.) on Jan. 2, 1909, in consultation with Drs. Earnshaw, Stengel and Pepper, during one of the severest attacks. The following description was made from notes taken at the bedside.

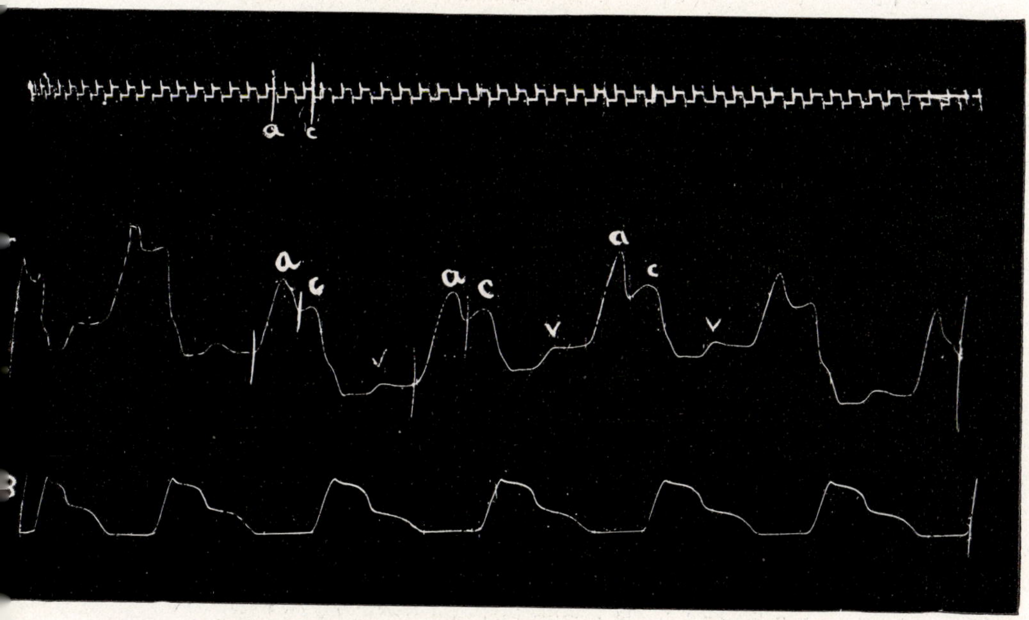


Tracing 2.—Case 1; March 1, 1909. Right jugular and brachial. Normal rhythm; *a-c* time averages 0.2 second.

At that time the patient was lying in bed, exceedingly pale, so pale that at times he looked as if he were actually dead. He appeared to be very weak, spoke but little, and then but a few words at a time. Any effort to speak was, as a rule, followed by a convulsion. As one observed the patient, who lay motionless, with his eyes closed, the pallor seemed to increase until the face was almost absolutely colorless, the respiration ceased and the appearance became truly that of a corpse. The breathing was slow and irregular, somewhat suggestive of the Cheyne-Stokes type; long pauses with occasional deep breaths between. The respiration seemed to have no effect on the radial pulse. At times several short respiratory movements, not particularly deep, followed one another in rather rapid succession. Twenty-three respirations were counted in three minutes. There were at times very long periods of apnea, which were usually associated with the long intermissions between ventricular contractions. The pulse was very irregular, often, indeed usually, occurring in groups of three beats, one or two strong beats followed by one or two feebler beats occurring in rapid succession, as if one, at any rate, of these beats were an extra-systole. There were between 20 and 30 beats to the minute. During four successive minutes there were 28, 25, 28, 23 beats, respectively. After unusually long pauses, sometimes amounting to as much as twenty seconds, during which there was often apnea, the patient turned his head slightly to the right, rolled his eyes upward, became rigid and showed slight convulsive movements as described above. Shortly after the beginning of the convulsive movements there was usually a general flushing, a deep breath and profuse sweating. The flush apparently coincided with the return of the radial pulse. The same flushing, sweating and deep respiration were associated with the return of pulsations after shorter periods of intermission and apnea, periods which had not been followed by convulsive movements. On this date Drs. Stengel and Pepper had taken several tracings of the radial and jugular pulse which showed, apparently, complete heart-block, the jugular pulsating at a rate of about a hundred and the radial showing no evident relation to the jugular beats.

A week later, Jan. 9, 1909, one of us (W. S. T.) saw the patient again in consultation with Dr. Earnshaw, when the following note was made:

"The patient has been on the whole better. The pulse at times has been fairly regular, between 50 and 60 to the minute, and the convulsions have been fewer. He has been able to take more food and there has been no vomiting. The condition to-day is entirely different from that of a week ago. He looks much better. His color is better and the rate of the pulse is now, at times, as high as 40 to the minute; at times, however, only 20 or 30. It occurs in groups of 6 to 10 beats at regular intervals with pauses amounting, sometimes, to as much as fifteen seconds. The auricular pulsations can be seen perfectly well in the neck. They cannot be heard either in the neck or over the heart. They occur regularly, or nearly so, at a rate of from 59 to 60 to the minute. With the hand on the apex impulse of the heart, or on the wrist, and the eye fixed on the jugular in which the *a* and *c* waves are easily distinguishable, it is clear that the ventricular beats nearly always follow the auricular contractions—that is, the impulse would appear to come through the auriculoventricular bundle. It is not an independent ventricular rhythm. The auricular impulses are so clearly defined in the neck that it is possible to see with certainty that during the period of observation, lasting perhaps half an hour, there were scarcely any ventricular beats that were not preceded by an auricular contraction. The only exceptions were occasional apparent extrasystoles which, however, were fewer than they were last week. The pallor developed in the same way as it did a week ago after longer pauses in the ventricular pulse, but it was not so marked. The resumption of the beats, after pauses which commonly amounted to as much as ten or fifteen seconds, were often preceded by a deep inspiration; but deep inspiration was not always followed by ventricular contraction, nor did swallowing affect the condition."

From this time the patient gradually recovered; the pulse intermissions became shorter and less frequent, and on February 2, the patient was removed from Philadelphia to Baltimore without ill effect. Here he remained at the Johns Hopkins Hospital under our observation until May 15.

The treatment consisted of rest, a light general diet, restricted in amount, and general massage with graded resistance movements. The patient was given small doses of atropin gr. 1/250 (0.00025 gm.) and strychin, gr. 1/40 (.0016 gm.) four times a day. Iodid of potassium was begun in doses of gr. x-xv (0.65-1 gm.), but as it was not well borne, it was abandoned. A Wassermann test later gave a negative result. The patient gradually improved and the pulse became regular, except for the periods at night when the nurse described waves of "weakness" of the pulse and occasional intermissions.

On February 20 the patient was allowed to sit up in a chair and take a few steps, the exercise being gradually increased. As a result the pulse rose occasionally to a little above 100.

On February 28 the nurse described one intermission of fifteen seconds during which there were but three or four pulse-beats.

On March 15 the patient suddenly felt rather weak, the face grew pale and the pulse, taken for a whole minute, showed about 29 beats. Immediately thereafter the pulse became regular, 80.

Three days later, March 18, the pulse again fell and became very slow, the rate ranging from 35 to 41, many of the beats coming in pairs with long pauses between. During the long pauses the jugulars could be seen to pulsate three or four times, but no auricular beats were audible. After about two hours, ten minutes after the patient had taken a small amount of whisky, the beats began to come through more often until soon the pulse became about 90, the jugular tracings showing a perfectly normal condition.

On the afternoon of March 20 the pulse suddenly became slow and irregular, 34 to 40, with pauses of three or four seconds, and frequent series of ventricular beats following one another in rapid succession. The jugular pulsations were fairly regular at about 100. Later in the evening the pulse became regular at 96. On the following morning at six there was suddenly a complete pause in the pulse of eight seconds' duration and again at 11 a. m., a period of slight irregularity, intermissions of three or four seconds without a beat and then one, two or sometimes three beats in rapid succession. At times one of us (F. W. P.) was able to hear the contractions of the auricle, the rate of which was clearly determinable by the visible jugular pulsations at about 100. After nearly five hours the pulse suddenly became 93 and then 88, every auricular impulse coming through.

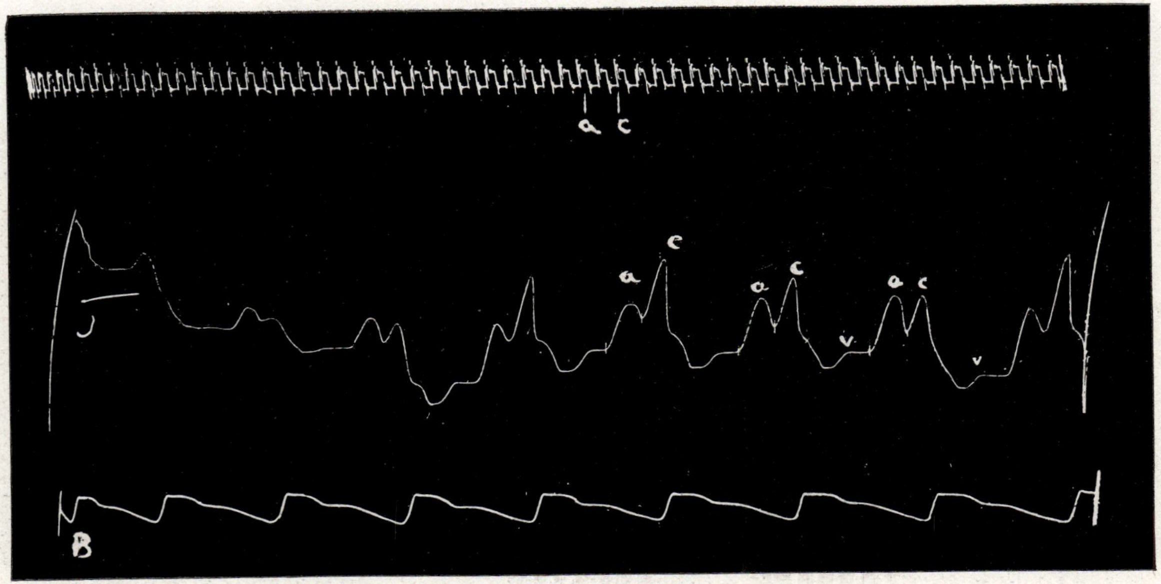


Tracing 3.—Case 1; March 15, 1909. Right jugular and brachial. Normal rhythm; *a-c* time averages 0.19 second.

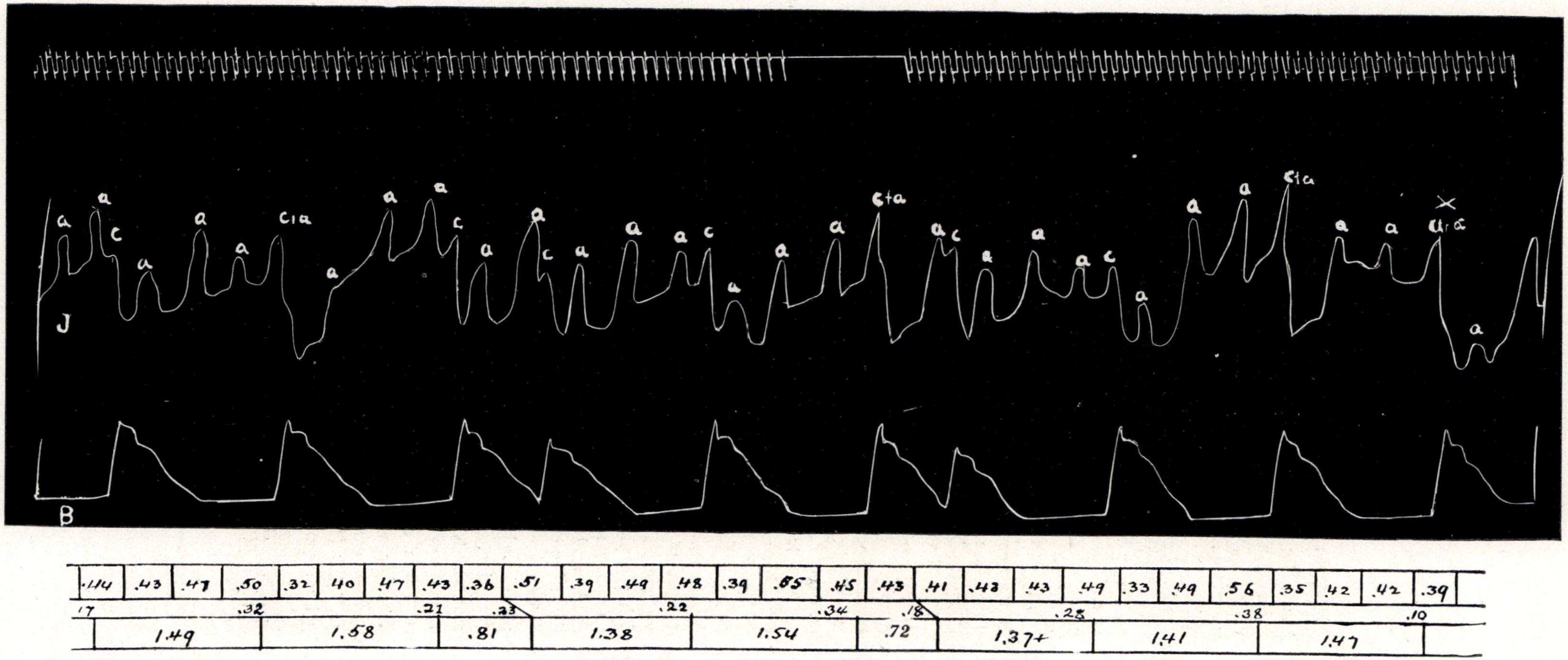

Tracing 4.—Case 1; March 18, 1909. Right jugular and brachial. Partial block.

At 9 a. m. the following morning, March 22, the block set in again. There were several complete pauses of as much as 10 seconds' duration. After a few minutes the pulse became regular again. At 10:10 at night there was a period of block lasting for ten minutes with long pauses of thirteen seconds, and at 11 p. m. a period lasting three hours and a half. The following note was made by Dr. Peabody: "During this period the pulse varied from 10 to 45 and the respirations from 8 to 15. The long pauses between beats were generally of about ten seconds' duration, but not infrequently they were as long as seventeen or even twenty seconds. During the pauses the face became very pale, the respirations became slow or ceased for long periods, perhaps twenty seconds, and at times in the long pauses there was twitching of the hands, feet and muscles of the face. On one occasion the patient had a fairly well-marked convulsion, throwing his hands up over his head. Sometimes he rolled his eyes upward, the pupils became dilated and there was loss of consciousness for a few seconds. Between long intermissions he was clear and comfortable. Early in the attack he vomited several times a dark liquid matter and now and again, in spite of morphin, there was vomiting or retching with an empty stomach. There was no nausea and the vomiting was violent, almost projectile. The abdomen was somewhat distended. After the only well-marked convulsion he said he saw yellow lights. Between the pauses the beats occurred singly, in pairs, in threes, or at times as many as 25 regular beats at a rate of about 80. There were frequent beats which seemed like extrasystoles. The beats were usually of good size and tension, sometimes rather feeble. Between 1 and 2 a. m. the pulse became more regular and the intervals shorter. At 3:20 the pulse suddenly became 88, the patient felt better and fell asleep."

On March 29 the patient was allowed to sit up in a chair. Shortly after this the pulse suddenly became slow, ranging from 30 to 40, and remained so for about fifty minutes, except for about three minutes, during which it was regular and at a rate of 70. The longest intervals during the attacks were twelve seconds. He was given atropin, gr. 1/60 (0.001 gm), hypodermically and ten minutes later the pulse became regular, 80 to the minute. Within an hour after the atropin was given the pulse-rate reached 100.

The patient remained in good condition until April 11, when suddenly, at 9:10 a. m., the pulse fell from 30 to 40, remaining slow for about twenty minutes.

Five days later, April 16, there were several periods during which the pulse was slow with complete pauses of from six to eight seconds, and in the evening, at 10:30, the pulse again fell to from 21 to 49, with pauses of ten, fifteen and eighteen seconds and a nearly regular pulse between. Atropin, gr. 1/60 (0.001 gm.), was given hypodermically at 11:22 p. m. Fourteen minutes later the pulse was 75, every beat coming through. At midnight, twenty-two minutes later, it was 88 with an occasional intermission. At 3:45 a. m. the block returned with a pulse 20 to 35, irregular, with periods of intermission amounting to from fifteen to seventeen seconds. The auricular rate was 96 to 100. Atropin, gr. 1/60 (0.001 gm.), was given hypodermically at 4:18 a. m. At 4:25 the pulse was 21, at 4:30, 74, all beats coming through. At 5:40 a. m. the block returned with pauses of fifteen seconds. Twice there was loss of consciousness. Often a series of 8 to 10 beats came through at a rate of about 80. There was vomiting. Strychnin, gr. 1/60 (0.001 gm.), was given at 7:01 a. m. and was followed almost immediately by stoppage of the block; pulse 80, regular. At 10:45 the pulse was 104.

At 12:35 p. m. the block returned with pauses of eight to twelve seconds; the auricular rate was about 100. Atropin, gr. 1/60 (0.001 gm.), was given at 1:13. The pulse at 1:18 was 32; at 1:23, 31; at 1:28, 27; at 1:32, 64; at 1:34, eleven minutes after administering the atropin, 82, regular, all impulses coming through. During this attack a long series of as many as 18 beats would come through regularly, only to be succeeded, at times, by a pause of about ten seconds. At 6 p. m. the pulse was 84 and the usual respiratory variations were observable in the pulse. At about 9 o'clock, however, the block returned again with pulse of 35 to 76.

At 2:35 the patient was seen by one of us (F. W. P.); he was then fairly comfortable; there were no long pauses between the beats and the pulse was for the most part fairly regular, but slow, averaging about 30 beats to the minute; auricular rate about 100; respiration irregular. Atropin, gr. 1/30 (0.002 gm.), was again given hypodermically at 5:52 a. m., but there was no great change in the pulse, which was 24 at 5:57; 25 at 6:15; 23 at 8:10; 43 at 9. Just after noon the block suddenly stopped and the pulse became regular at 92. During the evening there were again pauses of five or six seconds.

From this time to the day of his discharge, on May 15, the patient remained perfectly well. The nurse reported an occasional momentary intermission in the pulse, but beyond this, nothing. The patient was up and about, walking without discomfort, the recorded pulse ranging from 70 to 98. The blood-pressure during the time spent in the hospital ranged from 140 to 175.

On May 14, examination of the heart showed that the outermost point of dulness to the left was 11.5 cm. from the median line in the fifth space; to the right dulness extended about 4 cm. from the median line. There was no change in the character of the sounds; the pulse was regular, 22 to the quarter.

On May 15 the patient returned to Philadelphia. In June there was another period of block, lasting off and on till the end of July when there were several syncopal and convulsive attacks. After this, with the exception of one brief attack in February, 1910, the patient remained well till the late spring, when he had another severe period of bradycardia with convulsions. From this he recovered, and is now (November, 1910) in apparent good health.

On October 29 the patient consulted one of us (W. S. T.). He was in excellent condition; the pulse was 84; blood-pressure, maximum, 156; cardiac area and sounds as on last note. Tracings taken at this time show a regular pulse with a normal jugular tracing, the *a-c* time averaging 0.2 second, or slightly less.

In May, 1910, I saw Mr. T. again, about a week after a grave attack. He was in bed, but appeared to be in excellent condition. The pulse was regular, of normal rate and there was no change in the character of the heart sounds or in the size of the heart.

## SUMMARY OF CLINICAL OBSERVATIONS

In a man of 53 with rather thickened arteries and a slightly enlarged heart with a rough systolic murmur of maximum intensity at the aortic area, the following manifestations occurred:

1. Syncopal and convulsive seizures associated with bradycardia with intermissions in the ventricular pulse amounting sometimes to nearly or quite half a minute in length, and a marked irregularity in the size and sequence of the beats which occurred often in groups of three or more in rapid succession. The auricular rate was always 100 or above. The longer intermissions in the ventricular pulse were usually associated with long periods of apnea.

2. Similar attacks, usually without convulsions, in which the auricular rate was slower, once as slow as 59, while the ventricular beats occurred in groups of from two or three to ten, always at the same rate, and apparently following the same impulses as the auricular beats, but separated by long intermissions amounting sometimes to as much as fifteen seconds. These groups of beats were frequently ushered in by an appar-

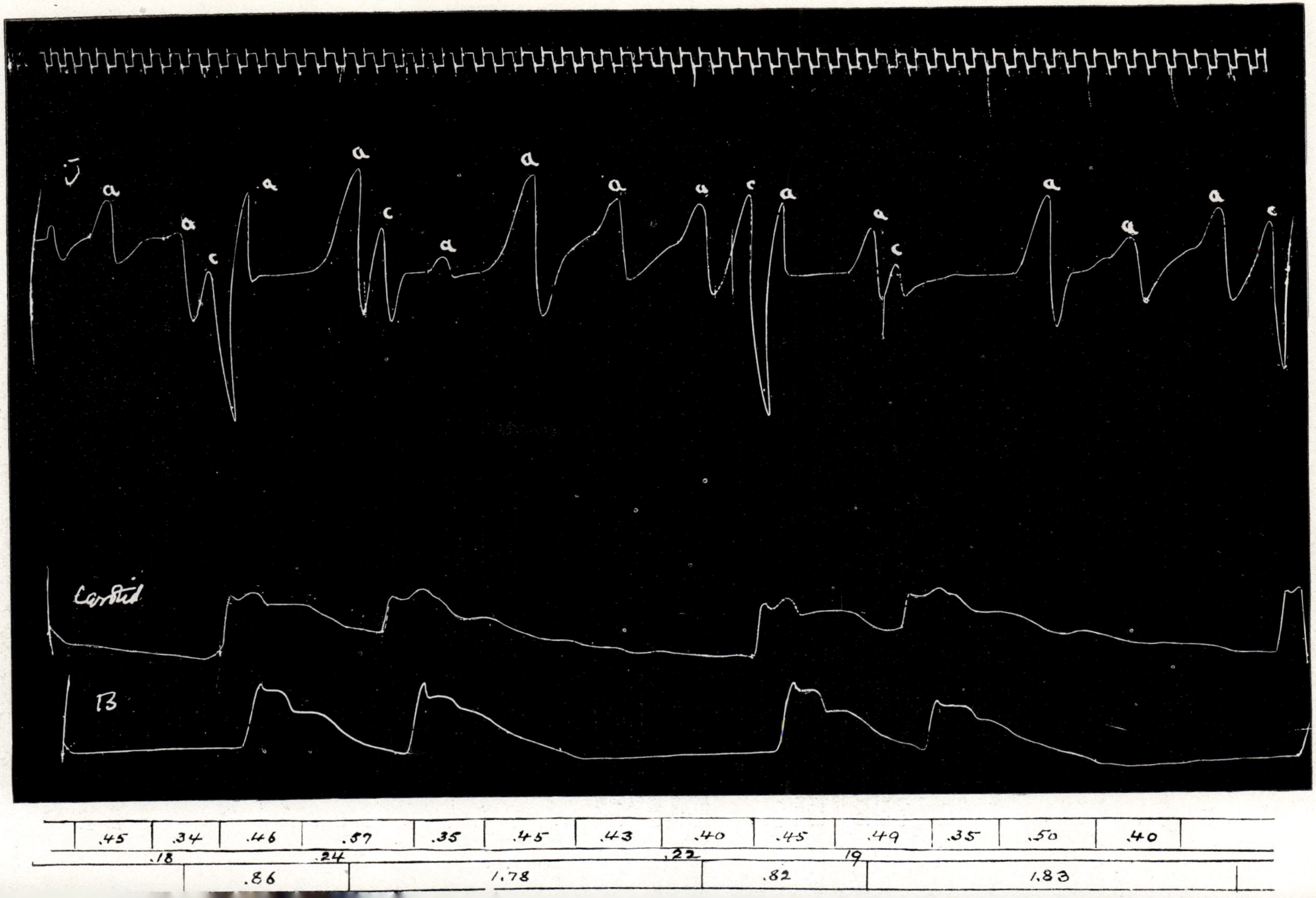
J
a
c
Carotid
B
.45
.34
.46
.57
.35
.45
.43
.40
.45
.49
.35
.50
.40
.18
.24
.22
19
.86
1.78
.82
1.83

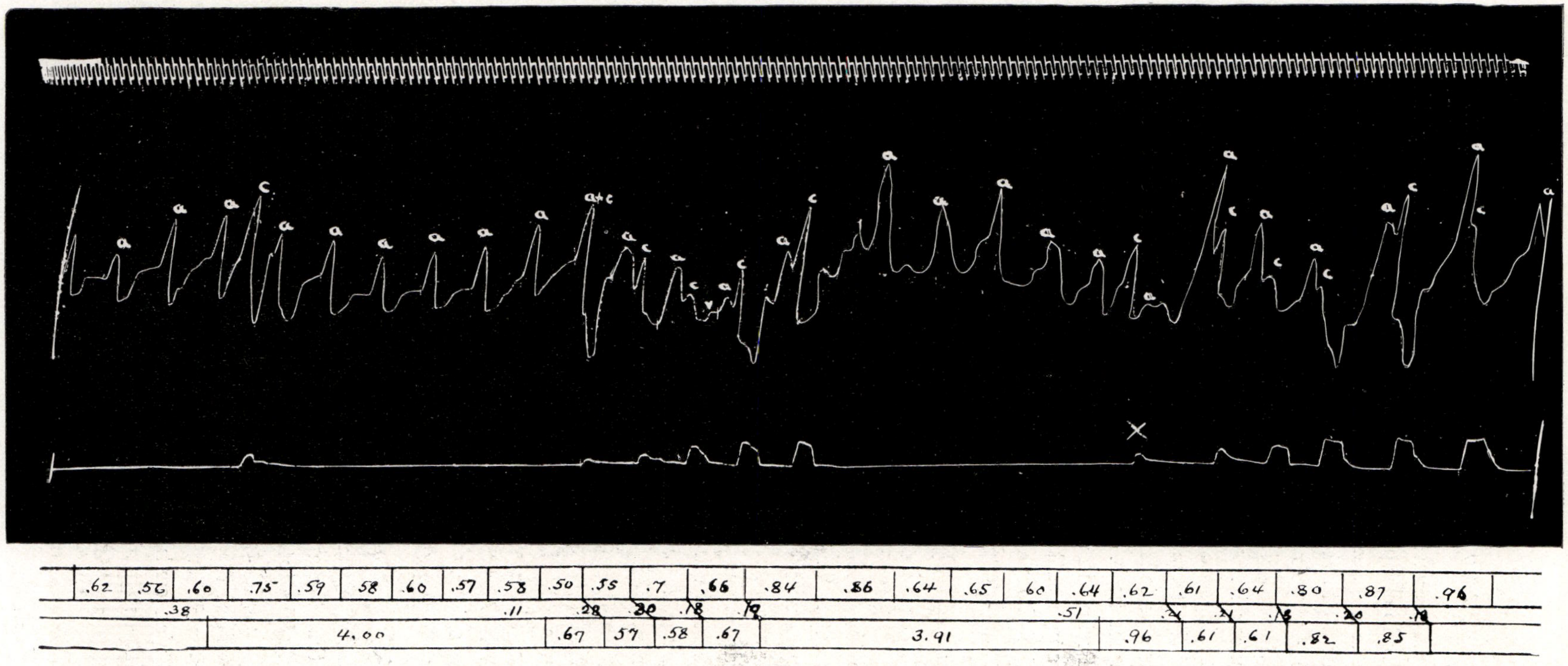

Tracing 6.—Case 1; April 16, 1909. Right jugular and brachial. Partial vagus (?) block. Ventricular contractions in groups with long intermissions.

ently spontaneous ventricular systole. Such attacks yielded in three instances to atropin, gr. 1/60 (0.001 gm.), injected hypodermically.

3. Periods during which there was a fairly regular ventricular rhythm of about 30 to the minute with an auricular rate of 100 to 120, giving one the impression of a complete auriculoventricular dissociation. One of these attacks failed to yield to atropin, gr. 1/30 (0.002 gm.), injected subcutaneously.

4. Periods during which there were intermissions of the ventricular pulse of shorter or longer duration, occurring at varying intervals. During these periods the waves of regular auricular contractions could be seen in the neck.

5. Periods in the intervals between these attacks in which the heart's action appeared to be regular and normal.

While the patient was in the Johns Hopkins Hospital numerous cardiographic and sphygmographic tracings were taken.

## CONSIDERATION OF SPHYGMOGRAPHIC TRACINGS

### *Tracings 1, 2, 3: Normal Rhythm*

Tracing 1, Nov. 28, 1908.—This is one of a number of tracings taken on this date. The record is of the brachial and jugular pulses which are apparently normal in all respects. The *a* wave is rather large, and the *a-c* time averages under 0.2 second. Tracings were taken at a slower rate of the drum and through longer periods of time, but no irregularities or abnormalities were noted.

Tracing 2, March 1.—This tracing was taken during an interval between attacks. The pulse was regular, 70. The jugular and radial tracings show no abnormalities. The *a-c* time, which averages 0.2 second, is occasionally, however, a trifle longer.

Tracing 3, March 15.—This tracing was taken four hours after an attack of dissociation in which the pulse had been irregular at a rate of about 29. At the time the tracing was taken, the rate of the pulse was 80 and regular. The jugular tracing is again normal, and the *a-c* time averages 0.19 second.

### *Tracings 4 and 5, March 18: Partial Block*

Tracing 4 was taken during an attack of block. The jugular curve shows that the auricles are contracting at the rate of about 130 to the minute. The intervals between the time of onset of the auricular beats vary from 0.32 to 0.56 second in length. Much of this discrepancy in the length of the intervals between the beats is due to the fact that it is very often difficult to determine the exact point of onset of the *a* wave. Ventricular contractions, as shown by the brachial curve, come either singly at a regular rhythm or in pairs. The occurrence of these beats in pairs does not follow with regularity. The longer intervals between ventricular beats are from 1.37 seconds to 1.58. The shorter intervals in the two instances on this tracing are, respectively, 0.81 and 0.72 second; that is, not far from one-half the longer intervals. Moreover, the time from the onset of an isolated contraction to the first of a following pair of contractions, or from the second of a pair to the following isolated contraction is from 1.37 to 1.58.

There are thus two distinct ventricular intervals, a long interval of from 1.37 to 1.58 and a short interval of from 0.72 to 0.81 second, the shorter being about one-half the longer interval. With the longer interval the ventricle is contracting at a rate of about 40 to the minute. If the shorter interval be taken as a standard, and the longer pause considered as due, perhaps, to a dropped beat, the ventricular rate is about 75 or 80. It will, however, be noticed on studying the tracing, that this apparent halving of the longer intermissions is only approximate. That the condition is not one of partial block with a regular 3 to 2 or 3 to 1 rhythm is shown by comparison with the jugular curve. There would seem to be little direct relation between the auricular and ventricular rhythms. While the relation of the *a* wave of the auricular contraction to the *c* wave of the ventricular contraction is in many instances such that one might fancy that the impulse had passed through the auriculoventricular bundle in the normal manner or with but slightly prolonged conduction time, at other points the *c* wave and the *a* wave fall at the same time and form one combined elevation on the jugular pulse. In one only of these combined waves is it possible to distinguish the *a* and *c* impulses with certainty. Here, at *x* on the tracing, a small wave superimposed on the summit of the larger elevation appears to correspond to the *c* wave, following the onset of the larger wave by 0.1 second. This apparent coincidence of the auricular and ventricular waves occurs three times in connection with an isolated ventricular contraction, once in connection with the first of a pair of ventricular contractions. In a tracing taken at the same time (Tracing 5), with a somewhat more rapid drum, there appears to be a more definite relation between the auricular and the ventricular contractions. The tracing includes two pairs of beats with the beginning of a third, and in all the *c* wave follows the *a* wave after an interval of 0.18 to 0.28 second. In the shorter ventricular pauses there is one auricular beat not followed by a ventricular impulse, and in the longer pauses three *a* waves without a succeeding *c* wave.

Do these tracings represent a partial auriculoventricular dissociation, or is the relation of the *c* waves to *a* waves only apparent? With short auricular intervals a large number of the ventricular beats must fall at such periods that they are within a normal or but moderately prolonged *a-c* time. Whether such ventricular beats are caused by the same impulses

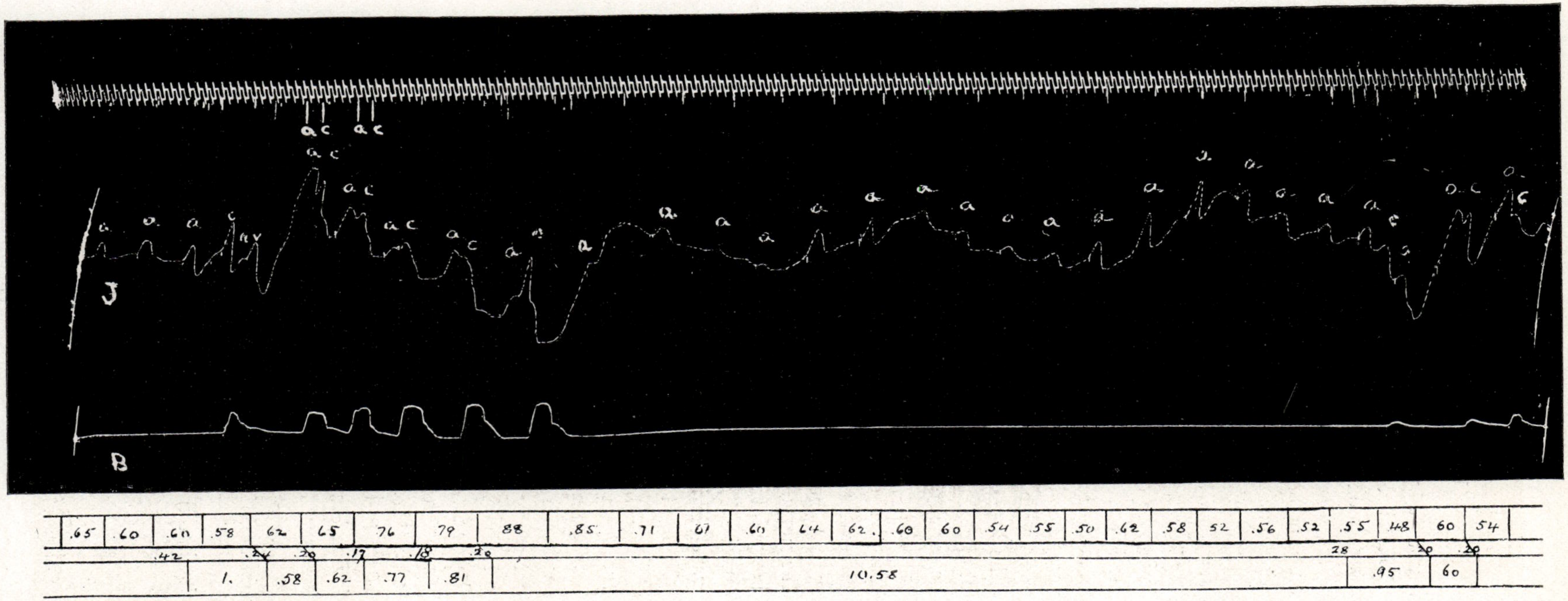


Tracing 7.—Case 1; April 16, 1909, 11:25 p. m. Right jugular and brachial. Partial vagus (?) block, showing an intermission of over ten seconds. Three minutes after the administration of atropin, gr. 1/60 (0.001 gm.).

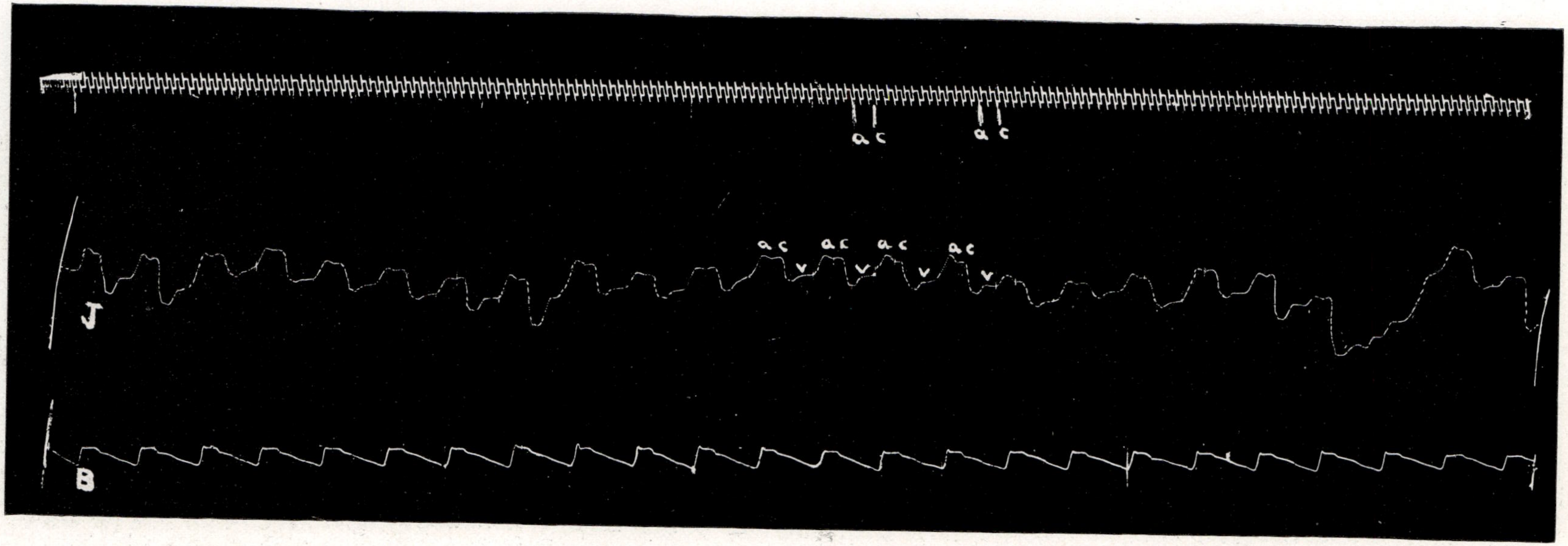


Tracing 8.—Case 1; April 16, 1909, 11:36 p. m. Right jugular and brachial. Normal rhythm. Fourteen minutes after administration of atropin, gr. 1/60 (0.001 gm.), during a period of partial block. The tracing was taken eleven minutes after Tracing 7.

which excite the preceding auricular contractions, or whether they are due to an independent contractility of the ventricle, their relation to the auricular contractions being purely one of chance, is often difficult to determine. Careful study of these two tracings, however, reveals an interesting point. Out of fifteen ventricular contractions three occur almost simultaneously with the auricular impulse, so that the two waves are fused, in one the *c* wave follows but 0.1 + second after the *a* wave, while in the other eleven beats, the *c* waves follow the *a* waves after a period of time varying from 0.17 to 0.28; but this is a period which might well represent in some instances a normal, in others a conduction time which is but slightly lengthened.

Now if, in the four instances in which *a* and *c* waves are practically combined, one compares the probable time of the onset of the *c* wave—which from comparison with the brachial pulse, would seem to represent the beginning of the combined waves—with the preceding *a* waves, we find that the periods of time between the two amount, so far as can be estimated, to 0.32, 0.34 and 0.38, respectively. Might these periods represent prolonged conduction time? It is conceivable, but it would assuredly be remarkable that the conduction should vary from 0.17, a normal period, to 0.38, a greatly lengthened period, in a wholly irregular manner during these fifteen beats. The improbability that these periods represent prolonged conduction time is rendered more evident by another consideration. As a rule, in disease of the bundle of His with partial block, the *a-c* time becomes longer with successive beats and is shorter with the first contraction following a blocked impulse. Here, on the other hand, the contrary is true. The longest *a-c* periods occur after long intervals in the ventricular beats, while the *a-c* interval in connection with the four beats occurring after the short intermissions, where one might have expected a prolonged *a-c* time, amounted to 0.23, 0.18, 0.24 and 0.19, respectively. We are, then, rather inclined to regard these beats with long *a-c* periods as spontaneous ventricular contractions.

Might it be that these tracings represent a total dissociation of auricle and ventricle, an automatic ventricular rhythm? Those beats which appear to be spontaneous ventricular systoles may well be evidence of an attempt on the part of the ventricle to initiate an independent rhythm. The occurrence, however, of so many other beats, each one of which follows an auricular systole after an interval of a length not far from the normal, would suggest that the stimuli giving rise to some of the ventricular contractions on these tracings, passed through the auriculoventricular bundle; that the condition, then, was one of partial dissociation.

Might one not fancy that these long intermissions are dependent on a lack of irritability of the ventricle, rather than on the blocking of stimuli? The first contraction of a pair, occurring either spontaneously or after a stimulus reaching it in the normal way, might conceivably be the result of a summation of stimuli which have individually failed to produce a response. As a result of such a summation of stimuli, spontaneously, or set off as it were, by the last impulse, a vigorous contraction occurs. This contraction, by improving the nourishment of the heart muscle and removing waste products, might render the rested ventricle readier for a time to respond to the subsequent regular stimuli.

*Tracings 6, 7, 8, April 16, 1909: Partial Dissociation Relieved by Atropin*

In Tracing 6 the jugular tracing shows the auricular waves occurring with fair regularity at intervals which average 0.66 seconds in length, giving an auricular rate of 90. The tracing from the brachial artery shows a very different condition from that which was noted in the previous tracings of March 18. The waves of ventricular contraction occur either singly or in series of three or more contractions, the individual beats of the series being in most cases equally spaced. The pauses without ventricular contractions sometimes amount to ten seconds (Tracing 7). After the pause the first beat is small and those succeeding become progressively larger, doubtless owing to the fact that the artery, empty at first, becomes fuller with each contraction. The average length of the intervals between the waves which occur in series on the brachial tracing, is 0.6 of a second, exactly the same as that of the auricular intervals. During these series of beats, then, the ventricles are contracting at the same rate as the auricles and the *a-c* intervals are essentially normal. In the two instances in which the *a-c* time is much longer than the normal, it is probable that the *v* wave from the preceding beat has masked the onset of the following *a* wave. The ventricles are, therefore, during these periods, responding to every impulse causing the auricular contractions. There is one exception to this rule. On all our tracings the interval between the first and second beats of a series is longer than that between the second and third. This is shown in Tracing 6, in which the first intervals are 0.67 and 0.96 second, respectively, and the second intervals, 0.57 and 0.61 second, and on Tracing 7, in which the first intervals are 1 and 0.95, respectively, the second 0.58 and 0.66 in each group. Moreover, the relation of the *c* waves associated with these contractions to the preceding *a* waves is not analogous to the relation between the succeeding *a* and *c* waves. While the *a-c* time of the beats which follow—with the exceptions above mentioned—is of about 0.2 second in each case, the *a-c* intervals of the first beats are 0.11 (time of *c* wave estimated from the brachial tracing) 0.51, 0.42 and 0.28, respectively. It is difficult to comprehend why, when a partial auriculoventricular block is beginning to give way, the *a-c* time of the first impulse

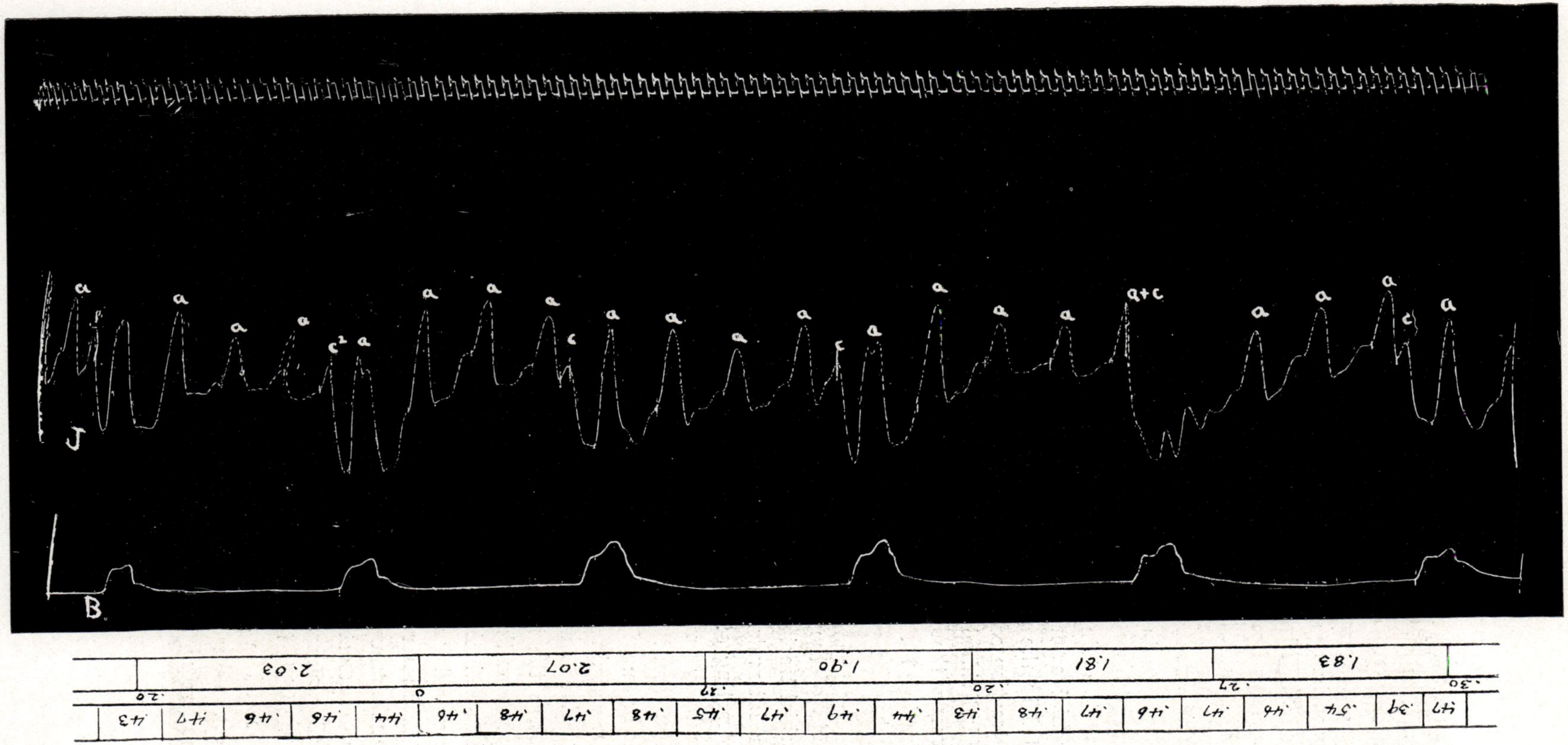


Tracing 9.—Case 1; April 18, 1909. Right jugular and brachial. Total block.

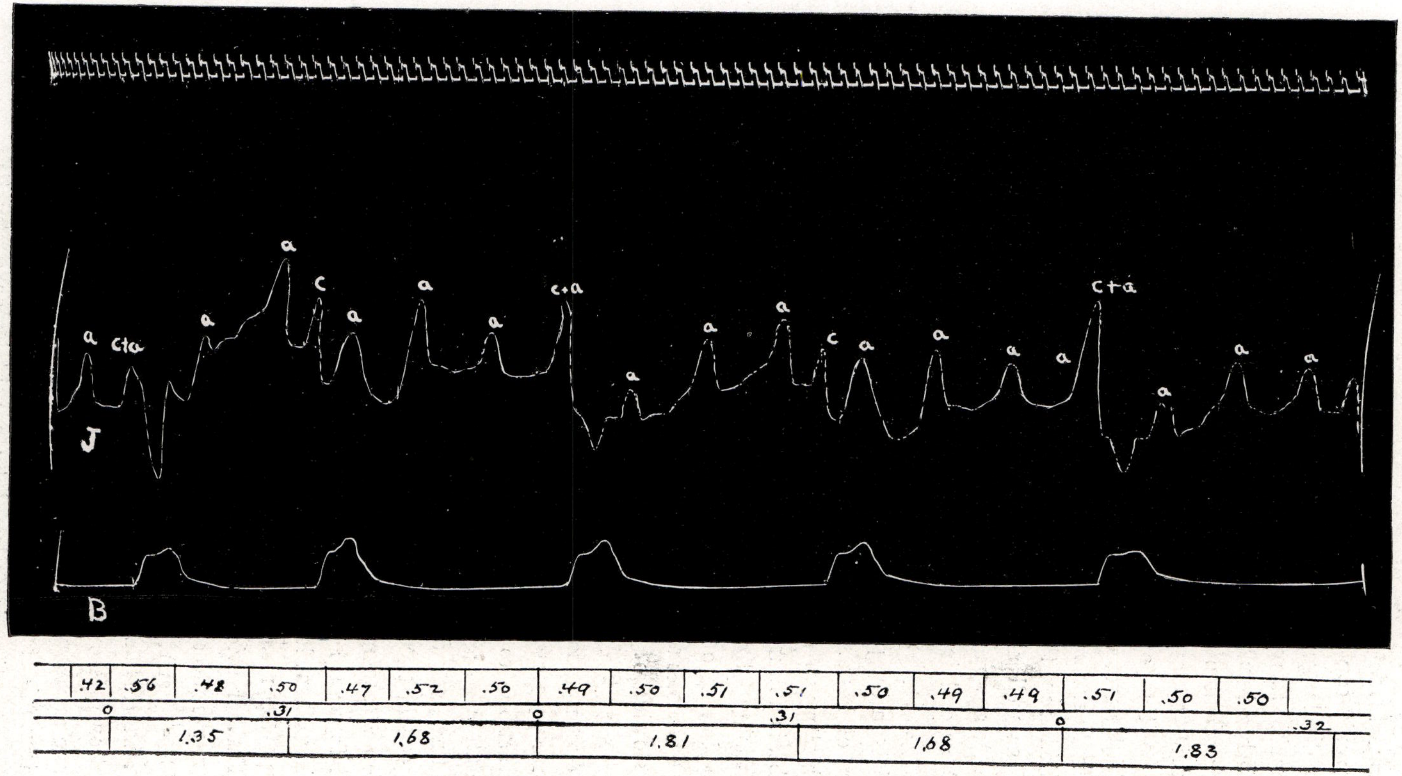


Tracing 10.—Case 1; April 18, 1909. Total block.

to come through should be longer than that with the following beats. One would expect exactly the reverse—a short *a-c* time at first, becoming gradually longer until the beats begin to drop out again. It seems more reasonable to regard these first beats as automatic systoles of a ventricle which has become irritable during the prolonged pause. The first ventricular beat of the first series on Tracing 6 occurs synchronously with an auricular impulse so as to cause a combined wave on the jugular pulse. The position of the *c* wave, calculated from the time of onset of the brachial wave, would make the *a-c* time 0.11 second, too short a period to justify the assumption that the auricular and ventricular contractions resulted from the same stimulus. One is then justified in regarding this beat, as well as the isolated beat which precedes it (*a-c* time = 1.38 second), as spontaneous ventricular systoles.

A second interesting peculiarity of the rhythm of both auricles and ventricles is shown in this and other tracings taken at this period. This consists in the progressive prolongation of the pulse intervals during each series of beats. Thus, in one instance, while the interval between the brachial waves at the beginning of the series is 0.5 second, that between the beats toward the end of the series of ten pulsations is 0.8 second. In Tracing 7 the intervals increase during five beats from .59 to .82. The same slowing of the rate applies to auricles as well as to ventricles; that is, the auricles are apparently subjected to the same influences. Moreover, this slowing of the auricular rate persists for a few beats after the ventricular contractions cease. The *a-c* time remains more or less constant and does not, as might be expected, if the lesion were one of conduction, become progressively prolonged. The relation of the isolated ventricular contractions to the contractions of the auricle cannot be determined absolutely. In some instances they occur at such times that it is possible that they may depend on the impulse which caused the preceding auricular contractions, but at other times they fall so far from a preceding auricular contraction that it would seem more reasonable, as has been said, to regard them as automatic ventricular systoles. A study of the tracings then, leads to the conclusion that the dissociation at this period was partial rather than complete.

Further evidence of this is given by the result of the atropin test. After the first tracings had been taken, atropin sulphate, gr. 1/60 (0.001 + gm.), was given subcutaneously. Three minutes later Tracing 7 was taken. This tracing shows an intermission of over ten seconds' duration. Shortly after the atropin was given the beats at the wrist became more frequent and the pauses became shorter. A tracing taken fourteen minutes after the injection (Tracing 8) shows that every auricular contraction is followed by a ventricular contraction with an *a-c* time of 0.2 second, which is well within normal limits. The heart's rate is 71.

The atropin test which was used by Dehio to distinguish between bradycardia of vagal origin and that dependent on changes in the heart muscle is generally regarded as being the best clinical test of complete organic heart-block. In typical cases of Adams-Stokes syndrome with permanently slow pulse the administration of atropin causes a rise in auricular rate without changing the ventricular rate. In case of partial block in which the dissociation is due in part, at least, to vagus influences, atropin usually accelerates the auricles and puts an end to the dissociation. It is noteworthy that while in this instance the dissociation was temporarily relieved, yet the rate of the heart when every impulse was coming through was only 70-80, somewhat slower than the previous rate of the auricles. This is extraordinary and, so far as we know, a unique feature of the case. And on the two other occasions on which the administration of atropin was followed by a disappearance of a partial dissociation, the same phenomenon—a diminution of the rate of the auricular pulse after atropin—was observed.

A point which is probably of some importance was, however, pointed out by Professor Howell; namely, the intervals between the auricular beats after the disappearance of the block, while longer than the average intervals before, are yet shorter than the intervals occurring just before and at the onset of the periods of long intermission in the ventricular pulse.

The action of atropin in dissipating the dissociation suggests strongly that at this time, at all events, vagus influences played a part, to say the least, in its causation. This is supported by the behavior of the respiration during the attacks. That the *a-c* time in this and in other tracings is so rarely prolonged beyond the normal limits justifies the query as to whether the defect may not be one of the irritability of the heart muscle rather than a disturbance of the mechanism of conduction.

One might fancy that the course of events during these periods is as follows: With a heart muscle the irritability of which is diminished, there occur, with waves of increased vagus action, a gradual slowing of the auricular rate and a diminution in the intensity of the stimuli passing to the ventricle without delay in their periods of transmission, or a further diminution, under the same influences, of the irritability of the ventricle, sufficient to result in the cessation of ventricular contractions. This increase in vagus action continues for a short time after the falling out of the ventricular contractions, as indicated by the delay in the several succeeding auricular beats. With the passing of this depressing influence and the resumption of a rapid auricular rate, the diseased and exhausted ventricle fails to respond to the succeeding

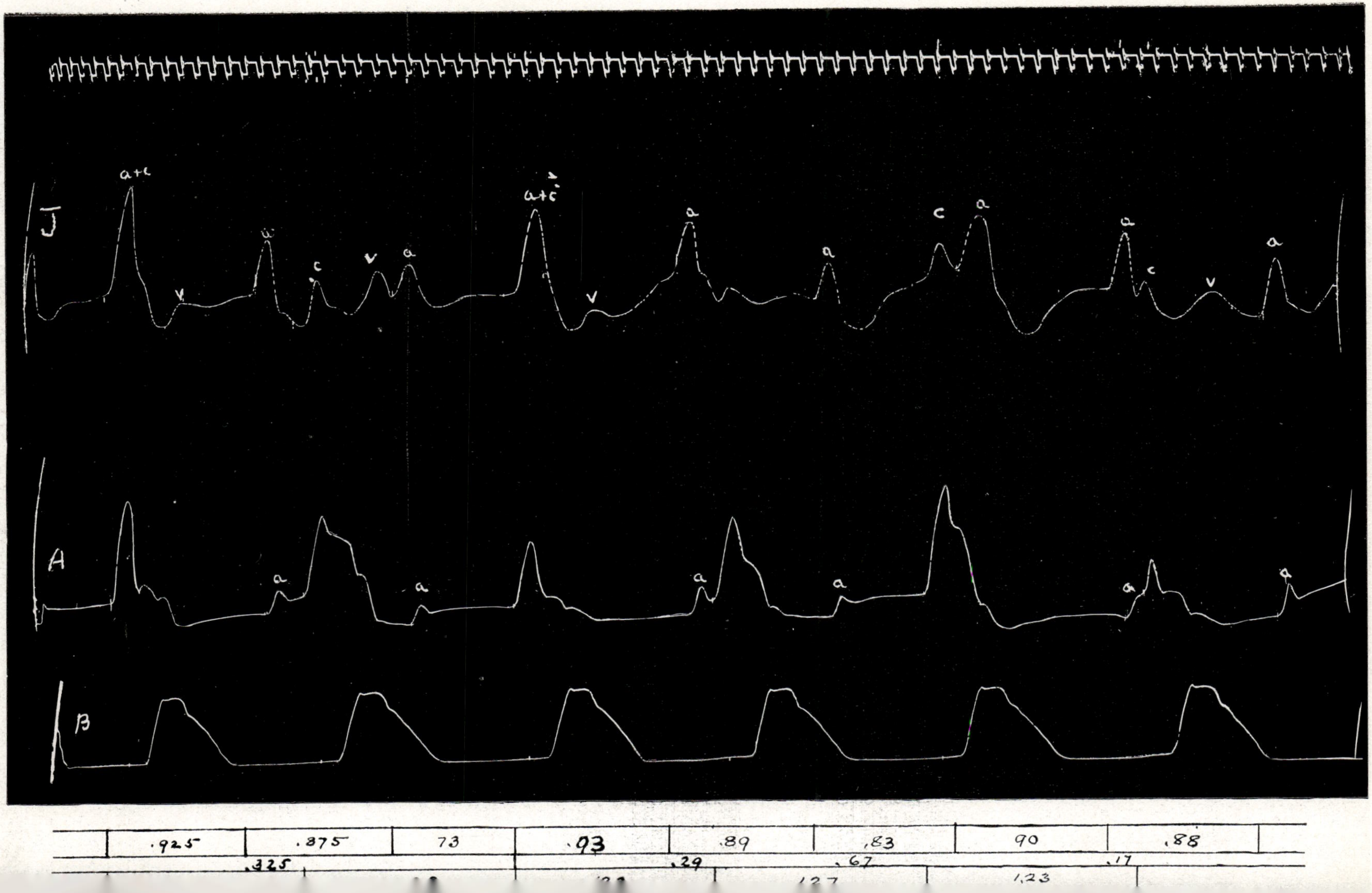
J
a+c
v
c
v
a
a+c
v
a
a
c
a
a
c
v
a
A
a
a
a
a
a
a
B
.925
.875
73
.93
.89
.83
90
.88
.325
.29
.67
.17
1.27
1.23

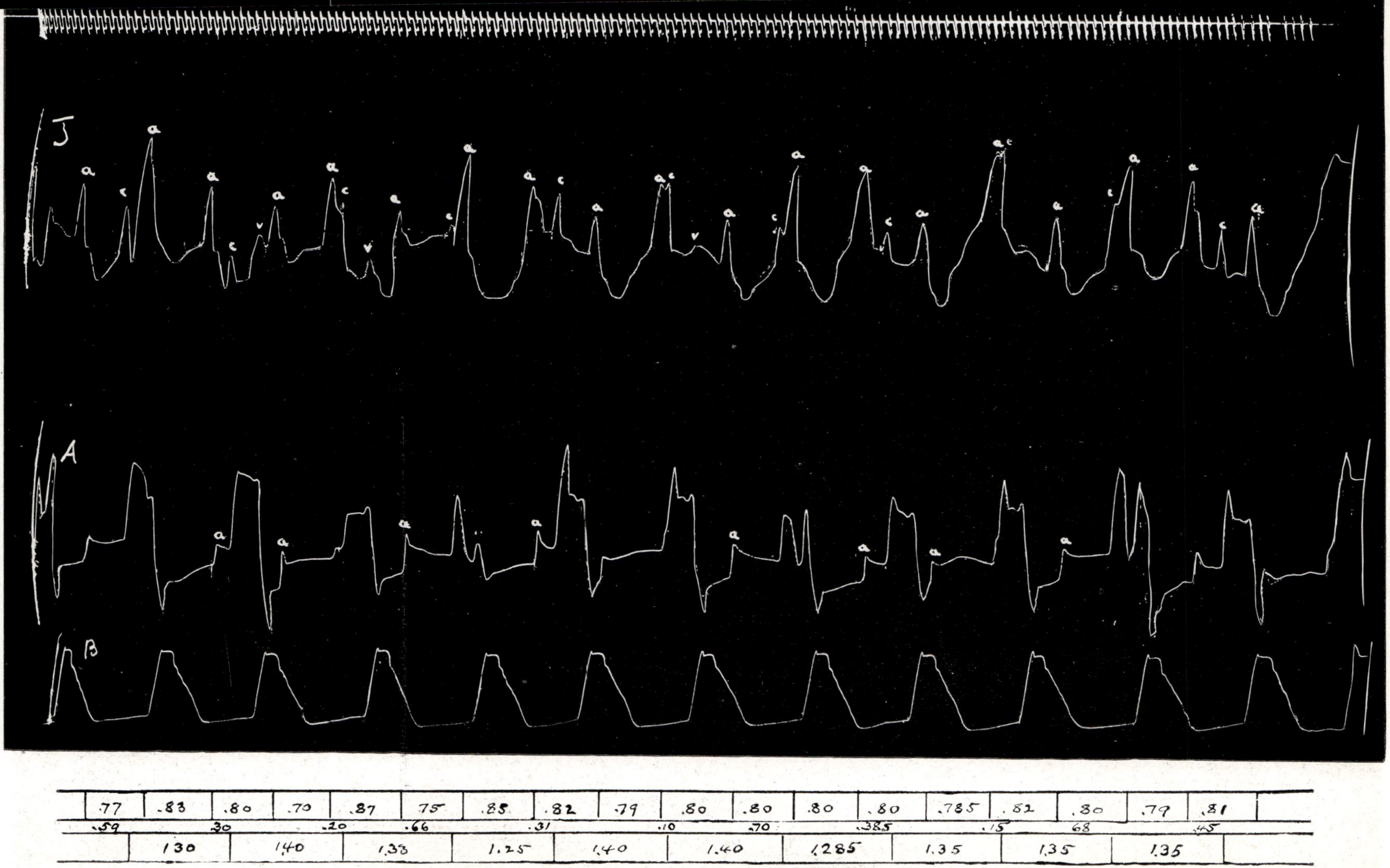


Tracing 12.—Case 2; April 21, 1909. Right jugular, apex and brachial. Relatively complete block.

individual stimuli. After a varying period, owing, perhaps, to a summation of stimuli (?) there occurs an apparently spontaneous ventricular contraction. This spontaneous contraction removes waste products and improves the circulation and nourishment of the heart muscle so that the rested ventricle is again able to respond to each stimulus as it arrives through the auriculoventricular bundle. But after a certain number of beats, with the return of a wave of vagus activity, the auricular rate is slowed and the ventricular contractions again fall out.

*Tracing 9, April 18: Complete Block Unaffected by Atropin*

Jugular tracings taken during this attack of block show auricular waves occurring at intervals averaging 0.5 second, a rate of 120 per minute. The ventricular rhythm, as determined by the brachial pulse and auscultation, showed that every ventricular beat was coming through to the wrist. The condition is quite different from that which is seen in Tracing 6. The ventricles are contracting regularly at intervals which average from 1.9 to 2.07 seconds, giving a rate of 31 + per minute. This is about the rate which is common in complete auriculoventricular dissociation with a permanently slow pulse. There is, however, an occasional beat with a shorter pulse period, as may be seen on Tracing 10, where the average rate is slightly more rapid. Comparison of the ventricular rhythm with that of the auricles shows that there is no apparent relation between them. The *c* waves occur at varying times after the *a* waves and, in some instances, fall synchronously with an *a* wave, so that one simple elevation is formed on the venous curve. It is, however, rather remarkable that out of twenty-one ventricular contractions studied on three good tracings, in which the interval between auricular waves averaged from 0.45 to 0.50 second, the *a-c* time was between 0.18 and 0.31 second in fifteen instances, 0.12 in one, while in five the *a-c* waves were fused.

Was this a complete *a-c* dissociation? In order to determine this question atropin, gr. 1/30 (0.0021 + gm.), was given subcutaneously. No change in the ventricular rate was observed. This result tends to confirm the view that, at this time, the dissociation was complete and suggests that vagus influences played little or no part in its production. About five hours after the atropin was given, and ten hours after the establishment of the dissociation, the attack ended spontaneously and the pulse became 92. It is worthy of note that during this attack, which was characterized by a slow regular pulse, the patient's general condition was quite different from that observed during the attacks in which the pulse was irregular. The unpleasant symptoms which accompanied the long pulse pauses—pallor, flushing, loss of consciousness and convulsions—were absent. Throughout the attack the patient was comfortable and undisturbed. He slept quietly, and ate his meals without any subjective discomfort. During the forty-eight hours preceding this attack of complete dissociation with regular pulse, he had five other attacks of irregularity with intermissions lasting from fifteen minutes to one and a half hours. Two of these were stopped by atropin. No atropin was given in the others. During the hour preceding the establishment of the slow regular rhythm the nurse's chart shows that the patient's pulse was very irregular, varying in rate from 36 to 76 with pauses of 8 to 10 seconds without beats. During this time he was aroused from his sleep and had frequent "flushes." With the establishment of a regular pulse the patient said that he felt a little short of breath, but was quite comfortable. The pulse-rate during the whole attack varied from 24 to 44 per minute. The urinary output was decreased. On the succeeding day there was another short attack lasting about eight minutes. After that, with the exception of occasional dropped beats, the pulse remained regular and at a normal rate until his discharge from the hospital four weeks later.

## SUMMARY OF THE TRACINGS AND GENERAL DISCUSSION

The tracings from this case show the following:

1. Regular normal rhythm with normal *a-c* conduction time. (Tracings 1, 2, 3, 7).

2. A dissociation of auricular and ventricular contractions (Tracings 4, 5), which, at first glance, appears to be complete, the auricles contracting regularly at the rate of over 130, the ventricles at a rate of about 50, somewhat irregularly owing to the occasional occurrence of beats in pairs with shorter intervals. Although no constant relation could be determined between the auricular and ventricular rates, yet it was found that a large proportion (11 to 15) of the ventricular beats followed the preceding auricular contractions within a period corresponding closely to the normal *a-c* time. We are, therefore, inclined to regard the condition as one of partial dissociation.

3. Partial dissociation of auricular and ventricular contractions (Tracings 6 and 7), both auricles and ventricles beating at a normal rate and in a normal sequence, with the exception of frequent long intermissions in the ventricular pulse. After these intermissions the first ventricular beat was apparently a spontaneous contraction bearing no definite relation to the preceding auricular systole. Then followed ventricular contractions occurring usually in groups of about six to ten in number, essentially regular in rate and bearing a normal relation to the action of the auricles. Slight slowing in the rate of both auricular and ventricular beats was noticed during the last several contractions before the periods of block, and in the first several auricular contractions after the onset of ventricular intermissions.

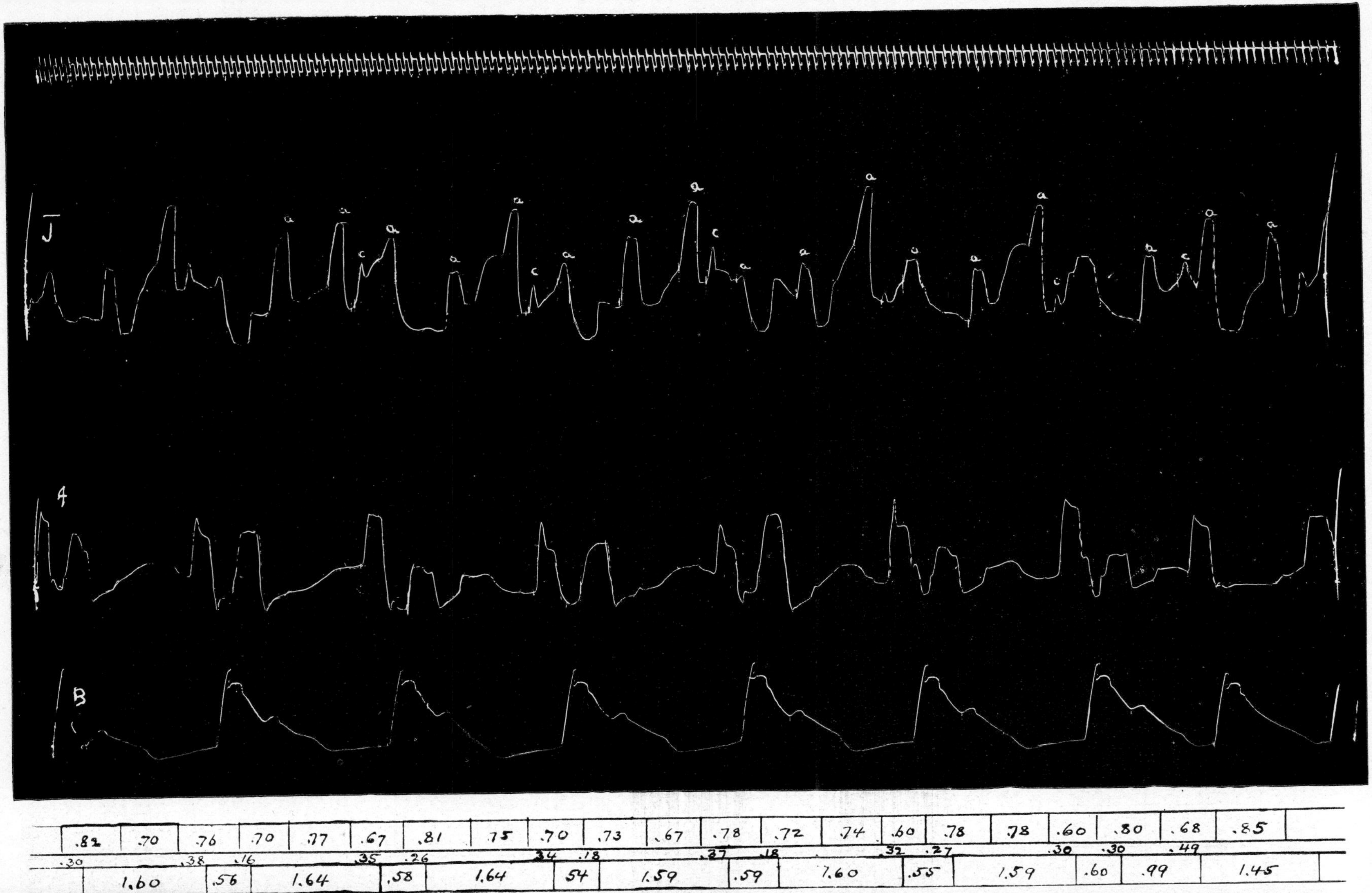

J
A
B
a
c
.82 .70 .76 .70 .77 .67 .81 .75 .70 .73 .67 .78 .72 .74 .60 .78 .78 .60 .80 .68 .85
.30 .38 .16 .35 .26 .34 .18 .37 .18 .32 .27 .30 .30 .49
1.60 .56 1.64 .58 1.64 .54 1.59 .59 1.60 .55 1.59 .60 .99 1.45

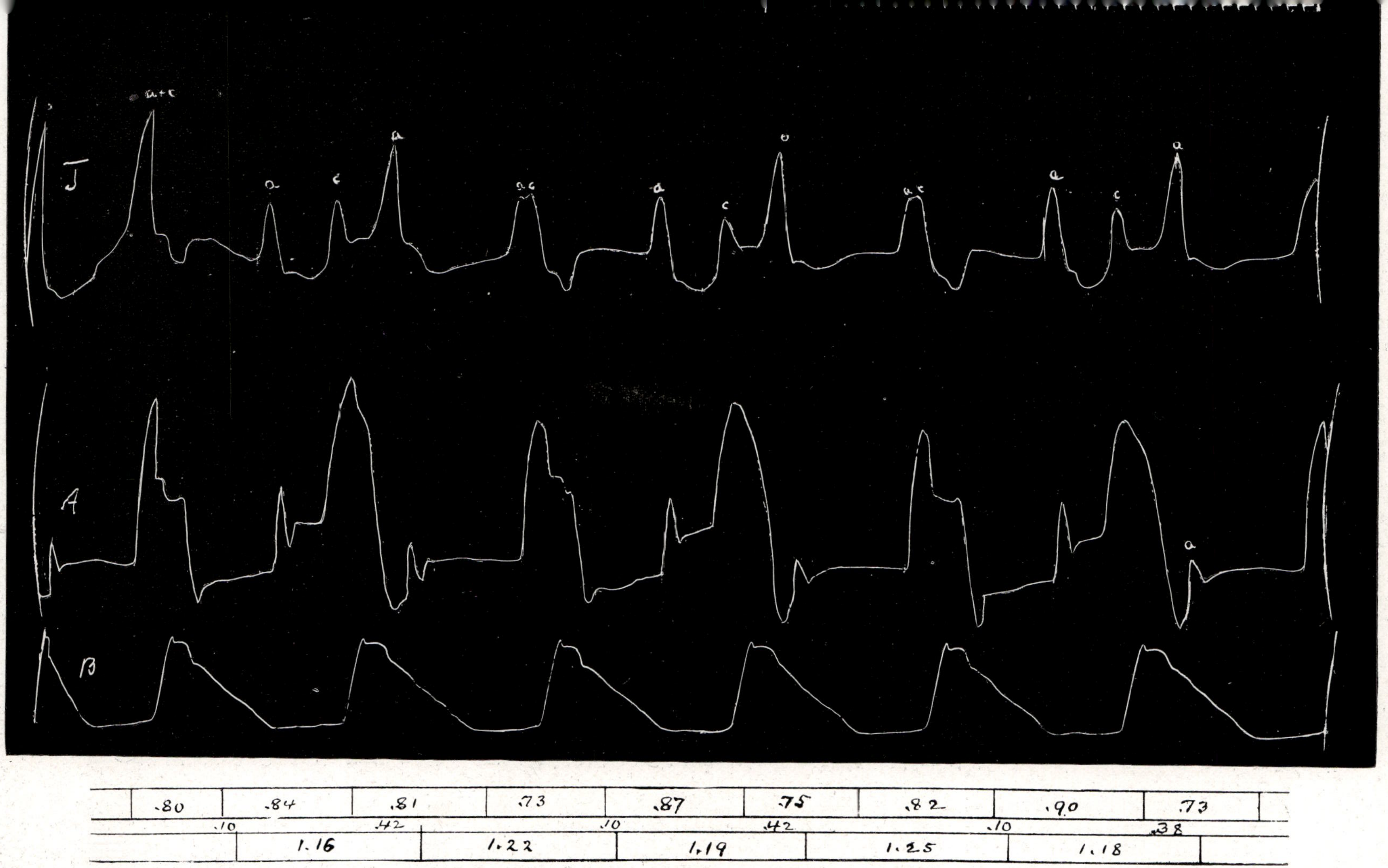


Tracing 14.—Case 2; April 22, 1909. Right jugular, apex and brachial. Relatively complete block.

This form of dissociation yielded, on three occasions, to the administration subcutaneously of atropin, gr. 1/60 (0.001 gm.). The auricular rate after atropin was, however, slower than it was before, but more rapid than the rate of the several slow beats at the time of onset of the periods of ventricular intermission.

4. Apparently complete auriculoventricular dissociation with a regular ventricular rhythm of 30 to 35 (Tracings 9, 10). This condition was not relieved by atropin, gr. 1/30 (0.0021 + gm.), injected subcutaneously.

It is unfortunate that we have not a good tracing taken during one of the attacks (see second paragraph under "Clinical Notes on Specific Attacks") with very long intermissions associated with convulsions and wholly irregular ventricular pulse. One tracing which we have studied (taken by Dr. Stengel) during the attack on January 2 suggests a complete dissociation. It is also very unfortunate that no graphic records of the respiration were made.

How are we to account for these various manifestations? One of the striking features of this case is the lack of essential lengthening of the *a-c* conduction time, even during periods of marked dissociation. The lengthening at several points where it appears is but slight and without regularity. This is unusual and raises the question as to whether a depressed excitability of the heart muscle may not play a part in the production of the symptoms. It would seem possible to account for most of the manifestations of the case on a hypothesis which supposes changes in or adjacent to the auriculoventricular bundle sufficient to cause (a) perhaps irritation of the bundle, (b) partial and at times, complete block but insufficient totally to destroy the bundle, (c) changes in the heart muscle which manifest themselves in a diminished irritability, (d) periods of increased vagus action occurring at times more or less regularly in waves.

At times there were periods of apparent complete block with rapid auricular action, irregular ventricular pulsations and long intermissions. At other times there were periods of total dissociation with a regular ventricular rhythm of about 30, and an auricular rate averaging about 120 to 130. Again, there were periods of partial dissociation with the occasional dropping of ventricular beats, the cause of which might have been diminished excitability of the ventricle or a diminution in the intensity of the impulse due to disease of the bundle or, perhaps, to vagus influence alone, or combined with this. Finally there were periods of partial block in which vagus influences must have played a part. In the absence of essential lengthening of conduction time at the periods in which the auricular rate became slower and the ventricular contractions fell out (Tracings 6 and 7), one would be tempted to suggest as an explanation that, under the influence of increased vagus action, the impulse passing through the diseased auriculoventricular bundle was insufficient to call forth a response from a ventricle of perhaps diminished excitability, either because of a diminution of the strength of the stimulus itself, or through some depressing influence on ventricular irritability.

That stimulation of the vagus by pressure, in the presence of disease of the bundle of His, may result in the falling out of ventricular beats with slowing of the auricular rate, but without notable prolongation of the *a-c* time was demonstrated experimentally by one of us (F. W. P.) in Case 2.

Of great interest is the apparent recovery of the patient after periods of dissociation so grave, at times apparently complete, and of such long duration, especially in the absence of any evidence of syphilis.

What may have been the nature of the disease of the bundle? It is difficult to answer the question with certainty. The physical signs—hypertrophied heart—rough aortic systolic murmur—point to a sclerosis at the aortic ring. One might suspect coronary changes arising perhaps at the root of the aorta with myomalacia followed by sclerosis, or a more gradual sclerosis due to similar changes in the neighborhood of and partially involving the auriculoventricular bundle.

One might, indeed, fancy that the disturbances depended on sclerotic changes in the artery of the bundle.

There are several cases in the literature of auriculoventricular dissociation with normal or nearly normal *a-c* time. In Hay's case,[2] during the periods of block, there was often appreciable prolongation of the *a-c* time which, however, was normal in the intervals. Nevertheless, there were times at which a sudden halving of the rhythm occurred without apparent lengthening of the intervening *a-c* periods. Wenckebach[3] reports a similar case and regards both instances as examples of intermission due to diminished irritability of the ventricles.

Gossage[4] reports a like instance with ventricular intermissions and, indeed, a tendency at times, to the establishment of an independent ventricular rhythm without prolongation of the *a-c* time.

One of us (W. S. T.) has recently observed a case in which physical effort was immediately followed by halving of the ventricular rhythm with a slight acceleration of the auricular rate, without prolongation of the *a-c* time. Vagus pressure in this case caused a single complete intermission of both auricle and ventricle (sino-auricular block?) followed by

---

2. Hay: Bradycardia and Arhythmia Produced by Depression of Certain of the Functions of the Heart, Lancet, London, 1906, i, 139.

3. Wenckebach: Beiträge zur Kenntniss der menschlichen Herzstätigkeit, Arch. f. Anat. u. Physiol., 1906, Physiol. Abth., p. 328.

4. Gossage: Independent Ventricular Rhythm; Heart-Block and the Stokes-Adams Syndrome, Without Affection of Conductivity, Heart, 1910, i, 238.

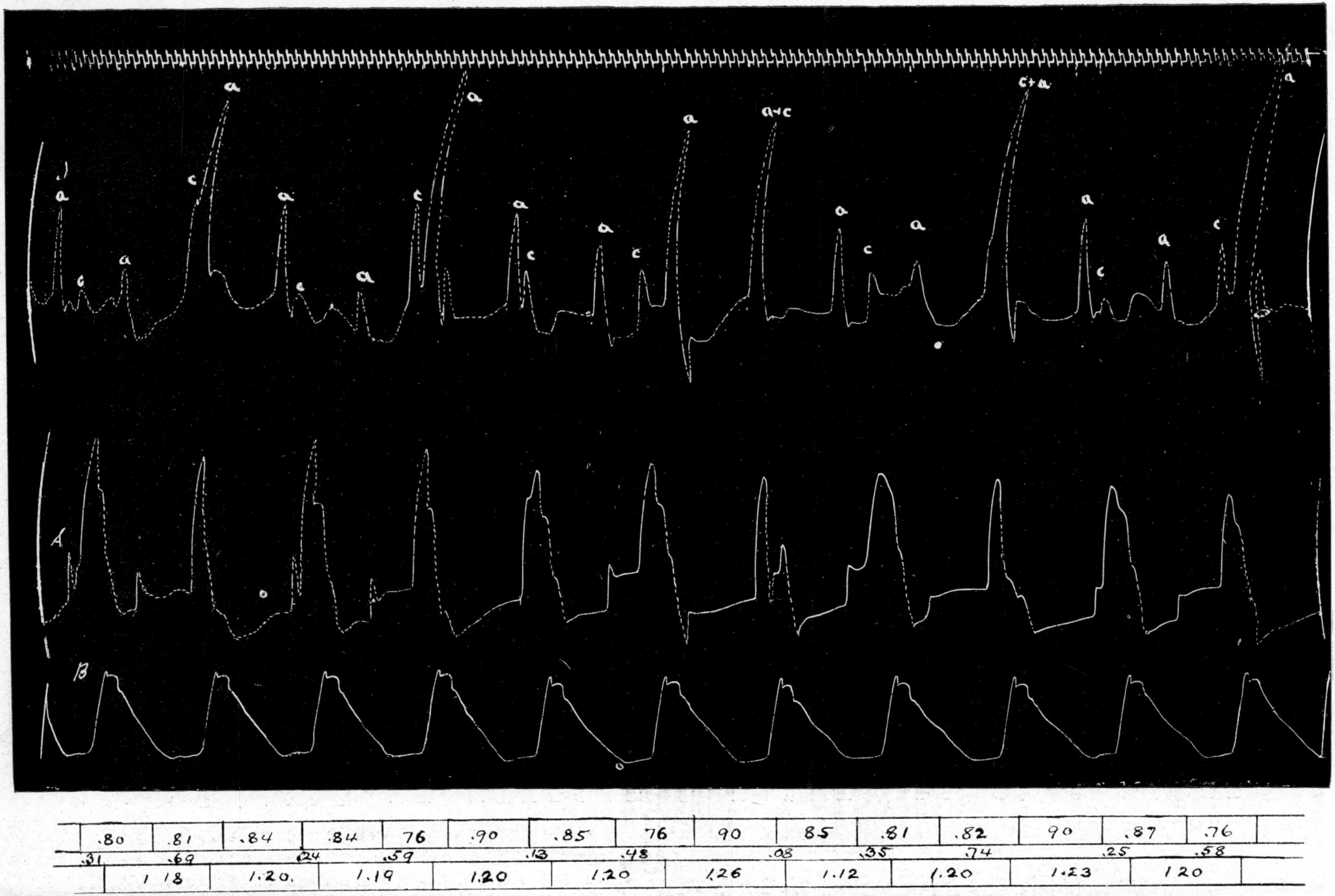

A
B
a
c
a+c
c+a
.80 .81 .84 .84 76 .90 .85 76 90 85 .81 .82 90 .87 .76
.31 .69 .24 .59 .13 .48 .08 .35 .74 .25 .58
1.18 1.20. 1.19 1.20 1.20 1.26 1.12 1.20 1.23 1.20

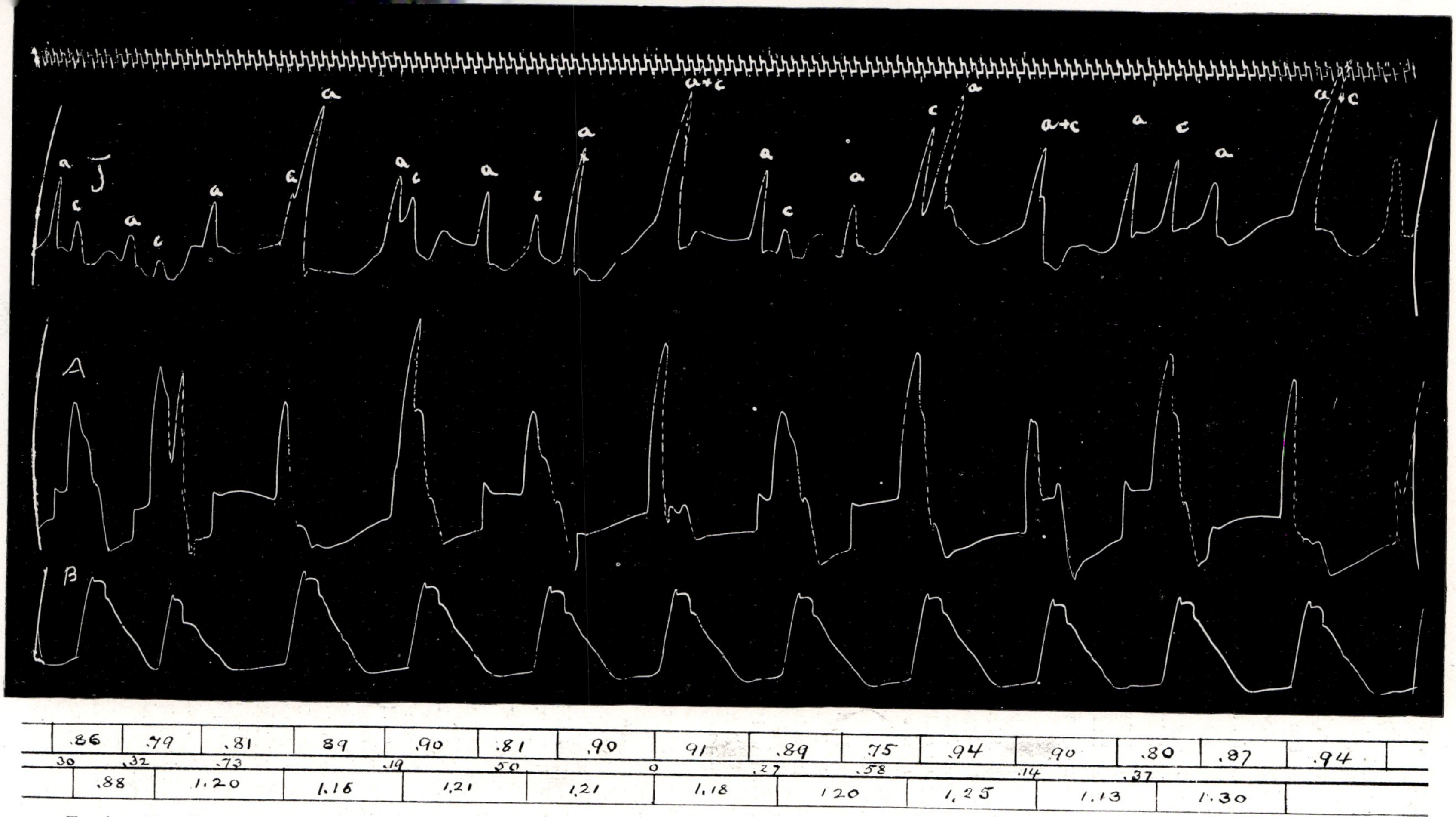


Tracing 16.—Case 2; April 22, 1909. Right jugular, apex and brachial. Relatively total block. Occasional response of ventricles to impulses passing through the auriculoventricular bundle.

a slowing of both auricular and ventricular rhythm without prolongation of the *a-c* time. During the period of pressure, after the first complete intermission there were occasional blocked auricular extrasystoles. The case was one of arteriosclerosis and chronic myocarditis.

In all these cases the most reasonable hypothesis for the explanation of the ventricular intermissions would appear to be that of a diminished irritability of the ventricles, and in all there were obvious cardiac defects. The autopsy of but one of these cases has been reported. In this case, that of Hay, there was definite involvement of the bundle of His, which was partly destroyed in a patch of fibrous myocarditis.

### *CASE 2*

*Adams-Stokes' syndrome; chronic myocarditis; hypertrophy and dilatation of the heart; partial and complete auriculoventricular dissociation with prolonged a-c intervals amounting, sometimes, to over 0.5 second; audible sound and visible and palpable impulse at cardiac apex with auricular systole; acceleration of cardiac rate with alternating pulse following atropin; development of 2 to 1 and 3 to 1 rhythm, following pressure on vagus, without essential change in auricular rate; improvement.*

H. J. (Gen. No. 68,051), colored, aged about 83, entered the hospital April 6, 1909, complaining of shortness of breath. There was nothing of importance in his family history. In 1906 he was operated on at the Johns Hopkins Hospital for trigeminal neuralgia. He had always been a heavy drinker of whisky and gin and a constant smoker; had had gonorrhea and syphilis.

*Present Illness.*—This was of about three years' duration. Since this time he had had occasional attacks of dizziness and fainting. During two of these, which occurred while he was walking along the street, he fell to the ground. He did not know how long he was unconscious. During November, 1908, the patient first noticed shortness of breath on slight exertion. At the same time his feet and legs became painful and swollen. In the last two weeks the dyspnea had become worse. He now had considerable pain in the right side of the chest, radiating toward the xiphoid process. The patient said that when he walked he became breathless and that if he did not stop he would fall. It was impossible to get a very satisfactory history.

*Physical Examination* (F. W. P.).—This showed a well-nourished old man. Thorax: Well formed; expansion, equal on the two sides. Lungs: Percussion note resonant over both fronts and axilla; marked diminution over the bases behind, where the fremitus was weak and breath sounds were barely audible. Forced inspiration was accompanied by numerous medium and fine moist râles. Heart: Point of maximum impulse visible and palpable in the seventh space, 11 cm. to the left of the mid-sternum; impulse, heaving, unaccompanied by a thrill. Dulness extended 4.5 cm. to the right in the fourth space and above to the third rib. On auscultation the heart's action was irregular with a definite pause between each three beats. There was a systolic murmur of considerable intensity at the apex, transmitted to the mid-axilla. At the base of the heart the first sound was barely audible; pulmonic second was loud and sharp. Aortic second was less distinct and followed at times by a very short diastolic blow. Pulse: Seventeen to the quarter, irregular in force and rhythm, large, at times slightly collapsing Vessel wall moderately thickened.

*Treatment and Course of Disease.*—The patient was put to bed; a diet, limited in quantity, and infusion of digitalis, 2 drams (8 c.c.), every four hours, were ordered. After several days the pulse was slower, between 50 and 60, falling on April 13 to between 40 and 50 to the minute. On April 20 it was noted that the pulsations of the veins of the neck were more frequent than those in the radial artery, but it was impossible to make out any definite relation between the two. The digitalis was omitted and atropin, gr. 1/120 (0.0005 gm.), to be injected subcutaneously twice daily was ordered. This was continued until April 25. The pulse ranged between 40 and 50, sometimes regular at a rate of about 40, sometimes showing distinct irregularities of rhythm. The jugular pulsations were obviously more frequent than those at the wrist.

On April 26 one of us (W. S. T.) noted that there were three impulses visible at the apex; one very distinct pulsation followed by two similar, but smaller ones. The impulse was visible in second, third and fourth spaces. There was no dulness over the manubrium. Point of maximum impulse was 9.5 cm. from the midsternal line. Dulness extended 10.5 cm. to the left at this point and 3 cm. to the right in the fourth interspace. The first sound was very faint, followed by a slight systolic murmur. The second sound at the apex was distinct; there was marked protodiastolic gallop. This was not audible over the right ventricle. The heart's action was regular, 72 to the minute.

On May 3, W. S. T. observed that "the pulse is beating at the rate of 76, sometimes quite regular. At other times there are intermissions at irregular intervals, but, if one feels at the apex carefully, a small impulse is always felt during intermissions and there is a visible pulsation in the neck. When one listens at the apex this is easily heard as a slight, soft sound. This sound is also heard, but rather more faintly, in the tricuspid area; it is undoubtedly an auricular sound. It is of entirely different character from the first sound and is not associated with a second sound. There is at times a slight, early diastolic gallop at the apex."

On May 29 the pulse was 80 and for the most part regular. Pressure over the vagus nerve in the neck, however, caused an almost immediate halving of the ventricular rate. On auscultation during the long pauses produced by pressure on the vagus, there was heard either a single sound or two dull sounds with a very short interval. The systolic murmur at the apex was louder at the slower rate than at the normal rate. At times the pulse assumed a bigeminal rhythm of its own accord. The second beat was then weaker than the first.

On June 1, shortly after 7 p. m., the patient complained of shortness of breath. Respirations were quick and shallow, 44 to the minute; the patient seemed in considerable distress. The pulse at the onset of the attack was 88 to the minute, but within a few minutes fell to 72. Continued pressure over the vagus on the right side of the neck resulted in a diminution of the respiratory rate to 28. The patient seemed very much relieved. The pulse-rate also diminished to a very perceptible extent.

June 16: It is now two weeks since the pulse has been as low as 50. The hourly pulse-chart shows that it has been usually regular, between 75 and 90. Slight pressure on the vagus is always followed by the establishment of partial block, generally a 2 to 1 rhythm, although one tracing shows two auricular systoles blocked by this means. The urine at no time showed more than a faint trace of albumin and an occasional granular cast.

The blood-pressure was at times as high as 180, but gradually dropped to about 140. The temperature was normal practically all the time.

The pulse-rate, from 70-90 during the first few days after admission, dropped to about 45 at which it continued for about a week. During the next four weeks the rate varied considerably. On the hourly pulse-chart, the rate, while often between 40 and 50, is shown at other times to have jumped to somewhere between 60 and 80. At either rate the rhythm was usually regular. Toward the end of the patient's stay the pulse-rate became more steadily high, at about 80 to 90. The condition improved so much that the patient was discharged on June 21, 1909.

The treatment, beyond that already mentioned, consisted of strychnin, gr. 1/30 (0.002 gm.), three times a day and, during the periods of especial irregularity of the pulse, iodid of potassium.

June 3, 1910: Several attempts were made to follow the course of events during the winter months, but without result. At last, however, we succeeded in

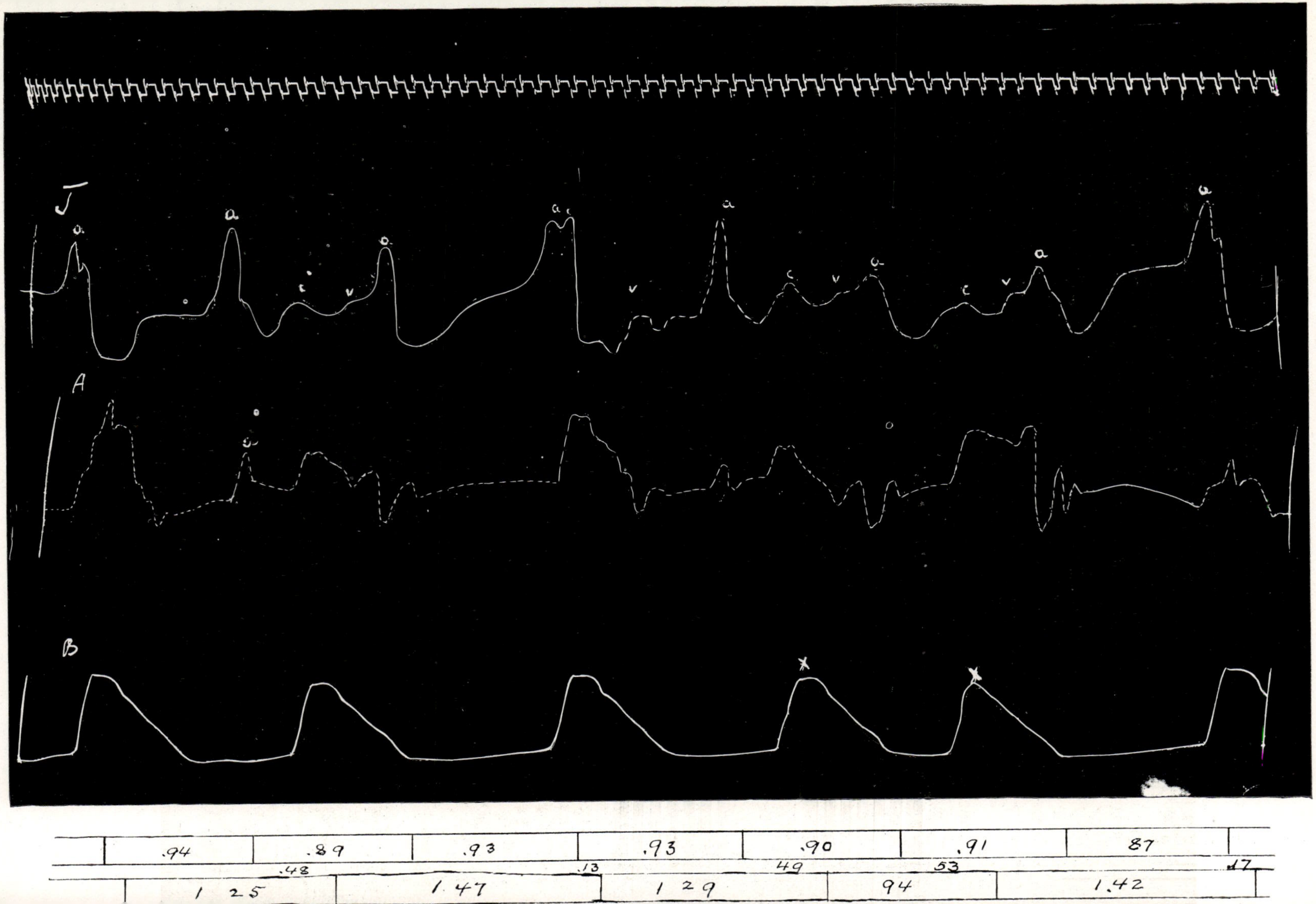
J
a
a
c
v
a
a c
v
a
c
v
a
c
v
a
a
A
B
x
x
.94
.89
.93
.93
.90
.91
87
.48
.13
49
53
.17
1 25
1.47
1 29
94
1.42

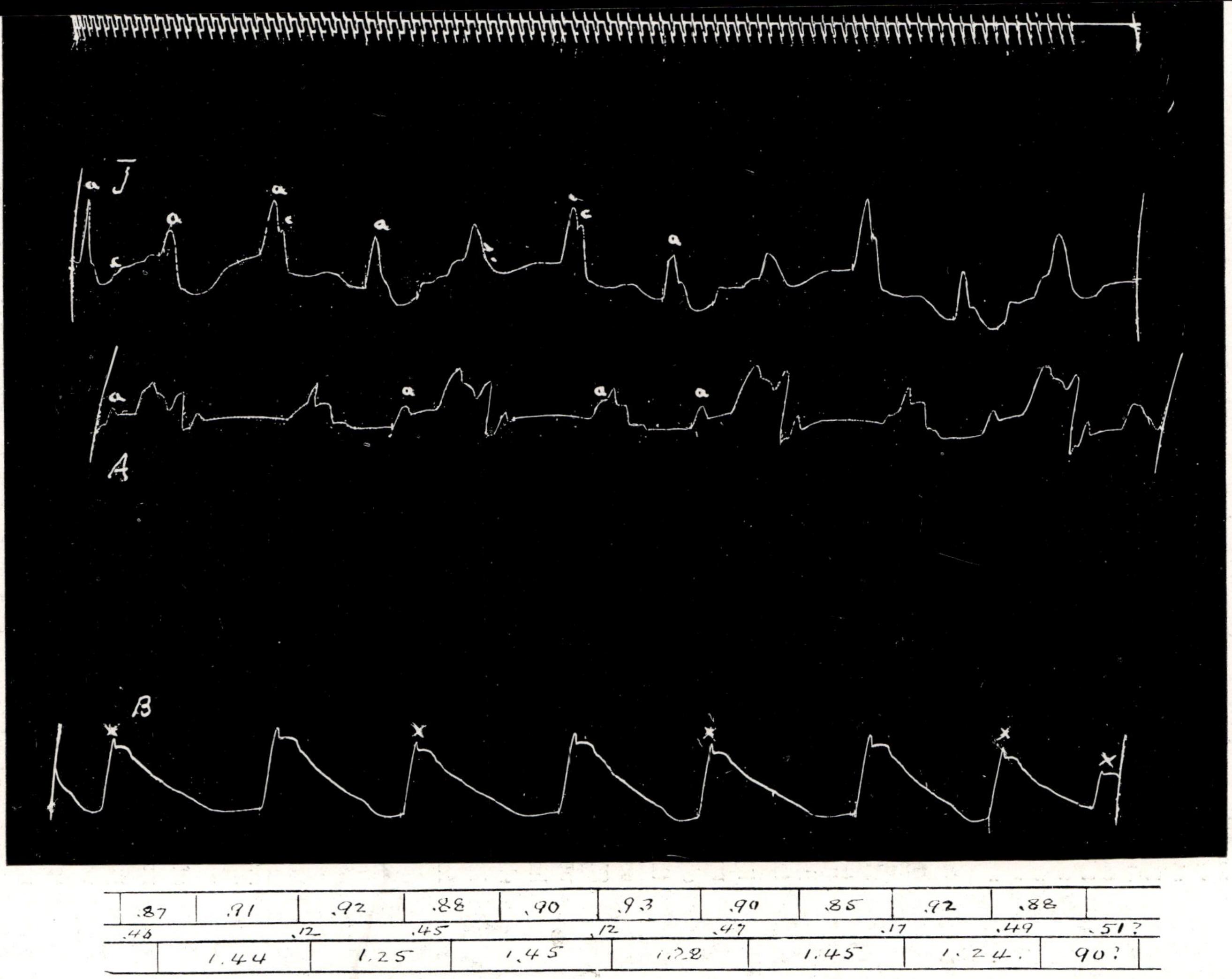


Tracing 18.—Case 2; April 24, 1909. Right jugular, apex and brachial. Partial block. Automatic ventricular rhythm modified by the occasional response of the ventricles to impulses passing through the auriculoventricular bundle.

finding the patient June 2, 1910. The attacks of dizziness and momentary loss of consciousness had been more frequent, the patient having fallen in the street many times. His general condition, however, was much as when last seen. He was rather short of breath and there was edema of the legs; the pulse was slow and at times quite regular at about 40, at other times showing occasional interpolated beats which were not followed by a compensatory pause. On morning of June 3 the cardiac impulse was visible and palpable in the fifth interspace, 11.5 cm. to the left of the median line, and occasional small impulses might be seen and felt at the apex between the regular ventricular contractions. The first sound at the apex was strong, fading out into a slight systolic murmur; the second clear at the apex and base. At times, at the apex, an extra sound was heard between ventricular beats. This sound was soft, just audible and obviously associated with auricular systole.

## SUMMARY OF THE CLINICAL MANIFESTATIONS

A man, aged 83, had dyspnea on exertion for three years, with several attacks of dizziness and faintness. Physical examination showed hypertrophy and dilatation of the heart with relative mitral insufficiency and probable aortic insufficiency. Following treatment with infusion of digitalis, but persisting for more than a month after its discontinuance, periods of bradycardia occurred, during which the pulse was sometimes regular at about 40, at other times irregular. The pulsation of the auricles, as observed in the neck, was evidently more frequent than that of the ventricles. Auricular pulsations were manifest by a slight audible sound and sometimes by a palpable and visible impulse at the apex. Slowing, usually halving, of the pulse-rate followed pressure on the vagus nerve. The pulse, during a period of somewhat over two months in the hospital, gradually returned to a rate of 80-90. A year later the patient showed a pulse, nearly regular, at a rate of about 40, with occasional interpolated beats. During the year there had been numerous attacks of faintness and momentary losses of consciousness.

## ANALYSIS OF CARDIOGRAPHIC AND SPHYGMOGRAPHIC TRACINGS

### *Tracings 11, 12 and 13: Relatively Total Block With 3 to 1 and 3 to 2 Rhythm*

Tracing 11, April 21, 1909.—The pulse is 44 to 48. The maximum blood-pressure is 190; minimum, 90. The venous pulsations in the neck appeared at the time to be more rapid than the arterial. Tracings of the brachial artery show that the ventricular contractions are nearly regular, at intervals averaging about 1.25 seconds, a rate of 48 per minute. The auricles are contracting more rapidly than the ventricles, at a rate of about 70, and there is no apparent simple ratio between their respective rates. Examination of the jugular pulse reveals the dissociation more clearly. The *c* waves appear to bear no constant relation to the *a* waves. They occur at different periods during the auricular intervals and at times synchronously with the *a* waves.

Under these circumstances, one combined wave appears on the jugular curve; this wave is frequently of unusual size, doubtless because the auricle, unable to open the atrioventricular valves during the ventricular systole, must, therefore, exert a strong back pressure into the veins. Further evidence of the auriculoventricular dissociation is shown by the tracings of the apex impulse. Here, the waves due to auricular contraction, which were easily visible and palpable, are shown clearly. The variations in their relations to the anacrotic wave of the cardiogram are clearly evident. This tracing then, might appear to reveal a condition of complete auriculoventricular dissociation. But another interpretation might be put on it.

One might fancy that, to begin with, the first *a-c* wave depended on an extremely prolonged conduction time which had resulted in the coincidence of a *c* wave corresponding to a preceding *a* wave, with a succeeding *a* wave which is blocked. The next *a-c* time is 0.325 in length; the next 0.73 +. Then follows a blocked *a* wave. This is again repeated, an *a-c* period of 0.29 being followed by one of 0.67 which, in turn, is followed by a blocked *a* wave, and then again by a shorter *a-c* interval. It might be asserted that it is quite unjustifiable to assume the possibility of an *a-c* period as long as 0.6 to 0.7, but, in a case in which the *a-c* time amounts sometimes unquestionably to over 0.5, such a fancy can hardly be regarded as wholly unreasonable. If this explanation be accepted, we have then, not a total block but a 3 to 2 rhythm. The strongest argument against this explanation would seem to be that the *a-c* time at the beginning of the second, fourth and sixth beats occurring on this tracing is 0.325, 0.29 and 0.17, respectively. But at no other period on the many tracings that we took of this case is there any certain *a-c* period as short as 0.17. In another tracing (Tracing 12) with a slower drum, the rate of the radial pulse is about 44 and regular. It seems impossible to determine any definite relation between the jugular and the radial pulse. The rate of the jugular pulsation is about 76.

There is apparently a complete dissociation of auricular and ventricular rhythms. The rate of the ventricle is, however, more rapid than the usual automatic rhythm. One might ask whether this were, perhaps, one of those instances described by Erlanger and Blackman[5] of "relatively complete block," where an automatic ventricular rhythm has arisen in a heart in which the auriculoventricular bundle is still capable of transmitting some stimuli. These stimuli are, however, usually of subminimal strength and incapable, ordinarily, of interfering with the established ventricular rhythm. It is not uninteresting, however, that the second, fifth and eighth ventricular beats following the preceding auric-

5. Erlanger and Blackman: Further Studies in the Physiology of Heart-Block in Mammals, etc., Heart, 1910, i, 214.

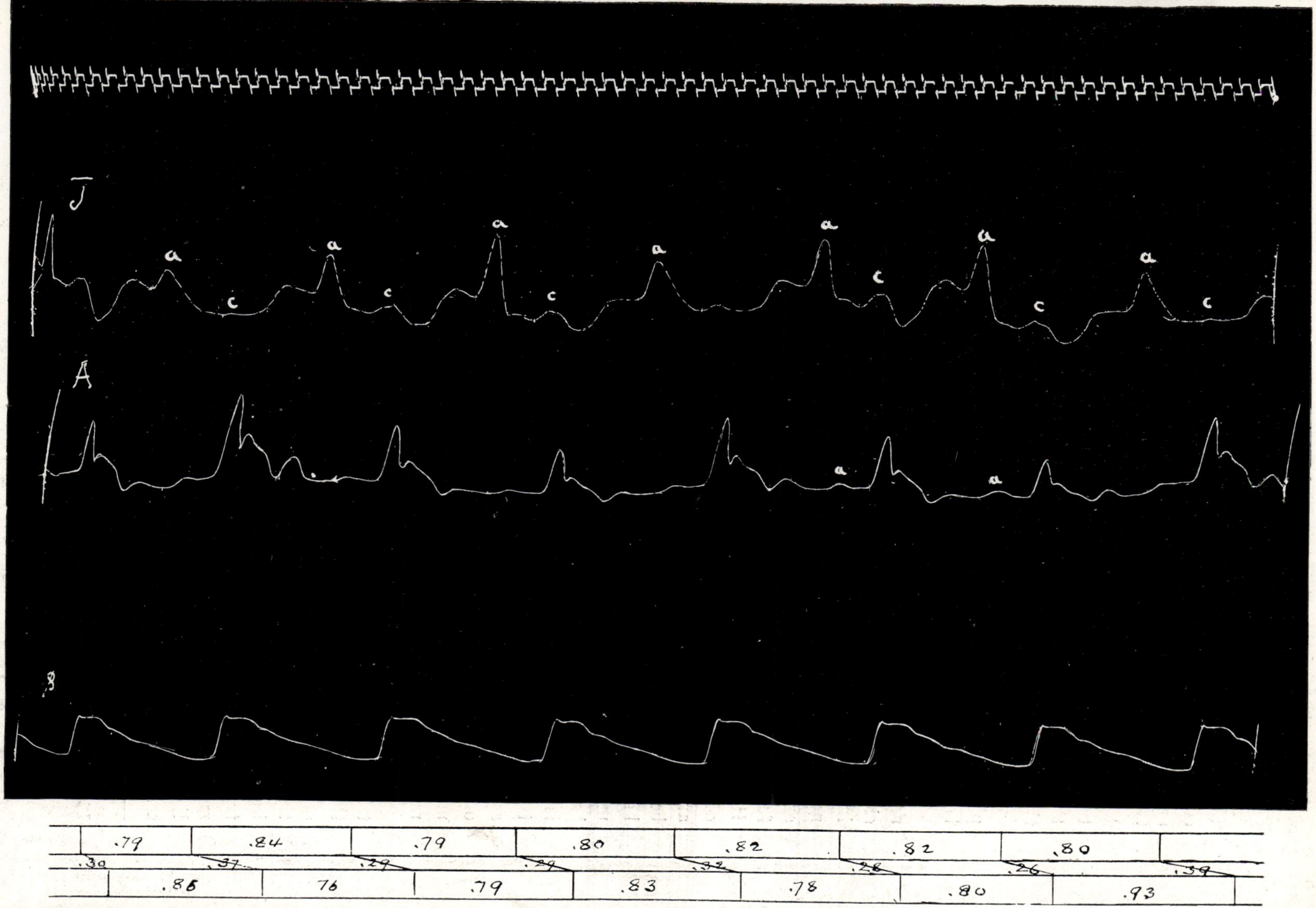


Tracing 10. Case 2; April 24, 1909. Right jugular, apex and brachial. Normal rhythm with prolonged *a-c* time. This tracing was taken

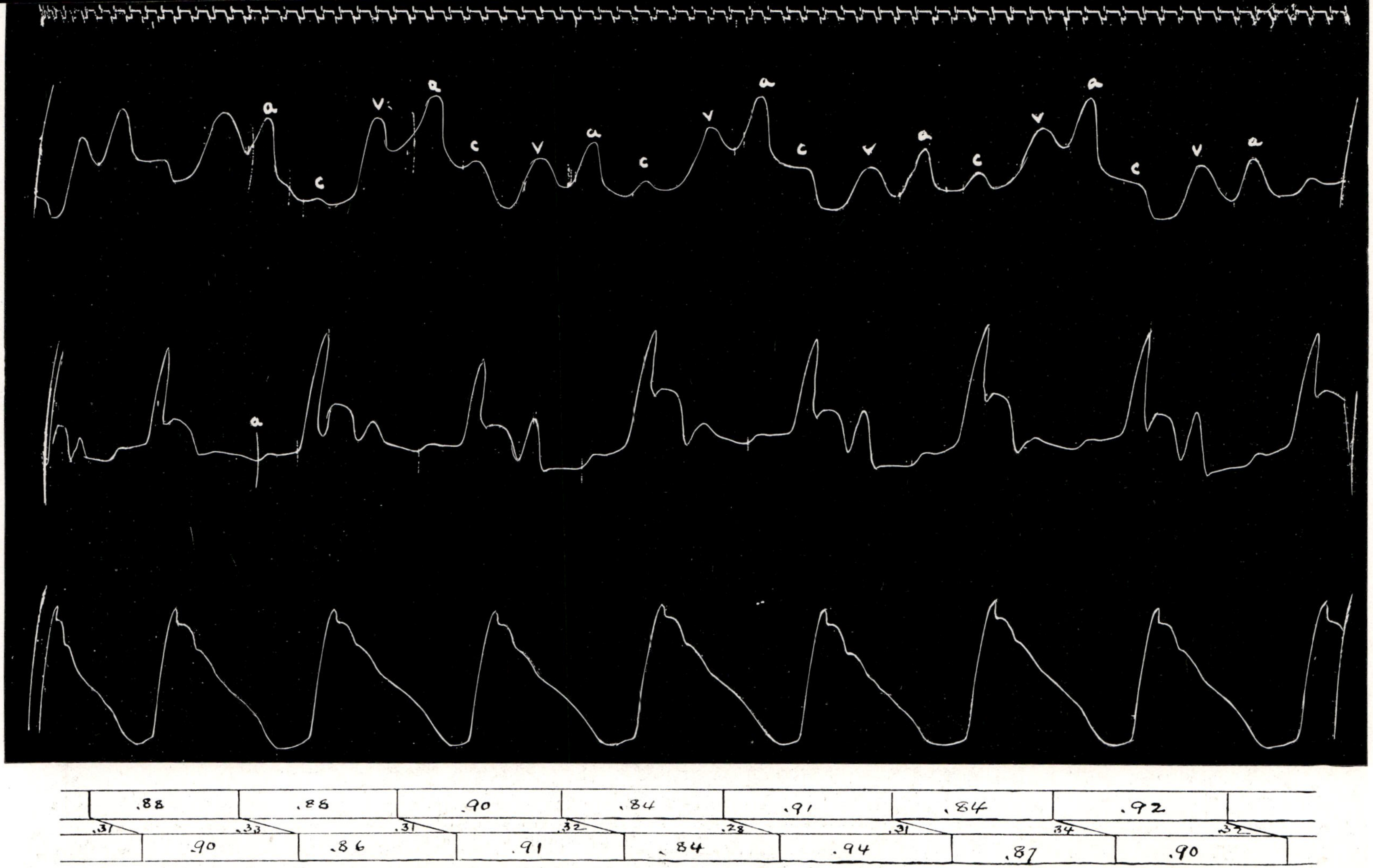


Tracing 20.—Case 2; April 25, 1909. Right jugular, apex and brachial. Normal *a-v* rhythm. Prolonged *a-c* time.

ular contractions by respectively 0.30, 0.31, 0.385 second are preceded by intermissions slightly shorter than the average. May it not be that in these instances the normal impulses reaching the ventricle at a time when it was nearly ready to contract from its inherent rhythmicity, have slightly hastened the contraction?

Another tracing (Tracing 13) taken on the same day does not apparently show a complete block. There is a bigeminal ventricular rhythm The *c* elevation corresponding to the first of each pair of ventricular beats follows an *a* wave after a fairly constant period, varying from 0.30 to 0.38, a conduction time similar to that observed in this case at other periods during a normal auriculoventricular rhythm. The second of each pair of contractions is, however, associated with a combined $a + c$ wave on the jugular pulse. By comparing the *a* wave with the brachial tracing, however, it is found that the *a*-brachial period suggests usually a normal, or but slightly increased conduction time. May these second ventricular contractions depend on the same stimuli as those causing the preceding auricular beats? The short *a-c* period in association with a contraction immediately following another with a lengthened conduction time, especially in a case in which at all other times the *a-c* period is markedly lengthened, would be difficult to explain, unless one assume that the impulse causing this contraction is ectopic, arising at a point farther down in the bundle than usual; but the auricular impulse follows the preceding after the usual period. Moreover, it is interesting to note that the second of each pair of ventricular contractions follows the first after an intermission which is almost constantly of about 0.6 second, a period more constant than that separating it from the preceding *a* wave. It would then seem probable that the second beat of each pair is a spontaneous ventricular systole to which the preceding ventricular beat bears some causal relation. The third auricular contraction associated with each group of beats is obviously blocked. There is one exception to this rhythm. The third auricular impulse in connection with the sixth pair of beats is followed after 0.49 second by a *c* wave and a radial pulse.

The tracing would, then, appear to represent a partial dissociation in which there is a fundamental 3 to 1 rhythm which becomes a 3 to 2 rhythm because of regularly interpolated ventricular extra-systoles which cause a bigeminal pulse.

### *Tracings 14, 15 and 16, April 22, 1910: Relatively Total Block, with Evidence of the Occasional Passage of Stimuli Through the Bundle of His*

In Tracing 14 the radial rate is about 50; auricular 78-79. The ventricular intervals are fairly regular, varying from 1.18 to 1.25 in length. The auricular intervals vary from 0.73 to 0.90. On studying the tracing one sees a combined $a + c$ wave in the jugular; an *a-c* interval of 4.2; a blocked wave. This is followed by a similar sequence twice, the lengthened *a-c* time averaging from 0.39 to 0.42. The combined *a* + *c* wave shows in two instances a double summit corresponding respectively to *a* and *c* waves. The *a-c* time is 0.10 in each case. In the third combined wave the onset of the *c* wave is not evident on the jugular pulse. The onset of the systolic elevation of the cardiogram corresponds exactly with the beginning of these three combined waves on the jugular curve and falls 0.10 second before the small notch indicative of the *c* wave where it is present. This is not much longer than the ordinary transmission time, apex to jugular. The character of these waves suggests, then, that the auricle and ventricle must have contracted almost simultaneously.

A second tracing (Tracing 15) with a slower drum, shows 11 ventricular beats to 16 auricular beats. On studying the tracing it is rather difficult on first glance to avoid the conclusion that it represents a complete dissociation. The comparative regularity of the auricular and ventricular rhythms and the great variations in the *a-c* periods would seem to be difficult to explain by another hypothesis. The rate of the pulse—between 49 and 50—is, however, rather more rapid than is common in essential ventricular rhythm.

On a third tracing (Tracing 16) showing 11 ventricular and 16 auricular beats, there appears to be in the main no definite relation between auricular and ventricular contractions. The intervals between the ventricular beats vary from 1.13 to 1.30 with the exception of one beat, which follows the preceding after an interval of 0.88. The intervals between the auricular beats are fairly regular, from 0.75 to 0.94. The regularity of the ventricular rhythm is here again suggestive of a total dissociation. It should, however, be noted that the ventricular rate on this tracing is not so regular as on the two preceding records, and it is significant that with the two ventricular contractions following the shortest intermissions (0.88 and 1.13) the *a-c* time is 0.32 and 0.37 second, respectively. Now, on tracings from this case at periods in which there is a regular auriculoventricular rhythm, for instance on Tracing 20, the *a-c* interval is often of about this length. It would, therefore, appear not improbable that these two beats have been hastened by the regular stimulus which has passed through the bundle. In other words we are probably in the presence of one of those instances of so-called relatively complete block in which, without total destruction of the *a-c* bundle, the ventricles have yet initiated an independent rhythm. The enfeebled stimuli coming through the injured bundle reach the ventricle as a rule either at a refractory period, or with a strength insufficient to call forth a response from a heart muscle, the irritability of which is diminished.

But here and there, as with the second beat on Tracing 16, an impulse may come through the bundle strength sufficient to call forth a ventricu-

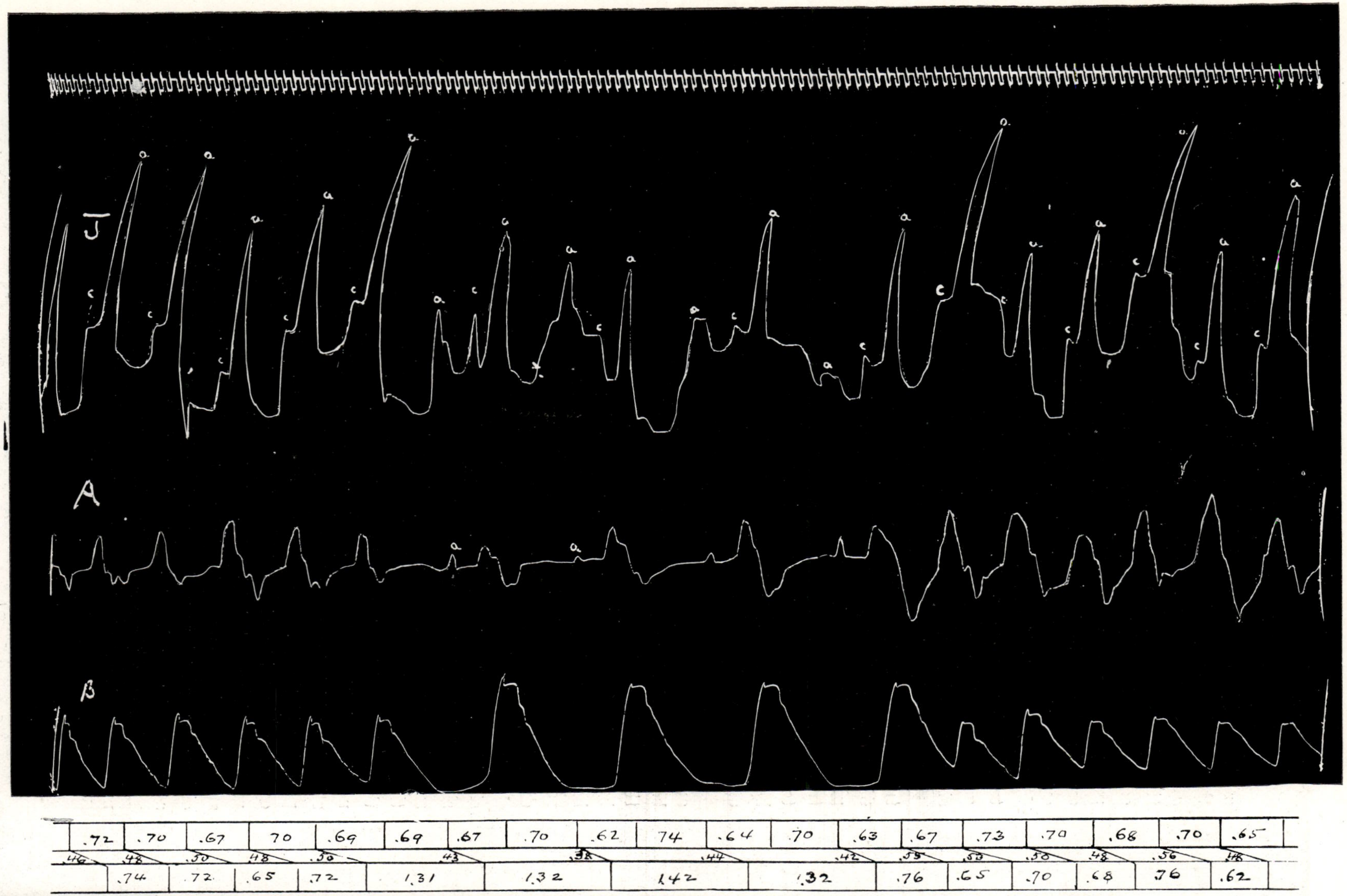
J
A
B
a
c
.72 .70 .67 70 .69 .69 .67 .70 .62 74 .64 .70 .63 .67 .73 .70 .68 .70 .65
.46 .48 .50 .48 .50 .43 .38 .44 .42 .55 .53 .50 .48 .56 .48
.74 .72 .65 .72 1.31 1.32 1.42 1.32 .76 .65 .70 .68 .76 .62

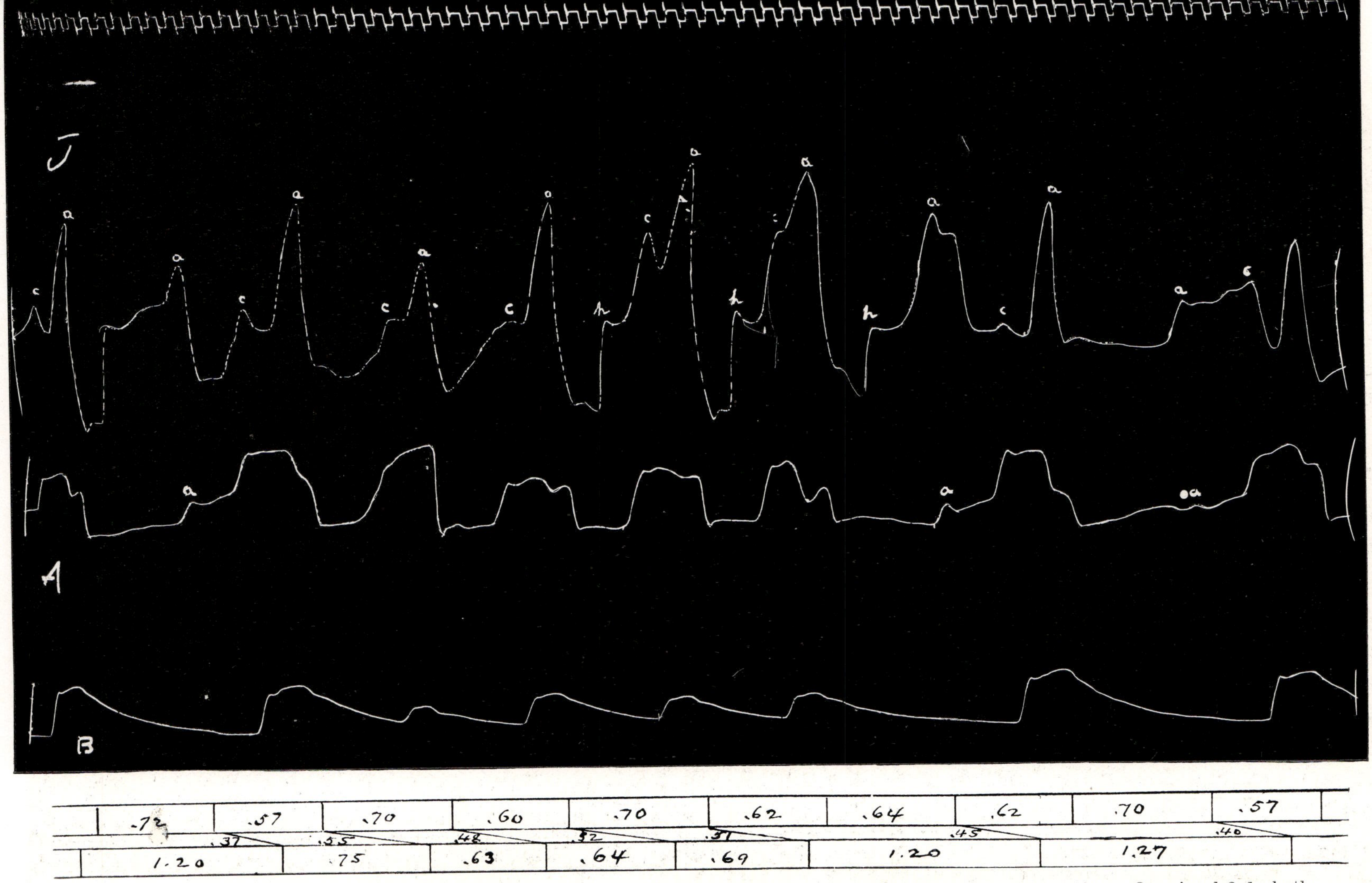


Tracing 22.—Case 2; April 29, 1909. Right jugular, apex and brachial. Normal *a-v* rhythm with prolonged *a-c* time. Occasional 2:1 rhythm.

lar response resulting in an occasional beat after a shorter interval. At other times an impulse reaching the ventricle at a moment when it is nearly ready to respond to the stimulus which one may regard as accumulating in itself, is sufficient to call forth a slightly precocious contraction. If, now, we turn back to Tracings 14 and 15 it is interesting to note that, in the shortest intervals between ventricular beats, the terminal *c* wave follows the preceding *a* wave after a period which is not far from that common in this case at times when stimuli are certainly passing through the bundle. This is seen on Tracing 14 in the intervals before the second, fourth and sixth *c* waves, and on Tracing 15 before the eighth *c* wave. We are, then, inclined to believe that although an independent, automatic ventricular rhythm at a rate of 40 to 50 has been initiated, yet the conduction through the auriculoventricular bundle is not wholly interrupted. The normal stimuli play a part at least in the excitation of some of the ventricular contractions.[6]

*Tracings 17, 18, 19, April 24, 1909: Partial Block Relieved by Atropin*

1. Before Atropin (Tracings 17, 18): The jugular tracing taken before the administration of atropin shows fairly regular contractions, the intervals averaging about 0.9 second, a rate of about 66 per minute. The analysis of the ventricular rhythm is less simple. The ventricular rate is much slower than that of the auricle, about 40 to the minute, and at first sight there might appear to be no relation between the two rhythms. It will, however, be noticed that the ventricular rhythm is not regular, the intervals varying between 0.9 and 1.47 in length. At two places on two tracings there are two short beats in succession and in each case the inter-

---

6. Another possible explanation of Tracings 14 and 15 occurred to us when we first studied these records, an explanation similar to that advanced by Griffith and Cohn (Quart. Jour. Med., 1910, iii, 136) to explain almost identical phenomena.

On Tracing 14 one might fancy that, after a transmission time of 0.42, the next impulse passed through the bundle so slowly that the ventricular response occurred after the succeeding auricular beat, which, as well as the following auricular contraction, is blocked. The cycle then begins over again. On Tracing 15, according to this hypothesis, we see an *a-c* time of 0.31, then of 0.69, then a blocked *a* wave. This is followed by an *a-c* time of 0.24, then one of 0.59, then an exceedingly long period of 1.03 and then a blocked *a* wave. Then comes an *a-c* time of 0.48 followed by one of .98 and a blocked *a*. The next cycle begins with a transmission time of 0.35, then one of 1.74 and then a blocked *a* and so on. In other words, the condition might be regarded as a 3 to 2 and occasionally a 4 to 3 rhythm.

In Tracing 16, except for the close sequence of the first two beats, a similar course of events may be made out. But such an explanation of these events we are inclined to discard for several reasons.

1. It is difficult to explain the comparative regularity of the ventricular action in a rhythm which changes from time to time from 3 to 2 to 4 to 3.

2. Just such a sequence of events as this might be expected to occur from the natural ratio one to another of the beats of two independent regular rhythms.

3. The possibility of an *a-c* period of over one second is not yet proved.

val is about 0.9 second, which is nearly the same as the auricular interval. The *a-c* periods in connection with the two beats following a short interval are each a trifle over 0.50 second.[7] The ventricular beats after the long pauses bear a less definite relation to the auricular beats and often occur on the jugular curve at nearly the same time as the auricular beats or at about 0.1 second later, so that one broad-topped double wave is formed. It is improbable that these latter beats depend on the stimulus causing the preceding auricular systole, for in this case the *a-c* time would amount to over 1 second. There are, however, six other ventricular beats in which the *a-c* period varies from 0.45 to 0.49. One of these initiates Tracing 18. The other five are preceded by intermissions of 1.25, 1.29, 1.25, 1.28 and 1.24 seconds, respectively. The intermissions preceding those ventricular contractions which, on the venous curve, occur synchronously with or shortly after the *a* waves, are of 1.47, 1.42, 1.44, 1.45 and 1.45; that is, appreciably longer in every instance than the intermissions preceding *a-c* periods of 0.45 and 0.49. Now an *a-c* conduction time as long as 0.45 to 0.49 second is shown in this case on Tracings 21, 22, 23. We are then inclined to regard these tracings as indicating a partial block in which the ventricle is attempting to initiate an intrinsic rhythm of 41 or 42 to the minute (intermissions averaging 1.446). With every third or fourth auricular systole the stimulus passing through the bundle after a prolonged conduction time, reaches the ventricle at a period when it is nearly ready to contract automatically. The result of this is a slightly precocious impulse such as is seen in the second and fourth beats on Tracing 7, and the third, fifth and seventh beats on Tracing 8. In addition to this, on two occasions, the succeeding normal impulse passing through the bundle, in each instance more slowly than the preceding, is yet sufficient to excite a ventricular contraction.

That the condition was not one of total block is shown by the result of the atropin test.

2. After Atropin: Atropin, gr. 1/30 (0.002 gm.), was given subcutaneously and Tracing 19 taken twenty-nine minutes after its administration. Here the ventricular rhythm is regular at a rate of 75. The auricular rate is the same; each auricular beat is followed after a transmission time of from 0.26 to 0.39 second, by a ventricular wave. As a result of the atropin, therefore, the ventricular rate has risen from 40 to 75; the *a-c* time has diminished materially in length; the auricular rate has risen from 66 to 75.

*Tracing 20, April 5, 1909: Normal Rhythm, Prolonged Conduction Time*

Tracings taken on this day show that the auricles and ventricles are contracting regularly and in normal sequence. The only abnormal point in the curves is that the *a-c* time is prolonged (0.28 to 0.34 second).

---

7. The position of the *c* wave in the second is estimated from the time of onset of the brachial pulse.

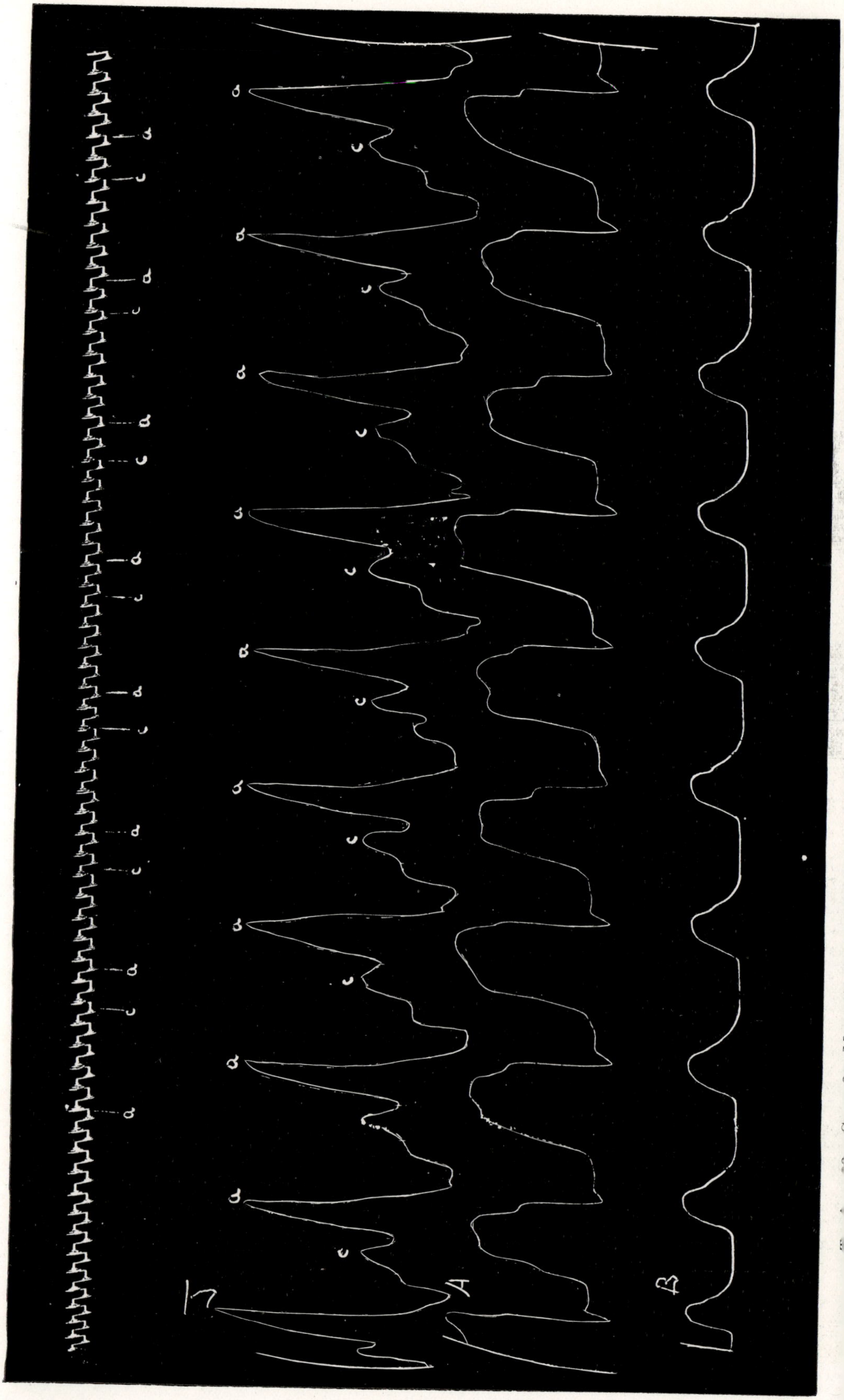

T
A
B

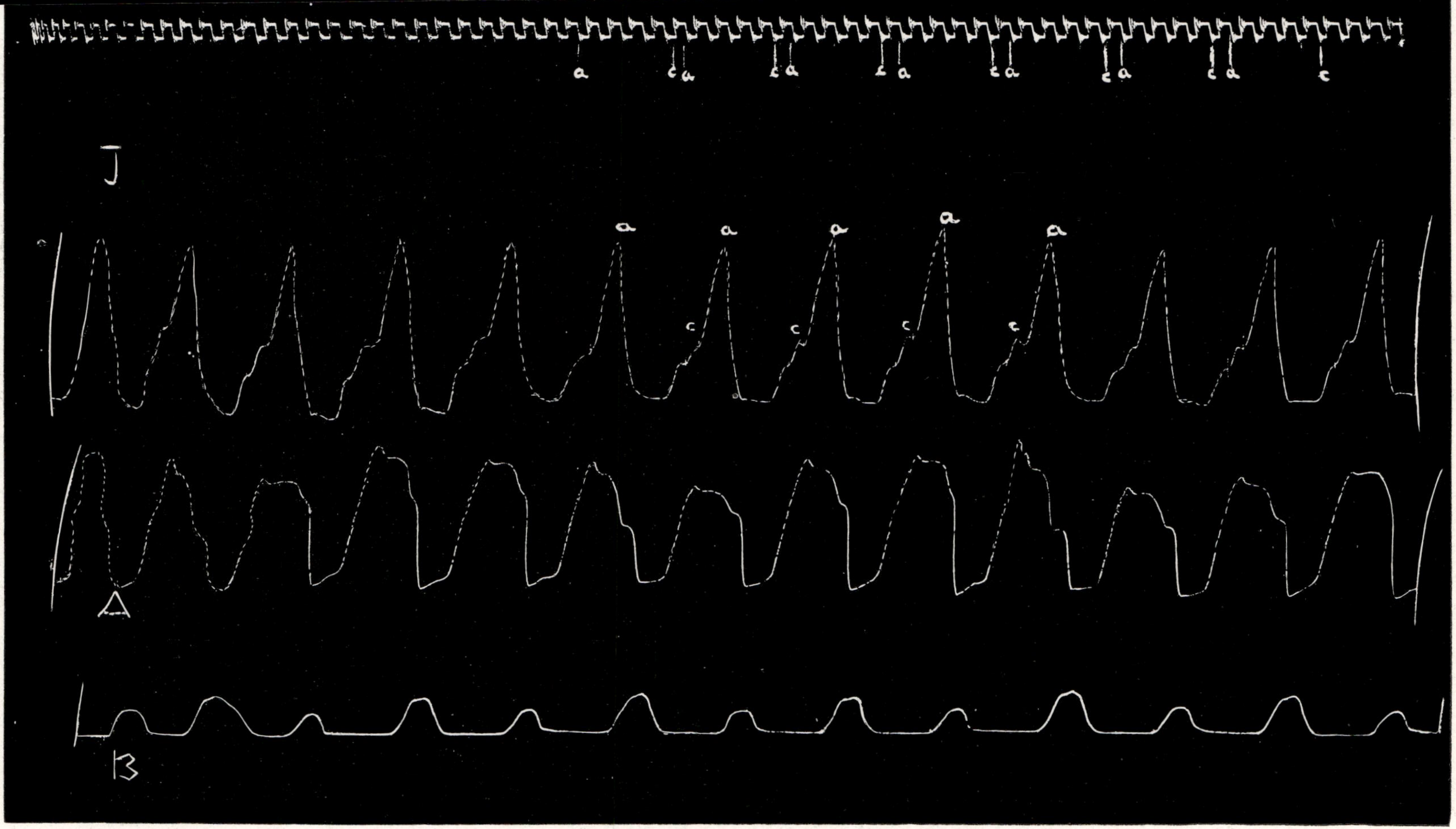


Tracing 24.—Case 2; May 17, 1909. Right jugular, apex and brachial. Tracing taken fourteen minutes after administration of atropin, gr. 1/30 (0.0021 gm.), given immediately after the recording of Tracing 23. Alternating pulse. Rapid cardiac action, *a-c* time slightly shorter than in Tracing 23.

*Tracings 21 and 22, April 29, 1909: Remarkably Prolonged Conduction Time; Occasional Halving of the Rate*

The auricles are contracting regularly at about 90 per minute. The ventricular pauses fall into two sets, one of which is approximately twice as long as the other. The long pauses are from 1.20 to 1.42 seconds long. The short are from 0.62 to 0.76 in length. During the period of rapid ventricular action every auricular systole is followed by ventricular systole with an *a-c* time which is from 0.48 to 0.56 second in length. During the period of slow ventricular rate there is a 2 to 1 rhythm. Every other auricular systole is blocked and the *a-c* time varies from 0.37 to 0.45 second. The shortening of the *a-c* time is probably due to the greater opportunity for the conduction fibers to regain their functional power during long pauses. During the shorter pauses the conduction time is so long that the *a* wave of the venous pulse follows immediately after the preceding *c* wave; it has an unusual height as the auricle is contracting at a time when the ventricle is also in systole. The condition present on this day was then a normal auriculoventricular rhythm with a long conduction time, changing at frequent intervals to a partial block with a 2 to 1 rhythm. The length of the *a-c* periods in these tracings is remarkable, the longest we believe that has been reported with the exception of the case of Griffith and Cohn.[6]

Of interest on this tracing are the distinct waves on the jugular curve, which we have marked *h*. These elevations occurring after the sharp auricular contraction which is combined with the *v*-wave, represent, probably, a centrifugal impulse associated with the closure of the mitral curtains incident to the sudden filling of the ventricles. They correspond fairly well to the position of the *h* (Gibson "*b*") wave on the normal jugular curve. The same condition is beautifully shown on Tracings 23 and 24, where the protodiastolic elevation of the cardiogram, which bears the same relation to this wave that it does in the normal tracing, is to be made out.

*Tracings 23, 24, May 17, 1909: Normal Rhythm, Prolonged Conduction Time, Acceleration of the Rate with Development of Pulsus Alternans Following Atropin, gr. 1/30 (0.0021 + gm.)*

The first tracing (23) shows auricles and ventricles beating regularly in normal sequence at a rate of 90. The *a-c* period is from 0.45 to 0.5 second. Atropin, gr. 1/30 (0.0021 + gm.), was given subcutaneonsly. Five minutes later the pulse was regular at 104. Twenty-three minutes after administration, another tracing was taken (24). The rate had then risen to 120. The pulse was regular. The conduction time averaged 0.41 second. There is a distinct *pulsus alternans* evident in the brachial tracing, one interval being slightly shorter than the preceding, the large beat following the short interval. The action of the atropin, therefore, has been to increase the rate of the auricles and ventricles, to shorten the *a-c* time slightly, and to produce *pulsus alternans,* so commonly present with an enfeebled myocardium.

*Tracings 25 and 26, May 19 and June 5, 1909: Heart-Block Induced by Pressure on the Vagus*

In Tracing 25 the rhythm is regular; the rate 71. The *a-c* periods vary in length from 0.32 to 0.36 second. As a result of light pressure on the vagus nerve in the neck, there was an immediate slowing of the radial pulse-rate due, as the jugular pulse shows, to the establishment of a partial block with 2 to 1 rhythm. The long ventricular intervals are about double the short ones. The beats after the long pauses are considerably larger than those following the shorter periods. The *a-c* time after the long pauses is slightly shorter than with the beats after the short pause. There is little, if any, effect on the auricular rate, although the average length of the auricular periods during pressure is 0.84, without pressure, 0.80 +. The dropping of alternate beats began almost immediately after pressure was applied to the neck, and continued more or less regularly until the pressure was removed. The change in rhythm was accompanied by no subjective symptoms.

A similar tracing taken on June 5 (Tracing 26) shows at one point the blocking of two successive *a* waves by vagus pressure. The *a-c* time after this long pause was 0.31 second as compared with 0.4 second before it. The auricular rate is slightly, but distinctly slower during vagus pressure, the intervals between beats averaging 0.765, as against 0.71 +.

These results are of real interest when considered in connection with certain of the events in Case 1. Here, it may be remembered, there were long pauses in the ventricular pulse, alternating with periods during which every auricular contraction was followed after a nearly normal interval by a ventricular beat. On several occasions the administration of atropin hypodermically resulted in the resumption, after about fifteen minutes, of normal auriculoventricular rhythm without essential change in the length of the *a-c* interval. In endeavoring to explain this phenomenon we advanced the hypothesis that, owing to alternating waves of vagus action, the strength of the impulses passing to auricle and ventricle was at times so far diminished as to fail to produce a response in a ventricle, the irritability of which was, perhaps, reduced, or that, through the same influence, the irritability of the ventricle was further affected. It is not uninteresting that an analogous condition should have been produced experimentally in this case, in which, in addition to disease of the auriculoventricular bundle, myocardial disease was clearly present as indicated by the hypertrophy and dilatation and the diminished contractility (alternating rhythm).

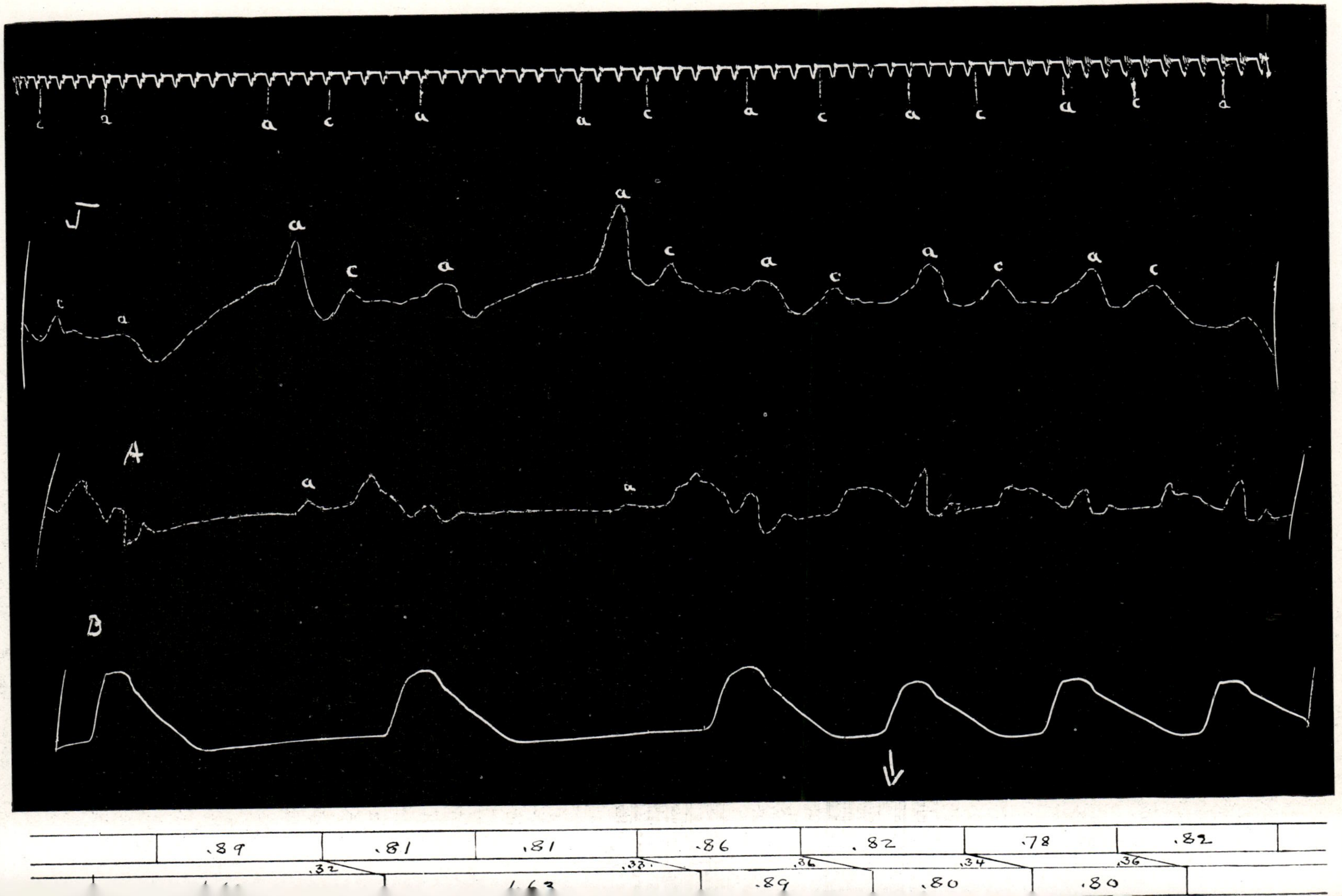
J
A
B
.89
.81
.81
.86
.82
.78
.82
.32
.33
.36
.34
.36
1.63
.89
.80
.80

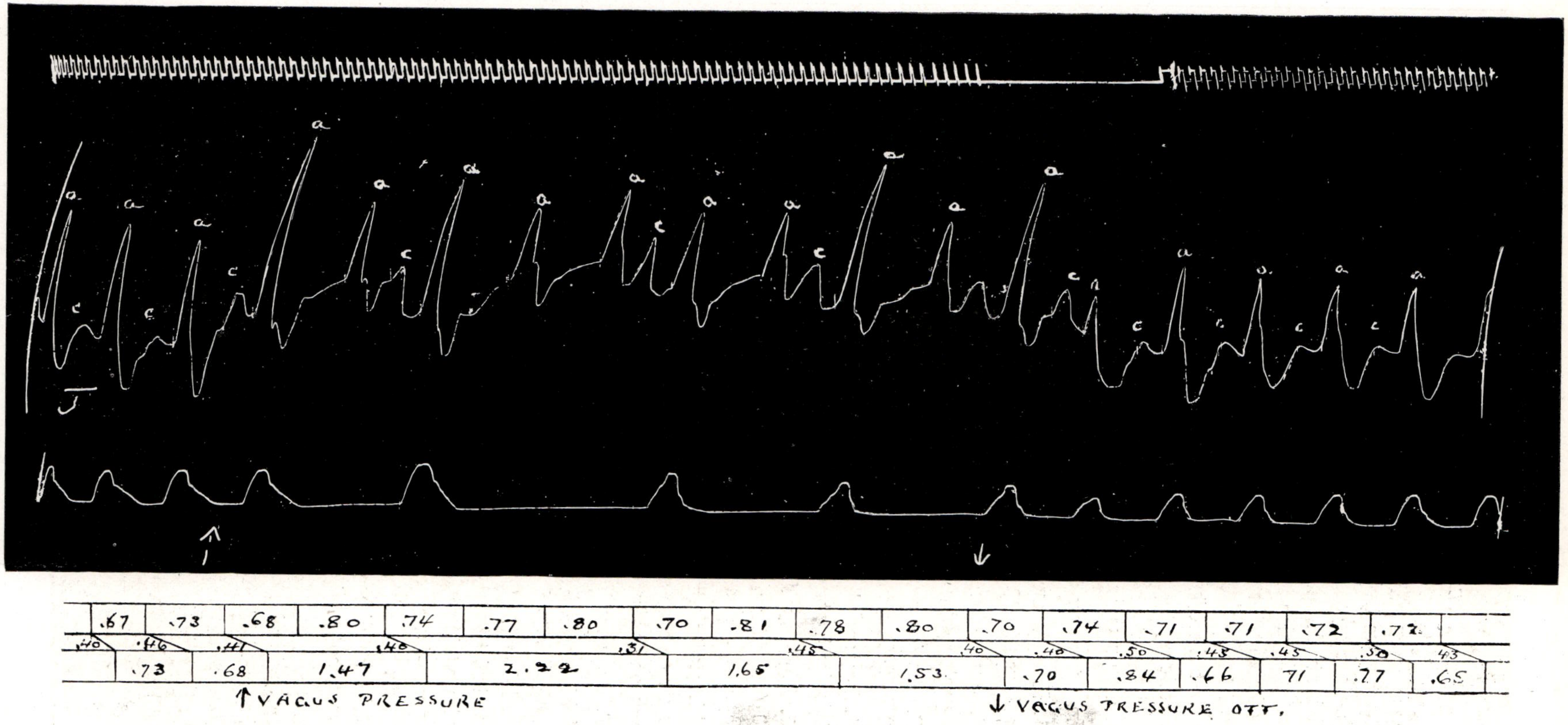


Tracing 26.—Case 2; June 5, 1909. Right jugular, apex and brachial. Effect of pressure on vagus, 2:1 and 3:1 rhythm.

*Tracing 27, June 3, 1910: Complete Auriculoventricular Dissociation*

Numerous tracings were taken on this date, but it was never possible to obtain a record of other than a regular pulse, the occasional interpolated beats disappearing as soon as the patient lay down. Tracing 27 shows auricular intervals varying from 0.78 to 0.99, averaging 90 +, a rate of about 66. The ventricular intervals vary from 1.55 to 1.61, averaging 1.585, a ventricular pulse of 38. On referring to the key it may be seen that there is no constant relation between auricular and ventricular contractions; there is apparently a complete dissociation.

### SUMMARY OF TRACINGS AND DISCUSSION OF THE CASE

In summary the tracings from this patient show:

1. Regular auriculoventricular rhythm with much prolonged *a-c* time (Tracings 20, 23).

2. Partial and relatively complete auriculoventricular dissociation with prolonged *a-c* time (Tracings 21 to 24).

3. Partial auriculoventricular dissociation relieved by atropin, gr. 1/30 (0.0021 gm.), given subcutaneously (Tracings 17, 18, 19).

4. Prolonged conduction time with occasional blocking of alternate ventricular beats (Tracings 21, 22).

5. Rapid cardiac action with alternating pulse following atropin, gr. 1/30 (0.0021 gm.), given subcutaneously (Tracings 23, 24).

6. The production of a 2 to 1 and a 3 to 1 rhythm as a result of the blocking of alternate and once of two successive auricular impulses by pressure on the vagus (Tracings 25 and 26), with little effect on auricular rate or on conduction (*a-c*) time.

7. Apparently complete auriculoventricular dissociation (Tracing 27).

This would seem to be a typical instance of disease of the auriculoventricular bundle with diminished conductivity in an hypertrophied and dilated heart. There was great prolongation of the *a-c* time with the characteristic falling out at times of alternate beats, at times of every third ventricular beat. At other times there were evident attempts on the part of the ventricle to initiate an independent rhythm. At no time, however, was the pulse-rate so slow as is common in complete auriculoventricular dissociation. These tracings appear to us to represent an independent auricular rhythm which has been set up in a heart in which the bundle of His is not wholly incapable of performing its functions. On a number of tracings those ventricular beats which follow the preceding auricular contractions after a period corresponding to the usual *a-c* transmission time in this case, are slightly precocious. This suggests to us that the impulses causing these beats have in reality passed through the auriculoventricular bundle (Tracings 22, 24, 25, 26, 27, 28).

An apparently spontaneous ventricular rhythm at a rate as rapid as 45 to 50 is a notable feature of this case. It would be interesting to know whether the last tracing represents a total or a relatively total block—whether the destruction of the bundle is complete. Further observation of the patient should give us the information. We had hoped to persuade the patient to allow us to pursue the study of his case by means of the electrocardiograph before the publication of these observations, but we have not as yet succeeded.

The production by vagus pressure of a partial block (Tracings 25, 26) with slight slowing of the auricular rate and no apparent lengthening of the *a-c* time suggests the possibility that the action may have consisted either in the diminution of the volume of the stimulus generated and conducted to the ventricle, or in the irritability of the ventricle itself. That the contractility of the ventricle was diminished at the outset is testified to by the alternating pulse with rapid auricular action after atropin (Tracing 24). After vagus pressure, however, there was no evidence of alternation.

The effect of vagus pressure in this case in producing a slight slowing of the auricle with occasional ventricular intermissions without apparent change in the *a-c* time is not without its analogies with the events which, in Case 1, we were inclined to ascribe to waves of vagus influence. In that case, it may be remarked in Tracings 6 and 7 that, following a slight slowing of the auricular rate without prolongation of the *a-c* time, there were frequently recurring intermissions in the ventricular contractions lasting often for long periods of time. The hypothesis which was advanced in explanation of this phenomenon was similar to that which would seem to explain the effect of vagus pressure in this case, namely, that by increased vagus action the amount of the stimulus conducted from auricle to ventricle was diminished to such an extent that it was unable to call forth a response from a ventricle, the irritability of which was, possibly, in itself diminished, or that the same vagus influence served to depress the ventricular irritability.

The lesion in this heart is probably a fibrous myocarditis seriously involving the His bundle without totally destroying it. The clinical phenomena are remarkably similar to those in the case reported by Griffith and Cohn.[8] In this instance there was also an exceedingly prolonged *a-c* interval, amounting once to 0.6 second. The tracings show intermissions, owing to the dropping of occasional beats, or a 2 to 1 rhythm due to the dropping regularly of alternate beats from failure of conduction. On another tracing, the dropping of every third beat causes an alternation of short and long pauses, a 3 to 2 rhythm. Occasional

8. Remarks on the Study of a Case Showing a Greatly Lengthened *a-c* Interval with Attacks of Partial and Complete Heart-Block, with an Investigation of the Underlying Pathological Conditions, Quart. Jour. Med., 1910, vii, 126.

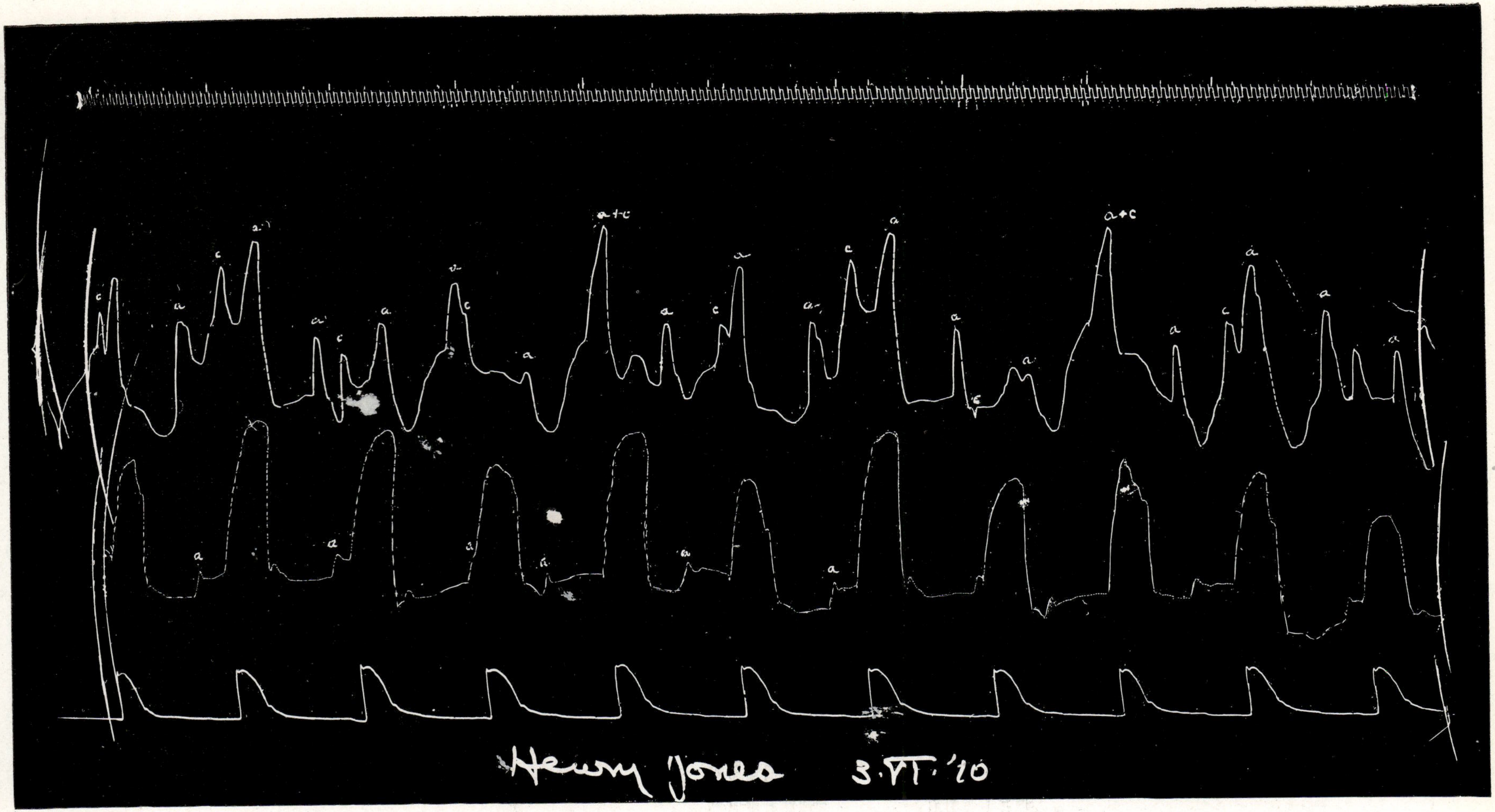


| | | | | | | | | | | | | | | | | | |
|---|---|---|---|---|---|---|---|---|---|---|---|---|---|---|---|---|---|
| .91 | .88 | .93 | .78 | .95 | .88 | .84 | .93 | .89 | .90 | .91 | .94 | .91 | .85 | .99 | .89 | .98 | .92 |

| | | | | | | | | | |
|---|---|---|---|---|---|---|---|---|---|
| .54 | .31 | .22 | .05 | .69 | .50 | .26 | .07 | .64 | .36 |

| | | | | | | | | | |
|---|---|---|---|---|---|---|---|---|---|
| 1.58 | 1.58 | 1.64 | 1.55 | 1.57 | 1.60 | 1.61 | 1.57 | 1.56 | 1.59 |

ventricular extrasystoles were noted, and finally, the establishment of a nearly regular ventricular rhythm of about 43, which the authors regarded as a 3 to 2 rhythm; this might, however, and we are inclined to believe, should be interpreted as we have interpreted Tracings 21 to 26 in Case 2; that is, as an automatic ventricular rhythm in which an occasional beat is hastened by an impulse which has passed through the *a-c* bundle. At other times there were periods of apparently total block with a rate of 26 per minute and once there was a characteristic alternating pulse. The lesion in this case proved to be an aneurysm of the right posterior sinus of Valsalva which had depressed the aortic cusp to such an extent that the septum membranosum was included in the aneurysmal pouch, severely compressing the main stem of the auriculoventricular bundle and cutting off the left branch.

## *GENERAL SUMMARY*

CASE 1.—A man of 53 with rather thickened arteries and a slightly enlarged heart, with evidences of sclerosis at the aortic ring (rough systolic murmur), showed:

1. Syncopal and convulsive seizures, associated with bradycardia and marked irregularity in the size and sequence of the beats. These occurred often in groups of three or more in rapid succession, followed by intermissions amounting sometimes to nearly or quite half a minute in length. The auricular rate, which could often be counted clearly in the neck, was usually 100 or above. Long intermissions in the ventricular pulse were usually associated with long periods of apnea. No wholly satisfactory tracings were taken during paroxysms of this sort. Those which we have suggest a complete dissociation.

2. Similar attacks, usually without convulsions, in which the ventricular beats occurred in groups of from two or three to ten, always at the same rate, and apparently following the same impulses as the auricular beats. These groups of beats were separated sometimes by intermissions amounting to as much as fifteen seconds. The auricular pulsations could usually be counted in the neck and were sometimes as slow as 59. Sphygmographic tracings showed that these groups of beats consisted of a primary ventricular contraction, apparently automatic, which was succeeded shortly by a series of beats which followed the preceding auricular contractions after an *a-c* conduction time of approximately normal duration. During these groups of beats the auricular rate became progressively slower without lengthening of the conduction time, until finally the ventricular impulses stopped. The retardation of the auricular impulses continued during the next several auricular contractions, after which it became more rapid.

Such attacks yielded on three occasions to the administration subcutaneously of atropin, gr. 1/60 (0.001 gm.). The auricular rate after atropin was slower than it was before, but more rapid than the rate of the several slow beats at the time of onset of the periods of ventricular intermission.

3. Periods during which there was a fairly regular ventricular rhythm of about 30 to the minute with a rather rapid auricular rate (100 to 120). The tracings show here an apparently complete auriculoventricular dissociation. One of these attacks failed to yield to atropin, gr. 1/30 (0.0021 gm.) given subcutaneously.

4. Periods during which intermissions in the ventricular pulse occurred at varying intervals and lasted for varying periods of time, followed usually by an apparently spontaneous ventricular contraction which was succeeded by one or more beats after a normal *a-c* conduction time. This condition, as shown in Tracings 4 and 5 would appear to be closely analogous to the condition described in paragraph 2. Indeed, it probably represents a lesser grade of the same condition.

5. Periods between these attacks in which the heart's action was regular, and the sphygmographic tracings revealed no abnormalities, the *a-c* interval remaining always normal.

Although there have been seven or eight grave attacks of Adams-Stokes' syndrome in a year and a half, the patient is to-day in good condition.

The remarkable features of this case appear to be the recurrence of long intermissions in the radial pulse, and the appearance at times of a total dissociation, with little or no evidence of a prolongation of the *a-c* conduction time, between attacks or during attacks in periods of partial block.

We have been inclined to regard the case as one of chronic sclerosis at the root of the aorta with partial involvement of the auriculoventricular bundle and a diminished irritability of the ventricle, many of the phenomena in the case being probably dependent on diminished ventricular irritability together with increased vagus influences. The cause of these waves of vagus action would appear to be wholly obscure.

Case 2.—A man, aged 83, had had for three or four years dyspnea on exertion and attacks of giddiness and faintness in which the had fallen to the street. Following treatment with infusion of digitalis, but persisting for more than a month after its discontinuance, there occurred periods of bradycardia, during which the pulse was sometimes nearly regular at about 40 and at other times irregular. The pulsations of the auricles observed in the neck were more frequent than those of the ventricles. The auricular pulsations further manifested themselves by a slight audible sound and sometimes by a palpable and even visible impulse at the apex. The cardiosphygmographic tracings showed a regular auriculoventricular rhythm with much prolonged *a-c* time, amounting sometimes to almost 0.6 of a second. At times, there is characteristic dropping out of ventricular beats associated with progressive prolongation of the *a-c* period and failure of conduction. At other periods, there is an attempt to set up a spontaneous ventricular rhythm at the rate of about 40, a rhythm, however, which is not quite regular because of an occasional precocious ventricular contraction, due, apparently, to the passage of a stimulus through the auriculoventricular bundle. The administration of atropin, gr. 1/30 (0.0021 gm.), resulted in the complete disappearance of irregularity and the development of a regular auriculoventricular rhythm with prolonged *a-c* conduction time.

Pressure on the vagus resulted in the dropping out sometimes of alternate and, occasionally, of two successive ventricular beats. There was slight slowing of the auricular rate with no apparent modification of the *a-c* conduction time.

On one occasion, the administration of atropin, gr. 1/30 (0.0021 gm.), was followed by rapid action of the heart with alternating pulse.

A year after the termination of our studies, the patient was seen again with an apparently complete auriculoventricular dissociation, the ventricular rate, however, being about 40.

This case we regard as a typical instance of disease of the bundle of His in a hypertrophied and dilated heart. The special points of interest are the extreme prolongation of the *a-c* conduction time, which at times was certainly as long as 0.56 second, and the evident efforts on the part of the ventricles to set up an automatic rhythm at a time when conduction was not completely blocked.

The many analogies between this case and that of Griffith and Cohn are also worthy of note.

406 Cathedral Street—13 Kirkland Avenue.

# A CASE OF POISONING DUE TO EATING POISON-HEMLOCK (CICUTA MACULATA)

## WITH A REVIEW OF REPORTED CASES *

ANFIN EGDAHL, M.D.
MENOMONIE, WIS.

The plant discussed in this paper, *Cicuta maculata* or, as it is more commonly called, water-hemlock or poison-hemlock, is a widely distributed plant in this country and has for centuries been known as a plant possessing a deadly poison. A number of cases of death have been reported by American and European physicians, but the cases undoubtedly are more numerous than those reported, as it is not always possible to ascertain the history of a case, a considerable number of the victims being children. The European form of the plant is called *Cicuta virosa*. It is found well distributed over the whole of Europe, but seems to vary somewhat in the activity of its poison in different localities.

It was not until the year 1876 that an approximate knowledge was obtained of the active agent in this plant. Boehm[1] published the results of a careful investigation into the characteristics of the poison and its action on certain animals and came to the conclusion that it was a resin. This was fatal to cats in doses of 5 cg. per kilo weight when given through the mouth and in doses of 7 mg. when given intravenously. The fatal dose for frogs was 2 to 3 mg. This substance Boehm has given the name of cicutoxin and regards it as the active agent of *Cicuta virosa*. The alkaloid coniin is also believed to be present. The poisons are found in all parts of the plant but chiefly in the root. When tried on animals it was found to be slowly absorbed through the intestinal tract; the effects at times would not appear until after the lapse of several hours. If vomiting took place it would very often save the life of the animal. Boehm was unable to find the exact place of absorption. When it was injected intravenously the action was very rapid, but absorption through the skin was slow. One observer states that it is popular knowledge in some parts of Europe that if slices of the roots of *Cicuta virosa* are placed on the backs of frogs convulsions will set in.

---

*This is not the poison-hemlock of historical interest. It is supposed that the cup of poison-hemlock drunk by Socrates was the *Conium maculatum*, a plant that has been introduced into this country.

1. Boehm: Arch. f. exper. Path. u. Pharmakol., 1876, v, 279.

The history of the case seen is characteristic of poisoning due to eating *Cicuta maculata.* The mother of the patient gave me the following details:

*History.*—The patient's family history was negative. She had always been well. There was no history of convulsions. While the patient was working with her father and younger brother in the field they found some strange-looking roots, which she tasted, and as they had a rather pleasant taste she chewed and swallowed some. (The exact quantity eaten could not be ascertained.) A few minutes afterward she fell over unconscious and had what her father called an attack of cramps. From this time on she was entirely unconscious and had convulsions every ten or fifteen minutes. She vomited several times and in the vomitus could be seen particles of the swallowed root. She was at once taken to the home.

*Examination.*—I first saw the patient about three quarters of an hour after the onset. She was entirely unconscious and slightly cyanotic; the eyes were dilated; the pupils did not react to light; there was loud, heavy breathing through nose and open mouth. Examination of mouth showed considerable amount of mucus and saliva, but was otherwise negative. The thorax was well formed. Fine râles were heard throughout both lungs. The heart was negative, 85 beats to minute. The pulse was of fair quality and force, normal in rate and rhythm, 85 to minute. The abdomen was negative.

*Course of Illness.*—Just after the completion of the examination the patient had one of her convulsive attacks of which three were observed. These began with twitching of the muscles around the mouth and eyelids, spreading rapidly to the muscles of the chest, arms, abdomen and lower extremities, until finally the muscles of the whole body were firm, hard and rigid, the forearms and hands slightly flexed and fingers clenched. The legs were extended and slightly parted; the head was slightly raised from the pillow, but the shoulders and buttocks rested on the bed. At the climax of the tonic convulsion the muscles of respiration appeared to be fixed, the face becoming markedly livid and cyanotic. Finally, when the patient appeared to be on the verge of suffocation, clonic convulsions would set in, the muscles would relax, and gradually the body would again come to rest. At the height of the attack the heart-beat would rise to 125-130 per minute.

The patient had no movements of the bowels or bladder during an attack, but froth and blood from a slight wound in the tongue appeared at the mouth.

These frightful convulsions were very different from any other convulsions that might be thought of under the circumstances, and when the mother showed me the root from which the child had eaten, it was decided at once to wash out the stomach. Dr. Heising was called in and with his assistance the stomach was emptied, though with the greatest difficulty on account of the violent convulsions.

At once the convulsions stopped, but a period of extraordinary restlessness appeared, lasting for about three hours, during which the patient tossed about aimlessly in bed from side to side and from one end to the other, striking her head against the bed or wall unless prevented from so doing. She was given doses of bromids and gradually became quiet; she remembered nothing, however, from the time the root was eaten at noon on Monday until the succeeding Wednesday evening. During this period she was very constipated and the bowels moved only by enemas. The stools presented nothing of particular interest. The bladder was unaffected. After the third day the patient made an uneventful recovery. The only thing worth mentioning was a stiffness and soreness of the whole body due, no doubt, to the convulsions.

It was learned that the father and the younger brother, a boy of 7, working with the patient had also tasted the roots. The father had chewed a bit of the root and spat it out, but shortly afterward felt dizzy and sick at the stomach. This passed over in a short time. The boy, however, shortly after eating a small quantity, became unconscious, had one convulsion and vomited the swallowed material. When seen he was conscious and resting quietly in bed but felt sick at the stomach. He made an uneventful recovery.

I sent the root shown me to Professor Ravenel, of the State Hygienic Laboratory at Madison, Wis. He kindly reported to me the results of an examination made by Dr. Dennison, of the department of botany of the

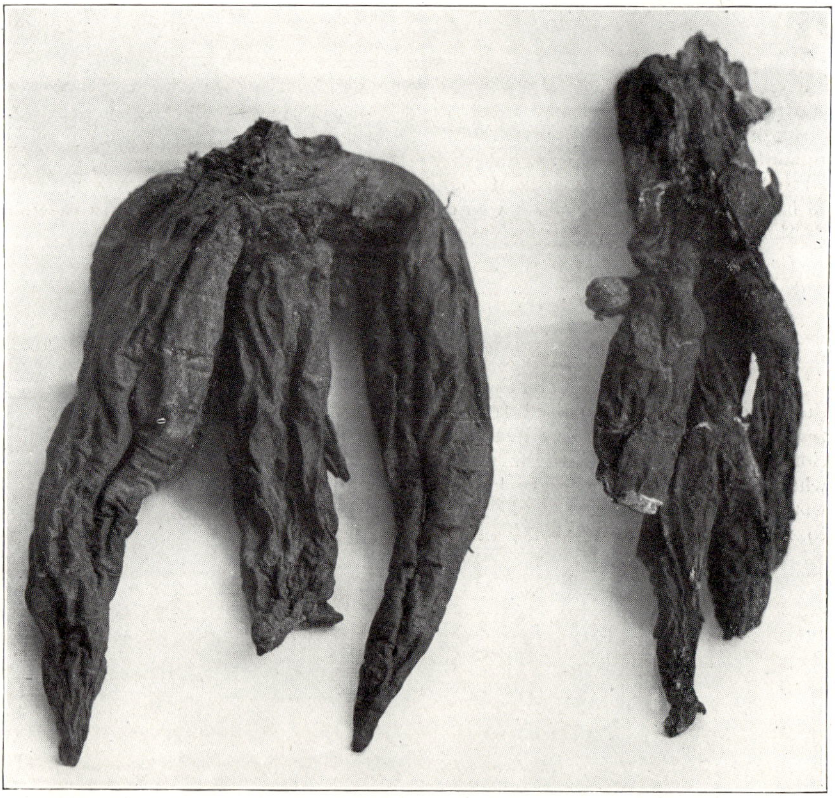

Partially dried roots of *Cicuta maculata.*

State University, who found that the root belonged to a plant popularly known as American water-hemlock, musquash-root, beaver-poison, children's bane, death of man, musquash-poison, poison-hemlock, poison snakeweed, spotted parsley, wild parsnip and wild hemlock, and botanically known as *Cicuta maculata.*

In the available literature forty-six cases of poisoning were found reported by European and American authors. The European physicians speak of the plant as *Cicuta virosa;* Professor Abel informs me, however, that those who have studied the two plants believe that they are very similar and possibly are identical. Certainly the clinical histories show no differences in symptomatology.

In looking over these histories the first point to be noticed is the great number of children among the victims, thirty-two out of a total of forty-six. This is to be expected, as few adult persons would eat the root except by mistake. A considerable number of the adult victims mistook the roots for spikenard, carrots, and a number of other edible roots. One person was given the roots cooked in a vegetable soup with homicidal intent. One other person had the root served with cooked vegetables with no knowledge of its toxic properties. The results seemed to be just as violent when the roots were eaten after cooking as when they are taken uncooked. Chevallier[2] reports five most interesting cases. A family of five was troubled with severe itching; for relief the skin was rubbed with *Cicuta aquatica*, with the result that all developed toxic symptoms and two of the children died. It has already been mentioned that it is possible to produce convulsions in frogs by rubbing the skin with slices of *Cicuta virosa*.

The symptoms of onset were very much the same in all the cases. Pain and discomfort in the region of the stomach were the first symptoms mentioned in five cases. This came on shortly after eating and varied in severity from a discomfort to severe pain; in one case the pain became a general distress.

The most characteristic and pronounced symptoms, however, were nausea, vomiting, and convulsions. These appeared in a few cases while the patients were still eating the roots; but in most of the cases from half an hour to two hours afterward. In several reports mention is made of the fact that the vomitus contained particles of the eaten root. The convulsions in typical cases are most violent and many of the observers speak of them as epileptiform. Bloody froth at the mouth is a usual occurrence, but no mention is made of involuntary movement of bowels or bladder. One adult person was killed by a fall sustained while in convulsions. A fatal termination occurred in twenty-one cases.

Of the minor symptoms may be mentioned:

| | |
|---|---|
| Dizziness is spoken of | in 4 cases |
| Buzzing in ears | in 2 cases |
| Arhythmia of heart | in 3 cases |
| Violent beating of heart | in 3 cases |
| Small and slow pulse | in 6 cases |
| Pulse fast (120-140 per minute) | in 1 case |
| Pulse moderate (90 per minute) | in 2 cases |
| Weak respiration | in 1 case |
| Uneven respiration | in 3 cases |
| Rapid respiration (40-45 per minute) | in 2 cases |

2. Chevallier: Jour. de chim. méd., 1836, series 2, ii, 606.

| | | |
|---|---|---|
| Paralysis and numbness of limbs | in | 2 cases |
| Stupor | in | 2 cases |
| Twitching of muscles | in | 1 case |
| Dryness of throat | in | 1 case |
| Feeble palate reflex | in | 1 case |
| Conjunctiva bloodshot | in | 1 case |
| Swollen abdomen | in | 1 case |
| Abdomen not rigid | in | 1 case |
| Pain in region of heart | in | 1 case |
| Fever | in | 1 case |
| Dilated pupils | in | 21 cases |
| Facial pallor and cold skin | in | 11 cases |
| Unconsciousness | in | 9 cases |
| General weakness | in | 2 cases |
| Anxious expression of face | in | 1 case |
| Skin warm and dry | in | 1 case |
| Very mobile eyeballs | in | 1 case |
| Trismus | in | 1 case |
| Hallucinations | in | 1 case |
| Deafness and confusion, etc | in | 1 case |
| Flushed face | in | 1 case |
| Pupils respond to light | in | 1 case |
| Pupils did not respond to light | in | 1 case |
| Diarrhea | in | 2 cases |
| Sweating | in | 3 cases |
| No sweating | in | 1 case |
| Polyuria | in | 1 case |
| Double vision | in | 1 case |

From this it will be seen that we have here a root containing a poison capable of producing a great variety of symptoms of varying degrees of importance. It is noteworthy that the observation made by Boehm experimentally that in cases in which early and free vomiting took place, often the life of the animal would be saved, is borne out clinically. Early and free vomiting is a most favorable occurrence and in the great majority of patients recovering, this took place either spontaneously or through the administration of emetics. There is some evidence to show that the vomiting is due to an action on a center in the brain.

Autopsies are reported in only five cases. The only findings worth mentioning are slight redness and injection of the gastric and upper intestinal mucosa and the presence of the eaten roots as the exciting agent. No change of particular significance can be pointed out. In one case a spotted condition of the spleen is mentioned.

The poisonous properties of the root are not lost by drying; but Boehm states that exposure to a temperature of 100 C. always diminishes its activity. Clinically, however, as has already been noted, cooked roots have produced death with all the important symptoms caused by eating the uncooked root. The ethereal or alcoholic solution of the poison may retain its toxic properties for years when kept at an ordinary temperature.

Boehm believes that the active principle acts on a center in the medulla oblongata, causing convulsions, stoppage of respiration, increase in blood pressure and vagus irritation. Experimentally cicutoxin has been found to produce in frogs: (1) violent clonic and tonic convulsions; (2) acceleration of respiration, which, however, ceases during the convulsive seizures; (3) slowing of the heart and, during the convulsive seizures, a long diastolic pause. All of these effects Boehm ascribed to an action on Heubel's center for convulsions, supposed to be located at the point of the calamus scriptorius.

The experimental effects on mammals may be summarized as follows: diarrhea, salivation, muscular twitchings, increased frequency of respiration appear shortly after administration of the drug; then there sets in violent convulsions affecting all the voluntary muscles of the body. During these convulsive attacks there has been noted a stoppage of respiration but a marked increase in the force of the heart-beats. Usually the contents of the urinary bladder are forced out, possibly owing to the violent contractions of the abdominal muscles. The convulsions last from about half a minute to two minutes. In the intervals the respirations are deep; the pupils are not always dilated but just before death dilatation appears. Death occurs usually at the height of a convulsive attack. Experimentally no characteristic local effects have been produced. Bennevitz[3] noted congestion of the blood-vessels of the brain in guinea-pigs. This, he concluded, might be due to a narcotic action of the poison.

The mode of action, and the toxic and pharmacological properties of the active agent or agents in this plant need to be studied over again.

Other poisons of the same group to which cicutoxin belongs are picrotoxin, obtained from *Anamirta paniculata,* œnanthotoxin, the active principle of *Œnanthe crocata;* coriamyrtin, which occurs in several species of *Coriaria;* phytolaccotoxin, prepared from a Japanese species of *Phytolacca,* which may possibly also be obtained from *Phytolacca decandra* or pokeberry. A number of the digitalis series contain bodies which may produce the same symptoms as cicutoxin and the other members of the picrotoxin group. Among these are toxiresin, obtained from digitoxin, digitaliresin, from digitalin, and oleandresin, from oleandrin. These bodies all produce powerful stimulation of the central nervous system, more especially of the areas around the medulla oblongata. Two alkaloids, samandarin and samandaridin, obtained from the skin of the newt, appear to resemble the members of the picrotoxin group in their effect.

Cushny[4] states that picrotoxin and its allies act chiefly on the medulla oblongata, while the spinal cord and the higher parts are little affected. He believes that there is no necessity for believing in the existence of a convulsion center, as intense stimulation of the medulla will produce clonic contractions of the muscles throughout the body. The medulla is

3. Bennevitz: Med. Ztg., 1836, v, 51.
4. Cushny: Pharmacology and Therapeutics, 1901, p. 425.

not, however, the exclusive seat of action for in many animals the reflexes are found to be increased when the medulla is severed from the cord and this indicates that the spinal cord is also more excitable than normally. Cushny states, in his text-book on pharmacology, that the action of the picrotoxin series on the spinal cord is best seen in the fish and reptile, but in the higher animals the action is more confined to the region of the medulla oblongata.

An interesting observation has been made by Christison,[5] in Scotland. He found that during the month of August the roots, leaves and fruit were almost without effect. This, Huseman[6] believes, is not due to climate, as in those parts of Scandinavia with almost the same climate the *Cicuta virosa* is decidedly poisonous during that month, so there must be other conditions affecting its activity.

Very meager data can be obtained as to the quantity of the root capable of producing death in an adult person. Prof. Charles Lee[7] states that a dram and a half has been known to destroy human life, but in view of Christison's observation just mentioned it may be that the activity of the poison varies with the seasons and with the locality. Lieutenant Carpenter,[8] U. S. A., states that two men who had eaten a whole root died in an hour and a half; a third who had eaten only a very small quantity recovered.

In the diagnosis of a case the following are the important points to be kept in mind, as shown in the case-histories quoted and the case of the patient observed.

1. The eating of parts of a strange plant and especially of the root, resembling that of the poison-hemlock.

2. The characteristic symptoms, pain in the region of the stomach, nausea, vomiting, and the frightful convulsions appearing usually within an hour. Especially significant is the presence of parts of the eaten plant in the vomitus. Unconsciousness is a condition seen in all of the cases of which I have had an oral description—four in number. In the cases reported in print, however, it is mentioned in only nine cases. Final proof is, of course, furnished by the demonstration of parts of the plant.

With a history of eating of a wild plant, with pain and discomfort in the region of the stomach, nausea and vomiting, and convulsions supervening within an hour or one hour and a half, the presumption is justifiable if the case is seen in this country, that the plant eaten is *Cicuta maculata*. Other poisonous wild plants found in the United States that are capable of causing convulsions are: black cherry (*Prunus serotina*);

---

5. Christison, quoted by Pribram: Arch. f. Krim.-Anthrop. u. Kriminalist, Leipsic, 1900, iv, 166.

6. Huseman, quoted by Pribram: Arch. f. Krim.-Anthrop. u. Kriminalist, Leipsic, 1900, iv, 166.

7. Lee, Charles: quoted in Tr. Minnesota State Med. Soc., 1871, Vol. I, 53-55.

8. Carpenter: Quoted in Tr. Minnesota State Med. Soc., 1871, I, 53-55.

Jamestown or jimson weed (*Datura tatula* and *Datura stramonium*); black nightshade (*Solanum nigrum*); and the sneeze-weed (*Helenium autumnale*). The convulsions produced by these plants are not, however, so severe as those produced by poison-hemlock.

In regard to the treatment there is not much to be said. Meyer[9] used a decoction of gallnuts in one case with very satisfactory results. Wine of antimony (tartar emetic) and zinc sulphate has been used in several, causing free emesis. The stomach-tube is, however, the most satisfactory on account of the quick and sure results obtained. It may also be well later to wash out the bowel thoroughly and give an active cathartic. The ordinary methods for the comfort of the patient, suitable bed-clothing, hot-water bottles to extremities where indicated, sponge baths, and bromids if the patient is very restless, are simple, efficient methods of treatment that have been used in many cases with good results. To control the very severe convulsions before the removal of the poison, chloroform and chloral have been suggested.

Considerable damage is done every year to cattle, which eat the tubers, or may be poisoned in marshes by drinking water contaminated by the juice of the roots, which may have been crushed by being trampled on. Melted lard is recommended for the treatment of cases of poisoning among cattle.

In regard to prophylaxis two thoughts will at once come to mind: (1) the education of the public to recognize our poisonous plants; and (2) the extermination of poisonous plants. Both of these methods can be employed, and as far as the *Cicuta maculata* is concerned the eradication of this plant in well-populated portions of the country would not be a difficult undertaking, if the people were taught to recognize it and to know its poisonous properties. In these days of preventive medicine, instruction in the recognition of our principal poisonous plants, about thirty in number, could be given in the departments of botany in our high schools, colleges, universities, and agricultural schools, and would undoubtedly result in the saving of a considerable number of human lives annually, as well as in the prevention of suffering experienced by thousands of people every year.

NOTE.—In addition to the authorities cited in the text, the following may be found of interest:

Caillard: Clin. d. hôp., Paris, 1829, iv, 33.

Chesnut: Principal Poisonous Plants of the United States, Bull. 20, U. S. Dept. Agri., Washington, D. C.

Hazeltine: New England Jour. Med. and Surg., 1818, vii, 219.

Henning: Mitt. a. d. Geb. d. Med., Altona, 1836, iv, 84.

Hwass: Upsala Lakaref. Förh., 1877-8, xii, 262.

Jawandt: Jour. d. pract. Arznk. u. Wundarznk., Jena, 1798, v, 588.

Kelp: Vrtljschr. f. gerichtl. Med., 1879, new series, xxx, 380.

---

9. Meyer: Med. Ztg., 1842, xi, 178.

Little: Clinic, Cincinnati, 1874, vii, 49.
Maly: Oesterr. med. Wchnschr., 1844, pp. 1065, 1097.
Matchett: Cincinnati Lancet and Obs., 1870, new series, xii, 462.
Stockbridge: New England Jour. Med. and Surg., 1814, iii, 334.
Trousdale: Brit.-Am. Jour., 1862, iii, 37.
Wilson: Lancet, London, 1871, ii, 396.
Folk: Tr. South Carolina Med. Assn., 1882, xxxii, 69.
Mossberg: Eira, Stockholm, 1889, xiii, 435.
Pohl: Arch. f. exper. Path. u. Pharmakol., 1894, xxxiv, 259.
Pribram: Arch. f. Krim.-Anthrop. u. Kriminalist, Leipsic, 1900, iv, 166.
Boehm: Arch. f. exper. Path. u. Pharmakol, 1874-5, iii, 216.

# THE OPSONIC INDEX IN THE DIAGNOSIS OF MIXED INFECTION IN PULMONARY TUBERCULOSIS *

ROSWELL T. PETTIT
OTTAWA, ILL.

The importance of mixed infection in tuberculosis is at present a much-disputed question. Some investigators believe that secondary invasion by pyogenic organisms is responsible for practically all the damage done in "consumption," while others believe that the tubercle bacillus alone is capable of producing all the pathological changes. Between these two extremes of opinion are found those occupying all possible positions in the middle ground. The reason for this great disagreement of opinion among investigators and clinicians is the inefficiency of the methods used in the diagnosis of mixed infection. Practically all of our data on the subject, up to the present time, have been obtained by: (1) animal experimentation; (2) post-mortem histological and bacteriological examination of the lung; (3) blood cultures before and after death; and (4) sputum examination.

The results obtained in animal experimentation are greatly at variance with each other. Sputum inoculated into rabbits and mice has resulted in a rapid septicemia due to the pyogenic organisms present; but Sternberg and Pasteur were able to produce septicemia with normal saliva. Prudden's[1] work in 1894 on the importance of streptococcus in cavity formation in guinea-pigs has been discounted since Marmorek[2] produced cavities by injecting tubercle bacilli in pure culture together with large quantities of tubercle toxins in 1907.

The results obtained by post-mortem examination of the lung are not reliable because of agonal and post-mortem bacterial invasion. The results of Ravenel[3] show many *Bacilli coli, Sarcinæ, Protei vulgares* and other organisms that undoubtedly invade the lung at the time of death or soon after. To just what extent streptococcus is an agonal invader, or at least a terminal infectious agent in these cases is difficult to determine.

Blood-cultures made from the heart's blood immediately after death show the presence of streptococci in a high percentage of cases. Repeated examinations of the blood in the same cases before death were negative.

---

* Work done under the Max Pam Research Fund.

1. Prudden, T. M.: New York Med. Jour., 1894, lx, 1.
2. Marmorek, A.: Compt. rend. Soc. d. Biol., 1907, lxii, 123.
3. Ravenel, M.: Rep. Henry Phipps Inst., 1907, iii, 216.

The streptococcus probably invaded the blood-stream in these cases during the agonal period, or soon after (Beco).

Blood-cultures during life have been positive only in far-advanced cases, and in most of the positive cases on record the organism was present as a terminal infection. Many of the early positive results reported are not reliable because sufficient precaution was not taken against contamination. More recently, however, with improved technic, organisms other than the tubercle bacillus have been isolated from the blood of tuberculous patients. In some of these cases the organism was not present as a terminal infection; one of Panichi's[4] patients did not die until seven months after the blood-culture was made (Panichi[5]).

The results obtained by sputum examination are very unsatisfactory. All the organisms of mixed infection found in the sputum of a patient suffering from pulmonary tuberculosis are found normally in the mouth, pharynx and trachea of the healthy individual. Whether they are present in the healthy lung is a disputed question. Cornet[5] says that they are not present in the atria and alveoli of the normal lung, and other investigators[6] say that they are. Because of the great variety of bacteria present normally in the upper air-passages, the sputum examined for organisms of mixed infection has been subjected to washing and the results obtained have varied greatly with the manner and intensity of this procedure. Most authorities advocate washing the fresh sputum in six changes of sterile salt solution. Sorgo[7] believes that this is insufficient, and says that the sputum should be whipped violently and broken into small bits, from a majority of which both the tubercle bacillus and secondary organisms can be cultivated. His results indicate that mixed infection is not so common as other observers have believed.

Our present methods of diagnosis of mixed infection are uncertain. Hence, a method of serum diagnosis, if reliable, would be of great value. The opsonic index, when introduced, promised to be such a method. Webb[8] has used it, but considers it too laborious a procedure for routine work. Yet he obtained abnormal indices to pyogenic organisms in cases suffering from pulmonary tuberculosis. He says:

> The third method of ascertaining the activity of these secondary organisms, testing the patient's resistance to them as measured by their opsonic indices, is a laborious and unnecessary procedure. In repeated instances patients have been found with a low index to their own staphylococcus and pneumococcus, and in febrile cases they have shown fluctuating indices to these as well as the tubercle bacillus.

---

4. Panichi: Berl. klin. Wchnschr., 1908, xlv, 1840.
5. Cornet, G.: Tuberculosis, edited by W. B. James, Philadelphia, 1905; W. B. Saunders Company, p. 583.
6. See references given by Norris and Pappenheimer: Jour. Exper. Med., 1905, vi, 48.
7. Sorgo: Ztschr. f. Tuberk., 1904, vi, 382.
8. Webb, G.: In Klebs' Tuberculosis, N. Y., 1909, D. Appleton & Co., p. 594.

Wirths[9] examined twenty-five cases of tuberculosis. He found no change in the opsonic index to *Diplococcus capsulatus, Micrococcus tetragenus catarrhalis,* the meningococcus, *Bacillus pneumoniæ,* the pseudo-diphtheria bacillus, *Bacillus coli,* or *Bacillus subtilis,* but he found abnormal variation in the opsonic index to the staphylococcus, streptococcus, pneumococcus and influenza bacillus. He considered the normal variation between 0.8 and 1.2. He also found that serums that gave a normal reading on drawing if allowed to stand twenty-four hours gave abnormal readings. He used the usual Wright technic and found the following:

2 abnormal opsonic indices (12 per cent.) out of 17 examined to *Bacillus influenzæ.*

2 abnormal opsonic indices (12 per cent.) out of 17 examined to staphylococcus.

18 abnormal opsonic indices (75 per cent.) out of 24 examined to pneumococcus.

6 abnormal opsonic indices (31 per cent.) out of 19 examined to streptococcus.

No change was found in five out of twenty-five cases, or 20 per cent. He found abnormal indices to both pneumococcus and streptococcus in six cases and abnormal indices to both pneumococcus and influenza in two cases, to staphylococcus and pneumococcus in one case. He found no change in the index in patients with hectic fever and he found normal temperatures in cases showing variation in the index to pneumococcus.

I have examined the opsonic index to streptococcus, pneumococcus, and staphylococcus in forty cases of pulmonary tuberculosis. I found the index to all of them between 0.8 and 1.2 in all cases but one and in this case the index to staphylococcus was 0.75. This case was complicated by a rectal sinus. Bacteriological examination of this sinus showed staphylococci. In several of these cases that were far advanced blood-cultures were made and Gram-positive cocci, undoubtedly streptococcus or pneumococcus, obtained. The blood-cultures were confirmed by finding Gram-positive cocci in blood-smears. Leukocyte counts were made in nearly all the cases. The usual Wright technic for the opsonic index was used on serums one or two days old.

In making the blood-cultures, blood (15–25 c.c.) was taken from the cubital vein in a sterile syringe; and 2 c.c. run over agar surfaces in each of two large flasks; and 5–10 c.c. introduced into each of two flasks containing 150 c.c. of litmus milk. Blood-smears were made by puncturing the lobe of the ear of the patient after washing the skin with alcohol and drying with sterile cotton, taking a drop of blood with a sterile loop and spreading between two coverslips. The smears were stained by Gram's method and counterstained with eosin.

---

9. Wirths, M.: Beitr. z. Klin. d. Tuberk., 1908, xii, 159.

Even in cases of undoubted mixed infection as shown by the fever, the leukocytosis, the positive blood-cultures and the findings of Gram positive organisms in blood-smears, there was no variation in the opsonic index to streptococcus, staphylococcus or pneumococcus.

The results are shown in the accompanying tables:

Table 1.—Opsonic Index to Various Organisms with Blood-Culture, Blood-Smears and Leukocyte Count

| No. | Classification. | —Opsonic Index to— Pneumococcus. | Staphylococcus. | Streptococcus. | Blood-Culture. | Blood-Smears. | Leukocytes. |
|---|---|---|---|---|---|---|---|
| 1 | Incipient, active........ | .94 | .96 | .92 | .... | .... | 8,200 |
| 2 | Far-advanced, passive... | .96 | .97 | .94 | .... | .... | 9,200 |
| 3 | Advanced, passive....... | .98 | .98 | 1.2 | .... | .... | 13,200 |
| 4 | Advanced, active........ | .91 | .95 | .88 | .... | .... | 17,000 |
| 5 | Advanced, active........ | .97 | .98 | 1.1 | .... | .... | 15,000 |
| 6 | Advanced, passive....... | .91 | .94 | .85 | .... | .... | 14,000 |
| 7 | Advanced, active........ | .90 | .95 | 1.1 | .... | .... | ..... |
| 8 | Advanced, active........ | .93 | .94 | 1. | .... | .... | 11,200 |
| 9 | Advanced, active........ | .95 | .98 | .95 | .... | .... | 17,000 |
| 10 | Advanced, active........ | .91 | .85 | .94 | .... | .... | 34,000 |
| 11 | Advanced, active........ | .97 | .93 | .84 | .... | .... | 22,000 |
| 12 | Advanced, passive....... | .95 | .98 | .87 | — | + | 33,000 |
| 13 | Advanced, passive....... | .98 | .97 | .95 | .... | .... | 17,400 |
| 14 | Incipient, passive....... | .96 | .92 | .98 | .... | .... | 11,000 |
| 15 | Advanced, active........ | .96 | .90 | .89 | .... | .... | ..... |
| 16 | Advanced, active........ | .90 | 1. | .92 | .... | .... | 18,000 |
| 17 | Advanced, passive....... | .90 | .92 | 1.2 | .... | .... | 19,000 |
| 18 | Advanced, passive....... | .93 | .98 | .95 | .... | .... | ..... |
| 19 | Advanced, active........ | .93 | .95 | .91 | .... | .... | ..... |
| 20 | Far-advanced, active.... | .96 | .94 | .85 | — | .... | 15,000 |
| 21 | Advanced, active........ | .97 | .93 | .86 | — | .... | 35,000 |
| 22 | Far-advanced ........... | .90 | .87 | .94 | + | + | 17,000 |
| 23 | Advanced, active........ | .87 | .92 | .89 | .... | .... | 15,000 |
| 24 | Advanced, active........ | .94 | .96 | .97 | .... | .... | 6,600 |
| 25 | Advanced, active........ | .89 | .91 | .84 | +(?) | .... | 13,400 |
| 26 | Incipient, passive....... | .98 | 1.2 | .96 | .... | .... | 7,000 |
| 27 | Advanced, active........ | .93 | .87 | .83 | .... | .... | 18,000 |
| 28 | Incipient, passive....... | .97 | .96 | .90 | .... | .... | ..... |
| 29 | Advanced, active........ | .96 | .85 | .92 | .... | .... | 9,800 |
| 30 | Advanced, passive....... | .96 | .96 | .98 | .... | .... | ..... |
| 31 | Advanced, passive....... | .94 | .96 | 1. | .... | .... | 21,000 |
| 32 | Advanced, passive....... | .97 | .94 | ... | .... | .... | ..... |
| 33 | Far-advanced, active.... | .93 | .88 | ... | — | .... | 8,400 |
| 34 | Far-advanced, active.... | .90 | .93 | .91 | + | .... | 19,000 |
| 35 | Incipient, passive....... | .98 | .94 | .89 | .... | .... | 23,000 |
| 36 | Advanced, active........ | .96 | .95 | .84 | .... | .... | 27,000 |
| 37 | Advanced, active........ | .96 | .97 | .84 | .... | .... | 29,000 |
| 38 | Advanced, active........ | .96 | .87 | .83 | + | + | 43,000 |
| 39 | Far-advanced, active.... | .94 | 1. | .83 | + | + | 18,000 |
| 40 | Advanced, active........ | .98 | .94 | .85 | .... | .... | ..... |

Table 2.—Characteristics of Organisms Isolated in Blood-Cultures

*Case 25.*—Plain Agar: White scattered colonies; small.
Potato: No growth.
Gelatin at 23°; growth along needle track; slight surface growth.
Litmus Milk: Acid production; fine granular curd; whey not separated.
Bouillon: Single; diplococci; clumps and short chains of Gram-positive cocci.

*Case 34.*—Plain Agar: No growth.
Potato: No growth.
Gelatin: No growth.
Bouillon: Very slight precipitate (?).
Dextrose Agar: No growth on surface; slight growth along needle track.
Blood-Agar: Clear, dew-like, greenish (?) colonies.
Gram-positive, single, diplococci and short chains, in smears from blood-agar.

*Case 39.*—Blood-Agar: Few clear colonies of definite greenish color.
Plain Agar: Slight growth, clear colonies.
Potato: No growth.
Litmus Milk: Acid production, coagulation.
Gelatin at 23°: No growth.
Gram-positive cocci in pairs from agar and milk.

*Case 38.*—Blood-Agar: Small grayish-white scattered colonies.
Plain Agar: Slight dew-like growth.
Potato: No definite growth.
Litmus Milk: Acid production, coagulation, no digestion.
Gelatin: Fine scant growth along needle track.
Gram-positive single and diplococci in milk.

*Case 22.*—Litmus Milk: Finely granular. Showed Gram-positive diplococci after five days.
Blood-Agar Plate: Small greenish (?) colonies.
No growth on any other media.

*Case 12.*—Blood-Agar: Profuse white growth.
Plain Agar: White extensive growth.
Potato: White powdery growth.
Litmus Milk: Acid production, coagulation, no digestion.
Bouillon: Profuse growth with precipitate.
Large single, and diplococci and cocci in clumps. Gram-positive.

In all cases, except Case 12, the organisms isolated from the blood show scant growth or none at all on the usual albumin-free culture media. For this reason I believe them to be streptococci and pneumococci rather than staphylococci and that they really came from the blood and were not present as contaminations from the skin or air.

Since this paper was written I have extended the blood-culture work and by certain modifications of technic have demonstrated conclusively that these sparsely growing Gram-positive cocci in pairs and chains come from the blood-stream and are not present in the cultures as contaminations. I have made blood-cultures in seventy-five cases of pulmonary tuberculosis and have found unquestionable streptococci or pneumococci in 45 per cent. of those examined. A report of this work will appear in another paper.

From these results I conclude that, in my hands at least, the opsonic index is not an accurate method of diagnosis of mixed infection in pulmonary tuberculosis.

# ENTAMŒBA TETRAGENA AS A CAUSE OF DYSENTERY IN THE PHILIPPINE ISLANDS *

CHARLES F. CRAIG, M.D.
WASHINGTON, D. C.

During the past seven years the researches of Schaudinn,[1] Viereck,[2] Hartmann and Prowazek,[3] Wenyon,[4] and others have demonstrated the existence of at least three species of amebas which are parasitic in the intestine of man. In 1903, Schaudinn extended the previous investigations of Casagrandi and Barbagallo,[5] and Jurgens,[6] and distinguished two species of amebas parasitic in the human intestine, placing them in the genus *Entamœba,* established by Casagrandi and Barbagallo. To one species, which he found in a large proportion of healthy individuals, as well as in diseases other than dysentery, he gave the name *Entamœba coli;* while to the other, which he found in patients suffering from dysentery, he gave the name *Entamœba histolytica.* In 1905, while working on the amebas present in soldiers invalided home from the Philippines because of amebic dysentery, I was able to confirm Schaudinn's work, and to show that the two species described by him were present in this group of islands,[7] and his conclusions have since been confirmed by nearly every student of the Protozoa. A few careful observers still maintain that the differentiation of these species is not based on sufficient evidence, but it is probable that they have confused the ameba which is the subject of this paper with the species described by Schaudinn, a mistake which is but natural when one remembers that *Entamœba tetragena* resembles both the species differentiated by Schaudinn and his followers.

---

* This paper, by Captain Charles F. Craig, Medical Corps, U. S. Army, is from the laboratory of the office of the Surgeon-General of the Army, Washington, D. C., Major F. F. Russell, U. S. Army Medical Corps, Director, and is published by authority of the Surgeon-General U. S. Army.

1. Schaudinn, F.: Arb. a. d. kais. Gsndhtsamt., 1903, xix, 563.

2. Viereck: Beiheft z. Arch. f. Schiffs- u. Tropenhyg., 1907, i, 1.

3. Hartmann, M., and Prowazek, S.: Arch. f. Protistenk., 1907, x, 312. Hartmann, M.; Beiheft z. Arch. f. Schiffs- u. Tropenhyg., 1908, v, 117.

4. Wenyon: Report Wellcome Research Laboratories, 1908, iii, 122.

5. Casagrandi, O. and Barbagallo, F.: Ann. d'ig. sper., 1897, new series, vii, 103.

6. Jurgens: Veröffentl. a. d. Geb. d. mil. San.-Wes., 1902, xx, 110.

7. Craig, C. F.: Am. Med., 1905, ix, 854, 897, 936; Jour. Infect. Dis., 1908, v, 324.

Briefly stated, the differentiation between *Entamœba coli* and *Entamœba histolytica* rests on differences in the appearance of the protoplasm and nucleus, and in the methods of reproduction. *Entamœba coli* presents no distinction between the ectoplasm and endoplasm, even when moving, save that the ectoplasm is free from granules; the nucleus is generally easily seen and possesses a definite nuclear membrane and is rich in chromatin; reproduction occurs by simple division; schizogony, with the formation of eight daughter amebas, and encystment, with the formation within the cyst of eight young amebas. *Entamœba histolytica,* on the other hand, presents a very great distinction between the ectoplasm and endoplasm, especially when moving, the ectoplasm being much lighter in color, more refractive, and glassy in appearance; the nucleus, while present, is generally invisible, has no well-defined nuclear membrane, and contains but a small amount of chromatin, while reproduction occurs by simple division, by gemmation or budding, and when conditions are unfavorable to vegetative existence, by the formation of minute spores which are formed by chromidia and a portion of protoplasm budding from the parent organism.

While studying amebas at the Army General Hospital, San Francisco, I had no difficulty in finding *Entamœba histolytica* in the feces of many of the patients suffering from dysentery, and *Entamœba coli* in the feces of healthy individuals. Since that time I have had the opportunity of studying these parasites in many hundreds of cases, and have found that Schaudinn's description of these species is correct. At the same time, an ameba was occasionally observed which could not be considered as typical of either of the species mentioned, in that it possessed a distinct ectoplasm, a well-defined nucleus containing much chromatin, and reproduced by simple division and the formation of cysts containing four daughter amebas. I have observed the same amebas both in soldiers suffering from dysentery contracted in the Philippines and in natives of those islands, and until the description by Viereck of *Entamœba tetragena,* I considered it as an atypical form of *Entamœba coli* or *Entamœba histolytica.*

In 1907, Viereck described an ameba occurring in patients suffering from dysentery contracted in Africa, and during the same year an independent description of the same organism was published by Hartmann and Prowazek. Viereck called the parasite *Entamœba tetragena,* and as his publication appeared before that of Hartmann and Prowazek, who had named it *Entamœba africana,* Viereck's name must be accepted as the proper zoological name of this species. As described by these authors, and since confirmed by Bensen[8] and others, *Entamœba tetragena* presents a very marked distinction between the ectoplasm and endoplasm when in

8. Bensen, W.: Arch. f. Schiffs- u. Tropenhyg., 1908, xii, 661.

motion; possesses a well-defined nucleus, rich in chromatin, and reproduces by simple division and the formation of cysts containing four young amebas.

At the time that I had the opportunity of studying amebas in San Francisco and in the Philippines the species now known as *Entamœba tetragena* had not been described, but on looking over my notes of cases observed during the past seven years I find frequent notations of the occurrence of an ameba corresponding to *Entamœba tetragena* in the feces of soldiers suffering from dysentery contracted in the Philippine Islands, and last winter, while demonstrating these parasites to the class at the Army Medical School, my attention was called to an ameba in one of the specimens which answered to the description of this species. The amebas in this instance were obtained from a discharged soldier who had contracted dysentery in the Philippine Islands and who had suffered from many recurrences. On careful study this ameba was found to agree in morphology and life-history with *Entamœba tetragena,* so that I have no hesitation in stating that this observation, taken in conjunction with my previous notes on a similar ameba observed in soldiers returning from the Philippines, proves to my mind that *Entamœba tetragena* is a frequent cause of dysentery in those islands. Moreover, I believe that much of the confusion and difficulty regarding the differentiation of *Entamœba coli* and *Entamœba histolytica* in the Philippines has been due to the presence in many cases of this third species which, possessing as it does morphological features common to both of the other species, has been confused with them and has furnished an argument against accepting Schaudinn's classification. Thus, while *Entamœba histolytica,* the dysentery ameba of Schaudinn, does not possess a well-defined nucleus, and does not encyst as does *Entamœba coli,* yet in certain cases of dysentery an ameba was observed not infrequently in which, as in *Entamœba histolytica,* there was a distinct differentiation of the ectoplasm and endoplasm but which contained a well-defined nucleus and formed cysts similar to those of *Entamœba coli.* Prior to the description of *Entamœba tetragena* it was impossible to classify such amebas properly, but the identification of this form with *Entamœba tetragena* explains the difficulty and will, I am sure, make the classification of the amebas found in man in the Philippines a much simpler task. From my observations I am convinced that there occur at least three species of amebas parasitic in the intestine in man in the Philippine Islands, two of them, *Entamœba histolytica* and *Entamœba tetragena,* causing dysentery, and one, *Entamœba coli.* a harmless commensal occurring in the intestine both in health and in disease.

The accompanying table gives the principal differential features of the species mentioned and will be found of service in differentiating them.

DIFFERENTIAL FEATURES OF ENTAMŒBA COLI, ENTAMŒBA HISTOLYTICA, AND ENTAMŒBA TETRAGENA

| *Name* | *Size* | *Pseudopodia* | *Motility* | *Protoplasm* | *Nucleus* | *Cyst Formation* | *Cultures* | *Methods of Reproduction* | *Pathogenesis* | *Staining* |
|---|---|---|---|---|---|---|---|---|---|---|
| *Entamœba coli,* Schaudinn, 1903. | 10 to 30 microns. Generally smaller than *Entamœba histolytica* or *Entamœba tetragena.* | Small, blunt and not clearly differentiated from rest of parasite. | Sluggish. | Ectoplasm not distinct except when moving, and then only because it is free from granules. Is grayish in color and not very refractive. Endoplasm is gray, finely granular, few non-contractile vacuoles. Is not generally phagocytic for red-blood corpuscles. | Distinct, having a well-defined nuclear membrane and much chromatin. Large karyosome. | Present. Eight young amebas developed within cyst. | Doubtful. | By simple division; autogenous sexual reproduction in cyst; and by schizogony with the production of eight daughter amebas. Eight amebas are produced within the cyst. | Is not pathogenic, occurring in a large percentage of healthy individuals. | With Wright's stain, ectoplasm, light blue; endoplasm, dark blue, and nucleus, red. |
| *Entamœba histolytica,* Schaudinn, 1903. | 10 to 70 microns. Generally from 15 to 40 microns. | Blunt or slender and finger-shaped. Very refractive and clearly differentiated from rest of the parasite. | Active. | Ectoplasm is very distinct and refractive, in some instances even when motionless. Glassy appearing. Endoplasm is granular, contains numerous non-contractile vacuoles and red-blood corpuscles, when latter are present in the feces. | Indistinct. No well-defined nuclear membrane and but little chromatin. Minute karyosome. | Minute spores developed by budding. Measure 3 to 5 microns. Possess a resistant membrane like a cystic covering. Development of the spores have not been studied. | Doubtful. | By simple division; gemmation; and by the budding of chromidial masses surrounded by protoplasm from the periphery of the mother parasite, forming minute spores. | Is the cause of a form of amebic dysentery. | With Wright's stain, ectoplasm, dark blue; endoplasm, light blue, and nucleus, pale red or pink. |
| *Entamœba tetragena,* Viereck, 1907. | 10 to 50 microns. About the size of *Entamœba histolytica* | Lobose or finger-shaped. Very refractive and well differentiated from rest of parasite. | Active. | Ectoplasm and endoplasm well differentiated. Ectoplasm hyaline in appearance. Endoplasm granular, containing numerous non-contractile vacuoles and red-blood corpuscles, when latter are present in the feces. | Distinct, having definite nuclear membrane formed by chromatin. Large karyosome. | Present. Four amebas develop within cyst. | Negative. | By simple division, and by autogamous sexual reproduction within cyst, four amebas being produced. | Is the cause of a form of amebic dysentery. | Does not stain well with Wright's stain |

A study of the table demonstrates that *Entamœba tetragena,* as regards its morphology and life-cycle, resembles both *Entamœba coli* and *Entamœba histolytica* and that until it was identified as a distinct species it must have caused great confusion in the differentiation of the species described by Schaudinn, either when it occurred alone in patients suffering from dysentery, or in combination with *Entamœba coli* or *Entamœba histolytica.* Further research on the amebas of the human intestine as observed in the Philippine Islands will decide how large a proportion of the amebic dysentery there present is caused by this parasite, but I believe that it will be found to be considerable and that this species of ameba has been responsible for most of the difficulty which some have experienced in the differentiation of Schaudinn's species, *Entamœba coli* and *Entamœba histolytica.*

# THE ACIDOSIS INDEX

## A CLINICAL MEASURE OF THE DEGREE OF ACIDOSIS

T. STUART HART, M.D.
NEW YORK

The detection of a condition of acidosis is usually a simple matter. The quantitative determination of the degree of acidosis, while most important from the clinical standpoint, is often neglected on account of the difficult and time-consuming procedures necessary to obtain accurate information.

### METHODS OF ESTIMATING THE DEGREE OF ACIDOSIS

The degree of acidosis may be determined in several ways. For the purpose of the present discussion, only those methods are considered which have for their object the determination of those forms of acidosis due to the presence of the acetone bodies, seen in their most severe types in diabetes mellitus.

1. The method of Stadelmann,[1] a classical chapter in the history of the discovery of the abnormal production of organic acids in diabetes, depends on the quantitative estimation of the bases (sodium, potassium, calcium, magnesium and ammonium) and of the inorganic acids of the urine. When organic acids are being excreted, it is found that the amount of bases excreted is in excess of the amount necessary to combine with the estimated inorganic acids. This excess of bases is excreted in combination with organic acids and therefore furnishes data upon which one may accurately estimate the amount of organic acids being eliminated. While this method is of great value, the amount of time required makes its employment prohibitive in ordinary clinical work.

2. Perhaps the most satisfactory procedure is the direct quantitative estimation of acetone and diacetic acid by the method of Messinger,[2] as modified by Huppert, or by the method of Hart,[3] combined with the estimation of oxybutyric acid by the method of Shaffer[4] or of Black.[5] These determinations give us most satisfactory direct information as to the degree of acidosis, but in turn must be discarded in clinical work on account of the time, skill, and facilities required for their execution.

---

1. Stadelmann: Arch. f. exper. Path. u. Pharmakol., 1883, xvii, 419.
2. Messinger: Analyse des Harns, 1898.
3. Hart: Jour. Biol. Chem., 1908, iv, 477.
4. Shaffer: Jour. Biol. Chem., 1908, v, 211.
5. Black: Jour. Biol. Chem., 1908, v, 207.

3. The levo-rotary properties of beta-oxybutyric acid make possible its quantitative determination by means of the polariscope, and while this gives us information of significant value, it is not a method of great accuracy and is one which can be used only with careful technic and a considerable expenditure of time.

4. Since the recognition of the fact that the organism protects itself from its excess of organic acids by the production of increased amounts of ammonia, the quantity of the ammonia excreted has been utilized to estimate the extent of the acidosis. The quantitative estimation of ammonia gives us much important information, not only as regards the degree of acidosis, but also as regards the effect of the therapeutic administration of alkalis, and its determination by Folin's[6] method is so simple and accurate that this should be a routine procedure in every advanced case of acidosis. One should, however, interpret the ammonia findings with due reference to the facts which are known to effect variations in its production, especially that it is regularly augmented on a diet rich in protein, and is produced in increased amounts for the purposes of neutralizing acids only when these acids are not already satisfied by the bases furnished by the body or taken in as food or medication. It is therefore evident that during the administration of alkalis the ammonia output is not a measure of the quantity of organic acids being excreted.

## NEW CLINICAL METHOD

Several years ago I proposed a simple test-tube method[7] for estimating the degree of acidosis in cases of moderate severity. I have used this with considerable satisfaction in following cases with the production of small amounts of acetone and diacetic acid, and I have sought to extend its usefulness by devising a simple method which should give us a rough clinical idea of the daily fluctuations of the organic acid output in cases of severe acidosis.

It should be clearly stated at the outset that there is no claim that this method accurately estimates the quantitative excretion of the acetone bodies. It does, however, afford real information in regard to the fluctuation of the total acidosis from day to day; it is certainly simpler and probably more accurate than the measure of acidosis which we obtain with the polariscope; and while it does not replace the information afforded by the determination of ammonia, it is of considerable value as a complement to this, especially when alkalis are being administered. In regard to all these points I hope to submit satisfactory proof.

---

6. Folin: Ztschr. f. physiol. Chem., 1902, xxxvii, 161.

7. Hart, T. S.: A Contribution to Our Knowledge of the Acetone Bodies, with a Clinical Method for the Quantitative Estimation of Diacetic Acid and Acetone, The Archives Int. Med., 1908, i, 218.

The method depends on the intensity of the color developed by adding ferric chlorid to urine containing the acetone bodies (Gerhardt's reaction). The solutions necessary are:

1. The "standard solution," consisting of ethyl acetate, 1 c.c.; alcohol, 25 c.c.; and distilled water to 1,000 c.c.

2. Ferric chlorid solution, consisting of 100 gm. of ferric chlorid dissolved in 100 c.c. of distilled water.

Take two test-tubes of equal caliber (one-half inch in diameter), put in one 10 c.c. of the "standard solution," and in the other 10 c.c. of the urine to be tested, add to each 1 c.c. of the ferric chlorid solution, allow the tubes to stand for a couple of minutes to permit the color to develop fully, and then compare the color of the two test-tubes when they are held between the eye and the sky. If the tube containing the "standard solution" is of a lighter shade than the urine mixture, dilute this with distilled water until the colors match, noting the volume to which it has been necessary to dilute the urine mixture.

By this means we obtain what we may call the "acidosis index per liter" in accordance with the following schedule:

| Volume of Urine Solution. | | Acidosis Index per Liter. |
|---|---|---|
| 10 c.c. | = | 1 |
| 15 c.c. | = | 1.5 |
| 20 c.c. | = | 2 |
| 25 c.c. | = | 2.5 |
| 40 c.c. | = | 4 |
| 100 c.c. | = | 10 |

(Intermediate volumes have a proportional index).

In order to obtain the "acidosis index" proper, we multiply the value of the "acidosis index per liter" by the amount of urine in liters passed in twenty-four hours.

For example: A patient passed 3,200 c.c. urine in twenty-four hours; when 10 c.c. of this was treated as described above, it was found necessary to dilute this to 75 c.c. in order to match the standard; his "acidosis index per liter" was therefore 7.5 and his "acidosis index" was 7.5 times 3.2 = 24.

## MATERIAL

This paper is based on observations made on forty-one cases of acidosis, varying in intensity from the mildest grades to those of extreme acid intoxication. By far the greater part were diabetics, but a few others have been included, viz., starvation, obesity, carcinoma of the stomach, febrile and post-operative cases. The material was drawn almost entirely from private practice, only a few hospital cases have been included. The patients were observed for varying periods, some seen in consultation were observed but once, while others have been followed personally for five or six years. The maximum number of observations made on a single case was 63.

EVIDENCE OF THE VALUE OF THE ACIDOSIS INDEX FOR ESTIMATING ORGANIC ACID ELIMINATION

In Table 1 is presented the record of a patient suffering from severe progressive diabetes terminating in coma July 6, 1909, who was seen at intervals for a considerable period.

I would call attention to the parallelism which exists between the degree of acidosis as estimated by the polariscope and the "acidosis index." This is shown graphically in Chart 1, which has been plotted from the values of Table 1. It will be noticed that the rise and fall of the two curves is very similar in direction, notwithstanding the fact that the curves tend to diverge in the higher values. This point will be referred to later.

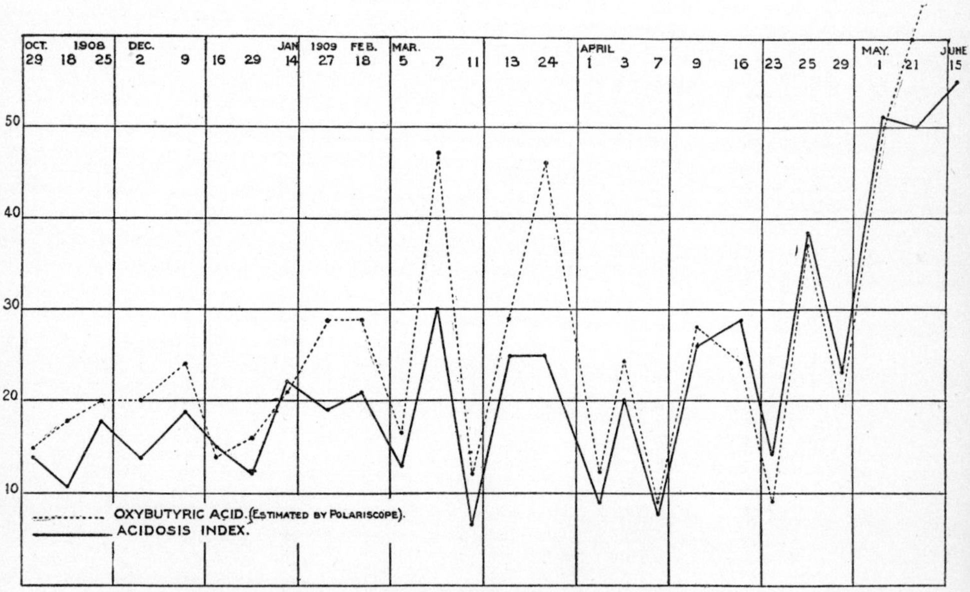


Chart 1.—Curve of oxybutyric acid estimated by polariscope, and acidosis index plotted from record of diabetic patient (Table 1).

Chart 2 is also plotted from Table 1. Here are compared the curves of the ammonia output and the "acidosis index." For this comparison only those days were selected from Table 1 on which the patient was taking no alkali, as on these occasions the ammonia more nearly represents the degree of acidosis.

Table 2 records the events of a severe diabetes in a boy aged 12; only those days are recorded on which no alkali was taken; this patient is still under occasional observation. Chart 3 is plotted from this record and shows a comparison of the curves of the ammonia output and the "acidosis index."

Cases of this kind could be multiplied, but they all show a very definite parallelism in the curves of the "acidosis index" and those of the acidosis estimated by the polariscope, and as calculated on the ammonia output.

In Table 3 will be found the record of the final month of a case of diabetes ending in collapse. In this case for a considerable period the total acidosis was accurately determined[8] by the method of Shaffer.

In Chart 4 the same case is recorded graphically. Here the ammonia curve is omitted, as this was modified by the administration of varying amounts of bicarbonate of soda by mouth and by infusion.

TABLE 1.—RECORD OF A DIABETIC PATIENT

| Date. | Urine Quantity c.c. | Ammonia gm. | Oxybutyric Acid, Estimated by Polarization gm. | Acidosis Index. | Bicarbonate of Soda gm. |
|---|---|---|---|---|---|
| 10/29/08 | 2,310 | .... | 15 | 14 | 0 |
| 11/10/08 | 1,920 | .... | .. | 10 | 0 |
| 11/18/08 | 2,100 | .... | 18 | 11 | 0 |
| 11/25/08 | 2,220 | .... | 20 | 18 | 12 |
| 12/ 2/08 | 2,220 | .... | 20 | 14 | 12 |
| 12/ 9/08 | 2,700 | .... | 24 | 19 | 16 |
| 12/16/08 | 2,100 | .... | 14 | 15 | 0 |
| 12/29/08 | 2,400 | 3.284 | 16 | 12 | 0 |
| 1/14/09 | 3,195 | 1.711 | 21 | 22 | 45 |
| 1/27/09 | 2,670 | 6.038 | 29 | 19 | 0 |
| 2/18/09 | 2,610 | 4.748 | 29 | 21 | 45 |
| 3/ 5/09 | 2,550 | 4.487 | 17 | 13 | 0 |
| 3/ 7/09 | 3,030 | 3.757 | 47 | 30 | 45 |
| 3/11/09 | 1,770 | 2.798 | 12 | 7 | 0 |
| 3/13/09 | 2,190 | 2.420 | 29 | 25 | 45 |
| 3/24/09 | 4,200 | 5.790 | 46 | 25 | 0 |
| 4/ 1/09 | 1,770 | 3.490 | 12 | 9 | 0 |
| 4/ 3/09 | 2,700 | 5.449 | 24 | 20 | 0 |
| 4/ 7/09 | 2,060 | 4.132 | 9 | 8 | 0 |
| 4/ 9/09 | 2,130 | 3.349 | 28 | 26 | 45 |
| 4/16/09 | 3,630 | 1.388 | 24 | 29 | 45 |
| 4/23/09 | 4,020 | 3.140 | 9 | 14 | 0 |
| 4/25/09 | 4,260 | 4.092 | 37 | 38 | 45 |
| 4/29/09 | 4,590 | 4.760 | 20 | 23 | 0 |
| 5/ 1/09 | 4,620 | 4.673 | 51 | 51 | 45 |
| 5/21/09 | 4,560 | 5.889 | 60 | 50 | 45 |
| 6/15/09 | 5,450 | 6.152 | 96 | 55 | 60 |

TABLE 2.—RECORD OF SEVERE DIABETES IN A BOY AGED 12

| Date. | Urine Quantity c.c. | Ammonia gm. | Acidosis Index. | Date. | Urine Quantity c.c. | Ammonia gm. | Acidosis Index. |
|---|---|---|---|---|---|---|---|
| 12/24/08 | 1,920 | 1,882 | 6 | 4/17/09 | 3,600 | 3,458 | 14 |
| 1/16/09 | 1,920 | 2.310 | 5 | 4/28/09 | 1,920 | 2.778 | 8 |
| 1/29/09 | 1,920 | 3.525 | 10 | 5/13/09 | 1,920 | 4. | 13 |
| 2/11/09 | 2,016 | 3.513 | 8 | 5/27/09 | 2,400 | 3.958 | 12 |
| 2/26/09 | 1,995 | 2.171 | 7 | 11/ 2/09 | 4,440 | 4.151 | 13 |
| 3/12/09 | 2,520 | 4.862 | 13 | 4/21/10 | 5,760 | 7.056 | 35 |
| 3/26/09 | 2,490 | 3.259 | 12 | 5/28/10 | 5,760 | 3.819 | 20 |

8. I am indebted to Dr. H. O. Mosenthal for assistance in making a part of these analyses.

TABLE 3.—FINAL MONTH OF A CASE OF DIABETES ENDING IN COLLAPSE

| Date. | Urine, Quantity. | Ammonia | Oxybutyric Acid Estimated by Polarization. | Total Acidosis as Oxybutyric Acid Determined Chemically. | Acidosis Index. | Bicarbonate of Soda, gm. |
|---|---|---|---|---|---|---|
| | c.c. | gm. | gm. | gm. | | gm. |
| 11/30/08 | 4,800 | 3.07 | 63 | .... | 58 | 60 |
| 12/ 2/08 | 4,680 | 3.51 | 62 | .... | 51 | 60 |
| 12/ 6/08 | 4,470 | 4.22 | 69 | .... | 47 | 24 |
| 12/ 8/08 | 4,050 | 3.90 | 62 | 38.13 | 36 | 50 |
| 12/10/08 | 3,150 | 3.24 | 55 | 24.67 | 30 | 25 |
| 12/13/08 | 2,040 | 1.89 | 31 | 21.25 | 20 | 25 |
| 12/15/08 | 1,800 | 3.35 | 24 | 16.11 | 16 | 0 |
| 12/17/08 | 1,800 | 3.59 | 20 | 16.40 | 14 | 0 |
| 12/21/08 | 2,310 | 4.02 | 36 | 17.73 | 17 | 10 |
| 12/24/08 | 2,550 | 4.45 | 28 | 19.27 | 20 | 10 |
| 12/29/08 | 3,360 | 3.55 | 15 | 12.70 | 13 | 5 |

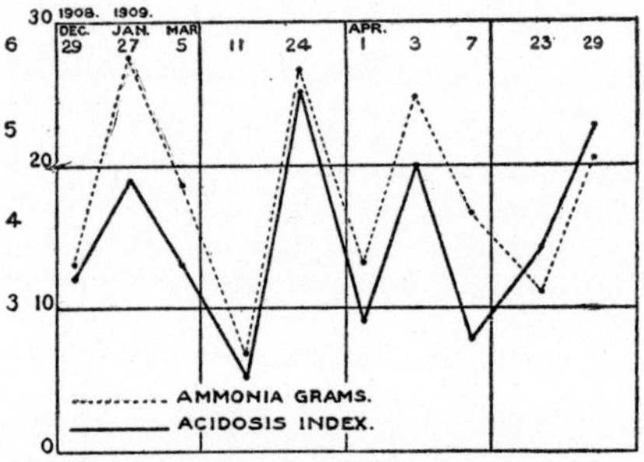


Chart 2.—Ammonia output and acidosis index, plotted from record of diabetic patient (Table 1).

It will be observed that there is a well-marked parallelism in the three curves. The similarity in the curves of the "acidosis index" and the total acidosis accurately estimated in grams of oxybutyric acid is extraordinary.

It is to be noted that while the parallelism of the three curves obtained by different methods is quite evident, the values estimated from the polariscopic readings are much too high, particularly in the larger amounts. This is entirely in harmony with the observations of Magnus Levy,[9] who has pointed out that the polariscopic estimations of beta-oxybutyric acid have given exaggerated values. This may explain the variations in the curves of Chart 1, where the polariscopic estimations are relatively very high when the acidosis is high. For this reason, and on account of the fact that the "acidosis index" corresponds much better with the ammonia output (see Chart 2), I am inclined to think that the

9. Magnus-Levy: Arch. f. exper. Path. u. Pharmakol., 1899, xlii, 149.

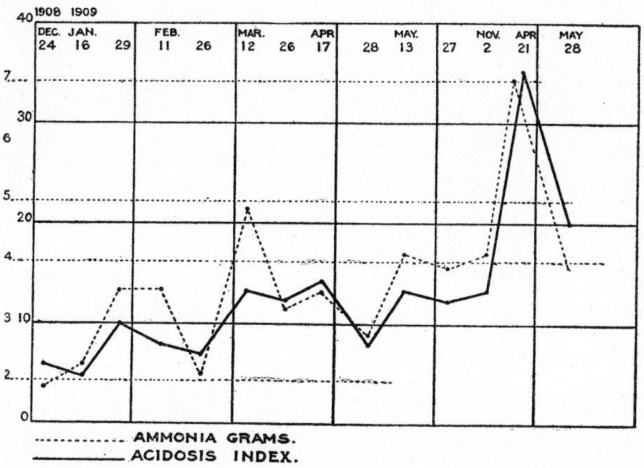


Chart 3.—Ammonia output and acidosis index, plotted from record of diabetic patient (Table 2).

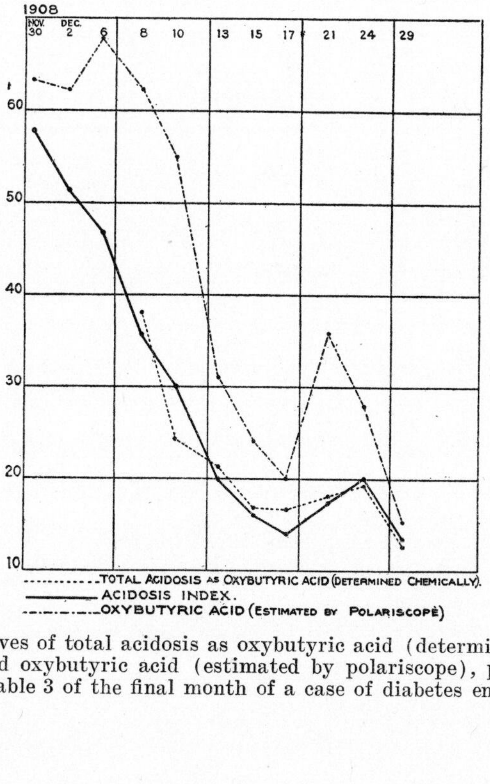


Chart 4.—Curves of total acidosis as oxybutyric acid (determined chemically), acidosis index and oxybutyric acid (estimated by polariscope), plotted from the record given in Table 3 of the final month of a case of diabetes ending in collapse.

"acidosis index" represents the actual degree of acidosis much more accurately than the polariscopic determination.

The "acidosis index" is of considerable value in those cases in which alkali is being administered. On the alkali days the ammonia output is usually greatly diminished and yet the "index" may be as great or even greater than on the non-alkali days. This denotes a large excretion of acetone bodies combined with the alkali, which has temporarily lessened the need for the large ammonia production. On these days the comparison of ammonia values and the "acidosis index" indicates the extent to which we have been able to replace ammonia by the ingested alkali.

### QUANTITATIVE VALUE OF THE ACIDOSIS INDEX

After observing the remarkable correspondence between the total acidosis accurately estimated and the "acidosis index" (see Chart 4), one is tempted to assign a quantitative value to the "acidosis index" (acidosis index 1 = 1 gram oxybutyric acid). This is the only case in which I have carried out a series of observations of the "acidosis index" checked by the total acidosis estimated by this method; but a few other isolated observations made in the same way tend to corroborate this value.

Moreover, Table 4, based on some 83 observations in fifteen individual cases, lends weight to this view.

TABLE 4.—ACIDOSIS INDEX IN 15 CASES, FROM 83 OBSERVATIONS

| Acidosis Index. | Ammonia 24 Hours—grams Averages. | Acidosis Index. | Ammonia 24 Hours—grams Averages. |
|---|---|---|---|
| 1 | 1.123 | 12 | 3.500 |
| 2 | 1.375 | 13 | 4.338 |
| 5 | 2.303 | 17 | 4.487 |
| 7 | 2.960 | 20 | 4.634 |
| 8 | 3.474 | 23 | 4.760 |
| 9 | 3.424 | 25 | 5.790 |
| 10 | 3.525 | 35 | 7.056 |

TABLE 5.—AMMONIA EQUIVALENTS FOR ACIDOSIS

| Oxybutyric Acid gm. | Ammonia—Grams: To Neutralize Acid. | From Food. | Total. |
|---|---|---|---|
| 6 | 1 | 1.5 | 2.5 |
| 12 | 2 | 1.5 | 3.5 |
| 18 | 3 | 1.5 | 4.5 |
| 24 | 4 | 1.5 | 5.5 |
| 30 | 5 | 1.5 | 6.5 |
| 36 | 6 | 1.5 | 7.5 |

In constructing Table 4, only those days were selected on which the patients were getting no alkali. The figures are for the most part averages. For example: In nine instances, each showing an "acidosis index" of 7, the ammonia output averaged 2.960 gm. If we assume that the high proteid diet of these days furnished 1.5 gm. of ammonia and that each additional gram of ammonia represents an acidosis of 6 gm. of oxybutyric acid,[10] we would obtain the values shown in Table 5.

If these figures are compared with those of Table 4, it will be seen that there is a very close similarity in the ammonia equivalent for an acidosis represented by a given amount of oxybutyric acid and the corresponding figures of the "acidosis index." When we recall, however, that the method of obtaining the "acidosis index" depends on the color reaction of diacetic acid, and that the relative amount of diacetic acid varies greatly,[11] inferences as to its quantitative value should be assumed with great caution and only after a much greater number of comparisons between the total acidosis (chemically determined by the more accurate methods) and the "acidosis index" have been made.

I think, however, that we are safe in concluding from the above studies that the "acidosis index" is of much value in following the daily fluctuations of the organic acid output, affording information well worth the three or four minutes necessary for its acquisition.

## CONCLUSIONS

1. The "acidosis index" is a measure of acidosis based on the depth of color obtained with the ferric chlorid reaction.

2. The values thus obtained run parallel with the degree of acidosis estimated by (a) the polariscopic method, (b) ammonia output, (c) chemical determination of the acetone bodies.

3. It is probably a better measure of acidosis than the polariscopic method.

4. It is a more accurate measure of acidosis during the administration of alkalis than the estimation of ammonia, and is a valuable complement to the estimation of ammonia.

5. It is a simple clinical means of following the daily fluctuations of the organic acid excretion.

6. The value of the information gained from a knowledge of this "acidosis index" is well worth the expenditure of the few minutes necessary for its acquisition.

130 West Fifty-Ninth Street.

10. Magnus Levy: Arch. f. exper. Path. u. Pharmakol., 1901, xlv, 389.
11. Hart: Jour. Biol. Chem., 1908, iv, 476.

# ACUTE YELLOW ATROPHY OF THE LIVER

## REPORT OF TWO CASES

EMIL NOVAK, M.D., and E. L. WHITNEY, M.D.
BALTIMORE

### CLINICAL AND PATHOLOGICAL STUDY, BY DR. NOVAK

Not only the rarity of this disease, but also the probable relation which it bears to certain other interesting conditions—the obstetrical toxemias, delayed chloroform poisoning, etc.—has induced us to report these two cases. According to Dr. J. Wickham Legg, who made a rather elaborate study of the history of this disease, the first description of the condition was given by Ballonius, who died in 1616. It was not, however, until 1843 that the name "acute yellow atrophy" was bestowed on the disease by Rokitansky. That the condition is a rare one can be appreciated from the fact that the total number of reported cases in all probability does not exceed 450. Out of 25,000 cases admitted to the London Fever Hospital during a period of nine years Murchison encountered only one case of this disease, while only three cases have occurred at the Johns Hopkins Hospital during its entire history, the third having been reported only recently by Thayer. So experienced a clinician as Osler stated in the third edition of his text-book (1898) that he had never observed a case up to that time, a statement which seemed to create some surprise among some of his contemporaries. The two cases which we are about to report have occurred within a period of about two and a half years, and are the only ones of which there is any record at the Maryland General Hospital.

Case 1.—The patient was a colored woman, aged 38, who applied for treatment at the gynecologic department of the dispensary on February 28, 1906, complaining of dysmenorrhea and increased frequency of micturition, which was accompanied by occasional stinging and burning pain. There was nothing of significance in her family history. She had always enjoyed good health, and no history of luetic infection was obtained. She had had no children, but gave a history of two miscarriages, the last having occurred about one year previously. The pelvic examination disclosed nothing of much significance, the uterus being small, moderately anteflexed, and freely movable, with no signs of existing or previous pelvic inflammation. Cystoscopic examination revealed the presence of a number of small ecchymotic areas over the lateral walls and fundus of the bladder, together with a mild grade of trigonitis. Examination of the catheterized specimen of urine showed the presence of bile pigments and the absence of albumin or casts. The presence of the jaundice next directed our attention to the liver. There was no history of gastro-intestinal symptoms, such as are usually observed in ordinary catarrhal jaundice, nor was there anything in the history to suggest a possible cholelithiasis. Examination of the liver was also negative, the liver dulness being of normal extent and there being no tenderness over any part of the liver region. The patient was instructed to return for further observation within a few days, but unfortunately she failed to do so, and we saw nothing of her until sixteen days later (March 16). At this time a message was sent to the hospital requesting that some one be sent to visit the patient at her home. The hospital intern who responded to the call found the woman comatose and evidently in a critical condition, and I was requested to see the patient with him. The woman was now intensely jaundiced, absolutely comatose, with a temperature of 101 F. and a pulse of 120. The rather unsatisfactory history elicited from the other occupants of the house was to the effect that the woman had been ailing from the time she had been at the dispensary. She had complained of pains over the entire body, especially in the limbs, and had vomited several times, while the yellowness of her eyeballs had been noticeable to those around her for some time. She had taken to her bed only the day before (March 15) at which time the vomiting had become very severe. During the night the patient had been restless and "out of her head," but by no means violent. Toward morning she had become quiet, and when I saw her, as stated above, she was in a condition of profound coma.

*Liver Dulness.*—Examination of the liver disclosed a most interesting condition, for there was a very striking decrease in the area of liver dulness, the lower border of which seemed to be almost a hand's breadth above the costal margin in the right mammary line. From the fact that the abdomen was soft and flat, and that there was no meteorism, there seemed to be no doubt that a very decided diminution in the size of the liver had occurred.

Both the clinical history and the physical examination seemed to point indubitably toward the diagnosis of acute yellow atrophy of the liver, and this diagnosis was therefore made. The patient was catheterized and a specimen of urine (90 c.c.) obtained for examination.

From this time the patient grew steadily worse and death occurred late in the afternoon of the same day (March 16), less than thirty-six hours from the time she had taken to her bed. With some difficulty I obtained permission to remove the liver through a small abdominal incision.

*Pathological Report.*—Macroscopic Examination: The liver is markedly diminished in size, weighing only 635 grams. Its consistency is very soft and flabby, so that if laid on a flat surface it tends to flatten out very decidedly. The capsule is loose and wrinkled, giving the organ a more or less shriveled appearance. The atrophy seems to be more marked in the left lobe, which is very small and tongue-like in appearance. On section the liver tissue is found to be moderately firm to the knife, the cut surface presenting a light yellowish background, studded with irregular splotchy areas of a reddish-brown appearance.

Microscopic Examination: The histological picture is on the whole one of such wide-spread degeneration that the section would scarcely suggest liver tissue. The normal lobular architecture of the liver is entirely lost. In some portions there is evident only a widespread necrosis of the liver cells, the nuclei staining poorly or not at all, and the protoplasmic outlines being very indistinct. Many of the cells appear to be much swollen and they are frequently vacuolated. Many of them, again, are filled with globular masses of a refractile appearance, suggestive of fat, although owing to the fact that osmic acid preparations are not available it is possible that this material may be glycogen. A considerable amount of brownish and orange-colored pigment is scattered throughout the liver cells, and a few plate-like crystals of cholesterin are seen.

In other areas the liver cells seem to some extent to have withstood the degenerative change and are gathered together in tube-like columns, suggestive of the tubular structure of the primitive liver. In these areas the nuclear staining is less impaired and the cell outlines are somewhat more distinct. Nowhere, however, can one observe anything approaching the normal histological structure of the liver.

The interstitial tissue seems to be present in greater amount than normal, although the increase may, in part at least, be relative, owing to the extensive destruction of the parenchyma. There is a very decided infiltration of small round cells, particularly in the neighborhood of the blood-vessels and bile-ducts, the infiltrating cells in some places being collected into clumps of rather lymphomatous appearance. There is a very decided proliferation of the bile-ducts, which show in some places a tendency to push into the degenerated lobules in the form of budding outgrowths. This is to be construed as an evidence of the regenerative changes which have been described as occurring in this disease by MacCallum and others. No mitoses are observed. The large bile-ducts show comparatively little pathological change.

On the whole, one of the most striking features is the varied appearance presented in different sections and even in different parts of the same section, so that the above picture must be considered as a more or less composite one.

CASE 2.—The patient, a colored woman, aged 20, was admitted to the Maryland Lying-In Hospital, at 10 p. m., on June 8, 1908 (service of Dr. J. M. H. Rowland, to whom I am indebted for the privilege of making this report). She had been in labor for a period of fourteen hours. Her family history was unimportant, but her previous history was of interest in that she had been pregnant twice before, her first labor, two and one-half years before, being complicated by a severe eclamptic attack, and her second pregnancy terminating prematurely at the seventh month. During the early months of her present pregnancy the patient had suffered with a moderate degree of vomiting, but this had not been excessive, nor was there any history of any other toxic manifestation during the course of this gestation. On the patient's entrance to the hospital she was examined by my colleague, Dr. Seegar, who found a moderate degree of pelvic contraction, and in view of the fact that after fourteen hours of pain the head was not yet well engaged, manual dilatation and version was decided on. Chloroform was used as an anesthetic, the duration of anesthesia being about 40 minutes. The operation itself presented no very unusual difficulties, and at its close (June 9, 1:30 a. m.) the patient was in good condition. Temperature a few hours afterward was 100.2 F., pulse 96.

I saw the patient for the first time on the day following delivery (June 10). At this time her temperature was 99.6 F., pulse 104, and her general condition seemed good, except that she was rather irritable and apathetic. This, however, we were inclined to attribute to her naturally surly temperament. The next day (June 11), it was noticed that her conjunctivæ were slightly icteric, and that the patient was even more somnolent than on the previous day. Evening temperature was 98.8 F., pulse 90.

On the morning of June 12, the patient was taken with severe vomiting, while the jaundice became much more marked. Constipation was obstinate, neither purgatives nor enemas being of any avail. The patient's mental condition was gradually growing worse. Questions put to her in an ordinary tone of voice received no response, and when she was spoken to in a loud voice only an indistinct mumbling reply was made. Percussion of the liver at this time seemed to show a slight decrease in size, but owing to the existence of a moderate grade of tympanites, too much importance could not be attributed to this sign. Temperature at this time 100.4 F., pulse 108.

From this time there was a steady progression of all the symptoms. The vomitus, which at first had consisted chiefly of a greenish-yellow fluid, now became tinged with altered blood, and later assumed the typical coffee-ground appearance. The temperature and pulse both rose as the patient grew worse, and the coma became absolute. There was no delirum. On percussion the area of liver dulness was found to be noticeably diminished, the lower border being about two finger-breadths above the costal margin. Death occurred on the afternoon of June 14, about five and one-half days after delivery, three and one-half days after the appearance of jaundice, and two and one-half days after the onset of the grave symptoms of the second stage of the disease. The temperature shortly before death reached 106.6 F., pulse 160.

The treatment in this case was largely symptomatic. Purgatives and enemas were given in an attempt to overcome the obstinate constipation, and when the heart action became rapid and feeble, strychnin sulphate was resorted to. In addition to this, salt solution was administered freely, both subcutaneously and by the rectum.

*Pathological Report.*—The following extracts from the autopsy protocol embrace the points of especial interest in this case:

Liver: The organ is appreciably decreased in size (weight 1,225 grams), the diminution, however, not being comparable to that seen in Case 1. The capsule is smooth throughout. The color of the liver is a very unusual shade of light yellow—almost an "ochre yellow." On section, however, the cut surface is seen to be studded everywhere with numerous small areas of a reddish-brown, hemorrhagic appearance. These areas, while they differ in size, are for the most part about 5 mm. in diameter.

Microscopically in all of the sections two main types of change may be observed among the liver cells, corresponding to the areas of yellow and red above described. In the former the principal change appears to be a wide-spread fatty metamorphosis, the protoplasm of the cells being filled with large and small fat globules, the cell outlines being indistinct and shadowy, and the nuclei in many places staining very poorly. One important exception, however, must be noted, for surrounding every portal space is a mantle of cells, usually one or two layers in thickness, which show very little fatty involvement. These cells are in a condition of parenchymatous degeneration, the granular protoplasm taking a good blue stain which brings these periportal collections of cells into rather bold contrast with the remaining cells of the lobule, which exhibit the fatty change above described. The unusually sharp demarcation between this peripheral zone of cells and the remainder of the lobule serves to make the lobular markings of the liver, if anything, more distinct than are seen in a healthy organ.

The portions of the sections corresponding to the reddish hemorrhagic areas seen on macroscopic examination can be outlined quite definitely under the microscope, the conditions found in these areas differing considerably from those just described. As might be expected, the most conspicuous changes are of a hemorrhagic nature. Numerous spaces are observed which resemble overdistended capillaries and which are filled with masses of faint yellow shadow corpuscles. Large clumps of brownish pigment are scattered about these areas, and numerous polymorphonuclear leukocytes are also seen. Nothing is seen of the normal structure of the liver except scattered clumps of fragmentary liver cells in advanced stages of degeneration. There is a considerable degree of small round-cell infiltration, but neither in the red nor in the yellow areas is there any evidence of regenerative attempts on the part of the liver-cells or bile-ducts.

Of the other organs, the kidneys show a severe type of acute parenchymatous nephritis, with a well-marked hemorrhagic tendency. This same hemorrhagic tendency is noted in the other organs, especially the spleen and lungs. The uterus presents a puerperal enlargement (length 18 cm.), its tissues are soft and succulent, and its cavity contains a quantity of offensive material. In addition, an important finding is the presence of several ounces of light yellowish pus in the pelvic cavity. The pelvic peritoneum is reddened and congested, but there are no adhesions, the pus having merely collected in a pool at the bottom of the pelvis. There is no extension of the pelvic peritonitic process to the general abdominal peritoneum.

406-7 Professional Building.

URINARY STUDY, BY DR. WHITNEY

The two cases reported by Dr. Novak present so typically the urine changes described first by Frerichs and his pupils that they are of more than ordinary interest, especially as the urinary studies were carried out according to the latest methods of investigating the distribution of the various nitrogenous bodies in the urine. The determinations were carried out according to the method of Kruger and Schmidt, with some very slight modification of the method suggested by an experience covering a period of about seven years. The urine is first precipitated with phosphotungstic acid in the presence of hydrochloric acid and the precipitated material filtered off. The nitrogen is determined first by the usual Kjeldahl method, while the nitrogen which is held in loose chemical combination is determined on another portion by heating for twelve or more hours to a temperature of 160 C. with half its volume of strong sulphuric acid on both the entire urine and on the filtrate from the precipitate produced by phosphotungstic acid. This gives us the total, and the loosely combined nitrogen of the entire urine and of the filtrate from the phosphotungstic acid separation. We thus obtain with a moderate expenditure of time the best insight into the relations of the various nitrogenous bodies present in the urine. Since these fractions contain certain bodies we can thus draw conclusions as to the relative increase or decrease of these bodies in the urine. The urea fraction is an especially definite one and to my mind one of the best methods we have to-day for the quantitative estimation of urea as a definite chemical compound, for which the hypobromite methods are absolutely untrustworthy.

The substances yielding their nitrogen in the different divisions as sketched above are as follows: The loose nitrogen of the precipitate comprises the entire nitrogen of ammonia, carbamic acid, and sulphocyanates and a portion of the nitrogen of uric acid, purin bases, creatinin, mucoid bodies, the protein bodies or nucleo-albumins of the normal urine and the proteins of pathological urine; the firm nitrogen of the precipitate contains the remainder of the nitrogen of the bodies enumerated above as yielding only a portion of their nitrogen and in addition the nitrogen of the diamines, the diamido acids and the ptomains if these be present. The loose nitrogen of the filtrate contains the entire nitrogen of urea, allantoin, and oxaluric acid with a part of the oxyproteic acid; the firmly combined nitrogen of the filtrate contains in normal urine glycocoll and its combinations, taurin and cystin derivatives; to which must be added in pathological urines the nitrogen of leucin, tyrosin, cystin and other amido acids.

The ammonia was determined separately by the method of Kruger-Reich, the uric acid by the Folin method.

The changes in the urine described by Frerichs and his pupils were at first supposed to be constant and of great diagnostic value, but the subsequent work of the other investigators showed that the changes were by no means so constant as at first supposed. The most marked alterations described in these first studies may be summarized as follows: A marked decrease in the proportion of nitrogen present as urea; in one case the urine showed but small amounts when first examined, while in the last examination, just before death, no urea was demonstrable by the method used, with a corresponding increase in leucin and tyrosin. In most cases an increase in the amount of ammonia was found, though in one case Frerichs states that ammonia was present only in traces.

Later studies have shown that these alterations may all be present in one case, that only a portion of them may present themselves, or that, in rare cases, the urine may present no marked changes from the normal. The leucin and tyrosin and other amido-acids are especially frequently missed, later observers failing to find them in most cases. This is no doubt partly due to the difficulty in isolating them in sufficient purity for their certain identification. Beyond this, however, a study of the conditions going on in the liver will give us a sufficient reason for the variations found, without ascribing them in all cases to errors in analysis.

In the first place we know that the liver is one of the organs which undergo autolytic changes to the greatest extent when removed from the body and kept under aseptic conditions. Under these conditions we find the proteins of the liver undergoing a digestion with the formation of leucin, tyrosin and other amido bodies, and also the formation of variable acid bodies, some of them belonging to fatty acids, some to the aromatic acids. These acids require a certain amount of alkali for their neutralization, which is furnished in part by the fixed alkali of the body and in part by ammonia, which is thus switched off from its normal transformation into urea. Add to this the acidosis, the result of hunger, which becomes very marked when the vomiting and comatose condition of the second stage come on, and we can readily understand the usual increase in the amount of ammonia in the latter stages without the assumption of an actual liver incompetency. Should the liver changes be focal, as according to the pathological picture appears most probable, we could understand why leucin and tyrosin might make their appearance in the urine late in the disease or not at all, depending on the stage at which death occurs and the amount of functionating liver tissue existing at the time of death.

The full report of the urinalyses in these two cases is as follows:

CASE 1.—Urine of March 15, 1906, in evening. Amount received, 90 c.c.
Acid reaction.
Dark brownish color with a tinge of greenish.
Albumin present (trace).
Sugar absent.
Specific gravity, 1,015.
Bile pigments present (marked reaction).

Freezing point, 0.79° C. Isotonic with 1.29% NaCl.
Conductivity at 15° C. = 127.40 x 10.[4]
Ammonia, 0.1037%.
Total nitrogen, 0.3485%.

NITROGEN SUBDIVISION

| | | % Total Substance | % Total Nitrogen |
|---|---|---|---|
| Total nitrogen P.T.A.* | Precip. | 0.1802 | 51.7 |
| | Loose | 0.1293 | 37.10 |
| | Firm | 0.0509 | 14.61 |
| Total nitrogen P.T.A. | Filt. | 0.1683 | 48.29 |
| | Loose | 0.1402 | 40.22 |
| | Firm | 0.0281 | 8.063 |
| Nitrogen of ammonia | | 0.08539 | 24.50 |

*P.T.A. signifies phosphotungstic acid.

The sediment was profuse, yellowish, flocculent. Microscopic examination showed a large number of pavement epithelial cells, numerous renal epithelial cells, few leukocytes, a few granular and a moderate number of hyaline casts. A few brownish crystals were present, arranged usually in rosette form, resembling the crystals seen in cold blood-clots and called hematoidin crystals. They were probably bilirubin crystals. No leucin or tyrosin crystals came down even on prolonged standing and the amount of urine was insufficient for a chemical test for them.

CASE 2.—Urine from 10:30 p. m., June 13, to 3 p. m., June 14, 1908, sixteen and one-half hours. Amount 300 c.c.
Brownish amber, aromatic, cloudy.
Specific gravity, 1,029.
Reaction acid, 10 c.c.; required, 8.3 c.c. N/10 KOH, indicator phenolphthalein.
Albumin present (trace only), globulin doubtful.
Sugar absent.
Indican normal.
Urea (Doremus), 1.9%.
Uric acid, 0.03656%.
Total nitrogen, 1.1105%.
Chlorin as NaCl, 0.1%.
Phosphates as $P_2O_5$, 0.093%.
Ammonia as $NH_3$, 0.3576%.

NITROGEN SUBDIVISION

| | | % Total Substance | % Total Nitrogen |
|---|---|---|---|
| Total nitrogen P.T.A. | Precip. | 0.4457 | 40.15 |
| | Loose | 0.3283 | 29.56 |
| | Firm | 0.1174 | 10.57 |
| Total nitrogen P.T.A. | Filt. | 0.6648 | 59.87 |
| | Loose | 0.4435 | 39.94 |
| | Firm | 0.2213 | 19.93 |
| Nitrogen of ammonia | | 0.2946 | 26.53 |
| Nitrogen of uric acid | | 0.01219 | 1.097 |

Bile pigments present, trace (Huppert). Diacetic acid, marked.
Blood and hemoglobin, absent.
Sediment profuse, yellowish, flocculent; microscopic examination shows the presence of a few pus cells, pavement and renal epithelium, numerous hyaline casts, few granular and epithelial casts, amorphous urates. No crystals of leucin or tyrosin, even after prolonged standing.

1103 Linden Avenue.

# ALLERGY*

C. E. VON PIRQUET, M.D.
BALTIMORE

(*Concluded from page 288*)

## DISEASES DUE TO HYPHOMYCETES

Fungi of several kinds, which are the causes of the different trichophytoses of man and animals, have been investigated recently by Bloch with regard to their allergic reactions. I wish to summarize and explain the results of his studies from my point of view.

*Action of a Primary Infection in Guinea-pigs.*—A small amount of pure culture of a trichophyton is rubbed vigorously into the shaved skin. After an incubation time of four to six days (the traumatic reaction disappears within the first two days), a circumscribed inflammatory redness appears, gaining in size during the next few days. The focus becomes intensely infiltrated and somewhat elevated, and from the sixth to the eighth day the first typical shields appear. These increase in size and depth, but finally become a compact, reddish plate on an infiltrated background. From the eigth to the twelfth days the acme of the disease is reached. After a few more days a spontaneous retrogression begins: the yellow masses fall off in large particles and with them the fungi. An ulcer is formed which is soon covered again with skin, and after three to four weeks the focus forms an even, hairless place with a ring of scales and some inflammatory nodules. In rabbits the course of the reaction is quite different.

*Reinfection.*—On revaccinating some weeks after the primary infection, on the same point or on any other point of the skin, no specific lesions can be discerned, and only the traumatic reaction occurs.

The train of events following a primary inoculation reminds us in its course very much of cowpox vaccination: complete latency for several days, slow progress of a local phenomenon, acme of lesions with intense local infiltration and redness from the eighth to the twelfth days, and afterward spontaneous involution. The apparent absolute immunity corresponds with the results of a revaccination after a short interval. The number of fungi brought into the skin does not suffice to give a toxic reaction exceeding in intensity the traumatic reaction.

---

* The manuscript of this article was received April, 1910. The delay in publication has been caused in part by the length of the paper and in part because the first proof was sent abroad and was lost in transit.

Bloch extended his studies to infection in man:

Dr. G. Inoculation of an agar culture of trichophyton. On the fifth day a slight redness appears. Sixth day: prominence and slight scaling. Eighth day: vaccination point larger, infiltrated and bears several typical yellow shields. Twelfth day: infiltration is more intense, shields are confluent. The further course does not follow a critical retrogression as in guinea-pigs; on the contrary, the inflammatory symptoms increase, a kerion Celsi is formed, beginning to heal after two months.

The outcome in the other three cases was more favorable, as no deep lesions were formed. In a reinfection, the one case which Bloch describes entirely, shows what I call "accelerated reaction."

Dr. M. four and a half months previously infected with trichophyton, slight affection. Second day: a slight redness. Fourth day: redness and slight elevation. Sixth day: distinct papules. Seventh day: papules very intensely red, infiltrated and scaling. Eighth day: intense scaling. Twelfth day: infiltration and redness have disappeared; no fungi could be detected at the point of vaccination. Whereas Dr. G., who had been infected the same day for the first time, showed a redness only on the fifth day, the redness appeared on Dr. M. as early as the second day, reaching its maximum on the seventh day, while the first infected reached its maximum on the twelfth day.

From analogy with cowpox it may be assumed that the micro-organisms have not all been destroyed immediately, but that a small number of them could develop themselves, being killed by antibodies which were formed in an "accelerated time." For the existence of a chronic disease, in spite of antibody formation, as in the case of Dr. G., we have an analogy in tuberculosis. Trichophyton seems to be able to exist in the human organism simultaneously with antibodies like the tubercle bacillus. The antibodies in guinea-pigs and rabbits, however, are powerful enough to kill the micro-organism, as the human antibodies do the cowpox micro-organisms.

*Allergic Reactions with Extracts of the Fungi.*—As early as 1902 Neisser and Plato, and in 1904, Truffi had demonstrated specific reactions analogous to the tuberculin reactions, by subcutaneous injections of the pressure extracts of the fungi and filtrates of cultures in individuals who had trichophyton diseases. They found fever and other general symptoms.

Bloch performed a cutaneous reaction with tuberculin, with filtrates made of bouillon cultures. "The vaccination was elicited with an undiluted trichophytin in conformity with the rules given by von Pirquet. After four hours, as the earliest time, more generally after twelve to twenty-four hours, a reaction appears in the form of a flat red papule of the size of a lentil or a pea. The papule, which causes intense itching, grows somewhat larger in the following twenty-four hours; after that it slowly becomes smaller, but sometimes is left visible for a long period." Very important is the experiment of Bloch concerning the first onset of cutaneous trichophytin reaction in the course of a first infection: After the infection, the skin was daily inoculated with trichophytin. These inoculations were found negative up to the sixth day. The vaccination of the seventh day gave rise to a small papule about 3 mm. in diameter. During the following days, the papule became successively larger and found this definite maximum with a diameter of 10 mm. These experiments show again a complete analogy with vaccinia, where I was able to demonstrate in successive daily revaccinations that the early reaction appears at the same time, when, after the end of a normal incubation period the general symptoms and the local area formation set in. Likewise in trichophytosis the altered cutaneous reactivity lasts a long time after the infection. Bloch found on himself an intense reaction two and one-half years after an experimental trichophyton disease. The intensity of the reaction seems to be greater the deeper the foci grow during the illness. After very superficial processes, there was slight or no reaction. The different fungi which cause hyphomycetic colonies do not yield trichophytons of a different character. It is as in tuberculosis, in which the tuberculin is made of different species of bacilli. The persons infected with cultures of trichophyton react also when tested with extracts of microsporon and achorion, and on the other hand, persons with favus react with trichophyton extract. In correspondence with this behavior—no specificity of the allergy of the skin of animals infected with one or the other fungus—animals infected with one of the fungi become immune against infection with the others.

Bloch was not able to obtain cutaneous reactions with extracts in animals. From what we know of tuberculin, I should suppose that these reactions could be found if the trichophytin be used intracutaneously. Very interesting and absolutely new and without analogy up to the present time is the experiment in which he grafted the skin of an allergic person on a non-allergic one and made a test on the grafted skin. Dr. Bloch made the experiment on himself. Two and one-half years after an artificial trichophytosis, he showed a very intense cutaneous reaction with trichophytin. He took skin from his own arm and transplanted it to an ulcus cruris of a patient who did not react with trichophytin. Ten days after the transplantation, a cutaneous test with trichophytin was made on the grafted skin, which had attached itself very well.

No papule was formed, but a necrosis of the transplanted layer followed with a diameter of about 10 mm. This necrosis, if it is to be ascribed to the trichophytin and not to a traumatic reaction, would prove (and this is the opinion Bloch advances) the existence of a cellular allergy.

## SPOROTRICHOSIS

Pautrier and Lutembacher gave two individuals infected with sporotrichosis, a subcutaneous injection of an extract of *Spororthrix schenkii*

(*Sporotrichon beurmannii*). The result was fever and a local reaction, while only two of fourteen control cases showed a slight reaction. Bloch used a cutaneous inoculation, de Beurmann and Gougerot the intradermal method. The results are not yet absolutely clear.

## TYPHOID FEVER

Pfeiffer's phenomenon, the lysis of typhoid bacilli by antibodies, occurring as a result of typhoid infection, induces Wolff-Eisner to think that the symptoms of typhoid fever are due to endotoxins. These endotoxins are liberated by the antibodies. Clinical phenomena of allergy are certainly to be expected in this disease, but are not yet known with certainty. Schick is of the opinion that a predisposition period must be recognized in typhoid fever as in scarlet fever. During this predisposition period there exists a hypersusceptibility and this indeed forms its characteristic feature. The recognition of this predisposition period may explain the occurrence of the relapses after certain intervals. Chantemesse saw characteristic inflammatory symptoms following the instillation of typhoid bacilli extract in the eye of patients suffering with typhoid fever. He asserts that this ophthalmic reaction occurs sooner in the course of the disease than the agglutination test. Kraus, repeating the experiments of Chantemesse, could not convince himself of the specificity of this reaction, stating that healthy individuals also give it to some extent, and that other bacterial extracts cause similar symptoms in typhoid fever patients. In addition he tried a cutaneous reaction, but without result. Zupnik, on the contrary, states that a cutaneous reaction is useful, while the ophthalmic reaction is not.

My own experiences have led me to believe that typhoid toxin is not to be considered analogous to tuberculin. An early reaction in the form of indefinite and slightly elevated papules is seen not only in typhoid fever patients, but likewise on the skin of healthy individuals, and especially on the skin of infants, while an active allergy can be excluded, where a previous infection can be eliminated. Convalescents from typhoid fever react, as a rule, somewhat more intensely, but the difference is only a quantitative one. A diagnostic use of the cutaneous reaction, as in cases of tuberculosis is, therefore, not possible in typhoid fever.

## DIPHTHERIA

In the course of the preparation of diphtheria antitoxin, Behring encountered a peculiar difficulty, furnishing one of the first examples of hypersensitiveness. Horses with a very high immunity against the toxin died sometimes after a relatively small dose of the toxin. In this instance certainly hypersensitiveness and immunity are in close affiliation and thus far this affiliation cannot be explained. A searching study of diphtheria poisoning is well adapted for the advancement of our theoretical knowledge of allergy. The observation of Wassermann proves the existence of allergy; we see that guinea-pigs immunized only to a certain degree by antitoxin injection have not acquired a complete protection against diphtheria, but respond to the introduction of toxin with a local inflammation. On injecting the toxin there appears on the place of inoculation an intense local inflammatory reaction, later becoming sharply defined and leading to a necrosis of the affected tissue. The animal, however, survives, while a normal guinea-pig receiving the same dose of diphtheria toxin does not show a local reaction at the place of inoculation, but dies quickly from the general effect of the toxin.

An allergy with regard to the time relations does not occur here. The effects are seen early, whether the animals have been treated previously or not. But the quantitative and qualitative change of the reaction is unmistakable.

Qualitative allergy: The animal not treated previously shows a general poisoning; the treated shows local inflammatory symptoms.

Quantitative allergy: Local hypersusceptibility of the treated animal combined with a lessened susceptibility with reference to the general effect. In this case we have a passive allergy produced by the injection of antitoxic serum, but we have likewise an active allergy in diphtheria, probably analogous to the results after injection of horse serum, etc.: Rist saw hypersusceptibility after the injection of the dead bodies of diphtheria bacilli without the toxin.

In conformity with the cutaneous tuberculin reaction, Schick investigated the cutaneous reaction with diphtheria toxin in man. He demonstrated that the reaction produced by vaccination with diphtheria toxin was not allergic, but due directly to the toxin, thereby distinguishing itself fundamentally from the cutaneous tuberculin reaction. It is very important to note that the reaction is much lessened by an addition of antitoxin or by a preliminary injection of antitoxin. Schick tried to use his results for the standardization of diphtheria antitoxin. Various amounts of antitoxin were mixed with a given amount of toxin, and then vaccinations were made with the different mixtures on the skin of man. In this way the amount of antitoxin necessary to suppress the reaction with a definite amount of toxin was determined. Roemer, in 1909, applied the intracutaneous method in guinea-pigs for the standardization of antitoxin in a way similar to the one Schick had used with the cutaneous method in man. His results were very satisfactory.

### SCARLET FEVER

The allergic manifestations of scarlatina differ from those in glanders and syphilis. It has been known a long time that the scarlatina nephritis appears as a rule in the third week. None of the hypotheses thus far advanced is able to account satisfactorily for the fact that the nephritis occurs just at that time. B. Schick, by an exact observation of very many cases of scarlatina, found two facts which throw a new light on the genesis of scarlatinal nephritis: 1. The nephritis is only one of the typical sequelæ. Equivalent and often very closely combined are: lymphadenitic affections of the regional glands, characteristic rises of temperature, without clinical findings, and finally, which is the most important point, real relapses of scarlet fever. 2. All these symptoms have in common the feature that they occur only at a certain time after the beginning of scarlatina. At the end of the second week a period of predisposition becomes manifest, reaching its maximum in the third week and ending with the sixth week. Table 4 records the occurrences of the different symptoms in the weeks from the onset of the scarlet fever rash:

TABLE 4.—OCCURRENCE OF SYMPTOMS BY WEEKS

| | Week after onset of scarlatina rash | | | | | | |
|---|---|---|---|---|---|---|---|
| | 1. | 2. | 3. | 4. | 5. | 6. | 7. |
| Lymphadenitis | .. | 2 | 37 | 22 | 6 | 1 | .. |
| Nephritis | .. | 2 | 18 | 7 | 3 | 3 | .. |
| Postscarlatinal fever | .. | 1 | 20 | 9 | 2 | 1 | .. |
| Scarlatina relapses | .. | 1 | 3 | 6 | 2 | 1 | .. |
| Total | .. | 6 | 78 | 44 | 13 | 6 | .. |

Typical relapses occurring at the same time at which other sequelæ make their appearance, make it very probable that these sequelæ are to be considered local relapses, or as a local repetition of the primary process. The sequelæ include the nephritis. Schick suggests that the micro-organisms which are the cause of scarlatina can remain in the organism after the disappearance of the rash, and are able to produce a new infectious or toxic action during the period of predisposition, which is to be explained as a hypersensibility of the organism.

## TUBERCULOSIS

The studies with regard to the changes of reactivity against the tubercle bacillus have been carried on by very many authors, and the literature is so extensive and increases so rapidly that I can only collect concisely the most important theories and clinical data. Arloing and Courmont, in 1881-91, had proposed the opinion, based on experiments with injection of tubercle bacilli, that these micro-organisms produce soluble bodies which deprive the organism of its natural powers of defence, so that it is left without protection against a later infection. Closely related to this *Ausschaltungstheorie* is the "aggressin" theory of Bail (1905). Koch and Babes had formed another theory, the *Additionstheorie.* They explained the tuberculin reaction by an addition of the injected toxin to the toxic bodies formed by the tubercle bacillus within the organism. Koehler and Westphal, in 1891, suggested that by a union of the tuberculin with products of the tubercle bacilli, a third new body was formed in the tuberculous focus. The theory of Marmorek (1904) is very similar. He thought that the tubercle bacilli secreted a fever-producing body under the influence of the injected tuberculin.

Von Pirquet and Schick (1903) regarded the tuberculin reaction from an entirely new point of view, finding an analogy between this reaction and the early reaction in serum disease and vaccinia. These authors explained it as a "vital antibody reaction." According to this conception, the tuberculous focus plays no part in the production of the reaction, but antibody-like substances produced by the organism and diffused through all the tissues enter into combination with the tuberculin, giving rise to a toxic substance in the general circulation, as well as at the point of the inoculation of the tuberculin. Schick studied the tuberculin reactions in the Children's Clinic in Graz, and confirmed in accordance with our theoretical forecast, the specificity of the *Stichreaktion.* This subcutaneous swelling and reddening had been considered as specific by Epstein as early as 1891, and Escherich had given it its name in 1892, but neither of them had drawn any theoretical conclusions, nor did Klingmueller, who studied this action histologically. My discovery of the cutaneous tuberculin reaction (1907) was a consequence of the former theory, and it served to establish a further analogy between cowpox vaccination and tuberculosis. Loewenstein, in 1904, and De Waele, in 1906, tried to bring the tuberculin reaction into analogy with the results of Behring and Knorr with regard to tetanus hypersusceptibility. Wassermann and Bruck, in 1906, worked along the same lines. They were the first who tried to solve the question as to the nature of the antibodies by exact biological experiments. These authors demonstrated in the tuberculous focus the presence of bodies giving a deviation of complement, and they were able to produce these bodies in the serum of the organism by consequent tuberculinization. They differ from von Pirquet and Schick in considering the antibodies as a kind of antitoxin, and explained the thermal reaction, ascribing their origin to the tuberculous focus. In recent years nearly all authors have agreed with von Pirquet and Schick in so far as they considered the tuberculin reaction due to antibodies. The relation of these to the complement-binding antibodies, however, is not yet clear. Wolff-Eisner considers the antibodies in question as lytic, dissolving the minute particles of the bodies of tubercle bacilli contained in the tuberculin, and delivering an endotoxin. He explains a lessened reactivity in the case of tuberculin by a different localization and saturation of receptors.

We will now regard the first experiment of Koch, in 1891, in the light of the allergy theory:

If a guinea-pig is inoculated with a pure culture of tubercle bacilli, the inoculation point, as a rule, seems to heal completely on the first day. After ten to fourteen days a little hard knot appears which soon opens and forms an ulcer, lasting until the death of the animal. Quite different is the effect if we inoculate a guinea-pig already tuberculous. For this purpose animals are best used which have been inoculated four to six weeks previously. In such an animal no knot is formed around the small inoculation point, but on the next or second day a singular change takes place. The point of inoculation becomes hard and of a dark color, and after some days it is seen distinctly that not only the point of inoculation itself has become necrotic, but the neighborhood in a diameter of 0.5 to 1 cm. Later on a necrotic-looking skin falls off and a flat ulcer is left which, as a rule, heals quickly and definitely without an infection of the neighboring lymph-glands.

In this experiment we can distinguish the three kinds of allergy:

1. *Time Allergy.*—After the first injection, ten to fourteen days elapse until the beginning of the clinical phenomena. After the second injection a necrosis appears within the first two days.

2. *Qualitative Allergy.*—The first inoculation leads to a hard knot, a chronic ulcer, and at the same time to a general infection. The second inoculation causes symptoms which remain entirely local and produces the superficial necrosis, not even giving rise to an infection of the regionary glands.

3. *Quantitative Allergy.*—Regarding the process in its entirety, the guinea-pig is certainly far more sensitive to the first injection than to the second, because the first injection leads to a general tuberculosis, the later only to an insignificant local lesion of short duration. But if we inoculate a normal and a tuberculous animal at the same time, and look at the effect on the second day, we shall consider the tuberculous animal as hypersensitive, because it shows a necrosis, whereas in the new animal, the vaccination has not yet caused any disturbance.

In a very evident way, Trudeau already, in the year 1897, showed the change of reactivity of the tuberculous and the non-tuberculous animal. After a first infection of the animal by inoculation of tubercle bacilli in the eye, no immediate results appear, but a caseation sets in after two weeks, which leads to a complete destruction. In an already tuberculous animal there is an immediate reaction which, however, disappears after some time. Trudeau, in his very excellent studies, was principally interested in the result more favorable for the animal, that is, the consequence of the second infection. My point of view, of course, is principally the time of reaction, and the other differences we see between the first and second one. I should like to cite Trudeau's own words:

In the controls, two days after the introduction of the virulent material into the eye, little or no irritation is to be observed, and little is to be noticed for two weeks when a steadily increasing vascularity manifests itself. Small tubercles appear in the iris, which gradually coalesce and become cheesy. Intense iritis and general inflammation of the structures of the eye develop, and in six or eight weeks the eye is more or less completely destroyed. . . . In the vaccinated animals the introduction of the mammalian bacilli at once gives rise to a marked degree of irritation. From the second to the fifth day the vessels of the conjunctiva are tortuous and enlarged, whitish specks of fibrinous exudation appear on the iris and in the anterior chamber, and more or less intense iritis supervenes; but, at the end of the second to the third week, when the eyes of the controls begin to show progressive and steadily increasing evidence of inflammatory reaction, the irritation in those of the vaccinated animals begins slowly to subside and the eyes to mend. . . .

In this instance we see the good side of allergy in tuberculosis, i. e., the protection against an infection, but this protection is only shown if, as in Trudeau's case, the infection is made with a small amount of bacilli. If instead of this, which we might call the physiological form of reinfection, we apply artificial methods of injecting large amounts of tubercle bacilli, we find again very intense and dangerous "anaphylactic" symptoms. They can be elicited either by an injection of living or dead bacilli, or by injection of the extract of tubercle bacilli.

1. *Injection of Living Bacilli* (Courmont, Detro and Bail).—After larger doses the tuberculous animals die within twenty-four hours. The deadly issue here is purely an accidental one. It is dependent entirely on the amount of the toxic product formed by the interaction of the antibodies of the tuberculous organism with the infecting material. If this amount produced in the early reaction is sufficiently great, the animals die; if the amount is small—and this naturally happens when a smaller number of bacilli is injected—the reaction disappears rapidly and the animals do not succumb. The fact that the severity of the toxic effect is entirely dependent on the quantity corresponds exactly with the above-mentioned findings of von Pirquet in revaccination with cowpox lymph. The size of the early reaction of a previously vaccinated individual was found to be dependent on the concentration of the lymph, while the amount of lymph inoculated does not influence the size of the reaction of a subject first vaccinated. With a very diluted lymph only the time is lengthened at which the vaccination effect develops. Hamburger has proved that the quantitative effect of a reinfection in tuberculosis is dependent on the quantitity of tubercle bacilli injected and his results were confirmed by Roemer.

2. *Injection of Dead Bacilli* (Strauss and Gamaleia).—Here, too, death occurs when a sufficiently large number of bacilli is injected.

3. *Injection of Tuberculin.*—The old tuberculin of Koch, a boiled, concentrated and filtered bouillon culture of tubercle bacilli kills tuberculous guinea-pigs in a dose of 0.5 gm., an amount which is borne without symptoms by an untreated animal. Tuberculous human beings are much more sensitive to tuberculin. Sometimes we see very severe symptoms after the injection of only 1 mg., and the same dose which is fatal for a guinea-pig could probably kill an adult human being. The reaction

after the injection of tuberculin consists first in general symptoms, especially fever; and secondly, in the focus reaction. This comprises inflammatory symptoms in the immediate neighborhood of tuberculous tissue. This type of reaction attracted the attention of Koch and up to the time of the discovery of the local tuberculin reactions, it formed the basis of all theoretical explanations.

After an intravenous injection these two forms of reaction only are seen, but if the injection is given into the subcutaneous tissue, we see furthermore the subcutaneous or *Stichreaktion* (Epstein, Escherich, Schick, Hamburger, Reuschel). F. Hamburger has proved that this subcutaneous inflammation is the most accurate test of tuberculous allergy. This reaction is generally positive in tuberculous children, with an injection of 0.10 mg. of tuberculin, sometimes with much smaller doses. The injection in the skin itself (intracutaneous reaction or intradermal reaction, tried by Mendel, Mantous, Moussu and Roemer) is of about the same accuracy. Here a minimal amount of tuberculin is introduced into the skin, so as to cause an infiltration of the skin. If minimal amounts are administered, both the subcutaneous and intracutaneous injections produce only local effects. Only if larger amounts are used, fever and other general symptoms are noticed.

The cutaneous vaccination with old tuberculin is not delicate but easier to perform (cutaneous test of von Pirquet). A papule of 5 to 20 mm. in diameter appears with all symptoms of local inflammation.

Even after simple contact of the outer skin with this old tuberculin, specific reactions appear (Lautier), but only when a very high degree of hypersensitiveness exists. On intense rubbing, however, with a tuberculin ointment (Moro's percutaneous test), the reaction is nearly as delicate as the cutaneous. The same may be said of the method described by Lignières and Berger, that of putting tuberculin on the shaved and rubbed skin.

The mucous membranes are more sensitive than the outside skin. Here simple applications of thin solutions of tuberculin lead to swelling, redness and secretion. This is the case on the conjunctiva (conjunctival test of Wolff-Eisner and Calmette), on the mucous membrane of the nose (rhino-reaction by Lafite, Dupont and Molinier), as well as on the mucous membranes of the urethra, the rectum and the vagina. Within the intestinal tract, local inflammatory phenomena cannot be noticed, but after an internal use of larger amounts of tuberculin, fever sets in, especially if at the same time the acid reaction of the stomach contents is neutralized by bicarbonate of soda (Freymuth). The mucous membrane of the respiratory tract also responds to an inhalation of evaporated tuberculin by a general reaction, manifesting itself in a rise of temperature (von Schroetter).

All these forms of reaction may be considered as identical in principle. It is only a matter of concentration that a given solution of tuberculin is able to produce a reaction on one part of the body and not on another. So, for instance, in a case which reacts feebly to a 5 per cent. instillation in the eye, undiluted tuberculin must be used on the skin in order to elicit slight symptoms.

*Time Elapsing until the Appearance of the Disease on First Inoculation and until the Establishment of Allergy.*—In the section on vaccination with cowpox, it was mentioned that the time of the appearance of the first symptoms is somewhat dependent on the concentration of the lymph, that is, the number of micro-organisms (Nourney, von Pirquet). This relation between the number of micro-organisms injected and the incubation time shows itself much more markedly in tuberculosis. In the experiments of Roemer, in cattle, with massive doses of tubercle bacilli, the temperature rose to a high level after an incubation recalling that of the first serum disease.

In four of his five temperature curves, recorded in *Beiträge zur Klinik der Tuberculose* (*Brauer's*), a very high fever is noted between the fourteenth and seventeenth days following the injection. This fever lasts until the death of the animal. In this final result tuberculosis differs from vaccinia and serum disease. In three of these cases slight elevations of temperature occurred, starting on the sixth and eighth days. Similarly, such slight elevations of temperature, preceding the real febrile state, are frequently met in cowpox. In one case of Roemer's the hyperpyrexia started as early as the seventh day.

On the other hand, after an infection with small amounts of tubercle bacilli, weeks or even months elapse before clinical symptoms are noticed. In view of such very prolonged periods of incubation, the question arises whether it is possible that the tubercle bacilli remain in the organism in a state of absolute rest, without multiplying and without stimulating the organism to react. I have observed similar occurrences in cowpox vaccination and attributed them to "sleeping germs." Here, the germs can be awakened later on by mechanical or by biological stimuli, for instance by the antibody formation following subsequent infection. Possibly the findings of Bartel in the lymphatic state could be explained in this way. In vaccinia the incubation time can be lengthened quite indefinitely by the sleeping of germs, whereas the simple differences in quantity cause only a delay of the reaction time from two to three days. It might be, however, that the lengthened incubation time in tuberculosis is more dependent on a very slow formation of antibodies which is not at all or very slowly instigated by very small amounts.

We shall now have to consider whether, as with serum, an incubation time of the allergy can be proved, and furthermore whether this incubation time coincides with that of the clinical symptoms. Immediately after a first injection, a tuberculin reaction can never be elicited. The shortest time after which Preisich and Heim found a positive reaction was five days, but on the whole about double this time is necessary after an infection with a large amount of bacilli. Roemer and Joseph found, with the intracutaneous test, that if small amounts are administered in guinea-pigs the allergy begins after a very long period, just as we have seen with regard to the clinical symptoms. Of their experiments I wish to cite only one, in which guinea-pigs were infected with various amounts of tuberculin from 0.1 mg. down to one billionth of a milligram, and were tested after three, five and eight weeks intracutaneously with 2 cg. of tuberculin. The guinea-pigs which had received 0.1 to 0.001 mg. showed an intense reaction after three weeks. The guinea-pigs with 10 micrograms and 1 microgram showed a weak reaction at that time, which became intense later on. The guinea-pigs, finally, which had received only 1/10 to 1/100 of a microgram began to react after five weeks.

In man also it is probable that there exists a time of incubation of several weeks at least, extending from the infection with a small number of bacilli to the beginning of the allergy, and an infection with a small number of bacilli may readily be the usual mode of infection. I should be inclined to assume that, as a rule, a period of one to three months elapses before the cutaneous reaction becomes positive, since its appearance signifies a rather intense sensitiveness. In this way the cases of tuberculosis in nurslings may be explained, where in the absence of a miliary tuberculosis, a very slight reactivity exists remaining below the threshold of a cutaneous reaction. I am of the opinion that these cases are in the first stage, having not yet attained their full power of reactivity. It is probable that after an infection with tuberculosis, the reactivity remains intense for several years, whether the tuberculosis has developed progressively, or whether it has been localized, and even after a decrease of this reactivity coupled with the disappearance of the antibodies, a slight reinfection or reinjection with tuberculous toxin arouses again the formation of the antibodies and reestablishes a higher degree of reactivity.

In one regard tuberculosis shows a difference from the serum disease, and that is that the tuberculin is not able to produce allergy in the normal organism. Neither with small nor large doses (F. Hamburger) is it possible to produce an allergy in an absolutely healthy and non-infected man. It seems that only the infection with living bacteria has this effect.

*Accelerated Reaction.*—All symptoms of allergy, of which we have spoken until now, belong to the group of immediate reaction, but we have as in analogy to the findings in vaccination and serum disease, also signs of "accelerated" reaction in tuberculosis, that is, symptoms which appear after an incubation time of four to seven days instead of a normal incubation time of eight to twelve days. To this class belong some cases of tuberculin reaction. In apparently healthy adults, which generally means individuals having a latent inactive tuberculosis of old date and of a localized character, we see not very rarely that the cutaneous reaction appears, not within twenty-four hours, but after a latent period of several days. This reaction may be explained on the assumption that at the time of the test, no more antibodies were present, but that the vaccination with the tuberculin stimulated a renewed formation of antibodies. This renewed formation of antibodies proceeds like the accelerated antibody formation to which I called attention when speaking about serum disease and precipitin formation. Among the same group of people, that is apparently healthy adults, we meet with "secondary" reaction which is closely related to the above-mentioned reaction. Continuing the test daily in cases in which the first cutaneous reaction was negative, a positive reaction appears after some days, and sometimes simultaneously the old vaccination points become positive. This is not a local phenomenon, but must be due to a general reformation of antibodies, because from that day on, tests made on different parts of the body have again positive reactions.

Roemer reinfected previously tuberculized cattle with large doses of tubercle bacilli. Among his cases I found good illustrations of accelerated reaction in the appearance of general symptoms.

In Animal 10, the high fever appears on the same evening, that is an immediate general reaction. In Animal 17, it appears on the fourth day: accelerated reaction. In Animal 20, on the first and then again on the fifth day: immediate and accelerated reaction, the double form I have described in the case of serum disease in man.

From this accelerated reaction we have to distinguish the early reaction. Here there is no evidence of a reformation of antibodies, but we see a very slow chemical action of the existing but diluted antibodies. The reaction appears not within twenty-four hours, but somewhat later, increasing steadily to a certain point, but not generally to a great intensity. We may gain a clearer understanding of these forms of reactions by recalling the results of my experiments in which the cutaneous reactions were made with different dilutions of tuberculin, and in which the different areas of the skin showed a different degree of sensitiveness, that is, some parts were highly sensitive, owing to a greater concentration of antibody at the place of vaccination, while others were slightly sensitive, having only small amounts of antibody. Using the tuberculin on parts of the skin rich in local antibody, the reaction appears rather suddenly after a very sharply defined period of latency, and attains its maximum within a few hours. On parts of slight sensitiveness, the reaction begins after the same period of latency, but increases very slowly. Finally the reaction proceeds to the same intensity, but at the beginning it can remain for a rather long time under the threshold of evidence, that is smaller than the traumatic reaction.

*Passive Allergy.*—The first experiments with regard to transferring the sensitiveness against tuberculin with the serum of tuberculous animals were made in 1902 by Preisich and Heim. In several instances they were able to obtain fever by simultaneous injection of tuberculin and the serum of tuberculous animals into animals free from tuberculosis, but as their experiments had not absolutely uniform results, they stopped the work, without reaching any conclusion. Von Pirquet, in 1907, sought to determine whether the cutaneous reaction was influenced in its character by mixing the tuberculin with the serum of an allergic person; he found, however, neither a lessening nor an increase of intensity. Pickert and Loewenstein, however, showed that the serum of tuberculous people, treated with tuberculin, exerted sometimes an inhibiting action on the tuberculin reaction of other allergic persons. Later on Pickert found this action also in cases which had not been treated with tuberculin. White and Graham confirmed these results, and in testing a large number of patients found a serum which had the contrary effect. Yamanouchi, Helmholz and Bauer made anaphylactic tests, injecting tuberculous serum in an animal and treating it afterward with tuberculin.

Yamanouchi took 5 c.c. of the serum of cadavers of tuberculous patients and injected it into rabbits. After twenty-four hours he injected 0.5 gm. of pure tuberculin in 5 c.c. of physiological salt solution. If death did not occur immediately, he repeated the tuberculin dose after twenty-four hours. Many of the animals died after these injections, but as the doses are very high, and as we should expect an antianaphylaxis to a second injection of tuberculin, his results cannot be regarded as conclusive. Helmholz injected 5 c.c. of defibrinated blood, and then made daily tuberculin reactions, which became positive from two to three days after the injection of the blood. The reaction appeared very clearly after a parabiotic[1] union of a tuberculous and healthy guinea-pig. The healthy guinea-pig sewed to the tuberculous one began to react after the fourth day. Bauer injected 2 c.c. of the serum of a tuberculous guinea-pig in man, and forty-eight hours later 0.125 gm. of tuberculin. In several but not in all cases the tuberculin injection was followed by fever.

*Lessened Susceptibility of Tuberculous Individuals Against Tuberculin.*—It is well known that some tuberculous individuals do not react with tuberculin, or better, react but very slightly. This occurs at different periods of the disease and for various reasons.

1. In the first state of infection. At this period the antibody has not been formed in sufficient amounts (experiments of Roemer and Joseph; findings on nurslings by different authors).

2. In the final stage of tuberculosis, especially in miliary tuberculosis. This fact had been known for a long time when von Pirquet was able to show in a number of cases by daily cutaneous vaccinations that the reactivity decreases progressively. It is a rule that older children lose their reactivity during the last two weeks of miliary tuberculosis. In children

1. Under parabiotic we here mean the joining of two animals. I mention this because the term parabiotic has been used in an altogether different sense by Wedensky [Arch. f. d. ges. Physiol. (Pflüger's), 1903, c, 1].

of the first years, however, it occurs that the allergy is retained up to the last day of life.

3. In cachexia. In the third stage of lung tuberculosis, it is very often seen that the tuberculin reaction is negative, or is attained only after injection of very high doses. In other cases we see a lessened cutaneous reactivity. Instead of an intense papilla formation, we find either colorless papules or reddish spots without exudation (cachectic reaction). As a rule, the tuberculin reaction does not change very much for several days, while this cachectic reaction presents a very different aspect already within some hours. These cachectic reactions may likewise precede the complete loss of reactivity in miliary tuberculosis.

4. During measles. Von Pirquet and Preisich demonstrated that in the first days after the eruption of the measles exanthem, the cutaneous reactivity always disappears, and it reappears only after about a week. Gruener showed that the tuberculin reactivity did not disappear entirely, as large doses of tuberculin injected subcutaneously, still produce a *Stichreaktion.* He calculated that the reactivity was about 100,000 times less than before. It is probable, but not yet proved, that other diseases act in the same sense on the tuberculous allergy. Diphtheria, scarlet fever and epidemic meningitis certainly do not act in this way. It has even been said (Heim and John), that scarlatina has a somewhat contrary action, since an old tuberculin reaction may reappear before the eruption of the scarlet exanthema. It has been supposed by several authors that typhoid fever could cause a tuberculin reactivity. This is certainly not the case. With the exception of leprosy, we know of no other process which could produce a tuberculin reaction, and in the case of typhoid fever, no other fact seems to have been proved but that comparatively many adults give a positive conjunctival reaction during that illness. The possibility exists that the typhoid infection acts as a stimulus to the production of tuberculous antibodies. The disappearance of the reaction during the eruptive state of measles may be explained on the assumption that during this time, owing to the morbid process of the disease, the tuberculous ergins are combined in some way, and therefore no more available for the reaction. Schick pointed out another possibility, suggesting that some other body necessary for the reaction, for instance, some complement-body, is lacking.

5. During continued treatment with tuberculin. In some of the cases an insensibility appears which first manifests itself in a negative result of the cutaneous test, and later on in the absence of fever and subcutaneous reaction. As in measles, it is not an absolute insensibility, but a gradually lessened one. One part of this anergy can certainly be brought into analogy with the antianaphylaxis experiments in serum disease. During the first days after the injection of larger amounts of tuberculin,

the reactivity is decreased to such an extent, that the cutaneous reaction becomes negative, reappearing only after some days (Vallée). This kind of anergy is to be explained by a saturation of the antibody (Hamburger). It can be continued by repeated injections of large doses (Schlossmann, Engel and Bauer). Soon after the last injection, the reactivity is reproduced and attains to the level of the cutaneous reaction after eight to fourteen days. Besides this kind of allergy, it is possible that another kind of immunity exists which may be due either to another antibody or to a different localization of the same antibody. In this way we could explain cases where several months after tuberculin treatment, a high degree of immunity or allergy still exists.

6. A long time after the onset of tuberculosis. If we make tests on people of different ages, we find progressively with the increase in age a growing percentage of clinically healthy people who show a very slight reactivity. (Subcutaneous reaction with high doses; no immediate cutaneous reaction.) Most of them become again susceptible several days after the test, and show then "secondary reactions." Post-mortem examinations of cases of this kind have revealed obsolete foci, for the most part small (E. Hamburger). We might, therefore, assume that in these cases we are confronted by a period of lessened reactivity several years after an acute stage.

7. Finally, there are some few cases in which we have a minimal reactivity, although none of the former explanations can be applied: Some cases of active tuberculosis have only a slight allergy, although they are not cachectic.

Is it possible to bring these facts into simple relation to the presence of antibodies in the serum of tuberculous individuals? Reviewing the properties of the organism and of the serum of tuberculous individuals with which we are at present familiar, we have the following:

1. Property of the body participating in the inflammatory reaction with tuberculin. This property appears as a result of an infection with tubercle bacilli after a period of incubation. It may be lessened by injection of large doses of tuberculin.

2. Properties of the serum of tuberculous individuals: A. In some cases the serum is able to carry the first-mentioned property to another organism, that is, to give a reaction with tuberculin (Preisich and Heim, Helmholz, Bauer and the case of Graham and White). B. In other cases the serum has an inhibiting effect on the tuberculin reaction (Pickert and Loewenstein). It has been noticed that this latter property is seen especially in those individuals who have been treated repeatedly with increasing doses of tuberculin. The precipitins, agglutinins and complement-fixing antibodies occur, we are told, under the same conditions, that is after repeated treatment with tuberculin. The agglutinins found by Arloing and Courmont and Koch never appear, according to Juergens,

when a human tuberculosis heals spontaneously, and rarely in the course of a spontaneous tuberculosis of guinea-pigs, but they occur regularly after the treatment of healthy or tuberculous animals with tuberculin. Salge, however, found agglutinins also in untreated children, and Schkarin especially in those suffering with scrofulosis. The results with regard to the precipitins (Bonome and Mangiagalli) are no more constant. Nor do the first reports concerning the antibodies which cause fixation of complement (Bordet and Gengou in 1903, Wassermann and Bruck in 1906) show any uniformity. Wassermann and Bruck and Luedtke found these especially after tuberculin treatment, whereas Morgenroth and Rabinovitsch could not confirm these results. Citron described their occurrence in different groups of cases, particularly in those which had been treated, and which had a high insensibility against tuberculin. Bauer never found such an antibody in tuberculous children before treatment, but they were formed regularly during the treatment. In non-tuberculous children it was, in spite of very large tuberculin doses, absolutely impossible to produce these antibodies. Investigations with regard to a possible relationship between tuberculin hypersensitiveness and the antibodies concerned in the fixation of complement seem to be beset with great difficulties. Armand Delille states that there exists a complete parallelism, while Wolff and Muesam, as well as Sigismund Cohn did not find this to be the case. Engel and Bauer, who have the largest experience, differentiate four groups of tuberculous children: (1) tuberculous cachexia: nearly absolute insensibility against tuberculin and no antibody formation during the treatment; (2) extensive tuberculosis, but with a better general state: high sensitiveness which cannot be lessened by tuberculin treatment; at the same time a large amount of complement-binding antibody is formed; (3) obsolete and inactive small foci in healthy children: slight reactivity which disappears very easily after ascending doses of tuberculin; at the same time very slight or no antibody formation; (4) finally middle cases: moderate sensitiveness, gradually decreasing during treatment, and a moderate formation of antibody.

It would be possible to explain these results on the basis of only one kind of ergins, if we select from the great variety of data only those which could easily be covered by such a theory. Supposing these ergins are present in small amounts, they unite with tuberculin with the formation of a toxic substance and give, therefore, inflammatory reactions within the tissues. Furthermore, on injecting serum containing these ergins in another individual, this individual will then react with tuberculin in a like manner. When present in large amounts, these ergins should be capable of neutralizing the formed toxin (or the reaction between ergin and tuberculin may proceed differently with little or no formation of toxin). I only mention this as one possibility of explanation, but it is much more probable that in reality these processes are of a far more complicated nature.

*Pulmonary Tuberculosis of Adults as an Allergic Phenomenon.*—Von Behring for the first time expressed the idea that pulmonary phthisis was not the consequence of an infection acquired a short time before the onset of the disease, but that the patients had been infected with tuberculosis in their early youth. His further ideas—that this first infection was brought about in the first year of life, and was caused by tubercle bacilli contained in cow's milk—were erroneous. But his conception that in the tuberculosis of the lungs we have to deal with a secondary, or rather a tertiary manifestation of the tuberculous infection has become very probable. Already extensive post-mortem examinations of adults have shown that nearly all men become infected with tuberculosis during their lifetime, as in nearly every one some slight residue of a smaller or larger tuberculous process is found (Naegeli). Since the local tests have been applied on large numbers of individuals, and since many statistics have been based on careful dissections of children of all ages (Ghon, Albrecht), we know that this large percentage of tuberculous lesions is not found during infancy. With very few exceptions, newly born infants have no signs of tuberculosis, and only about 5 per cent. become infected during the first year of life. Even these are not included in the number of tuberculous adults, because nearly all infants infected so early in life die some months after the infection, but we see that after the first year, there is a constant increase in the percentage of slight tuberculous lesions, and therefore, of infections which do not lead to death. It may be stated that at least about 5 per cent. of the children of the poorer classes become infected each year in cities in which tuberculosis of the lungs is prevalent among adults, as in Vienna and probably New York. Therefore, when these children reach the age of twenty years, nearly all of them have been infected with tuberculosis (F. Hamburger). The first infection in early childhood is hardly ever followed by an excavating tuberculosis of the lungs. We find either a small local infection of the lung only, and some foci in the regionary glands, or we find a dissemination especially in the lymphatic system and the bones, often concomitant with a tendency to catarrhal symptoms of the mucous membranes and the outer skin (scrofulosis). In cases of generally disseminated tuberculosis occurring during the first years of life, the upper parts of the lungs are not especially affected and a cavity is hardly ever found. In the adult, on the contrary, the upper parts of the lungs form a seat of predilection for the tuberculous process. No doubt there exists a very interesting difference in the localization of the disease. The fact that the apices of the lungs of adults are places of predilection has been explained on anatomical and physiological grounds (ventilation deficient). Bantel thinks that the lung tissue in itself is less resistant than the other tissues. One might ask whether the lungs acquire a disposition to that special kind of infection with advancing age. I am rather inclined to think that the reason may be that an infection in childhood has left an allergic condition to tuberculosis, producing a tendency to new forms. As in discussing vaccinia, I shall consider the effect of a renewed infection with tuberculosis in individuals who have become allergic in consequence of an infection during childhood. When a tuberculous animal is injected with a large number of tubercle bacilli, it shows sudden symptoms within twenty-four hours, leading to an immediate death, or at least to a high fever beginning immediately after the injection. When a small amount is injected, this second slight injection leads to an early but rapidly healing local lesion (Koch).

Trudeau, in 1902, injected guinea-pigs with virulent cultures of tuberculosis and paid special attention to the post-mortem findings in the lungs. He found that guinea-pigs which had before been infected with an attenuated strain of tubercle bacilli showed, after the second infection, a far more marked reaction in the lungs than the controls, "so much so as to give the impression that the protected are more susceptible than the controls, but the immunity is shown by the fact that the lesion so rapidly produced tends in the protected animals to remain localized, to retrograde and become absorbed.

This has been proved, furthermore, by F. Hamburger, who showed that cutaneous infections in allergic animals made a very fugitive impression on the skin. The result of the reinfection, whether it leads to death or to a local lesion of short duration is entirely dependent on the amount used. A small number of bacilli cause reinfections from the outside, but it can readily be conceived that a reinfection with a somewhat larger number may take its origin from foci inside the body. The glands can harbor living tubercle bacilli for a long time. If such a focus should be opened, for instance, by traumatism or an operation, it discharges a large number of bacilli into the veins. The bacilli would, for the most part, be filtered out in the lungs. If the bacilli are single, they may be killed and produce a very slight toxic reaction in their neighborhood like a tuberculin test or like the early reaction in vaccinia, but if they occur in larger aggregations, those in the center of the mass may not be killed but may remain alive. In their neighborhood a zone of inflammatory reaction is maintained which goes through a process of pus-formation or caseation and leads, later on, to cavity-formation. The latest experiments in this line have been done by Roemer. He injected chronic tuberculous guinea-pigs with small amounts of tubercle bacilli. The course of the primary tuberculosis was practically not affected by the reinfection, for the animals died after a term which corresponded to the slow progress of the first infection. But a marked allergy was shown to the second infection: after very small doses (which, however, were many times larger than the smallest dose necessary to give a fatal tuberculosis to a normal guinea-pig) a second infection showed no lasting results at all. Increasing the dose ten times, indurations occurred at the point of injection, caseation of the regionary lymph-glands, and—a point which interests us especially—a cavity formation in the lungs. Roemer furthermore conducted experiments with the object of determining whether this cavity formation resulted only on reinfection with bacilli derived from a source outside of the body ("additional infection" of Behring), or whether bacilli grown in the same organism could also produce this lesion. He took a tuberculous gland from a tuberculous guinea-pig, made an emulsion of the gland, and injected it subcutaneously into the same guinea-pig. Again, besides slight local changes, a cavity formation in the lung resulted; thus it is proved that a "metastatic auto-infection" (Roemer) can produce tuberculosis of the lungs.

In the human organism such an auto-infection could be brought about not only by the mechanical opening of a gland containing an old culture of tubercle bacilli. A second possibility is given when a latent tuberculosis exists and the organism passes through a period of "anergy." This supposition is thus far purely theoretical and rests solely on my demonstration of anergy in measles. In the last chapter it was mentioned that the sensitiveness to tuberculin drops to a minimum for about a week following an eruption of measles exanthema. In the sense of our theory this means that the antibodies necessary for this reaction are absorbed—that is, are not free to combine with the tuberculin—or that some condition necessary for their interaction with the tuberculous virus no longer exists. For the explanation of the auto-infection on the basis of anergy we shall keep in mind, first, the diminished sensitiveness during the eruptive stage of measles, and second, the old clinical experience that during the same period a latent tuberculosis may disseminate itself acutely throughout the whole body. I therefore advance the hypothesis that tubercle bacilli, which are located in the center of foci surrounded by reactive zones, can grow within the reactive zones, penetrate them and enter the general circulation during the period when the antibodies are lacking or unable to display their function with regard to the tubercle bacilli. After the period of anergy reactivity begins again, and foci are formed at every point where tubercle bacilli have been located.

I should suppose, although it is not yet proved, that similar periods of anergy will be found in the course of other diseases, and that the influence which some periods of life possess in the spreading of tuberculosis, according to clinical experience, will be explained in the same way. It is a remarkable analogy between measles and pregnancy that, in the latter, cavity formation in the teeth progresses often acutely; likewise we see in measles the invasion of the body by various affections of the mucous membranes and the skin.

In view of the foregoing we may distinguish three states of tuberculosis analogous to syphilis: (1) primary tuberculosis; primary effect on place of infection with participation of the regionary lymph-glands; (2) secondary tuberculosis: a more or less general spreading of the tuberculosis some time after, but in direct connection with the primary infection; and (3) tertiary tuberculosis, a spreading of the tuberculous process, occurring years after the primary infection, with intense reactive processes, and especially cavity formation.

When the first infection takes place during certain favorable periods of life (childhood, not infancy), the disease does not pass the primary localized lesions. An infection in infancy, especially in the first year of life, is nearly always followed by a fatal secondary state. Some individuals develop a non-fatal secondary state of long duration (scrofulosis).

All individuals who have passed through a primary or a secondary state in their youth, possess for the rest of their life some resistance against a new infection from outside. But they are in danger of passing into a tertiary state of tuberculosis by auto-infections with bacterial cultures contained within some old lesions in their own body. These cultures can enter the circulation either by a mechanical opening of their capsules or during anergic periods (disappearance of antibodies) in which the bacilli can penetrate the reactive zones.

## *CONCLUSIONS*

Having passed in review all the details of our knowledge in connection with each group of diseases, it now remains to give the result of our investigations. In order to study the change of reaction, we had to study what the clinical reaction in itself means to the body. We have seen that in most of the diseases which we have here considered, the clinical reaction was not an immediate consequence of the infection, but that it was a phenomenon of a more complicated nature, a phenomenon which could not be explained simply by the action of a micro-organism of some other foreign substance on the tissues, but involving the existence of a third factor. This third factor appears only some time after the first infection. In order to arrive at some explanation of this third factor, it first of all appeared essential to study the time in which the reaction appears, and here we may distinguish between the following groups:

### GROUP I.—THE REACTION APPEARS AFTER EIGHT TO TWELVE DAYS

We have found a number of diseases in which a period of eight to twelve days elapsed between the infection and the clinical reaction. This is true not only of spontaneous infectious diseases, like smallpox, measles, whooping-cough, chicken-pox and others; we see it also if we produce an artificial infection on the skin with a micro-organism belonging to that group, that is with vaccinia. The same phenomenon is seen after the injection of horse-serum in man: in the serum sickness of man we have an example of a non-infectious disease following the same rules of time.

But the clinical appearance of disease is not the only reaction following this law. The formation of certain antibodies and the appearance of a change in the reactivity are two other phenomena following the same law. Between the injection of horse-serum in the circulation of rabbits and the appearance of precipitating antibodies in their blood a period of eight to twelve days is consumed. The same period furthermore elapses between the injection of different proteins in the guinea-pig and the appearance of a state of hypersusceptibility against the identical kind of protein.

### GROUP II.—THE REACTION APPEARS AFTER THREE TO SEVEN DAYS

Under certain conditions it has been noted that the time of the reaction was between three and seven days. A man revaccinated ten years after his first vaccination does not require eight to twelve days for the development of the reaction; on the contrary, the clinical manifestations appear after the short period above mentioned. Similar phenomena seen after the injection of horse-serum in man after a long interval, while finally, the time of precipitive formation is shortened also on reinjection. When an animal which has been injected several months previously, but has already lost its precipitating antibodies, is injected again, the antibody then reappears at this early date.

### GROUP III.—THE REACTION APPEARS IMMEDIATELY

The third type of reaction with regard to its time relationship is the immediate reaction. Clinically the most striking examples of this are seen when a child previously treated with antidiphtheria serum receives another injection some weeks later and shows within a few minutes a general rash of urticaria, edema, and signs of collapse. Even more impressive is the behavior of guinea-pigs, when a second injection given intravenously or intracerebrally leads to immediate death. We have seen a similar type of reaction occurring within twenty-four hours in vaccinia, in tuberculosis and in several other diseases.

### QUANTITATIVE AND QUALITATIVE CHANGES OF THE REACTION

It has been shown that we can clearly distinguish between three groups of reactions with regard to the time at which they appear. But aside from the differences observed in this regard, there are changes in the reactions with regard to their intensity and their quality. First, infections with a small amount of micro-organisms were followed by a far more intense reaction than the subsequent infections. On the other hand we generally found that if the injection was performed a second time, the immediate effect of it was of startling intensity. We then found also differences in the quality of reaction. Instead of a generalized effect of the infection with tuberculosis, for instance, a second infection leads only to a local inflammation. Besides these, two other phenomena have been noted:

1. The change in the reaction can be transmitted with the serum of one animal to another: if, for instance, the serum of a rabbit, which, by a former injection, has acquired the property to react immediately, is injected into a guinea-pig, this guinea-pig becomes for a short time nearly as susceptible as the rabbit was.

2. Somewhat in contrast to the production of altered reactivity is the following phenomenon: if an animal which has acquired the property of the immediate reaction is injected with a large amount of the material to which it is susceptible, it is not able to react for several days. For instance, tuberculous cattle, after having received an excessive amount of tuberculin, do not give any tuberculin reaction for a short time.

Table 5 contains in an abridged form the different diseases with their allergic phenomena described in the first part, with the name of the observers and the date of publication.

## EXPLANATION OF THE PHENOMENA

In the preceding sections I have limited myself more or less to stating the facts and to drawing my conclusions on the basis of these facts. In the following pages it is my intention to give an explanation of the phenomena in a more subjective manner, calling to my aid many suppositions not as yet quite proved scientifically. I wish it distinctly understood that this effort at an explanation does not claim to rest entirely on facts, and that I reserve the right to changes whenever new investigations may make it necessary. The sketches I use for illustration are not made with the intention of creating the opinion that everything therein contained is mathematically proved. They should be accepted only for what they are intended, that is as a scheme to make myself clearly understood.

The incongruity between the generally accepted theories with regard to the incubation time of infectious diseases and the phenomena I had observed in serum diseases first led me to question these theories taught *ex cathedra.* I had been taught that the incubation time was dependent on the development of the micro-organism, and that only after its toxins had reached a certain point of evolution within the human body, was it powerful enough to elicit symptoms of a general reaction. I should have supposed that in a body which by a previous infection had acquired some resistance against a disease, the micro-organism would grow more slowly, and reach that limit later; therefore a second attack if it developed at all might be expected to appear after a longer incubation time than the first.

Table 5.—Allergic Phenomena of Various Diseases

| | Altered Reactivity—Allergy. | | | | | | | | | | | | | |
|---|---|---|---|---|---|---|---|---|---|---|---|---|---|---|
| | First Reaction After Incubation time of 8-12 days. Appearance of | | Incubation of 4-7 days. "Accelerated Reaction." | No Incubation Time—*Immediate Reaction*—Produced by | | | | | | | | | Transmission of Allergy (passive A.) by Injection of Allergic Serum. | Suppression of Allergy (Antianaphylaxis) by injection of Allergen. |
| | | | | Injection. | | | | Vaccination. Outer Skin. | | | Application—Mucous Membrane | | | |
| | | | | Intravenous. General Reaction | Subcutaneous. | | | | | | | | | |
| | Disease. | Allergy. | | | General Reaction. | Local (Stich) Reaction. | Focal Reaction. | Intracutaneous. | Cutaneous. | Percutaneous. | Conjunctiva. | Digestive Tract. | | |
| Serum disease: Man | v. Pirque | t and Schi | ck, 1903 | ........ | v. Pirquet and Schick, '03. | v. Pirquet and Schick, '03. | | | | | | | | |
| Rabbit | ........ | or von Pirquet and Schick. | ........ | Arthus, 1903. | Arthus, 1903. | Arthus, 1903. | ........ | ........ | ........ | ........ | ........ | ........ | v. Pirquet and Schick 1905: Nicolle,'07. | Nicolle,'07. Besredska, 1907. |
| Guinea-pig | ........ | Rosenau and Anderson, 1906. | ........ | Otto, '06. Rosenau and Anderson, 1906. | Theo. C. Smith,'03, Rosenau and Anderson,'06 | Lewis, '08. | ........ | ........ | ........ | ........ | ........ | ........ | Otto, 1907.. | Otto, 1907. |
| Urticaria: Man | ........ | Landman, 1908. | ........ | ........ | ........ | ........ | ........ | ........ | H. Lee Smith, 1909. | Clinic... | ........ | Clinical experience. | Bruck,1909. | |
| Hayfever: Man | ........ | ........ | ........ | ........ | Dunbar, 1903. | Dunbar, 1903. | ........ | ........ | Blackley 1873. | ........ | Blackley 1873; Wolff-Eisner, 1904. | | | |
| Cowpox: Man | Clinical experience. | v. Pirquet, 1903. | v, Pirquet, 1907. | ........ | Knoepfelmacher, 1906. | Knoepfelmacher, 1906. | ........ | ........ | von Pirquet, 1903. | | | | | |
| Tuberculosis: Man | ........ | ........ | ........ | Koch, '91 | Koch, 1891. | Epstein,'01 Escherich, 1892. | Koch,'91. | Mendel, 1908. | von Pirquet, 1907. | Moro,'07. | Wolff-Eisner, 1807; Calmette 1907. | Freymuth. | ........ | F. Hamburger, 1908. |
| Cattle | Roemer, 1908. | ........ | (Roemer, 1909.) | Koch, '91 | Koch, 1891. | ........ | Koch,'91. | Mantoux 1908. | Vallée, 1907. | Lignièraes,'07 | Vallée, 1907. | ........ | ........ | Vallée, '07. |
| Rabbit and guinea-pig | ........ | Preisich and Heim, 1902. | ........ | Koch, '91 | Koch, 1891. | ........ | Koch,'91. | Roemer, 1909. | ........ | ........ | ........ | ........ | Yamanouchi, Bauer, Helmholz, '09. | |
| Glanders: Horse and man | ........ | ........ | ........ | ........ | Helman and Kalming, '91. | Helman and Kalming, '91. | ........ | ........ | Vallée, 1907. | Schnurer 1907. | Schnurer 1907. | | | |
| Lepra: Man | ........ | ........ | ........ | ........ | De Beurman and Gougens. | De Beurman and Gougens. | De Beurman and Gougens. | | | | | | | |
| Syphilis: Man | Clinic.- | ........ | ........ | ........ | ........ | Finger and Landstrum,'04 | ........ | | | | | | | |
| Trichophytia: Man, rabbit | Bloch, | 1909. ...... | (Bloch, '09) | ........ | Neisser and Plato,'04 | Neisser and Plato,'04 | ........ | ........ | Bloch, '09 | | | | | |

But I had seen that the symptoms of serum disease appeared more than a week after a first injection of horse-serum in man, while, after a second injection, these symptoms appeared immediately. This was entirely contrary to every rule with which I had been familiar. It appeared to me, therefore, that the whole question should be approached from an entirely new point of view. The first outbreak of serum disease could not be due to an evolution of any constituent of the injected serum; it must be that the organism had to take part in the reaction by the formation of an antibody. The presence of this antibody might then lead immediately to a reaction on a second injection. The reaction in either case resulted from a combination of the antibody with the horse-serum, forming a toxic compound, and this toxic compound was the cause of the symptoms of the disease. This explanation involved also quite a new conception of an antibody. Thus far the antibodies were numbered among the protective substances, which is just the contrary of the supposition. Diphtheria antitoxin was considered as a typical antibody. The action of this antibody is to neutralize completely the antigen, i. e., the diphtheria toxin, while in my hypothesis these other antibodies form a new toxic body with the antigen. The principal new conception consisted in the suggestion that a disease might be due indirectly to an antibody, an idea to which at that time adherents of the school of Ehrlich, like Kraus, took strong exception.

I shall illustrate my idea by the following example: A man takes an insoluble salt not decomposed in the digestive tract. The salt particles will slowly pass through the whole intestine and leave the body without any action. But now let us suppose that the invaded organism has the property of changing the gastric juice according to the foreign bodies which enter the stomach. Let us suppose that this salt would elicit after a period of eight to twelve days a specific gastric juice, able to dissolve the salt. If after that time a part of the salt has been left within the intestinal tract, it will now be dissolved. Now it may act as a poison in either of two ways: First, the salt itself in solution is a poison; second, a new body formed by a chemical union of the stomach juice and the salt may be a poison. Granted our suppositions, the general symptoms would appear after eight to twelve days, a time analogous to that at which serum disease appears after the first injection of horse-serum. Two weeks later the stomach will still secrete this specific juice. If the man now takes this insoluble salt again, it will be dissolved immediately after it has passed into the stomach and will elicit an immediate intoxication, analogous to the early reaction after the second injection of serum. The degree of the intoxication will be dependent on the amount of salt taken. In the first instance, the degree of the intoxication is not so much dependent on the amount of salt taken, as on the amount still in existence when the secretion of the special juice sets in.

We may take another example, in which the intestinal canal figures, in order to explain my conception with regard to the infectious diseases. A man takes milk containing a small number of bacteria which cannot be attacked by any of the intestinal juices, but which find a good medium in the walls of the intestinal canal. The bacteria will form colonies wherever they settle, and each of these colonies will grow slowly. Now we suppose again that the bacteria stimulate the secretion of a specific ferment in the beginning of the second week. With the appearance of this ferment the digestion of the bacteria, the absorption of toxic products, and therewith the disease begins. Again there are two possibilities: the ferment may be able to dissolve the bacteria and the colonies will be killed *in toto;* a large amount of toxin would be produced at once, the disease will be intense but will come to an end after a very few days. Or the ferment acts only on the products of the bacteria or on their dead bodies; then the disease will not set in so acutely but will last for a long time. The first example corresponds to the acute infectious diseases, especially to cowpox, and the second to chronic infections and especially to tuberculosis. In both cases the question remains whether the contents of the bacteria or their products are toxic in themselves, or whether the combination of these with the ferment constitute the agent harmful for the organism.

We can study an example of an acute infection very well on the skin in vaccinia. To make myself clearly understood I shall have to repeat some of the data given in the first chapter. A colony of the micro-organism is formed on the skin. We can observe its growth from day to day, and we see that it follows the same rule of growth as a colony on an agar plant (Fig. 1, first row, *A*). On the eighth day this colony is filled with an enormous number of micro-organisms. We can take the contents of a vaccination blister and make new colonies on thousands of other arms. But one or two days later the ferment-like antibody appears. The colony is attacked, its contents digested and a toxic body is formed by that digestion. This is diffused in the neighborhood and elicits the intense local inflammation which we call area. In addition the toxin enters the general circulation and produces fever. At the same time the micro-organisms are killed, and we can no longer vaccinate with the contents of the now yellow pustule. After two or three days the struggle with the micro-organisms is finished, but the organism contains the new antibody for a long time.

Now we revaccinate. As long as the antibody is present, the micro-organism introduced into the scarification of the skin is attacked and digested immediately. The micro-organisms have not the time to multiply and therefore only an extremely small amount of toxin is formed.

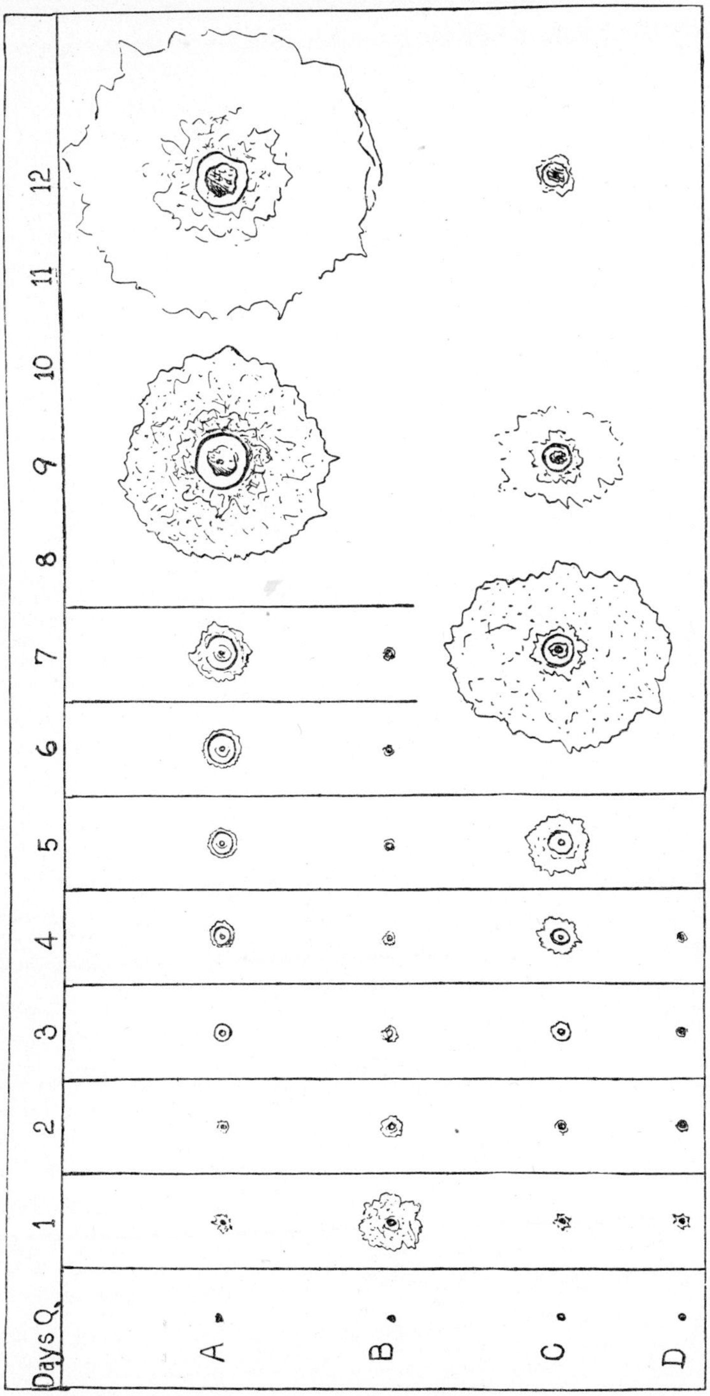


Fig. 1.—Effects of cowpox vaccination in man watched from day to day: A, first vaccination with cowpox. B, revaccination after short interval; early reaction. C, revaccination after long interval. D, traumatism alone.

This is the immediate reaction designated "early reaction" in vaccinia (Fig. 1, second row, *B*). If a number of years have elapsed between the first vaccination and the second, the antibodies are no longer present but the organism has retained the property to form them more quickly than on the first occasion. Here we see that during the first days the organisms multiply (Fig. 1, third row, *C*) as in a first vaccination, the antibodies are produced more quickly and attack the micro-organisms after only four or five days. Since the micro-organisms have not had time to multiply in sufficient numbers, the amount of digestion products is rela-

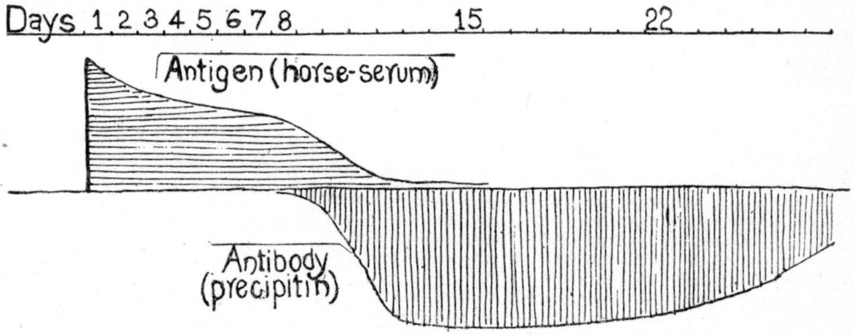


Fig. 2.—Formation of precipitin in rabbits after injection of horse-serum.

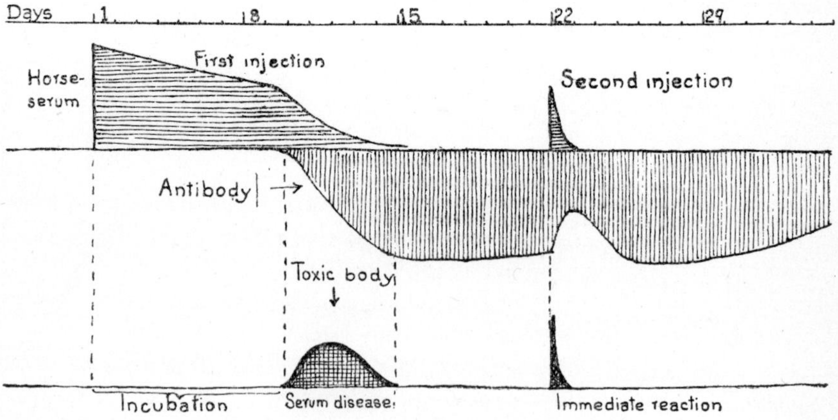


Fig. 3.—Effects of horse-serum in man.

tively small. The result is a comparatively small local inflammation, and practically no general symptoms.

In the following pages I shall pass in review the whole subject, illustrating it with diagrams. This will give me the opportunity to touch on several other points and will aid in making the subject clear. In all the figures the time is indicated as abscissa. The antibody is indicated by vertical shadings below the abscissa, and the antigen (or allergen) is shown by horizontal shadings above it. By this antigen (Detre's term) I understand a substance which is able to give rise to an antibody in the organism. Figure 2 shows in a very schematic manner the formation of precipitin in rabbits. On the first day a considerable amount of horse-serum is injected. This horse-serum does not disappear immediately. Its presence can be shown by a daily test with antihorse-serum of another animal. We see then that the amount of the antigen present in the vessels of the rabbit diminishes slowly from day to day. On the tenth day, with another test (that is, mixing the serum of the rabbit with horse-serum), we detect the formation of a precipitin. The precipitin increases to a considerable amount within some days and then remains at about the same height for a longer period.

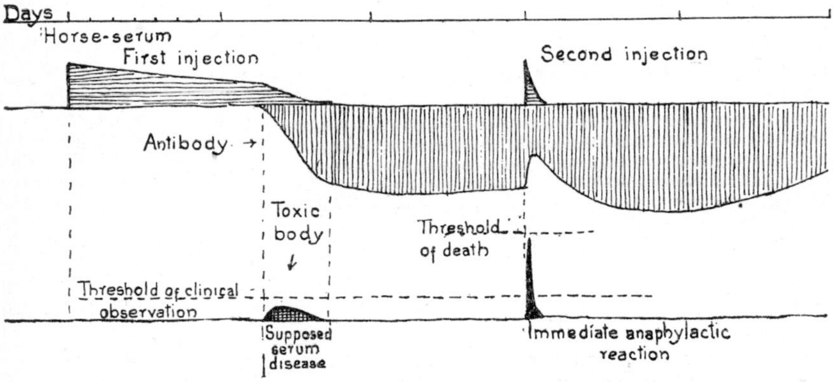


Fig. 4.—Effects of horse-serum in guinea-pigs or rabbits.

EFFECTS OF HORSE-SERUM IN MAN

In Figure 3 we meet one fact encountered in Figure 2, i. e., the connection between the antigen and its antibody. Here we have injected the horse-serum not into a rabbit but into man, and are able to observe the effects of the toxic body formed when antigen and antibody meet, that is, the serum disease. We see that at the time when the antibody arises, and therefore the antigen disappears, symptoms of general disease occur. The supposed connection is that these symptoms are due to toxic bodies formed by this digestion of the allergen through the antibody. To the right of the figure we see in a schematic way the effect of a reinjection. With the first injection, the horse-serum was present at first and the antibody arose later. Here we have the contrary: the antibody is present and the horse-serum comes later, but the effect is a similar one, except that the toxic body is formed immediately and elicits what we call an immediate reaction.

In Figure 4 we return to the rabbit, in order to show what the reinjection means. We suppose that after the first injection there must also be some serum disease after an incubation time. This is only a supposition, because the clinical phenomena of it could not be so easily proved as in man. I say, therefore, that the phenomena due to the toxic body are below the level of clinical observation. This level is shown by a broken horizontal line. On reinjection the immediate reaction rises far above this line, and if we apply the horse-serum to a very sensitive part of the body, for instance, if we inject into the brain, it even reaches a second broken line, i. e., the limit of death.

In Figure 5 we assume that we injected with horse-serum a rabbit which had been injected several months before and which had already

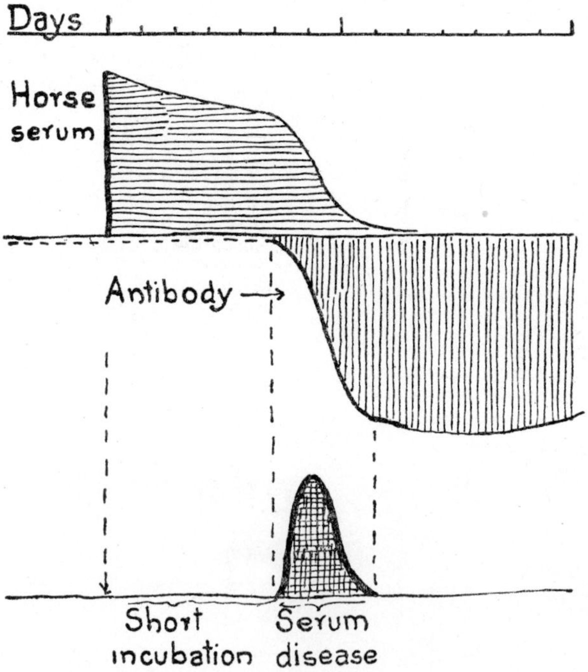


Fig. 5.—Accelerated serum disease.

lost the precipitin in its blood. We see here that the antibody appears as early as the sixth day, and consequently the horse-serum disappears at the same time. This is the accelerated reaction. In rabbits, however, we are not able to observe the clinical phenomena seen in man, indicated by the lower part of the figure. The serum disease appears after an incubation time as short as five days.

Figure 6 adds one more complication to the process. A man is injected who had been injected before and who still contains antibodies. The horse-serum reacts first with the existing antibody. The toxic substance produced at that time causes an immediate reaction, but the

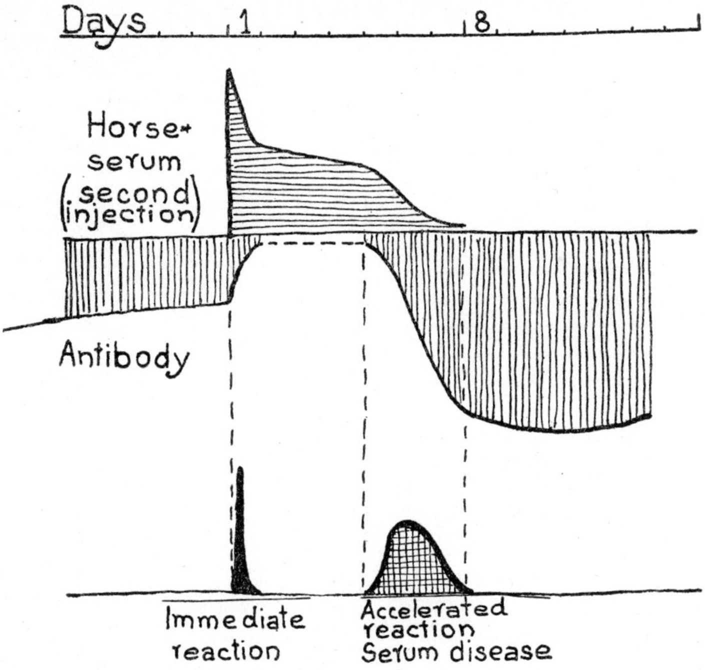


Fig. 6.—Double reaction after reinjection in man.

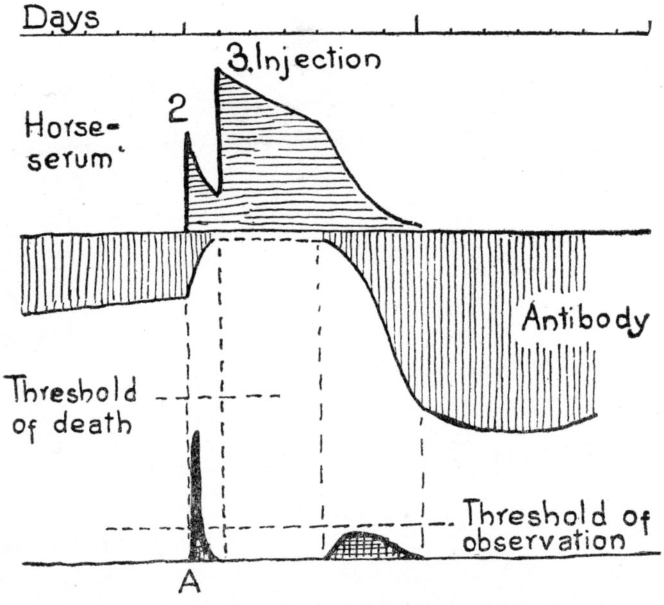


Fig. 7.—Anergy (antianaphylaxis).

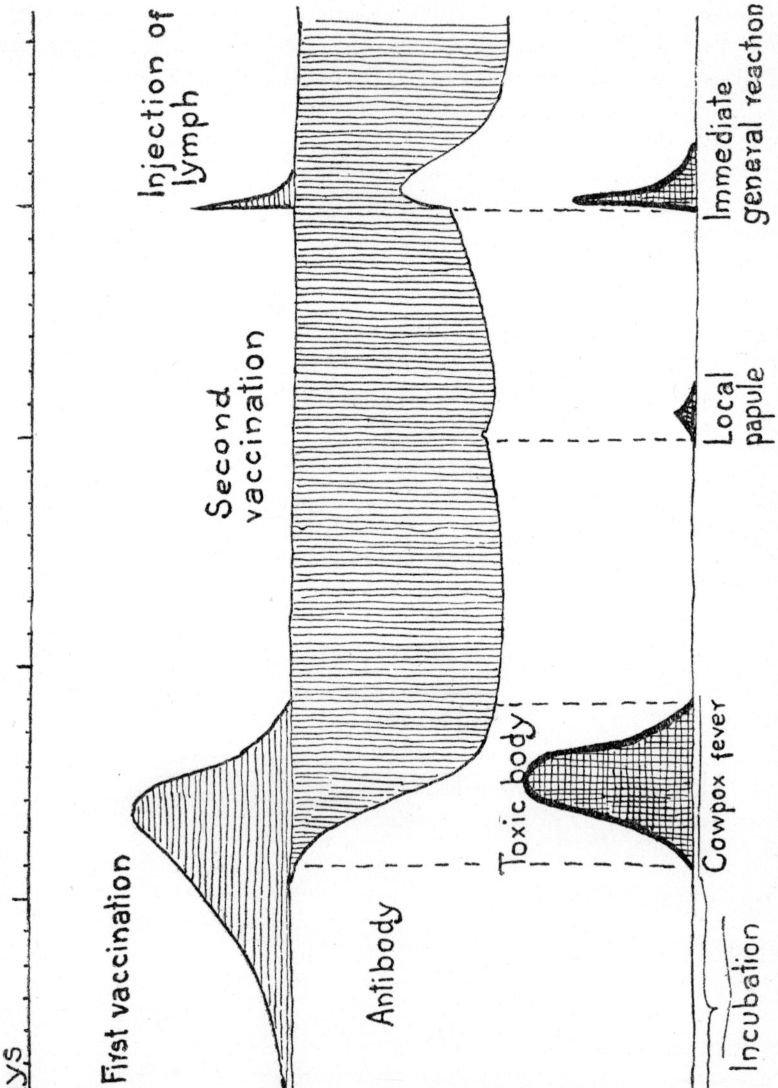


Fig. 8.—Effects of first and repeated cowpox vaccination in man.

amount of horse-serum is relatively larger than the amount of antibody, and after the union has taken place, no free antibody is left. After a period of four days a new formation of antibody begins. The antibody destroys the remainder of the horse-serum, and the result is again a toxic action, an "accelerated serum disease." I have described these cases of a combined early and "accelerated reaction" in the chapter on serum disease in man. During the time the antibody is lacking a repetition of the horse-serum injection has no immediate effect, because the horse-serum finds no antibody to unite it. This is shown in Figure 7, which shows an experiment on a rabbit several weeks after the first injection of horse-serum. It contains antibody. A second injection (a) is performed. The horse-serum injected unites immediately with the exist-

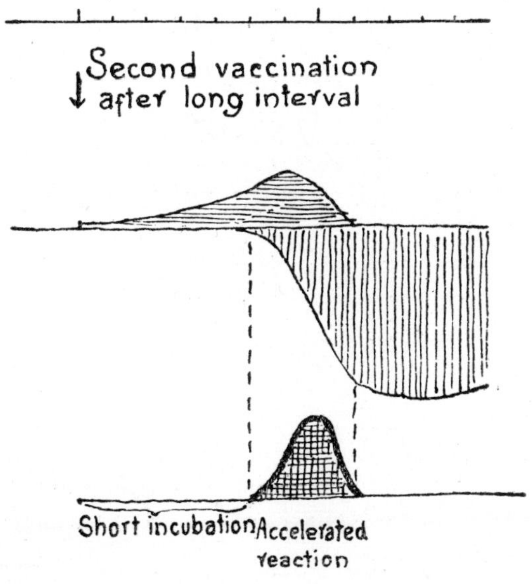


Fig. 9.—Second cowpox vaccination after long interval.

ing antibody, thus forming the toxic body, and so elicits acute symptoms. If they do not reach the death limit, the animal survives. On injection twenty-four hours later of a third amount of horse-serum, no symptoms occur. This phenomenon is called by Nicolle "antianaphylaxis." The animal requires some time for a renewed production of antibody and when this is accomplished, it becomes susceptible again. The serum disease which ought to be concomitant with that reformation of antibody does not reach the threshold of clinical observation.

Now we come to the infectious diseases (Fig. 8), and take as an example vaccination. The difference from the former examples lies in the fact that the allergen is not introduced directly in a maximum amount, but develops gradually during the incubation time. Therefore, the curve above the line reaches its maximum on the tenth day; when its further growth is checked by the appearance of the antibodies it decreases rapidly. The digestion of the allergen again gives rise to general symptoms which are noted as a feverish state of vaccinia. Two other experiments are noted on the same figure. The one is revaccination in the usual method. A minimal amount of allergen is put into the skin, producing a slight local reaction, while the general reaction does not reach the threshold of clinical observation. But if we inject the lymph of vaccinia, thereby introducing a large amount of allergen in the body, a greater amount of toxic body is formed, eliciting an intense local reaction and general symptoms, both disappearing rapidly.[2]

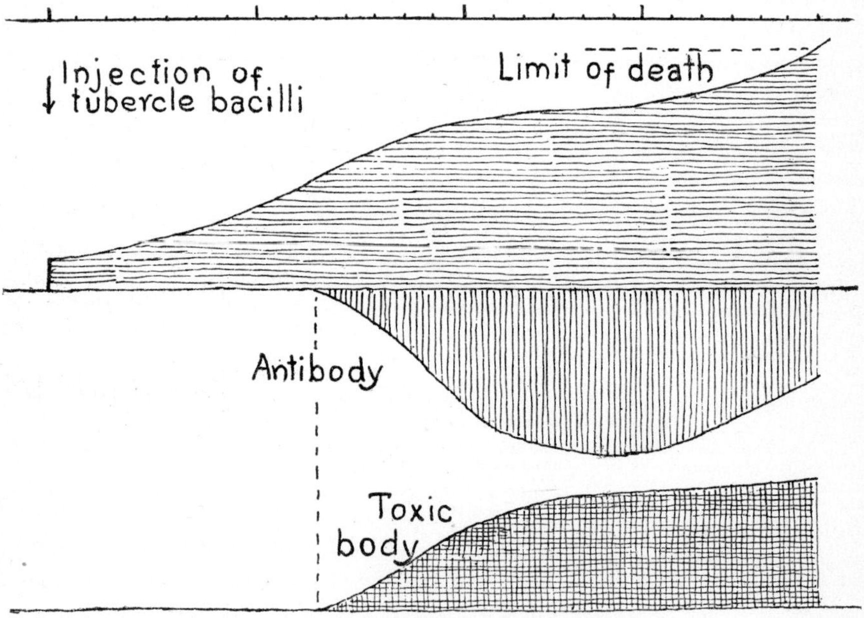


Fig. 10.—Injection of large amount of tubercle bacilli.

Figure 9 shows an accelerated reaction in vaccinia. The early reappearance of the antibody is analogous to the phenomenon shown in Figure 5. The difference from a first vaccination (Fig. 8) is that the vaccinia micro-organisms have not had time to develop to any considerable extent during the short time required for the production of the antibody. The toxic body formed is therefore too small in amount to give rise to an intense general reaction. It hardly reaches the threshold of clinical manifestation, and the only phenomena seen are of a local nature.

2. Certain phenomena of lessened reactivity during the time of the first vaccination are left out purposely, because the time is not yet ripe for the discussion of these complications. They are treated more explicitly in my book.

Figure 10 shows the condition in an infection with a large number of tubercle bacilli, as in Roemer's experiments on cattle. As in vaccinia, with the appearance of the antibody, a toxic substance is formed leading to fever, but in tuberculosis unlike vaccinia the allergen is not destroyed: the tubercle bacilli keep on growing and after some weeks cause the death of the animal.

Second injections of horse-serum in animals may also be followed by death, but in the case of tuberculosis the death limit is reached by wholly different means. In the reinjection of horse-serum it is simply a question of the penetration of the foreign serum into the central nervous system whether the death limit be reached or not. If the allergen be digested locally at the point of application and do not reach the central organs, the animal survives the shock. In tuberculosis after ample infection, the death limit is reached of necessity, and it is only a question whether death will occur sooner or later.

In tuberculosis it is exceptional to see an acute clinical phenomenon so early as is shown in Figure 10. As a rule the incubation time both

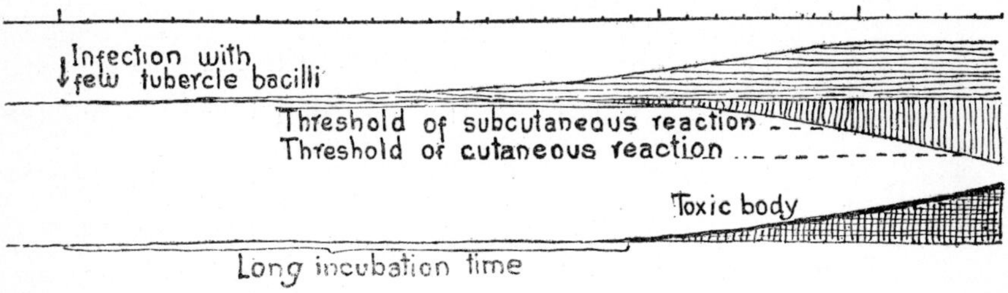


Fig. 11.—Slow antibody formation after infection with few or attenuated tubercle bacilli.

of the clinical phenomena and of the manifestation of allergy is a far longer one. To understand this we must revert again to vaccination, to those cases in which we use a very diluted lymph. We see then that the incubation period is lengthened. Extremely small amounts of allergen seem to elicit the antibody formation only very slowly, a phenomenon which we also met with in the experiments with horse-serum on guinea-pigs. And Roemer's experiments with tuberculosis show that the antibody formation can occur very late after an infection with few or with attenuated germs (Fig. 11). In these cases the human organism is able to resist the infection and to overcome it in time. Clinical facts to which I allude are the bronchial infections of older children, and Figure 12 explains the train of events. In this figure the time is marked in months instead of days. The antibody, although slowly formed, precedes the growth of large masses of tubercle bacilli and so is able to overwhelm them. After some time the allergen begins to decrease; that means that the bacilli are localized. A very small amount of toxic body is produced;

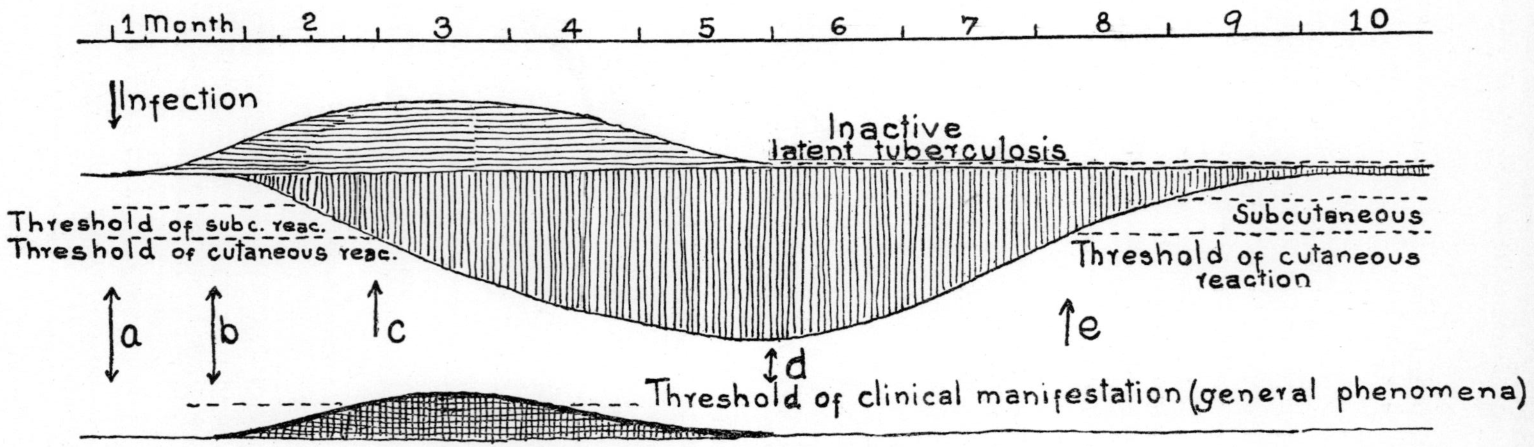


Fig. 12.—Course of benign infection of man with tuberculosis.

the clinical symptoms hardly reach the threshold of manifestation. After several months practically no more free allergen is present in the organism; the antibodies, however, are present for a much longer time and decrease only slowly.

We can distinguish several periods in this type of weak tuberculous infection. During the first weeks (*a* to *b* in Fig. 12) tubercle bacilli are slowly growing with no clinical reaction. This is a period in which tubercle bacilli may be found only microscopically, or by injection of the tissues in animals (Bartel's lymphatic state). Between *b* and *c* the antibodies slowly increase just as the tuberculous process does, but the formation of toxin is a slight one, so that the general symptoms do not reach the threshold of clinical manifestation. Between *c* and *d* the struggle is at its height, leading for some time to general symptoms, such as loss of appetite, anemia, fever, but is terminated by the successful fight of the antibodies against the bacilli. In the period *d* to *e* therefore the allergen, i. e., the tubercle bacillus, does not play any rôle in the general system, but the existence of the antibodies can be proved by the tuberculin

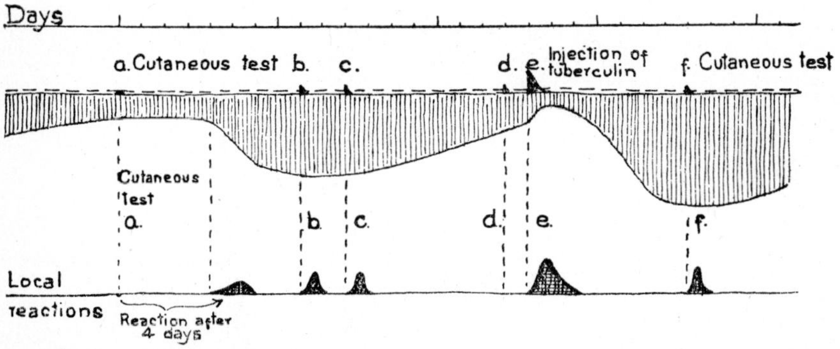


Fig. 13.—Cutaneous and subcutaneous reaction in a case of healed tuberculosis ("latent inactive tuberculosis").

reaction. After *e* the antibodies fall below the level of the cutaneous reaction. With this level I introduce a new conception. The antibodies must be present in the tissues of the skin in a certain concentration, in order to give a positive cutaneous test with undiluted tuberculin. If we inject the tuberculin into the subcutaneous tissue, we can still elicit positive reactions. The level of the subcutaneous reaction is a lower one, as is shown in Figure 13, which is supposed to form the continuation of Figure 12 after point *e*. A minimal amount of antibodies is present, an amount not only below the cutaneous but even below the subcutaneous level. An application of tuberculin in any way arouses a renewed formation of the antibodies in the same way as is seen in Figures 4 and 8. When the new-formed antibodies enter the circulation, we expect to see some phenomena corresponding to the "accelerated reaction." This is exactly what happens if we make a skin test; we find local papule formation occurring between the fourth to the seventh day. If after that date we make again a cutaneous test (point *b* Fig. 13), we get an early reaction ("secondary reaction"). Generally the organism cannot be stimulated to further production of antibodies by means of the cutaneous inoculation, and a following cutaneous test *c* elicits the same size of papules. After some time the antibody content of the organism decreases again. Let us suppose that it stands between the level of the cutaneous and the subcutaneous reactivity. If we make a cutaneous test at point *d,* Figure 13, we would get no reaction, but if we inject say 1 mg. of old tuberculin subcutaneously, we get a *Stichreaktion.* This procedure stimulates a renewed antibody formation, and at point *f* the cutaneous reaction will again become positive.

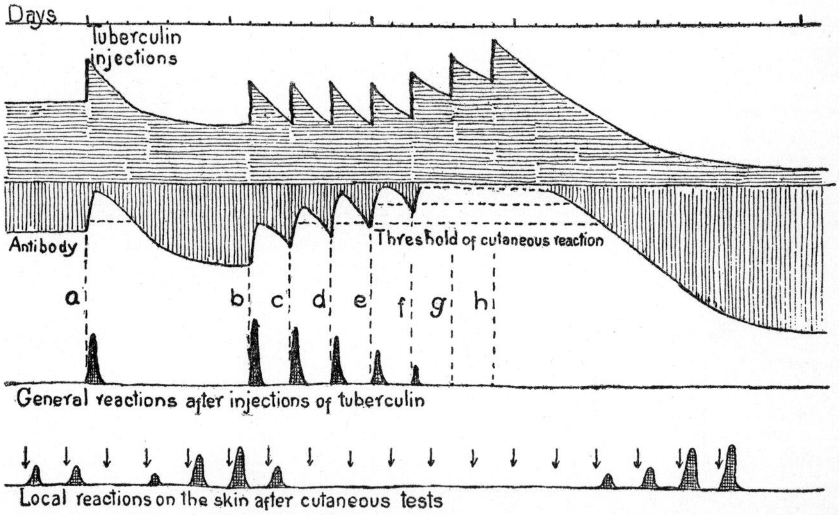


Fig. 14.—Tuberculous "immunity" (better "anergy") by repeated large doses of tuberculosis.

In Figure 14 an explanation of the effects of the administration of large amounts of tuberculin is tried. Two base lines differentiate between the general and local reactions. At point *a* an intravenous injection of tuberculin is given. A general reaction takes place. The amount of antibody falls but is restored shortly. Now we test the reactivity every other day with a cutaneous test (lowest base line), and then we inject six times large doses of tuberculin, say 1 mg. The cutaneous tests do not lessen the general content of antibody, on account of the minute amount of tuberculin introduced (about 0.000001 gm). The injections, however, lead to a continuous diminution of the antibodies, since they are spaced at such short intervals that the antibodies have no time to rise to their original level. Consequently they are exhausted more and more until after the injection *f*, the zero point is approached. As the tuberculin injections can only elicit a general reaction if the tuberculin meets with the antibody, the general reactions are lessened every time, and at point *g* no reaction at all occurs. After the last injection the antibodies have again time to enter the circulation. This is clearly shown in the effect of the cutaneous tests. The cutaneous reactions before *a* are equal; after *b*, however, the test is made at a time when the antibody is present only in amounts a little over the threshold of cutaneous reactivity, therefore the reaction is small. The next time the reactions are completely negative, and only several days after the last injection of tuberculin the reaction reappears with the rising of the antibody content over the threshold of cutaneous reactivity. In the special section on tuberculosis

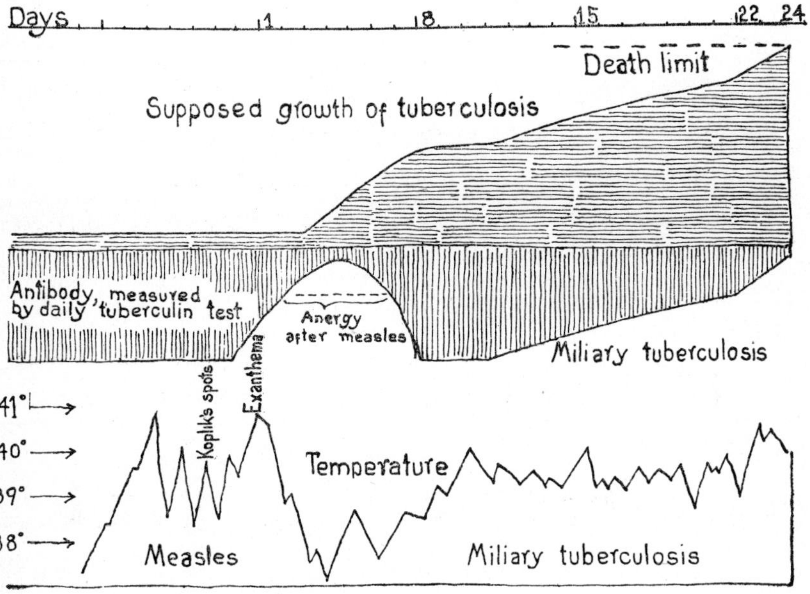


Fig. 15.—Influence of measles on tuberculosis.

we became acquainted with two other reasons for a lessened reactivity to tuberculin. These are the conditions existing in measles and miliary tuberculosis. Figure 15 gives a scheme illustrative of both of these processes. It is constructed on the basis of a case observed by myself. The antibody is measured with daily cutaneous tuberculin tests; the fever curve, indicating the amount of the secondary toxic body, is copied from the chart. The growing of the tubercle bacilli is hypothetical but confirmed at the end by the post-mortem examination. The amount of tuberculin antibody remains unchanged for the first days of the fever of measles; it begins to decrease rapidly with the appearance of the exanthem. My hypothesis is that the tubercle germs, kept in check until now by the antibodies, grow unobstructedly and spread during that period of anergy. After that period, owing to measles, the antibodies return to their former height only for three days; then, a second slow decrease begins, corresponding to the symptoms of the miliary tuberculosis: exhaustion of antibodies, followed by death on the twenty-fourth day after the eruption of measles.

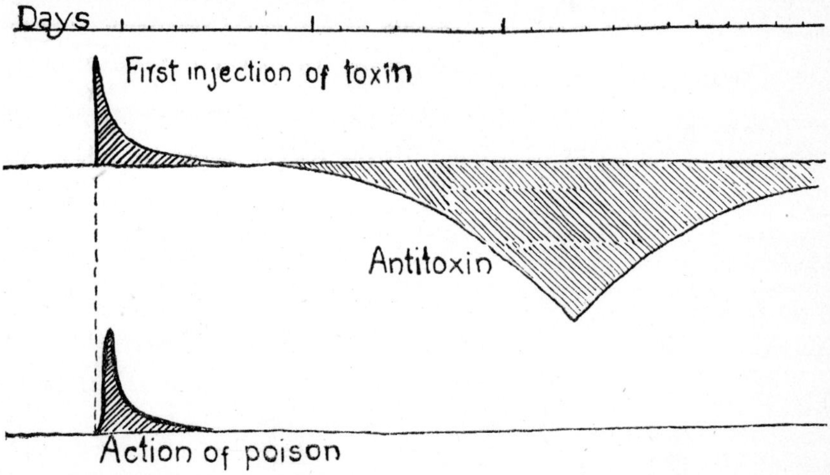


Fig. 16.—Antitoxin formation after single injection of a primary toxic antigen.

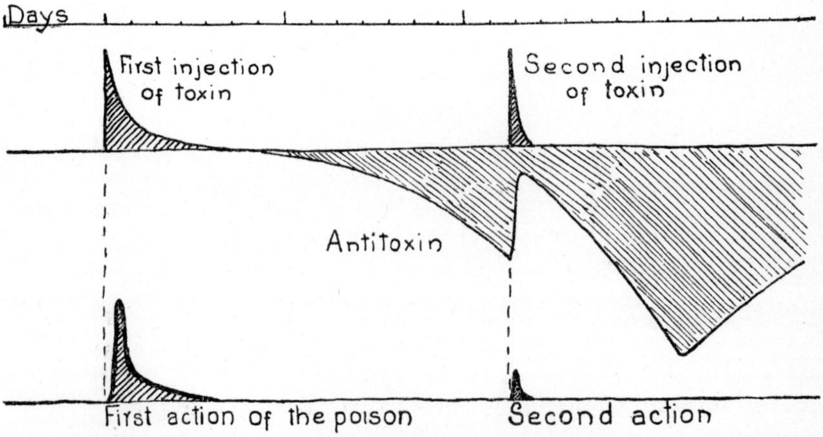


Fig. 17.—Effects of repeated injections of a primary toxic antigen.

MORE COMPLICATED EXPLANATIONS

In the special section on tuberculosis I pointed out that this explanation does not seem to cover all types of tuberculin immunity any more than does the explanation of the effects of vaccinia in this simple manner embrace every feature. The reason seems to be that besides the one antibody which we have considered until now, other antibodies are also involved in the process. The relation of these different antibodies to one another has not as yet been sufficiently studied. Thus far we can point to but one example, indicating the lines we shall have to follow in order to come to a clearer understanding of these more complicated events. This example is that of the effects of eel-serum which have been studied by Doerr and Raubitschek.

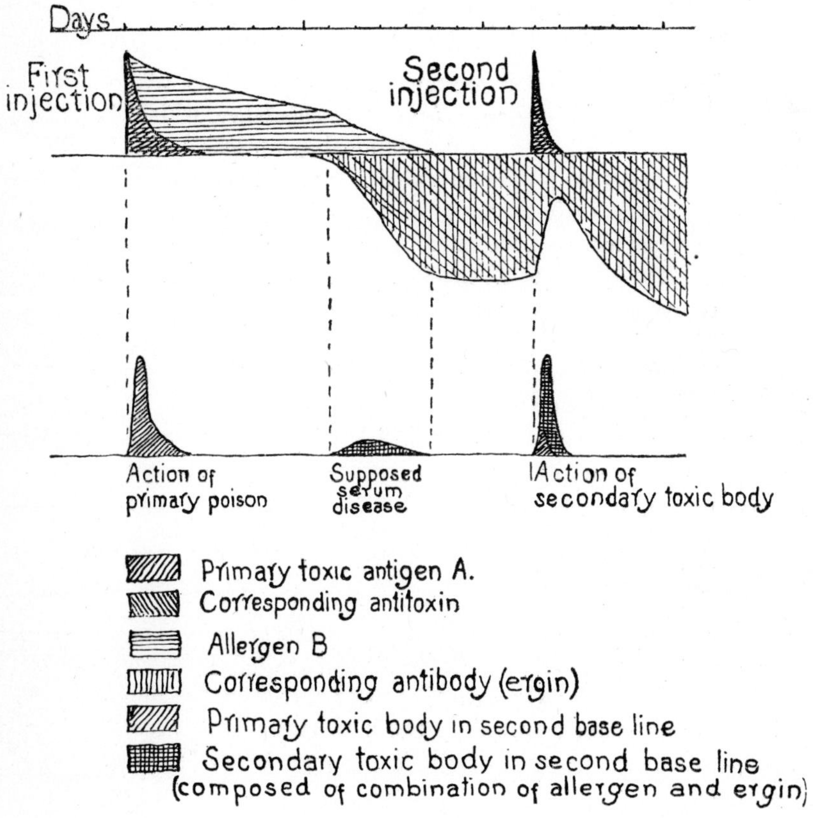


Fig. 18.—Action of eel-serum.

Before approaching this complication, however, we shall have to consider in a few words and two figures the action of a primary toxin, which has at the same time the property of acting as an antigen, that is, of eliciting an antitoxic antibody.

Figure 16 shows on the upper base line, the injection of a certain quantity, and, below the line, the appearance of antitoxic qualities in the serum of the animal. On the lower base line, the immediate toxic action of the poison is indicated.

Here we see the effects of a second administration of the same toxin: it combines with the antitoxin, and only a minimal action on the organism can be noticed clinically.

Now let us return to the eel-serum (Fig. 18). This figure is an attempt at an explanation of the phenomena described by Doerr and Raubitschek. On injection of eel-serum, we must distinguish two different effects. One substance, *A*, in the eel-serum is in itself toxic. This substance is thermolabile and is destroyed by a temperature of 56 C. But there is another substance, *B*, which acts like horse-serum, i. e., it is not primarily toxic, but gives rise to an "ergin" or anaphylactic "antibody." We have to suppose that this allergen coming in contact with the newly-formed antibody produces a secondary toxic substance, which, however, is not concentrated enough to produce clinical symptoms of serum disease. At the second injection of the unheated eel-serum, the effect is a complex one. The primary toxic part, *A*, of the eel-serum meets the antitoxin and therefore has almost no clinical action as it is to the greatest extent neutralized. The allergen, *B*, meets its anaphylactic antibodies and produces a secondary poison which manifests itself in an "immediate reaction."

Probably certain phenomena in diphtheria have to be explained in a similar complicated manner. Here the toxin which plays the main part in diphtheria intoxication is a primary poison. The amount of this poison depends on the number of diphtheria bacilli grown in the organism. At the same time the bacteria contain substances which give rise to ergins (Rist). We are not yet able to determine clinically which of the symptoms are due to the secondary toxins.

In scarlatina, for instance, we shall have to recur to similar explanations. The primary effects of scarlatina occur within a very short time; they have no incubation period. So we can assume that we are dealing with a primary poison. On the other hand, the fact that nephritis and a number of other sequelæ appear between the third and seventh weeks, as Schick pointed out, speaks in favor of an allergic process as the basis of these sequelæ.

### THEORY OF THE VARIOLA AND MEASLES EXANTHEMATA

Another complicated process is the exanthem formation after a long incubation period. I have tried to form a hypothesis as to the exanthemata bringing them into connection with the formation of antibodies. Supposing from an analogy with vaccinia that the exanthem of variola appears on the tenth or eleventh day after infection I tried to determine what time the micro-organisms of variola settled in the skin. As we know that the first symptoms of exanthem appear two to four days after the rise of the temperature, we can determine when the variola germ enters the skin. If we infect the skin from outside with variola, the papule appears two or three days after the infection. In variola living germs enter the skin, certainly not from the outside, but by way of the blood, by arterial distribution. This arterial distribution, therefore, must take place two to three days before the beginning of the first nodules; that is, coincidently with the first rise of temperature. Now we know, from the analogy between vaccinia and variola, that the rise of temperature means the entrance of the antibodies into the general circulation (Figure 8). If the deposition of the variola germs in the skin occurs at the same time with the entrance of the antibodies, it is most probable that there exists a causal relation between the two phenomena. The possibility suggested itself that the antibodies concerned in the deposition of the germs in the skin belonged to the agglutinins. This view gained in strength through the old findings of Weigert and Zuelzer. I do not wish to enter here more deeply into a discussion of this hypothesis which I have treated fully in my book on vaccination. The agglutination hypothesis plays a minor part in my theory. The most important point of this theory is that the exanthem formation is due to an effect of antibodies. I entertain the same conception for all infectious exanthemata which appear after a similar incubation time, especially for measles, German measles and chicken-pox.

I wish to call attention to another phenomenon: the relation of the leukocytes to the appearance of the fever in these diseases, although the study of this relationship is not sufficiently far advanced to permit definite conclusions. In small-pox a leukocytosis exists during the incubation time; with the outbreak of the disease the number of leukocytes drops sharply to reach the lowest figures two or three days later. The same is true in measles and to some extent also in vaccinia. Similar observations have been made in serum disease. As long ago as 1903 I drew attention to these facts, but as yet thorough studies have not been made in this connection.

## CONCLUSION

This whole study has been directed toward the establishment of new conceptions with regard to the clinical phenomena of certain diseases. I have deviated from the methods by which an explanation of these phenomena has been sought, disregarding to a great extent microscopical studies and test-tube experiment. I have replaced these methods by studying the changes in reactions which occur in an organism during an infection, or after having passed through an infection or an intoxication of some kind, studying these changes in the organism itself. As a result it is seen that in a great many diseases it has been possible to demonstrate an altered reactivity of the organism, which I have called "allergy." To recapitulate briefly what manner of alterations I refer to, reference may be made to the following table, which shows the different kinds of allergy which have been discussed:

### Divisions of Allergy

I. ALTERED REACTIVITY ACCORDING TO TIME, COMPARED TO A FIRST REACTION AFTER EIGHT TO TWELVE DAYS

1. Early reaction (immediate reaction) within twenty-four hours. This can be obtained by:
   - (a) Intravenous injection: associated with general symptoms (death).
   - (b) Subcutaneous injection. Here we have to distinguish:
     - (*a*) General symptoms (fever, exanthema).
     - (*b*) Local symptoms (*Stichreaktion*).
     - (*c*) Co-reaction of other foci.
   - (c) Cutaneous vaccination.
   - (d) Conjunctival application.
2. Torpid early reaction—second to fourth day.
3. Accelerated reaction—fourth to seventh day.

II. ALTERED REACTIVITY ACCORDING TO QUANTITY

1. Re-enforced reactivity (hypersensibility, paradoxical reaction, anaphylaxis).
2. Lessened reactivity (hyposensibility).
3. Abolished reactivity (insensibility, immunity).

III. REACTIVITY ALTERED ACCORDING TO QUALITY. (CHANGES REGARDING COLOR, MICROSCOPICAL OBSERVATIONS, ETC.).

This study prompted me to advance new theories of a general character. The old ideas, especially with regard to the symptoms of disease, were abandoned. It has been shown that the symptoms for instance of infectious diseases are not entirely due to the action of the micro-organisms *per se*, but that in many diseases the organism itself takes an active part in the production of most of the symptoms by an interaction of products of its own with products derived from the infecting agent. The products by which the organism participates in the reaction are the so-called antibodies. The total reaction taking place such as production of antibody, interaction of the antibody with the micro-organisms, etc., must be of a chemical nature. Up to the present time the antibodies have generally been considered apart from the organism. Their action has been studied in the test-tube or under the microscope. The method I have introduced to prove the existence of antibodies dispenses entirely with the microscope and the test-tube and depends solely on the vital reaction. I have found that by determining the altered reactivity it is possible to judge of the existence of an antibody just as well as through certain phenomena of hemolysis, precipitation or agglutination, which heretofore have attracted the attention.

In this way, for instance, the phenomena on the skin in which antibodies are concerned have been studied far more carefully than before. And what is more important, the new method has led to an extension of our knowledge of other diseases in which the micro-organisms or other foreign substances have no primary action on the organism, but elicit symptoms only after the formation of a secondary toxic body. With the study of serum disease and vaccinia as a basis, practical results have been obtained. The altered reactivity could be used for diagnosis, a point which attracted the attention of the medical profession.

The fundamental idea leading to an application of the altered reactivity for diagnostic purposes was gained from vaccinia. It was noticed that an early reaction after a vaccination, i. e., a papule formation within twenty-four hours after the application of a drop of vaccinia into a scratch on the skin, was found only in persons who had been vaccinated previously. If, for instance, we should like to find out, without seeing the scars, how many children out of a hundred had been vaccinated before and how many had not, it could be done simply by vaccinating all the children. Those who show an early reaction are children who have had this infection before. This practical conclusion was applied to tuberculosis, and the cutaneous tuberculin reaction was found just as reliable as the cutaneous reaction in vaccinia. A man showing local inflammation within twenty-four hours on the spot where the tuberculin is applied behaves differently from a normal individual; he is able to give this reaction only because he has formed antibodies against tuberculosis on a former occasion. It has been shown furthermore that this early reaction on the skin rests on the same foundations as Koch's febrile reaction with tuberculin, and that the antibody theory therefore could be applied to the latter. Similar results have been obtained in glanders, leprosy and in the diseases caused by hyphomycetes. Finally, the observations of altered reactivity and the antibody theory which resulted from these observations have led to a new explanation of immunity in a number of infectious diseases. In vaccinia, smallpox and other diseases the immunity is not based on an acquired insensibility against the virus, but it is based on antibody formation and on the early reaction. It has been shown that here two kinds of protection exist; the one is due to still existing antibodies. The micro-organism comes immediately into contact with the antibody and is destroyed, forming with the antibody at the same time, a digestion product which acts as a poison to the neighborhood. But owing to this immediate destruction, it is deprived of the time necessary for its development to an extent sufficient to give rise to general symptoms. The other kind of protection is seen when a long period has elapsed between the first and the second infection. The antibodies are no longer present, but the cells of the organism retain the property to form the antibodies in a shorter time, i. e., in four to seven days instead of eight to twelve days; therefore, the micro-organism, while not immediately destroyed, yet does not develop to the same degree as in an organism not previously infected so that the amount of toxin produced by the interaction of antibody and micro-organism is comparatively small.

It is to be hoped that the continuation of studies along this line will not only advance our theoretical knowledge with regard to the exanthemata of infectious diseases, and enable us to distinguish different periods in tuberculosis, etc., but that the practical method of diagnosis by the allergic reactions will be extended to other diseases. It is especially to be hoped that it will furnish us with the means of a short and practical diagnosis of syphilis, and aid us in the explanation of its phases and localizations.

118 West Franklin Street.

BIBLIOGRAPHY

Achard and Aynaud: Les globulins dans l'anaphylaxie, Compt. rend. Soc. de biol., 1909, lxvii, 83.

Anderson, J. F.: Transmission of Resistance to Diphtheria Toxin by the Female Guinea-Pig to Her Young, Jour. Med. Research, 1906, xv, 241; Stimultaneous Transmission of Resistance to Diphtheria Toxin and Hypersusceptibility to Horse-Serum by the Female Guinea-Pig to Her Young, Jour. Med. Research, 1906, xv, 259; Maternal Transmission of Immunity to Diphtheria Toxin; Maternal Transmission of Immunity to Diphtheria Toxin and Hypersusceptibility to Horse-Serum in the Same Animal, Bull. 30, Hyg. Lab. U. S. P. H. and M.-H. S., 1906.

Anderson, J. F., and Rosenau, M. J.: Anaphylaxis, The Archives Int. Med., 1909, iii, 519.

Armand, Delille and Huet: Contribution à l'étude du poison tuberculeux, Jour. de Physiol. et de Pathol. gener., 1906, viii, 1056.

Arthus, M.: Injections répétées de sérum de cheval chez le lapin, Compt. rend. Soc. de biol., Paris, 1903, lv, 20; Sur le séro-anaphylaxie du lapin, Compt. rend. Soc. de biol., 1906, lx, 1143.

Axamit: Ueberempfindlichkeitserscheinungen nach Hefeinjektion, Arch. f. Hyg,. 1907, lxii, 15.

Babes, V., and Proca, G.: Untersuchungen über die Wirkung der Tuberkelbazillen und über gegenwirkende Substanzen, Ztschr. f. Hyg., 1896, xxiii, 331.

Bail: Ueberempfindlichkeit bei tuberculösen Thieren, Wien. klin. Wchnschr., 1904, xvii, 30; Der akute Tod von Meerschweinen an Tuberkulose, Wien. klin. Wchnschr., 1905, xviii, 15.

Bartel, J.: Probleme der Tuberkulosefrage, Vienna, Deuticke, 1909.

Battelli and Mioni: Leucopénie et leucocytose par injection de sang héterogène chez le chien, Compt. rend. Soc. de biol., 1904, lvi, 760.

Bauer, J.: Die Immunitätsvorgänge bei Tuberkulose, Beitr. z. klin. Tuberk. (Brauer's), 1909, xiii, 383; Die passive Uebertragung der Tuberkuloseüberempfindlichkeit, München. med. Wchnschr., 1909, lvi, 1218.

Bauer and Engel: Tuberkuloseimmunität und spezifische Therapie, Beitr. z. klin. d. Tuberk. (Brauer's), 1909, xiii, 427.

Beclère, A., Chambon and Menard: Etude expérimentelle des accidents postsérothérapiques, Ann. de l'Inst. Pasteur, 1896, x, 567.

Von Behring, E., and Kitashima, S.: Ueber Verminderung und Steigerung der ererbten Giftempfindlichkeit, Berl. klin. Wchnschr., 1901, xxxviii, 157.

Belfanti and Carbone: Produzione di tossiche nel siero di animali inoculati con sangue eterogeneo, Gior. della r. accad. di med., Turin, 1898.

Besredka, A.: De la toxicité des sérums thérapeutiques et du moyen de la doser, Compt. rend. Soc. de biol., 1907, 477; Comment peut-on combattre l'anaphylaxie? Ann. de l'Inst. Pasteur, Paris, 1907, xxi, 950; Du mécanisme de l'anaphylaxie vis-à-vis du sérum du cheval, Ann. de l'Inst. Pasteur, Paris, 1908, xxii, 496; Des moyens d'empécher les troubles anaphylactiques, Compt. rend. Soc. de biol., 1909, lxvi, 125; De l'anaphylaxie lactique, Compt. rend. Soc. de biol., Paris, 1908, lxiv, 888-889.

Besredka, A., and Steinhardt, Edna: De l'anaphylaxie et de l'antianaphylaxie vis-à-vis du sérum de cheval, Ann. de l'Inst. Pasteur, Paris, 1907, xxi, 117; Du mécanisme de l'antianaphylaxie, Ann. de l'Inst. Pasteur, Paris, 1907, xxi, 384.

De Beurmann and Gougerot: Contribution a l'étude bactériologique de la lèpre, Le léproline de Rost, Bull. et mém. Soc. méd. d. hôp. de Paris, 1907, series 3, xxiv, 1397.

Biedl, A., and Kraus, R.: Experimentelle Studien über Anaphylaxie, Wien. klin. Wchnschr., 1909, xxii, 363.

Bienenfeld, Bianca: Das Verhalten der Leukocyten bei der Serumkrankheit, Jahrb. f. Kinderh. u. phys. Erziehung., 1907, lxv, 174.

Bier, A.: Beeinflussung bösartiger Geschwülste durch Einspritzung von artfremden Blut, Deutsch. med. Wchnschr., 1907, xxxiii, 1162.

Bingel: Ueber die Einwirkung einer intrakutanen Injektion von Diphtherietoxin auf die Haut, und den Antitoxingehalt des Serums beim Menschen, München. med. Wchnschr., 1909, lvi, 1326.

Blackley, C. H.: Experimental Researches on the Causes and Nature of Catarrhus Æstivus, London, Baillière, Tindall & Cox, 1873; ref. Am. Jour. med. Sc., 1874, lxvii, 181.

De Blieck, L.: Vergelijkende Onderzoekingen naar de Onderkenningsmiddelen van Kwaden Droes, Buitenzorg, 1909.

Bligh, W.: Hypersensitization to Antidiphtherial Serum, Brit. Med. Jour., 1908, i, 501.

Bloch and Massini: Studien ueber Immunität und Ueberempfindlichkeit bei Hyphomyzetenerkrankungen, Ztschr. f. Hyg. u. Infektionskr., 1909, lxiii, 68.

von Bokay, J.: Die Heilserumbehandlung gegen Diphtherie in dem Budapester "Stefanie"-Kinderspitale, Jahrb. f. kinderh., 1897, xliv, 133.

Boernstein, Felix: Ueber Anaphylaxie durch Fütterung gegenüber Fütterung, Centralbl. f. Bakteriol., Abt. I, 1908, i, 374.

Bourlier, P.: Les éruptions sériques; maladie du sérum; symptomes et pathogénie, Thèse de Paris, 1906-1907.

Brieger: Weitere Erfahrungen über Bakteriengifte, Ztschr. f. Hyg., 1895, 101.

Bruck, C.: Experimentelle Beiträge zur Ætiologie und Pathogenese der Urticaria, Arch. f. Dermat. und Syph., 1909, xcvi, 241.

Buttersack: Immunität und Heilung im Lichte der Physiologie und Biologie, Virchow's Arch. f. path. Anat., 1895, cxlii, 248.

Cabannes, E.: Recherches au sujet de la toxicité des sérums héterogènes, Compt. rend. Soc. de biol., Paris, 1907, lxii, 809.

Calmette: Sur un nouveau procédé de diagnostic de la tuberculose chez l'homme par l'ophthalmoréaction à la tuberculine, Compt. rend. Acad. d. sc., Paris, 1907, cxliv, 1324.

Chantemesse: L'ophthalmo-diagnostic de la fièvre typhoïde, Deutsch. med. Wchnschr., 1907, xxxiii, 1572.

Cheney, Henry W.: The Serum Disease, Illinois Med. Jour., 1907, xii, 248-253.

Citron, J.: Ueber Tuberkuloseantikörper und das Wesen der Tuberkulinreaktion, Berl. klin. Wchnschr., 1907, xliv, 1135.

Courmont, P.: Etudes sur les substances solubles prédisposant a l'action pathogène de leurs microbes producteurs, Rev. de. méd., 1891, xi, 843.

Currie, J. R.: Examples of the Immediate and of the Accelerated Reaction Following Two Injections of Antidiphtherial Serum, Jour. Hyg., 1907, vii, 61; On the Supersensitization of Persons Suffering from Diphtheria by Repeated Injections of Horse-Serum, Jour. Hyg., 1907, vii, 35; The Serum Disease in Man After Single and Repeated Doses, Glasgow Med. Jour., 1908, lxix, 277; Abnormal Reactions to Horse-Serum in the Serum Treatment of Cerebrospinal Fever, Jour. Hyg., 1908, viii, 457.

Currie, J. R., and MacGregor, A. S. M.: The Serum Treatment of Cerebrospinal Fever, Lancet, London, 1908, ii, 1073.

Dallera: Considerazioni e casi clinici di trasfusione del sangue, Morgagni, Napoli, 1875, xvii, 512.

Davidsohn, Heinrich, and Friedemann, Ulrich: Untersuchungen über das Salzfieber bei normalen und anaphylaktischen Kaninchen, Arch. f. Hyg., 1909, lxxi, 9.

Dehne and Hamburger, F.: Experimentelle Untersuchungen über die Folgen parenteraler Einverleibung von Pferdeserum, Wien. klin. Wchnschr., 1904, xvii, 807.

Detre-Deutsch: Superinfektion und Primäraffekt, Wien. klin. Wchnschr., 1904, xvii, 764.

Doerr, R.: Die Anaphylaxie, Handbuch der Technik und Methodik der Immunitätsforschung, ii, 856.

Doerr, R., and Raubitschek, H.: Toxin und anaphylaktisierende Substanz des Aalserums, Berl. klin. Wchnschr., 1908, xlv, 1525.

Doerr, R., and Russ, V. K.: Studien ueber Anaphylaxie. Die Identität der anaphylaktisierenden und der toxischen Substanz artfremder Sera, Zeitschr. f. Immunitätsforsch. u. exper. Therap., 1909, ii, 109; Der anaphylaktische Immunkörper und seine Beziehungen zum Eiweissartigen, Ztschr. f. Immunitätsforsch. u. exper. Therap., 1909, iii, 181.

Dunbar: Zur Ursache und Heilung des Heufiebers, Münch., Oldenbourg, 1903.

von Dungern: Die Antikörper, Jena, Fischer, 1903.

Engel: Ueber das Verhalten der kindlichen Tuberkulose gegen Tuberkulin, Beitr. z. klin. d. Tuberk. (Brauer's), 1909, xiii, 245.

Epstein: Ueber die Anwendung Koch'scher Injektionen im Säuglings und ersten Kindesalter, Prag. med. Wchnschr., 1891, xvi, 5.

Escherich: Die Resultate der Koch'schen Injektion bei Scrofulose und Tuberkulose des Kindesalters, Jahrb. f. Kinderh., 1892, xxxiii, 369.

Ferrand and Lemaire: Etude clinique et histologique de la cutiréaction chez l'enfant, Presse méd., 1907, xv, 617.

Finger and Landsteiner: Untersuchungen über Syphilis am Affen, Sitzungsb. Ber. d. k. Akad. d. Wissensch. in Wien., 1906, cxiv, 3 Abt., 497.

Floyd, Cleaveland, and Barker, W. W.: General Susceptibility in Typhoid and Colon Infection as Shown by the Ophthalmic Test, Jour. of. Med. Research, 1909, xx, 95.

Francioni, Carlo: La diminuzione del complemento nella malattia de siero, Riv. di clin. pediat., 1908, vi, 321; La malattia da siero, Sperimentale, 1904, 767; Perdita dell' immunita passiva in seguito alla malattia de siero nella difterite, Riv. di clin. pediat., 1907, v, 601.

Friedberger, E.: Kritik der Theorien ueber die Anaphylaxie, Ztschr. f. Immunitätsforsch. u. exper. Therap., 1909, ii, 208.

Friedberger and Nassetti: Ueber die Antikörperbildung bei parabiotischen Thieren, Ztschr. f. Immunitätsforschung, 1909, ii, 509.

Friedemann, Ulrich: Ueber passive Ueberempfindlichkeit, München. med. Wchnschr., 1907, liv, 2414; Weitere Untersuchungen ueber den Mechanismus der Anaphylaxie, Ztschr. f. Immunitätsforschung u. exper. Therap., 1909, ii, 591.

Friedemann, U., and Isaak, S.: Ueber Eiweissimmunität und Eiweissstoffwechsel, Ztschr. f. exper. Path. u. Therap., 1905, i, 513; 1906, iii, 209; Weitere Untersuchungen über den parenteralen Eiweissstoffwechsel, Immunität und Ueberempfindlichkeit, Ztschr. f. exper. Path. u. Ther., 1907, iv, 830.

Gay, F. P., and Adler, H. M.: The Chemical Separation of the Sensitizing Fraction (Anaphylactin) from Horse-Serum, Jour. Med. Research, 1908, xviii, 433.

Gay, F. P., and Southard, E. E.: Serum Anaphylaxis in the Guinea-Pig, Jour. Med. Research, 1907, xvi, 143.

Gessner: Ueber das Verhalten des Menschen bei paragenitaler Zufuhr artgleichen Spermas, Zentralbl. f. Gynäk., 1906, xxx, 794.

Goodall, E. W.: The Supersensitization of Persons by Horse-Serum, Jour. Hyg., 1907, vii, 607.

Gruener, Ottokar: Die kutane Tuberkulinreaktion im Kindesalter, Wiener klin. Wchnschr., 1908, xxi, p. 986; Ueber die Herabsetzung der Tuberkulinempfindlichkeit Tuberkulöser während der Masern, München. med. Wchnschr., 1909, lvi, 1681.

Hamburger, F.: Zur Frage der Immunisierung gegen Eiweiss, Wiener klin. Wchnschr., 1902, xv, 1188; Arteigenheit und Assimilation, Vienna, Deuticke, 1904; Ueber den Wert der Stichreaktion nach Tuberkulininjektion, Ref. München. med. Wchnschr., 1908, lv, 688; Ueber Tuberkulinimmunität, München. med. Wchnschr., 1908, lv, 2174; Die Tuberkulose als Kinderkrankheit, München. med. Wchnschr., 1908, lv, 2702.

Hamburger, F., and Moro, E.: Ueber die biologisch nachweisbaren Veränderungen des menschlichen Blutes nach Seruminjektion, Wien. klin. Wchnschr., 1903, xvi, 445.

Hamburger, F., and von Reuss: Die Folgen parenteraler Infektion von verschiedenen genuinen Eiweisskörpen, Wien. klin. Wchnschr., 1904, xvii, 859; Ueber die Wirkung artfremden genuinen Eiweisses auf die Leukocytes, Ztschr. f. Biol., 1905, xlvii, 24.

Hartung: Die Serumexantheme bei Diphtherie, Jahrb. f. Kinderh., 1896, xlii, 72.

Heilner, Ernst: Ueber die Wirkung grosser Mengen artfremden Blutserums im Tierkörper nach Zufuhr per Os und subkutän, Ztschr. f. Biol., 1907, i, 26; Ueber die Wirkung künstlich erzeugter physikalischer (osmotischer) Vorgänge im Tierkörper auf den Gesamtstoffumsatz mit Berücksichtigung der Frage von der Ueberempfindlichkeit, Ztschr. f. Biol., München. u. Berl., 1908, xxxii, 476; Versuch eines indirekten Fermentnachweises (durch Alkoholzufuhr), zugleich ein Beitrag zur Frage der Ueberempfindlichkeit, München. med. Wchnschr., 1908, lv, 2521.

Heim, P., and John, K.: Das Wiederaufflammen einer bereits abgelaufenen Cutanreaktion während einer Scharlachinfektion, Wien. med. Wchnschr., 1908, lviii, 1831.

Helman, C.: Diagnose des Rotzes mittels subkut. Injektionen von Rotzbazillenextrakten, Bote f. öffentl. Veterinärwesen, 1891 (quoted by Wladimiroff).

Helmholz, Henry F.: Ueber passive Uebertragung der Tuberkulin-Ueberempfindlichkeit bei Meerschweinchen, Ztschr. f. Immunitätsforschung u. exper. Therap., 1909, iii, 371.

Johannessen, Axel: Ueber Injectionen mit antidiphtheritischem Serum und reinem Pferdeserum, Deutsch. med. Wchnschr., 1895, xxi, 855.

Kalning: Zur Diagnose des Rotzes, Arch. f. Veterinäer-Wissensch., 1891 (quoted by Wladimiroff).

Kassowitz: Metabolismus und Immunität, Wien. med. Wchnschr., 1906, lvi, 909.

Klingmueller, V.: Beiträge zur Tuberkulose der Haut, Arch. f. Dermat., 1904, lxix, 167-206.

Knoepfelmacher: Subkutane Vaksineinjektionen am Menschen, Verhandl. d. Gesellsch. f. Kinderh., Dresden, 1907; Ztschr. f. exper. Pathol. u. Therap., 1907, iv, 880.

Knorr: Experimentelle Untersuchungen ueber die Grenzen der Heilunsmöglichkeit des Tetanus, Habilitationsschr., Marburg, 1895, 31 pp., 8 pls., 8 vo.

Koch, R.: Ueber bakteriologische Forschung, Verhandl. d. x. internat. med. Cong., 1890, Berlin, 1891, x; Weitere Mitteilungen ueber ein Heilmittel gegen Tuberkulose, Deutsch. med. Wchnschr., 1890, xvi, 1029; Fortsetzung der Mitteilungen ueber ein Heilmittel gegen Tuberkulose, Deutsch. med. Wchnschr., 1891, xvii, 101.

Kraus, R., and Doerr, R.: Ueber Bakterienanaphylaxie, Wien. klin. Wchnschr., 1908, xxi, 1008.

Kraus, R., Doerr, R., and Sohma: Ueber Anaphylaxie hervorgerufen durch Organextrakte (Linsen), Wien. klin. Wchnschr., 1908, xxi, 415.

Kraus, Lusenberger, and Russ: Ist die Ophthalmoreaktion nach Chantemesse zu diagnostischen Zwecken bei Typhus verwertbar? Wien. klin. Wchnschr., 1907, xx, 1335.

Kraus, R., and Volk, R.: Zur Frage der Serumanaphylaxie, Ztschr. f. Immunitätsforsch. u. exper. Therap., 1909, i, 731.

Kretz, R.: Ueber die Beziehungen zwischen Toxin and Antitoxin, Ztschr. f. Heilk., 1902, xxiii, 400.

Landmann, P.: Ein seltener Fall von Idiosynkrasie gegen Hühnereiweiss, etc., München. med. Wchnschr., 1908, lv, p. 1079.

Lautier: Eine neue Art von Tuberkulin-Haut-Reaktion beim Menschen; ref. München. med. Wchnschr., 1908, lv, 773.

Lefmann, G.: Zur Kenntniss der Giftsubstanzen des artfremden Blutes, Beitr. z. chem. Physiol. u. Path. (Hofmeister's), 1908, xi, 255.

Lehndorff: Serumkrankheit nach wiederholter Seruminjektionen, Monatsschr. f. Kinderh., 1905-6, iv, 545.

Lemaire, Henri: Recherches cliniques et expérimentales sur les accidents sérotoxiques, Thèse de Paris, 1906.

Levaditi, C., and Reijchman: Sur l'adsorption des protéines anaphylactisantes de sérum par les éléments cellulaires, Compt. rend. Soc. de biol., 1909, lxvi, 1078.

Lewis, Paul A.: The Induced Susceptibility of the Guinea-Pig to the Toxic Action of the Blood-Serum of the Horse, Jour. Exper. Med., 1908, x, 1-29.

Lignières: Sur un nouveau mode de réaction de la peau à la tuberculine et son utilisation dans le diagnostic de la tuberculose, Compt. rend. Acad. d. sc., Paris, 1907, cxlv, 727.

Löwenstein and Kauffmann: Ueber die Dosierung des Alttuberkulins zu diagnostischen Zwecken, Ztschr. f. Tuberkul., 1906, x, 17.

Löwenstein and Rappaport, E.: Ueber den Mechanismus der Tuberkulinimmunität, Ztschr. f. Tuberk., 1904, vi, 566.

Lucas, W. P., and Gay, F. P.: Localized Anaphylactic Intoxication in Children Following the Repeated Injection of Antitoxin, Jour. Med. Research, 1909, xv, 251.

Mantoux, C., and Lemaire, J.: Intradermo-réaction à la tuberculine chez 300 enfants non malades de un a quinze ans, Compt. rend. Soc. de biol., 1909, lxvii, 356.

Marfan and Lemaire, H.: Contribution à l'étude des accidents sérotoxiques; L'erythème marginé aberrant, Rev. mens. d. mal. de l'enf., 1907, xxvi.

Marfan and Le Play: Recherches sur la pathogénie des accidents sérothérapiques, Bull. et mém. Soc. méd. d. hôp. de Paris, 1905, series 3, xxii, 274.

Marmorek: Antituberkuloseserum und Vaccin, Berl. klin. Wchnschr., 1903, xl, 1108.

Mendel: Ueber intrakutane Tuberkulinanwendung zu diagnostischen Zwecken, Beitr. z. klin. d. Tuberk. (Brauer's), 1909, xiii, 139.

Meirowsky, E.: Ueber die diagnostische und spezifische Bedeutung der von Pirquetschen Hautreaktion, Arch. f. Dermat. u. Syph., 1909, xciv, 335.

Michaelis, L.: Zur Frage nach dem Zusammenhang zwischen toxischer, sensibilisierender und praezipitogener Substanz bei der Anaphylaxie, Ztschr. f. Immunitätsforsch., 1909, ii, 29.

Moll, Leopold: Ueber das Verhalten des jugendlichen Organismus gegen artfremdes Eiweiss und über seine Fähigkeit, Antikörper zu bilden, Jahrb. f. Kinderh., 1908, lxviii, 1.

Moro, E.: Ueber eine diagnostisch verwertbare Reaktion der Haut nach Einreibung mit Tuberkulinsalbe, München. med. Wchnschr., 1908, lv, 216.

Moro, E.: Klinische Ueberempfindlichkeit, München. med. Wchnschr., 1908, lv, 2025.

Moro and Doganoff: Zur Pathogenese gewisser Integumentveränderungen bei Scrofulose, Wien. klin. Wchnschr., 1907, xx, 933.

Moussu, G.: Cultures de tuberculose "in vivo," Compt. rend. Soc. de biol., Paris, 1905, lix, 409.

Moussu, G., and Mantoux, C.: Sur l'intradermo-réaction à la tuberculine chez les animaux, Compt. rend. Acad. d. sc., Paris, 1908, cxlvii, 502.

Nadejde, G.: Hypersensibilisation à la tuberculine des cellules nerveuses situees au voisinage d'un foyer tuberculeux intracérébral, Compt. rend. Soc. de biol., 1909, lxvi, 994.

Nakayama, H.: Impfversuche mit Aktinomyces astéroides, Arch. f. Hyg., 1906, lviii, 207.

Netter, Arnold, and Debre, Robert: Les éruptions sériques après injections intrarachidiennes de sérum antiméningococcique, Compt. rend. Soc. de biol., 1909, lxvi, 976.

Nicolle, Maurice: Contribution à l'étude du "phénomène d'Arthus," Ann. de l'Inst. Pasteur, Paris, 1907, xxi, 128.

Nicolle, M., and Abt: Les anticorps des albuminoides et des cellules, Ann. de l'Inst. Pasteur, 1908, xxii.

Nicolle, M., and Pozerski, E.: Une conception générale des anticorps et de leurs effets, Ann. de l'Inst. Pasteur, 1908, xxii, 26; 237.

Nourney: Experimentelle Beiträge zur Lehre von der Impfung, L. D. Strassburg, 1881.

Otto, R.: Das Theobald Smith'sche Phänomen der Serum-Ueberempfindlichkeit, Von Leuthold Gedenkschrift, 1905, i; Zur Frage der Serum-Ueberempfindlichkeit, München. med. Wchnschr., 1907, liv, 1665; Ueber Anaphylaxie und Serumkrankheit, Handbuch der pathogenischen Mikroorganismen (Kolle and Wassermann), 1908, ii, 255.

Pautrier, L. M., and Lutembacher: Sub-cuti-réaction positive obtenue chez deux sporotrichosiques par l'injection sous-cutanée de cultures jeunes de sporotrichose, broyées, diluées dans du serum et sterilisées, Compt. rend. Soc. de biol., 1909, lxvii, 24.

Pfeiffer, Hermann: Ueber die nekrotisierende Wirkung normaler Serum, Wien. klin. Wchnscshr., 1905, xviii, 465.

Pick, E. P., and Yamanouchi, T.: Chemische und experimentelle Beiträge zum Studium der Anaphylaxie, Ztschr. f. Immunitätsforsch. u. exper. Therap., 1909, i, 676.

Pickert, M.: Ueber natürliche Tuberkulinresistenz, Deutsch. med. Wchnschr., Leipz. u. Berlin, 1909, xxxv, 1013.

Pickert, M., and Loewenstein, E.: Eine neue Methode zur Prüfung der Tuberkulinimmunität (Vorläufige Mitteilung), Deutsch. med. Wchnschr., 1908, xxxiv, 2262.

von Pirquet, C.: Zur Theorie der Infektionskrankheiten (Vorläufige Mitteilung), April 2, 1903, Veröffentl. d. k. Akad. d. Wissensch. Wien., Feb. 13, 1908, Akad. Anzeiger, 6; Zur Theorie der Vakzination, Verhandl. d. Gesellsch. f. Kinderh., Kassel, 1903! Die frühzeitige Reaktion bei der Schutzpockenimpfung, Wien. klin. Wchnschr., 1906, xix, 855; Allergie, München. med. Wchnschr., 1906, liii, 1457; Ist die vakzinale Frühreaktion specifisch? Wien. klin. Wchnschr., 1906, xix, 1407; Eine Theorie des Blatternexanthems; Wien. klin. Wchnschr., 1907, xx, 271; Klinische Studien ueber Vakzination und vakzinale Allergie, Leipzig, Deuticke, 1907, 194; Demonstration z. Tuberkulindiagnose durch Hautimpfung, Berl. klin. Wchnschr., 1907, xliv, 699; Die Allergieprobe zur Diagnose der Tuberkulose im Kindesalter, Wien. med. Wchnschr., 1907, lvii, 1369; Der diagnostische Wert der kutanen Tuberkulinreaktion auf Grund von 100 Sektionen, Wien. klin. Wchnschr., 1907, xx, 1123; Die kutane Tuberkulinprobe; Med. Klin., 1907, iii, 1197; Kutane und konjunktivale Tuberkulinreaktion, Handbuch der Technik und Methodik der Immunitätsforschung (Kraus and Levaditi), 1908, i, 1035; Das Verhalten der kutanen Tuberkulinreaktion während der Masern, Deutsch. med. Wchnschr., 1908, xxxiv, 1297; Allergie, Ergebn. d. inn. Med. u. Kinderh., Julius Springer, Berlin, 1908, i, 420; Quantitative Experiments with the Cutaneous Tuberculin Reaction, Jour. Pharmacol. and Exper. Therap., 1909, i, 151.

von Pirquet and Schick, B.: Zur Theorie der Inkubationszeit (Vorläufige Mitteilung), Wien. klin. Wchnschr., 1903, xvi, 758, 1244; Zur Frage der Aggressins, Wien. klin. Wchnschr., 1905, xviii, 531; Die Serumkrankheit, Leipsic, Deuticke, 1905; Ueberempfindlichkeit und beschleunigte Reaktion, München. med. Wchnschr., 1906, liii, 66.

Portier and Richet, C.: De l'action anaphylactique de certains venins, Compt. rend. Soc. de biol., Paris, 1902, lxiv, 170.

Preisich, K., and Heim, P.: Ueber das Wesen der Tuberkulinreaktion, Centralbl. f. Bakteriol., 1902, xxxi, 681.

Ranzi, Egon: Ueber Anaphylaxie durch Organ- und Tumorextrakte, Ztschr. f. Immunitätsforsch. u. exper. Therap., 1909, ii, 12.

Remlinger, P.: Contribution a l'étude du phénomène d'anaphylaxie, Compt. rend. Soc. de biol., Paris, 1907, lxii, 23-25.

Reuschel, F.: Vergleichende Bewertung der Tuberkulinreaktionen im Kindersalter, München. med. Wchnschr., 1908, lv, 326.

Richet: Arbeiten über die Anaphylaxie beim Aktiniengift, Compt. rend. Soc. de Biol., 1902, liv, 170; 1903, lv, 246; 1904, lvi, 302; 1905, lviii, 112; 1907, lxii, 358, 643; Ann. de l'Inst. Pasteur, 1907, xxi, 497; De l'anaphylaxie et des toxicogénines, Ann. de l'Inst. Pasteur, Paris, 1908, xxii, 465; Du poison contenu dans la sève du kura crepitans (ou assaku), Compt. rend. Soc. de biol., 1909, lxvi, 763; L'anaphylaxie crée un poison nouveau chez l'animal sensibilisé, Compt. rend. Soc. de biol., 1909, lxvi, 810; De la réaction anaphylactique in vitro, Compt. rend. Soc. de biol., 1909, lxvi, 1005.

Rist, E.: Sur la toxicité des corps de bacilles diphtéritiques, Compt. rend. Soc. de biol., 1903, lv, 978.

Roemer, Paul H.: Weitere Versuche über Immunität gegen Tuberkulose durch Tuberkulose, Beitr. z. klin. d. Tuberk. (Brauer's), 1909, xiii, 1; Spezifische Ueberempfindlichkeit und Tuberkulose-Immunität, Beitr. z. Klin. d. Tuberk. (Brauer's), 1908, xi, 2.

Roemer, P. H., and Joseph, K.: Zur Verwertung der intrakutanen Reaktion auf Tuberkulin, Beitr. z. Klin. d. Tuberk. (Brauer's), 1909, xiv, 1.

Rosenau, M. J., and Anderson, John F.: A Study of the Cause of Sudden Death Following the Injection of Horse-Serum, Bull. 29, Hyg. Lab. U. S. P. H. and M.-H. S., 1906; Studies on Hypersusceptibility and Immunity, Bull. 36, Hyg. Lab. U. S. P. H. and M.-H. S., April, 1907; The Specific Nature of Anaphylaxis, Jour. Infect. Dis., 1907, iv, 552; Further Studies on Anaphylaxis, Bull. 45, Hyg. Lab. U. S. P. H. and M.-H. S., June, 1908; Further Studies Upon the Phenomenon of Anaphylaxis, Bull. 50, Hyg. Lab. U. S. P. H. and M.-H. S., 1909.

Rosenhaupt, H.: Klinischer Beitrag zur Serumkrankheit, München. med. Wchnschr., 1905, lii, 2019.

Rovere: Sur la présence de précipitines dans le sang de sujets atteints d'accidents consécutifs à des injections de serum antidiphtherique, Arch. gén. de méd., 1906, vi.

Saeli: Sulle fine alterazioni di struttura degli organi per injezioni di siero di sangue eterogene, Ref. med., 1905, i, 2.

Salge: Einige Bemerkungen zu dem Thema "arteigenes und artfremdes Eiweiss" in Bezug auf die Säuglingsernährung, Monatsschr. f. Kinderh., 1906, v, 213.

Salus, Gottlieb: Ueber das Wesen der biologischen Phänomene in der Medizin und ueber die natuerlichen Grenzen ihrer Verwertbarkeit, Med. Klinik, B., 1907, iii, 1525; Wirkungen normaler Sera auf den Organismus, Med. Klinik, 1908, iv, 1033; Versuche über Serumgiftigkeit und Anaphylaxie, Med. Klinik, 1909, v, 509.

Schick: Zu von Pirquet's Vortrag, Verhandl. d. Gesellsch. f. Kinderh. in Cassel, Wiesbaden, T. F. Borgmann, 1903, p. 161; Die diagnostiche Tuberkulinreaktion in Kindesalter, Jahrb. f. Kinderh., 1905, lxi, 811; Die Nachkrankheiten des Scharlachs, Jahrb. f. Kinderh., 1907, lxv, 132 (Ergängungshaft); Kutane Reaktion bei Impfung mit Diphtherietoxin, München. med. Wchnschr., 1908, lv, 504; Ueber Diphtheriekutanreaktion, Verhandl. d. 25 Versamml. d. Gesellsch. f. Kinderh., xxx, Deutsch. Naturf. u. Aerzte, 1908, Wiesb., 1909, xxv, 330.

Schlossmann: Vergiftung und Entgiftung, Monatsschr. f. Kinderh., 1905, iv, 207.

Schlossmann and Moro: Zur Kenntnis der Arteigenheit der verschiedenen Eiweisskörper der Milch, München. med. Wchnschr., 1903, i, 597.

Schnuerer, J.: Allergie bei Rotz, Ztschr. f. Infektionskr. d. Haustiere, 1908, iv, 210; Die Diagnose der ansteckenden Tierkrankheiten mittels der neueren Immunitätsreaktionen mit Ausnahme des subkutanen Einverleibens von Tuberkulin und Mallein, Verhandl. 9, intern. tierärztl. Kong. Haag, 1909, p. 11.

Sleeswijk, J. G.: Untersuchungen über Serumhypersensibilität, Ztschr. f. Immunitätsforsch. u. exper. Therap., 1909, ii, 133.

Smith, Henry Lee: Buckwheat-Poisoning, THE ARCHIVES INT. MED., 1909, iii, 350.

Smith, Theobald: Discussion on Hypersusceptibility, Jour. Am. Med. Assn., 1906, xlvii, 1010.

Stadelmann and Wolff-Eisner: Ueber Typhus und Kolisepsis und über Typhus als Endotoxinkrankheit, München. med. Wchnschr., 1907, liv, 1161, 1237.

Strauss and Gamaleia, N.: Recherches expérimentales sur la tuberculose, Arch. de méd. expér., 1899.

Trudeau, E. L.: Remarks on Artificial Immunity in Tuberculosis, Brit. Med. Jour., 1897, ii, 1849; Artificial Immunity in Experimental Tuberculosis, New York Med. Jour., 1903, lxxviii, 105; Antibacterial or Antitoxic Immunization in Tuberculin Treatment, Jour. Am. Med. Assn., 1909, lii, 261; Tuberculin Immunization in the Treatment of Pulmonary Tuberculosis, Am. Jour. Med. Sc., 1907, cxxxiii, 813.

Trudeau, E. L., and Baldwin, E. R.: Experimental Studies on the Preparation and Effects of Antitoxins for Tuberculosis, Am. Jour. Med. Sc., 1898, cxvi, 692; 1899, cxvii, 56.

Uhlenhuth: Zur Kenntnis der giftigen Eigenschaften des Blutserums, Ztschr. f. Hyg., 1897, xxvi, 384.

Vallée, H.: Sur un nouveau procédé de diagnostic expérimental de la tuberculose et de la morve, Bull. Soc. centr. de méd. vét., Paris, 1907, lxi, 308.

Vaughan, V. C.: Discussion of Rosenau and Anderson's paper on Hypersusceptibility, Jour. Am. Med. Assn., 1906, xlvii, 1009.

Vaughan, V. C., and Wheeler, S. M.: The Effects of Egg-White and its Split Products on Animals; A Study of Susceptibility and Immunity, Jour. Infect. Dis., 1907, iv, 476.

Verliac, H.: Recherches expérimentales sur les toxins de l'actinomycose, Thèse de Paris, Steinheil, 1907.

De Waele, H.: La réaction à la tuberculine, Ann. Soc. de méd. de Gand, 1906, lxxiv, 84; Etude sur l'immunité conferée par la méthode des sacs de cellulose et sur les produits microbiens dialysants, Centralbl. f. Bakteriol., 1906, xlii, 636, 760; Contribution a l'étude de l'anaphylaxie, Bull. Acad. roy. de méd. de Belge, 1907, 4 s., 715.

Wassermann, A.: Wesen der Infektion, Kolle and Wassermann's Handbuch der pathogenen Mikroorganismen, 1903, i, 223.

Wassermann and Bruck, C.: Experimentelle Studien über die Wirkung von Tuberkelbazillen-Präparaten auf den tuberkulös erkrankten Organismus, Deutsch. med. Wchnschr., 1906, xxxii, 449.

Wassermann and Citron, J.: Die lokale Immunität der Gewebe und ihre praktische Wichtigkeit, Deutsch. med. Wchnschr., 1905, xxxi, 573.

Weaver, George H.: Serum Disease, THE ARCHIVES INT. MED., 1909, iii, 485.

Wechselmann: Ueber Satinholzdermatitis, eine Anaphylaxie der Haut, Deutsch. med. Wchnschr., 1909, xxxv, 1389.

Weichardt, W.: Ueber spezifisches Heufieberserum, Verhandl. d. Physik-med. Soc., Erlangen, 1905, p. 209; Paradoxe Reaktion bei Kenotoxin, Fol. Haemat., 1907, iv, 1.

Weil-Hallé, B., and Lemaire, H.: Quelques conditions de l'anaphylaxie sérique passive chez le lapin et le cobaye, Compt. rend. Soc. de biol., Paris, 1907, lxiii, 748.

Wells, H. Gideon: The Nature of the Poisonous Element of Proteins That is Concerned in the Reaction of Hypersensitization, Jour. Am. Med. Assn., 1908, i, 527; Studies on the Chemistry of Anaphylaxis, Jour. Infect. Dis., 1908, v, 449-483.

Werbitzky, F. W.: Contribution a l'étude de l'anaphylaxie, Compt. rend. Soc. de biol., 1909, lxvi, 1084.

White, William C., and Graham, D. A. L.: Studies on the Action of Sera on Tuberculin Cutaneous Reaction, Jour. Med. Research, 1909, xxi, 261.

Wladimiroff, A.: Immunität bei Rotz, Kolle and Wassermann's Handbuch der pathog. Mikroorganismen, 1904, iv, 1020.

Wolff-Eisner, A.: Ueber Grundgesetze der Immunität, Ztschr. f. Bakteriol., 1904; Berl. klin. Wchnschr., 1904, xli, 1105, 1131, 1156, 1273; Die Endotoxinlehre, München. med. Wchnschr., 1906, liii, 217; Das Heufieber, sein Wesen und seine Bedeutung, Munich, L. L. Lehmann, 1906; Ueber die Urticaria vom Standpunkte der neueren Erfahrungen, Dermat. Zentralbl., Leipz., 1907, x, 164; Ueber Eiweissimmunität und ihre Beziehungen zur Serumkrankheit, Centralbl. f. Bakteriol., 1906, xl, 378; Typhustoxin, Typhusantitoxin und Typhusendotoxin, Die Beziehungen zwischen Ueberempfindlichkeit und Immunität, Berl. klin. Wchnschr., 1907, xliv, 1216; Discussionsbemerkung, Berl. klin. Wchnschr., 1907, xliv, 703; Die Ophthalmo- und Kutandiagnose der Tuberkulose, Würzburg, Stuber., 1908.

Yamanouchi, T.: Ueber die Anwendung der Anaphylaxie zu diagnostischen Zwecken, Ref. München. med. Wchnschr., 1908, lv, 2506.

Zupnik: Ophthalmoreaktion bei Typhus, Wiss. Ges. Deutscher Aerzte in Boehmen, April 12, 1907, Ref. München. med. Wchnschr., 1908, lv, 148.

Note.—In this paper the very recent contributions to the subjects under discussion could not be considered. It must be remembered that a considerable time has elapsed between the writing of this paper and its publication.

# BOOK REVIEW

INNERE SEKRETION. Ihre physiologischen Grundlagen und ihre Bedeutung für die Pathologie. Von Dr. Artur Biedl, Wien. Mit einem Vorwort von Dr. R. Paltauf, Wien. Cloth. Price, $5.50. Pp. 538. Berlin: Urban and Schwarzenberg (Rebman Co., New York, American Agents), 1910.

No other branch of medical science owes its progress to so uniformly divided a participation by physiologist, pathologist, and clinician, as does this ever-fascinating subject of the internal secretions. We may, indeed, venture the suggestion that perhaps one of the most valuable achievements made in this field is that it has served to bring together these interests, which tend always, to their very great detriment, to drift apart. Although each of the many subdivisions of the field has been the subject of monographic treatment, yet a thorough and extensive review of the entire ground has not previously been available, although the evident interrelationship of all the internal secretions indicates that only such a correlated review can be adequate. Professor Biedl, who has been an active investigator of various problems concerning internal secretions, has succeeded in the colossal task of meeting this need in our literature, in a manner which must receive our sincere commendation. In a book with 412 large pages of solid text he has taken up the following topics:

First a general discussion of the history of the subject, with an analysis of our present understanding of the limits and the underlying principles of the production and action of the internal secretion. This relatively brief general section is followed by a *spezieller Teil,* in which the internal secretions of the following organs are considered: thyroid and parathyroid glands (78 pages), thymus, the adrenals and the chromaffin system (161 pages), the hypophysis, pineal gland, sexual glands, pancreas, gastro-intestinal tract and kidneys.

Our criticism of the book as a whole may be made very brief. It is a characteristically German, thorough analytical review of the literature, by a man who is an active and careful investigator in the problems of the subject he discusses, and not a mere library investigator, as the writers of books in other languages too frequently are.

The author has preserved splendidly the proper balance between the enthusiasm of the investigator and the conservative judgment with which personal experience endows maturity; original ideas are abundantly expressed, but personal impressions are never confused with demonstrated facts, and the entire book is based on a broad knowledge and unprejudiced view which gives it full face value. We are perhaps especially pleased to note that American work, which in this field has been far from insignificant, has received much more consideration than we are accustomed to find in German medical literature, and the names of Cushing, Abel, Howell and other American investigators are treated as respectfully as if they were spelled with umlauts; even so, however, much worthy American work fails to be mentioned in the text or to appear in the bibliography of 126 pages which forms a valuable part of the book. In short, the degree of thoroughness, reliability, and good judgment expressed on the pages of this work warrant its being accepted as the standard publication on the subject it covers, and until replaced by a newer work it should be the starting-point for every search into the literature of any phase of internal secretion. This is not to be interpreted as meaning that there are no errors of omission and commission, or that there is not room for difference of opinion as to the relative amount of space the different subjects should have received; but, all in all, such faults are not common and seldom are they glaring; for, always appreciating the difference between subjective and objective, the author saves himself from leading the reader astray.

There being so many unsolved and debated problems concerning the internal secretions fresh in the thoughts of all of us, it may be justifiable to take the space necessary to present the author's mature judgment concerning them, and other such matters as this book may offer of special interest.

In the first instance we find a novelty in that the consideration of the various secretions is based on a special conception of hormone action, which serves to bring them together on a common ground and to satisfy our knowledge of their mutual cooperations and antagonisms. The hormones, as Biedl shows, may be divided according to their function into assimilatory and disassimilatory, the former favoring anabolic phases of metabolism and generally causing inhibition of tissue activity, while the disassimilatory hormones increase catabolic change and, in consequence, increase functional activities. To the latter class belongs especially the thyroid secretion, which in most cases causes rapid tissue breakdown when in excess; and Biedl looks on the production of this hormone as the chief function of the thyroid, advising us to discard entirely the old theory that the chief value of the thyroid is as a detoxicating organ. He considers the evidence of the essential dependence of tetany on the parathyroids to be convincing and he has himself observed relief of the symptoms from the administration of calcium to animals with tetany from parathyroid extirpation, but without prolongation of life. The evidence of a relationship of some sort between the parathyroids and the thyroids seems to be conclusive, but Biedl is unable to tell just what the nature of this relationship is; it certainly is not an antagonism, and the use of thyroid extract in all cases of postoperative tetany is urged in view of the undoubted clinical results. The chemistry of the thyroid is inadequately considered, and it is not up to date.

So contradictory and incomplete is the testimony on the functions of the thymus that there is found no sufficient ground on which to hazard any conclusions; even the evidence that the thymus is itself responsible for the so-called "mors thymica," or its relation to the entire picture of "status lymphaticus," seems to Biedl to be inconclusive.

The adrenals are looked on as consisting of two entirely distinct tissues. The medulla is discussed with the rest of the chromaffin organs under the title of the "adrenal system," and the cortex is taken up as a chief part of the "interrenal system," since it is only in the higher vertebrates that the chromaffin tissue is enclosed in the lipoid-rich cells of the interrenal tissues; elsewhere in the animal kingdom the two structures are as distinct anatomically as functionally. Of the two parts of the adrenal the cortex alone is essential to life, for there is enough chromaffin tissue in the remainder of the "adrenal system" to compensate for loss of the adrenal medulla. However, so far as Addison's disease is concerned, the evidence does not seem to be sufficient to determine which of the two parts of the suprarenal is responsible for which symptoms, but probably it is the destruction of cortex tissue which is the most important, since even when all the adrenal medulla is destroyed, there still remains more than half of all the chromaffin tissue of the body.

Biedl believes that there have been enough successful experimental transplantations of adrenal tissue to warrant the hope of an eventual successful transplantation therapy in adrenal disease. Much attention is given to the action of epinephrin on each of the tissues of the body; as to the problems of experimental epinephrin arteriosclerosis, the author believes that the hypothesis that the vascular lesions are due to high blood-pressure is untenable in view of the fact that the dextrorotary epinephrin, which has no pressor action, causes typical arteriosclerosis. The results of recent studies on the presence of epinephrin in the blood are summed up with the statement that exophthalmic goiter is the only disease in which there is constantly an increased amount of epinephrin in the blood. The special properties of the adrenal cortex, and especially its relation to the generative organs, are particularly well covered. No less than fifteen pages are devoted to the chemistry of the adrenal cortex, with its interesting collection of lipoidal substances; and the importance of the cholin, which also is found there, once a topic of active investigation, is entirely discredited. No conclusions are reached as to what may be the purpose of this abundant production of lipoids, although recent hypotheses of their relation to immunological processes receive due attention. It seems probable that the interrenal system, which includes the adrenal cortex and the so-called accessory and aberrant adrenal tissue, produces in common with the thymus, hypophysis, thyroid and sex glands, hormones with assimilatory influence, which are of significance in the somatic and psychic development of the individual.

The available information concerning the carotid gland requires but two pages for its exposition, and the contention of Kohn that this organ is merely a part of the adrenal system seems to be established. On the other hand, the coccygeal gland, commonly placed in the same group, would seem to be merely an inactive mass of rudimentary caudal blood-vessels.

Experimental work of the author on the hypophysis supports Cushing's work, which shows that removal of the anterior lobe alone is fatal, excision of the posterior lobe causes no evident effect, while merely cutting across the infundibular stalk is as certainly fatal as removal of the entire gland. This is in striking contrast to the marked physiological activity of extracts of the posterior lobe and the relative inactivity of anterior lobe extracts. As to the controversy concerning the importance of the hypophysis in relation to acromegaly, the favorable results of operative removal of hypophyseal tissue seem to settle the question affirmatively; on the other hand it seems to be entirely undetermined whether the changes in the hypophysis in this disease are primary or secondary to some other unknown condition. Biedl suggests that in acromegaly the hypophyseal changes are primary, while in giantism the hypophysis becomes enlarged secondarily because of a primary defect of some sort in the sex glands, and he recommends experimental therapeutic use of generative tissue preparation in the treatment of acromegaly and gigantism.

Little positive enlightenment has been found in the literature on the pineal gland. The evidence afforded by clinical cases seems to be reliable enough to show that in early life this organ has an influence, probably inhibitory, on the sex glands. Biedl states that he has succeeded in removing the pineal gland from experimental animals, and that in adults, at least, no effects were observed.

The internal secretions of the sex glands receive an unusually extended consideration of 50 pages. Starling and Lane-Claypon found that extracts of the fetus, and not extracts of the placenta or generative tissues, cause mammary gland hypertrophy, and Biedl has been able to confirm this observation. He further builds up a theory of lactation based on the existence of antagonistic assimilatory and disassimilatory hormones. The theory of Bouin and Ancel that the interstitial organ (or Leydig's interstitial cells) is responsible for the secretion of a hormone by the testicle seems to be established, although it is probable that the gland cells also have an internal secretion, the former being more associated with sexual development and the latter with fat metabolism. To Biedl the most plausible hypothesis of ovarian function is that the interstitial cells, which in this organ undoubtedly form a specialized tissue, influence the periodic processes of the female generative organs, while the other tissues (corpus luteum and germinative epithelium) secrete hormones with opposite and inhibitory influence. Leo Loeb's important studies on the sexual cycle in the female are not considered.

As to the relation of the pancreas to diabetes, Otto Cohnheim's theory of a hormone stimulating glycolysis in the muscles seems to be looked on as unproved, and indeed Biedl goes so far as to reject the idea that diabetes depends on defective glycolysis. Rather, he believes, excessive glycogenolysis is responsible in pancreatic diabetes, the pancreatic hormone, which he has demonstrated to pass through the thoracic duct, may owe its effect to an inhibition of the nervous apparatus which regulates glycogenesis. He takes no decided stand on the question of whether the islands of Langerhans alone, or the acinar epithelium alone, or both, are concerned in the production of this hormone.

The Archives of Internal Medicine

Vol. VII APRIL, 1911 No. 4

# BLOOD-PRESSURE IN TUBERCULOSIS *

HAVEN EMERSON, M.D.
NEW YORK

The presence of the tubercle bacillus, a local injury of tissue and diminished bodily resistance are accepted as a necessary trio of conditions which determine tuberculous infection. Clinicians for many centuries have recognized the third factor as important, while the first two have been accepted only in the present age of exact pathology. It is the hope of the modern student so to analyze the elusive complex of bodily or general resistance as to put preventive medicine, as applied to the individual, on a sound basis.

One method of attacking this problem is to determine the functional changes which accompany or facilitate infection. In tuberculosis, the functions of the special tissue affected, of nutrition and of the circulation suffer chiefly. Of these three the local repair and correction of the error in nutrition are so dependent on efficient circulation that study of the functional errors of the cardiovascular system should help us in the treatment of the disease, and may throw light on the conditions which predispose to, or accompany, infection.

The picturesque descriptions by the ancients of the classes predisposed to tuberculosis can be condensed into the three phrases, "delicacy of constitution, incomplete growth, and imperfect development." The people who live in an environment which we recognize as predisposing to tuberculous infection, and yet do not succumb to it, can be separated by no means yet devised from the early subjects of tuberculosis, as far as the efficiency of their circulation is concerned. Functional tests of the circulation are not yet delicate enough to establish a diagnosis. Potain and his followers assert that when we record a persistent abnormally low pressure for which we can find no other cause, we must consider the case as probably one of incipient tuberculosis, and that such a condition of the circulation may precede local signs or temperature elevation. This opinion has not been accepted generally, or verified fully, and yet, for

*Read before the Section on Pharmacology and Therapeutics of the American Medical Association, at the Sixty-First Annual Session, held at St. Louis, June, 1910.

generations, one of the earliest signs characteristic of tuberculous infection has been the alteration in the rate and quality of the arterial pulse. The most reliable proof we have of functional disturbance of the circulation is an alteration in the relation between pulse-rate and blood-pressure, a manifestation of the so-called Marey's law. General arterial blood-pressure cannot fall without a corresponding increase in the heart-rate, if the neuromuscular mechanism of the heart is unimpaired, and a rise in blood-pressure is normally met by a compensatory slowing of the heart rate. General blood-pressure cannot fall below a certain normal limit for more than brief periods without impairing the nervous, glandular and muscular efficiency of the body.

The positive opinions of the German writers that physical or other definite signs of tuberculous infection always precede any characteristic alteration of the blood-pressure, and the enthusiastic convictions of the French writers that they often make a correct diagnosis on finding a characteristic hypotension before physical signs of the disease are observable, led me to make clinical tests to see if any help could be had from the sphygmomanometer in the early diagnosis of pulmonary tuberculosis.

This series of observations and the ample discussion in the literature of the cause of the commonly observed hypotension led to experimental studies on mammalian tissues with various tubercle products.

In the Seton Hospital at Spuyten Duyvil, N. Y., for advanced pulmonary tuberculosis, and at the Bellevue Hospital Tuberculosis Dispensary in New York, I have made observations of the pulse-rate and blood-pressure in 200 cases of pulmonary tuberculosis, chiefly in the later stages of the disease. In the laboratories of the College of Physicians and Surgeons of Columbia University, I have tested the effects of the tubercle products on various animals and by perfusion tests on isolated tissues.

The tests on patients were all made in the following manner: the patient lay in the horizontal position on an examining table, and the pulse was counted for consecutive periods until the rate ceased to vary. The systolic blood-pressure (with the Janeway instrument), and the pulse-rate were then taken. The patient then stood erect, and after waiting for the pulse to assume a constant rate, the blood-pressure and pulse were again taken. All the observations were made between 3 and 5 in the afternoon, the midday meal having been eaten between 12 and 1. The hospital patients were either bed patients or those who had been resting for one or two hours immediately preceding the test. The dispensary patients had been seated in the waiting-room for an hour, and often longer, preceding the test. I was familiar with all the patients tested and they were accustomed to the use of the instrument and did not exhibit any emotional phenomena which might cause errors in the observations.

No attempt to record diastolic pressure was made, as I am convinced of my own unreliability in reading a fluctuating mercury column, and facilities were not available for using any graphically recording instrument. The pressures here reported are all systolic pressures, the mean of several consecutive observations.

The normal individual in a rested condition will usually have a slightly higher blood-pressure in the vertical than in the horizontal position, to meet the need of competent blood-supply to the brain under more difficult hydrostatic conditions. Under ideal conditions this is accomplished by a general, and especially splanchnic vasoconstriction, and there may be at the same time a slowing of the heart-rate. It is not abnormal, however, to have a slight increase in the heart-rate on taking the erect position in healthy individuals. According to Crampton, and from the report of Barach recently published, young men trained for athletic contests are apt to show some increase in heart-rate on assuming the erect position, in a small per cent. of cases, but what is very significant is that after such exertion as a "Marathon race" a great increase is found in the percentage who show quickened heart-rate in the standing position. Fatigue brings out the lack of sufficient vascular support, and the heart compensates.

If then we find either a stationary or a falling blood-pressure or a marked increase in the heart-rate on a change from the horizontal to the erect position, we may properly assume that there is a lack of proper tone, or vasoconstrictor control. Such a condition is not uncommon in undernourished, fatigued people of sedentary habits, and in those who have been for some weeks bedridden or have recently recovered from an infectious disease. It is rare to find a person in good health who will exhibit any but a slight increase in the heart-rate, or a fall in blood-pressure, or a rise in blood-pressure with a marked increase in the frequency of the pulse in this test. H. Chon, in 1904, in a detailed study of the pulse in tuberculous patients, makes especial note that while in health a change from the horizontal to a sitting or standing position is accompanied by a slight, if any, increase in the pulse-rate, in the tuberculous subject this minimum exertion is accompanied by so exaggerated an increase that it can be used as an early diagnostic sign. He includes an essential toxic hypotension among the causes of the tachycardia in tuberculosis.

The result of my observations is as follows:

Of the 200 patients, 119 were male and 81 female.
20 were under 20 years of age,
166 were between 20 and 50 years,
14 were over 50.

No relation was found between the sex or age of the patients and the tachycardia, hypotension or the abnormal response to change of position.

24 were in the first stage (National Association classification)
65 in the second stage,
108 in the third stage.
3 were found to be non-tuberculous.

Of the 24 in the first stage
11 showed entirely normal circulation, neither tachycardia nor abnormally low pressure, nor a fall in pressure on assuming the vertical position, with or without marked increase in the pulse rate.
13 showed marked abnormalities in the circulation as indicated just above.

In other words, physical examination seems to be more reliable for early diagnosis than are the circulatory tests.

Of the 65 in the second stage
28 showed normal circulation,
37 showed abnormal.

Of the 108 in the third stage
28 normal,
80 abnormal.

Of the three non-tuberculous, all were normal.

Thus of the 200, we find 130 in whom there were easily recognized errors of circulation, characterized by low blood-pressure, with or without rapid pulse, and a fall in pressure on assuming the erect posture.

There were in addition twenty-seven more in whom I found a marked increase in the pulse-rate (an average of fifteen beats in the minute) on assuming the erect position, but in whom there was a normal blood-pressure or a marked hypertension, due in the majority of cases to an accompanying nephritis or arteriosclerosis.

This increased rapidity of pulse should, I think, be considered an abnormal functional reflex, an evidence of increased vasomotor irritability or weakness.

If we study the 157 who showed what I shall for purposes of discussion describe as abnormal circulation, we find on dividing our 200 patients into groups on the basis of clinical progress that

Of the 98 who were progressing unfavorably, that is to say, were failing steadily,
90 had an abnormal circulation,
8 had a normal circulation.

Of the 75 who were improving
55 had abnormal circulation,
20 had normal circulation.

Of the 20 who were stationary in condition, *i. e.*, whose cases for the time being were arrested,
10 had abnormal circulation,
10 had normal circulation.

Of the four subjects of incipient tuberculosis
2 had abnormal circulation,
2 had normal circulation.

Of the 3 non-tuberculous subjects
all had normal circulation.

TABLE 1.—Circulation of Patients Divided into Groups on the Basis of Clinical Progress

| Patients | Circulation: Abnormal No. | Circulation: Normal No. | Normal % |
|---|---|---|---|
| 98 Progressing unfavorably | 90 | 8 | 8.8 |
| 75 Progressing favorably | 55 | 20 | 36.3 |
| 20 Stationary or arrested | 10 | 10 | 50. |
| 4 Incipient | 2 | 2 | 50. |
| 3 Non-tuberculous | 0 | 3 | 100. |
| 200 | 157 | 43 | |

From which figures it would appear that the disorders of the circulation are in a general proportion to the clinical severity of the disease.

If we divide our cases on the basis of their nutrition, we find of the eighty-seven who were losing weight, eighty-four had abnormal circulation and three normal.

TABLE 2.—Circulation of Patients Divided into Groups on the Basis of Nutrition

| Patients | Circulation: Abnormal No. | Circulation: Normal No. | Normal % |
|---|---|---|---|
| 87 losing weight | 84 | 3 | 3.5 |
| 60 stationary in weight | 41 | 18 | 30.0 |
| 50 gaining weight | 32 | 19 | 38.0 |
| 3 non-tuberculous | .. | .. | ..... |
| 200 | 157 | 40 | ..... |

Again we see a rough parallel between abnormal circulation and poor nutrition.

TABLE 3.—Circulation of Patients Divided into Groups on the Basis of Temperature

| Patients | Circulation: Abnormal No. | Circulation: Normal No. | Normal % |
|---|---|---|---|
| 63 running T. over 100° F. | 61 | 2 | 3.1 |
| 62 running T. between normal and 100° F. | 53 | 9 | 14.5 |
| 70 running normal T. | 41 | 29 | 41.4 |
| 2 running subnormal T. | 2 | 0 | 10.0 |
| 3 non-tuberculous | .. | .. | ..... |
| 200 | .... | .. | ..... |

As was to be expected, we find (Table 3) that fever, one indicator of toxic condition, is highest in cases in which we find lowest percentage of normal circulation, another toxic result.

TABLE 4.—CIRCULATION OF PATIENTS DIVIDED INTO GROUPS ON THE BASIS OF OCCURRENCE OF HEMORRHAGES

| | Circulation | | |
|---|---|---|---|
| | Abnormal | Normal | |
| Patients | No. | No. | % |
| 57 having had hemorrhages | 47 | 10 | 17.6 |
| 140 having had no hemorrhages | 110 | 30 | 21.4 |
| 3 non-tuberculous | .. | .. | ..... |

A large proportion of the cases recorded as having hemorrhages (Table 4) were Class III cases with frequent hemorrhages.

TABLE 5.—CIRCULATION OF PATIENTS DIVIDED INTO GROUPS ON THE BASIS OF MEDICATION

| | Circulation | | |
|---|---|---|---|
| | Abnormal | Normal | |
| Patients | No. | No. | % |
| 162 receiving none | 130 | 32 | 20.3 |
| 28 receiving dilator or depressor drugs | 25 | 3 | 14.2 |
| 7 receiving constrictor or pressor | 2 | 5 | 71.3 |

What little we can conclude from this classification according to medication is that we must distrust the apparent benefit from any drugs which have any tendency to diminish vascular tone, or to allow of dilatation, as for example, alcohol, potassium iodid and coal-tar depressants.

Although the number of cases is too small to permit a sound conclusion to be drawn, I think that it is probably safe to say that much benefit can be expected from the use of such drugs as caffein, digitalis and spartein over long periods for the sake of establishing or maintaining a general blood-pressure which will more nearly approach the normal than can be established by general hygienic measures as usually adopted, although cold air and abundant nutrition are of marked value.

The inability of tuberculous patients, whether they show hypotension, normal pressure or hypertension, to respond by a rise of pressure to a change from horizontal to vertical condition is, I believe, good evidence of an abnormal circulatory condition which I think can be shown by the accompanying summary (Table 6) which expresses a general picture, although the figures are rather misleading.

TABLE 6.—BLOOD-PRESSURE OF TUBERCULOUS PATIENTS IN THE VERTICAL AND HORIZONTAL POSITIONS

| In the horizontal position | | In the vertical position | |
|---|---|---|---|
| No. Patients | Pressure mm. | No. Patients | Pressure mm. |
| 99 | under 120 | 91 | under 120 |
| 63 | between 120-140 | 66 | between 120-140 |
| 38 | over 140 | 38 | over 140 |

Of the forty-nine in whom the blood-pressure was over 140 mm. in the horizontal or vertical position or in both

40 were gaining or in an arrested state.................................81.6%
9 were losing in weight and condition.

Of the sixty-six in whom the blood-pressure was 110 mm. in the horizontal or vertical position or both

16 were gaining or in arrested state.................................24.2%
50 were losing in weight and condition.

This summary of the extremes of the list of blood-pressures indicates the relation between general condition and blood-pressure in tuberculosis in a rather striking way. In general, the patients with high pressure, even though the cause of the increased pressure was an arteriosclerosis, primary or secondary to a chronic nephritis, did better than patients with subnormal blood-pressure.

Of the 200, 104 (52 per cent.) showed a stationary or falling pressure, eighty-six (43 per cent.) showed a rise of pressure in changing from horizontal to erect position.

One hundred and fifty-five (77 per cent.) showed a rise of pulse-rate on assuming erect position, with an average increase of fifteen beats to the minute.

Twenty-seven showed a stationary pulse-rate on taking erect position, and of these twenty-three had a pressure under 120. Of these twenty-seven, sixteen showed with the stationary pulse a constant or a rising pressure; in other words, they showed a normal reaction to change of posture. The remaining eleven showed a fall in pressure in two instances of 10 mm.; in one 18 mm., and another 20 mm., with the stationary pulse-rate evidently not a favorable picture.

There were eleven who showed a fall in pulse-rate, on assuming the erect position, of an average of eleven beats to the minute. Of these, six showed a drop in pressure as well as a drop in the pulse-rate, and apparently obesity in three and arteriosclerosis in three explain this paradoxical result. The marked difficulty in breathing in the horizontal position due to undue pressure of a heavy abdominal weight against the diaphragm causes a high arterial pressure in the horizontal position and a more nearly normal pressure in the seated or standing position in the obese. The inelasticity of the arteries in the arteriosclerotic accounts for a fall in pressure on standing.

The other five showed rises of pressure with the falling pulse-rate and as theirs were all favorable, improving or early cases, we must consider this as in the nature of a physiological occurrence although it is unusual.

Of the 200, 157 showed either a fall in pressure or a stationary pressure, or a marked increase (over fifteen beats to the minute) in pulse-rate, or both, on changing from recumbent to erect position.

There were ninety in whom there was a fall or stationary pressure, with a rise in pulse-rate on assuming erect position.

If we accept this test as an indication of functional weakness of the vascular system or heart muscle or both, we find that among tuberculous patients there is a very high percentage who show a marked functional disturbance of the circulation. The constant acceleration of the pulse-rate has been an accepted proof of this for many years. It is less well understood that this acceleration may be in response to a lack of vascular tone, and not to any inherent changes in the heart-muscle or its nervous mechanism, and that the accompanying fall in blood-pressure may occur with an increased heart-rate, and that this can be brought out by a simple change of position in the way described above.

It is well to remember that excessive rapidity of heart action will of itself suffice to cause a fall in arterial blood-pressure, for as has been repeatedly shown by physiologists, Yandell Henderson and others, the output of the heart diminishes with an increase of the heart-rate beyond a certain acceleration, the increase in the rate being at the expense of the diastolic filling of the heart, and hence a diminished volume outflow at each systole.

Although I cannot claim that the results here reported are sufficiently definite or that they can be relied on to indicate positively a diagnosis, I think that they do demonstrate value in associating our observations of pulse and blood-pressure in the way described for the sake of gauging less indefinitely a functional disorder which must have our consideration in the treatment of the disease.

## II. EXPERIMENTAL REPORT

There may be said to be three main possibilities to consider as causes of the phenomena of hypertension and rapid heart-rate which we have observed. One is the theory that the heart-muscle is directly and chiefly responsible by its altered myocardium, atrophy, atony, or degeneration due to the toxins of the bacillus and to the malnutrition incident to the disease. Another reasonable theory is that the blood-vessels are chiefly responsible by a vasodilatation caused by the tubercle toxins, for the hypotension, and that the tachycardia is a compensatory effort on the part of the heart.

The third possibility is that the nervous control of both blood-vessels and heart is interfered with by the toxic action of the bacterial product on the vasomotor and cardiac centers and that neither the heart-muscle nor the vessel-walls are directly affected, but that both vasodilatation and tachycardia are of nervous origin.

Until the recent studies by orthodiagraphic methods have been verified and the evidence presented by Bouchard duplicated, we cannot accept his statements as final, but it seems very likely that they are correct, namely, that hypertrophy of the heart occurs in the early stages of

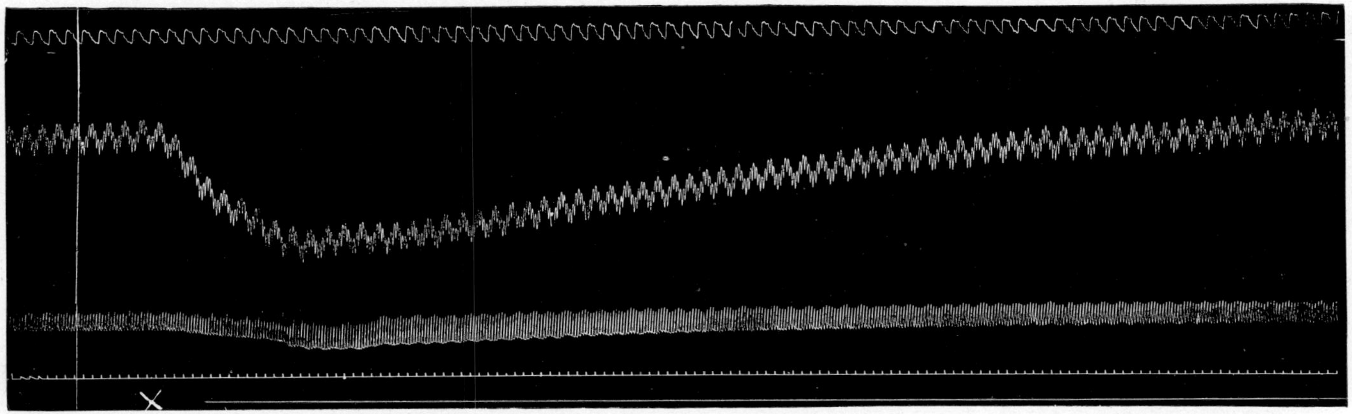


Fig. 1.—Effect of 1 gm. of old tuberculin administered intravenously on etherized cat. Records from above downward are, respiration, carotid blood-pressure (mercury manometer), carotid blood-pressure (Hürthle membrane manometer), time in 2-second intervals, abscissa. The break in the abscissa at X represents the period of injection. Read from left to right.

the disease when the rapid heart action succeeds in maintaining a fair to normal pressure, and that later there is a marked atrophy and degeneration of the heart. This would account for the discrepancies in the conclusions of the pathologists as to whether the heart of the tuberculous individual is large for the body weight or small. It depends, according to Bouchard, on whether the autopsy is performed in the stage of physiological compensation or in the period of degeneration. That there is no marked increase in size of the heart even when circulatory compensation is established is seen from Brown's figures from the Adirondack Cottage Sanitarium, where he found only eight of 1,289 patients who showed cardiac hypertrophy, and of these eight there were six with chronic valvular disease.

Where cardiac hypertrophy with or without perfect compensation has developed in response, for instance, to a mitral stenosis, we find either a very low incidence of tuberculosis or a high percentage of recovery where infection has occurred (Tileston).

Even exact methods of physical examination supplemented by thorough autopsy will never settle the origin of the circulatory disturbances of tuberculosis, however much agreement there may be as to end-results.

We must resort to experimental work in the lower animals for an analysis of the cause of hypotension and tachycardia in tuberculosis.

By exclusion we can go far to indicate the site of the injury by a bacterial toxin which we see take effect on the peripheral circulation, but we have no positive direct evidence for diphtheria toxin, pneumococcus toxin or for tubercle toxin. Finding a dearth of experimental evidence of any kind in relation to the effect of tubercle products, I offer the following as a step toward an explanation:

The materials used were provided by Dr. Isaac Levin of the Rockefeller Institute, by the Department of Health of the City of New York and by the Saranac Laboratory.

Two frogs were so arranged that the capillary blood-flow in the urinary bladder-wall could be watched through a microscope fitted with a micrometer eye-piece. To each was given 1 c.c. of ether in five equal doses in the dorsal lymph-sac. In the ether given to one was dissolved 1 mg. of bacillary fat extracted from the dry tubercle powder. In the course of an hour and a half, at the end of which time both frogs died, the capillaries of the frog which received ether alone were chiefly small and blanched, while the other one showed marked dilatation of the capillaries, an increase of 25 per cent. in the caliber of the small vessels having occurred. To reason from a single observation on cold-blooded animals as to conditions in human beings would not be justified, but what evidence there was pointed to a vasodilator effect.

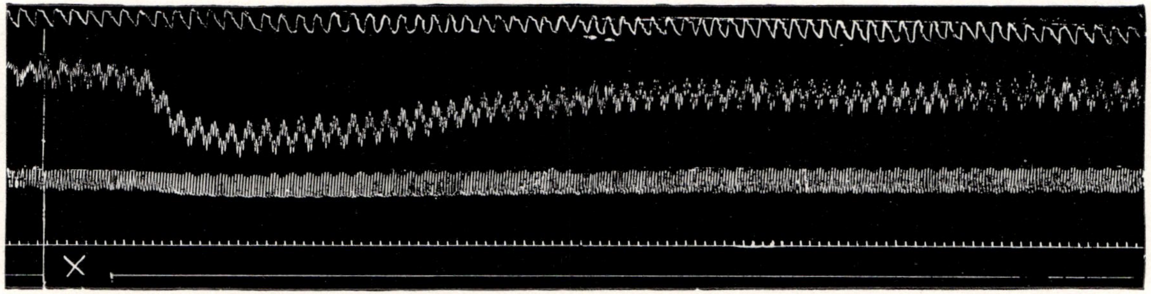

Fig. 2.—Effect of 0.5 gm. of old tuberculin administered intravenously on etherized cat. Records as in Figure 1. No change in heart action with the drop in carotid pressure.

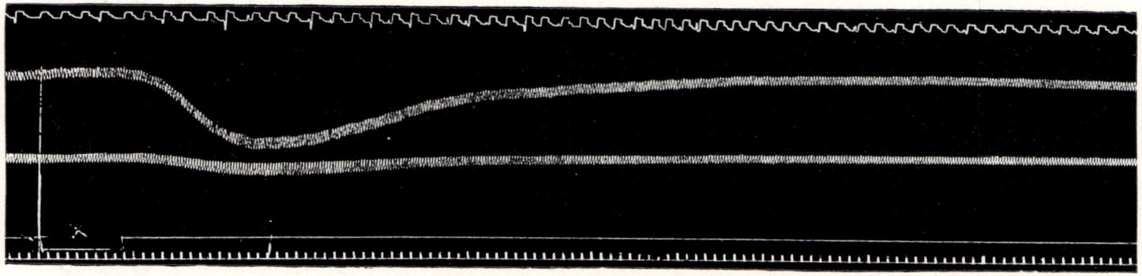

Fig. 3.—Effect of same dose as in Figure 2. Records as in Figure 1, but abscissa above time record. Distinct increase in heart action.

An etherized dog was then used, and continuous graphic records of respiration by pleural cannula, and blood-pressure by mercury manometer and membrane manometer were made, while various doses of ether and a solution of bacillary fat or wax of the tubercle bacillus were given by the jugular and femoral veins.

Although the ether solution of the bacillary fat appeared to depress the blood-pressure and relax the arterial tone for a much longer period than did an equal dose of ether alone, still the effect of the fat was not sufficiently striking to be free from doubt.

An etherized cat was then used and records made as in the previous experiment. *Bacillen-Emulsion* was then injected intravenously in doses from 0.005 mg. to 5 mg. of solid substance. Following this, old tuberculin was used in doses from 1 mg. to 0.5 mg. of solid substance. Lastly solutions of mannite culture of tubercle bacillus in normal salt solution was used from 0.01 gm. to 0.1 gm. at a dose. Even the largest dose, 5 mg. of *Bacillen-Emulsion,* gave no change in blood-pressure or in heart-rate.

The old tuberculin gave a marked fall in general blood-pressure, with an increase in the pulse-pressure, as recorded by the Hürthle membrane manometer, and a very brief acceleration amounting to five heart-beats to the minute when 1 gm. was given (Fig. 1). Milder effects were obtained with the smaller doses (Figs. 2 and 3). An error which must be considered is that in the evaporating to one-tenth of the original bulk of the culture, there is a concentration of the veal extractives, peptone, and sodium hydrate in the old tuberculin, which may be responsible for some of the depressing action on the circulation. However, as the dose of 1 gm. of old tuberculin contains but a very small amount of the extractives, and as their first effect is usually to constrict the blood-vessels and stimulate heart action, and only later develop a depressant action, and as our effect from old tuberculin was always a marked vasodilatation with no previous cardiac or vasoconstrictor stimulation, it is fair to assume that the cause of the fall in blood-pressure is some substance contained in the bacterial products.

Small doses of the mannite culture gave no result, and large doses gave the characteristic inhibition of respiration and heart action and prolonged depression of blood-pressure, which usually follow the administration of sodium carbonate and sugar solutions. The effects observed could not be ascribed to the tubercle products in the culture, but rather to the materials of which the culture medium was compounded.

Two etherized cats were used and the observations with *Bacillen-Emulsion,* Old Tuberculin and mannite culture were repeated, and then a series of tests was made with an alcoholic extract of the dried tubercle powder, and with a watery suspension of tuberculinic acid. The only new error to be tested for or explained in this experiment was the use of alcohol in the solution of the dried tubercle powder. As a control, alcohol, in the amounts used in testing the dissolved extract, was injected in 50 per cent. and 95 per cent. strengths into the veins, and records were taken (Fig. 4). One c.c. of 95 per cent. alcohol caused a drop in carotid pressure from 120 mm. to 106 mm. Hg, and a depressed heart action with a complete recovery in fifty-five seconds from the time of the injection.

One c.c. of the alcoholic extract of tubercle powder in 95 per cent. alcohol caused a drop in carotid pressure from 148 mm. to 106 mm., with extreme arterial relaxation and a return to normal only after five minutes (Fig. 5).

Five-tenths of a cubic centimeter of the alcoholic extract caused a drop from 135 mm. to 106 mm. in carotid pressure, and a return to previous pressure and arterial tone only after one and a half minutes (Fig.

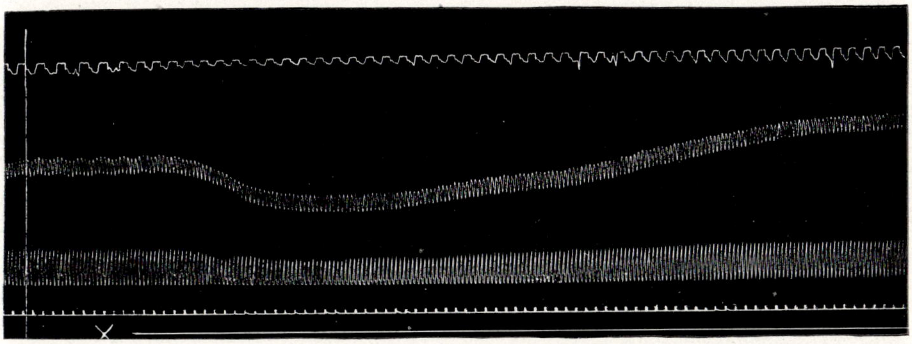

Fig. 4.—Effect of 1 c.c. 95 per cent. alcohol administered intravenously on etherized cat. Note the depressed heart action accompanying the fall in carotid pressure. The records are as described in Figure 1.

6). Even 0.1 c.c. of the alcoholic extract showed a fall in carotid pressure from 140 mm. to 134 mm. in thirty seconds.

No effect was observed as a result of the use of tuberculinic acid; 0.0045 gm. in suspension in 1 c.c. of water.

A last experiment was made with an etherized dog. No result was obtained from a solution of tuberculinic acid; 0.0046 in 1 c.c. decinormal sodium hydroxid.

The same marked vasodilator effect was observed from the use of alcoholic extract of the dry powder, as was seen in the previous experiment with the cat. The usual extreme depression was noted with a mannite culture.

The use of 5 mg. of *Bacillen-Emulsion* proved effective in giving a marked fall from 110 mm. to 86 mm., with evidences of vasodilatation, although smaller doses gave no result (Fig 7).

Bacillary fat (0.05 mg.) was partly emulsified and partly dissolved at 37 C. in 1 c.c. of olive oil, and injected intravenously, but no effect was observed.

Further to test the effect of tubercle products on the circulatory apparatus some perfusion experiments were made on the isolated dog's heart, and on the blood-vessels of the dog's leg. A dog was etherized and the heart and great vessels were rapidly removed and placed in a warmed, moist chamber, and the aorta was connected with a supply of Ringer's solution, thoroughly oxygenated, and warmed to a temperature of 34 to 40 C. and supplied at a pressure which varied from 60 to 86 mm. Hg. The various products were injected into the artificial circulation fluid through the rubber tube connected with the aorta. The apex

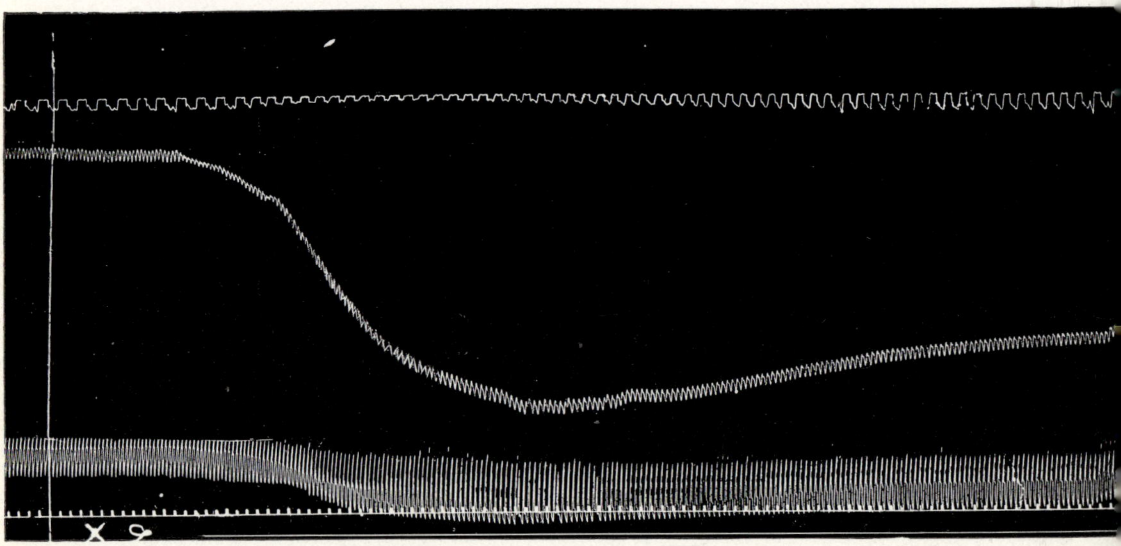

Fig. 5.—Effect of 1 c.c. of extract of tubercle powder in 85 per cent. alco

of the left ventricle was attached to a lever arranged to write on a smoked drum.

When the leg was used the same perfusion fluid under a pressure of 80 to 100 mm. Hg was supplied through a cannula tied to the femoral artery. The outflow from the veins of the leg was measured by the use of a recording tip-bucket.

The results of the tests on the perfused heart were as follows: the culture media, without bacteria, evaporated to one-tenth its volume, giving the same strength of veal extractives, peptones, and sodium hydrate as is found in the old tuberculin, was used as a control, and its effect was to stimulate the rapidity of the heart action and cause an increase of the extent of diastolic relaxation and systolic contraction, with later a distinct loss of cardiac tone.

When small doses of the old tuberculin were given, a noticeable slowing of the heart was sometimes recorded, but with larger doses, and frequently with small doses, cardiac acceleration was found, and a loss of tone similar to that produced by the concentrated bouillon alone.

There was no constant variation in the effects of these two substances by which any conclusion as to a specific action of the tubercle products could be determined.

A new preparation called *Eisen-Tuberculin* was tested without any result on the heart action.

*Bouillon filtré* was used and in each instance an acceleration and increased systolic excursion was observed, similar to, but milder than the results from equal bulk of old tuberculin and old tuberculin culture

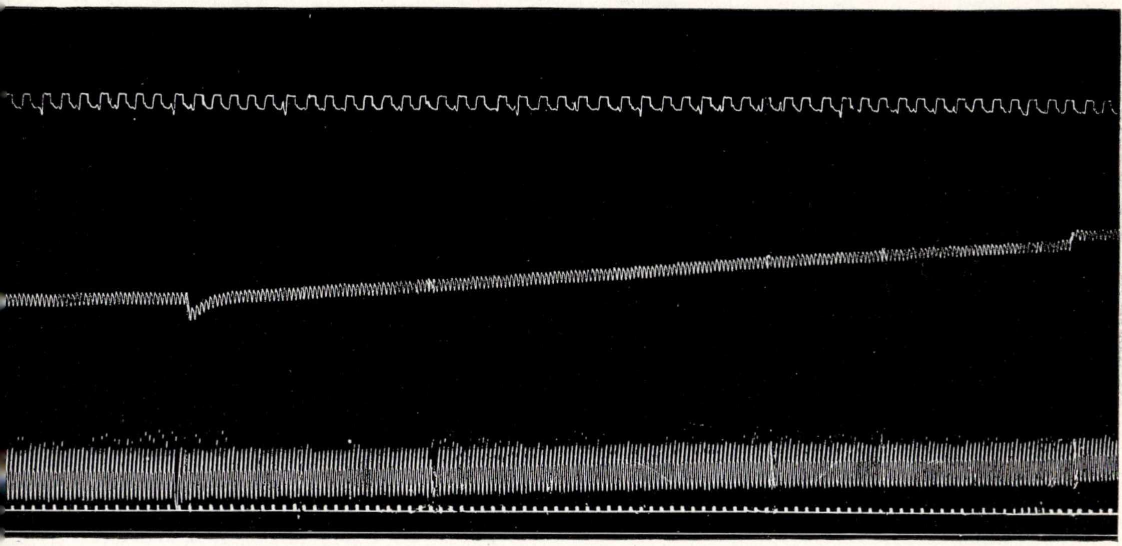

ainistered intravenously, on etherized cat. Records as described for Figure 1.

medium. It was apparent that the effect was that of the extractives used in the medium, and was not due to tubercle products.

Mannite culture caused marked depression of force and frequency of heart action—in all probability due to the substances of the culture medium, as explained above.

An aqueous extract of the dried powder gave no change in the heart action. It is correct to say, then, that doses of various tubercle products many times larger than the largest dose used with safety in human beings have no specific action on the heart muscle of dogs when thrown directly into the circulation of the heart in an artificial circulating fluid.

The tests on the leg preparations showed with the concentrated broth culture medium an increase in the flow during and immediately after the injection, followed by a diminished flow for two minutes. This is a characteristic vasoconstrictor effect, the first increase being due to emptying of the larger vessels and the delay to an obstruction to the flow.

Old tuberculin gave the same results in exact proportion to the bulk used.

The *Eisen-Tuberculin* caused a slight delay in the flow.

The mannite culture in water caused marked decrease in the flow.

*Bouillon filtré* had no effect.

Aqueous extract of the dry tubercle powder had no effect.

It would appear from these tests that there is no specific action of the tubercle products on the musculature of the blood-vessels.

Briefly then, from the foregoing observations on patients suffering from pulmonary tuberculosis, and from manometric tests of the effect of tubercle products on the circulation of mammals, in all of which cases we find evidence of a tendency to loss of vasomotor tone and a depression of general blood-pressure, and from the perfusion tests on the heart and

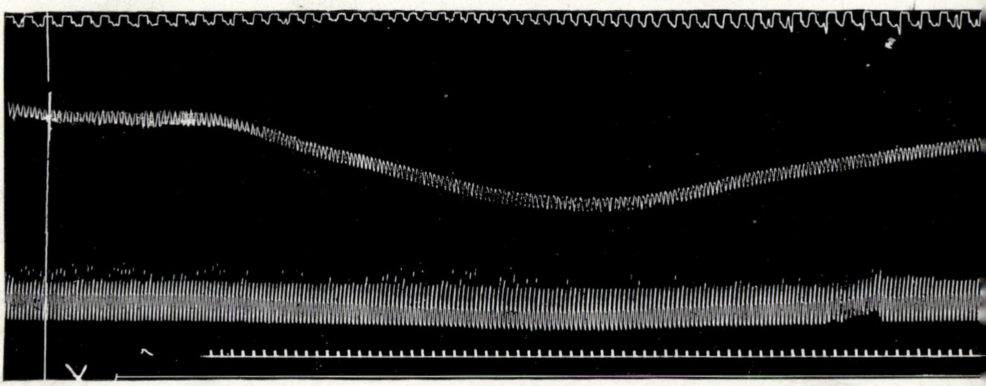

Fig. 6.—Effect of 0.5 c.c. of extract of tubercle powder in 95 per cent. alco

peripheral circulation of dogs in none of which do we find evidence of direct or local action on the heart or blood-vessels, we may properly consider that when the products of the tubercle bacillus are distributed through the circulation to various parts of the body, their effect on the circulation is probably due to some action on the central nervous system and not to any direct effect on the heart or vessels.

With the difficulty of proving a variation from normal limits in the blood-pressure, and with the increasing exactness of specific tests for tuberculosis to help our diagnosis as based on the history and examination of patients, it is not likely that the functional test above described will displace any of the well-recognized proofs of early tuberculosis, but it may confirm them.

As a measure and indication of the need of rest in the course of treatment, and as evidence when exercise has exceeded safe limits, it appears to me a useful test.

Whether specific treatment of tuberculosis infection shall prove universally successful or not, certainly the understanding and treatment of the severe and persistent circulatory disturbance that always accompanies the disease will play a large part in abbreviating the course of treatment and our knowledge will encourage us to insist on absolute rest when rest is indicated, and to control and graduate the exercise that is allowed during convalescence in proportion to the ability of the blood-vessels to maintain an adequate blood-pressure without undue and prolonged rapidity of the heart-rate.

## III. HISTORICAL DISCUSSION

Personal experience, even when it is of much wider range than what I have offered, must be subject to correction by the observations of others before it can be accepted as final. Therefore, a review of the literature will be given, to summarize previous studies.

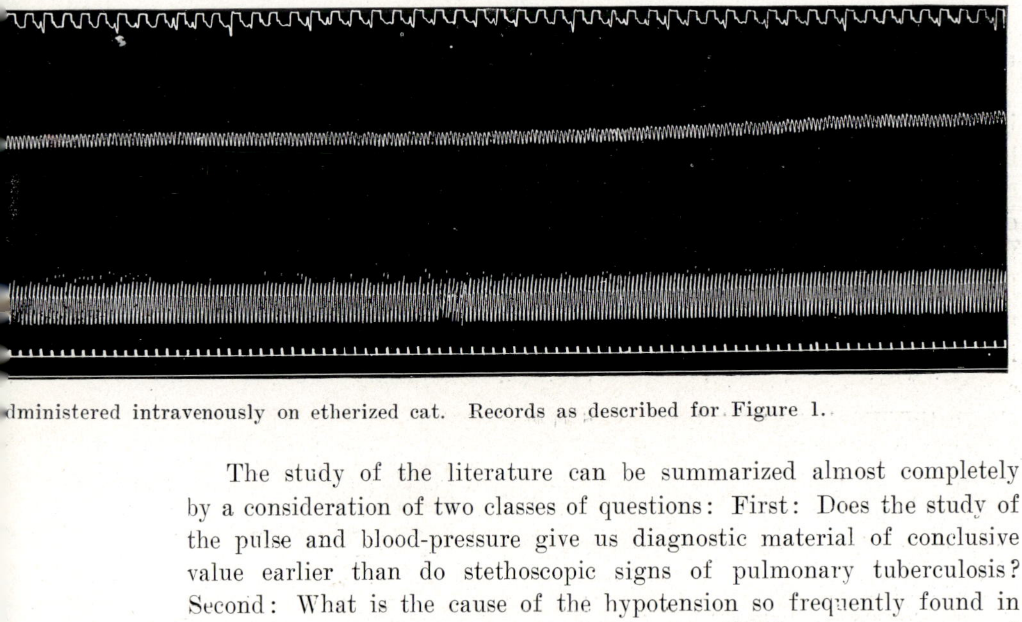

dministered intravenously on etherized cat. Records as described for Figure 1.

The study of the literature can be summarized almost completely by a consideration of two classes of questions: First: Does the study of the pulse and blood-pressure give us diagnostic material of conclusive value earlier than do stethoscopic signs of pulmonary tuberculosis? Second: What is the cause of the hypotension so frequently found in tuberculosis and can this hypotension be remedied by treatment or used as a prognostic indication?

As to the diagnostic usefulness of tachycardia and hypotension, we find that the French writers in general consider that persistent hypotension, unexplained by other causes, is a fact of definite diagnostic value, and they assert that it precedes stethoscopic signs of pulmonary tuberculosis (Potain, Regnault, Faisans, Papillon, Homolle, Renaud, Teissier, Fourmeaux, Fagart, Ledoux, Bosc and Vedel, Lamy and Strandgaard). There is so much agreement among these authors that it is unnecessary to quote largely from their writings. From clinical observations with

various kinds of blood-pressure machines and under a variety of conditions as to time and position of the tests, these writers agree that low blood-pressure is a constant, early, diagnostic sign in pulmonary tuberculosis, whether the case is febrile or not, and whether stethoscopic evidence is present or not. As a differential point between the chloroanemia of adolescence and incipient tuberculosis, they consider persistent hypotension as a reliable sign of the latter. As a means of detecting latent tuberculosis, they rely on it. They find that the fall in pressure is in proportion to the susceptibility of the individual and the severity of the infection. They find that the pressure falls with the advance of the disease, with the development of new foci of disease, increase in fever, and with the degree of accompanying cachexia. For example, Regnault says: "Low blood-pressure is a phenomenon, constant in tuberculosis, increasing with rise of temperature or advance of cachexia but present in early or afebrile cases, and present from the beginning and throughout the disease in spite of treatment. It is of early diagnostic value and those who recover are those in whom the pressure is nearest to normal."

Renaud says: "Recognition of the symptom of hypotension is of incontestable value in doubtful cases of pulmonary tuberculosis, even before stethoscopic signs, in pleurisy with effusion, in making a differential diagnosis and in atrophic cirrhosis of the liver with ascites, to determine the origin of the fluid."

Teissier finds "hypotension a constant and precocious sign before local or general symptoms and noted in those with an hereditary predisposition and in those with latent tuberculous lymph-nodes"; "a most important and valuable sign, indicating a tuberculizable field or an actual infection; not a pathognomonic sign." "Carefully made pressure observations, well controlled, taken with general and physical signs, give valuable diagnostic and prognostic results in tuberculosis."

Strandgaard, the one writer not in any way associated with the French school, agrees in the main with their conclusions. He finds "hypotension a valuable aid in diagnosis suggesting tuberculosis in general or an active process in particular." "The pressure is low in proportion to the stage of the disease."

The precautions used in arriving at these conclusions are in most cases so carefully reported and the details are so fully covered that one must credit these statements with being based on close observation. The chief defect in these, as indeed in most so-called clinical reports, is the scantiness of the material studied. Regnault reports thirty-five cases, Reynaud nineteen, Ledoux thirteen, Lamy nine, Fagart eight, and although the value of their statements lies in the prolonged periods of months and even years over which they have watched their cases, still

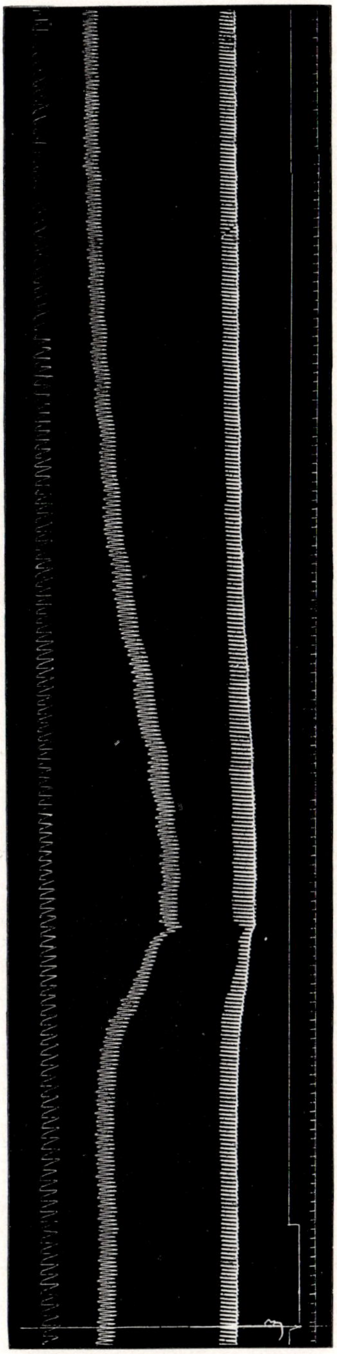

Fig. 7.—Effect of 5 mg. of Bacillen-Emulsion intravenously upon an etherized dog (weight 8 kilos). Records as described for Figure 1, except that in this case the time record is below the abscissa or base line.

the conclusions are rather more positive and general than the number of cases warrants. In the reports of Potain, Teissier, and Papillon, evidently large hospital experience and an abundance of clinical material was drawn on for the studies and yet they fail to tell the exact number of patients whom they examined. On the other hand, Strandgaard's work at the Boserup Sanatorium in Denmark is of the greatest value, since he studied 622 patients under continuous observation over long periods. The conditions for study were ideal, and his conclusions, although more guarded than those of the French writers, show definitely his feeling that "hypotension is a valuable aid in diagnosis."

Reitter in a very careful prolonged study of ten cases of renal tuberculosis found that all but two ran a pressure always 100 mm. or lower. One of the others ranged from 110 to 105. The other had a pressure of 160 and was the subject of chronic valvular disease and marked cardiac hypertrophy.

In six cases of pyuria suspected of being tuberculous in origin, he found pressures of 110 mm. or over, and in all of them the cause was proved to be non-tuberculous.

His conclusion is excellent: "Hypotension shares the fate of so many other symptoms of disease which are not always found in every case, but when they do occur are of marked value in differential diagnosis; e. g., if hypotension occurs in a case of nephritis or renal lit[illegible]ere is probably a renal tuberculosis. Hypotension should make [illegible]ect tuberculosis even if the lesion found is a renal one."

The other side of the picture is presented by Burckhardt, [illegible] Igersheimer, John, Naumann, Battistessa and Mathes. While most of them admit the occurrence of hypotension in pulmonary tuberculosis, they pretty generally agree that it cannot be determined constantly enough to serve as an early sign, or at any event before physical signs of the disease can be made out. Burckhardt finds no constant hypotension in twenty-three patients of Class I (Turban), at Davos, and even among thirteen patients of Class II he can reach no conclusion from the blood-pressure.

Hensen finds blood-pressure about normal until just before death.

Igersheimer found among twenty-four patients no constant relation between the degree of the disease and blood-pressure.

John found, in 120 cases, a normal blood-pressure and pulse rate in all the incipient cases.

Naumann in 100 cases found normal and subnormal pressures equally distributed among all three classes of patients.

Battistessa in thirty cases concludes that sphygmomanometry can give no help in early diagnosis and that arterial pressure in pulmonary tuberculosis does not show any constant modification.

Mathes in 100 cases found normal pressure in early or light cases. Hypotension, he finds, is not an early sign but is the result of emaciation.

We cannot attribute this discrepancy in opinions to the instruments used, nor to the standards of normal pressure adopted by the different observers, as similar although not identical pressures were considered normal by both groups of observers, and similar instruments were used. The Riva-Rocci instrument or one of its modifications was used by observers of both groups, the Gaertner more often by the Germans and the Potain instrument oftener by the French.

From my own observations, I should say that at present more reliance could be placed on the results of a thorough physical examination of the chest than on blood-pressure tests, but I have no doubt that many more cases of early, unsuspected or well-developed cases would be identified as tuberculous if it were as much a matter of routine to make careful blood-pressure tests as it is to observe pulse-rate and temperature. Any case of hypotension should put us on our guard at once. If it persists and no other cause is found to explain it, such a hypotension should probably be treated on much the same hygienic principles as is suspected early tuberculosis.

[illegible] of the hypotension which is almost universally found in [illegible] tuberculosis, there is a good deal of speculation among the writers [illegible] quoted, but there are scanty sources from which one can draw any safe conclusions.

At least one cause we may abandon, namely, cachexia. Several writers who deny the presence of hypotension except in advanced cases consider the cause to be merely the wasting accompanying the disease. So many observers have found hypotension in early cases and in cases where there is no loss of strength or weight that this explanation can well be ignored.

For the rest, the causes may be summed up in two general statements: first, that the hypotension is primary and the direct result of the action of the toxins of the tubercle bacillus and of the associated bacteria of ulcerating tissue on the neuromuscular mechanism of the peripheral circulation; second, that the hypotension is secondary to some essential disturbance, as of the diminished solid contents of the blood (Cazes), irritation of gastric and pulmonary terminals of the pneumogastric nerve, excess of carbon dioxid in the blood, secondary anemia (Ledoux), fever which causes tachycardia, this causing hypotension, which in its turn causes cerebral anemia thus stimulating the accelerans center in the brain (Krehl), diminished respiratory surface and compression of the vagus by bronchial lymph-glands (Gibson).

As none of the theoretical explanations given, except that of Krehl and of those who believe in the direct toxic origin of the hypotension, is supported by any facts of value, or has been subjected to the test of experimental verification, I shall consider them only as they may be incorporated in the more satisfactory, even if not positively proved, theory of toxic origin.

Bouchard, in 1891, found that Koch's tuberculin caused a dilatation of the rabbit's retinal vessels which lasted for days. He considers this proof that there is a substance produced by the tubercle bacillus which acts on the vasodilator center. He asserts that the result of this vasodilatation is the albumin, blood and peptone he finds in the urine in tuberculosis; pulmonary and renal congestion being the usual result of general vasodilatation.

Arloing, Rhodet and Courmont, in 1892, found that the injection of 2,000 to 2,500 mg. of tuberculin caused a fall in blood-pressure in dogs and goats after thirty seconds, the pressure rising presently but not to the previously normal. They publish no tracings of their experiments. Charrin and Le Noir, in 1893, noted dilatation of vessels of rabbits' ears after injecting urinary extracts of tuberculous patients. The dilatation was found to be more marked if the urine was taken during high fever. They concluded that it was evident that some dilator substance was produced by the tubercle bacillus and that this substance was excreted by the kidneys.

Arloing and Guignard isolated four substances from Koch's tuberculin, and one of these substances caused dilated vessels, with a fall in blood-pressure, and rapid heart action. They publish no graphic records of their work in rabbits and do not describe their technic.

My own experiments on lower animals point to a distinct vasodepressant effect of the tubercle products, the actual manner of such toxic action remaining undetermined, but the indications being that the central rather than the peripheral, the nervous rather than the muscular mechanism of circulation is the sufferer.

On the other hand, Bauer, using curarized guinea-pigs, found that old tuberculin (Koch) caused no fall in blood-pressure. But he obtained no fall from the culture medium used as control, and there is reason in this to suppose there was an error in his method, for the peptones of the standard culture medium have always in my hands caused some fall in pressure.

On testing twenty patients with 0.005 to 0.001 doses of old tuberculin he found no fall in pressure except occasionally when a reaction occurred, and his conclusions are very positive that old tuberculin causes no fall in blood-pressure in animals or human beings. The weight of evidence seems to be against him.

The opinions of clinical observers are of value to a limited degree in drawing conclusions in such a complicated matter as the causes of tachycardia and hypotension. But such as they are, the sentiment is strongly in favor of a primary toxic origin of low pressure with various later contributory causes.

For instance, Papillon, Levy and Geisbock find that fall in blood-pressure always follows tuberculin injections and that the fall is in proportion to the dose of tuberculin and may last from three or four days up to three weeks.

Igershcimer alone finds a primary and constant rise in pressure on administering tuberculin, and that this rise which occurs in twelve or twenty-four hours after a dose of from 1 to 5 mg. is independent of change of pulse or temperature. His observations were made at Davos.

A long list of authors come out strongly for the theory that hypotension in tuberculosis is primarily the result of the tubercle toxins, e. g. Regnault, Teissier, Ledoux, Norris, Gibson, Bosc and Vedel, Turban, Homolle, Battistessa, Pottenger, Max, Faisans, and Strandgaard. Max considers as a contributory cause also the diminished albumin and hemoglobin content in the blood of tuberculous patients.

Bouchard and Balthazard consider primary cardiac dystrophy the cause of low pressure.

Inasmuch as the observers who note hypotension as an early or diagnostic sign in tuberculosis also generally allude to hypotension as a predisposing cause to tuberculous infection, we may expect to find empirical or logical treatment advised, directed to improving the circulation.

Galecki at Brehmer's sanatorium at Goerbersdorf, and Strandgaard at the Boserup Sanatorium, found that the rest-cure with abundant alimentation and regulated exercise raised the pressure in hypotension cases, kept normal pressure cases normal and delayed the fall in pressure if advancing cases were benefited by the treatment.

Igersheimer found that in only 32 per cent. of thirty-seven cases allowed one hour exercise did the pressure rise; in 58 per cent. it fell and in 8 per cent. it remained the same after exercise. Pressure in a normal person rises on exercise or stays normal, but does not fall. He finds that overfeeding helps to raise low pressure.

Faisans urges that all causes of tachycardia be avoided, such as tea, coffee, preparations containing coca or kola and especially alcohol, also exposure to direct sunlight, all being contributory causes of hypotension. He states that the pressure can be raised by rest, fresh air, moderate alimentation and carefully regulated exercise.

Fourmeaux advises treatment by gentle exercise and nourishment, and states that if cure or arrest is to be accomplished, the blood-pressure must be raised to normal.

The reliance placed by clinicians on the rapidity of the pulse is an indication of the probable prognostic value of hypotension, for it is found that the tachycardia is a fair measure of the hypotension, and as has been explained above, tachycardia is a necessary physiologic sequel to hypotension. Schneider, after observing a thousand cases over a period of four years at the Goerbersdorf Sanatorium, says that he considers the rapidity of the pulse a most reliable means of prognosis in tuberculosis. The following authors came out quite as strongly in favor of hypotension as a safe guide in prognosis: Regnault, Burchhardt, Galecki, Max, Naumann, Reynaud, Battistessa, Grosset, Marfan, Fagart and Strandgaard.

### IV. SUMMARY

Hypotension or subnormal blood-pressure is universally found in advanced pulmonary tuberculosis, in which condition emaciation may play a part in its causation. Hypotension is found in almost all cases of moderately advanced tuberculosis, or in early cases in which the toxemia is marked except when arteriosclerosis, the so-called arthritic or gouty diathesis, chronic nephritis, or diabetes complicate the tuberculosis and bring about a normal pressure or a hypertension. Occasionally the period just preceding an hemoptysis or during an hemoptysis may show hypertension in a patient whose usual condition is that of hypotension.

Hypotension has been found by so many observers in early, doubtful or suspected cases with or before physical signs of the disease in the lungs, and is considered by competent clinicians so useful a differential sign between various conditions, and tuberculosis, that it should be sought for as carefully as it is the custom at present to search for pulmonary signs.

Hypotension when found persistently in individuals or families or classes living under certain unhygienic conditions should put us on our guard against at least a predisposition to tuberculosis. Most unhygienic conditions, overwork, undernourishment and insufficient air, are of themselves causes of a diminished resistance, and it seems likely that a failure of normal cardiovascular response to exercise or change of position may be found to indicate this stage of susceptibility, especially to tuberculous infection.

The difficulty of proving a subnormal pressure is so much greater than that of determining an increase of pulse-rate or of temperature that some means such as the one I suggest in the tests I have made personally should be tried before considering a patient normal just because a single systolic reading shows a pressure within normal limits.

Hypotension, when it is present in tuberculosis, increases with an extension of the process. Recovery from hypotension accompanies arrest or improvement. Return to normal pressure is commonly found in those who are cured. Continuation of hypotension seems never to accompany improvement. Prognosis can as safely be based on the alteration in the blood-pressure as on changes in the pulse or temperature.

The causes of low blood-pressure in tuberculosis are probably primarily a toxic action on the vasomotor center in the medulla, allowing of a vasoparesis or stimulating an active vasodilatation, and secondarily, progressive cardiac atrophy or degeneration. Toxic action on the vasomotor nerves or their motor terminals or on the nervous mechanism of the heart cannot be positively denied, although there is no proof of it at present. Toxic action of tubercle products has not been demonstrated on the muscle of the vessel-wall or heart, although with regard to the latter, the degenerated heart-muscle found in advanced cases may play a large part in causing hypotension. Rapid heart action is a usual and necessary sequel to low blood-pressure and will, if extreme, aggravate the hypotension by the very act of its shortened diastole. It has been suggested, but not proved, that lack of vagus inhibition owing to pressure by enlarged bronchial lymph-nodes and presence of sympathetic excitation from similar or reflex causes such as pulmonary or gastric irritation, are responsible for the tachycardia and hypotension.

"Fever will cause rapid heart action by effect on accelerans nerve endings in the heart. Diminished general pressure results in lower cerebral pressure which of itself stimulates the cerebral origin of cardiac accelerans nerves especially when the low pressure is due to vasoparesis" (Krehl).

The secondary anemia, with its diminished albumin, salts and hemoglobin content serves to add to the hypotension from purely physical causes in the blood-stream.

Diminished area of lung tissue, resulting in an increased carbon dioxid content of the blood, is suggested as a contributory cause of hypotension.

Displacement of the heart, which is so common a result of retracted lung tissue or loss of expansion due to cavity formation or adhesive pleurisy, is spoken of as a cause of tachycardia accompanying hypotension, and it certainly seems to be a contributory cause in some cases.

Marked vasomotor irritability is recognized as a frequent phenomenon in pulmonary tuberculosis and is supposed to result in tachycardia and hypotension, but it is not easy to see exactly what is meant by this term unless a certain functional instability, for which we have no proof of any definite local cause.

Disease of the adrenal bodies is to be mentioned as a possible factor, only to be set aside for lack of any consistent pathologic proof.

Primary cardiac atrophy, congenital or acquired, can no longer be considered as a factor in the presence of modern orthographic *x*-ray examinations, and in the absence of agreement among pathologists.

The result of hypotension in tuberculosis or in any other condition is insufficient capillary pressure, more or less venous stagnation and insufficient nourishment, with resulting atrophy or degeneration of the essential organs of the body.

The treatment of tuberculosis in all its stages should take into consideration the need of assisting in every way the return to normal pressure, first by relieving the relaxed vessels of the load put on them during the vertical position or exercise, and later by assisting the heart by abundant nutrition, moderate exercise and the stimulating effect on cardiac and vascular tone of cold fresh air, to meet the extra work put on it by the loss of vascular tone. Thus will the heart be able to maintain its normal bulk and strength or even to gain from the atrophy or small size of the early disease, to a normal size, so that brain, kidneys, lungs and body at large may be properly nourished, until the disease is arrested and the toxic products of the tubercle bacillus are no longer distributed from the site of the lesion.

The following bibliography is, I believe, complete at present:

BIBLIOGRAPHY

Arloing and Guinard: Cong. p. l'étude de la tuberc. chez l'homme et chez les animaux, 1898, 4th Session, p. 707.

Arloing, Rhodet and Courmont: Compt. rend. Cong. de la Tuberc., Paris, 1892, p. 32.

Auclair: Thèse, Paris, 1897.

Barach, J. H.: Physiological and Pathological Effects of Severe Exertion (the Marathon Race) on the Circulatory and Renal System, The Archives Int. Med., 1910, v, 382.

Barbary, F.: Cong. internat. de la tuberc., 1906, i, 566.

Battistessa, P.: Gaz. med. ital., 1907, lviii, 91, 101.

Bauer, F.: Ztschr. f. klin. Med., 1907, lvii, 368.

Bosc, M. F. J., and Vedel, M.: Cong. franç. de méd., 1904, vii, i, 208, 337.

Boschi, G.: Gaz. d. osp. e d. clin., 1906, xxvii, 1545.

Bouchard: Compt. rend. Acad. d. sc., Paris, 1888, cvi, 1582; 1891, cxiii, 524.

Bouchard and Balthazard: Rev. de la tuberc., 1903, x, i; Cong. Internat. de la tuberc., i, 550.

Brown, L.: Am. Jour. Med. Sc. Phila., 1908, cxxxvi, 819.

Burckhardt: Ztschr. f. Tuberk., 1906, viii, 459; Deutsch. Arch. f. klin. Med., 1901, lxx, 236.

Cazes, F.: Thèse, Paris, 1889-1890, No. 236, Chap. V, p. 56.

Charrin and Le Noir: Compt. rend. Soc. de biol., Paris, July 22, 1893, series 9, 769.

Chon. H.: Thèse, Lyon, 1904-05, No. 32.

Crampton, C. W.: Med. News, 1905, lxxxviii, 529.

Fagart: Thèse, Paris, 1906, No. 141.

Faisans: Semaine méd., Paris, 1898, xviii, 305.

Fourmeaux: Cong. internat. de la tuberc., 1906, i, 564.

Galecki: Beitr. z. Klin. d. Tuberk., 1905-06, iv, 269.

Geisbock: Cong. f. inn. Med., 1904, xxi, 97.

Gibson, A. M.: Tr. Am. Climat. Assn., 1906, xxii, 96.
Grancher: Semaine méd., 1890, x, 315.
Grosset, M.: Rev. de la tuberc., 1905, series 2, ii, 243.
Henderson, Y.: Am. Jour. Physiol. 1906, xvi, 325.
Hensen: Deutsch. Arch. f. klin. Med., 1900, lxvii, 436.
Homolle: Rev. de méd., 1881, i, 252.
Igersheimer: Inaug. Diss. Tübingen, 1904.
John, M.: Ztschr. f. diät. u. physik. Therap., 1902, v, 275.
Krehl, L.: Pathologische Physiologie, 1904, p. 77.
Lamy, H.: Tribune med., 1904, new series, ii, 725.
Ledoux, S. A.: Thèse, Paris, 1902, No. 128.
Levy, L.: Beit. z. Klin. d. Tuberk., 1905, iv, 99.
Maragliano, G.: Presse méd., 1896, iv, 273.
Marfan, A. B.: Rev. d. méd., 1907, xxvii, 1005.
Mathes: Thèse, Paris, 1905.
Naumann, H.: Ztschr. f. Tuberk., 1903, v, 118.
New, M.: Inaug. Diss., Heidelberg, 1902.
Norris, G. W.: Ztschr. f. Tuberk., 1905, vii, 295.
Papillon: Thèse, Paris, 1898.
Potain: La pression arterielle de l'homme à l'état normal et pathologique, Paris, 1902, Masson.
Pottenger, F. M.: The Effect of Tuberculosis on the Heart, The Archives Int. Med., 1909, iv, 306.
Regnault: Thèse, Paris, 1898.
Reitter: Ztschr. f. klin. Med., 1907, lxii, 358.
Reynaud, G.: Thèse, Paris, 1901.
Strandgaard, N. J.: Hosp.-Tid., 1907, xv, 1041.
Schneider, H.: Deutsch. Aerzte-Ztg., 1904, xxiii, 533.
Teissier, P.: Cong. Internat. de la Tuberc., 1906, i, 554.
Tileston, W.: Passive Hyperemia of the Lungs and Tuberculosis, Jour. Am. Med. Assn., 1908, L, 1179.
Turban, K.: Diagnosis of Tuberculosis of the Lungs, N. Y., 1906, Wm. Wood & Co.
Vialard, M. F.: Bull. gén. d. therapeutique, 1903, cxlv, 277.

120 East Sixty-Second Street.

# PYROGENIC ACTION OF SALT SOLUTIONS IN RABBITS

HENRY F. HELMHOLZ, M.D.
CHICAGO

The recent publications of Meyer,[1] Schloss,[2] Friberger,[3] and others have brought non-bacterial fevers again into the foreground. Numerous articles have appeared from the clinic of Finkelstein, which have shown that sugar and various salts given hypodermically or by mouth produce fever in young infants suffering from the acute gastro-intestinal disturbance called dyspepsia. In 1907 Schaps[4] showed that, by the hypodermic injection of even so small an amount as 5 c.c. of physiological salt solution, a febrile temperature could be produced. Although these observations were denied by Weiland[5] they have since been substantiated by a number of observers. Meyer and Rietschel[6] showed that in about 40 per cent. of the cases which reacted to physiological salt solution, no reaction could be obtained by the injection of the same amount of a modified Ringer's solution. These were not the first experiments, however, on the pyrogenic action of salts. In 1895 Krehl[7] published, in an article on fevers, a series of observations on the effect of salt solution given subcutaneously to rabbits; 0.4 gm. of the salt given in 5 per cent. solution produced reactions varying from 0.9° to 1.3° C. Lüdke,[8] in a recent publication, states that he was entirely unable to produce fever with 1 to 3 per cent. solutions of sodium chlorid in adults suffering from gastro-intestinal disturbances.

The pyrogenic action of salt solutions when given by mouth was demonstrated for the first time by Meyer last year, when he showed that a large percentage of infants under 4 months of age with dyspeptic stools would react to the oral administration of a 1 per cent. solution of

---

1. Meyer, L. F.: Experimentelle Untersuchungen zum alimentären Fieber, Deutsch. med. Wchnschr., 1909, xxxv, 194.

2. Schloss, E.: Studien über Salzfieber, Biochem. Ztschr., 1909, xviii, 14.

3. Friberger, H.: Untersuchungen über das sogenannte Salzfieber, München. med. Wchnschr., 1909, lxi, 1946.

4. Schaps, L.: Salz- und Zuckerinjectionen beim Säugling, Berl. klin. Wchnschr., 1907, xliv, 597.

5. Weiland, R.: Kochsalz- und Zuckerinfusionen beim Säugling, Berl. klin. Wchnschr., 1908, xlv, 1309.

6. Meyer, L. F., and Rietschel, H.: Giftwirkung und Entgiftung des Kochsalzes bei subcutaner Infusion, Berl. klin. Wchnschr., 1908, xlv, 2217.

7. Krehl, L.: Versuche über die Erzeugung von Fieber bei Tieren, Arch. f. exper. Path. u. Pharmakol., 1895, xxxv, 222.

8. Lüdke, H.: Ueber Ursachen und Wirkungen der Fiebertemperature, Ergebn. d. inn. med. u. Kinderh., 1909, iv, 493.

sodium chlorid with a rise in temperature. He showed that this action was a property of sodium halogen compounds. Schloss later showed that potassium salts also possess this pyrogenic property, but to a much less degree, and that calcium salts on the other hand cause subnormal temperatures. The work of Friberger substantiated in the essentials that of Meyer; it differed quite widely, however, in the relative number of cases which reacted.

The experiments that follow were undertaken to determine whether or not similar reactions to salt solution could be obtained in rabbits. The essentials in the technic used were as follows:

1. All animals were brought to the laboratory one day before using and the temperature was controlled at regular intervals. The highest temperature on this day was taken as the control, above which temperatures were considered as febrile.

2. The animals were fed liberally on carrots.

3. Temperatures were taken at regular intervals of one to three hours, depending on the experiment. The thermometer was always introduced 2.5 cm. into the rectum and allowed to remain for five minutes.

4. Sterilized solutions were introduced subcutaneously under the skin of the abdomen, intravenously into a vein of the ear or orally by means of a stomach-tube.

Before passing on to other methods of administering the salt solution it seemed advisable to repeat the experiments of Krehl. The results of the experiments, however, were not in agreement with those of Krehl, so a large number of injections were made to prove the point. Of eight subcutaneous injections of 5 per cent sodium chlorid, the average reaction was 0.2° C. above the highest temperature recorded the day before. The highest reaction in an unused animal was 0.35°; in an animal that had been injected before, 0.4°. Two unused animals were injected with a 2.5 per cent. solution of sodium chlorid. The one with 10 c.c. reacted with a rise of 0.2°, the other with 50 c.c. failed by 0.2° to reach the highest temperature of the day previous. The administration of 0.5 gm. of sodium chlorid in a 1 per cent. solution subcutaneously failed in three experiments to produce fever. The time between the injection and the fastigium varied from five to twelve hours. For particulars of individual experiments see tables appended.

The reactions with sodium bromid were very similar, except that they averaged a little higher. The average rise in temperature in seven experiments was 0.33° C.; the highest temperature reached was 0.65° above the control temperature, and the time between injection and fastigium varied from five to twelve hours.

With the sodium iodid the greatest differences were observed, not only between the used and unused animals, but also between different

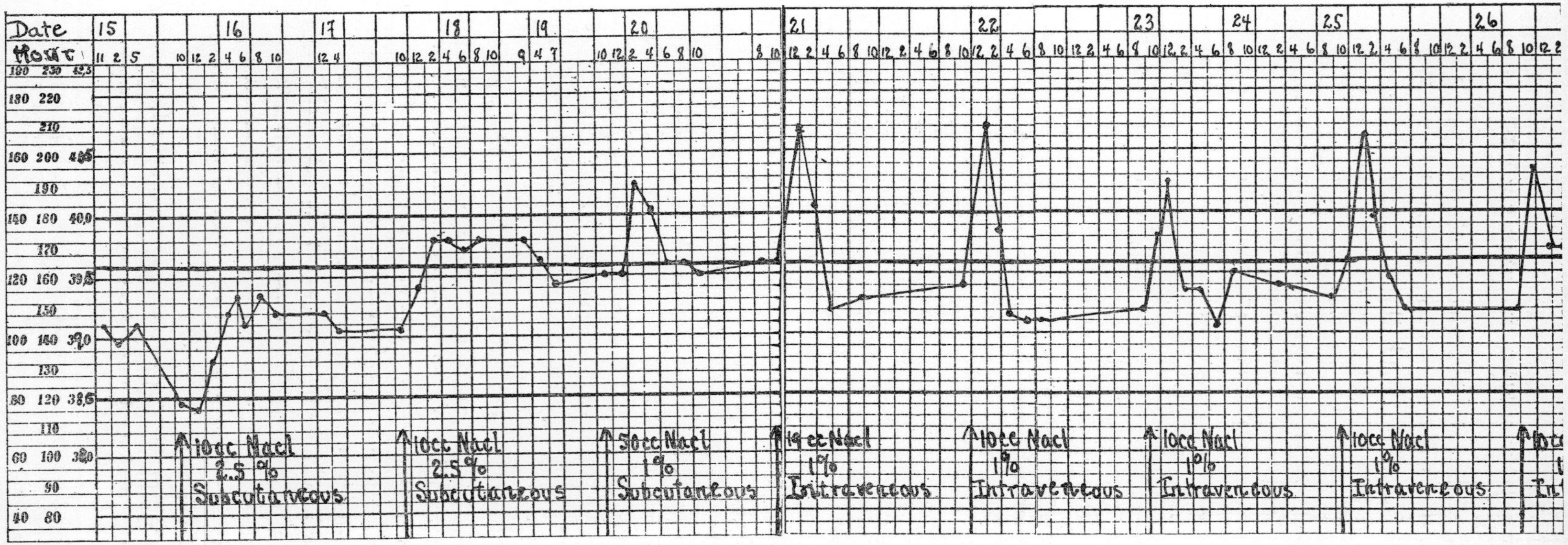


Chart showing effect of halogen salts.

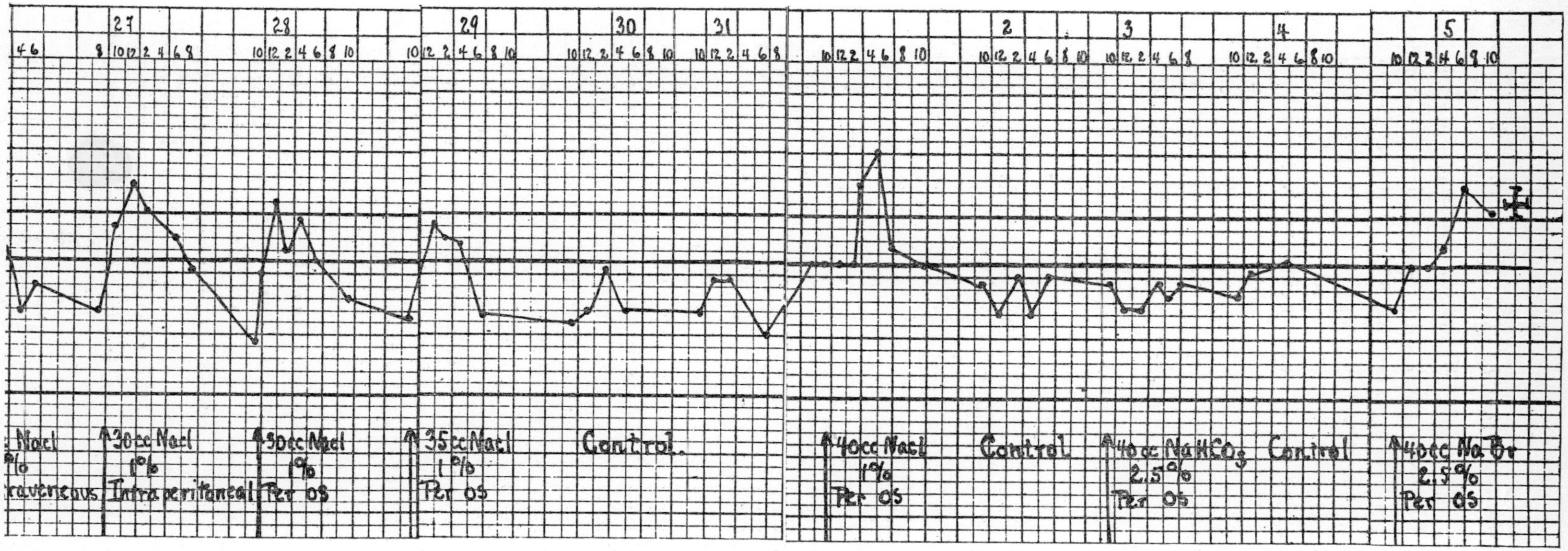


Chart showing effect of halogen salts, continued.

animals of the used group and between different animals of the unused group. Several of the unused animals reacted quite definitely with 0.5°, 0.7° and 1.1°; a fourth failed by 0.1° to reach the maximum of the previous day. The general average of ten experiments was, however, only 0.32°.

TABLE 1.—SUBCUTANEOUS INJECTIONS

| Number of experiments. | Salt used. | Concentration in per cent. | Quantity used in c.c. | Time to fastigium in hours. | Highest temperature. | Rise above control. | Animal.* |
|---|---|---|---|---|---|---|---|
| 1a | NaCl | 5 | 10 | 9 | 39.7 | 0.1 | F |
| 1b | NaCl | 5 | 10 | .. | 39.35 | —0.25 | G |
| 1c | NaCl | 5 | 25 | .. | 39.6 | 0.00 | G |
| 2a | NaCl | 5 | 10 | 5 | 39.65 | 0.35 | F |
| 2b | NaCl | 5 | 25 | .. | 39.5 | 0.20 | G |
| 3a | NaCl | 5 | 10 | .. | 38.9 | —0.1 | G |
| 3b | NaCl | 5 | 10 | 6 | 39.4 | 0.4 | G |
| 4 | NaCl | 5 | 10 | 9 | 39.75 | 0.4 | G |
| | | | | | | Av. 0.18 | |
| 1 | NaCl | 2.5 | 10 | 5 | 39.35 | 0.25 | F |
| 2 | NaCl | 2.5 | 50 | .. | 39.4 | —0.2 | F |
| | | | | | | Av. 0.12 | |
| 1a | NaCl | 1 | 50 | .. | 39.45 | —0.55 | F |
| 1b | NaCl | 11 | 50 | .. | 39.5 | —0.5 | G |
| 1c | NaCl | 11 | 50 | .. | 39.6 | —0.4 | G |
| | | | | | | Average | |
| 1 | NaBr | 5 | 10 | 12 | 39.1 | 0.1 | F |
| 2 | NaBr | 5 | 10 | 6 | 39.6 | 0.40 | F |
| 3 | NaBr | 5 | 10 | 6 | 39.3 | —0.1 | G |
| 4a | NaBr | 5 | 10 | 6 | 39.55 | 0.65 | G |
| 5a | NaBr | 5 | 10 | 5 | 39.75 | 0.6 | G |
| 5b | NaBr | 5 | 10 | 9 | 39.85 | 0.65 | G |
| 4b | NaBr | 5 | 10 | 6 | 39.35 | 0.45 | G |
| | | | | | | Av. 0.33 | |
| 1a | NaI | 5 | 10 | 6 | 40.1 | 0.7 | F |
| 1b | NaI | 5 | 10 | 3 | 39.2 | —0.2 | G |
| 2 | NaI | 5 | 10 | 6½ | 40.0 | 1.1 | F |
| 3 | NaI | 5 | 10 | 5 | 39.75 | 0.4 | G |
| 4a | NaI | 5 | 10 | 3½ | 39.55 | —0.1 | F |
| 5a | NaI | 5 | 10 | 7 | 40.2 | 0.5 | F |
| 6 | NaI | 5 | 10 | 7 | 39.85 | 0.05 | G |
| 7 | NaI | 5 | 10 | 6 | 39.2 | 0.2 | G |
| 4b | NaI | 5 | 10 | 9 | 39.4 | —0.25 | G |
| 5b | NaI | 5 | 10 | 6 | 39.25 | —0.4 | G |
| | | | | | | Av. 0.32 | |

* F, unused animal; G, used animal.

In thirty experiments there was just one febrile reaction of 1° or more, and there were five reactions of 0.5° or more; of these six reactions three were produced by sodium bromid and three by sodium iodid—in spite of the fact that almost one-half of the experiments were performed with sodium chlorid without a reaction of even 0.5°. With only 20 per cent. of the experiments showing anything like a definite reaction it does not seem justifiable to hold the salt alone responsible for the reaction, but rather secondary causes which are variable.

Having determined that the sodium salts injected subcutaneously produced fever only exceptionally, the intravenous method of injection was tried.

In order to see what water alone would do, five animals were injected with amounts of distilled water varying from 3 to 10 c.c. The resulting febrile reaction varied from 0.5° to 1.3° and occurred from one and one-half to two hours after injection. The average rise was 0.85°, the greatest average rise of any of the experiments. The action here must be due to the destruction of the blood-cells and the setting free of pyrogenic substances.

If, instead of water, a 1 per cent. solution of sodium chlorid was used, the reactions were very much less, averaging only 0.3°. One animal

TABLE 2.—INTRAVENOUS INJECTIONS

| Number of experiments. | Salt used. | Concentration in per cent. | Quantity used in c.c. | Time to fastigium. | Highest temperature. | Rise above control. | Animal.* |
|---|---|---|---|---|---|---|---|
| 1 | Aq. distill ........... | .. | 10 | 1½ | .... | 0.5 | G |
| 2 | Aq. distill ........... | .. | 10 | 1 | .... | 1.35 | F |
| 3 | Aq. distill ........... | .. | 5 | 2 | .... | 0.5 | F |
| 4a | Aq. distill ........... | .. | 3 | 2 | .... | 0.6 | F |
| 4b | Aq. distill ........... | .. | 6 | 2 | .... | 1.3 | G |
| | | | | | | Av. 0.85 | |
| 1a | Locke's sol. .......... | .. | 10 | .. | 39.1 | —0.25 | F |
| b | Locke's sol. .......... | .. | 19 | 2 | 39.6 | 0.25 | G |
| c | Locke's sol. .......... | .. | 10 | 1 | 39.4 | 0.05 | G |
| d | Locke's sol. .......... | .. | 20 | .. | 39.1 | —0.25 | G |
| 2a | Locke's sol. .......... | .. | 10 | .. | 39.15 | —0.2 | F |
| b | Locke's sol. .......... | .. | 10 | .. | 39.2 | —0.15 | G |
| c | Locke's sol. .......... | .. | 10 | .. | 39.35 | 0.0 | G |
| d | Locke's sol. .......... | .. | 10 | .. | 39.25 | —0.1 | G |
| 3 | Locke's sol. .......... | .. | 10 | 2 | 39.95 | 0.65 | G |
| | | | | | | Av. 0.04 | |
| 1a | NaCl .............. | 1 | 19 | 2 | 40.7 | 1.1 | G |
| b | NaCl .............. | 1 | 10 | 2 | 40.7 | 1.1 | G |
| c | NaCl .............. | 1 | 10 | 2 | 40.3 | 0.7 | G |
| d | NaCl .............. | 1 | 10 | 2 | 40.6 | 1.0 | G |
| e | NaCl .............. | 1 | 10 | 2 | 40.35 | 0.75 | G |
| 2 | NaCl .............. | 1 | 55 | .. | 39.25 | —0.1 | G |
| 3 | NaCl .............. | 1 | 10 | 2 | 39.35 | 0.00 | G |
| 4a | NaCl .............. | 1 | 10 | 2 | 39.7 | 0.35 | G |
| b | NaCl .............. | 1 | 20 | 2 | 39.75 | 0.4 | G |
| 5 | NaCl .............. | 1 | 10 | 2 | 39.4 | 0.25 | G |
| 6 | NaCl .............. | 1 | 10 | .. | 39.15 | —0.5 | G |
| 7 | NaCl .............. | 1 | 10 | 2 | 39.5 | —0.2 | G |
| 8 | NaCl .............. | 1 | 10 | 1 | 40.05 | 0.75 | G |
| | | | | | | Av. 0.3 | |

* F, unused animal; G, used animal.

TABLE 3.—INTRAPERITONEAL INJECTIONS

| Number of experiments. | Salt used. | Concentration in per cent. | Quantity used in c.c. | Time to fastigium. | Highest temperature. | Rise above control. | Animal.* |
|---|---|---|---|---|---|---|---|
| 1 | NaCl .............. | 1 | 30 | 3 | 40.25 | 0.65 | G |
| 2 | NaCl .............. | 1 | 40 | 9 | 39.95 | 0.6 | G |
| 3 | NaCl .............. | 1 | 50 | 7 | 39.75 | 0.4 | G |
| 4a | NaCl .............. | 1 | 30 | 6 | 46.55 | 1.05 | F |
| 4b | NaCl .............. | 1 | 30 | 9 | 40.05 | 0.55 | G |
| 4c | NaCl .............. | 1 | 30 | 8 | 40.1 | 0.6 | G |
| 5 | NaCl .............. | 1 | 25 | 6 | 40.2 | 1.0 | F |
| 6 | NaCl .............. | 1 | 10 | .. | 39.1 | —0.25 | G |
| 7 | NaCl .............. | 1 | 10 | .. | 39.2 | —0.00 | G |
| 8 | NaCl .............. | 1 | 20 | .. | 39.0 | —0.65 | G |
| 9 | NaCl .............. | 1 | 20 | .. | 39.2 | —0.5 | G |
| | | | | | | Av. 0.36 | |

* F, unused animal; G, used animal.

which showed practically no reaction to subcutaneous injection, reacted very markedly to intravenous and oral administration. The temperature reached its highest point two hours after the injection. The five reactions of the animal mentioned above varied from 0.7° to 1.1°; those of the other animals from minus 0.5° to 0.75°. In most of the experiments, 10 c.c. were injected, in one 20 c.c. and one 5 c.c., without any apparent difference in the resulting reaction. For instance, one animal after an injection of 19 c.c. of a 1 per cent. solution showed a rise of 1.1°; on the day following, with 10 c.c. the reaction was just the same. In this series of thirteen experiments all of the animals had been injected before.

TABLE 4.—ORAL ADMINISTRATION

| Number of experiments. | Salt used. | Concentration in per cent. | Quantity used in c.c. | Time to fastigium. | Highest temperature. | Rise above control. | Animal.* |
|---|---|---|---|---|---|---|---|
| 1 | NaCl ............... | 1 | 100 | .. | 38.55 | —0.6 | F |
| 2a | NaCl ............... | 1 | 30 | 3 | 40.1 | 0.6 | G |
| b | NaCl ............... | 1 | 30 | 3 | 39.9 | 0.3 | G |
| c | NaCl ............... | 1 | 40 | 6 | 40.5 | 0.9 | G |
| 3 | NaCl ............... | 1 | 50 | 12 | 39.5 | 0.15 | G |
| 4 | NaCl ............... | 1 | 50 | 12 | 39.5 | —0.2 | G |
| 5 | NaCl ............... | 1 | 40 | 9 | 39.5 | 0.3 | G |
| 2d | NaCl ............... | 1 | 50 | .. | 39.3 | —0.3 | G |
| e | NaCl ............... | 1 | 30 | 9 | 39.95 | 0.2 | G |
| 1 | NaCl ............... | 2.5 | 50 | .. | 39.4 | 0.05 | G |
| 2 | NaCl ............... | 2.5 | 50 | 12 | 39.2 | 0.00 | G |
| 1 | NaCl ............... | 3 | 30 | 8 | 39.6 | 0.25 | G |
| 6 | NaCl ............... | 1 | 50 | 6 | 39.15 | 0.15 | G |
| 7 | NaCl ............... | 1 | 50 | 8 | 39.6 | 0.05 | G |
| 8 | NaCl ............... | 1 | 50 | .. | 39.25 | —0.35 | G |
| 9 | NaCl ............... | 1 | 50 | .. | 38.4 | —0.5 | G |
| 10 | NaCl ............... | 1 | 50 | 5 | 39.5 | 0.35 | G |
| 11 | NaCl ............... | 1 | 50 | 8 | 39.4 | —0.2 | G |
| 12 | NaCl ............... | 1 | 50 | 5 | 39.1 | —0.0 | G |
| 13 | NaCl ............... | 1 | 50 | 5 | 39.05 | —0.5 | G |
| 14 | NaCl ............... | 6 | 50 | .. | 39.15 | 0.2 | G |
| 15 | NaCl ............... | 6 | 50 | .. | 39 | —0.5 | G |
| | | | | | | Av. 0.19 | |
| 1 | $NaHCO_3$ ............ | 2.5 | 40 | .. | 39.45 | —0.15 | G |
| 1 | NaBr ............... | 2.5 | 40 | 9 | 40.25 | 0.65 | G |
| | After Butyric Acid Feedings | | | | | | |
| 1 | NaCl ............... | 1 | 25 | 6 | 39.2 | 0.1 | G |
| 2 | NaCl ............... | 2 | 30 | 7½ | 39.65 | 0.5 | G |
| 3 | NaCl ............... | 2 | 50 | 6 | 38. | 0.05 | G |
| 4 | NaCl ............... | 2 | 30 | 7 | 39.0 | 0.45 | G |
| 5 | NaCl ............... | 2 | 10 | .. | 38.6 | —0.7 | F |
| 6 | NaCl ............... | 2 | 10 | .. | 38.15 | —0.1 | F |
| 7 | NaCl ............... | 2 | | | | | |
| | and sugar ......... | 5 | 10 | 6 | 39.35 | 0 | F |
| 8 | NaCl and sugar....... | .. | 10 | .. | 39 | —0.3 | G |
| 9 | NaCl and sugar....... | .. | 10 | .. | 38.5 | —0.2 | G |
| 10 | NaCl and sugar....... | .. | 10 | 6 | 38.95 | 0.2 | G |
| | | | | | | Av. 0.12 | |

* F, unused animal; G, used animal.

For comparison with this series, nine experiments were made, using Locke's solution instead of 1 per cent. sodium chlorid. Of the nine, only two gave a positive reaction, one 0.65° and the other 0.25°. The general average for the reactions was 0.04°, which is practically nil.

Three experiments in which 5 per cent. sodium chlorid was injected intravenously resulted in reactions of 0.55°, 0.4° and 0.4°, when the amounts injected were 25 c.c., 10 c.c. and 18 c.c., respectively. The action here seems to be related to the difference in concentration between the injected solution and the blood rather than to any direct action of the salt. Three experiments with 5 per cent. sodium chlorid averaged 0.45°—only half as great as the reactions produced by the distilled water, so that there is no reason to suppose that the action of the salt in hypertonic solution is any other than that of the hypotonic distilled water, that of being a solution which, introduced into the blood, there produces products of destruction which have pyrogenetic powers.

Intraperitoneal injections were next tried in a series of eleven experiments, using 1 per cent sodium chlorid. Of these, two were on used animals which, injected with 25 and 30 c.c., reacted by rises in temperature of 1.05° and 1.0°; of the seven remaining animals which had been used before, five reacted with an average of 0.54°, the other four failed to reach the normal of the day before. One animal that died in the course of the experiment showed on section considerable clear fluid in the peritoneal cavity, which coagulated soon after removal, showing that the injection caused considerable exudation. The average reaction was 0.36°.

In full knowledge that injecting salt solution by mouth into an adult rabbit is not comparable to the giving of salt solution to sick infants, a series of experiments was nevertheless tried to see if the temperature could be influenced. Seventeen experiments were made with 1 per cent., two with 2.5 per cent., one with 3 per cent. and two with 6 per cent. solutions of sodium chlorid.

Of the seventeen experiments with the 1 per cent. solution, nine reactions were positive, varying from 0.2° to 0.9°. Of these, three were in one animal with reactions of 0.3°, 0.6° and 0.9° after the injection of 30, 30 and 40 c.c. The experiments on this animal are perhaps the most interesting of all, because of the very definite reactions to salt solutions given by mouth, corresponding, as they do, very closely to the reactions in infants. The animal received three injections subcutaneously, five injections intravenously and one injection intraperitoneally before the solutions were given by mouth. The first two oral administrations were given on succeeding days and the results were very nearly alike. In order to make sure that the animal was not running a daily fever temperature, the temperature was taken during the next two days and the highest control temperature was 39.6°; exactly the same as the highest control temperature taken at the beginning of the experiments. Forty c.c. of a 1 per cent. solution of sodium chlorid given the following day caused a rise of 0.9°. The day following was again controlled and no temperature over 39.6° was obtained, making it almost positive that the reaction was due in some way to the salt solution. The very marked difference between the sodium halogen salts and the other sodium salts in their ability to produce fever, as was first shown by Meyer and since verified by Schloss, made it seem of value to see whether it would hold in this case. Forty c.c. of a 2.5 per cent. solution of sodium bicarbonate were given by mouth without producing the slightest reaction. The day following, 40 c.c. of a 2.5 per cent. solution of sodium bromid produced a reaction of 0.65°. The animal unfortunately died the day following, so that the experiments could not be repeated. Autopsy revealed nothing to account for the death of the animal. The intestines were unfortunately so damaged by post-mortem decomposition that histological studies could not be made. The chart shows at a glance the very definite character of the reactions. In stronger concentration sodium chlorid gave very slight reactions or negative ones. Giving 50 c.c. of a 2.5 per cent. solution the reactions were 0 and 0.25°; giving 3 per cent. in similar amounts, 0.25°, and giving 6 per cent., minus 0.2° and minus 0.5°.

Great emphasis is laid on the fact that in order to obtain positive reactions in infants, it is necessary that the gastro-intestinal lining be in the condition accompanying dyspepsia. In order to produce an irritable condition of the bowel, increasing amounts of butyric acid were given to the rabbits by mouth several days before the salt was given. Bokai[9] was the first to show that the group of fatty acids had a very marked effect on the intestinal linings, producing diarrheas, hyperemia, hemorrhages and ulcerations. Czerny and Keller[10] lay great emphasis on these experiments and consider the acute symptoms in the conditions which they term toxicose, Finkelstein's intoxication, cholera infantum, etc., as due in large part to the fatty acids produced. Myerhoefer and Pribram[11] showed that the rate of absorption through the intestinal wall was markedly increased during acute digestive disturbances. By means of repeated doses of butyric acid, an attempt was made to produce a condition of the intestinal canal most favorable for rapid absorption. Ten experiments on young rabbits which had been treated with butyric acid gave some positive and some negative results. Twenty-five c.c. of a 1 per cent. solution of sodium chlorid gave a reaction of 0.1°; 2 per cent. sodium chlorid in doses from 10 to 50 c.c. gave three reactions of 0.05°, 0.5° and 0.45° and two negative reactions. Adding to the 2 per cent. sodium chlorid 5 per cent. of glucose gave only one positive reaction of 0.2° out of four experiments.

---

9. Bokai: Experimentelle Beiträge zur Kenntnis der Darmbewegungen, Arch. f. exper. Path. u. Pharmakol., 1888, xxiv, 153.

10. Czerny, A., and Keller, A.: Des Kindes Ernährung, etc., ed. 1, Leipsic, F. Deuticke, ii, 155.

11. Meyerhoefer, E., and Pribram, E.: Das Verhalten der Darmwand als osmotische Membran bei akuter und chronischer Enteritis. Wien. klin. Wchnschr., 1909, xxii, 875.

Let us return now and compare the results of these experiments with those of others working along the same line. The difference in the subcutaneous experiments is so marked that they will be considered first. Inasmuch as Krehl does not give the entire set of temperatures and controls, but merely the actual rise in temperature, it is impossible to say whether his control is the highest temperature of the previous twenty-four hours or merely the temperature taken just before the administration of the salt. The pyrogenic action of the above-mentioned salts, when given subcutaneously in the concentration of a 5 per cent. solution is very slight, and in the great majority of instances does not influence the temperature of the animal to any definite extent. Four-tenths of a gram of sodium chlorid given subcutaneously produces an average rise of 1.3°, according to Krehl; the greatest rise above the normal that was recorded in a series of eight experiments was 0.4°, and the average reaction was 0.18°, a little more than a tenth of the Krehl average. For sodium bromid, he observed an average reaction of 1.2°. The average reaction for my experiments was only 0.33°, with no reaction more than one-half that of his average reaction. For sodium iodid, his reaction average is 0.9°. In my series of ten experiments there was a single reaction of 1.1°, exceeding his average. The average of the ten, however, was only 0.32°.

Out of the series of thirty experiments there is only a single reaction which is to be compared to the reactions obtained by Krehl. It seems very probable, therefore, that some secondary factor is necessary to produce fever and that the salts *per se* in this concentration very rarely produce a definite febrile rise in temperature.

The intravenous injections varied according to the tendency of the injected solution to produce destruction of the formed elements of the blood. Distilled water had the most marked effect, a 5 per cent solution of sodium chlorid less than one-half as much and Locke's solution practically no effect. Van den Velden[12] was unable to produce a rise in temperature by injecting intravenously from 3 to 5 c.c. of from 5 to 10 per cent. solution of sodium chlorid in adults.

As was to be expected, the giving of salt solutions by mouth produced fever only exceptionally; the exception, however, proved to be perhaps the most interesting experiment. The animal on three occasions reacted with fever of from 0.6° to 0.9°, the temperature being controlled the day before and the day after. As to why this animal should have reacted and the others not have reacted in like manner, as to whether it was the salt *per se* or toxic products swept into the circulation with the salt, it is impossible to say.

---

12. Van den Velden, R.: Zur Wirkung intravenöser Zufuhr hypertonischer Kochsalzlösungen, Verhandl. d. Cong. f. inn. Med., Wiesbaden, 1909, xxvi, 155.

## SUMMARY

1. Five per cent. solutions of sodium chlorid, bromid and iodid, when injected into rabbits subcutaneously, produced no rise in temperature in the great majority of experiments.

2. Sodium chlorid produces a slight rise in temperature when given in high concentration intravenously and practically no rise when modified according to Locke.

3. One per cent. sodium chlorid may in exceptional instances produce a febrile rise in temperature when given by mouth.

1449 Dearborn Avenue.

# THE RETENTION OF ALKALI BY THE KIDNEY WITH SPECIAL REFERENCE TO ACIDOSIS *

HERMAN M. ADLER, M.D., AND GERALD BLAKE, M.D.
HATHORNE, MASS. BOSTON

For some time now the conception of an acid intoxication has been familiar to every student and practitioner of medicine. Since the first work of Naunyn on this subject in which many of the pathological phenomena of diabetes were explained by the demonstration of an acid intoxication to which the name "acidosis" was given, a great many facts have been collected and which support in all essentials the original investigations of Naunyn and his pupils. And it has become more and more evident that disturbances, both quantitative and qualitative, in the ability of the body to deal with varying amounts of acid, are not only important but by no means infrequent occurrences. Contrary to the assumption of the early investigators, whose views are to some extent maintained by many at the present time, it may be stated as a demonstrated fact that the reaction of the blood, and probably of the tissues, varies under all conditions during life within such very narrow limits that it may be called constant and neutral. Instead, therefore, of speaking of the "alkalinity" of the blood it will be more accurate to speak of the "neutrality" of the blood. The reasons for this interpretation are of such a nature that we can merely refer to them here, but those interested may find explanation at length in the literature.[1] Since, therefore, the constancy of reaction of the blood seems to be a fundamental condition of life there must necessarily exist some provision by means of which the neutrality may be maintained in spite of the introduction, either pathologically or experimentally, of acid or alkaline substances. Such a mechanism has been demonstrated in recent years by the investigations of Friedenthal, Henderson, and others. Briefly, this consists of a more or less complicated equilibrium between acid substances on one hand, and bases, chiefly bicarbonates and alkaline phosphates, on the other hand. When acid and base are present in suitable proportions the reaction will be neutral no matter what the actual quantities of the various substances may be. From this it will be apparent that it is quite possible to have a variation in titratable acidity or alkalinity without any variation in reaction. This explains the reason for the discrepancy between the results obtained by titrating sam-

---

* From the Laboratory of the Department of Theory and Practice of Physic, Harvard Medical School.

1. Henderson, L. J.: Ergebn. d. Physiol., 1909, viii, 254-325, Bibliography.

ples of blood or of serum and those obtained by determining the reaction of the blood by means of the concentration cell or by indicators. We assume then that in order to maintain the neutrality of the blood, the organism will meet the introduction of an acid by an increase of base, and that the only important change that we need at present to consider will be a slight increase in concentration. This increase is met by the kidney by an increased excretion. The function of the bases of the blood, therefore, is in the main twofold: in the first place to transport acid, and in the second place to help to maintain the proper concentration. The most important acid which the bases of the blood are called on to transport is carbonic acid. If for any reason more acid is introduced into the circulation than the bases present and in reserve in the tissues are able to neutralize, acid intoxication will result. The stronger, chemically speaking, an acid is, the more readily will it combine with base. Carbonic acid is a weak acid, and will, therefore, be readily replaced by a number of stronger acids which may occur in large quantities under pathologic or experimental conditions. In cases of extreme acidosis in which all available alkali is required to counteract the effect of the pathological increase in acid substances, such as beta-oxybutyric and diacetic acid, the organism is unable to transport a sufficient quantity of carbonic acid from the tissues to the lungs, and a condition will result in the patient which may vary from lethargy to coma and finally end in death. There is one mechanism of which the organism avails itself in extreme cases to combat the effect of an increase of acid; and this mechanism serves at the same time to liberate a certain amount of bases to carry on the carbonic acid transport. In acidosis the organism no longer combines all its ammonia to form urea, but uses the ammonia directly to neutralize the acid substances. The ammonia thus combined is excreted in the urine and the estimation of the amount thus excreted has been the only available means of determining the degree of acid intoxication. While this method has proved of great help, it gives us an index of only one part of the conditions existing within the organism, and leaves us entirely without information in regard to the very important question of the reserve of alkali within the body. While the individual differences in alkali content of the blood and tissues in living beings is at present quite beyond our methods of investigation, it appears that a considerable amount of useful information might be obtained if we could measure, in our acidosis patients, not only the amount of ammonia that is excreted but also the amount of alkali that is retained.

The following investigation was undertaken in order to determine, first, whether any variations occurred in acidosis between the amount of ammonia and the amount of base excreted; second, whether such variations, if they occurred, would give us information in regard to the acid neutralizing power of the organism; third, whether the method employed

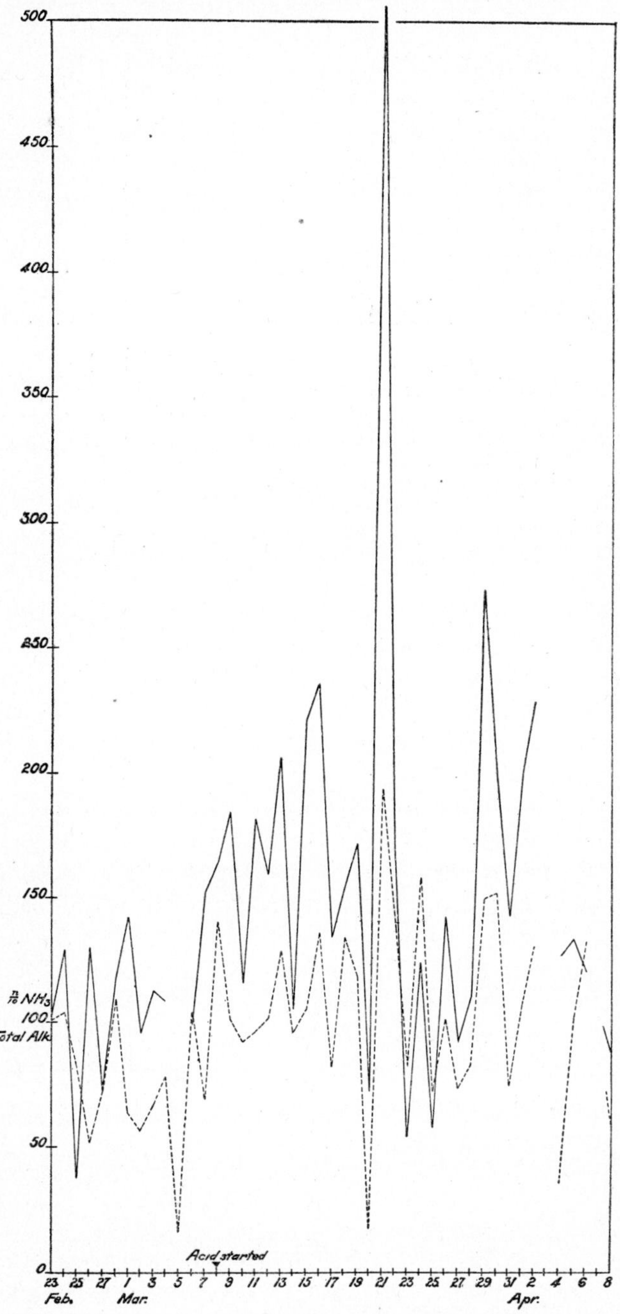


Chart 1.—Diagram of ammonia excretion and alkali retention, Experiment 1, Table 1.

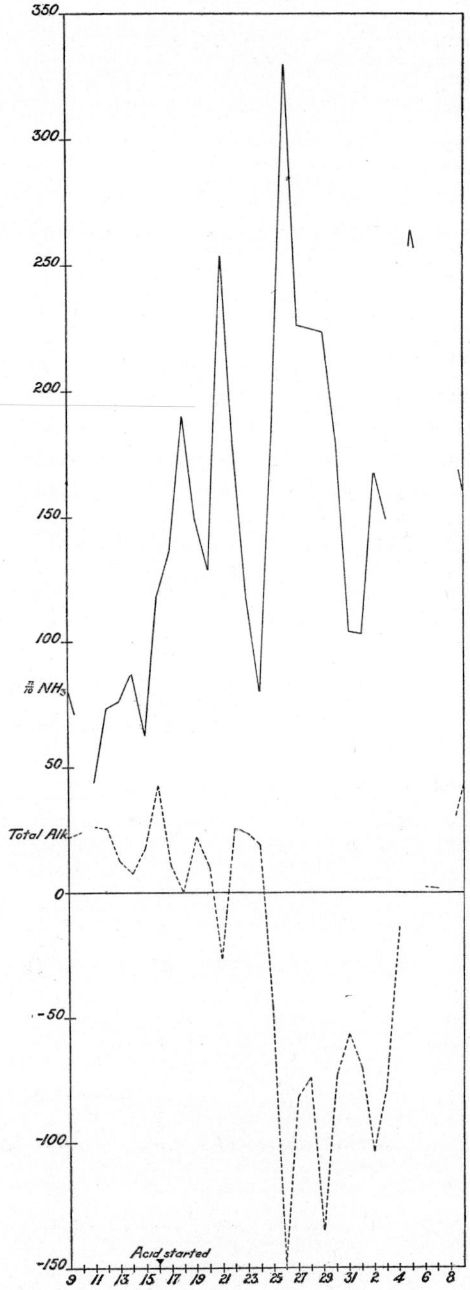


Chart 2.—Diagram of ammonia excretion and alkali retention, Experiment 2, Table 2.

was of sufficient accuracy and simplicity to make it of use in the clinical laboratory.

## I. METHOD

The method employed in this investigation is the one reported by Henderson and Adler.[2] It consists in comparing the properly prepared urine with a standard solution so made up as to correspond in concentration and reaction to blood. The method depends on the facts that neutral red changes color at the exact point of reaction of the blood;[3] and furthermore, that this change, while a fairly rapid one, shows intermediate shades of color between the full red of acid and the lemon-yellow of alkali. At the reaction of the blood the neutral red in solution is a reddish yellow; at the ordinary reaction of urine it approaches a light burgundy. If then a solution corresponding to blood in reaction be used as the standard, with neutral red as an indicator, a second specimen of urine made up under similar conditions as regards dilution and the quantity of neutral red used, may be titrated with a one-tenth normal sodium hydrate until the color of the urine specimen corresponds exactly to that of the standard solution. Obviously in titrating back to the reaction of the blood it is necessary to add to the acids of the urine precisely the amount of alkali which, formerly combined with them in the blood, has been retained by the kidney in the preparation of the urine. In addition to this retention of alkali another portion of base has been saved to the body by the substitution of ammonia for fixed alkali. Clearly, these two quantities are additive. Together they measure the effective work of the kidney in saving basic substances for the further neutralization of acid and transport of carbonic acid.

The solutions required are as follows:

1. A stock solution containing 36.2 gm. anhydrous di-sodium phosphate and 5.4 gm. anhydrous mono-sodium phosphate per liter. This solution when diluted in the ratio 1 to 80 gives the reaction of normal blood and is used for comparison of colors with the indicator.
2. A 25 per cent. aqueous solution of neutral red.
3. A solution of potassium oxalate approximately normal.

The procedure is as follows:

Three c.c. of the phosphate solution are placed in a 300 c.c. flask.

One c.c. of the neutral red solution is added and water to 240 c.c. This is the standard.

Ten c.c. of urine are treated with 1 c.c. of the oxalate solution and allowed to stand ten minutes. The urine is then filtered into a 300 c.c. flask, the precipitate washed, 1 c.c. neutral red solution added and the whole made up to about 240 c.c. One-tenth normal hydrate sodium solution is then run into the urine from a burette until the color matches that of the standard. The number of cubic centimeters of alkali thus used are calculated to the total volume of urine and the figure thus obtained represents the alkali retention.[4]

---

2. Henderson, L. J., and Adler, H. M.: Jour. Biol. Chem., 1909, vi, p. xxii.
3. Salm, E.: Ztschr. f. physik. Chem., 1906, lvii, 471.
4. Folin, O.: Am. Jour. Physiol., 1903, ix, 265.

EXPERIMENTS

Three sets of experiments were performed. In the first the animals were kept on a constant diet of dog biscuit and water and were given varying quantities of a 0.8 per cent. hydrogen chlorid solution by the

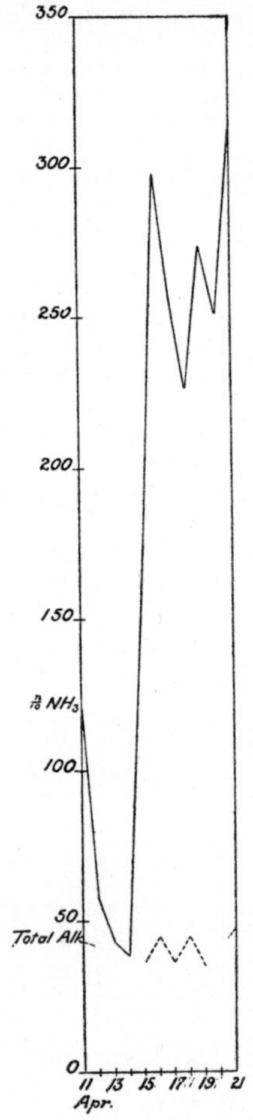


Chart 3.

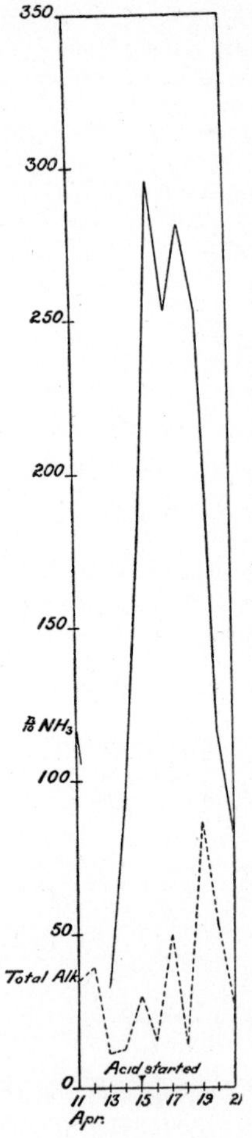


Chart 4.

Chart 3.—Diagram of ammonia excretion and alkali retention, Experiment 3, Table 3.

Chart 4.—Diagram of ammonia excretion and alkali retention, Experiment 4, Table 4.

stomach-tube. In the second series a constant diet of flour was substituted for the dog biscuit in order to reduce the amount of nitrogen and salts and thus the available alkali. In the third series the animals were given no food or acid and only a measured amount of water. In all the experiments the urine was examined daily and the total quantity, the ammonia content, and the titratable bases were determined. The urine was furthermore examined for albumin or sugar, acetone and blood. At no time did we find either albumin or sugar, and, as was to have been expected in dogs, at no time did acetone appear in the urine even in the severest, fatal, case. The ammonia determinations were made according to the method of Folin.[5]

EXPERIMENT 1 (Table 1).—Feb. 23, 1909. Large male mongrel dog. Constant diet of 250 gm. dog biscuit and 600 c.c. of water mixed together and made into thick paste. In addition the dog received water of which he took varying amounts as indicated in the table. The acid feeding was begun March 8 and continued until the 23d. From March 18 he was given two feedings of acid a day. On March 19 diarrhea set in and persisted until the end of the experiment.

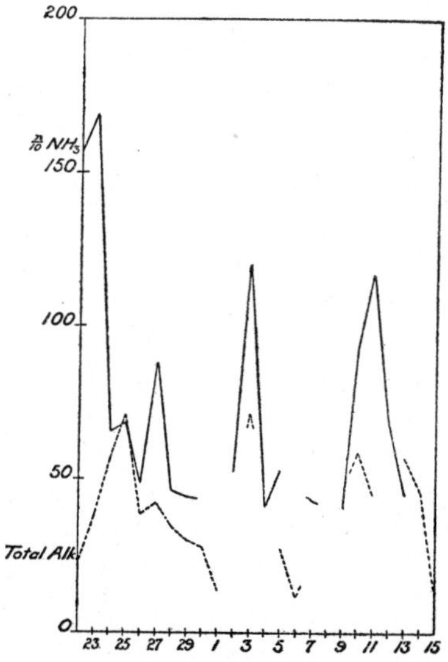


Chart 5.—Diagram of ammonia excretion and alkali retention, Experiment 5, Table 5.

On March 26 the dog vomited shortly after the acid feeding and continued this until the end of the experiment. Vomitus consisted at first from 10 to 20 c.c. of mucus mixed with the acid solution. Later small amounts of food appeared in the vomitus.

EXPERIMENT 2 (Table 2).—March 8, 1909. Small fox terrier bitch. Same amount of food given and under the same conditions as in Experiment 1. The acid feeding was begun on March 15 and continued daily until April 9. The animal appeared well and was very lively during the entire experiment. On March 21 diarrhea set in and continued until the end of experiment, but this did not seem to interfere with the general health. About March 20 it was noted that she was in heat and the table and the curve show that the amount of alkali excreted rose to enormous proportions. Although this entirely vitiated the

5. Folin, Otto: Ztschr. f. physiol. Chem., 1902, xxxvii, 161.

experiment the results seem to us of sufficient interest to warrant continuing the experiment and to record the results. The dog showed a gain of one-quarter of a pound during the experiment.

Experiment 3 (Table 3).—April 9, 1909. Same dog as in Experiment 1. Dog was kept on a constant diet of 250 gm. of wheat flour, which was made up into a dough with water and without other additions baked into a dry biscuit. This was fed to the dog daily, together with 600 c.c. of water, of which the dog took varying amounts as shown in the table. A double feeding of 0.8 per cent. hydrogen chlorid was given daily throughout the experiment. The dog had soft movements from the beginning and vomited about 10 to 20 c.c. of mucus once or twice a day, usually shortly after the acid feeding. Practically no acid, however, was lost in this way. The dog kept constant weight throughout the experiment.

Experiment 4 (Table 4).—April 9, 1909. Male bull terrier pup, about four months old. The condition of the experiment was as in Experiment 3. The acid feeding began on April 14 and continued once a day until the 20th. The dog was lively throughout the experiment and did not vomit. He had soft move-

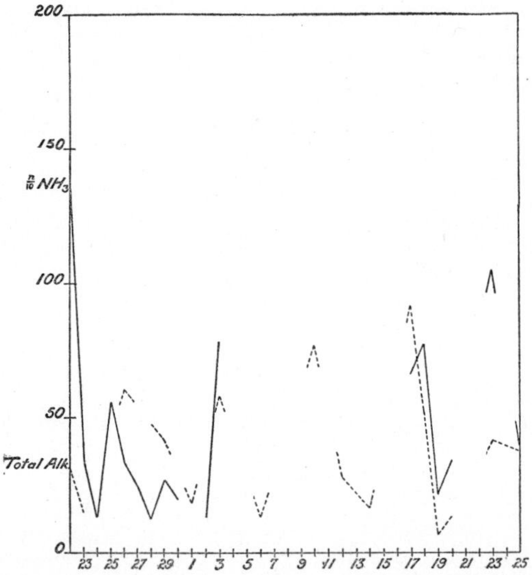


Chart 6.—Diagram of ammonia excretion and alkali retention, Experiment 6, Table 6.

ments during the period of acid feeding. The weight throughout the experiment remained the same.

Experiment 5 (Table 5).—April 22, 1909. The same dog as used in Experiments 1 and 3. Neither food nor acid was used during this experiment, but the starvation depended on to aggravate the acidosis induced by immediately preceding acid feeding. The stools throughout the experiment were normal. There was no vomiting. There was a rapid loss of weight throughout the experiment from 19½ pounds at the beginning to 12 pounds at the end. On May 13 the animal appeared languid and indifferent. On the 15th he died in coma. The urine early became scanty in amount in spite of the fairly large quantities of water that the dog consumed. This necessitated the omission of either the ammonia or the alkali determinations on certain days.

Experiment 6 (Table 6).—April 22, 1909. The same dog as in Experiment 4. Same conditions as in Experiment 5. Dog weighed at the beginning of the experiment 13¼ pounds and weighed 8¼ at the end of the experiment on May

25. The movements were normal throughout the experiment. The same difficulty as in Experiment 5 was met in obtaining an adequate quantity of urine. The animal was weak and torpid at the end of the experiment, but rapidly recovered on being fed.

## DISCUSSION

From the comparison of the curves, omitting the second, it is apparent that the results of this method of determining the alkali retention not only vary with the conditions in the organism as indicated in the ammonia output, but are sufficiently regular and sufficiently large to be of value by themselves in estimating the capacity of the organism for withstanding acid. When the results obtained thus are added to the ammonia determinations we get a very much more accurate idea, not only of how much acid the organism has to combat, but also how far the alkali reserve has been involved in the struggle. The clinical material that we have been

TABLE 1.—EXPERIMENT 1, ACIDOSIS IN DOG WITH DIET OF DOG BISCUIT, WATER AND 0.8 PER CENT HYDROGEN CHLORID

| Date | Water c.c. | Acid c.c. | Urine c.c. | Total $NH_3$ c.c. | $n/10NH_3$ c.c. | Total Alk. c.c. | $n/10NH_3$ + Total Alk. c.c. |
|---|---|---|---|---|---|---|---|
| 2/23 | 565 | 0 | 140 | .1827 | 103.1 | 100.8 | 203.9 |
| 2/24 | 565 | 0 | 160 | .2197 | 129.2 | 104.0 | 233.2 |
| 2/25 | 625 | 0 | 80 | .0636 | 38.0 | 83.2 | 121.2 |
| 2/26 | 605 | 0 | 70 | .221 | 130.0 | 51.6 | 181.6 |
| 2/27 | 555 | 0 | 120 | .123 | 72.3 | 72.8 | 145.1 |
| 2/28 | 550 | 0 | 140 | .199 | 117.5 | 109.2 | 226.7 |
| 3/1 | 750 | 0 | 100 | .243 | 142.9 | 64.0 | 206.9 |
| 3/2 | 545 | 0 | 130 | .167 | 95.2 | 56.5 | 151.7 |
| 3/3 | 500 | 0 | 95 | .193 | 112.9 | 66.5 | 179.4 |
| 3/4 | 615 | 0 | 105 | .184 | 108.2 | 78.7 | 186.95 |
| 3/5 | 610 | 0 | 15 | ..... | ..... | 15.7 | short day |
| 3/6 | 525 | 0 | 120 | .1688 | 99.2 | 104.4 | 203.6 |
| 3/7 | 0 | 0 | 125 | .259 | 152.3 | 69.7 | 222.05 |
| 3/8 | 100 | 72 | 180 | .279 | 164.1 | 140.4 | 304.5 |
| 3/9 | 750 | 72 | 130 | .313 | 184.1 | 101.4 | 285.5 |
| 3/10 | 575 | 70 | 105 | .196 | 115.2 | 92.4 | 207.6 |
| 3/11 | 500 | 70 | 115 | .309 | 181.7 | 96.6 | 278.3 |
| 3/12 | 580 | 72 | 90 | .271 | 159.4 | 101.7 | 261.1 |
| 3/13 | 475 | 70 | 140 | .351 | 206.4 | 129.0 | 335.4 |
| 3/14 | 550 | 70 | 85 | .179 | 105.2 | 96.0 | 201.2 |
| 3/15 | 995 | 72 | 110 | .377 | 221.7 | 105.6 | 327.3 |
| 3/16 | 645 | 74 | 160 | .401 | 235.8 | 136.0 | 271.8 |
| 3/17 | 705 | 72 | 65 | .228 | 134.1 | 82.2 | 216.35 |
| 3/18 | 800 | 153 | 140 | .263 | 154.1 | 134.4 | 288.5 |
| 3/19 | 630 | 155 | 110 | .291 | 171.7 | 118.8 | 290.5 |
| 3/20 | 505 | 147 | 50 | .123 | 72.3 | 17.5 | 89.8 |
| 3/21 | 175 | 153 | 215 | .860 | 505.8 | 193.5 | 699.3 |
| 3/22 | 945 | 155 | 115 | .277 | 162.9 | 138.0 | 439.9 |
| 3/23 | 665 | 156 | 70 | .092 | 54.1 | 83.3 | 137.4 |
| 3/24 | 575 | 100 | 140 | .211 | 124.8 | 158.2 | 283.0 |
| 3/25 | 525 | 149 | 75 | .0994 | 58.5 | 72.7 | 131.2 |
| 3/26 | 720 | 152 | 85 | .251 | 142.8 | 102.0 | 244.8 |
| 3/27 | 225 | 78 | 70 | .157 | 92.9 | 74.2 | 167.1 |
| 3/28 | 445 | 161 | 100 | .188 | 111.2 | 84.0 | 195.2 |
| 3/29 | 585 | 156 | 200 | .464 | 273.6 | 150.0 | 423.6 |
| 3/30 | 595 | 160 | 160 | .336 | 198.4 | 152.0 | 350.4 |
| 3/31 | 480 | 160 | 60 | .241 | 142.6 | 75.0 | 217.6 |
| 4/1 | 600 | 160 | 80 | .338 | 199.6 | 107.2 | 306.8 |
| 4/2 | 490 | 78 | 105 | .389 | 229.3 | 131.2 | 360.5 |
| 4/3 | 595 | 82 | 16 | .... | .... | .... | .... |
| 4/4 | 360 | 164 | 240 | .214* | 126.7 | 36.0* | 162.7 |
| 4/5 | 235 | 160 | 110 | .226* | 133.7 | 102.3* | 236.0 |
| 4/6 | 450 | 160 | 120 | .204* | 120.9 | 133.2* | 254.1 |
| 4/7 | 490 | 170 | 16 | .... | .... | .... | .... |
| 4/8 | 420 | 161 | 40 | .150 | 88.8 | 60.0 | 148.8 |

*Part lost.

TABLE 2.—EXPERIMENT 2, ACIDOSIS IN DOG UNDER SAME CONDITIONS AS EXPERIMENT 1

| Date | Water c.c. | Acid c.c. | Urine c.c. | Total $NH_3$ c.c. | n/10$NH_3$ c.c. | Total Alk. c.c. | n/10$NH_3$ + Total Alk. c.c. |
|---|---|---|---|---|---|---|---|
| 3/ 8- 9 | 545 | 40 | 0 | .136 | 80.0 | 22.0 | 102.0 |
| 3/ 9-10 | 350 | ... | 0 | .... | .... | .... | .... |
| 3/10-11 | 350 | 90 | 0 | .074 | 44.2 | 26.1 | 70.3 |
| 3/11-12 | 405 | 80 | 0 | .124 | 73.6 | 25.6 | 99.2 |
| 3/12-13 | 430 | 50 | 0 | .129 | 76.0 | 12.5 | 88.5 |
| 3/13-14 | 445 | 75 | 0 | .147 | 87.7 | 7.5 | 95.2 |
| 3/14-15 | 460 | 65 | 0 | .106 | 62.8 | 17.5 | 80.3 |
| 3/15-16 | 450 | 110 | 72 | .200 | 118. | . 42.9 | 160.9 |
| 3/16-17 | 420 | 80 | 75 | .221 | 136. | 10.4 | 146.4 |
| 3/17-18 | 460 | 150 | 76 | .323 | 190. | 0 | 190.0 |
| 3/18-19 | 385 | 110 | 75 | .253 | 149. | 22. | 171.0 |
| 3/19-20 | 420 | 100 | 75 | .219 | 129. | 10. | 139.0 |
| 3/20-21 | 200 | 110 | 78 | .425 | 254. | — 26.4 | 227.6 |
| 3/21-22 | 575 | 90 | 75 | .300 | 177. | 25.2 | 202.2 |
| 3/22-23 | 320 | 65 | 77 | .188 | 117. | 24.0 | 141.0 |
| 3/23-24 | 305 | 65 | 77 | .134 | 79.4 | 18.8 | 98.2 |
| 3/24-25 | 330 | 60 | 78 | .306 | 182.4 | — 45.0 | 137.4 |
| 3/25-26 | 290 | 120 | 77 | .561 | 330. | —148. | 182.0 |
| 3/26-27 | 220 | 75 | 74 | .384 | 226. | — 81.7 | 144.3 |
| 3/27-28 | 260 | 85 | 75 | .382 | 225. | — 73.9 | 151.1 |
| 3/28-29 | 290 | 75 | 69 | .379 | 223. | —135. | 88.0 |
| 3/29-30 | 200 | 55 | 74 | .307 | 181. | — 72.6 | 108.4 |
| 3/30-31 | 200 | 45 | 76 | .176 | 104. | — 56.2 | 47.8 |
| 3/31- 1 | 200 | 35 | 76 | .180 | 103. | — 70.0 | 33.0 |
| 4/ 1- 2 | 200 | 55 | 75 | .285 | 168. | —103.4 | 64.6 |
| 4/ 2- 3 | 200 | 50 | 77 | .253 | 149. | — 78.5 | 70.5 |
| 4/ 3- 4 | 200 | 40 | 77 | .... | .... | — 13.6 | .... |
| 4/ 4- 5 | 200 | 110 | 76 | .448 | 264. | .... | .... |
| 4/ 5- 6 | 200 | 20 | 77 | .... | .... | 2.0 | .... |
| 4/ 6- 7 | 200 | 10 | 80 | .... | .... | 1.7 | .... |
| 4/ 7- 8 | 200 | 65 | 57 | .... | .... | .... | .... |
| 4/ 8- 9 | 600 | 60 | 62 | .272 | 160. | 43.2 | 203.2 |

TABLE 3.—ACIDOSIS IN DOG WITH DIET OF DRY BISCUIT, WATER, AND 0.8 PER CENT. HYDROGEN CHLORID

| Date | Water c.c. | Acid c.c. | Urine c.c. | Total $NH_3$ c.c. | n/10$NH_3$ c.c. | Total Alk. c.c. | n/10$NH_3$ + Total Alk. c.c. |
|---|---|---|---|---|---|---|---|
| 4/ 9-10 | 120 | 161 | lost | .... | .... | .... | .... |
| 4/10-11 | 140 | 163 | 90 | .205 | 120.5 | 43.2 | 163.7 |
| 4/11-12 | 365 | 0 | 30 | .098 | 57.6 | .... | .... |
| 4/12-13 | 340 | 155 | 25 | .074 | 43.5 | .... | .... |
| 4/13-14 | 290 | 163 | 30 | .065 | 38.2 | .... | .... |
| 4/14-15 | 380 | 158 | 110 | .265 | 155.8 | 36.3 | 192.1 |
| 4/15-16 | 210 | 156 | 155 | .506 | 297.6 | 44.9 | 342.5 |
| 4/16-17 | 260 | 164 | 130 | .435 | 255.8 | 36.4 | 292.2 |
| 4/17-18 | 300 | 151 | 180 | .384 | 225.8 | 45.0 | 270.8 |
| 4/18-19 | 450 | 0 | 160 | .465 | 273.5 | 35.2 | 308.7 |
| 4/19-20 | 0 | 163 | 135 | .426 | 250.5 | .... | .... |
| 4/20-21 | 580 | 76 | 190 | .535 | 314.7 | 47.5 | 362.2 |

TABLE 4.—EXPERIMENT 4, ACIDOSIS IN DOG UNDER SAME CONDITIONS AS EXPERIMENT 3

| Date | Water c.c. | Acid c.c. | Urine c.c. | Total $NH_3$ c.c. | n/10$NH_3$ c.c. | Total Alk. c.c. | n/10$NH_3$ + Total Alk. c.c. |
|---|---|---|---|---|---|---|---|
| 4/ 9-10 | 100 | ... | 10 | .... | .... | .... | .... |
| 4/10-11 | 150 | ... | 100 | .199 | 117.0 | 35.0 | 152.0 |
| 4/11-12 | 320 | ... | 110 | .... | .... | 39.6 | .... |
| 4/12-13 | 220 | ... | 40 | .054 | 31.7 | 11.2 | 42.9 |
| 4/13-14 | 300 | ... | 80 | .159 | 93.5 | 12.8 | 106.3 |
| 4/14-15 | 295 | 80 | 200 | .306 | 180.0 | 30.0 | 210.0 |
| 4/15-16 | 205 | 77 | 195 | .503 | 295.8 | 15.6 | 311.4 |
| 4/16-17 | 140 | 72 | 125 | .430 | 252.9 | 50.0 | 302.9 |
| 4/17-18 | 300 | 80 | 210 | .479 | 281.7 | 14.0 | 295.7 |
| 4/18-19 | 590 | 0 | 310 | .428 | 251.7 | 86.8 | 338.5 |
| 4/19-20 | 600 | 75 | 230 | .198 | 116.4 | 52.9 | 169.3 |
| 4/20-21 | 195 | ... | 135 | .142 | 83.5 | 27.0 | 110.5 |

TABLE 5.—ACIDOSIS IN DOG UNDER STARVATION REGIME

| Date | Weight c.c. | Water c.c. | Urine c.c. | Total $NH_3$ c.c. | n/10$NH_3$ c.c. | Total Alk. c.c. | n/10$NH_3$ +Total Alk. c.c. |
|---|---|---|---|---|---|---|---|
| 4/21-22 | 19½ | 460 | 125 | .266 | 157. | 23.7 | 180.7 |
| 4/22-23 | ...... | 365 | 160 | .287 | 169. | 38.4 | 207.4 |
| 4/23-24 | ...... | 350 | 85 | .111 | 65.6 | 56.2 | 121.8 |
| 4/24-25 | ...... | 300 | 75 | .116 | 68.6 | 71.2 | 139.8 |
| 4/25-26 | ...... | 450 | 51 | .083 | 49.0 | 39.0 | 88.0 |
| 4/26-27 | ...... | 320 | 65 | .151 | 89.0 | 42.2 | 131.2 |
| 4/27-28 | 16 5/16 | 220 | 50 | .078 | 46.8 | 35.0 | 81.8 |
| 4/28-29 | ...... | 335 | 40 | .074 | 44.8 | 30.8 | 75.6 |
| 4/29-30 | ...... | 225 | 40 | .073 | 43.8 | 28.4 | 72.2 |
| 4/30- 1 | ...... | 200 | 20 | .... | .... | 14.4 | .... |
| 5/ 1- 2 | ...... | 300 | 40 | .088 | 52.4 | .... | .... |
| 5/ 2- 3 | ...... | 600 | 55 | .204 | 120.3 | 71.5 | 191.8 |
| 5/ 3- 4 | ...... | 225 | 35 | .069 | 41.1 | .... | .... |
| 5/ 4- 5 | 15 | 180 | 40 | .090 | 53.7 | 28.0 | 81.7 |
| 5/ 5- 6 | ...... | 245 | 20 | .... | .... | 11.8 | .... |
| 5/ 6- 7 | ...... | 135 | 30 | .074 | 43.9 | .... | .... |
| 5/ 7- 8 | ...... | 80 | ... | .... | .... | .... | .... |
| 5/ 8- 9 | ...... | 150 | 30 | .066 | 39.2 | .... | .... |
| 5/ 9-10 | ...... | 90 | 75 | .158 | 93.2 | 59.2 | 152.4 |
| 5/10-11 | ...... | 220 | 65 | .198 | 117.0 | 45.5 | 162.5 |
| 5/11-12 | 12¾ | 240 | 80 | .115 | 68.8 | .... | .... |
| 5/12-13 | ...... | 90 | 60 | .076 | 45.6 | 57.0 | 102.6 |
| 5/13-14 | ...... | 100 | 80 | .... | .... | 46.4 | .... |
| 5/14-15 | ...... | 60 | 15 | .... | .... | 12.9 | .... |

TABLE 6.—ACIDOSIS IN DOG UNDER SAME CONDITIONS AS EXPERIMENT 5

| Date | Weight c.c. | Water c.c. | Urine c.c. | Total $NH_3$ c.c. | n/10$NH_3$ c.c. | Total Alk. c.c. | n/10$NH_3$ +Total Alk. c.c. |
|---|---|---|---|---|---|---|---|
| 4/21-22 | 13 5/16 | 130 | 125 | .229 | 135.5 | 31.2 | 166.8 |
| 4/22-23 | ...... | 135 | 115 | .0578 | 34.0 | 14.9 | 48.9 |
| 4/23-24 | ...... | 120 | 30+ | .0219+ | 12.9+ | .... | .... |
| 4/24-25 | ...... | 290 | 85 | .093 | 55.7 | .... | .... |
| 4/25-26 | ...... | 50 | 55 | .056 | 33.8 | 60.4 | 94.2 |
| 4/26-27 | ...... | 80 | 30 | .048 | 24.7 | .... | .... |
| 4/27-28 | ...... | 40 | 30 | .020 | 12.3 | .... | .... |
| 4/28-29 | 11 5/16 | 100 | 40 | .045 | 27.3 | 42.0 | 69.3 |
| 4/29-30 | ...... | 135 | 35 | .032 | 19.8 | .... | .... |
| 4/30- 1 | ...... | 80 | 20 | .... | .... | 18.6 | .... |
| 5/ 1- 2 | ...... | 290 | 25 | .0204 | 12.3 | .... | .... |
| 5/ 2- 3 | ...... | 410 | 40 | .132 | 78.8 | 58.0 | 136.8 |
| 5/ 3- 4 | ...... | 140 | ... | .... | .... | .... | .... |
| 5/ 4- 5 | ...... | 40 | ... | .... | .... | .... | .... |
| 5/ 5- 6 | 10 5/16 | 100 | 15 | .... | .... | 13.5 | .... |
| 5/ 6- 7 | ...... | 65 | ... | .... | .... | .... | .... |
| 5/ 7- 8 | ...... | 65 | ... | .... | .... | .... | .... |
| 5/ 8- 9 | ...... | 205 | ... | .... | .... | .... | .... |
| 5/ 9-10 | ...... | 60 | 50 | .... | .... | 77.0 | .... |
| 5/10-11 | ...... | 115 | 5 | .... | .... | .... | .... |
| 5/11-12 | ...... | 100 | 25 | .... | .... | 28. | .... |
| 5/12-13 | 9 1/16 | 120 | ... | .... | .... | .... | .... |
| 5/13-14 | ...... | 150 | 15 | .... | .... | 16.2 | .... |
| 5/14-15 | ...... | 100 | ... | .... | .... | .... | .... |
| 5/15-16 | ...... | 175 | ... | .... | .... | .... | .... |
| 5/16-17 | ...... | 300 | 70 | .112 | 65.8 | 91.7 | 157.5 |
| 5/17-18 | ...... | 275 | 100 | .132 | 78.0 | 52. | 130.0 |
| 5/18-19 | 9.0 | 375 | 50 | .0374 | 22.0 | 7.0 | 29.0 |
| 5/19-20 | ...... | 300 | 125 | .057 | 34.6 | 13.7 | 48.3 |
| 5/20-21 | ...... | 300 | 25 | .... | .... | .... | .... |
| 5/21-22 | ...... | 225 | 120 | .... | .... | .... | .... |
| 5/22-23 | ...... | 440 | 230 | .170 | 104.8 | 41.4 | 146.2 |
| 5/23-24 | ...... | 440 | 125 | .... | .... | .... | .... |
| 5/24-25 | ...... | 440 | 90 | .066 | 39.6 | 37.8 | 77.4 |

TABLE 7.—ACIDOSIS IN HUMAN SUBJECTS

| Subject | Date | Urine cc. | Acetone | Total $NH_3$ | $n/10NH_3$ | Total Alk. | $n/10NH_3$+ Total Alk. |
|---|---|---|---|---|---|---|---|
| C | Apr. 1-2 | 1301 | + | 1.18 | 697.3 | 78.0 | 775.3 |
| .. | May 4-5 | 1520 | + | 1.30 | 826.0 | 15.2 | 841.2 |
| .. | May 4-5 | 1552 | + | 1.26 | 744.0 | 77.6 | 821.6 |
| .. | May 16-17 | 1171 | + | .906 | 533.0 | 156.3 | 689.3 |
| B | May 10-11 | 243 | .. | .297 | 174.9 | 102.0 | 276.9 |
| .. | May 10-11 | 870 | .. | .887 | 522.0 | 252.0 | 774.0 |
| R | May 12-13 | 1555 | .. | .792 | 466.0 | 279.0 | 745.0 |
| .. | May 12-13 | 874 | .. | .666 | 392.0 | 183.5 | 575.5 |

C. Severe case. Diacetic acid constantly present with a minus carbohydrate balance of about 30 during most of the time. Given 30 gm. soda bicarbonate daily.

B. Moderately severe case. No diacetic acid for nine months. Never given soda bicarbonate. Has a plus carbohydrate balance of about 30-50.

R. Moderately severe case with diacetic acid present occasionally. Given 20 gm. soda bicarbonate up to May 3, none after May 3. Diet contains about 16 gm. carbohydrate; about 9 gm. nitrogen.

able to observe has necessarily been scanty, but as can be seen in the specimens presented in Table 7, the same general observations that were made experimentally hold here as well. In the curves it will be observed that the higher the ammonia curve reaches above the base line the higher ordinarily the alkali retention line runs. In these cases, as a rule, while the acidosis is severe, the organism is in no immediate danger of coma. The starvation experiment, which ended fatally, is not absolutely corroborative of this, because the animal died undoubtedly from exhaustion due to the previous acid intoxication. Even here, however, it will be observed that toward the end this alkali retention curve falls considerably below the ammonia curve. It is interesting to note that in Experiment 2 the alkali retention is decreased instead of increased almost proportionately, as the ammonia is increased. Whether this be due to alkaline secretion from the vagina entirely or in part also to the added condition of acidosis, it is clear that we are dealing here with an unfermented urine which is more alkaline than the blood, a condition which, except in those cases in which large amounts of alkali have been fed, has been considered by many an impossibility.

## CONCLUSIONS

1. The amount of base excreted in the urine in acidosis, while following in general the variations in the amount of ammonia, may show differences which are of importance in estimating the power of the organism to resist intoxication.

2. Whether the amount of base excreted varies with the amount of ammonia or not, it is important to determine both quantities as they represent two distinct mechanisms of defense.

3. The method employed in this investigation is of such simplicity and accuracy as to recommend itself as a valuable aid to the clinician.

We wish to thank Dr. Francis A. Benedict of the Carnegie Institution Nutrition Laboratory, and Dr. Elliot P. Joslin for the clinical material used; Dr. L. V. Henderson for his kind interest, and Mr. R. S. Titus for assistance in the preliminary work.

Danvers State Hospital, Hathorne—212 Beacon Street, Boston.

# THE EFFECTS OF CERTAIN INTERNAL SECRETIONS ON MALIGNANT TUMORS *

G. L. ROHDENBURG, M.D., F. D. BULLOCK, M.D., AND P. J. JOHNSTON, M.D.
NEW YORK

Several isolated observations have been made in connection with the effects of internal secretions on malignant tumors. Thus Cahen[1] records cases of carcinoma of the breast in which after an incomplete breast amputation, the ovaries, too, were taken out. Of these cases he reports in some, a total disappearance of axillary nodes with gain in weight, the best results being obtained in young women, while the operation was valueless in women over 49 years of age. The significance of such absence of germ glands is somewhat diminished by the observations of Stickler,[2] who reports 200 cases of tumors in bovines, 100 of which were in castrated animals; and 120 tumors in equines, ninety-one of which were in castrated animals. In connection with other secretions Gwyer[3] has administered the thymus gland in cases of tumor and reports decrease in rate of growth, decrease in pain, decrease and in some cases disappearance of enlarged glands. The thyroid also seems to have some connection with malignant growth; thus Stuart-Low[4] removed the thyroid in five cases of malignant tumor and records cessation of growth, decrease of pain, increase of weight and softening of nodes; while Bell[5] reports atrophy of the thyroid in cases of carcinoma.

With the idea of throwing some light on the relation of some of the internal secretions to malignant tumors, the following scheme of work was laid out: first, to note the effect on infectivity and malignancy of tumors of the removal of internal secreting glands of rats; second, to try to destroy immunity by removal of different internal secreting glands; third, to ascertain the effect of gland extracts on tumors in mice; fourth, by the use of gland extracts to endeavor to produce immunity in mice; fifth, to ascertain the effect of gland extracts on pieces of tumor in the test-tube; and sixth, to note the results of treatment of human beings with gland preparations.

---

*From the Cancer Laboratory of the Department of Zoology, Columbia University, N. Y.; under the auspices of the George Crocker Special Research Fund.

1. Cahen: Deutsch. Ztschr. f. Chir., 1909, xcix, 415.
2. Stickler: Arch. f. klin. Chir., 1902, lxv, 616.
3. Gwyer: Ann. Surg., 1907, xlvi, 86; 1908, xlvii, 506.
4. Stuart-Low, W.: Lancet, London, 1909, ii, 1138.
5. Bell: Med. Rec., 1907, lxxii, 306.

## I. EFFECTS PRODUCED BY INOCULATING RATS WITH TUMOR AFTER CERTAIN GLANDS ARE REMOVED

One hundred and ninety rats were taken and divided into five equal groups. As nearly as it was possible to select them, all rats were of one size (full-grown), and from a common stock. One group of thirty-eight animals was used as a control. In the remaining groups we removed the testes from one, the thymus from a second, the thyroid from a third, and the spleen from a fourth; while we started with an equal number of animals in each group the death of some of the animals left us with unequal numbers at the end of the experiment. After allowing a varying period of time (from seven to forty-five days) for the absence of the missing internal secretion to affect metabolism, an equal number of each group and of the controls were inoculated at the same time with rat carcinoma.

All of our operations were performed under ether anesthesia. The tumor was of Flexner-Jobling origin. The trocar method of inoculation was employed and all rats of a given group were inoculated at one time from the same tumor. The tumors were measured on the day of appearance, and on the fifteenth, twentieth, and thirtieth days following inoculation. At the end of forty days of tumor growth the animals showing an immunity were set aside for another section of the work and the others killed and examined. It was found that in the thyroid and thymus group, only one-third to one-half, on the average, of the gland in question had been removed. The results of this set of experiments are summarized in Table 1.

TABLE 1.—GLAND-FREE ANIMALS INOCULATED WITH TUMOR*

| | Control | Thyroid removed | Spleen removed | Thymus removed | Testes removed |
|---|---|---|---|---|---|
| Number of animals in series | 29 | 29 | 24 | 23 | 38 |
| Average interval between operation and inoculation in days | 0 | 21 | 13 | 14 | 12 |
| Average interval between inoculation and appearance of tumor in days | 11 | 11 | 7 | 5 | 6 |
| Total number of takes including spontaneous cures | 24 (83%) | 23 (78%) | 20 (81%) | 18 (78%) | 32 (81%) |
| Number of positive tumors on 30th day | 21 (72%) | 14 (47%) | 17 (70%) | 13 (56%) | 23 (60%) |
| Number of animals in which there were no takes | 5 (17%) | 6 (20%) | 4 (16%) | 5 (21%) | 6 (16%) |
| Number of spontaneous cures up to 30th day | 3 (12%) | 9 (39%) | 3 (15%) | 5 (27%) | 9 (27%) |
| Number of spontaneous cures up to 40th day | 4 (16%) | 12 (52%) | 3 (15%) | 8 (44%) | 12 (37%) |
| Average size of tumors on— | | | | | |
| 1st day | 6×6 | 4×4 | 3×3 | 3×4 | 4×3 |
| 15th day | 8×8 | 6×7 | 7×8 | 5×6 | 6×7 |
| 20th day | 10×11 | 8×9 | 8×9 | 8×8 | 7×8 |
| 30th day | 12×13 | 10×10 | 12×14 | 11×12 | 10×12 |

* In this and the following table all measurements are given in millimeters. Fractions have been discarded in computing averages and percentages.

In considering the results, several factors figure in drawing conclusions. A first factor is the normal condition of tumor infectivity and malignancy for that portion of the history of the tumor during which our experiments were conducted. A second factor is the effect of narcosis on these phases of tumor life. A third factor is the specific action of the absence of one of the internal secretions. A fourth factor is the small number of rats in each group. The fourth factor is a weakness that can be overcome by further experiments along the same lines.

Although the number of animals operated on is too small for safe generalization we believe that the variations shown in the table are probably attributable to the absence of the internal secretion. It would appear from our results that the rate of tumor growth or "malignancy" is not affected while the "infectivity" appears to be, as shown by the number of spontaneous cures and "no takes." The influence on infectivity, if there is any, is not restricted to one gland but is apparently shared by at least two of the glands in the series. In passing it may be said that our observations bear out, to a certain extent, various clinical observations on the human being.

## II. EFFECT ON IMMUNITY OF REMOVAL OF SOME OF THE INTERNAL SECRETORY GLANDS

Table 1 shows a varying percentage of animals immune to tumor inoculations. The immunity indicated was of two types. In some rats no tumor appeared on inoculation (called in Table 2, Type 1), in others a tumor grew for a time, and then disappeared (called in Table 2, Type 2). To the immune rats set aside in Section 1, we added others which had been previously inoculated with sarcoma and which had shown an immunity. According to Ehrlich and others[6] rats immune to sarcoma are also immune to carcinoma.

At the beginning of this experiment some of the rats were normal, while some had one or another of the glands removed. From the latter and from the normal rats we removed one gland so that we had single gland-free and combination gland-free rats. For example we had rats thyroid-free, and others with a combination of spleen-and-thyroid-free, spleen-and-thymus-free, etc. After allowing an interval for recovery, these rats were inoculated for a second time, this time with carcinoma. The remark concerning incomplete thyroid and thymus removals, as made in the first section of this article, applies here with the exception of those animals starred (*) in Table 2, in which the removal was complete. It will be noted that immunity was destroyed in the three starred animals with complete removal of certain glands. This is such a small

6. Lewin: Ergebn. d. inn. Med. u. Kinderh., 1908, ii, 168.

number that the results may be accidental, perhaps owing to previous faulty inoculation.

In considering the results the possibility must be borne in mind that, *ex hypothesi,* through previous unsuccessful inoculations the several internal secretions may have been stimulated to such a degree that a long period of time is necessary before the immunizing substance disappears from the body. It will be noted that, out of eighteen animals showing Type 1 of immunity, eleven developed tumors which disappeared after varying periods of time; and that of fourteen animals of Type 2 of immunity, nine developed tumors of which but six disappeared. This we have interpreted as showing a lessened degree of immunity.

TABLE 2.—RESULTS OF A SECOND TUMOR INOCULATION OF GLAND-FREE ANIMALS

SINGLE GLAND-FREE ANIMALS

| Origin of animal | Type of immunity | Operation Removal of | Results following operation Tumor | Disappeared in |
|---|---|---|---|---|
| Immune sarcoma .......... | 1 | Thyroid | 5×6 | 10 days |
| Immune sarcoma .......... | 1 | Thyroid | 2×4 | 10 days |
| Immune sarcoma .......... | 1 | Thyroid | 4×3 | 15 days |
| Immune sarcoma .......... | 2 | Spleen | 7×9 | 30 days |
| Immune sarcoma .......... | 1 | Spleen | 2×2 | 15 days |
| Immune sarcoma .......... | 1 | Spleen | 2×4 | 15 days |
| Immune sarcoma .......... | 1 | Spleen | No tumor developed | |
| Immune sarcoma .......... | 1 | Spleen | No tumor developed | |
| Immune sarcoma .......... | 1 | Thymus | 2×3 | 10 days |
| Immune carcinoma ........ | 1 | Spleen | 7×8 | 30 days |
| Immune carcinoma ........ | 1 | Spleen | 3×3 | 10 days |
| Immune carcinoma ........ | 1 | Spleen | No tumor developed | |
| Immune carcinoma ........ | 1 | Spleen | No tumor developed | |
| Immune carcinoma ........ | 1 | Testes | 3×4 | 10 days |
| Immune carcinoma ........ | 1 | Testes | No tumor developed | |
| Immune carcinoma ........ | 1 | Testes | No tumor developed | |

COMBINATION GLAND-FREE ANIMALS

| Origin of animal | Type of immunity | Operation Removal of | Results following operation Tumor | Disappeared in |
|---|---|---|---|---|
| Immune thyroid-free ....... | 1 | Thymus | 5×4 | 30 days |
| Immune thyroid-free ....... | 1 | Thymus | 5×5 | 20 days |
| Immune thyroid-free ....... | 2 | Testes | 4×5 | 15 days |
| Immune thyroid-free ....... | 2 | Testes | 2×3 | 10 days |
| Immune spleen-free ........ | 1 | Thymus | No tumor developed | |
| Immune spleen-free ........ | 2 | Testes | 2×2 | 10 days |
| Immune thymus-free ....... | 2 | Testes | No tumor developed | |
| Immune thymus-free ....... | 2 | Testes | 2×3 | 10 days |
| Immune thymus-free * ...... | 2 | Testes | 10×15 | Did not disappear |
| Immune thymus-free * ...... | 2 | Testes | 5×7 | Did not disappear |
| Immune thymus-free * ...... | 2 | Testes | 10×11 | Did not disappear |
| Immune testes-free ........ | 2 | Thymus | 2×2 | 10 days |
| Immune testes-free ........ | 2 | Spleen | No tumor developed | |
| Immune testes-free ........ | 2 | Thymus | No tumor developed | |
| Immune testes-free ........ | 2 | Thymus | No tumor developed | |
| Immune testes-free ........ | 2 | Thymus | No tumor developed | |

## III. THE EFFECT OF INJECTIONS OF GLAND EXTRACTS ON TUMORS IN MICE

This phase of the work had to do with the effect of various extracts of the glands and other tissues on tumors in mice. If one goes over the literature of the various reported immunizing and curative agents in carcinoma one is struck with their wide diversity. The question of a common active substance is one that naturally arises. With this in view a method of isolating such a substance was devised, the details of which will appear later.

Following this method, substances were prepared from human tissue (uterine fibroid), from the entire tissues of a macerated mouse, from the entire tissues of a macerated rat and from the spleen, thyroid, thymus, testes, pancreas, and pituitary glands of cattle. A number of mice with tumors of different sizes and ages were given subcutaneous injections of these various extracts in five-minim doses every other day. The injections were made in a region away from the tumor.

Our results showed that small tumors up to 5 by 5 mm. treated with any of the extracts disappeared in from five to ten injections. Large tumors were but slightly affected by the gland extracts, but were markedly affected by the rat and mouse extracts. A tumor 18 by 21 mm. treated with rat extract diminished in size to 8 by 7 mm. within five days. In several mice, tumors of about 18 by 21 mm. in size disappeared absolutely in from seven to twelve days. At times we saw slight to marked local reaction, as evidenced by redness and heat in the tumor area, while those tumors which were examined under the microscope showed marked areas of degeneration.

## IV. THE EFFECT OF GLAND EXTRACTS ON MICE PREVIOUS TO INOCULATION WITH CARCINOMA

This section of the work had to do with an attempt to produce immunity by injecting gland and other extracts in mice previous to inoculation with carcinoma. Mice of approximately the same size and age and from the same stock were divided into groups of four each and received injections of 5 minims of the extract every other day for three injections. After the last injection an interval of two days elapsed, and the animals were then inoculated by the trocar method, all at one time, and with pieces of the same tumor. Four animals were inoculated as a control group at the same time.

TABLE 3.—RESULTS OF TUMOR INOCULATION ON MICE PREVIOUSLY INOCULATED WITH CARCINOMA

| | No. positive tumors on 30th day | No. spontaneous cures | No. no takes |
|---|---|---|---|
| Controls | 3 | 1 | 0 |
| Human extract | 0 | 0 | 4 |
| Rat extract | 0 | 0 | 4 |
| Mouse extract | 0 | 0 | 3* |
| Thyroid | 1 | 0 | 3 |
| Spleen | 0 | 0 | 4 |
| Testes | 0 | 0 | 4 |
| Pituitary | 0 | 0 | 4 |
| Thymus | 0 | 0 | 4 |
| Pancreas | 0 | 0 | 4 |

* One animal died before end of experiment. The one mouse in thyroid group showing tumor may be due to the fact that most of the injection given escaped on two of the three injections.

Table 3 records the data of each group, from which it may be seen that all of the extracts used produced a high percentage of immunity.

This rather puzzling result we interpret as due to the action of a specific (?) chemical compound which may be derived from all tissues put through the same chemical process.

## V. THE EFFECT OF GLAND EXTRACTS ON PIECES OF TUMOR IN THE TEST-TUBE

Walker[7] in his paper on the effects of certain serums on carcinoma in mice, has shown that if pieces of tumor are placed in the serum of a rat which has been injected with an emulsion of testes, degeneration of the cancer cells takes place. The cells are, according to his observation, invaded and replaced by white blood-cells.

Following his idea we took pieces of healthy tumor tissue from a mouse carcinoma and cut it into pieces about 2 by 2 mm. in size. The undegenerated tumor tissue can readily be distinguished from the necrotic in the gross and particular care was taken to secure only the non-necrotic portions of the tumor. The gland extracts were prepared as before. About 3 c.c. of each of the gland extracts were placed in a separate test-tube and a portion of the tumor placed in each. As control we used a piece of tumor to which nothing had been done and which was placed in a solution of glycerin one part and water two parts, while another piece was placed immediately in fixative. The test-tubes were then placed in the incubator at 40 C. for forty-eight hours. The pieces of tumor were then removed and placed in sublimate-acetic acid solution and stained with iron hematoxylin. All of this was done immediately after killing the mouse, the interval between killing and action of the gland extracts being not more than fifteen minutes.

The results of this work were negative. It was found that all of the gland extracts caused necrosis of the tumor material as did the glycerin control. The necrosis involved the entire piece of tumor and as far as could be seen there was no greater necrosis in one piece than another. We saw no replacement or invasion of the cells by white blood-cells.

## VI. THE TREATMENT OF MALIGNANT GROWTHS IN HUMAN BEINGS WITH VARIOUS GLAND EXTRACTS

The first section of this paper shows that removal of the testes and thyroid has an influence on tumor infectivity and that removal of the thymus also has some effect. In the second section evidence was given to indicate that immunity was destroyed in three animals by complete removal of the testes and thymus. While this last may be a coincidence, still it deserves some consideration. Some evidence further is given in the fourth section to show that there is present in many of the internal

7. Walker: Lancet, London, 1908, ii, 797.

secretory glands a substance which confers immunity. The thymus, testes, and thyroid are a group of glands intimately connected. Removal of the testes causes an increase in size of the thymus and *vice versa.* In many women the thyroid increases in diameter during menstruation, and in most women the size of the gland is decidedly increased during pregnancy.

In 1905, Bayliss and Starling announced that they had perfected a method by which they could extract from the fetus of a rabbit a definite chemical, which when injected into a virgin female rabbit produced some of the changes seen in pregnancy, i. e., enlargement of the breast with secretion of milk. Since then they and others have announced from time to time the discovery of hormones isolated from different structures which had a decided influence on some of the vital processes of the body. A hormone may be defined, then, as a definite chemical compound, or class of compounds, the exact chemical nature of which is at present not clear, which possesses the power of causing, or is necessary to many of the biologic and chemical changes of life.

At the risk of being overspeculative we would explain our results as due to the fact that the three glands, the thymus, the testes, and the thyroid, acting together, produce such a hormone which may be the immunizing or curative agent and that removal of one of the glands causes temporary overactivity of the other two, producing an increase of hormone and a corresponding increase of immunity. We have had no means of obtaining this hypothetical hormone in concentrated or pure state; we therefore tried the effects of the glands in various combinations on human carcinomata.

All of the patients treated were surgically inoperable and the growths were positively malignant, both clinically and microscopically. We are indebted for the cases to Drs. Fischer, Grant, Gwyer, Kammerer, Kiliani, Krug, Manheimer, Meyer, Murphy, Neef, Oppenheimer, Stetten, Stieglitz, Tovey, Tuthill and Stein. In administering the thymus gland alone or in any of several combinations we have come to the same conclusions as Gwyer, the pioneer in this field. In agreement with his experience, we have found that nutrition is markedly improved, patients gaining in weight from 1 to 14 pounds. The hemoglobin and red cells markedly increase and the patients feel stronger, while pain is greatly diminished. The discharge and bleeding, if any, were lessened, and in a majority of cases stopped. The local changes were variable, in some a marked local reaction being present, in others none. The glands diminished in size and in some cases disappeared. The tumors themselves showed a cessation of growth, and in some cases a temporary decrease in size. In one case recorded below a complete disappearance occurred.

Our conclusions, based on forty-eight cases, are as follows: The thymus, when given for a period of from three to five weeks, markedly influences malignant tumors by relief of pain, gain in weight, reduction in size of glands, and cessation of growth of tumor. After this comes a period of quiet with neither progress nor retrogression for about two weeks. Then the tumor either gradually increases in size, or remains for a long period stationary, or, as in one case in which the growth was small, may completely disappear with no recurrence.

Mrs. Q., referred by Dr. Stieglitz, six years ago had a radical breast amputation for carcinoma by Dr. Lilenthal; two years later an operation for gall-stones. About one month before commencing treatment she complained of severe intercostal neuralgia. Examination revealed a local recurrence about three inches long by two inches wide. Because of a very severe nephritis only a partial removal under local anesthesia was attempted. The remaining mass measured about 1.5 by 1.5 inches, projecting into an intercostal space. The patient was placed upon thymus extract given hypodermically in five-minim doses daily. The pain was relieved after three injections. The mass grew steadily smaller and after fifteen injections disappeared. There has been no recurrence to date, which is nine months after treatment.

This patient also had three fulguration treatments.

The administration of the thyroid extract alone showed results similar to those of thymus but to a less degree: slight decrease in gland involvement, decrease in rate of tumor growth, and slight relief of pain, but no gain in weight.

The administration of testes was followed by no decrease in glandular involvement, and apparent increase in size of the tumor and rate of growth; no gain in weight and no relief of pain.

The combination of thymus and testes gave the results produced by thymus alone, but not more marked. It was noted in three cases which had stopped improving under thymus that administration of testes in conjunction with thymus, produced a further but temporary improvement.

The combination of thymus and thyroid was no better than thymus alone. That of testes and thyroid was no better than thyroid alone; while the combination of all three glands again proved to be no more active than the thymus gland alone.

## CONCLUSIONS

planned, we cannot draw positive conclusions at present. The evidence,
In this preliminary report on the scheme of work as originally however, drawn from the various lines of experimentation, is sufficiently encouraging to justify us in pursuing these lines of research. Briefly summarizing this evidence, we would point out (1) that removal of certain glands (i. e., thyroid, thymus and testes) appears to decrease the susceptibility to cancer; (2) that removal of single glands or combination of glands in immune animals leads to lessened immunity to cancer;

(3) that extracts of thymus, thyroid, spleen, pancreas, pituitary, and testes on injection tend to increase immunity against cancer and that extracts of certain other tissues produce like effects; (4) that similar extracts, on injection in cancerous organisms, alleviate pain, reduce tumors, or even cause them to disappear; and finally (5) that our results, combined with those of other observers, tend to the conclusion that many tissues contain some common element, possibly of the nature of a hormone, which is capable of producing immunity.

In conclusion we would express our gratitude to Drs. Fred. Gwyer and Gary Calkins, without whose help in material, chemical investigations, and suggestions, this investigation would not have been possible.

Department of Zoology, Schermerhorn Hall, Columbia University.

# THE DURATION OF TRYPANOSOME INFECTIONS

JOHN L. TODD, M.D.
MONTREAL, CANADA

## I. INTRODUCTION

It is well known that trypanosomes may be absent for long periods from the peripheral blood of an animal or of a person suffering from an infection by trypanosomes, and that although no treatment has been given. It also frequently happens that the parasites may reappear, after a more or less lengthy absence, in the blood of persons or of animals who have apparently been cured by appropriate treatment of an infection by trypanosomes. It is important to collect instances of such disappearances and recurrences of the parasites in order that an opinion may be formed as to the length of time during which a recurrence is possible in cases of apparent recovery from trypanosomiasis or apparent cure.

## II. HUMAN TRYPANOSOMIASIS

The following observations prove that symptoms may be absent for long periods from persons who are infected with trypanosomes, and that those infected may die from the disease many years after the date at which it was acquired.

There are many records of negroes who have died of sleeping-sickness five or eight years after leaving the district in which the disease was contracted.[1]

One of five subjects of early trypanosomiasis in Africans who were seen in the Gambian Protectorate[2] during the winter of 1902, died from definite sleeping-sickness in 1905; the four other subjects were alive and well in May, 1904, but they were all dead, from unreported causes, in 1909.

The records of 102 infected persons who were seen in the Congo, at an early stage of their disease, when no symptoms beyond glandular enlargement were perceptible, indicate that one-third of such persons will live on without treatment for from thirty to forty months.[3] It has not been possible to keep track of all of these negro patients, but five of them, without treatment, were well and working at forty-eight months after they were first observed to be infected.

The symptoms disappeared, without treatment, from three Europeans who were infected with trypanosomes; they recurred after fifteen months in one case

---

1. Nabarro, D.: Trypanosomes and Trypanosomiasis, transl. by Laveran and Mesnil, London, 1907, Ballière, Tindall & Cox, p. 370.

2. Dutton, J. E. and Todd, J. L.: First Report of the Trypanosomiasis Expedition to Senegambia (1902), Liverpool School of Tropical Medicine, Memoir XI, London, 1903, Williams and Norgate.

3. Todd, J. L.: A Review of the position of Gland Palpation in the Diagnosis of Human Trypanosomiasis, Jour. Trop. Med. and Hyg., London, 1908, xi, 229.

and after three years in another. The third patient was still well two years after the commencement of the disease.[4]

A consideration of these facts makes it easy to understand why some observers hold that untreated human trypanosomiasis is, in the end, invariably fatal; while others believe that spontaneous recovery may occur, especially in localities such as the Gambia and Sierra Leone, where the disease is endemic and apparently less virulent than it is in areas where it is epidemic.

Before 1905, preparations of inorganic arsenic, especially liquor arsenicalis, were the most efficient trypanocides known. In 1905, the value of para-amido-phenyl-arsenic acid (atoxyl) was discovered. Since then other valuable trypanocides, such as the antimony preparations and various anilin compounds, have been described.

It was observed during the very earliest attempts at the treatment of trypanosomiasis, that the parasites frequently recurred and caused the death of animals which were supposed to have been cured.

The results have been published of the treatment of a large number of Europeans infected with trypanosomiasis; a number of these cases are mentioned in a recent number of the Bulletin of the Sleeping-Sickness Bureau.[5] The history of several of these persons strongly indicates that recovery may occur in cases of trypanosomiasis if the patients be well cared for and efficiently treated. Many of these patients are in good health at more than three years after the commencement of their disease, while one is well nine years after the date on which symptoms were first observed.

Martin and Darré[6] report four Europeans who were apparently cured out of twenty-two patients treated by atoxyl alone, or by atoxyl combined with orpiment or with tartar emetic; these four patients are in absolute health three and one-half to four years after the commencement of their disease.

Although the records of the treatment of these Europeans are so encouraging, the following facts should not be forgotten:

In some unfortunate instances, the disease has been entirely resistant to the therapeutic measures which have been successful in the treatment of other Europeans.

It has happened, not infrequently, that the trypanosomes have recurred and that the patients have died of trypanosomiasis in instances in which the disease was not treated early, or in which the treatment was not as energetic, or as constant, as it should have been. Even in patients who received early, energetic and constant treatment, signs of trypanosomiasis have been observed for so long as from three to five years after the commencement of the disease.[5,6]

One patient, a European, who became infected in 1902 was treated and, in 1908, seemed to have been cured of the disease; in 1910 he died of it.[7]

---

4. Nattan-Larrier, L.: Sur les résultats du traitement de la trypanosomiase chez le blanc, Bull. Soc. de path. exotique, Paris, 1908, i, 620.

5. Todd, J. L.: Trypanosomiasis in Europeans, Bull. Sleeping-Sickness Bureau, London, 1910, ii, 314.

6. Martin, L. and Darré, H.: Résultats éloignés du traitement dans la trypanosomiase humaine, Bull. Soc. path. exotique, Paris, 1910, iii, 333.

7. Martin, L., and Darré, H.: Résultats éloignés du traitement dans la trypanosomiase humaine, Bull. Sleeping-Sickness Bureau, London, 1910, ii, 212.

Many Africans affected by trypanosomiasis have been treated by various methods. Unfortunately, careful records have not always been kept of the results of their treatment. The most important attempts at treatment on a large scale have been made since 1905. The commissions sent out by Great Britain, France, Portugal, Spain and Germany have all reported on the results of their attempts at treatment; while Broden and Rodhain at Léopoldville, Thiroux in Senegal, and Ayres Kopke at Lisbon, as well as other workers, have treated patients in smaller numbers. In spite of the warnings given by those who made the experiments and observations, which led to the employment of atoxyl and its derivatives in the treatment of trypanosomiasis, some of the investigators who have employed these trypanocides in the field have been carried away by the almost miraculous benefit which they bring to persons even moribund from sleeping-sickness: consequently, unduly favorable reports have sometimes been made concerning these drugs. Yet, although the records have not been published of even a small proportion of the patients treated by these commissions and workers, it does seem probable, from the reports which have been published, that a proportion of the negroes treated have been cured of the disease.

Hodges[8] reviews the results of the treatment of several hundred cases in Uganda since 1906. He concludes that the percentage of apparent cures is extremely small (about 2 per cent. of the total number of patients treated at all stages of the disease). The probability of the treatment being successful depends upon the earliness with which it is commenced; and the number of recurrences increases with the length of time elapsed since the discontinuance of the treatment.

The cases are reported of two sick sepoys who were apparently cured five years after they were found to be infected.[8]

A negro,[9] who seemed to be cured of trypanosomiasis, had a recurrence of the disease after fifteen months of, apparently, perfect health.

Kopke[10] reports the results obtained in 52 cases of trypanosomiasis in Africans, who were treated by him since July, 1905; atoxyl was given alone, or in combination with other drugs. Six of the patients are possibly cured; the trypanosomes have been absent, without a recurrence, from the blood of one of them for two and a half years. It seemed practically impossible to cure patients whose cerebrospinal fluid contained trypanosomes; thirty-four such patients died within a year after the commencement of treatment.

The records of these last cases tend to support the assertion that the appearance of the third stage of sleeping-sickness and of its accompany-

---

8. Hodges, A.: Progress Report on the Uganda Sleeping-Sickness Camps from December, 1906, to November, 1909, Bull. Sleeping-Sickness Bureau, London, 1910, xix, 260.

9. Martin, G., and Leboeuf: Les rechutes dans le traitement de la trypanosomiase humaine; De l'association de la couleur de benzidine Ph. (Afridol violet) à l'atoxyl. Bull. Soc. pathol. exotique, Paris, 1909, ii, 54.

10. Kopke, A.: Traitement de la trypanosomiase humaine; Rapport présenté au XVI Congrès International de Médecine, Trav. de l'Ecole de méd. trop. de Lisbonne, Lisbonne, 1909.

ing symptoms is caused by the penetration of the trypanosomes into the cerebrospinal canal. It also supports the assertion that patients whose cerebrospinal fluid contains trypanosomes invariably die, and that it is useless to attempt to treat them.

The following case is of interest in this connection. Its chief interest is that it scarcely agrees with the above assertions, since symptoms of nervous derangement were never present and the patient lived, in spite of very inadequate treatment, for four years and seven months after trypanosomes were found in his cerebrospinal fluid.

The patient, a male negro, aged 23, seen July 7, 1904, lived in the missionary station at Bolobo. He had been ill for a year and had lost a little weight; he complained of weakness and there had been intermittent insomnia and headache; no change had been noticed in his character and there had been no pathologic sleep.

The patient was well nourished and muscular. A careful physical examination disclosed nothing abnormal save a spleen which extended 10 c.c. below the costal margin. When the sole of the foot was stroked the great toe was extended. The pulse-rate was 84 and the temperature was normal. The glands were not definitely enlarged.

Trypanosomes were not found in the blood; the cerebrospinal fluid was distinctly cloudy and on examination was found to contain a few trypanosomes together with scanty leukocytes.

A short course of liquor arsenicalis was commenced at once; no record was kept of the way in which it was administered but it was not given constantly. After that time the patient, occasionally, had slight fevers. On Feb. 6, 1909, trypanosomes could not be found in the blood but the patient was not as strong as he had been and his friends feared that he had sleeping-sickness.

## III. TRYPANOSOMIASIS IN ANIMALS

Each of the trypanosomes which cause a disease in animals has been shown to be pathogenic for every mammal into which it has been subinoculated. It is true that the intensity of the infection produced varies in accordance with the virulence of the parasite and with the susceptibility of the animal inoculated.

For example, *Trypanosoma gambiense* produces a severe infection in some monkeys, (*Cercopithecus patas*), while baboons are almost resistant to it.

The virulence of the infection produced by each parasite in the experimental animal employed is usually constant.

For example, *Trypanosoma brucei* always kills rats and other small animals quickly, but the disease produced by it in cattle may last for, certainly, several months.

*Trypanosoma dimorphon* always kills small laboratory animals rather less quickly than does *Trypanosoma brucei*, while cattle infected by it may live in perfect health for several years.

Although the type of infection produced by each trypanosome in each experimental animal is more or less constant, yet exceptions do occur and an infection may run an unusually acute, or an unusually chronic course.

For example, rats and other small animals are easily infected with *Trypanosoma gambiense* and they usually die of the infection within a month or two;[11] but an infection has been observed to last in a rat for 388 days and infected animals occasionally recover.[12]

Monkeys, infected with *Trypanosoma gambiense*, have remained for 150 days without showing symptoms of the disease.

*Trypanosoma dimorphon* usually kills horses infected by it; but the disease caused by it sometimes runs a chronic course and horses may even recover as in the following instance.

A horse, Case VI,[2] found naturally infected with *Trypanosoma dimorphon* in the Gambia in 1902, and brought to England; it was carefully observed until January, 1907. Then, since the animal had always been in apparently excellent health and since its blood was never found to be infected with trypanosomes, in spite of the most careful examinations, it was thought to be cured. The horse was reinoculated in February, 1907, and again in July with *Trypanosoma dimorphon*, in order to ascertain whether an immunity had been acquired. The animal sickened; trypanosomes were constantly in its blood, and in spite of treatment with antimony, it died a year later of trypanosomiasis.

Another horse, Case X,[2] observed to be infected at the same time, remained in the Gambia. It was still alive and well in February, 1909. Subject VI was not treated; Subject X, which remained in the Gambia, received liquor arsenicalis from time to time and it was well cared for although it was constantly worked.

Many attempts have been made in animals of various species to treat natural and artificially produced infections of many different trypanosomes. Because *Trypanosoma brucei* produces a disease of short duration and of constant type in experimental animals, it has been used most frequently in these attempts.

Because of the absolute control under which they are treated and because of the large doses of trypanocidal drugs which they tolerate, a large number of animals, especially laboratory animals, have certainly been cured of experimental infections by the parasites of nagana and of other trypanosomiases.

Many rats cured of nagana, by various methods, have lived uninfected, for from 200 to 519 days after the cessation of treatment.

Monkeys treated by atoxyl and mercury for an experimental infection with *Trypanosoma gambiense* have remained healthy for over a year.[13]

Much caution should be used, however, before an animal is accepted as cured; for it has frequently happened that trypanosomes have recurred after an exceedingly long period and have led to the death of an apparently cured animal.

---

11. Dutton, J. E., Todd, J. L., and Kinghorn, A.: Cattle Trypanosomiasis in the Congo Free State, Ann. Trop. Med. and Parasit., Liverpool, 1907, ii, 233.

12. Thomas, H. W., and Linton, S. F.: A Comparison of the Animal Reactions of the Trypanosomes of Uganda and the Congo Free State Sleeping-Sickness, with those of *Trypanosoma gambiense*, Liverpool School Trop. Med., Memoir xiii, London, 1904, Williams and Norgate.

13. Breinl, A.: Experiments on the Combined Atoxyl-Mercury Treatment in Monkeys Infected with *Trypanosoma gambiense*, Ann. Trop. Med. and Parasit., Liverpool, 1909, ii, 345.

A rat died of an infection by *Trypanosoma brucei;* the parasites had appeared in its blood 222 days after they had been driven from it by a dose of atoxyl.[14] Recurrences after about 100 days are frequently recorded: *Trypanosoma brucei* reappeared, for the third time, in the blood of a rat which had been treated by arsenophenylglycin[15] after an interval of 148 days. Another dose of the drug caused the parasites to disappear; they are still absent 264 days later.

*Trypanosoma equiperdum* reappeared after intervals of 105 to 126 days in the blood of rats treated by orsudan,[16] a preparation similar to atoxyl.

## IV. CONCLUSIONS

The good results which followed the treatment of human trypanosomiasis usually have been so immediate and the patients have remained in good health so long, that it seems exceedingly probable that some can be cured; but it is evident, from a consideration of the records of patients treated that, to be successful, the treatment must be energetic and must commence early in the course of the disease. Since the disease has recurred after eight years in persons who had apparently recovered from it, or had been apparently cured of it, it is evident that it would be rash, with our present knowledge, to state definitely that a patient is cured, until that length of time has elapsed since the commencement of treatment. During that period, the case should be carefully observed in order to recognize and combat any recurrence. Similar conclusions may be drawn from the records of the treatment of animal trypanosomiases.

NOTE.—In addition to the authorities previously cited, the following will be found of interest:

Bruce, D.: Further Report on the Tsetse-Fly Disease or Nagana in Zululand, London, 1897, Harrison & Sons.

Thomas, H. W. and Breinl, A.: Trypanosomes, trypanosomiasis and sleeping-sickness, Liverpool School Trop. Med., Memoir XVI, London, 1905, Williams and Norgate.

---

14. Moore, B., Nierenstein, M., and Todd, J. L.: The Treatment of Experimental Trypanosomiasis, Part II, Ann. Trop. Med. and Parasit., Liverpool, 1908, iv, 265.

15. Campbell, R. P., and Todd, J. L.: The Action of Arsenophenylglycin on *Trypanosoma brucei.* Montreal Med. Jour., 1909, xxxviii, 794.

16. Kinghorn, A., and Montgomery, R. E.: Human Trypanosomiasis in Rhodesia and Nyasaland, Ann. Trop. Med. and Parasit., Liverpool, 1909, ii, 277.

# THE PATHOLOGICAL ANATOMY OF THE HUMAN THYROID GLAND *

DAVID MARINE, M.D., AND C. H. LENHART, M.D.
CLEVELAND, OHIO

## *INTRODUCTION*

Our conception of a satisfactory anatomical classification of thyroid changes is a scheme, composed of the major types of changes observed, arranged in the order of their manifestation and in which all separate or individual observations may find proper grouping. It is universally admitted that such a classification does not exist. It is, however, in connection with that group of anatomical changes embraced under the general term "goiter" that the greatest confusion exists.

Studies based on large series of thyroids from the lower animals are still too few, though fortunately they are increasing because observers are realizing that human material is too complicated, and that the cataloguing of the almost infinite variety of possible histological variations has not simplified existing classifications or established the sequential relations of these changes. The multiplicity of terms now in use for each type of thyroid change is merely the result of this cataloguing process to which Virchow[1] a half century ago called attention in the following words: "With reference to true goiter the opinion has long been held that it comprises a series of definite varieties (struma lymphatica, cystica, ossea, vasculosa, etc.) which can develop independently of each other. This is wrong. All these so-called varieties are only different modes of development of essentially the same form of goiter. They (the so-called varieties) mean only different forms of terminal conditions or metamorphoses which can be combined with one another in the same tumor, and a very large and striking variety of these metamorphoses may exist in the same tumor (goiter)."

While numerous and complicated anatomical classifications of human goiter have appeared since Virchow thus wrote, and while the literature has been enriched by many detailed descriptions of histological changes, it does not appear that the really fundamental types of change and their sequential relations are yet established.

Several factors have been and are still operating to retard our fuller appreciation of these fundamental or major anatomical groups. Among these factors may be mentioned the following:

---

* From the H. K. Cushing Laboratory of Experimental Medicine, Western Reserve University.

1. Virchow: Die krankhaften Geschwülste, 1863, iii, 4.

1. We are still ignorant of the essential cause of goiter.

2. Human surgical material is so complicated and pure types of thyroid changes are so rarely observed in man that it has been impossible to reconstruct the primary changes from these terminal conditions. The recognition and appreciation of the primary or fundamentally important changes can be brought about only by the extensive study of autopsy thyroid series or series from the lower animals.

3. In order to interpret the anatomical changes it is necessary to correlate them with the functional activity of the thyroid, and definite criteria of such functional activity are by no means easy to determine. The best that can be done at present is to compare the iodin contents with their corresponding histological structures in large series of glands.

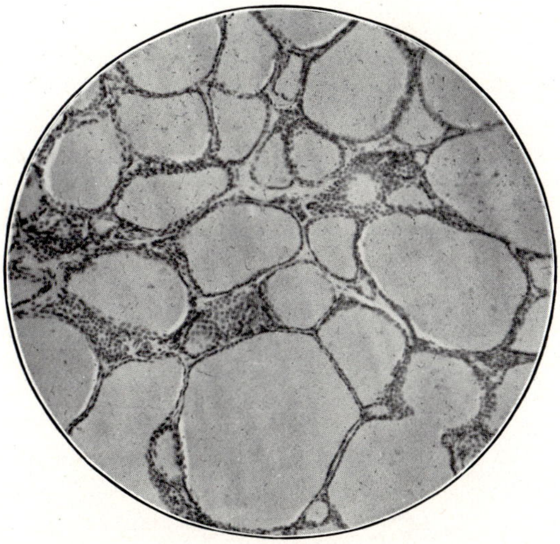

Fig. 1.—Normal human thyroid. Note the uniform colloid; the low cuboidal epithelium; the scanty stroma; the small, rounded follicles.

4. In the correlation of the clinical manifestations of goiter with the anatomical findings the probability has not been borne in mind that the thyroid changes are the result of a systemic disturbance instead of the cause of the systemic disturbance.

5. It does not seem possible at the present time to distinguish or to separate, solely by anatomical studies, those thyroid hyperplasias which should be considered as tumors from those which should be designated as physiological or compensatory hyperplasias. This fact is implied in the use of such terms as "adenomatous" or "adeno-parenchymatous goiters."

6. The thyroid undergoes exceedingly rapid histological changes the causes for which are still ill understood. Thus an active hyperplasia with high columnar epithelium and no stainable colloid may change to

a colloid gland with low cubical epithelium and abundant colloid in from two to three weeks.

All these factors introduce grave difficulties in the way of establishing the major and fundamental types of thyroid changes. Nevertheless, by the utilization of material from human autopsies and from the lower

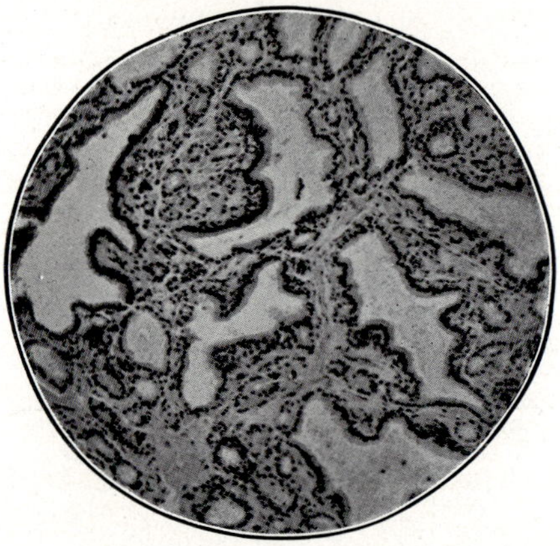

Fig. 2.—Marked glandular hyperplasia (human). Note the reduced colloid; the high columnar epithelium; the increased stroma; the enlarged and irregular follicles.

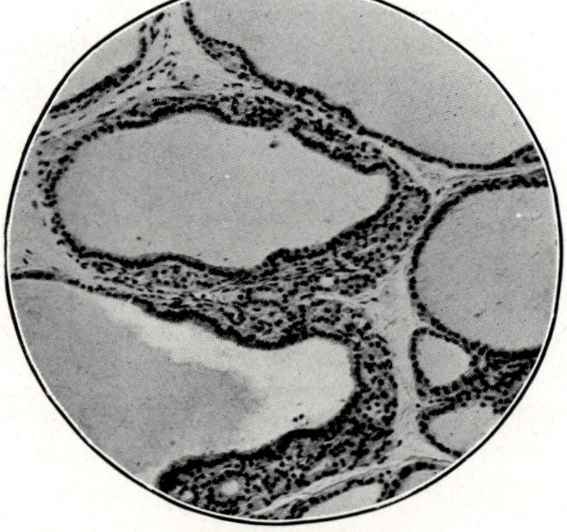

Fig. 3.—Colloid-moderate glandular hyperplasia, i. e., a hyperplasia occurring on an old colloid goiter. Note the slightly reduced colloid; the high columnar epithelium; the increased stroma, the enlarged follicles.

animals, together with our present accumulation of experimental data, it is possible to overcome the major difficulties and to separate the essential and major types of anatomical changes from the minor and secondary changes which thyroids in common with other tissues may undergo.

## CLASSIFICATION

The classification which we present has already appeared in outline,[2] but only those divisions concerned with the development of goiter were discussed in detail. Here we shall give connected, though necessarily brief, descriptions of all the individual divisions. These descriptions embody the results obtained from our anatomical material, both comparative and human, together with conceptions gained from our experimental observations with many animal species from fish to man.

Throughout all the work we have made mention of the general similarity of the various types of changes in the several animal groups studied; this we wish again to emphasize.

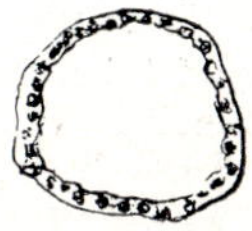

Fig. 4.—Diagrammatic sketch of normal follicle.

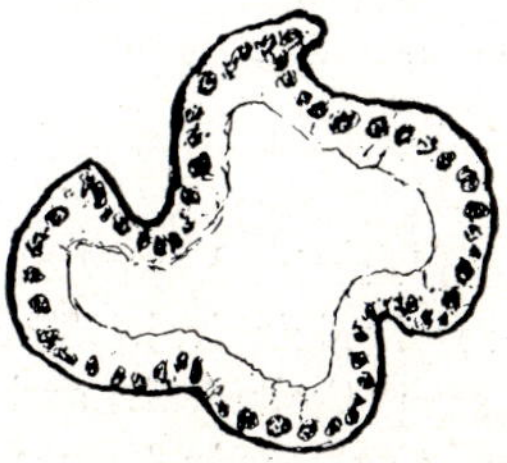

Fig. 5.—Diagrammatic sketch of actively hyperplastic follicle originating from the normal follicle.

The classification follows:

I. Normal Thyroid.
II. Active Hypertrophies and Hyperplasias (goiter).[3]
  1. Developing from the normal thyroid.
  2. Developing from the colloid gland (goiter).
III. Colloid Glands (Goiters).
IV. Regeneration (Hyperplasias).

---

2. Marine and Lenhart: Relation of Iodin to the Structure of Human Thyroid, etc., The Archives Int. Med., 1909, iv, 440.

3. The term "goiter," being clinical, embraces several anatomical groups. These different groups represent different "stages" in the common process and it is therefore important to establish the sequence and logical order of these anatomical changes. In this way one can eliminate many of the terms now in use by demonstrating that they represent only minor or accidental changes. For the physiological stages of goiter this has been established.

V. Atrophies:
  1. Premature atrophies
    (a) of obesity
    (b) of cretinism
    (c) of myxedema
  2. Senile
VI. Degenerations:
  1. Hyaline
  2. Amyloid
  3. Calcareous, etc.
VII. Inflammations:
  1. Acute thyroiditis
  2. Chronic thyroiditis
VIII. Tumors:
  1. Benign
    (a) Fetal adenoma
    (b) Simple adenoma
  2. Malignant
    (a) Carcinoma from fetal adenoma (carcinoma simplex)
    (b) Glandular carcinoma
    (c) Sarcoma
    (d) Endothelioma
IX. Complications:
  1. Hemorrhage
  2. Cyst formation
    (a) From hemorrhage
    (b) From fetal adenoma

We have made nine major anatomical divisions, in the belief that they represent different physiological or pathological stages. The first four divisions, viz., normal thyroid, active hypertrophy or hyperplasia, colloid gland and regeneration, are physiological. The remaining five divisions are properly designated as pathological, and are only the generally accepted groupings common to all body tissues.

In the broadest conception, there are no anatomical changes seen in the thyroid which have not their counterpart in other tissues. The anatomical changes accompanying both physiological and pathological processes are pronounced in the case of the thyroid, while in the case of some other tissues as the brain, striped muscle, liver, kidney, etc., functional variations are accompanied by comparatively slight anatomical changes. This, however, is only the visible expression of the wider range or cycle of functional adaptability with which the thyroid, and blood and lymphatic tissues as well, are endowed.

Just as there is no group of anatomical changes specific for the thyroid, so one may also add that there is as yet no evidence of any disease entity, with the possible exception of tumor, arising in and due primarily to changes in the thyroid. All the data at present available indicate that the thyroid changes, with whatever symptom-complex associated, are secondary to, and the result of, some more general systemic disturbance (probably nutritional).[3]

## I. NORMAL THYROID

The wide variations in the functional activity and the corresponding anatomical variations make it difficult specifically to define the normal thyroid. But, aside from these differences clearly dependent on physiological variations, histologists generally are in agreement in regard to the limitations of normal structure. The normal gland must always be the base line or point of departure, and without a definition of the limits of normal variations one cannot have a clear conception of the departures from normal. For this reason, then, we consider the normal thyroid the most important of the nine groups.

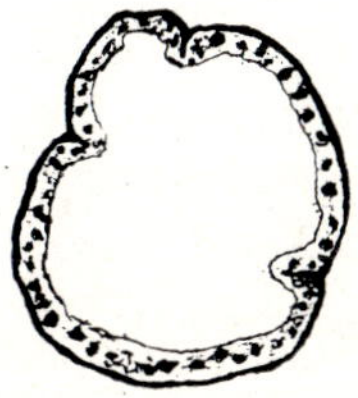

Fig. 6.—Diagrammatic sketch of colloid involution of an actively hyperplastic follicle. Compare with the normal follicle (Fig. 4).

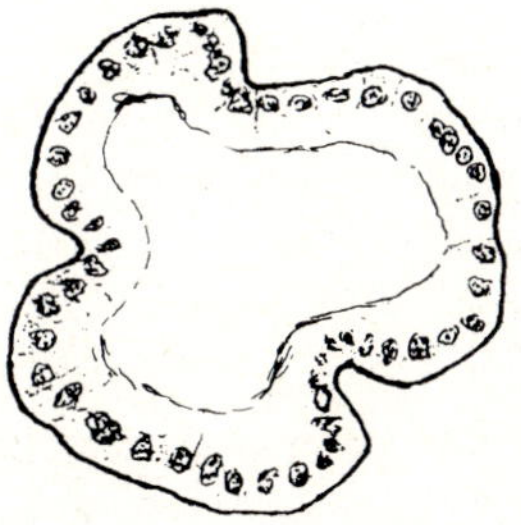

Fig. 7.—Diagrammatic sketch of an actively hyperplastic follicle originating from the colloid follicle (Fig. 6).

The weight of the normal thyroid in all animals studied, from fish to man, is the lowest and represents the smallest amount of thyroid tissue compatible with normal body functions. The normal adult human thyroid weighs between 20 and 27 gm. (This applies to the seacoast type. It is lower than the weight usually stated. There can be no doubt that in goitrous districts much larger glands are considered as normal, although from our experiments and observations we believe that all such glands have at one or more times shown hypertrophic changes, and if the histological examination shows any evidence to that effect, we class them as colloid glands.) The lateral lobes are in general symmetrical and of uniform size, though slight variations are common. The isthmus is

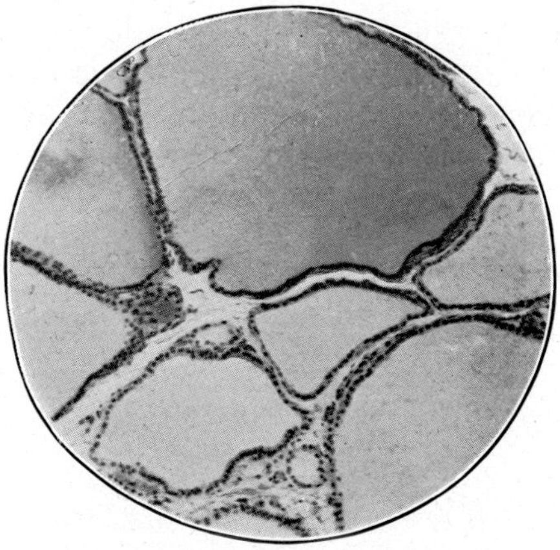

Fig. 8.—Colloid goiter (human). Note the enlarged follicles; the low cuboidal epithelium; the uniform colloid; the slightly increased stroma.

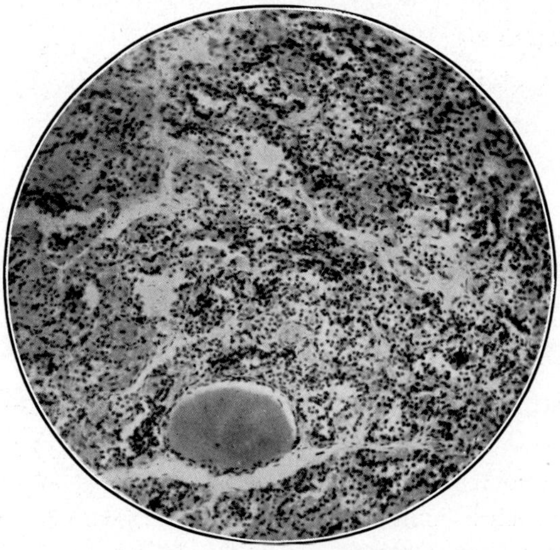

Fig. 9.—Senile atrophy. Note the disappearance of recognizable follicles; the occurrence of old desiccated colloid masses in atrophic follicles; the hyaline transformation of the stroma.

rarely absent, while the pyramidal portion is variable as to its presence, shape and size. The entire gland is invested in an outer fibrous areolar capsule, which strips easily, leaving a slightly lobulated smooth surface. The inner or proper capsule is thin and translucent. Thickened portions (trabeculæ) of the true capsule, constituting the stroma, extend into the gland, mark out the lobules and support the blood-vessels and lymph-vessels. In some lower vertebrates, including the bony fish, the gland has no capsule. The color of the thyroid is similar in all animals examined, and varies from a pale amber red to a bright amber red. The consistency is firm and somewhat elastic. On section the follicles can be distinguished with the naked eye in all the larger mammals. They vary considerably in size, although the normal follicles vary the least, and measurements of from 0.3 to 0.8 mm. would include most of the follicles of

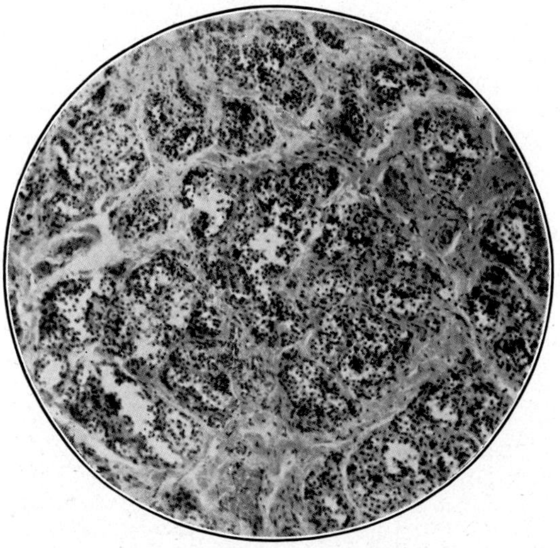

Fig. 10.—Premature atrophy (cretinoid) of childhood. Note the generalized increase in the stroma; the compressed follicles; the desquamation and perhaps piling up of the epithelial elements; the absence of colloid.

the normal human thyroid. All the follicles are filled with clear, amber yellow, viscid colloid, which gives to the thyroid its specific characteristic.

The microscopical appearance of the thyroid unit—the alveolus or follicle—is similar in all animals from fish to man. The follicles are in general round or oval, closed spaces lined with a single layer of low cuboidal or at most cuboidal epithelium. (High cuboidal or columnar epithelium always indicates hypertrophy.) The cells are quite regular in size although one can often distinguish the so-called "chief" and "colloid" cells described by Langendorff and others. Whether there is any difference in the physiological activity of these cells is doubtful. They

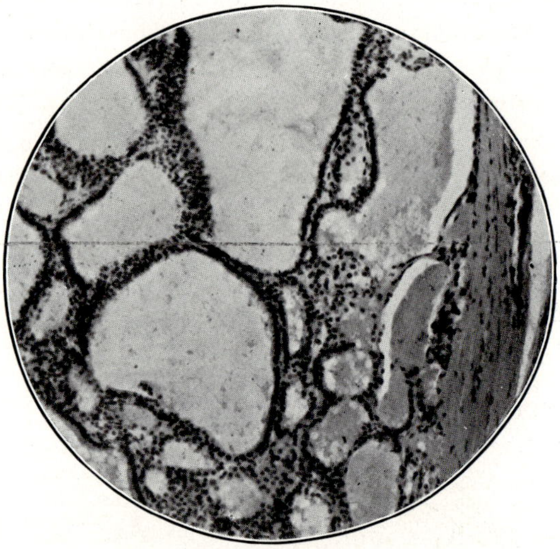

Fig. 11.—Simple adenoma. Note the well-differentiated tissue; the capsule; the reduced colloid; the irregular-sized follicles; the low columnar epithelium.

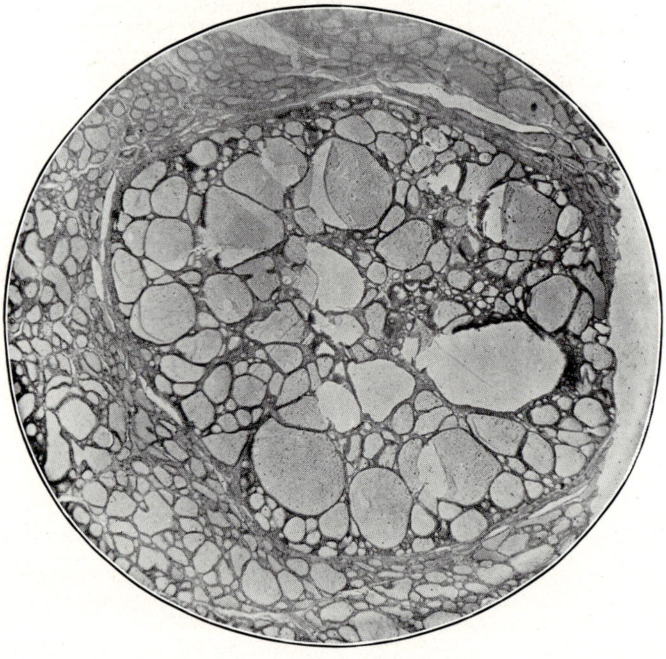

Fig. 12.—Low magnification to show a circumscribed and encapsulated mass of thyroid hyperplasia which reacted with iodin just as the surrounding hyperplasia with resulting colloid gland.

probably represent different stages of secretory activity of the same cells. The nuclei are small, basal and vesicular. The colloid lies in contact with the free border of the epithelial cells and completely fills the follicle save for an occasional vacuole-like area. It is homogeneous and following metallic or alcoholic fixation stains deeply with acid dyes. The colloid of adjacent follicles may not stain with the same intensity and colloid-like material is frequently to be seen in the lymphatic spaces—an observation usually taken as anatomical evidence that the lymphatics form the normal paths of exit for the colloid.[4] The blood and lymph capillaries form richly anastomosing networks about each follicle and give to the thyroid tissue a relatively larger blood-supply than any other body tissue.

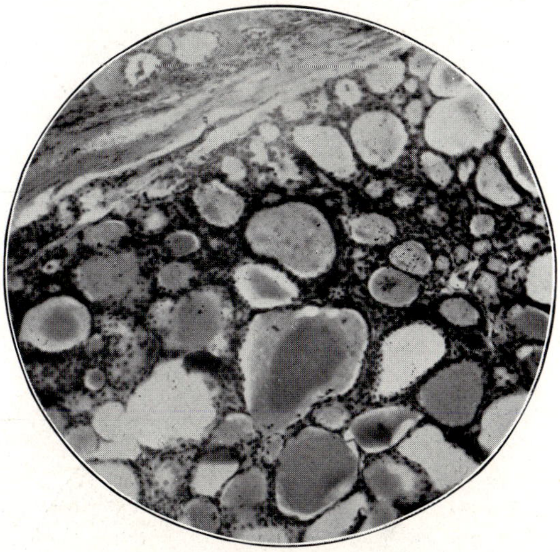

Fig. 13.—Adenoma representing intermediate type between fetal adenoma on one hand and simple adenoma on the other; note the capsule, the small follicles and the colloid.

## II. ACTIVE HYPERPLASIAS (GOITERS)[5]

### 1. *Primary*

### (Hyperplasia Developing from the Normal Gland)

As a result of increased physiological activity, from whatever cause and in whatever animal, the thyroid undergoes changes characterized by

4. Carlson and Woelfel (Am. Jour. Physiol., 1910, xxvi, 32) were unable to obtain any physiological evidence that the lymphatics form the paths of exit of the secretion. Hunt and Seidell (Jour. Pharmacol. and Exper. Therap., 1910, ii, 15) have aptly pointed out that Carlson's findings with such methods in no way disprove the view that the thyroid secretion passes out by the way of the lymphatics.

5. "Active" is used to distinguish this, the growing stage, from the colloid or quiescent stage.

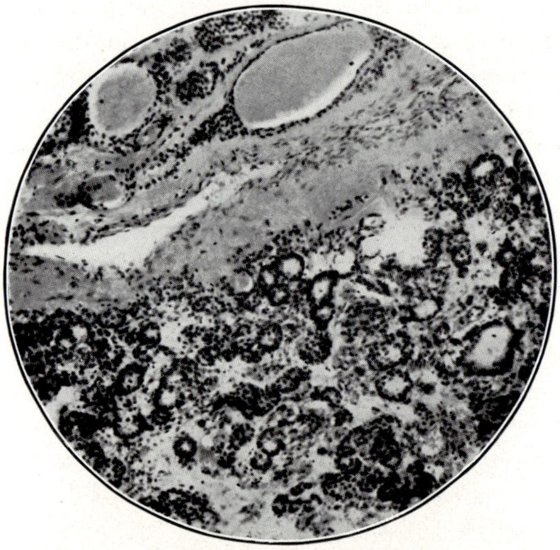

Fig. 14.—Adenoma of intermediate type but closely approximating the true fetal adenoma. Note the capsule with the tumor tissue on one side and the original thyroid on the other side.

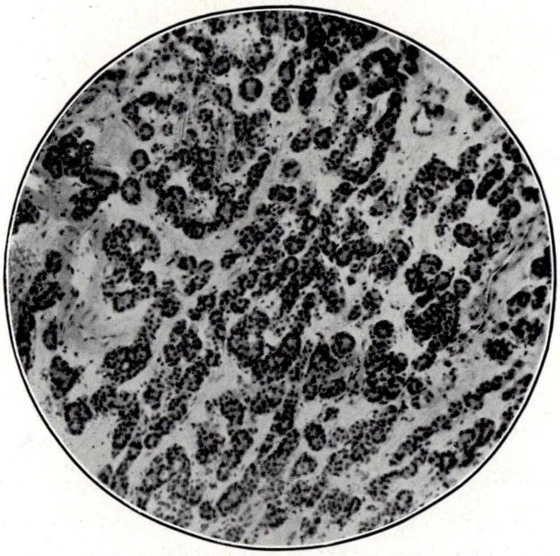

Fig. 15.—True fetal adenoma. Section taken from central part of tumor where follicles are more separated. Note size, shape and arrangement of follicles, the lining epithelium and the absence of colloid.

a general increase in its blood-supply, a general decrease in the stainable colloid and a general change from cuboidal to columnar epithelium. If these changes continue to the stage of cell proliferation, the condition is properly designated as hyperplasia. There are all degrees of the abnormal cell growth from the slightest departure from normal (hypertrophy) to the marked proliferation (hyperplasia).

Hyperplasia is the anatomical evidence of increased physiological activity of the gland, and the instances in which visible goiters appear are only accidents, so to speak, since the great majority of all hyperplasias in all animals never reach that degree of proliferation which could be clinically diagnosed as goiter. Clinically, therefore, goiter is relatively rare, while anatomically it is extremely common if one uses the term "goiter," as we believe it should be used, in its anatomical-pathological sense. All

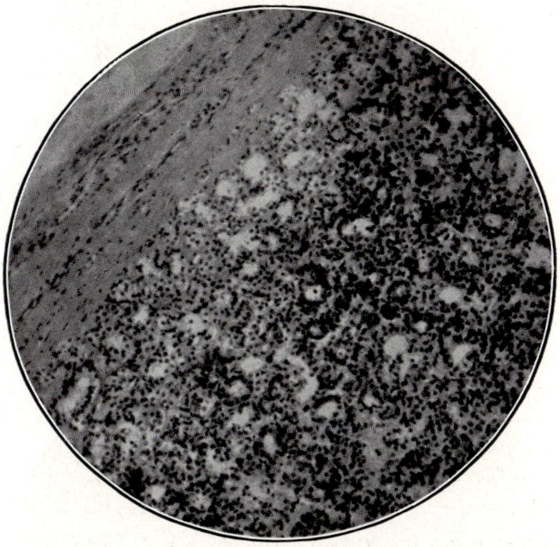

Fig. 16.—True fetal adenoma showing relation to capsule.

these degrees of hyperplasia are to be considered as stages in the common process of goiter development. In previous publications[6] we have emphasized the great frequency of active hyperplasia in dogs, sheep, cattle, hogs, fish and man.

Tracing the development of hypertrophy and hyperplasia from the normal gland, the first change noticed in the thyroid is its increased blood-supply. The capsular vessels dilate and hypertrophy and become tortuous. The capillaries surrounding the follicles are dilated. The gland becomes larger, softer and takes on a brighter red color. Micro-

6. Marine and Williams: The Archives Int. Med., 1908, i, 349. Marine and Lenhart, ibid., 1909, iii, 66; 1909, iv, 440; Jour. Exper. Med., 1910, xii, 311.

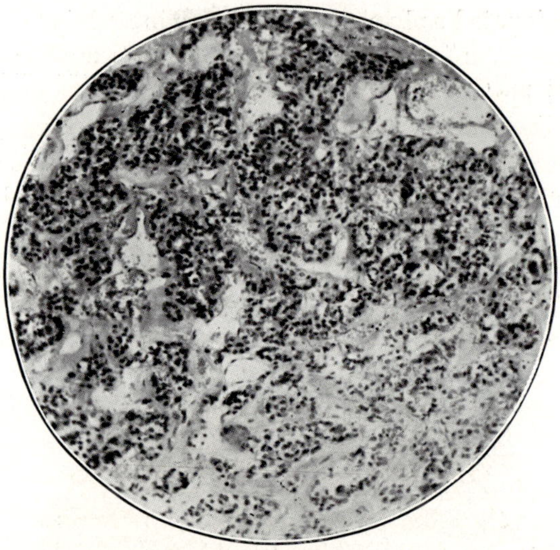

Fig. 17.—Fetal adenoma undergoing degeneration; note the broad hyalinized stroma bands, the distorted follicles, the swollen and degenerating epithelial cells. Histologically it somewhat resembles carcinoma.

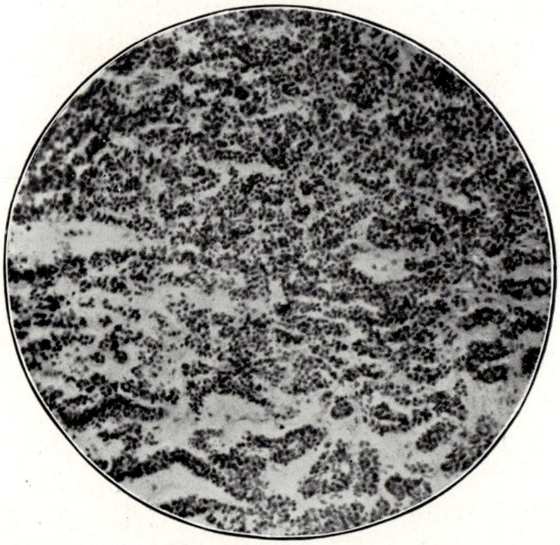

Fig. 18.—Carcinoma with metastases. Fetal adenoma type. Difficult of differentiation from fetal adenoma histologically.

scopically there is lessening of the stainable colloid, at first but palely staining; later vacuolization and finally actual disappearance of the true colloid, its place being taken by a granular albuminous débris in which may be seen leukocytes and shed epithelial cells. As the colloid disappears the epithelial cells change from the normal cuboidal to high cuboidal, to columnar and finally to high columnar. With the disappearance of the colloid and the growth in size and number of epithelial cells, the color of the gland changes from the normal—amber red—to reddish translucency, to grayish red and finally to the soft, fleshy, gray red and opaque color of the marked hyperplasia as is classically seen in developing exophthalmic goiter. As true hyperplasia of the epithelial cells takes place, the follicles enlarge, and infoldings and plications of the lining epithe-

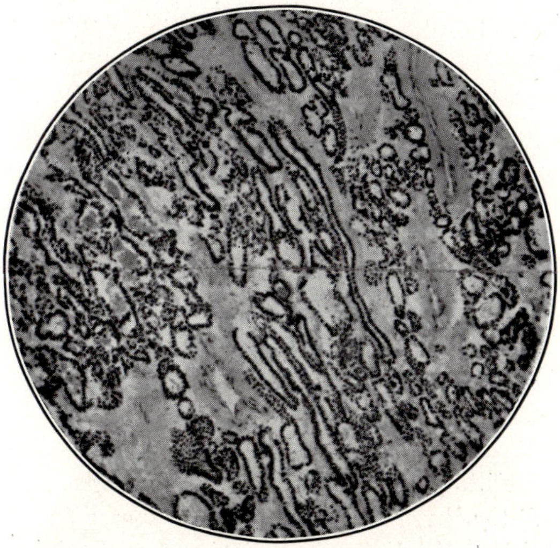

Fig. 19.—Carcinoma with lung metastases showing some differentiation. Follicles tend to grow out in tubules. Some stainable colloid.

lium begin to appear in all encapsulated thyroids. These infoldings are less marked in non-encapsulated glands, as in the bony fish.

The gland capsule and stroma hypertrophy parallel with the epithelial proliferation and the increased blood-supply. In the early stages of hyperplasia this hypertrophy is slight, while it may be unusually prominent in the late stages, especially of exophthalmic goiter, as will be discussed more fully under "Atrophies."

In the advanced stages of active hyperplasia and notably in exophthalmic goiter there are scattered throughout the stroma smaller or larger groups of lymphoid cells. These groups of lymphocytes are interpreted by some observers as evidence of a chronic inflammatory process, while others look on them as the local manifestation of the general lymphoid hyperplasia that is so commonly associated with thyroid hyperplasia. The latter view would appear to be the more logical, as these lymph foci are never seen in the thyroid apart from a systemic lymphoid hyperplasia.

### 2. *Secondary*

### (Hyperplasia Developing from Colloid Glands)

Active hyperplasias developing from colloid glands are not essentially different from those developing from normal glands. Their interpretation offers more difficulties on account of the wider range of possible morphological changes and the more complicated life-history. It is rare to find secondary hyperplasias free from other morphological changes, while with primary hyperplasias this is the rule. The extent of these additional changes, such as hemorrhage, cyst formation, degeneration, enlarged follicles, etc., depends on the duration of the thyroid enlargement, the number of times hyperplasia and involution to the colloid state have occurred, and on many other minor factors as trauma, treatment, pregnancy, locality, intercurrent diseases, food, etc.

We have often seen the statement: "It is difficult to understand why some goiters have large colloid cysts while others do not." The explanation for this is simple, and may be represented graphically, as in Figures 4 to 7. These diagrams illustrate the fundamental point in the interpretation of the so-called "cystic goiters" or "papillary cystic goiters." Simply stated, then, our studies have led us to believe that all goiters with enlarged colloid follicles are the result of previous periods of hyperplasia alternating with periods of more or less complete return to the colloid state. These secondary hyperplasias, or hyperplasias developing from colloid glands, are illustrated clinically in the so-called "secondary exophthalmic goiters," the thyroid enlargements of succeeding pregnancies, the enlargements with succeeding menstruations, or finally, in any thyroid which has undergone hyperplasia and involution more than once. Each period of active hyperplasia as a rule further enlarges the follicles, since follicles, once enlarged, do not return again to their original size, although in all cases they tend to do so and most cases do become somewhat smaller as the active hyperplasia returns to the colloid or quiescent state.

The important anatomical changes are similar to those occurring in the primary hyperplasias and are found in the blood-vessels, colloid and epithelium. The blood-supply is increased. The stainable colloid is lessened, but slightly in the milder degrees, while it may be entirely absent in the marked degrees of hyperplasia. The epithelium changes from cuboidal to high cuboidal, and finally, to high columnar. These changes are not so uniform throughout the gland as in primary hyperplasias. The reasons for this are simple. It means that a human thyroid rarely completes the cycle of hyperplasia and involution without accompanying complications such as calcification, endarteritis, hemorrhage, lymph obstructions, etc., which interfere with or modify the tissue's activity. This is commonly observed in all long-standing goiters. It is well known that in all goiters regeneration is most marked in the peripheral zone, and Ribbert[7] was the first observer to point out that in the experimental regenerations of dogs' thyroids following partial removal, the changes occurred earlier in the peripheral zone. Frequently one sees large central areas, or it may be but a few follicles, that fail to join in the active hyperplasia. In such follicles or groups of follicles the epithelium may be completely atrophied leaving only the hyaline stroma about the desiccated hard colloid masses. Thus it may be seen that there are varied histological pictures presented in these secondary hyperplasias, but the process is as simple and straightforward as in the primary hyperplasias.

### III. COLLOID GLANDS (GOITER)

The pure type of colloid gland may be defined as that anatomical state of the thyroid which is present when an actively hyperplastic gland ceases further growth and returns to the condition nearest normal that such a gland can assume. True colloid glands are physiologically normal and only anatomically abnormal. The extent of the abnormality depends on the size of the gland, the size of the follicles, the number of times the gland has undergone hyperplasia and involution. There are all grades of the colloid glands depending on the degree of active hyperplasia preceding the involution. Thus, if only an hypertrophy has preceded the involution it would be difficult or impossible to distinguish such a gland from normal. We have called such glands "normal-colloid" in order to complete the picture of the process, although practically these glands would be considered as normal. The opinion is often expressed that colloid glands are the result of passive dilatation of the follicles, which in turn is due to some obstruction of the paths of exit for the colloid. Our experience has led us to believe that this process is not the common or usual mode of origin of colloid glands; it is our opinion that the process of thyroid enlargement is always initiated as an active hyperplasia.

Colloid glands (goiters) are often classified as "cystic degenerations." In pure form they have nothing in common with "degeneration," as this term is ordinarily used in pathology. They are properly classified as involutions or physiological atrophies, since they are capable of all the biological reactions of the normal gland so far as these are at present known. In man pure types of colloid gland (goiter) are rarely available, for several reasons, among which may be mentioned the longer life-history, treatment, trauma, etc. Colloid glands (goiters) may be produced experimentally in from two to three weeks by giving small doses of iodin

7. Ribbert: Virchow's Arch. f. path. Anat., 1889, cxvii, 151.

to animals with active hyperplasias. Their spontaneous production, while tending to take place in all active hyperplasias, extends over months or years, depending on age, sex, locality, treatment, etc.

Pure colloid glands (goiters) are not essentially different, anatomically, in any animal thus far studied, from fish to man. They differ essentially from normal glands in all these animals only in size (although as has been pointed out this may not be a means of differentiation), and in showing the vestiges of previous hyperplasia. The prominence of these vestiges in any given specimen depends on the degree and duration of the preceding hyperplasia and the length of time since the involution occurred. They are most evident in the quickly induced involutions from marked hyperplasias. These changes are to be found in the size and shape of the follicles, in the presence of sprig-like projections into the follicles in the more recent involutions, in the blood and lymph-vessels, and in the capsule and stroma. The epithelium is normal (cuboidal). The stroma is increased, although there are exceptions to this statement, depending on the extent of the fibrosis occurring during the stage of active hyperplasia and the extent of its absorption, which normally occurs during the process of involution. The thickened thyroid capsule is likewise an inheritance from the preceding hyperplasia. The arterial walls are always thickened and tortuous, and histologically show an obliterating endarteritis similar to that seen in the involuting uterus or thymus. Calcification is very common in these thickened walls and even the vein walls may contain calcareous deposits. The most striking gross change in the veins and lymph-trunks is the great lessening in their caliber. This is associated with some thickening of their walls. The stainable colloid, like the epithelium, is normal in appearance and distribution in the follicles. The follicles are in general much larger than in normal glands, but their size depends on the degree of active hyperplasia preceding the involution and perhaps on other minor factors as duration of the process of involution, mechanical obstruction, etc.

Briefly summing up the discussion of the three divisions of normal, actively hyperplastic and colloid glands, we have attempted to emphasize their relative importance, their sequential relations and their anatomical characteristics. We have pointed out that the difficulties to be overcome in reducing these changes to three major divisions arise from the fact that several types of morphological changes are frequently combined in the same gland. The physiological processes which start these changes are comparatively simple, and by using them as guides one can avoid the confusion which has arisen from attaching separate names to each histological variation, irrespective of its relative importance.

IV. REGENERATION

The thyroid cells are well endowed with the power of growth and division. It is one of the best adapted of mammalian tissues for the demonstration of physiological cell growth and division. Halsted[8] was the first to demonstrate clearly this marked characteristic of the thyroid in the dog and since then it has been found true for all animals examined. Regeneration follows partial removal or partial destruction of the gland from any cause. No sharp line of separation can be made between the spontaneous active hyperplasia (goiter) and regeneration either anatomically or physiologically. Both are associated with growth and division of the cells and we believe both are compensatory processes. If any differentiation were possible it would be to restrict the term "regeneration" to the cell growth following partial removal or partial destruction of the gland. Some observers have stated that regeneration ceases when the gland reaches its normal volume, but this is of little aid, since the amount of thyroid normally needed by the organism cannot be measured quantitatively for the reason that the smallest number of thyroid cells capable of performing the thyroid functions under favorable conditions of environment and nutrition is so small as compared with the degree of thyroid proliferation that may occur under unfavorable conditions of environment or nutrition. In other words, the amount of thyroid depends on the physiological requirements of the animal, and these may be altered by a variety of means.

The histological characteristics of regeneration are identical with those described under "Hyperplasias." The process is initiated as an enlargement of the existing cells from the normal cuboidal to columnar. As cell division takes place, infoldings and plications of the lining epithelium occur. There is a disappearance of the colloid and the blood-supply increases. Under normal and constant environment, cell growth ceases when the physiological balance is attained, and then the hyperplastic tissue slowly returns to the colloid or quiescent state. Normal gland growth occurs without any departure from the normal histological structure, as can be demonstrated experimentally in pups with the use of iodin, while in either regeneration or spontaneous hyperplasia the above-described cycle of changes occur.

The rapidity of the process of regeneration depends on the known factors of age, the amount of gland removed, the iodin content, and most certainly on other factors probably of the nature of chemical coordination with which we are not as yet familiar.

Summing up, it may be stated that regeneration is a compensatory and reparative process which is identical anatomically and probably physiologically as well, with the spontaneous hyperplasias (goiters). Separa-

8. Halsted: Johns Hopkins Hosp. Rep., 1896, i, 373.

tion of regeneration from spontaneous hyperplasia in the light of our present knowledge is impossible and unjustified for reasons other than completeness, convenience and clearness of description.

## V. ATROPHIES

### 1. *Senile Atrophy*

The thyroid is physiologically active throughout the life of the organism. This activity is most pronounced during youth and early adult life and gradually lessens with age. The senile thyroid is reduced in size—sometimes by half its original volume. This reduction in volume is due mainly to the epithelial and colloid losses. The gland is firmer to the touch. The vessels undergo sclerosis, which is frequently accompanied by calcification. The stroma is relatively prominent. The follicles are smaller and more irregular in size. The epithelial cells are less uniform in size and shape. Desquamation is the rule. The nuclei lose their uniform, rounded, vesicular form and become irregular in size, shape and staining intensity. These changes are commonly associated with other secondary changes, as scar formation, pigment of hemorrhagic origin both in the stroma and in the colloid, small cysts often containing cholesterin, calcification, etc., indicating the wide range of physiological activity and the complicated life-history.

### 2. *Colloid Glands*

Mention may be made of colloid glands (goiters) since they are slightly related to the atrophies. Their relation to atrophy lies in the fact that they represent the quiescent state following a period of hyperactivity, but as this atrophy ceases when the stage of normal activity is reached such a process is better designated as "involution."

### 3. *Atrophies From Disease*

Mild degrees of atrophy of the senile type are sometimes seen in certain chronic wasting diseases, as tuberculosis in particular, also in marasmus, diabetes, cancer, etc.

### 4. *Premature Atrophies*

A. Often in cases of young obese individuals and practically constantly in the special form of obesity described by Dercum, one finds well-marked atrophic changes of the myxedema type. It is a widely held opinion that there is a definite relationship between the thyroid atrophy and the clinical symptom-complex.

B. The atrophy seen in endemic cretinism and myxedema is a special form, in that it occurs in association with or supervenes on active hyperplasia of the gland. In other words, it is a form of atrophy occurring despite the attempts of the gland cells to regenerate, and is best regarded as the result of sustained thyroid activity without intervening periods of physiological rest. Whether these changes result from some toxin acting directly on the cells, or whether it is an exhaustion from overwork consequent on a lack or deficiency of some element of nutrition needed by the organism, is not established, although the evidence favors the latter view. Thus in cretin pups we have been able to cause the atypical columnar thyroid cells to return to a cuboidal form with the accumulation of colloid in the follicles, by the administration of small doses of iodin, and later, by partial removal, to cause these cells to grow and divide regularly.

Seventy-five per cent. of all cretins have clinically enlarged thyroids, and, if careful anatomical examinations could be made before the clinical manifestations of cretinism supervened, there can be little doubt that a well-marked active hyperplasia would be found in all cases in which thyroid tissue was present. It would thus seem that the same nutritional deficiency or disturbance which causes the thyroid cells at first to grow and divide, later causes their death when their work and growth energy is exhausted. This process is more evident in myxedema, in which the age of the individual allows earlier detection through more careful observations during the early or developmental stage. Thus exophthalmic goiter is the most frequent forerunner of myxedema in adults and doubtless, as Ord[9] has pointed out, all cases of myxedema are preceded by an active thyroid hyperplasia with or without the symptom-complex of exophthalmic goiter. Again, it appears certain that the same deficiency which causes the thyroid to react with cell proliferation will, if unrelieved, finally induce the death of these cells from exhaustion. Just as there is anatomical overlapping, so to speak, between hyperplasia and atrophy, so also there is clinical overlapping. Thus the exophthalmic goiter symptom-complex frequently coexists with the myxedema symptom-complex.

The anatomical changes in cretinism and myxedema are similar. Taking a typical case of myxedema following exophthalmic goiter, the anatomical changes are briefly as follows: there is usually a history of the gland becoming smaller and perhaps somewhat firmer to the touch. It is still very vascular. The colloid is practically absent. The epithelial cells have lost their regular and uniform columnar type characteristic of the early stage of active hyperplasia and are irregular in size and shape. There is perhaps some piling up of the epithelial cells and desquamation of the partially degenerated cells. The nuclei are in general large, often hyperchromatic and irregular in size and outline. Nuclear figures are still observed, but the new formation of cells is not sufficient to offset the cell-death, and the follicles become smaller, though still preserving the infoldings of the well-developed hyperplasia. The surrounding fibrous stroma is relatively, perhaps absolutely, increased, and as the

9. Ord: Brit. Med. Jour., 1898, ii, 1473.

follicles become smaller from the death of their secreting cells the fibrous bands appear wider, and finally give the appearance of a generalized cirrhosis in which are nests of compressed epithelial cells with or without the outlines of follicles. This interstitial cirrhosis is secondary to and consequent on the death of the epithelial elements. Lymphoid foci are scattered here and there throughout the stroma. Milder types of these changes are frequently seen in exophthalmic goiter[10] when there is but little clinical suspicion of developing myxedema. This is the simplest picture of the anatomical changes in the thyroid in myxedema, and those occurring in the cretin thyroid are similar. Most cases, either of myxedema or of cretinism, in man do not present so simple an anatomical picture for the reason that other processes as cyst formation, hemorrhage, calcification, adenoma, groups of enlarged follicles filled with desiccated colloid, etc., may all be crowded into the same gland.

Summing up, then, the type of atrophy supervening on active hyperplasias and clinically associated with myxedema or cretinism is a cell-death due to exhaustion from overwork and malnutrition. The process is simple, but the anatomical changes in such glands, especially in long-standing cases, are often highly complex. This type of atrophy, we believe, is the usual end stage of all active hyperplasias unless terminated by death or recovery of the individual, and considering the total number of active hyperplasias from all causes and in all animals, it is a rare sequel.

## VI. DEGENERATIONS

In thyroid histopathology the term "degeneration" has been loosely used. Thus one often meets such terms as "colloid," "hemorrhagic," "fibroid" or "cystic degeneration." We believe its use should be limited to the commonly accepted types of degeneration or infiltration, such as hyaline, calcareous, amyloid, parenchymatous, fatty, etc.

Hyaline transformation of both the vessel-walls and the stroma accompanies normal senile atrophy. It is especially seen in the stroma

10. Mac Callum, W. G. (Jour. Am. Med. Assn., 1907, ii, 1158, 1160) has made specific mention of these changes in certain cases of exophthalmic goiter occurring in Professor Halsted's clinic at the Johns Hopkins Hospital but attempted no explanation. His description is as follows: "It is in these extreme cases that peculiar alterations in the epithelial cells are sometimes found. In several instances we have observed areas in which the epithelium was enormously swollen so as to practically obliterate the lumen of the alveolus. These large irregular cells no longer preserve the columnar form but are shapeless masses of finely granular protoplasm which take an intense pink stain with the eosin, and in which the nuclei are also irregular in form and size and stain very deeply, almost black, with hematoxylin. Usually one or two alveoli only show such a change in their epithelium; or there may be only a few cells of this form intercalated among others of the usual type in the alveolar wall, but sometimes over considerable areas all the alveoli are packed with such cells. Their significance is far from clear."

of long-standing colloid goiters with marked arterial changes and in the interior of old fetal adenomata, giving a yellowish color to the cut surface. Microscopically, the stroma becomes thicker and stains homogeneously so that the thyroid follicles may appear as rings of epithelial cells embedded in a hyaline matrix with but few blood-vessels remaining and no recognizable basement membranes.

Calcareous deposits are of frequent occurrence in human goiters, and are particularly to be seen in the capsule and stroma, vessel-walls, the scars of old hemorrhages, in cyst walls or in the interior of fetal adenomata. The deposits may be very extensive and particularly in scar tissue may take the structure of bone. Such conditions have given rise to the terms, "calcareous and osseous goiter."

Amyloid degeneration is usually observed in connection with similar deposits in other organs but may occur independently,[11] particularly in the benign tumors.

Cloudy swelling has not, to our knowledge, been included among the thyroid lesions. It has seemed to us in the examination of many glands from individuals dead of acute intoxications that the condition usually designated as "toxic reaction" is analogous to the cloudy swelling of such tissues as the kidney epithelium, the hepatic cells, or the muscle cells. The anatomical changes are hyperemia, enlargement and granulation of the cytoplasm of the epithelial cells with corresponding nuclear enlargement, loss of colloid substance and perhaps desquamation. In extreme cases the epithelial cells have ragged, granular free borders, as if undergoing disintegration. We have looked on these changes as the anatomical evidence of increased functional activity of the thyroid and the precursor of true hypertrophy and hyperplasia if the tissue is able to cope with the intoxication, or of thyroid atrophy if it be overwhelmed by it. (See "Inflammation.")

All these types may be present in the same gland, while hyaline and calcareous changes are commonly associated.

## VII. INFLAMMATIONS: THYROIDITIS, STRUMITIS

The infectious theory of goiter gave origin to the view that all true goiters were chronic inflammatory reactions. This conclusion is based on the occurrence of a general increase in fibrous tissue, which, as already pointed out under "Atrophies," may practically replace all the epithelial elements, and the occurrence of foci of lymphocytes and scattered small round cells in the stroma. The connective tissue increase is more rationally explained as part of the general thyroid reaction during active hyperplasia and its persistence after the epithelial elements have died. The foci of lymphocytes are, as already suggested, the local manifestations of

11. Stoffel: Virchows Arch. f. path. Anat., 1910, cci, 245.

the general systemic lymphoid hyperplasia which accompanies the thyroid hyperplasia. Wandering cells, and sometimes plasma cells, may be seen in the stroma about cysts, hemorrhagic or degenerated areas, and are most likely present because of the local irritation.

True inflammatory reactions are rare. They are never primary. Many of the so-called acute forms of thyroiditis are scarcely more than active hyperemias or cloudy swellings. These conditions are not infrequently seen in food intoxications, drug rashes, intestinal exanthems and following skin burns, syphilis, etc.[12]

Suppurative thyroiditis may occur in the course of puerperal infections, ulcerative endocarditis, scarlet fever, measles, typhoid fever, influenza, pneumonia, tonsillitis, etc., and may be the result of extension from adjacent tissues as well as originating within the gland. It occurs more frequently in thyroids which have undergone goitrous enlargement or which contain tumors. Injuries, as in the old iron or iodin injections, were frequently followed by areas of necrosis and abscess formation. In generalized tuberculosis the thyroid is commonly involved. Solitary or caseous tubercle is rare. Gummata have been reported in seventeen instances, according to Davis.[13]

## VIII. TUMORS

We are not in possession of sufficient facts to draw sharp lines between physiological hyperplasia and regeneration on the one hand and tumor growth on the other. In some tissues, such as brain, cartilage, muscle, etc., whose capacities for regeneration are more limited, the distinction can usually be made with accuracy. But in tissues whose regenerative capacities are pronounced, as bone-marrow, lymphoid tissue, thyroid, etc., the distinction is difficult indeed, and in many instances impossible at the stage when such a distinction would be of the greatest scientific value.

---

12. De Quervain (Mitt. a. d. Grenzgeb. d. Med. u. Chir., 1906, xv, 297) and Sarbach (ibid., 1906, xv, 213), however, include under the term "thyroiditis simplex" the reaction of the gland in the acute fevers. This reaction is characterized anatomically by enlargement of the gland, hypertrophy of the epithelial cells, occasionally desquamation, disappearance of the colloid and, as Aesbacher (ibid., 1906, xv, 269) and others have shown, by a lessening of the iodin content. This is the usual reaction of the gland under any increased functional demands, whether the result of known bacterial toxins, such as typhoid fever, or of unknown toxins of metabolic origin. A similar type of thyroid change is that commonly noted in chronic pulmonary tuberculosis (Roger and Garnier: Arch. gén. de méd., 1900, clxxxv, 385). Early in the disease the so-called "thyroiditis simplex" or "toxic reaction" occurs with increased functional activity of the thyroid—often even to a definite goitrous enlargement and later, as the general nutrition of the patient fails, sclerosis and atrophy supervene. In typhoid fever a toxic reaction with active thyroid hyperplasia is usual. It ordinarily subsides as the patient's nutrition improves, but under unfavorable conditions the hyperplasia may persist with manifestations of exophthalmic goiter or later of myxedema.

13. Davis: Tr. Chicago Path. Soc., 1906-09, vi, 273.

The microscope is our most accurate means of differentiation, but of late, since effort has been concentrated on the tumor problem, its limitations have become more evident. Of the tissues in the examination of which we are confronted with this difficulty, the thyroid should be given prominent consideration. Here experience has taught us that the microscope is only an aid, and that some method to augment its value must be devised in order sharply to differentiate physiological hyperplasia from true tumor. The thyroid also illustrates the danger of applying without reserve criteria true for one animal or one tissue to another animal or another tissue. Thus the thyroid of the bony fish is not encapsulated, and the appearance of invasion ordinarily strongly in favor of malignancy in localized or encapsulated tissues may be highly misleading when applied to the fish thyroid, where any growth would give the microscopical appearance of invasion. Some biological reaction must be devised to supplement the anatomical observations before we can safely say that certain growths are true tumors. This end might best be attained by taking advantage of the generally held opinion that the tumor cell during succeeding generations loses more and more of its original physiological attributes, and therefore is less and less capable of physiological function and physiological control. Evidence is being adduced that many kinds of physiological activity are controlled chemically, and that if any agency can be isolated that either physiologically increases a tissue's activity or physiologically decreases its activity, then the problem of more accurately defining tumor is by so much simplified.

In the case of the thyroid one cannot be certain whether its physiological activity results from the presence or the absence of some agent (probably chemical), but it has long been known that iodin will *lessen* the anatomical manifestations of the thyroid's activity, and since Baumann discovered its normal presence in chemical combination with thyreoglobulin, efforts have been made to define its physiological importance. The results of this work have suggested the use of iodin as a means of determining the limits of the physiological activity of the thyroid at a stage when the microscope is of slight value. To what extent iodin may serve as a physiological test for thyroid hyperplasia cannot at present be stated. We have been using the iodin reaction for some years, but progress is limited for the reason that our ordinary laboratory animals do not develop thyroid adenomata. Some light will doubtless be shed on the relation of tumor to physiological hyperplasia by utilizing the goiter material from artificially reared fish where goiters are so readily produced in large numbers.

Our observations with the iodin reaction in tumors are as yet confined to human goiter and the results will be used in the descriptions to follow. In general, we consider all hyperplasias as physiological which react with iodin in from two to six weeks.

### *1. Adenoma*

Adenomata are the most common tumors of the human thyroid. Like uterine fibromyomata, they develop during the organ's period of greatest physiological activity and are not seen apart from a general thyroid hyperplasia.

We have not observed these tumors in the thyroids of dogs, cats, sheep, pigs, horses, cattle, rabbits or guinea-pigs. They are present in nearly all long-standing human goiters. In man, two groups may be made for convenience: (A) fetal adenomata and (B) simple adenomata.

A. Fetal adenomata were so named by Billroth from their histological resemblance to the normal fetal thyroid. These tumors are usually small, frequently multiple, and may attain to the size of one's fist. They may occur in any part of the thyroid and are always rounded, completely encapsulated masses. If one examines large series of these tumors it will be found that, although the general architecture is the same, there are wide limits in the amount of colloid and the height of the epithelial cells. These changes are in general comparable to the changes seen in physiological hyperplasia. Thus these tumors have a period of active growth, followed by a period of cessation of growth, and finally pass into what might be called a colloid or resting state. This cycle of changes is similar anatomically to the cycle observed in the physiological hyperplasia but with this difference, that while iodin will constantly induce the colloid change in ordinary hyperplasia it has no manifestly similar action in the fetal adenomata. For this reason we look on these growths as tumors, but of the benign type, since after variable periods of active development they cease further growth and return to the colloid or resting state.

In the growing stage, these tumors are round, rather soft masses of highly cellular, friable tissue and grayish red in color. Histologically the tumor is composed of small, round, more or less closely packed follicles undistended with colloid, in a delicate stroma, and each follicle is lined with cuboidal or high cuboidal epithelium. This is the classical picture as described by Billroth,[14] Bloodgood[15] and others.

The colloid or resting stage is characterized in the gross by being a firm, elastic, yellowish, translucent mass. Histologically, while preserving the general architecture of the growing stage, the follicles tend to be larger; they all contain colloid; the epithelium lining the follicles is low cuboidal and the stroma compressed to thin strands, or in older tumors to hyaline bands of connective tissue.

These descriptions represent the typical growing stage and the typical resting stage. There are all intervening gradations, and in most

---

14. Billroth: Müllers Arch. f. Anat. u. Physiol., 1856, p. 144.
15. Bloodgood: Surg. Gynec. and Obst., 1906, ii, 121.

instances, additional pathological processes are present, as hyaline degeneration, calcification or cyst formation.

B. Simple adenomata include those rounded encapsulated growths composed of more differentiated thyroid tissue. They are not seen apart from a generalized active hyperplasia. Nevertheless, they are partially independent of the reactions of the generalized or physiological hyperplasia, as evidenced by the fact that one finds these areas in spontaneous colloid goiters and, while frequently affected by iodin, they are not constantly affected as are the ordinary hyperplasias. Thus these masses have many of the attributes of ordinary hyperplasia and some features common to tumors. Here is where the difficulty above mentioned arises in sharply differentiating between tumors and ordinary hyperplasia. We have tentatively called these growths "tumors," because morphologically all of them are circumscribed encapsulated masses, but it is certain that many of them should be grouped under the physiological hyperplasias.

Histologically, these masses are composed of irregular-sized follicles, often with infoldings and plications of the lining epithelium, which is columnar during the growing stage and cuboidal during the resting or colloidal stage. The stainable colloid varies as in ordinary hyperplasia with the degree of cell proliferation. Additional pathological processes, such as hyaline degeneration, hemorrhage, calcification, cyst formation, etc., occur, but less frequently than in the true fetal adenomata.

To sum up, the "fetal adenomata" group is well defined and properly classed as consisting of benign tumors. The simple adenoma group includes a rather wide list of circumscribed masses of thyroid hyperplasia which have characteristics in common with both tumor and ordinary hyperplasia. There are many gradations between the true fetal adenoma and the so-called simple adenoma, but tentatively and to avoid unnecessary confusion we believe all these growths can be classified in one or the other group.

*2. Carcinoma*

Carcinoma of the thyroid is relatively a rare tumor. The microscopical diagnosis is uncertain, since, apart from the difficulty of distinguishing between physiological hyperplasia and tumor, there is the additional factor of malignancy. The cell picture is often of little aid, and other factors, as the gross appearance of the tumor (Langhans), the clinical history, metastases, and the reaction with iodin should always be considered. One not uncommonly sees puzzling histological appearances in the premature atrophies of early myxedema and also in involuting adenomata. The same is true of the so-called thyroid cancer of fish. Although this is still disputed, the available evidence would indicate that true cancer is relatively as rare in fish goiter as in mammalian goiter.

Goiter, in some unknown way, favors the development of cancer just as it favors the development of benign tumors. Cancer developing in an otherwise normal thyroid must be exceedingly rare. Reports of such cases are to be found in the literature, as well as reports of thyroid metastases, especially in bone or lung where no evidence of a primary growth in the thyroid could be found (Cohnheim). We have never observed thyroid cancer apart from preexisting goiter, and since the histological distinction between benign tumors, ordinary hyperplasias and true cancer is an exceedingly difficult one, we are rather inclined to believe that mistakes are not uncommon.

We have seen nine cases of thyroid cancer in dogs, and were able to make experimental observations in two cases. We administered iodin and removed portions of the gland every two weeks. The cancerous tissues in both the thyroid lobes and the lung metastases were not morphologically changed by iodin, while the original simple hyperplasia was changed to the colloid state.

Human thyroid cancers may be divided anatomically into two groups (1) in which the growth has more of the characteristics of fetal thyroid and (2) in which the follicles are more differentiated as evidenced by their larger size and more abundant colloid.[16]

The fetal or simplex type is the more common. It may arise from a preexisting fetal adenoma (*Die wuchernde Struma* of Langhans). Histologically these cancers are characterized by the general absence of colloid, the tendency of the follicles to form solid and closely packed

---

16. Langhans (Virchows Arch. f. path. Anat., 1907, clxxxix, 69) describes five forms of malignant epithelial tumors of the thyroid: (1) proliferating struma; (2) carcinomatous struma; (3) metastasizing colloid struma; (4) small alveolar, large-celled struma; (5) papilloma. Our Group 1 includes Langhans' Forms 1, 2 and 4, while our Group 2 includes his Forms 3 and 5. Langhans points out that his Form 1 (proliferating struma) is not true cancer for the reason that metastases occur through the blood-stream. Only two of Langhans' fifteen cases had metastases. This form (proliferating struma) includes the borderline tumors and is Langhans' largest group. We have classed these tumors with the benign fetal adenomata unless there were demonstrable or very clear histological evidence of malignancy for the following reasons: (1) They occur in any decade of life but especially in the third and fourth decades. (2) They do not occur apart from a generalized hyperplasia. (3) They are always completely encapsulated masses, and shelling them out usually effects a cure. (4) They may be primarily solitary but are frequently multiple. (5) Demonstrable metastases are rare. (6) Histologically the metastasizing tumor is not distinguishable from the nonmetastasizing tumor either in its general architecture or any irregularity of cell type. Langhans lays stress on the history of rapid growth, the presence of epithelial tissue in the clefts of the capsule and the relation of the epithelial elements to the blood-vessels in determining the malignant nature of these tumors. We have been led to attach no very great importance to these factors, because mechanical effects play a great rôle in determining the morphological differences and because age of the tumor, usually an undeterminable factor, also modifies the structure.

columns of cells in which the cells are irregularly columnar and the arrangement of the nuclear material greatly disturbed.

The second type sometimes called "papillary cystic cancer" is characterized anatomically by larger rounded or elongated follicles with infoldings and plications, each follicle containing colloid. The epithelial cells may be cubical but are more often columnar. The irregularities in the size of the cells and their nuclei may not be prominent.

Summing up then, we would insist on two major types of human thyroid cancer, the infrequency of cancer as compared with ordinary goiter and benign tumors, the difficulty of histological diagnosis and, in consequence, the need of other criteria in making the differentiation.

### *3. Other Tumors*

Several types of sarcoma, including endothelioma, have been reported and, in rare instances, cases of combined carcinoma and sarcoma. Inasmuch as these tumors are easily recognized, further discussion will be omitted.

## IX. COMPLICATIONS

### *1. Hemorrhage*

Hemorrhages are the most frequent pathological changes in the thyroid. While one occasionally sees small hemorrhagic areas in otherwise essentially normal glands, they are *par excellence* complications of goiters. They rarely occur during the developing stage of goiter but during its colloid phase. We have never observed long-standing human colloid goiters without hemorrhages. Why hemorrhages should occur during the colloid phase is not difficult to understand when one recalls the fact that the developing hyperplasia is soft, compressible and elastic, while in the colloid phase the gland is firmer and the follicles distended with colloid so that slight trauma or manipulation, or even the follicular distention, is sufficient to cause their stretched walls to rupture. Perhaps sudden rises in blood-pressure, as in violent exertions, are causal factors. Hemorrhages are very common in dogs' thyroids, and fighting or other forms of exertion doubtless strain the capillaries and thinned follicular walls to the point of rupture.

The thyroids of all animals thus far examined are subject to hemorrhages. Anatomically the hemorrhage may appear only as a reddish, brownish, greenish or yellowish discoloration of the colloid. Larger areas of hemorrhage tend to encapsulate, and the cavities contain brownish material, sometimes viscid from colloid admixture, while at times it is more fluid. In general, however, in the small hemorrhagic areas, colloid forms the body of the mass while the extravasated blood produces the discoloration. The term "hemorrhagic goiter" is commonly used to describe old nodular and varicolored goiters, the result of multiple small and large areas of hemorrhage of different ages. We do not consider the term descriptive, since hemorrhage is not an essential part of goiter but always a secondary and complicating factor. Areas of hemorrhage are frequent causes of scar formation. These scars make up many of the so-called capsular adhesions so commonly encountered in old human goiters.

Owing to the normal architecture of the thyroid, hemorrhage forms the starting-point for most thyroid cysts.

### *2. Cysts*

Some observers use the term "cyst" to include enlarged colloid-filled follicles, and designate all colloid goiters as "cystic goiters." We believe that this is wrong, first for the reason that cyst formation is no essential part of goiter formation, and secondly, because there is no clear anatomical separation between colloid glands (goiters) and normal glands.

True thyroid cysts are common for the reason that hemorrhage is common. Thus while two or three types of intrinsic cysts may be differentiated, they are all closely related to hemorrhage.

A. Cysts Dependent on Hemorrhage into Follicles: These are the usual thyroid cysts. They vary in size from a few millimeters to 6 or 8 cm. in diameter. The smaller ones have the slightly thickened follicular walls as their cyst walls, while the larger cysts include in addition to the follicular walls, portions of the gland capsule or trabeculæ, together with a new formation of connective tissue. In such cyst walls calcification is frequently seen. As mentioned above, the cyst contents consist of blood in various stages of decomposition, mixed with more or less colloid. Sometimes the material is pasty, sometimes viscid, sometimes watery. In color the contents vary from dark brown to clear amber yellow. Cholesterin is frequently present in these cysts.

B. Cysts Originating from Adenomata: In human goiter cyst formation in adenomata is common. The exact mode of development of these cysts is not clear. The primary change probably is an interference with the nutrition of the interior of the tumor resulting in central necrosis. Hemorrhage then takes place, and this may extend the softening quite to the capsule. More often one sees in these cystic adenomata a zone of living tissue beneath the capsule.

The original capsule of the adenoma makes the cyst wall. Calcification of the fibrous capsule is frequent. Cysts of this origin make up the largest cysts of the thyroid and are those usually treated surgically. The adenomatous origin of these cysts can usually be made out from the operation specimen, since they are frequently not shelled out as is possible, but are in truth amputated together with more or less of the original thyroid stretched and flattened against the cyst wall.

The contents of these cysts are as a rule more fluid than the primarily hemorrhagic cysts; this is due doubtless to the lessened colloid contents of fetal adenomata and the denser cyst wall preventing absorption. The material is frequently brownish in color and may contain small masses or clumps of tissue débris suspended in a more fluid medium. In long-standing cysts of this origin a clear yellow or greenish fluid is not uncommon.

# STUDIES ON WATER-DRINKING

## IV. THE EXCRETION OF CHLORIDS FOLLOWING COPIOUS WATER-DRINKING BETWEEN MEALS * [1]

S. A. RULON, JR., M.D., AND P. B. HAWK, PH.D.
URBANA, ILL.

Considerable investigating has been done on the influence of copious water ingestion on the chlorid excretion of fasting animals. The work of Forster[2] is often quoted in this connection. In one instance this investigator increased the urinary chlorid output from 0.175 gm. to 0.992 gm. by causing a dog to ingest 3 liters of water on the eighth day of the fast. This is the most pronounced increase in the chlorid excretion yet reported as following the ingestion of large volumes of water. From a series of investigations on dogs in which different animals were subjected to the influence of external hemorrhage or to the influence of poisoning by phosphorus or by carbon monoxid Kast[3] later came to the conclusion that there was a very close relationship between increased protein catabolism and the augmented chlorin output accompanying such catabolism. Inasmuch as the procedure of Kast rendered his experimental animals abnormal the results obtained therefrom cannot be considered on a comparative basis with the data obtained from a study of the course of the metabolic processes of normal subjects. Heilner[4] in a more recent study of copious water-drinking failed to secure any uniform relationship between the increased catabolism of protein matter, as measured by the increased output of nitrogen, and the accompanying rise in the chlorid excretion. In one experiment the ratio of chlorin to nitrogen was 1 : 16.7, whereas in a second test the ratio was 1 : 6.9. Benedict† has also found that the intensity of protein catabolism cannot be correctly judged from a consideration of the chlorin output.

### REPORT OF EXPERIMENTS

#### EXPERIMENT I

The purpose of this investigation was the study of the influence on the chlorid excretion of large amounts of water taken between meals. The subject of the

---

* From the laboratories of physiological chemistry of the University of Illinois and of the department of medicine of the University of Pennsylvania.

1. For I, II and III of this series of studies see, respectively: Hawk: Univ. Penn. Med. Bull., 1905, xviii, 7; Fowler and Hawk: Jour. Exper. Med., 1910, xii, 388; Rulon and Hawk: Jour. Am. Chem. Soc., 1910, xxxii, 1686.

2. Forster: Ztschr. f. Biol., 1873, ix, 364.

3. Kast: Ztschr. f. physiol. Chem., 1888, xii, 267.

4. Heilner: Ztschr. f. Biol., 1906, xlvii, 538.

†Benedict: Carnegie Publication, No. 77.

experiment was a young man 24 years of age who was a third-year student of medicine. His body weight was 60.6 kg. The plan adopted was to place the subject on a uniform diet containing a moderate amount of water and to continue this diet until nitrogen equilibrium was attained. After the course of the normal nutrition of the equilibrium plane had been noted it was then proposed to cause the subject to ingest a large volume of water through a period of four days and to note the influence of this increased ingestion of fluid on the urinary concentration of chlorids. Following this water period it was proposed to place the subject again on the original diet fed at the time nitrogen equilibrium was being attained in order to observe any metabolic variations which should follow the copious ingestion of water. The three periods of the experiment, i. e., the preliminary, water and final periods, were three, four and two days in length respectively.

The meals were taken at 7:30 a. m., 12:30 p. m. and 5:30 p. m., the menu for each meal being 700 gm. of whole milk, 40 gm. of butter and 100 gm. of soda crackers. During the entire experiment 100 c.c. of water was taken with each meal. This water ingestion was supplemented during the preliminary and final periods by the ingestion of 100 c.c. additional at 10 p. m. During the water period, however, 400 c.c. of water was taken hourly from 8 a. m. to 9 p. m. and 300 c.c. at 10 p. m. Moderate exercise of a uniform character was taken by the subject each day.

The body weight was accurately determined each day before breakfast and immediately following the emptying of bladder and rectum. The urine was collected in twenty-four-hour samples during the first two days of the preliminary period and the last day of the final period. During each of the other days of the investigation the urine was collected in four three and one-half-hour periods beginning at 8 a. m. and in a fifth period ten hours in length beginning at 10 p. m. Powdered thymol was used as urine preservative. The method of Volhard was used in the quantitative determination of the chlorids.

*Discussion of Data from Experiment I.*—The data obtained in the quantitative determination of urinary chlorids in this experiment are given in Table 1. It will be observed that the excretion of chlorids for the first day of the preliminary period was equivalent to 10.66 gm. of sodium chlorid, this value being increased to 11.04 gm. and 10.90 gm. on the other days of the period. The average output of chlorids by way of the urine for this preliminary period was equivalent therefore to 10.87 gm. of sodium chlorid. On the first day of the water period, however, when the ingestion of water was increased from 400 c.c. per day to 5,900 c.c., the chlorid outgo was slightly increased. The excretion for this day aggregated 11.49 gm. expressed as sodium chlorid. The day following, however, that is, the second day of increased fluid intake, the urinary concentration of chlorids decreased somewhat from the value observed on the first day of the period and very nearly approached the average value for the preliminary period. In fact, this value for the day in question was practically identical with the average value for the last two days of the preliminary period. The excretions in question were an average of 10.97 gm. for the last two days of the preliminary period as against 10.96 gm. for the second day of the water period. Following this return to the normal plane the chlorids again increased on the third day of copious water ingestion, as is shown by an output of 11.33 gm. expressed as sodium chlorid. The excretion on the fourth and last day of this period (11.19 gm.) was somewhat above the normal plane, but less than the previously mentioned excretions observed on the first and third days.

TABLE 1.—CHLORID EXCRETION—EXPERIMENT I

| Period | Day of Period. | Day of Experiment. | No. of Subperiod. | Urine Examination: Volume, Subperiod, c.c. | Urine Examination: Volume, Total for Day, c.c. | Urine Examination: Chlorid Excretion, Subperiod, gm. | Urine Examination: Chlorid Excretion, Total for Day, gm. |
|---|---|---|---|---|---|---|---|
| Preliminary (400 c.c. of water per day) | 1 | 1 | . | ... | 900 | .... | 10.66 |
| | 2 | 2 | . | ... | 1330 | .... | 11.04 |
| Preliminary (400 c.c. of water per day) | 3 | 3 | 1 | 140 | 1350 | 1.82 | 10.90 |
| | | | 2 | 235 | | 2.18 | |
| | | | 3 | 260 | | 3.00 | |
| | | | 4 | 360 | | 1.63 | |
| | | | 5 | 355 | | 2.27 | |
| Water (5900 c.c. of water per day) | 1 | 4 | 1 | 720 | 6720 | 2.05 | 11.49 |
| | | | 2 | 1750 | | 2.63 | |
| | | | 3 | 1580 | | 2.35 | |
| | | | 4 | 1360 | | 1.84 | |
| | | | 5 | 1310 | | 2.62 | |
| Water (5900 c.c. of water per day) | 2 | 5 | 1 | 680 | 6320 | 1.60 | 10.96 |
| | | | 2 | 1750 | | 2.54 | |
| | | | 3 | 1400 | | 2.17 | |
| | | | 4 | 1320 | | 2.31 | |
| | | | 5 | 1170 | | 2.34 | |
| Water (5900 c.c. of water per day) | 3 | 6 | 1 | 730 | 6530 | 1.64 | 11.33 |
| | | | 2 | 1670 | | 2.39 | |
| | | | 3 | 1200 | | 1.92 | |
| | | | 4 | 1380 | | 2.28 | |
| | | | 5 | 1550 | | 3.10 | |
| Water (5900 c.c. of water per day) | 4 | 7 | 1 | 620 | 5530 | 1.51 | 11.19 |
| | | | 2 | 1800 | | 2.52 | |
| | | | 3 | 840 | | 1.81 | |
| | | | 4 | 1300 | | 1.95 | |
| | | | 5 | 970 | | 3.40 | |
| Final (400 c.c. of water per day) | 1 | 8 | 1 | 140 | 1025 | 1.54 | 12.25 |
| | | | 2 | 185 | | 2.32 | |
| | | | 3 | 170 | | 1.98 | |
| | | | 4 | 215 | | 2.76 | |
| | | | 5 | 315 | | 3.65 | |
| Final (400 c.c. of water per day) | 2 | 9 | . | ... | 790 | .... | 9.80 |

On the eighth day of the investigation the water ingested was reduced in volume to that taken during the preliminary period. An examination of Table 1 will indicate that the decreased fluid intake was not followed by a decreased chlorid output. In fact, it will be observed that the chlorid excretion for this day was not only higher than that for any day of the preliminary period, but moreover it exceeded by a comparatively wide margin that registered for any day of the water period. It is of considerable interest that an excretion of 12.25 gm. should be obtained on this day, when all the dietary factors were the same as those which obtained during the preliminary period, when the average excretion was but 10.97 gm. This excretion of 12.25 gm. embraced a larger increased output of chlorids than was secured during the entire four days of the water period. During the four days in question the chlorid output was increased 1.08 gm. above the normal, whereas the 12.25 gm. represents an increase of 1.28 gm. above the preliminary level. The increased excretion on this single day at the opening of the final period therefore exceeded the total increase of the entire water period by more than 18 per cent. This high value of 12.25 gm. was succeeded on the following day, the last of the experiment, by an output of 9.8 gm. of chlorids expressed as sodium chlorid.

### EXPERIMENT II

The chlorid data discussed in this connection were obtained from the analysis of urines collected during an investigation already reported.[5] The subject was a young man 29 years old possessing a body weight of 61.5 kg. The daily schedule was similar to that in Experiment I except that the hours for meals were different, breakfast being at 9 a. m., luncheon at 1 p. m. and dinner at 6 p. m. The three uniform meals each included 25 gm. of butter, 110 gm. of crackers and 600 gm. of whole milk. The extra volume of water ingested during each day of increased water ingestion was 4,500 c.c., one liter being taken at 11 a. m., 12 m., 3:30 p. m. and 8 p. m., and 500 c.c. at 10 p. m. This experiment was nine days in length, three days being devoted to the preliminary period, two days to the water period and four days to the final period.

TABLE 2.—CHLORID EXCRETION—EXPERIMENT II

| Period | Day of Period | Day of Experiment | Urine Data: Volume c.c. | Urine Data: Specific Gravity | Urine Data: Chlorid Content gm. |
|---|---|---|---|---|---|
| Preliminary (500 c.c. of water per day) | 1 | 1 | 1090 | 1018 | 7.90 |
| | 2 | 2 | 997 | 1020 | 8.82 |
| | 3 | 3 | 770 | 1023 | 7.23 |
| Water (5,000 c.c. of water per day) | 1 | 4 | 5250 | 1005 | 11.55 |
| | 2 | 5 | 5800 | 1005 | 10.44 |
| Final (500 c.c. of water per day) | 1 | 6 | 1275 | 1016 | 7.39 |
| | 2 | 7 | 1160 | 1018 | 8.23 |
| | 3 | 8 | 1140 | 1020 | 8.77 |
| | 4 | 9 | 885 | 1024 | 7.34 |

*Discussion of Data from Experiment II.*—During the preliminary period of three days 400 c.c. of water above that contained in the 1,800 c.c. of milk was daily ingested. On this diet the chlorid output was 7.9 gm., 8.82 gm. and 7.23 gm. respectively. The average output for this three-day period, therefore, was 7.98 gm. On the day of the increased water ingestion, i. e., when 4,500 c.c. of water above that normally taken was introduced into the body, the chlorid excretion increased to 11.55 gm. On the following day on a similar water ingestion the chlorid output aggregated 10.44 gm., a value far above the preliminary level but somewhat lower than that registered on the first day of the water period. The chlorid excretion for the four days of the final period ranged from 7.34 gm. to 8.77 gm., yielding an average daily output of 7.93 gm. This average output agrees very closely with that obtained for the preliminary period, i. e., 7.98 gm. The data for this experiment are given in Table 2.

5. Hawk: Loc. cit. These analyses were made by Dr. F. D. Crowl.

### EXPERIMENT III

The data here discussed were obtained from urines collected in an experiment on the cryoscopic characteristics of urine following copious water ingestion.[6] The experiment was similar to Experiment II, already discussed. The experimental periods were divided as follows: preliminary, four days; water, three days; final, two days. The general plan of the experiment as well as the character and arrangement of the meals and the volume of extra water ingested each day of the water period were similar to those in Experiment II. The diet, however, contained about the same quantity of chlorid as the one fed in Experiment I. The subject of the experiment was a young man 22 years of age who was a third-year medical student.

TABLE 3.—CHLORID EXCRETION—EXPERIMENT III

| Period | Day of Period | Day of Experiment | Urine Data: Volume c.c. | Urine Data: Chlorid Content, c.c. |
|---|---|---|---|---|
| Preliminary (500 c.c. of water per day)... | 1 | 1 | 1500 | 16.43 |
| | 2 | 2 | 1300 | 11.71 |
| | 3 | 3 | 900 | 10.88 |
| | 4 | 4 | 900 | 11.48 |
| Water (5000 c.c. water per day).......... | 1 | 5 | 4100 | 15.58 |
| | 2 | 6 | 5550 | 25.14 |
| | 3 | 7 | 4370 | 15.64 |
| Final (500 c.c. of water per day).......... | 2 | 9 | 1150 | 11.21 |
| | 1 | 8 | 1220 | 13.63 |

*Discussion of the Data from Experiment III.*—The data concerned are given in Table 3. The data there given indicate that the chlorid output for the first day of the experiment (16.43 gm.) was considerably influenced by the diet ingested previous to the experimental time. This value is therefore not taken into consideration. The remaining three days of the preliminary period show values of 11.71 gm., 10.88 gm. and 11.48 gm. respectively for the urinary chlorid concentration. On the first day of the period of copious water-drinking the excretion of chlorids was increased to 15.58 gm., an increase of 4.22 gm. above the average daily output (11.36 gm.) of the preliminary interval. This indicates an increase of over 37 per cent. in the total chlorid output. The maximum chlorid excretion, however, occurred on the next day, the second of the water period. On this day the excretion aggregated 25.14 gm. as against 15.58 gm. for the first day of the period[7] and as compared with a daily average of 11.36 gm. for the preliminary period. This increase of over 121 per cent. above the normal output and of over 61 per cent. above the total output for the first day of copious water ingestion is very surprising and far exceeds that recorded in any of our experiments on any other day of copious water ingestion. The third day of the water period shows a total of 15.64 gm. of chlorids in the urine, a value closely comparable to

6. We are indebted to Dr. C. N. Sturtevant for specimens of these urines.

7. Heilner (loc. cit.) in one experiment on a fasting dog made a similar observation when he secured an excretion of 0.44 gm. of NaCl on the first day of increased water ingestion and 0.572 gm. on the second day.

the value of 15.58 gm. secured on the first day of the water period. During the final period the excretion for the first twenty-four-hour interval fell to 13.63 gm. and underwent a still further decrease to 11.21 gm. on the second day. It will be observed that the excretion for this day was very nearly the same as the daily average excretion for the preliminary period, thus indicating that the course of the excretion had returned to the normal.

## GENERAL DISCUSSION AND INTERPRETATION

Let us first consider the data from Experiment II (see Table 2). In this study we have a pronounced increase in the chlorid excretion on the first day of copious water-drinking, with an excretion nearly as great on the second and last day of the water period. With the opening of the final period with its low water ingestion, we observe a return to the conditions which obtained during the preliminary period, when a similar water ration was fed. Such influence as was exerted by the water on the chlorid output was apparently limited to the two days in which it was ingested in large amount. When we consider the data from Experiment III as given in Table 3, we find a situation very similar to that already mentioned under the second experiment. We have the same preliminary period of fairly uniform output followed by a period of copious water-drinking in which the chlorid output was markedly increased. The data from these two experiments (II and III) differ, however, in that the former showed the maximum output on the first day of increased water ingestion, whereas the maximum in the latter experiment came on the second day of the water period. We have here, then, two experiments on two different subjects and each of these experiments shows a marked increase in the concentration of the urinary chlorids during the period of copious water-drinking with a return to the normal course as soon as the daily ingestion of the large volume of water is discontinued. The pronounced increases in the chlorid output observed during the water periods of Experiments II and III we would interpret as due principally to the stimulation of gastric secretion through the introduction of the large volumes of water into the stomach. The flushing of the tissues and the stimulation of protein catabolism may have been contributing factors. (These points are further discussed later.)

When we turn to the data from Experiment I (Table 1), we find a condition rather different from the conditions existing in the experiments just discussed. Instead of a period of marked increase in the output of chlorids during the interval of copious water-drinking, we find the excretion but slightly increased during this interval. After the period of copious water-drinking is completed, however, and a return is made to the low water ingestion we observe a pronounced increase in the output of chlorids. This increase is of such magnitude as to carry the total output for the day over 18 per cent. above the total increased output for the four days of the water period. How are we to explain the rather unusual course of the chlorid excretion observed in this instance following the ingestion of large volumes of water between meals? The small increased output of chlorids observed during the period of time through which the large volume of water was being ingested might be explained from three different standpoints.

In the first place, we may infer that the pronounced flushing of the tissues by means of this increased fluid ingestion might have caused the observed increase in the urinary chlorin concentration. In fact, we might perhaps expect a decidedly more pronounced stimulation in the chlorin excretion than our data indicate when it is remembered that a volume of water 5,900 c.c. in excess of that customarily ingested was introduced into the body of the subject on each day of the water period.

In the second place, the catabolism of protein matter which has been shown to follow the ingestion of large volumes of water[1] might explain a part of the rise in the chlorid output. However, that the percentage thus accounted for probably was small will be seen from a consideration of the following calculation:

Protein catabolism during water period represented by loss of 0.68 gm. of N.
N. in fresh muscle = 3.2 per cent.
Muscular tissue equivalent to 0.68 gm. of nitrogen = 21.3 gm.
Chlorin in muscle = 0.069 per cent.‡
Chlorin content of 21.3 gm. of muscle = 0.0144 gm.
Blood content of fresh muscle = 7 per cent.
Blood in 21.3 gm. of muscle = 1.491 gm.
Chlorin in human blood = 0.26 per cent.
Chlorin content of 1.463 gm. human blood = 0.0039 gm.
Chlorin content of 21.3 gm. of muscle and 1.491 gm. of blood = 0.0183 gm.
Increased output of chlorin during four days of water period = 0.825 gm.
Portion of increased chlorin excretion of water period due to protein catabolism = 2.22 per cent.

If we consider the increased nitrogen excretion of the water period as arising from stimulated protein catabolism, we find that the increased chlorin output for the corresponding period was about fifty times too large to be accounted for on that basis. We might perhaps be permitted to assume in this connection that the increase in the nitrogen and chlorid concentrations of the urine arose principally from the catabolism of nitrogenous body tissues, the chlorin being excreted in its entirety whereas the greater part of the resulting nitrogen was resynthesized within the organism[8] in some way, thus permitting the excretion of but a small portion of the total amount which resulted from the catabolic processes.

‡This value, according to some investigators, should be 0.04 per cent.

8. Paton: Jour. Physiol., 1910, xxxix, 485.

In the third place, we may look on the increased chlorid output in the urine of the water period as due to the fact that the introduction of this large volume of water into the stomach has furnished sufficient stimulation to produce an increased outpouring of gastric juice. This excess hydrochloric acid, we may suppose, appears in the urine as ammonium chlorid, thus raising the chlorid content of that excretion. That water does possess the stimulatory power mentioned above has been shown by Pawlow[9] and more recently by Foster and Lambert.[10] These latter investigators furnished very convincing proof of the fact that the entrance of water into the stomach does not dilute the gastric juice as formerly believed but acts as a stimulant and is followed by a more copious outpouring of gastric juice possessing a higher acid concentration. We have recently obtained experimental evidence in corroboration of these findings.[11] When the combined evidence from these different sources is taken into consideration with the further fact that Walter[12] has shown that hydrochloric acid fed to dogs is excreted in the urine mainly in the form of ammonium chlorid, we have a very strong foundation for the claim that at least a portion of the increased output of chlorids observed during the water period of our experiment was due directly to the stimulation of the gastric secretion through the agency of the excess water ingested.

It is apparent from the above discussion that rather logical arguments may be deduced for the explanation of the increased output of chlorids following copious water ingestion on the basis of either of three distinct theories. Does the cooperation and coordination of these three factors discussed above bring about the conditions observed to surround the chlorid output or does the efficient force reside in one individual factor? It would be difficult to divorce ourselves entirely from the belief that the flushing of the tissues of a man's body with 5 liters of water does not to some small degree, at any rate, increase the content of urinary chlorids. When we search the records for experimental verification of our belief, however, we fail to find such verification. On the other hand, we have definite and convincing experimental evidence that increased protein catabolism as well as an increased flow of gastric juice accompanies copious water ingestion.[1, 10] It is possible, therefore, for the chlorin output to be augmented from these two sources. But which of these two factors are we to consider the more efficient in this regard?

On the basis of mathematical calculation we have shown that a very small part of the increased output of chlorids following copious water-drinking arose from increased protein catabolism, unless we are to accept

9. Pawlow: The Work of the Digestive Glands, p. 125.
10. Foster and Lambert: Jour. Exper. Med., 1908, x, 820.
11. Wills and Hawk: Unpublished data.
12. Walter: Arch. f. exper. Path., 1877, vii, 148.

the theory that the major portion of the resulting nitrogen was not excreted in the urine. Therefore with no experimental evidence in favor of the "flushing" hypothesis and with only a small part of the output accounted for on the basis of increased protein catabolism we must logically turn to the stimulated gastric secretion for a solution of the problem. Experimental evidence already mentioned has demonstrated conclusively that the ingestion of large volumes of water is accompanied by the outpouring of an increased volume of gastric juice which possesses a hydrochloric acid concentration higher than normal. We would, therefore, interpret our data as indicating an increased chlorid output brought about through the fact that the unusually large volumes of water ingested have caused a pronounced stimulation of the gastric function. The excess hydrochloric acid thus produced is reabsorbed from the intestine and is mainly excreted in the urine as ammonium chlorid, thus increasing the chlorid concentration of the urine. It is entirely possible that all three factors previously mentioned (flushing of tissues, catabolism of protein matter, increased flow of gastric juice) are contributing forces in increasing the chlorin output, but we believe the major part of the increase is due to the increased flow of gastric juice.

None of the theories just advanced as explanatory of the increased output of chlorids observed during the period of copious water ingestion, however, can well explain the reason for the very pronounced increase in the chlorid excretion on the day following the four-day period of high water intake of Experiment I. We cannot explain this finding on the basis of the tissue-flushing properties of the ingested fluid, inasmuch as the volume of water ingested on this day was only 400 c.c. as compared with an ingestion of 5,900 c.c. for each day of the water period. That there was no "latent period," causing the water ingested on the last day of the water period to be mainly retained within the tissues and organs of the body until the next day and thus by means of its flushing activities cause a pronounced increase in the chlorid output for the first day of the final period is also apparent. This is clearly shown by the observation that on an ingestion of 2,100 c.c. of milk and 400 c.c. of water the total urine volume was only 1,025 c.c., or 41 per cent. of the fluid ingested.

The hypothesis that the increased chlorid output was due to protein catabolism is not in keeping with the facts shown by the analytic data, as the day in question, although showing the maximum chlorin output, was somewhat below normal in its nitrogen excretion. Likewise, it will be found that the stimulatory power of the water, in causing an additional outpouring of gastric juice and thus directly increasing the chlorid concentration of the urine, is also incompetent to explain the large percentage increase in the chlorid output for the first day of the final period.

In order to accept this factor as explanatory of the observed phenomenon, we must admit that a small volume of water has a more pronounced stimulatory action than a large volume of the fluid. Evidence adduced by Pawlow[9] and by Foster and Lambert[10] as well as the data from certain experiments made by one of us in the laboratories of the University of Illinois,[13] indicates very clearly that such a theory is untenable. How, then, are we to explain this increased excretion of chlorid, which is nearly 13 per cent. above that observed during the normal period and about 9 per cent. above the average daily output for the water period? We would suggest the following explanation: the absorption of the large volume of water from the intestine causes a temporary increase in the volume of blood within the vessels of the circulatory system. In order to maintain this augmented volume at the proper chlorid concentration, the excess chlorin resulting from the stimulation of gastric secretion is utilized and in addition chlorids are withdrawn from the body tissues, either by a process of flushing or as a result of the protein catabolism induced by the copious water ingestion. Finally, however, the excess fluid is withdrawn from the blood and eliminated from the body by way of the urine. The withdrawal of this water causes a gradual increase in the chlorin content of the blood, and therefore, in order to reduce this content to the normal concentration, the withdrawal of the excess water is followed by the passage of some of this excess chlorin into the urine.

On the basis of the above theory there would be a small increased output of chlorids on each day of increased water ingestion and a more pronounced outpouring of chlorids on the first day following the period of water ingestion. The large increase in the chlorin concentration of the urine of this day would be due to the fact that the large volume of water is suddenly eliminated from the diet at a time when the blood-vessels contain an excessive volume of blood whose chlorin concentration has been maintained through the utilization of gastric juice chlorin and the abstraction of tissue chlorids. This excess water is eliminated from the blood and no excess water is present to be absorbed from the intestine and thus maintain the conditions which were in force during the water period. In this dilemma the entire blood-stream transfers its burden of excess chlorids to the urine and the normal equilibrium is restored. The rate of this process would be regulated somewhat by the office exerted by the body tissues in furnishing water to the blood in order to properly dilute the concentrated menstruum. This factor would tend to delay, to some degree, the passage of the blood chlorids into the urine.

The abnormally low excretion of chlorids on the second day of the final period is apparently simple of explanation. Throughout the water period, as well as during the first day of the final period, the body has

13. Wills and Hawk: Unpublished data.

been excreting undue quantities of chlorids in the urine. This excess chlorin has been furnished by the gastric juice and the body tissues. The thing of prime importance now for the organism is to restore to the tissues the chlorids they yielded to the blood-stream when needed to maintain the normal concentration of that medium. The blood is now possessed of its normal chlorin content whereas the tissues are subnormal in this respect. On the ingestion of the usual daily quota of chlorin, therefore, the tissues abstract sufficient of the element to replace that previously lost. On this theory the excretion of only 9.8 gm. of chlorids, expressed as sodium chlorid, on the second day of the final period, is easy of explanation. The demands of the tissues are probably not satisfied in a single twenty-four-hour period, however, but in a comparatively short time they regain their normal chlorin content.

When we examine the chlorin output for the different three and one-half hour periods of the various days an interesting feature is noted. On every day of the water period the maximum excretion of chlorids occurred during the second period of the day, i. e., from 11:30 a. m. to 3 p. m. The data from the days of the preliminary and final periods in which the urine was collected in these short periods do not show any such uniformity. In the preliminary period the maximum output was excreted during the third three and one-half-hour period, i. e., from 3 p. m. to 6:30 p. m., whereas in the final period the urine passed between 6:30 p. m. and 10 p. m. showed the highest chlorid concentration. If we now examine the data for the urine flow during the water period we shall observe that the periods of maximum chlorid excretion were also periods of maximum urine flow. This fact apparently lends some emphasis to the theory that the excess output of chlorids noted during the water period originated through the flushing of the tissues. When we consider, however, the further fact that between 11:30 a. m. and 3 p. m. occurred the mid-day meal we are confronted with the possibility that the chlorin excess may have been due to the water acting as a stimulant to the gastric secretion. But why should this period between 11:30 a. m. and 3 p. m. show a larger output of chlorids and of urine than the period from 3 p. m. to 6:30 p. m. or the one from 8 a. m. to 11:30 a. m., inasmuch as each of these periods also includes one of the three uniform meals?

Let us consider the factors tending to influence the urine flow during the different three and one-half-hour periods. We notice, in the first place, that the opening period of the day, i. e., from 8 a. m. to 11:30 a. m., exhibits the lowest urine volume on every day of the experiment. This low volume no doubt results from the fact that a period of nine and one-half hours (10 p. m. to 7:30 a. m.) has elapsed since the last water was ingested. Hence the tissues absorb and retain a certain percentage of the water ingested during this first period. For this reason the volume of urine is low. The next period, i. e., from 11:30 a. m. to 3 p. m., opens therefore with the tissues possessing a relatively high water content. Under these conditions the major portion of the ingested water is ejected thus causing a high urine volume. The second meal of the day comes in the early part of this period (12:30 p. m.) and the urine flow for this three and one-half hour period is therefore augmented by a large part of the extra fluid ingested at that time. The third period of the day, i. e., from 3 p. m. to 6:30 p. m., also opens with the tissues well supplied with water but the conditions in this case differ from those in force during the previous period in the relative position of the meal within the period. In this case the meal comes near the close of the period and therefore the excess fluid is not eliminated quickly enough to permit any considerable portion of it being included in the period urine volume. From the above discussion it must be apparent that we might logically expect the maximum urine flow during the interval from 11:30 a. m. to 3 p. m. on each day of copious water ingestion.

An argument similar to the above may be advanced to account for the maximum chlorin output during the second period of the day, i. e., from 11:30 a. m. to 3 p. m. One-third of the chlorid ingested in the food during the day is introduced into the body during the early portion of this period. It enters at a time when the vessels of the circulatory system and the tissues are water laden and are endeavoring to maintain the blood at its normal concentration. Under these circumstances a portion of this ingested chlorin would naturally be utilized in adjusting the osmotic relations between the blood and the body tissues and the greater part of the excess would be eliminated from the body in the urine.

RELATION BETWEEN THE VOLUMES OF INGESTED AND EXCRETED FLUIDS

This relation, as found in Experiment I, has been shown in tabular form in Table 4. From an examination of the data recorded in this table it will be seen that the daily ingestion of fluid (water and milk) during the preliminary period was 2,500 c.c., no correction being made for milk solids. On this fluid ingestion there was excreted by the subject on the opening day of the test 900 c.c. of urine, or only 36 per cent. of the fluid volume ingested. On the next two days of this period the values rose to 53.2 per cent. and 54 per cent. respectively.

With the opening of the water period the relation observed during the preliminary period was considerably altered. For example, on the initial day of this period 84.0 per cent. of the ingested fluid was excreted, the intake aggregating 8,000 c.c. followed by an outgo of 6,720 c.c. On the remaining three days of the period when similar volumes (8,000 c.c.)

TABLE 4.—RELATION BETWEEN THE VOLUMES OF INGESTED AND EXCRETED FLUIDS

| Period | Day of Period. | Day of Experiment. | No of Subperiod. | Fluid ingested (per day), c.c. | Urine Volume: Subperiod, c.c. | Urine Volume: Total for Day, c.c. | Percentage of Ingested Fluid Recovered. | Specific Gravity: Subperiod Sample. | Specific Gravity: Daily Composite Sample. |
|---|---|---|---|---|---|---|---|---|---|
| | 1 | 1 | . | 2500 | ... | 900 | 36.0 | .... | 1023 |
| | 2 | 2 | . | 2500 | ... | 1330 | 53.2 | .... | 1019 |
| | | | 1 | | 140 | | | 1025 | |
| | | | 2 | | 235 | | | 1021 | |
| Preliminary.......... | 3 | 3 | 3 | 2500 | 260 | 1350 | 54.0 | 1024 | 1020 |
| | | | 4 | | 360 | | | 1014 | |
| | | | 5 | | 355 | | | 1023 | |
| | | | 1 | | 720 | | | 1008 | |
| | | | 2 | | 1750 | | | 1003 | |
| Preliminary.......... | 1 | 4 | 3 | 8000 | 1580 | 6720 | 84.0 | 1005 | 1006 |
| | | | 4 | | 1360 | | | 1005 | |
| | | | 5 | | 1310 | | | 1010 | |
| | | | 1 | | 680 | | | 1007 | |
| | | | 2 | | 1750 | | | 1004 | |
| Preliminary.......... | 2 | 5 | 3 | 8000 | 1400 | 6320 | 79.0 | 1003 | 1005 |
| | | | 4 | | 1320 | | | 1006 | |
| | | | 5 | | 1170 | | | 1008 | |
| | | | 1 | | 730 | | | 1005 | |
| | | | 2 | | 1670 | | | 1004 | |
| Preliminary.......... | 3 | 6 | 3 | 8000 | 1200 | 6530 | 81.6 | 1004 | 1005 |
| | | | 4 | | 1380 | | | 1005 | |
| | | | 5 | | 1550 | | | 1006 | |
| | | | 1 | | 620 | | | 1006 | |
| | | | 2 | | 1800 | | | 1005 | |
| Preliminary.......... | 4 | 7 | 3 | 8000 | 840 | 5530 | 69.1 | 1006 | 1006 |
| | | | 4 | | 1300 | | | 1005 | |
| | | | 5 | | 970 | | | 1008 | |
| | | | 1 | | 140 | | | 1019 | |
| | | | 2 | | 185 | | | 1020 | |
| Preliminary.......... | 1 | 8 | 3 | 2500 | 170 | 1025 | 41.0 | 1021 | 1021 |
| | | | 4 | | 215 | | | 1021 | |
| | | | 5 | | 315 | | | 1024 | |
| Preliminary.......... | 2 | 9 | . | 2500 | ... | 790 | 31.6 | .... | 1027 |

were ingested the urine contained volumes equivalent to 79 per cent., 81.6 per cent. and 69.1 per cent. of that ingested. We thus see that on each day of the water period a higher percentage of the ingested water was excreted than on any day of the preliminary period. The percentage excretion for the final period, when the same volume of fluid was ingested as during the preliminary period, i. e., 2,500 c.c., was 41 per cent. for the first day and 31.6 per cent. for the second day of the period, the last day of the experiment.

From a consideration of all the data on fluid ingestion and excretion it is evident that on the days of low fluid intake a small percentage of the fluid ingested was excreted in the urine. On the other hand, during the water period when large volumes of fluid were being introduced into the organism a higher percentage of the ingested fluid was eliminated in the urine. These data confirm those obtained by one of us (Hawk) in a previous experiment. Certain fasting studies made at the University of

Illinois[13] as well as certain experiments reported by Benedict[14] indicate a similar relation between the volumes of the ingested and excreted fluids.

The specific gravity of the urine specimens ranged between 1019 and 1027 for the preliminary and final periods and between 1005 and 1006 for the water period. The urine was acid in reaction to litmus throughout the experiment.

## SUMMARY

Three experiments are described in which the topic under investigation was the influence of copious water-drinking between meals on the excretion of chlorids. The subjects were young men ranging in age from 22 to 29 years. Each experiment was divided into three periods, a preliminary period during which nitrogen equilibrium was attained through the feeding of a uniform ration of low water content, a water period during which the uniform ration was supplemented by the drinking of large volumes of water between meals, and a final period in which the conditions of the preliminary period were in force.

In two of the experiments there was a pronounced increase in the output of chlorids on the days of added water intake with a return to normal during the final period. This augmented excretion of chlorids is interpreted as indicating that the large volume of water ingested during this period has markedly stimulated the secretion of gastric juice. The excess hydrochloric acid thus passed into the intestine has been reabsorbed and appears, at least in part, in the urine as ammonium chlorid. The main bulk of the increase in the chlorid excretion we believe to have originated in this way. The flushing of the tissues and the stimulation of protein catabolism brought about by the copious water-drinking may have been contributing forces in causing the increased output of chlorids observed.

In one experiment there was a small increase in the chlorid output on each of the days of increased water ingestion followed by a pronounced rise in the output on the first day following the water period. Neither the flushing properties of the water nor its stimulating efficiency as regards protein catabolism or gastric secretion offers a satisfactory explanation for the high chlorid concentration observed on the day following the period of copious water-drinking. It is evident, in the case of this subject, that the water period ended with the vessels of the circulatory system rather fully distended through the excessive water-drinking. The chlorid content of this large volume of blood has been maintained at the normal level partly through the withdrawal of tissue chlorids. As the period of low water ingestion opens the fluid volume within the blood-vessels is quickly decreased to the normal quota, and this withdrawal

13. Howe, Mattie and Hawk: Unpublished.
14. Benedict: Carnegie Publication, No. 77.

forces the excretion of the corresponding chlorids. This attempt of the body to maintain the blood at the proper chlorid concentration may, therefore, have caused the elimination of a relatively large quantity of chlorids on the day after the copious water drinking between meals had been discontinued.

If we attempt to account for the increased output of chlorids noted during the period of copious water ingestion on the theory that this increase originated through a stimulated catabolism of protein matter within the organism we find it possible to account for only 2 per cent. or less of the increased chlorin output on this basis.

In every instance in which a portion of the urine of each day of the water period was collected in four subperiods three and one-half hours in length (see Table 1) it was observed that the maximum chlorid output and urine volume occurred during the second period of the day, i. e. from 11:30 a. m. to 3 p. m. It was also observed that the highest percentage of ingested fluid (84 per cent.) was excreted during the periods of copious water intake.

# THE USE OF DIGIPURATUM IN HEART-DISEASE

WILLIAM F. BOOS M.D., L. H. NEWBURGH, M.D.
AND HENRY K. MARX, M.D.
BOSTON

Digitalis leaf preparations from different localities show great differences in pharmacologic strength. This variation in pharmacologic efficiency is due to the fact that there are a number of factors, variations in which will modify the amount of the active substances contained in the leaves. Among these factors are the soil, the gathering season, the methods of collecting and drying the leaves and the methods used in preserving the dried product. Carefully trained apothecaries may render the conditions fairly constant for one locality, but even then the leaves themselves are found to vary greatly from year to year. This variation in strength will of course be found also in the Galenic preparations made from the dried leaves.

In 1902 Fraenkel[1] studied the strength of digitalis and strophanthus preparations obtainable in Heidelberg and the surrounding towns, that is, the leaf and seed preparations of practically one section. His material consisted of samples of the tincture and infusion of digitalis and the tincture of strophanthus from six different sources. As his unit of strength he used the minimum amount of each preparation which was necessary to produce systolic stoppage of the heart in 100 gm. of frog in one hour. As a result of his tests Fraenkel found that the samples of the infusion of digitalis varied from 100 to 275 per cent. in strength, the samples of the tincture of digitalis varied from 100 to 400 per cent. and those of the tincture of strophanthus showed variations in strength of from 100 to 6,000 per cent.

What these figures mean is best shown by a table giving the total weight of frog in which the maximal daily dose for the human adult, of the strongest and the weakest preparation respectively, will produce systolic standstill of the heart in one hour.

Buehrer[2] studied the fluidextract of digitalis obtainable throughout one section of Switzerland and found the preparations to vary from 100 to 400 per cent. He also tested the fluidextract of two successive years from one apothecary and found the two preparations to show a difference of 200 per cent. in strength, both extracts being tested within a few days of their preparation.

---

1. Fraenkel: Therap. d. Gegenw., 1902, iv, 106.
2. Buehrer: Corr.-Bl. f. schweiz. Aerzte, 1900, xxx, 617.

Total Weight of Frog in Which Maximal Daily Dose for the Human Adult, of Strongest and Weakest Preparation Respectively, Will Produce Systolic Standstill of the Heart in One Hour

| Maximal dose for twenty-four hours | | | Systolic standstill of heart in weight of frog from weakest prep. | strongest prep. |
|---|---|---|---|---|
| | c.c. | | gm. | gm. |
| Tinct. digit...... | 5.0 | | 200 | 830 |
| Infus. digit...... | 100.0 | (1 gm. powd. leaves) | 1.450 | 4,000 |
| Tinct. stroph..... | 1.5 | | 150 | 10,000 |

Since the German apothecary is probably the most carefully trained apothecary in the world, these figures represent about the best results obtainable under the old system of unstandardized preparations. They will serve to explain in a great measure the almost proverbial uncertainty of digitalis medication in the past. This variation in strength of digitalis

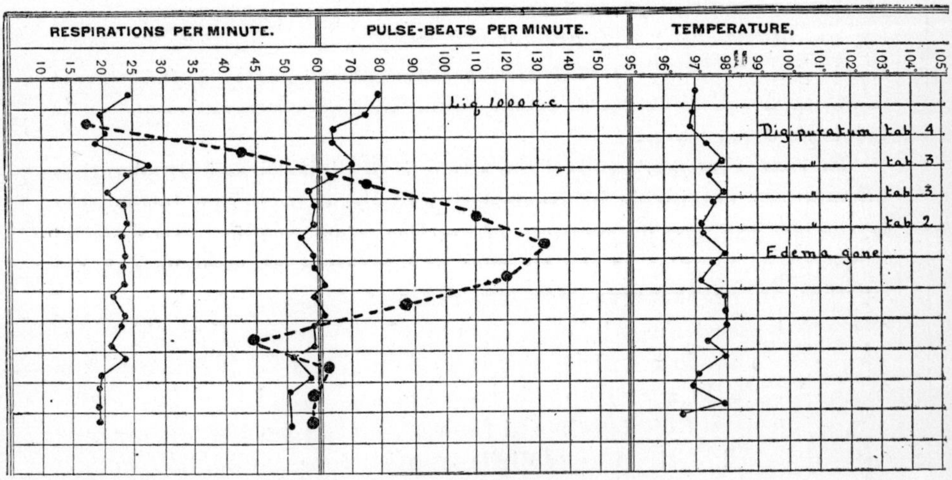


Chart 1.—Case 1 (Hosp. No. 165,337). Man, aged 39; mitral and aortic regurgitation, enlarged liver, marked brawny edema of legs, no dyspnea, mild break in compensation. In this and the following charts, the line of dashes represents the urinary output in ounces.

preparations, particularly of the tincture, which is undoubtedly the most reliable Galenic preparation, makes systematic treatment with unstandardized preparations an impossibility. The physician is obliged to feel his way, to test the strength of his preparation on the patient himself, as it were. If he is cautious his results may be negative, or at least unsatisfactory; if, on the other hand, the physician, relying on former experience, "pushes" the drug he may be suddenly confronted with a case of pronounced digitalis intoxication.

The use of the pure active principles of the digitalis group makes exact dosage possible, and therefore many French physicians, following the lead of Huchard, use pure crystalline digitoxin (digitaline Nativelle). In Germany, too, digitoxin (Schmiedeberg) and digitalin (digitalinum verum, Kiliani) are used to a limited extent. The therapeutic value of the active principles as compared with that of the leaf extracts was fully discussed at the nineteenth congress for internal medicine (Wiesbaden, 1901). At this congress many prominent clinicians spoke strongly in favor of the leaf extracts. They asserted that neither digitalin nor digitoxin alone could produce the true digitalis effect obtainable from the leaf preparations. In a recent paper by one of us[3] the properties of digitalin and digitoxin are discussed at some length, and it is shown that stro-

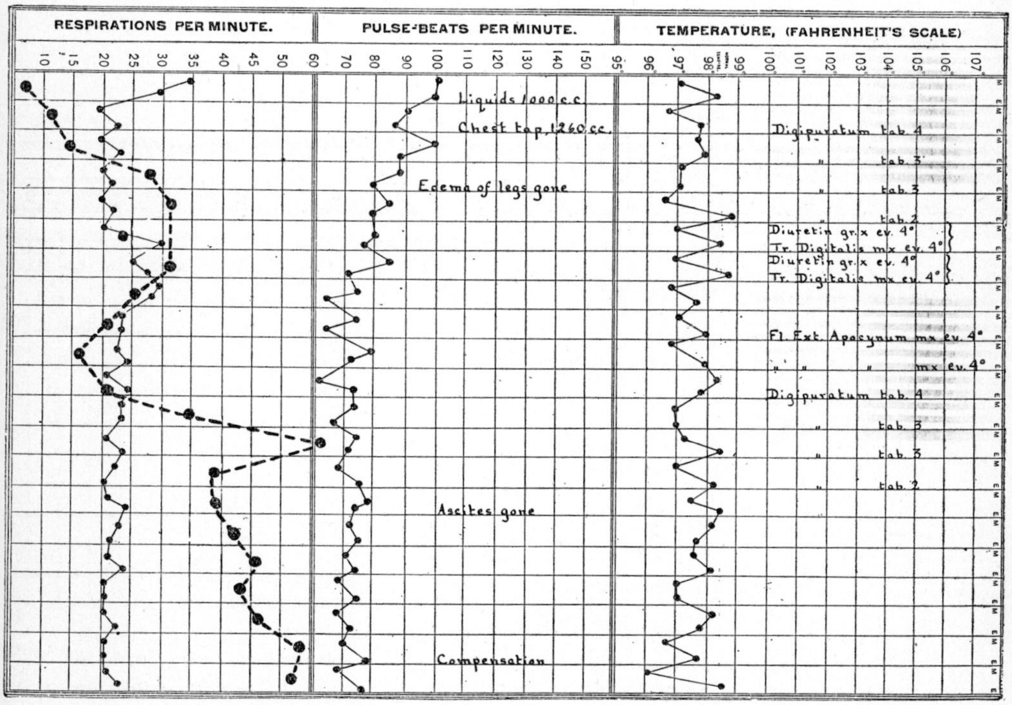


Chart 2.—Case 2 (Hosp. No. 165,545). Man, aged 38. Myocardial weakness, broken compensation, general anasarca, dry pericarditis and pleuritis. The effect on the pulse was prompt. The first digipuratum cure had little effect on the diuresis; the pronounced diuresis which began on the tenth day was probably started by the fluidextract of apocynum and continued by the second digipuratum treatment.

phanthin is probably a better substitute for digitalis leaf preparations than either of the digitalis bodies. But strophanthin is specially suited for intravenous application; it is not adapted for long-continued digitalis medication. In his lectures on digitalis Schmiedeberg himself warns his

3. Boos: Boston Med. and Surg. Jour., 1909, clxi, 589.

pupils against the use of pure digitoxin, on account of the insolubility and the great toxicity of this drug.

These facts all show that the need of leaf preparations of known strength is very great, and the introduction of physiologically standardized preparations of the tincture and fluidextract was therefore a decided step in advance. But these preparations are reliable only if they have been recently standardized, since it seems to be very difficult to render liquid preparations of digitalis permanent in point of pharmacologic strength. That is why German physicians prefer to use the powdered leaves, preparations of these being considered more nearly permanent.

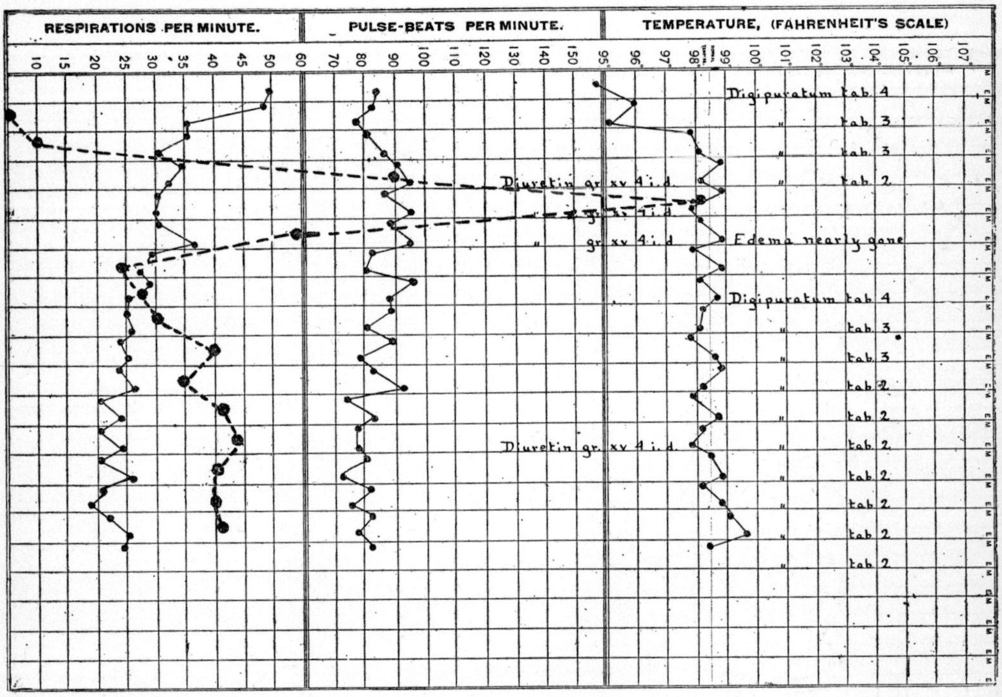


Chart 3.—Case 3 (Hosp. No. 166,588). Man, aged 67. Senile heart, failing compensation for six months. Had not slept in bed for two weeks. At entrance: cyanosis, urgent dyspnea, edema of lungs, enlarged, tender liver, massive brawny edema of legs and genitals, general anasarca. Blood-pressure 150 mm. Hg. Fifth day after entrance, striking improvement. Patient sleeping well at night without morphin; color good, edema very slight.

Focke[4] made a special study of these leaf-powders. His experience was that leaf-powders, which he obtained from various reliable German druggists, deteriorated in some cases more rapidly than the fluid preparations. The cause of this deterioration he found to be an excessive moisture con-

4. Focke: Therap. d. Gegenw., 1904, xlv, 250.

tent of the powdered leaves. As a result of his tests Focke concludes that the deterioration in strength which occurs in the course of one year is proportional to the amount of moisture above 3 per cent. which is contained in the leaf-powder. Some powders which contained as much as 8 per cent. moisture showed a loss in strength of over 60 per cent. Focke prepared permanent leaf-powders in the following manner: he dried the leaves quickly with artificial heat at a temperature just below 100 C. until the moisture content was below 1.5 per cent.; he then removed the thick stems, coarsely powdered the leaves and preserved them in air-tight tins. All the samples of leaf-powder prepared and preserved in this manner showed no diminution in strength after one year.

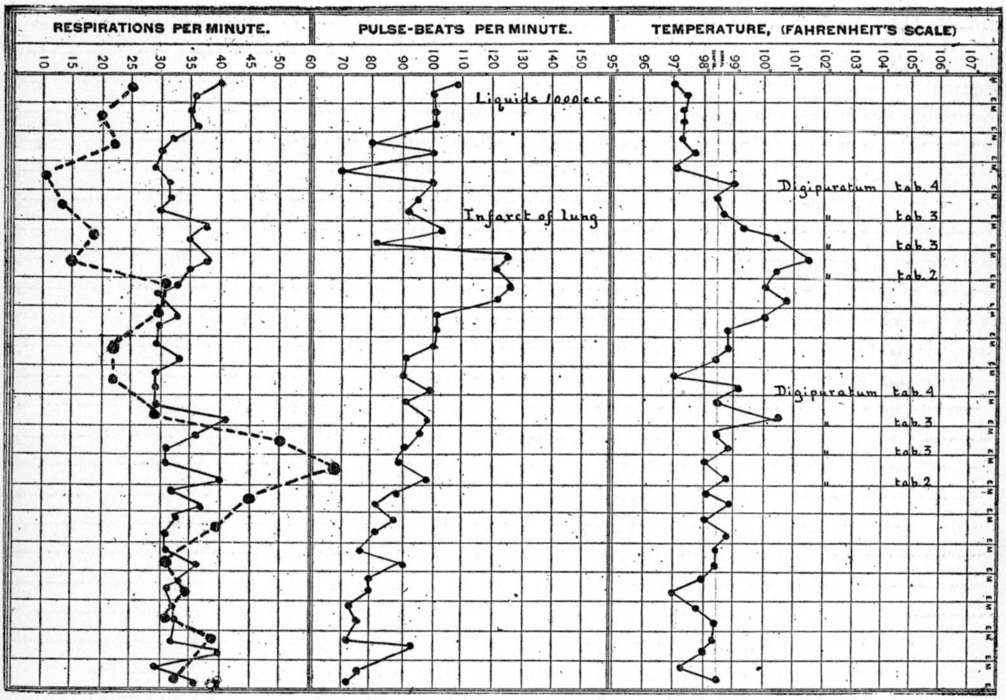


Chart 4.—Case 4. (Hosp. No. 165,693). Man aged 47. Myocardial insufficiency, mitral regurgitation (relative), broken compensation, edema of lungs, enlarged liver, edema of legs, infarct of lung involving whole right lower lobe. Marked general improvement and efficient diuresis with second digipuratum cure. Discharged with fair compensation.

Standardized leaf-powders prepared according to Focke's method may therefore be used for accurate dosage. There is, however, another factor which often renders digitalis medication difficult and at times even impossible, namely, the tendency of leaf preparations to produce in many patients gastro-enteric disturbances. Such disturbances are due, no doubt, in part if not wholly to the presence in the leaves of digitonin, a constituent of the digitalis leaf which is pharmacologically a saponin, the saponins and sapotoxins being characterized by their irritant action on the gastro-enteric tract. It was with the hope of lessening this irritant action of digitalis that Gottlieb essayed by chemical means to remove the digitonin from the leaf-extract. He succeeded in obtaining a product which is free not only from digitonin, but also from 85 per cent. of the other bulky and inactive matter which ordinarily passes into a leaf-extract. When Gottlieb compared the action of his purified product with that of the original leaves he found that he had recovered practically all the digi-

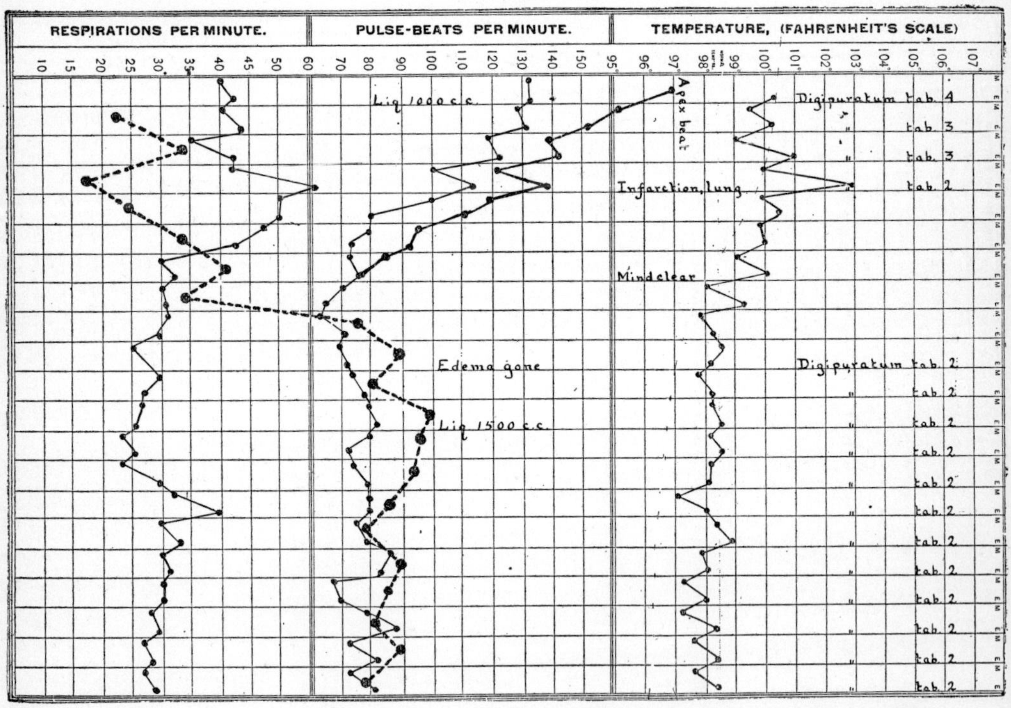


Chart 5.—Case 5 (Hosp. No. 165,949). Woman, aged 23. Mitral stenosis and regurgitation, aortic regurgitation. At entrance the apex and the radial pulse were 50 beats apart; patient was delirious; cyanosis and dyspnea were marked; patient had been vomiting badly and looked as if she would die. The apex and the radial pulse became synchronous on the seventh day; the pulse-rate fell and the urine increased. No vomiting after entrance. In a week patient was rational and comfortable; the ascites and the edema were gone.

talin and digitoxin contained in the crude leaves. To this purified product Gottlieb gave the name of "digitalis depuratum," or "digipuratum," for short.

This purified digitalis extract is a yellow liquid. The active principles contained in it are insoluble in cold water and acids, but easily soluble in dilute alkalies, a property which insures their ready absorption from the intestine. The yellow fluid is standardized physiologically and is then taken up with sugar of milk to form a powder. The powder obtained is further diluted with sugar of milk until the resulting product has a definite and constant pharmacologic strength. In his physiologic tests Gottlieb uses *Rana temporaria* (the German field frog), obtained during the months of July to October and kept in captivity as short a time as possible before use. His unit of strength is the minimum amount of the extract which in thirty minutes will cause systolic stoppage of the heart of a frog weighing 30 gm. This quantity Gottlieb calls a "frog

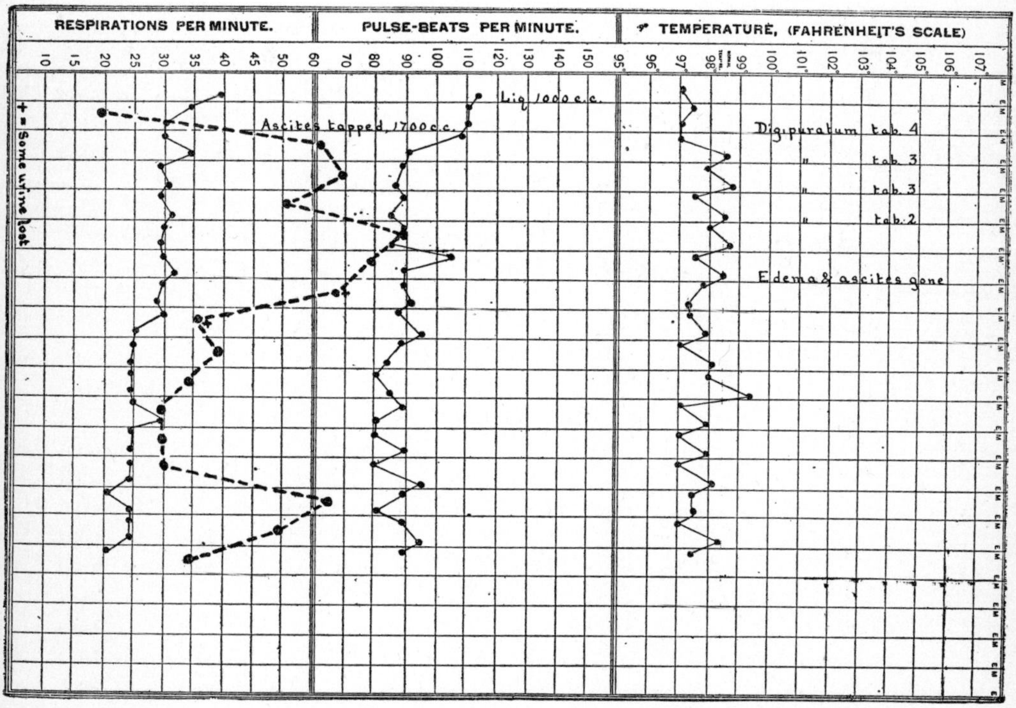


Chart 6.—Case 6 (Hosp. No. 166,029). Man, aged 44. Chronic glomerulonephritis, hypertrophy and dilatation of the heart, broken cardiac compensation, old syphilis. Blood-pressure 190 mm. Hg; very large ascites; extremely firm dema of legs; edema of lungs; pleural anasarca; Cheyne-Stokes respiration; very severe break in compensation. Tapping of ascites gave marked relief. The early diuresis was probably due to the tapping; it cannot possibly be attributed to the digipuratum because only two tablets of the drug had been taken when it began. The digipuratum diuresis began on the fourth day of the medication.

unit." By standardizing a large number of the best leaf-powders obtainable, Gottlieb found that the ordinary dose of the powdered leaves, 0.1 gm., varied in strength in the different samples from 4 frog units to 12. Eight frog units being the average, Gottlieb chose this strength for his purified extract. Digipuratum is therefore prepared as a powder having the constant strength of 8 frog units to each 0.1 gm. of the powder, corresponding to the average strength of a single dose (0.1 gm.) of the crude powdered leaves. For greater convenience of dosage digipuratum is usually dispensed in tablet form, each tablet containing 0.1 gm. of the powder. These tablets have an agreeable vanilla flavor and are taken readily by all patients.

The very favorable results obtained with digipuratum by Hoepfner,[5] Mueller,[6] Tissot,[7] Clemens[8] and others encouraged us to try the preparation in the medical services of the Massachusetts General Hospital.

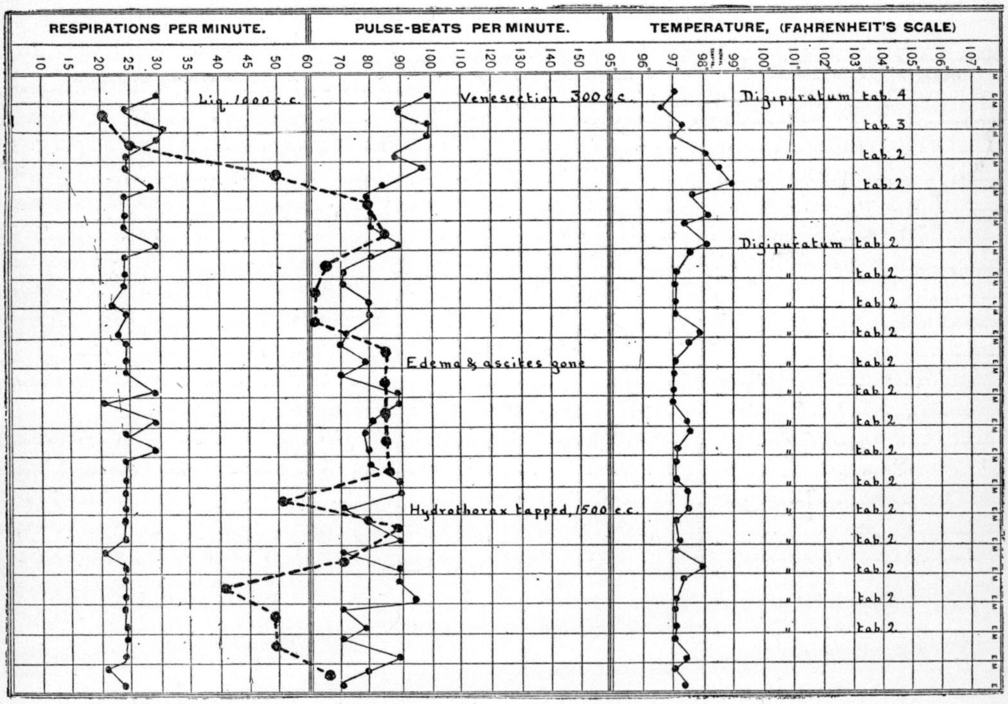


Chart 7.—Case 7 (Hosp. No. 166,254). Man, aged 49. Chronic glomerulonephritis (blood-pressure 240 mm. Hg), hypertrophy and dilation of heart, broken cardiac compensation (rather acute, very severe break in compensation), edema of lungs, right hydrothorax, slight ascites, enlarged liver, marked brawny edema of legs, general anasarca. Venesection at entrance gave immediate relief to subjective symptoms. On the fifth day after entrance the edema of legs was practically gone.

---

5. Hoepfner: München. med. Wchnschr., 1908, lv, 1774.
6. Mueller: München. med. Wchnschr., 1908, lv, 2651.
7. Tissot: Folia Serol., 1909, iii, 1.
8. Clemens: Fortschr. d. Med., 1908, xxvi, 1057.

In the treatment of broken cardiac compensation we gave the drug as suggested by the clinicians mentioned, namely, in the form of so-called treatments; that is to say, we employed the ideal digitalis medication, giving large doses in as short a time as possible. We were enabled in this way to determine if the drug, when it is given in sufficient quantity rapidly to produce its physiologic effect, is really free from the irritating substances which usually make similar dosage of the crude drug an impossibility, and to determine if under these circumstances this drug exhibits a lesser tendency to produce cumulation than the crude preparations. We gave digipuratum as a rule in treatments of twelve tablets in four days; four tablets the first day, three the second day, three the third and two the fourth day (that is, 1.2 gm. or 18 grains in four days).

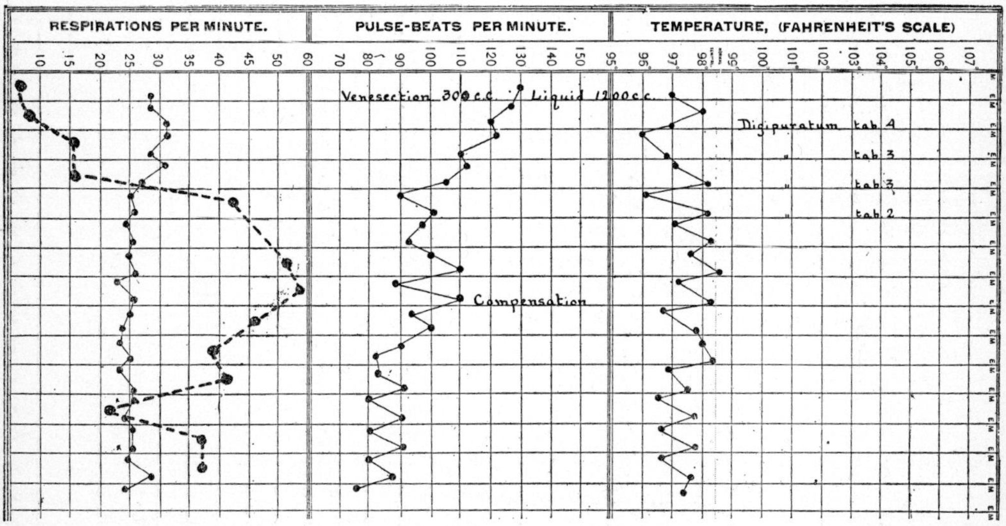


Chart 8.—Case 8 (Hosp. No. 166,451). Man, aged 36. Aortic insufficiency, aortic roughening, Cheyne-Stokes respiration, acutely dilated heart. Venesection, rest, digipuratum. Discharged, with compensation, in fifteen days.

In many of the more serious cases we were obliged, of course, to continue the drug in doses of one or two tablets for a longer or shorter period.

In order to show in a purely objective way what the drug will do, we shall report in brief (see charts and legends) eight cases taken from the first fifteen cases of heart disease treated at the hospital with digipuratum. The cases which we reported were chosen with a view to illustrating the action of digipuratum alone, as well as in combination with other therapeutic measures. To make the picture more graphic we reproduce the charts with as little text as possible.

Each of the eight cases shows interesting features. The diuresis is efficient in all the cases. In Case 3 the diuretin probably played little or no part in producing the phenomenal urinary output. Cases 1, 2, 5 and 8 show the marked effect of digipuratum on the pulse-rate. Case 5 is perhaps the most remarkable case of all. This patient was sent into the hospital in a moribund condition and we felt but little hope of her life. She reacted very quickly to digipuratum, however, and compensation was established in a week. The patient has been under the care of one of us since leaving the hospital. At first she needed two tablets of digipuratum daily for several months; after that the dose could be gradually diminished until now, after one year, she takes on the average only four or five tablets a week. At times she goes a week or ten days without the drug. She is comfortable, looks after her household duties and makes many visits, although she lives up one flight of stairs. The physical signs are the same as when she left the hospital.

In some of the cases the first digipuratum treatment gave little or no result, while the second was very efficient. Cases 2, 6, 7 and 8 illustrate the good results which may often be obtained by combining digipuratum medication with venesection or the removal of fluid from the body by tapping. In Case 2 the efficient diuresis which began on the tenth day was due to a combination of digipuratum with the fluidextract of apocynum. The blood-pressure was rarely affected. There was no vomiting or diarrhea in any of the cases.

Digipuratum has now been in use at the Massachusetts General Hospital for over a year and more than 180 cases of primary heart disease or secondary cardiac involvement have been treated with it. The effect on the urinary output has been very prompt in most instances. There was not a single case of vomiting or diarrhea; in fact, the vomiting of a number of cardiac patients at entrance was promptly stopped by digipuratum. Cumulative poisoning has never been observed. One of the early patients, a boy of 16, was given 106 tablets in six weeks; at no time was there any suggestion of digitalis poisoning. In one or two instances the house officers were made uneasy by sudden drops of forty or more beats in the pulse-rate, but no disagreeable consequences followed in any case. It must be borne in mind, however, that digipuratum is a digitalis preparation, and that as such it must necessarily have a tendency to produce poisoning by cumulation. In the case of digipuratum this tendency is merely much diminished, so that it is possible by means of this drug to push digitalis therapy in a manner heretofore unknown.

374 Marlboro Street—Massachusetts General Hospital.

# A CASE OF STRONGYLOIDES INTESTINALIS WITH LARVÆ IN THE SPUTUM *

JOHN G. GAGE, M.D.
NEW ORLEANS

Although infection with *Strongyloides intestinalis* is by no means uncommon in the South, patients with larvæ in the stools being frequently observed by physicians, nevertheless the number of reported cases is not large and is not a true index of the prevalence of the disease. This is probably due to the fact that this parasite is usually considered harmless.

In the case here reported the larvæ were discovered first in the sputum. The patient entered the hospital with a diagnosis of pneumonia. His temperature promptly dropped to normal but, because his general condition did not improve and because of impaired resonance and later expectoration, tuberculosis was suspected and his sputum examined.

I saw the first larvæ while examining the fresh sputum, and thought they might be a contamination of some sort, because the patient had vomited that day and the sputum contained food particles and milk; but, on the following day, Dr. Dock found them in a fresh bit of sputum just coughed up by the patient. Fresh sputum was examined almost daily during the patient's stay in the hospital and on careful search larvæ could always be found, so the idea that the larvæ came from elsewhere than the respiratory tract was abandoned.

They were slender worms, measuring 0.43 mm. to 0.45 mm. in length by 0.02 mm. in breadth, and having a long cylindrical esophagus which occupied nearly all the anterior half of the worm. The idea that they were hookworm larvæ was ruled out at once, and, after a short search through the books, it was decided they were some variety of strongyloid, and as such they were reported by Dr. Dock before the Orleans Parish Medical Society. Later, after they had been studied in connection with the larvæ obtained by incubating the stools, they were identified as the filariform larvæ of *Strongyloides intestinalis*. The larvæ in the sputum did not have the characteristic serpentine motion of filariform larvæ, their movements consisting of coiling and uncoiling. This was probably due to the tenacity of the sputum and the pressure of the cover-glass. I saw one or two larvæ in which the sexual anlage was present, which would point to their being but a few hours old.

---

*From the Medical Clinic of Dr. George Dock, and the Charity Hospital, New Orleans.

Examination of the stools showed enormous numbers of larvæ, identified as the rhabditiform larvæ of the *Strongyloides intestinalis.*

Nematodes and their larvæ are described as occurring in various parts of the body of man and animals. Braun[1] speaks of instances in which they have been found in the skin, heart, blood, eye, urethra, subcutaneous tumors, and bronchial lymph-glands. Richard,[2] in discussing Siler's paper on uncinariasis, mentions a patient with chronic bronchitis whose sputum contained hookworm larvæ.

## REPORT OF CASES

*History.*—The patient, H. G., white man, age 48, a painter by occupation, entered Charity Hospital Oct. 16, 1909, complaining of chills and fever. Family history was negative. The patient was born in New Orleans and lived here until about 16 years of age, when he went to work on board a ship. He said he "followed the seas for four years and was all around the world"; came back to New Orleans and had not been out of the city since. He used tobacco and was a heavy drinker. He had worked at his trade as a painter for twenty years. He said that he had always eaten all the green vegetables he cared for and drank "all kinds of water and whenever I can get it." He had had the usual diseases of childhood; had malaria when young. He never had scarlet fever, typhoid fever or diphtheria. He denied venereal disease; had always been healthy. He said that he had not lost a day's work because of illness in thirty years. He had been feeling ill for a week or ten days and, two or three days before coming to the hospital was taken with a chill while on his way to work and felt so miserable that he went home. A physician was called who told him he had "typhoid-pneumonia" and advised him to enter the hospital. He entered at the crisis of a lobar pneumonia involving both upper lobes.

The signs rapidly cleared and, November 22, there was merely slight dulness above, with dull tympany below, feeble breath sounds, piping râles, and, on cough, abundant moist râles. At the right base crackling persisted. The patient was emaciated, with harsh, dry skin and muddy complexion.

*Laboratory Findings.*—Sputum: About 5 c.c.; pale yellow; mucopurulent; tenacious; blood-streaked in places; slightly fetid odor. No tubercle bacilli; many large cocci and short thick rods. No elastic tissue. One imperfect spiral. Many food particles and much detritus from mouth. Fifteen or twenty larvæ were seen.

Blood: Red cells 3,020,000. White cells 13,300. Hemoglobin 70 per cent. (Tallqvist). Differential count, 500 cells counted: Small lymphocytes 13.2 per cent.; large lymphocytes 2.0 per cent.; transitionals 1.4 per cent.; polymorphonuclears 79.8 per cent.; eosinophils 3.2 per cent.; mast cells 0.4 per cent. Few microcytes, no macrocytes, few poikilocytes. No nucleated red cells.

Urine: Turbidity marked. Specific gravity 1013. Reaction alkaline. Color pale yellow. With heat and nitric acid, very small precipitate. With acetic and potassium ferrocyanid, slight precipitate. Fehling's test no reduction. Foam white. Sediment large. Large amount of pus. No larvæ.

Stool: Small light brown, semisolid. Odor fecal. Enormous numbers of larvæ. No flagellates, no amebas. One trichocephalus egg. One Charcot crystal.

*Course of Disease.*—Three times during the patient's stay in the hospital I found eggs in the fresh stool. On two occasions the egg contained dead embryos, once well preserved, the other time brown, granular and badly disintegrated.

1. Braun: Animal Parasites of Man, 1899.
2. Richard: Post-Grad., 1909, xxiv, 475.

None of the eggs seen in the stools was in segmentation nor were they likely to have been mistaken for hookworm eggs.

Because of the weakened condition of the patient, and in view of the fact that nearly every one agrees that it is useless to try to get rid of the worms in the intestine, our patient received no anthelmintic.

When he entered the hospital he had fever of 101-105 F., which lasted about two days, after which time he was afebrile during his stay, with the exception of two slight flurries, each lasting about a day, the temperature rising to 101 on one occasion and to 100 on the other.

At first the patient had no cough and no sputum, but later a slight cough developed with scarcely any sputum, so that it was difficult to get any for examination, but finally a specimen was obtained in which larvæ were found. At first the sputum had somewhat the appearance of material from bronchiectatic cavities, but had not the foul odor. Later the sputum became more abundant and bronchitic in character. While the sputum was scanty the larvæ were fairly abundant, several could be found in looking over a few low-power fields, but as the sputum became more copious a longer search was required; sometimes one had to look over as much as 5 c.c. before one larva could be found. But one could always find them after a long enough search.

As Teissier has reported filariform larvæ in the circulating blood, large amounts of this patient's blood were examined, but no larvæ were found.

The patient's appetite was very poor and he ate scarcely anything, but previous to this illness he had always been a hearty eater. After he had been in the hospital about three weeks he had attacks of vomiting for three or four days, apparently without much nausea. After this time he would take no nourishment except a small amount of tea or soup and a few crackers.

After he had been in the hospital about one week he developed a diarrhea, passing from ten to twelve stools in the twenty-four hours. The diarrhea was most marked in the early morning hours, when he would pass seven or eight stools between 4 and 6 a. m. This lasted but a few days and then for a week or ten days he was free from diarrhea, with but one or two soft stools per day. During the rest of his stay in the hospital, periods of diarrhea occurred about every two weeks. The stools were always soft and when the patient had diarrhea they were thin but never dysenteric in character.

He had one other symptom which is common in infection with *Strongyloides intestinalis*, namely, the desire to go to stool was very urgent, and he had to defecate at once, even when the stool was of normal consistency. He said that he had never been troubled with diarrhea, but after drinking bouts his stools were more numerous and thinner than usual. This never lasted longer than one day. He had noticed this for the last four years.

The patient was personally very filthy, and the sheets were always wet and smeared with feces. The skin over his back and buttocks was red and irritated, and a bed-sore developed over the sacrum.

The patient grew weaker, his cough worse and sputum more abundant and, although during the last few days he complained of some shortness of breath, he had no fever and examination of his chest showed nothing other than signs of a diffuse bronchitis.

He died Dec. 17, 1909, after having been in the hospital two months.

The histological findings in this case are recorded in a paper read before the meeting of the American Pathologists and Bacteriologists at Washington.† Briefly, the findings were as follows:

*Macroscopic Post-Mortem Examination.*—There was catarrhal inflammation and superficial ulceration of the small intestines. Mucus from the duodenum contained large numbers of adult worms, active rhabditiform larvæ and eggs in all

†Gage: Jour. Med. Research, 1910, xxiii, 177.

stages of development. The eggs, while numerous, were few in proportion to the number of larvæ. There were many larvæ, a few eggs, but no adult worms in the mucus from about the middle of the ileum. There were numerous areas of fresh bronchopneumonia throughout the lower lobes of both lungs. Sputum taken from the trachea and bronchi contained a few larvæ. The pelves of both kidneys were distended with pus. The other organs were apparently negative.

*Microscopic Post-Mortem Examination.*—Sections of the small intestine showed adult worms, eggs and larvæ in the lumen of the intestine and in Lieberkühn's glands, as has been described by many others. In addition to this I found larvæ in lymph-spaces and lymph-vessels, in the muscularis mucosæ, submucosa, between the muscle coats and beneath the serosa. I could find none in blood-vessels. In the sections of lung I found one larva in an antevesicular tube, another in the perivascular tissue between two lobules, and a third in an air-vesicle.

In addition to the above case I have seen larvæ in stools from fourteen other persons: four students (two from Louisiana, one from Mississippi, and one from Tennessee); one patient in Charity Hospital who has always been a resident of Louisiana; three other patients in Charity Hospital and two in Touro Infirmary who left the hospitals before I had an opportunity to get histories from them; three children under the care of Dr. Irwin, who kindly sent me specimens of their stools, and one other person whose stool was sent by a medical student to the Clinical Laboratory for examination. The following case report was sent to me by Dr. Allan C. Eustis and is included by his permission:

CASE 2.—Patient, Mrs. G., white woman, aged 41, wife of a farmer and mother of six children, was a resident of Lafourche Parish until six years ago, when she moved to Vermilion Parish. Family history is negative. She had been in good health all her life and never complained until July, 1907, when she began having headaches, edema of the face and ankles, weakness and pains in the limbs and gradual emaciation. I first saw her on Oct. 11, 1907, in consultation with Dr. Cushman.

*Examination.*—This showed a flabby condition of the muscles, sunken eyes and considerable weakness. There was no tenderness of any of the abdominal viscera and the heart and lungs were negative. Liver and splenic dulness were not noticeably increased. The abdominal wall was very much relaxed. There was no history of diarrhea and the stools were normal in appearance. Pulse was 120 and of low tension; respiration 18 per minute. Temperature was normal and had been so from the beginning of the attack. No plasmodia. Hemoglobin 80 per cent. Tallqvist. Leukocytes 11,500. Red blood cells 4,625,000. The patellar reflexes were entirely absent, but there was no Romberg's symptom or Argyll Robertson pupil. Closer examination of the muscles of the lower limb showed the peroneal group of muscles absolutely non-reactive to the faradic or galvanic current.

The differential blood-count at this time showed 56 per cent. eosinophils and this led to an examination of the stools, which at first were negative but, after administration of a full dose of Epsom salts, showed myriads of rhabditiform embryos of *Strongyloides intestinalis.* They were at first mistaken by me for trichinæ and a proper anthelmintic was sought. Thymol and the others having no clinical effect, the embryos were subjected to various solutions while under the microscope. Among these were thymol, santonin, male-fern, calomel, quinin bisulphate, glycerin, liquor formaldehydi and salicylic acid. Only two had any effect. Liquor formaldehydi was found to kill the embryos, but had to be used in such strong solution that the intestinal canal would not tolerate it. Phenyl salicylate (salol) was then tried with excellent results.

*Treatment and Course of Disease.*—The patient was put on three-grain doses of salol every three or four hours and kept on the following soluble diet for one month and a half; chicken, beef and oyster bouillon, gelatin, fruit-juices, sugar-candy and a dozen raw eggs per day. The patient never lost weight. In addition she was given enemas of a gallon of salt solution containing one of the mild antiseptics. The number of embryos began to diminish from the time we placed the patient on phenyl salicylate and they finally disappeared. The muscles were treated by daily applications of the faradic current with complete recovery. Today the patient is absolutely well and, while I have made examinations of her stools, even after the administration of a saline, I have not been able to find the eggs or embryos since she was discharged. The eosinophils have diminished also, showing only 2 per cent. at the last count made, about a month ago. Jan. 17, 1910, patient is still in perfect health and careful examination of the stools fails to reveal the presence of any embryos.

## RESULTS OF CULTURES

I attempted to grow the larvæ found in the stools and to repeat the work of others along this line. Stools containing larvæ were placed in an incubator at 37 C., on top of the incubator at about 30 C., and at room temperature; but a temperature of 30 C. was most suitable. Portions of the stool were put in moist sterile sand and on moist filter-paper, but the larvæ grew quite as well in the stools themselves. I soon found that the larvæ grew best when the stool was the consistency of a thick paste; that when it was too firm or too fluid they did not do so well; also that the amount of air present had to be considered, for, if the stools were placed in closed containers, most of the larvæ died, either from lack of oxygen or because of the high gas pressure developed by fermentation. The work with the larvæ from the first case was carried on by incubating the stools themselves in open dishes at 30 C.

As it was not possible to follow accurately the development of any given larva when growing the larvæ in the stools, I adopted the following technic, after many modifications: By means of a capillary pipette the larvæ were picked out of smear preparations and placed in distilled water in a watch-glass, and, after a second washing, were put on the medium and incubated at 32 C. in a moist atmosphere. In this way I got rid of the fecal matter and the greater part of the bacteria and could plant as many larvæ as desired. This method is especially desirable when stools contain few larvæ.

This prevents contamination with other nematodes and avoids the criticism brought forward by Leiper[3] concerning Ozzard's observations on *Ankylostoma duodenale*. Leiper rejected Ozzard's results because sufficient precautions against contamination had not been taken. He suggests that the cultures may have been contaminated by the water or sand used, or that the source of contamination had passed through the alimentary canal of the patient. He says:

3. Leiper: Brit. Med. Jour., November, 1909, p. 1332.

When we remember that free-living nematodes abound in all soil and vegetables, that their eggs and larvæ are able to withstand a considerable degree of drying and that they multiply exceedingly in the course of a few days, we should be very loth to accept results of experiments that do not rigorously exclude the possibility of their presence.

Watch-glasses are more convenient than Petri dishes, because the larvæ are kept within a smaller compass and because the sides of the Petri dishes prevent the examination of the edge of the medium. It is convenient to use a very low-power objective, which has the advantage of a large field and plenty of room between the objective and the stage. Slides 2 by 3 inches are much better than the usual 1 by 3 because more material can be examined and much time saved.

The following medium, a modification of the Hiss semisolid medium, was suggested by Dr. Duval, and was found most suitable, because in it the larvæ can move about freely and can be followed through all stages of development.

1000 c.c. distilled water.
80 gm. gelatin.
10 gm. agar.
5 gm. beef extract.
Boil, clear and titrate to 2 per cent acid.

When incubated at 32 C. the sexes can usually be distinguished in about twelve hours and are fully developed in twenty-four hours: however, it sometimes happens that twice that length of time is required. Development may be greatly retarded by a more thorough washing of the larvæ before planting them on the medium, or by incubating them at 25 C. instead of 32 C. I was not able to hasten their development by incubating them at 37 C. When a large number of larvæ are planted it is often noticed that they do not all develop uniformly, that some have already coupled and the females contain eggs well-advanced in segmentation before others have shed their skins. Often there are a few which develop much more slowly and, instead of maturing in twenty-four hours, require forty-eight or more, often dying before fully developed. Those which survive usually develop into filariform larvæ.

I noticed, in growing the larvæ from different cases, that the larvæ in some cases will nearly all develop into filariform larvæ, the proportion of sexual forms being about 1 to 100, and the sexual forms all males. In other cases the sexual forms predominate, the proportion of filariform larvæ being 1 to 25; and in these cases there are more females than males, the proportion being 1 to 6 or 8. This has been noted by others and is discussed in Thayer's article, but no satisfactory explanation has been offered. I believe that it is possible to determine into which of these groups a given case will fall, by careful examination of the larvæ in the stool. In those which develop into sexual forms the sexual anlage is more prominent; it appears larger, more hyaline and refractive, and is easily seen with a low power objective. In those which develop into filariform larvæ the sexual anlage appears somewhat smaller, less refractive, and more difficult to see, often a high-power objective being required to find it.

I have followed Thayer[4] very closely in describing the rhabditiform and filariform larvæ, because his description is excellent.

*Rhabditiform Larvæ.*—In the fresh stools these measure all the way from 0.225 to 0.45 mm. in length, by 0.02 to 0.03 mm. in breadth. The worm diminishes slightly in size toward the head and gradually tapers down to a sharp-pointed tail. The periphery is somewhat refractile, while within, the substance is filled with glistening, refractive, fat-like granules which are much larger toward the head than toward the tail. The mouth of the worm appears, as far as it can be made out, to consist of a simple funnel-shaped depression. The esophagus, between one-third and one-fourth the length of the worm, shows a long bulb-like enlargement at the head, followed by a constriction, which is succeeded by a second round or ovoid enlargement, in the middle of which is a triangular opening; the outlines of this opening are glistening and refractive, indicating clearly the tridentate, chitinous armature described by other observers. The outlines of the cells bordering the digestive tract, of which in some instances a slight suggestion can be made out, are as a rule entirely hidden by the glistening granules above mentioned. The anal outlet is situated at a distance equaling about one-tenth the length of the worm from the tip of the tail. The anterior lip of the anal outlet is slightly raised. A little below the middle of the worm, on the same side as the anal opening, is a small clear elliptical area, the rudiment of the sexual apparatus. The worms manifest a very active serpentine motion and, in many, repeated and violent muscular contractions of the esophagus are observed; these are especially marked about the tridentate opening, which appears to open and shut with considerable force.

*Filariform Larvæ.*—These are longer and more delicate in structure, measuring 0.4 to 0.55 mm. in length, and from 0.016 to 0.022 mm. in breadth. The distinct esophageal enlargements are lost and all trace of the rudiment of the sexual gland has disappeared. Though the parasite is more delicate as a whole than the younger embryo, the tail is blunter and more truncated. They are more active, showing most striking serpentine movements.

I have noticed that when larvæ from a case in which filariform larvæ predominate are planted, they collect at the edge of the medium in ten to twelve hours and one often sees writhing masses of from ten to thirty or more. Even in this short time the sexual anlage has disappeared, one

4. Thayer: Jour. Exper. Med., 1901, vi, 75.

is seldom seen, and never in a fully developed filariform larva. Braun's picture[1] of the filariform larvæ shows the sexual anlage, but there is no reference to it in the original article. The larvæ remain at the edge until they molt, which they do in from twenty to twenty-four hours, after which they are found all through the medium. Probably they collect at the extreme edge because the medium is firmer there and their skins are more easily shed. These larvæ are much more active than the sexual forms and are not often seen lying quiet until they are several days old. When placed in a drop of water under a cover-glass their movements are much more violent and in a short time the worms are to be found at the extreme edge. I have never been able to observe them feeding. They are more resistant, live longer, and grow under conditions which would be unfavorable to the development of the sexual forms. On only one occasion were they found in the fresh stool and then but three were seen.

My own observations, except for a few points mentioned below, agree so completely with Strong's,[5] that I quote his description of the free-living adult males and females:

*Free-Living Adult Females.*—"The females are longer than the males; their bodies also taper more in the posterior portion. They measure generally from 1 mm. to 1.4 mm. in length, and from 0.05 mm. to 0.075 mm. in breadth. In the adult free-living generation the esophagus has the same form as that of the larvæ, except that it shows a relatively smaller increase in length, measuring now about 0.16 mm. Of the three portions of the esophagus the buccalic is the longest. It measures 99 microns and represents in consequence a little more than half of the entire apparatus. The cephalic extremity is rounded and pierced by the mouth, about which, on careful examination, three or four papillæ can be made out. Next to the mouth comes a vestibule, which for a short length presents a gradual enlargement. It is much better developed than in the larvæ, and enters the anterior extremity of the esophagus, which juts from its interior in the form of a smooth cone. This part of the esophagus is continuous with the bulbous or terminal portion, which encloses an apparatus for trituration consisting of three chitinous teeth. .... The intestine of the female is somewhat longer than that of the male. It ends, as in the larvæ, in a papilla at the right side of the body at the base of the tail and often protrudes a little. In the females the posterior extremity of the body stretches itself out into a tapering, thin, fine tail, often lightly coiled into a spiral. A little below the middle of the body and on the right side is the vulval opening, marked by a slight contraction and giving access to a double uterus, the horns of which extend, the one anteriorly, the other posteriorly. Each of these ends in an ovary. The eggs measure 70 by 45 microns. They are elliptical; the shell is delicate and the vitellus contains a few granules. The eggs are often more or less segmented when laid. Indeed, not infrequently they hatch in the body of the adult, and one can then see the embryos moving within the body of the mother. As a rule, hatching is completed in twenty-four hours. At first the worms are thin, the tails are tapering, and the bulbous swelling of the esophagus and the chitinous teeth are apparent. They soon change and pass from the rhabditiform to the strongyloid stage."

In my observations I never saw the tail of the female coiled into a spiral, as described above. After coupling, eggs appear first at the vulva

---

5. Strong: Johns Hopkins Hosp. Rep., 1902, x, 91.

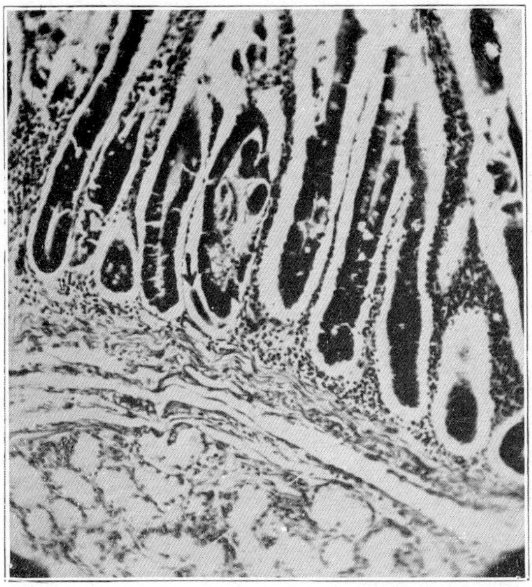

Fig. 1.—Larva at the bottom of one of Lieberkühn's glands just inside the basement membrane on its way to the close-meshed system of lymphatics in the mucous membrane. The arrows indicate the location of the larvæ. This and the following illustrations show sections of intestine and lung from Case 1.

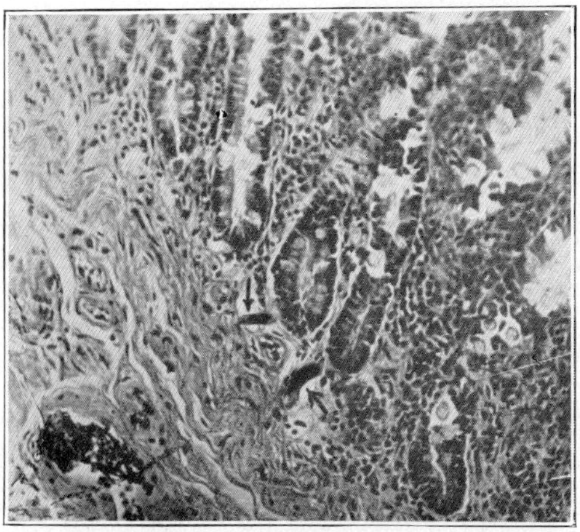

Fig. 2.—Larva breaking through into the muscularis mucosæ probably in a lymph-vessel.

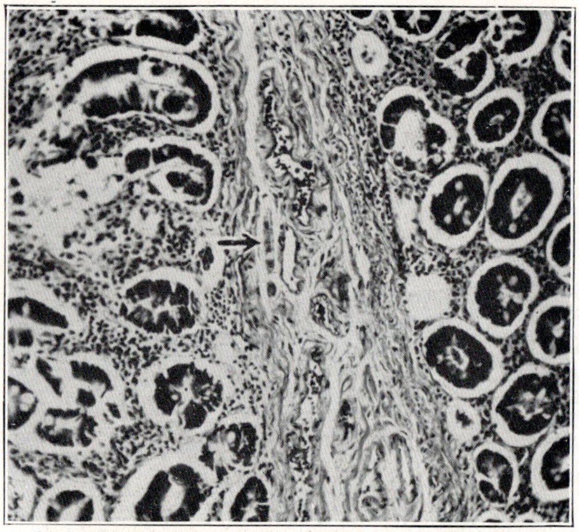

Fig. 3.—Larva in a lymph-vessel in the muscularis mucosæ of a valvula connivens.

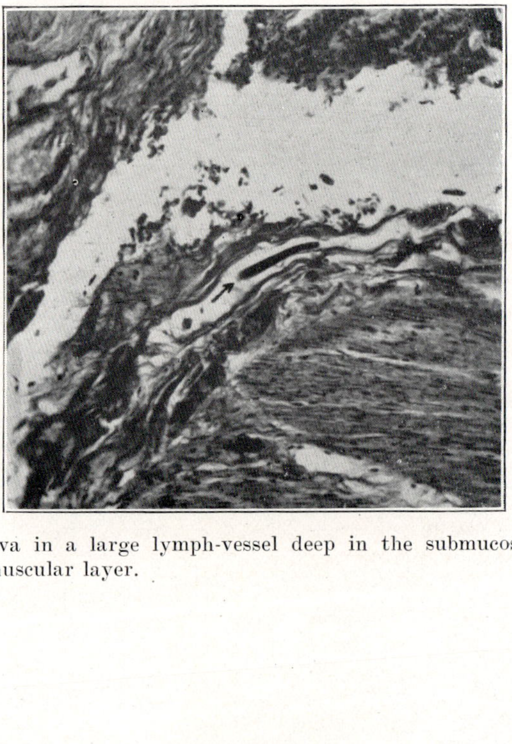

Fig. 4.—Larva in a large lymph-vessel deep in the submucosa, close to the inner circular muscular layer.

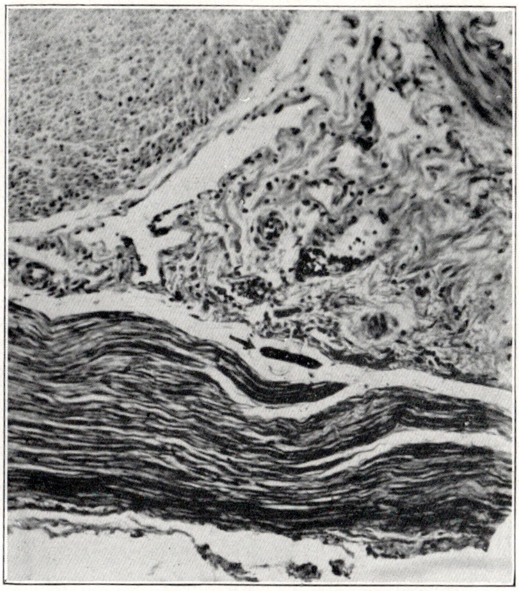

Fig. 5.—Larva just inside outer longitudinal muscular coat of the duodenum.

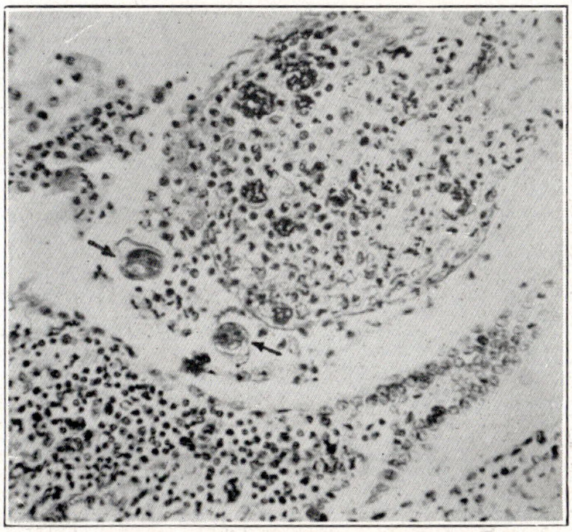

Fig. 6.—Larva, cut in two places, in an antevesicular tube of the lung. The larva is surrounded by inflammatory exudate.

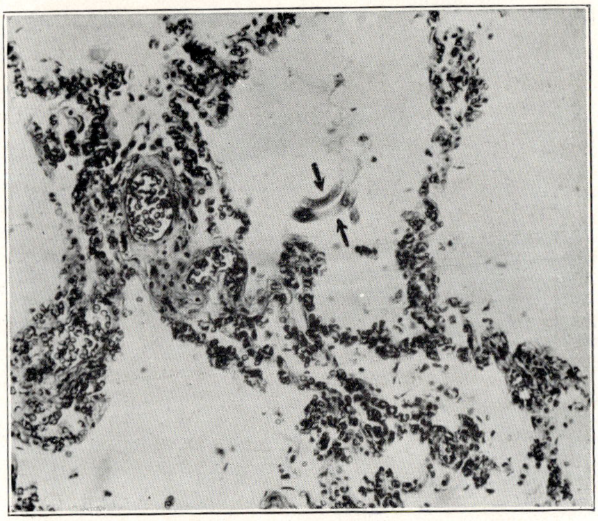

Fig. 7.—Larva coiled up in an air-vesicle. Portions of two coils shown.

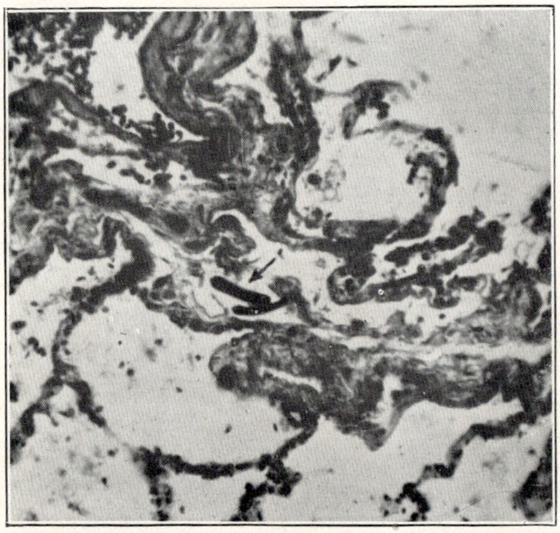

Fig. 8.—Larva in the interlobular connective tissue of the lungs.

and develop rapidly in both directions until there are sometimes as many as twenty-six, closely packed and lying transversely, which is quite different from the arrangement of the eggs in the body of the parasitic mother worm in the intestine. Those nearest the vulva are most developed and often contain embryos, and one can trace all stages of segmentation as either extremity is approached. The eggs when laid usually contain embryos. Unfertilized eggs segment to the mulberry-mass stage but no further. The females produce but one batch of eggs and I have never seen them couple the second time.

*Free-Living Adult Males.*—"The males are shorter and thinner than the females, measuring from about 0.75 to 1 mm. long by 0.04 to 0.06 mm. wide. The esophagus is a little shorter than in the female. The caudal extremity measures about 70 microns; it tapers quickly and is curved on itself in a manner quite different from the spiral coils in the tail of the female. Just at the base of the tail one can readily distinguish two cone-shaped and curved spicules, which represent the copulatory organ."

Cline describes a long gland made up of globules which is situated in the posterior third of the male and terminates at the base of the tail. I have often seen this; the globules appear to be small granular cells, larger and more granular at the posterior end. The gland extends through the middle third of the worm, but at this place is hard to see, and is sometimes indistinct. I have often seen the worm rupture at the base of the tail and the gland cells flow out. This is most often observed in old males. Between the posterior end of the gland and the spicules are two clear oval cavities. When placed under a cover-glass the males are sometimes seen to protrude and retract the spicules, one at a time. This occurs just before they die. On the tip of the tail is a delicate flagellum which is 30 to 40 microns long, 5 microns broad at the base and tapers to a fine point. This is easily seen when the worms are in the yellowish semisolid medium but, when placed in water, it is very easily overlooked. I have never seen this described, nor have I seen it represented in drawings.

Both sexes shed their skins and couple in from twenty to twenty-four hours. When about to couple the female lies quiet except for a movement of the head and a rapid rhythmic contraction of the second bulb of the esophagus. The male crawls around the female five or ten minutes before grasping her, stopping often and coiling his tail. He then coils the posterior half of the body around the female, so that the body of the male lies in a plane at right angles to the body of the female. Often two and sometimes three males are coiled around the female at the same time. After coiling his tail loosely around the female near the head the male begins to move around and around, feeling with the spicules while the female crawls slowly through the loop until the vulva is reached, when the coils tighten and the spicules are pressed in. The female does not struggle to get away as described by Perroncito,[6] who says, "She makes an effort as if to disengage herself." The worms remain in this position from three and one-half to five minutes; then the male uncoils and lies quiet for five to seven minutes and the female crawls away. Again my observations disagree with Perroncito who says, "The act has a short duration of from forty to fifty seconds." I have seen copulation many times and the time required for it was never less than three minutes. After a female has coupled she is not again approached.

In twenty-four hours after coupling the young larvæ are found free in the medium. These have an esophagus with a double dilatation, an oval sexual anlage—in fact, the same structure as in the larvæ found in the stools. This generation always died, so I was unable to watch its further development.

The larvæ feed on the bacteria or their products and not on the medium. When transferred to fresh medium they remain among the bacteria transferred with them and move away from the point of inoculation as the bacterial growth spreads. While feeding, the worms lie quiet, except the anterior end, which is in constant motion. The second dilatation of the esophagus shows strong rhythmic contractions which extend forward to the mouth and the entire esophagus moves up and down within the worm with each contraction. When the bacterial growth becomes too profuse, the worms die, if not transferred to fresh medium. By transferring them every day or every second day I have been able to keep the females alive four to six days after reaching maturity, but the males lived only half as long.

## PREVALENCE AND DISTRIBUTION

Baetjer,[7] in a recent article, expresses the opinion that strongyloides infection is apparently quite uncommon in this country; but I agree with Stiles, who believes that it is common, especially in the Southern States. Baetjer found but fourteen cases reported in the United States which, with his case and six others in the Johns Hopkins hospital statistics, made a total of twenty-one. I find twenty-nine cases mentioned which, with Baetjer's seven, Eustis' one and my fifteen, make a total of fifty at the present time: Strong,[5] one case; Thayer,[4] two additional ones; Ohlmacher,[8] one; Price,[9] one; Moore,[10] one; Brown,[11] three; Hall,[12] one;

6. Perroncito: Quoted by Strong.

7. Baetjer: Bull. Johns Hopkins Hosp., 1910, xxi, 118.

8. Ohlmacher: Am. Med., 1903, v, 816.

9. Price, Marshall Langton: Occurrence of the *Strongyloides Intestinalis* in the United States, Jour. Am. Med. Assn., 1903, xli, 651.

10. Moore: Am. Med., 1903, v, 876.

11. Brown: Boston Med. and Surg. Jour., 1903, cxlviii, 583.

12. Hall, J. N.: A Case of Infection by Strongyloides Intestinalis. Jour. Am. Med. Assn., 1907, xlviii, 1182.

Stiles, in discussing Price's paper, mentions four; Moore, in discussing the same paper, mentions two others; Brush,[13] three; Cline,[14] one; Daland,[15] one; Baetjer,[7] seven; Dock,[16] one; Simon,[17] five; and Patterson,‡ two. The distribution of the reported cases shows that the disease is found in nearly every one of the southern states; and some imported cases are seen in the North. The disease is far more prevalent than the number of reported cases would lead one to believe. I examined the stools of 200 students of Tulane University and found 2 per cent. of them infected with this parasite, which may be taken to indicate the prevalence among apparently healthy individuals. The prevalence among sick people must be much greater. Statistics showing the prevalence among patients at the Charity Hospital are not at hand, but the men who examine the stools, chiefly for the hookworm eggs and amebas, find the larvæ so often that they attach little importance to their presence. Mild infections are easily overlooked in the ordinary examination of the stool, since examination of several preparations is necessary. I have often noticed that, for several days at a time, a long search is required to find the larvæ in stools in which ordinarily they are easily found. I have also noticed, especially when the stools are firm, that larvæ are more numerous in the portion of the stool passed last.

### THE MANNER IN WHICH LARVÆ GAIN ENTRANCE TO THE BODY

It has been proved conclusively that infection occurs both by mouth and through the skin. Wilms[18] infected a patient by feeding the larvæ, and animals can be infected in this way, although this method sometimes fails with animals (Schlüter[19]). It has been shown by Van Durme,[20] Marzocchi,§ and Daland, that the larvæ penetrate the skin and that animals can be infected in this way, and that the penetration of the skin by the larvæ causes a lesion similar to ground itch in man. In 1904 Looss[21] succeeded in infecting himself with *Strongyloides* by placing larvæ on the skin. He applied several hundred larvæ to the skin of his forearm and, on the sixty-fourth day, found the first larvæ in his stools;

13. Brush: South. Med. Jour., 1908, i, 248.
14. Cline: Post-Graduate, 1908, xxiii, 451.
15. Daland: New York Med. Jour., 1908, lxxxvii, 761.
16. Dock: New York Med. Jour., 1909, xc, 53.
17. Simon, Sidney K.: Amebic Dysentery, Jour. Am. Med. Assn., 1909, liii, 1526.

‡Patterson, H. S.: Parasites Found in New York City, THE ARCHIVES INT. MED., 1908, ii, 185.

18. Wilms: Schmidt's Jahrb., 1897, cclvi, 272.
19. Schlüter: Med. Klin., 1905, i, 1305.
20. Van Durme: Thompson Yates Lab. Rep., Liverpool, 1902, iv, 471.

§Marzocchi, V.: Gior. d. r. Accad. di med. di Torino, 1907, series 4, xiii, 3.

21. Looss, A.: Compt. rend. du 6 Cong. Internat. de Zool., Berne, 1905, p. 225.

larvæ were present on all subsequent examinations, as many as two or three in every 4 c.mm. of the feces. His conclusions are as follows:

For the species of the genera *Ankylostoma* and *Strongyloides* there is a possible mode of entrance through the skin in addition to that by way of the mouth, by which the mature larvæ can make their way into their host. The larvæ, after boring into the skin, penetrate the superficial lymph-vessels or veins and are carried through the heart into the lungs in that way. In the lungs they pass from the blood-vessels into the air-tubes and finally wander through the trachea, larynx and esophagus to the intestines. In the lymph-glands apparently a number of larvæ are kept back and rendered harmless. The larvæ get to their goal all the more easily and in larger numbers, the younger the affected individual of the species of host. In old hosts a larger or smaller number of larvæ are kept back in the tissues where they wander around under the skin producing the skin disease known as the "creeping eruption," etc. They are able to live as long in the form of wandering larvæ as the adult worm; that is to say, about five years.

It is difficult to say which is the more common mode of infection. The frequent occurrence of strongyloides larvæ in the stools of patients suffering from amebic dysentery might be taken to indicate that infection by way of the mouth is the usual one. But, since they do easily penetrate the skin and reach the intestines and are sometimes found in patients who also have hookworm disease, it seems likely that infection through the skin is a common, if not the usual, manner of infection, as it is in hookworm disease, and that some of the ground-itch in the South is due to the penetration of the skin by strongyloides larvæ.

## DURATION OF INFECTION

It is impossible to tell accurately how long man harbors this parasite, but patients are known to have had larvæ in the stools for several years. From the enormous number of larvæ in some cases it seems that these patients must reinfect themselves. It has been suggested by Grassi,[22] and later by Ward,[23] that the direct transformation of rhabditiform larvæ into filariform larvæ and then back to the parasitic mother worms may occur inside the intestine. The finding of three filariform larvæ in a fresh stool from one of my cases would seem to bear this out, but this cannot be a common occurrence, or at autopsy there would be found all the stages between the filariform larvæ and the adult worm, which is not the case.

The finding of larvæ in the sputum in Case 1 here reported, after the patient had been in bed two months, indicates that he was reinfecting himself. Because of his personal filthiness and the irritation of the skin over his buttocks and back, I thought that the larvæ were gaining entrance through the skin at this place, and probably some did. However, the

22. Grassi: Gior. di r. Accad. di med. di Torino, 1883 series 3, xxxi, 119.
23. Ward: Reference Handbook of Medical Sciences.

presence of larvæ in the lymph-spaces and lymph-vessels of the intestinal wall suggests another plausible explanation—that the larvæ pierce the intestinal walls, enter the lymph-stream, pass up the thoracic duct into the subclavian vein, thence through the right heart to the lungs, appear in the sputum and, when swallowed, develop into adult parasites. This idea is strengthened by the fact that some of the larvæ in the sputum were young, as shown by the presence of the sexual anlage. In this way a vicious circle is set up and the infection grows steadily worse, and, as the number of worms in the intestine increases, more larvæ penetrate the intestinal walls and pass over the route above described. This must be a slow process and extend over many years, since there were comparatively few larvæ in the sections of the intestine and in the sputum, and this was a severe case as to stools.

## SYMPTOMS

*Strongyloides intestinalis* was first described in cases of Cochin-China diarrhea and was regarded as the cause. However, this point has been under discussion and the reader is referred to the articles by Thayer[4] and Strong,[5] in which the pathogenicity is fully discussed. Noc,[24] in a recent article, asserts that the diarrhea in Cochin-China is in reality amebic dysentery. Whatever the cause of the so-called Cochin-China diarrhea, there can be no doubt that *Strongyloides intestinalis* is pathogenic and is the cause of some of the diarrhea in the United States, especially in the southern states. While not all persons harboring this parasite have diarrhea, the proportion of those who do is large enough to convince physicians who see many cases that the diarrhea is due to *Strongyloides.*

During the last six months I have seen fifteen cases, and of these, in thirteen there was diarrhea more or less marked. In one case in which there was no diarrhea there was a tendency to constipation, but a small dose of cathartic caused profuse evacuations; in the other case there were so few larvæ in the stools that none could be found by the ordinary method of examination and only a few by the method described by Bass.[25] One of the thirteen with diarrhea also had amebic dysentery and so cannot be considered, which leaves twelve in which *Strongyloides intestinalis* was the only obvious cause. Many of these patients will deny having diarrhea, in fact, will say they are constipated; but further questioning will bring out the fact that they have periods lasting a day or two, when the stools are soft, unformed, even fluid, and of increased frequency. In the interval the stools are normal or there is constipation. This has

---

24. Noc: Ann. de l'Inst. Pasteur, 1909, xxiii, 177.
25. Bass, C. C.: Mild Uncinaria Infections, The Archives Int. Med., 1909, iii, 446.

been my experience with the university students whose stools contained the larvæ.

The severity of the symptoms is not always in proportion to the number of larvæ present in the stools. One of my patients presenting no diarrhea at all had many times more larvæ in the stools than had others presenting a moderate diarrhea.

The diarrhea is chronic and intermittent and often very suggestive of amebic dysentery. The attacks occur from once every few days to once a month, and last one or two days; in severe cases the diarrhea may be almost continuous. Usually there is no pain. The desire to go to stool is often sudden and very urgent, even when the stools are of normal consistency and this sometimes may amount to incontinence. As a rule more stools, two or three or more, depending on the severity of the symptoms, are passed during the early morning hours than during the rest of the day. The stools are very seldom dysenteric in character, unless associated with amebas, and in mild cases are not even fluid. Except in severe cases the general condition of the patient is not greatly affected; however, while none of the students harboring the parasite considered themselves ill, all were poorly nourished and anemic-looking individuals.

All of my patients had a mild anemia, the hemoglobin ranging from 70 to 90. The highest eosinophil count was 13.2 per cent., the lowest 2.5 per cent. There is usually a mild eosinophilia, although this may be absent. Sometimes a marked eosinophilia is present. Eustis, in the report previously cited, records a case showing 56 per cent.; Baetjer's case showed 45 per cent., and Daland's case 38.2 per cent.

## TREATMENT

Opinions differ as to the value of treatment, for while some report successful results, the majority report failures. Eustis, in the above paper, reports a cure and attributes his success in part to the soluble diet given. On the other hand, Cline treated a patient for several months and, while the number of larvæ diminished, they did not disappear entirely. His patient received the following treatment: large doses of thymol preceded by a twenty-four hour fast, one dose per week for six weeks; bismuth-beta-naphthol daily for six weeks, except on the days thymol was administered; male-fern for two days in succession each week for six weeks; large doses of calomel and santonin for three days, followed by castor oil for three weeks. In addition he took at different times phenyl salicylate (salol) and castor oil equal parts, 60 cg., three times a day; mineral acids, iron and strychnin. Regulation of diet.

The ipecac treatment, as used in amebic dysentery, was tried in one case by Simon,[26] of New Orleans, but was not effective. In none of my

26. Simon: Personal communication.

cases was treatment administered. Since the infection is so common it is worth while trying various drugs in the hope that an effective one may be found.

The reinfection described here easily accounts for the failure to get rid of the parasites. Larvæ which had penetrated the intestinal walls would not be affected by an anthelmintic, and on again reaching the intestines would develop into adults, so in a short time larvæ would appear in the stools even though all the adults were killed at the time the anthelmintic was administered. The treatment indicated is comparable to that for malaria; it should be repeated at intervals for a long time in order to kill those parasites which were beyond the reach of any single course of treatment.

I wish to express my gratitude to Dr. Dock, at whose suggestion I began this work, and who directed my work throughout; I wish to thank him especially for his valuable assistance in reviewing the recent literature.

I am also deeply indebted to Dr. C. W. Duval for the use of his laboratory and many valuable suggestions.

# BOOK REVIEW

THE ELEMENTS OF THE SCIENCE OF NUTRITION. By Graham Lusk, Ph.D., Sc.D., F.R.S. (Edin.), Professor of Physiology at Cornell University Medical College, New York City. Second Edition. Cloth. Price, $3 net. Pp. 402, with 13 illustrations. Philadelphia: W. B. Saunders Co., 1909.

Among those familiar with its predecessor, this second edition of Lusk's work will find a ready acceptance. The new volume differs from the other mainly in its consideration of facts which have been discovered during the past three years, and although there has been some increase in size, the book retains its compactness and character. Even more than before one is impressed by the fact that in this work we have to do with an unusual and significant type of American medical writing. Its character may be gleaned from the following excerpts from the preface, which are a true index of what follows in the text:

"The aim of the book is to review the scientific substratum on which rests the knowledge of nutrition, both in health and in disease." Throughout no statement has been made without endeavoring to give proof that it is true. "The widespread interest in the subject of nutrition at the present time leads the author to hope that this book may prove of value to the student of dietetics and to the clinical physician."

Concerning the manner in which the material is handled, it may be said that there are fifteen chapters. The first, devoted to a historical review of the development of our knowledge of metabolism and the fundamental laws on which it is based, is permeated with a fine spirit of respect for the work of the men who broke the ground and built up what has become famous as the "Munich school," of which the author is a disciple and to the main tenets of which he closely adheres to his thinking. The second chapter deals with the metabolic phenomena as seen in starvation, uncomplicated by foods or other agencies, and the third with regulation of temperature. With these chapters as a background, the effects on the metabolism of the various foods (protein, fat, and carbohydrate) of mechanical work and of the better studied pathological conditions, fever, diabetes, gout, Basedow's disease, etc., are taken up in separate sections. Chapters on "The Food Requirements During the Period of Growth," "A Normal Diet," and "Theory of Metabolism" complete the list. An appendix of ten pages contains food composition tables from Bryant and Atwater; a table from Langworthy's report shows the comparative cost of protein energy as purchased in different forms of food; and a table of urinary composition after Folin is given.

From the standpoint of the theoretical worker, this book is especially valuable by virtue of the data which have been supplied from the laboratory of the writer himself, and because of the critique which this first-hand knowledge enables him to exercise, this advantage being most in evidence in the chapter on the influence of the protein foods, in the discussion of fats and carbohydrates, and in the brilliant interpretations which are made of the phenomena seen in phosphorus poisoning and diabetes. Fatty infiltration and lactic acid excretion are handled with notable originality and insight. Owing, however, to a constant recognition of clinical problems, the continuity between laboratory and bedside work is kept steadily in mind, and the volume is full of suggestions which are valuable from the clinical standpoint. The chapter on regulation of temperature brings the principles of bodily heat control into intimate relationship with such manifestations as "acute intoxication" during infancy, with the rational handling of fever, with problems of ventilation, and the like, while such chapters as those devoted to gout and diabetes make excellent clinical reading. All in all, this book does more to show the inseparability of theoretical laboratory and bedside work than any work which has yet been published in this country.

The Archives of Internal Medicine

Vol. VII MAY, 1911 No. 5

# ORIENTAL SORE IN PANAMA

S. T. DARLING, M.D.
ANCON, C. Z.

The following account of an autochthonous case of Oriental sore in Panama adds one other to the list of regions to be included in the geographical distribution of this disorder. The lesion followed the bite of a fly which was undoubtedly a tabanid; and as the case is a solitary one, it raises again the question of the specificity of the different strains of *Leishmania tropica* causing Oriental sore.

## REPORT OF CASE

*History.*—The patient, J. A. C., negro, aged 44, was born in Demerara. He had lived in Paramaribo for three years, in Nickeri for eighteen months and in Trinidad subsequently for twenty-four years. In September, 1909, he came to the city of Panama where he lived one month. Since October, 1909, he has been living on a cacao and rubber plantation out in the bush several miles from Empire. The residents at the plantation are native Colombians and Jamaican negroes. There are no natives of, or visitors from, the Levant, India or other regions of the Old World where Oriental sore is endemic. The patient states that he has never seen anywhere a sore similar to his.

*Present Illness.*—One day in May of this year, while sitting under a wild cashew tree, the man was bitten on the right forearm by a large fly which, from his description, was a tabanid.[1] The wound was scratched and the resulting sore exuded a watery fluid. The patient, to relieve the itching, continually scratched and pinched the sore. After a month's duration it increased in size and a very hard, thick crust formed on its surface. The itching now ceased, but the margins of the sore became quite tender, and the epitrochlear and axillary lymph-nodes also became tender at this time. During the past three months the sore has been from 20 to 30 mm. in diameter. One month ago (duration of sore three months) a small nodule appeared under the skin 4 cm. above the ulcer, but it did not break down and the skin has remained normal.

*Examination.*—The patient presented himself at the laboratory on August 17. The sore was located on the right forearm, near the wrist, on the ulnar aspect. It was circular and covered with a raised, flat, granular, grayish-yellow crust, which was very hard and thick. At that time, after four months' duration, the outside diameter, including the raised skin margin, was 22 mm.; the diameter of the crust was 17 mm. On lifting the crust, a circular fossa was seen, separating the raised skin margin from the granulating and healing surface of the ulcer. The appearance and location of the ulcer were so unique that the diagnosis of Oriental sore was at once suggested. Portions of the crust were removed and smears made from the granulating surface. A few microorganisms, exactly resembling *L. tropica,* were found.

1. His description is of some value as he had occasionally collected material for the laboratory, including tabanids.

*Infecting Organisms.*—On August 26 the patient entered the hospital for treatment. The ulcer was excised well beyond the raised margins and below to normal subcutaneous tissue (Dr. Herrick). Smears from its granulating surface contained free and intracellular microorganisms, resembling *L. tropica.* Most of them were oval, one end being obtuse, the other acute. All contained a trophonucleus and a kinetonucleus; a few presented small achromatic spaces in the pale blue cytoplasm. A refractile capsule was not detected. Some were in intracellular groups of two, four, five and eleven or more.

DIMENSIONS OF THE MICROORGANISMS

| Length. microns. | Breadth. microns. |
|---|---|
| 6 | 3.5 |
| 5 | 3.5 |
| 6 | 3. |
| 9 | 4.25 |

Length of kinetonucleus...... 1.5 microns.
Diameter of trophonucleus.... 2.75 microns.

The microorganism, while slightly larger than some of those described elsewhere, presented the same morphology noted in cases from

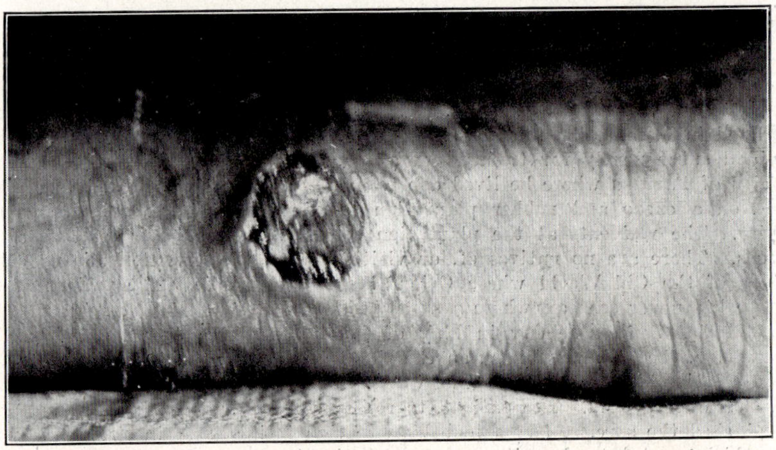

Fig. 1.—The ulcer.

the Old World and it closely resembled the gregarine phase of *Crithidia* found in representatives of *Tabanus* and other invertebrates. It is not impossible that the case described here, following, as it does, the history of a bite by a tabanid, is the result of an inoculation with an invertebrate intestinal flagellate (*Crithidia?*), which was able to take up a parasitic existence in the tissues of man.

Smears from the ulcer were stained for the presence of acid-fast bacilli, but none was found.

*Histology.*—The ulcer is covered with a thick eosin-staining mass of desquamated epithelium containing a few polymorphonuclear leukocytes. Beneath this the granuloma is nearly covered with squamous epithelium showing much metaplasia of the rete, which extends downward deeply into the corium and papillæ, dividing it into elongated chambers. Here and there the stratum corneum is carried downward with the rete and is pinched off into cell nests. The corium and papillæ are uniformly and richly infiltrated with newly formed cells of the lymphoid and plasma type; there are numerous proliferated endothelial and epithelioid cells and several giant cells also. The endothelium of the capillaries, particularly that of the papillæ, is swollen and proliferated. There are no areas of necrosis. With the highest powers a few microorganisms (*L. tropica*) are seen in groups of from one to a dozen individuals imbedded in the cytoplasm or placed alongside the nucleus of an endothelial, epithelioid or other cell. In the deeper portions of the skin the cellular proliferation is limited to perivascular collections of small, round cells of the lymphoid type, surrounding blood and lymphatic vessels and sweat-glands.

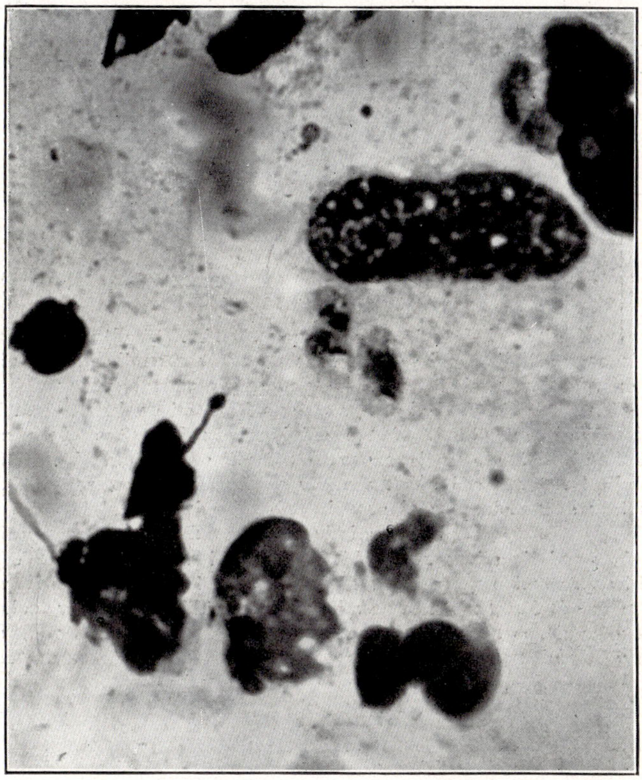

Fig. 2.—*L. tropica* in a large endothelial cell with oblong nucleus.

Oriental sore is an ulcerating[2] skin granuloma caused by a protozoon, *Leishmania tropica,* or by allied forms.

The lesion has been given various names, of which the following are among the commonest; Lahore, Multan and Delhi sore; Oriental sore;

2. Non-ulcerating types have been described by R. M. Carter (Oriental Sore of Northern India, A Protozoal Infection, Brit. Med. Jour., 1909, ii, 647); by D. B. Thompson and A. Balfour (Two Cases of Non-Ulcerating "Oriental Sore," Better Termed, Leishman Nodules, Tr. Soc. Trop. Med. and Hyg., London, 1910, iii, 107) and by Cambillet (Un cas de Bouton d'Orient à Flatters [Alger], Bull. Soc. Path. Exot., Paris, July 21, 1909).

Delhi boil; Aleppo boil; Biskra boil; Gafsa boil; pian bois; ulceras de Baurú; mycosis cutis chronica; lupus endemicus; granuloma endemicum. Better terms, no doubt, would be those expressing the relation to the pathogenic agent and the location of the lesion, as "dermal leishmaniosis" or "ulcerating leishmaniosis."[3]

As its many names indicate, the disease is found chiefly in the Orient and Levant—Delhi, Lahore, Punjab, in India; Persia, Arabia, Transcaucasia, Turkey, Morocco, Algeria and Egypt. Strong's[4] case of skin ulceration of the first type in the Philippines seems to have been one of mycotic skin infection.

Very few cases have been reported from the New World. Juliano Moreira,[5] in 1896, reported its occurrence in Bahia, Brazil.

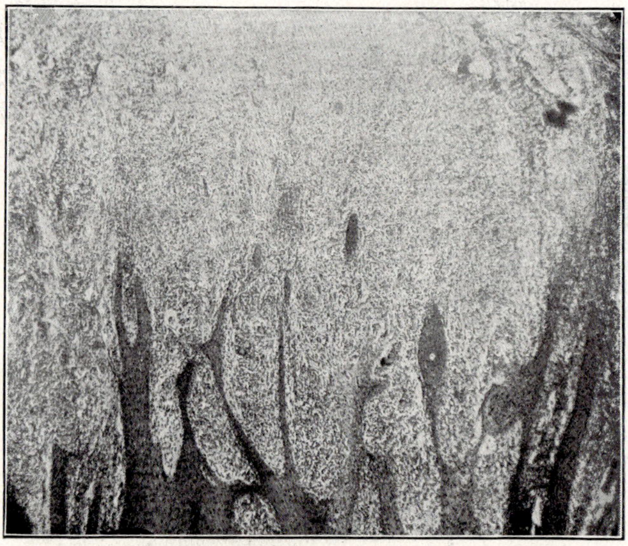

Fig. 3.—Section of ulcer showing metaplasia of the rete and cellular proliferation in the corium.

Carini and Paranhos[6] reported cases seen among Syrian, Portugese and Brazilian laborers at Baurú, São Paulo, Brazil. A case has also been reported occurring in French Guiana.[7]

3. Lindenberg at São Paulo, Brazil, has found *L. tropica* in *le ulcére de Bauru* and he has designated the disease as *Leishmaniose ulcéreuse*.

4. Strong: Philippine Jour. Sc., 1906, i, 91.

5. Scheube, B.: The Diseases of Warm Countries, Ed. 2, Philadelphia, 1904, P. Blakiston's Son and Co.

6. Carini, A., and Paranhos, O.: Identification de l'ulcera de Baurú avec le bouton d'Orient, Bull. Soc. path. exot., Paris, May 12, 1909; Rev. med. de São Paulo, Brazil, March 31, 1909.

7. Nattan-Larrier, Tonin and Keckenroth: Bull. Soc. path. exot., Paris, 1909, ii, 587.

According to Castellani and Chalmers[8] the disease was first recognized and described by Russell in 1756. At that time it was thought to be caused by bad drinking-water. Between that period and 1903, when Wright's paper[9] appeared, various microorganisms, parasites, ova of parasites, fungi, etc., were regarded as the etiologic factors. The contagious character of its virus had been recognized at an early date, for the Jews of Bagdad were in the habit, at one time, of inoculating their children with the disease so that they would not later get a disfiguring scar on the exposed parts.

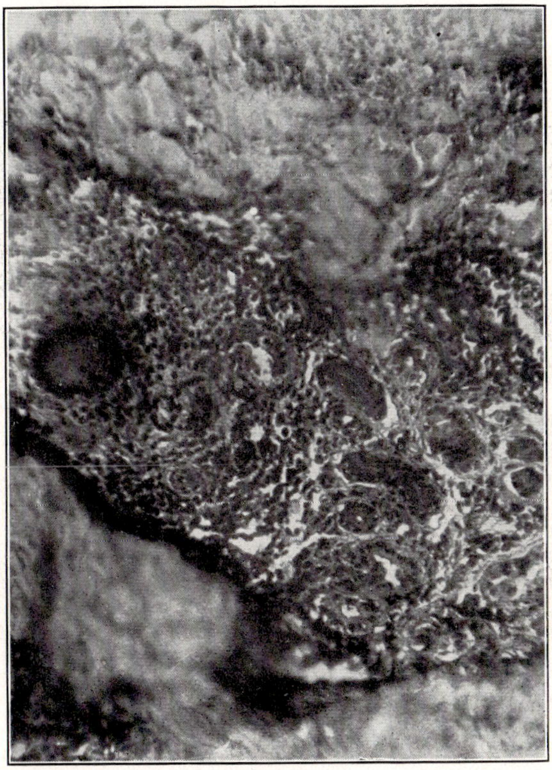

Fig. 4.—Section of ulcer deeper than that shown in Figure 3, showing cellular proliferation, chiefly of the round cell type, around the sweat glands. A large giant cell is seen.

It is possible that the patient in the case described here became infected while on an errand to the city of Panama. On the other hand, there is an emphatic history of a bite by a tabanid while in the bush.

8. Castellani, A., and Chalmers, A. J.: Manual of Tropical Medicine, New York, 1910, Wm. Wood & Co.

9. Wright: "Protozoa in a Case of Tropical Ulcer (Delhi Sore)," Jour. Med. Research, 1903, x, 472.

The population of the Canal Zone comprises men from nearly every region of the world, and an infected native from a region in which Oriental sore is endemic might have come here in an infective condition. A tabanid, *Stomoxys,* or one other of the muscid flies, mechanically by biting or sucking could then infect from such a person a second individual.

Since early in 1905 I have examined material here in Panama for the detection of *L. tropica* in cases of chronic skin ulceration, but until the case described here was seen, nothing of a positive nature had been encountered.

During the year 1904 and early in 1905 every village in the Canal Zone and the cities of Panama and Colon contained many fine examples of tropical ulceration. In one of the villages near Colon, for example, nearly every native had a tropical ulcer. These were usually undressed,

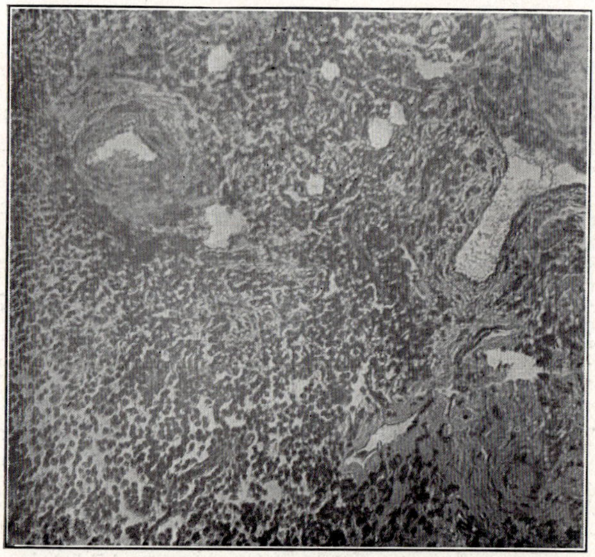

Fig. 5.—Section of ulcer near that shown in Figure 4. There is much perivascular round cell proliferation.

or imperfectly dressed, and were exposed to flies and bugs, which undoubtedly acted as agents of transfer for the virus, for the disease was stamped out by surgical cleanliness and the use of dressings. The sloughing ulcers of the lower limbs and other forms of ulceration are now more rarely found, except among natives and those who are living in the bush beyond the pale of sanitary measures.

On first view, then, it might seem rather extraordinary that an isolated case of Oriental sore should have been found, but it must be remembered that whereas in the Canal Zone within the limits of efficient sanitation most tropical diseases have been wiped out, a different condition prevails in the bush and jungle where no attempt has as yet been made to alter the primitive and insanitary mode of life of the natives; here one may expect to encounter a relatively richer pathological fauna and flora.

The case described here is not so inexplicable when it is known that the patient was not an employee of the commission and did not live in commission quarters, but lived on a cacao and rubber plantation several miles out in the bush outside of the zone of sanitation, from which region few patients are ever received into the hospitals.

Bagdad, where Oriental sore is endemic, has about the same latitude as Charleston, S. C.; and it would not be surprising to find cases reported in the southern states in the future. A careful examination of stained films and sections of tissue from chronic granulomata of the exposed parts would undoubtedly reveal some examples of this type of ulceration.

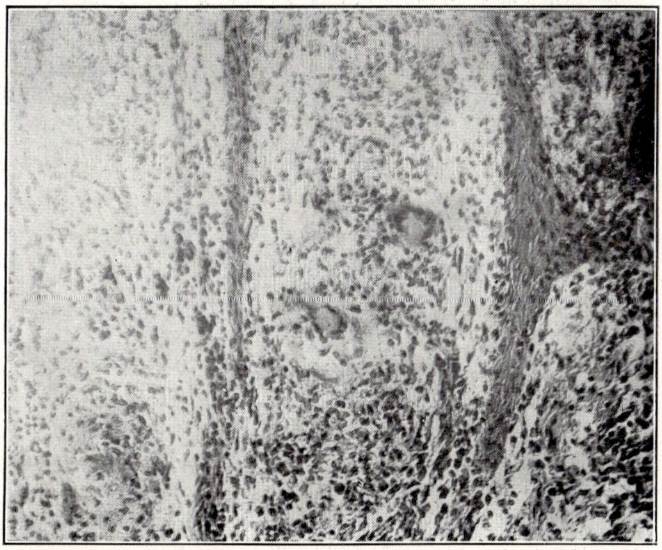

Fig. 6.—Section of ulcer from the same location as that shown in the upper third of Figure 3. There is much cellular proliferation in the papillæ, and between two attenuated metaplastic down-growths of the rete two giant cells are seen.

EPIDEMIOLOGY

Carter states that age, sex, food, race, constitution and hygienic conditions play no part in the etiology. This is borne out by Manson[10] and Laveran's experience, the former stating that in Delhi, in 1864, from 40 to 70 per cent. of the resident Europeans were affected with the local sore, while Laveran remarks that the slightest wound tends to become transformed into the *bouton*. At Bagdad it is said that few escape an

10. Manson, P.: Tropical Diseases, Ed. 4, N. Y., Wm. Wood & Co.

attack at particular times of the year; visitors even for a few days are almost certain to contract it.

The disease is confined to certain endemic regions, as Delhi, Bagdad, Lahore, etc. Hirsch has noted a seasonal variation in that the disease is most prevalent at the beginning of a cool rainy season, and in more temperate climates at the end of summer—fly season?

### LOCATION OF THE SORE

The lesion is nearly always on an exposed part, the face, arms or legs, suggesting that the disease is transmitted by a fly rather than by a bedbug or flea. Carter,[2] in a series of cases of Oriental sores seen in South Arabia, noted the following distribution: Out of the 1,154 sores, 914 were on the lower limbs, 113 were on the upper limbs, most of them being near the elbow-joint, and twenty-six were on the face, forehead, side of nose, outer or inner canthus of the eye, or side of cheek.

This location of sores about the elbow-joint and lower limbs is identical with the location of the bite of *Stegomyia calopus*.

### ETIOLOGY

Cunningham,[11] in 1885, described bodies found in sections of tissue from a case of Delhi boil. The sections were made with a freezing microtome and had been stained with gentian violet. The bodies described and measured by Cunningham could hardly be the bodies now recognized as the cause of Oriental sore, for they were entirely too large, 12.6 by 8.8 microns, the largest measuring 12.8 by 25.6 microns, the smallest 6.4 by 6.4 microns. Such minute specimens as the latter were, however, rare. It would seem more likely that Cunningham was describing *Blastomyces*, or the results of cell degeneration.

Wright of Boston[9] published an account of protozoa in a case of tropical ulcer ("Delhi sore"). The patient was not a native of America, but was a "female child, 9 years of age, born in Armenia. . . . The lesion had made its first appearance before the child left Armenia." Wright found intracellular protozoa—*Helcosoma tropicum*, Wright, 1903 —in large endothelial cells in scrapings from the ulcer. Wright's observations established the etiologic nexus of Oriental sore with a protozoon. His work was confirmed by Mazinowsky, Borgow, James, Plehn and others.

### THE PATHOGENIC AGENT

*Leishmania tropica* is found in stained films or sections of tissue invading large mononuclear endothelial cells. It is also found occasionally in the large mononuclear lymphocyte and in the polymorphonuclear

11. Cunningham: Scientific Memoirs by Medical Officers of the Army of India, Part 1, 1884, Calcutta, 1885.

leukocyte. The microorganism is round, oval, or oat-shape, with a large purple-staining mass, the trophonucleus, placed at the periphery, and a smaller deeply staining rod or dot, the kinetonucleus. This is always placed a short distance from the trophonucleus and when rod-shaped at different angles with respect to it and the long axis of the parasite. The cytoplasm stains blue as in the malarial parasite, and there are small achromatic spaces, in some specimens exactly like those in the gregarine phase of *Crithidia.* The microorganisms are commonly 2 to 4 microns in diameter. In smears many are free, others are imbedded in a matrix, while others are intracellular in mononuclear cells, chiefly of the endothelial type.

The intracellular parasite resembles very closely *L. donovani* and *L. infantum,* and also the gregarine phase of many flagellates found in the intestinal tracts of invertebrates such as *Crithidia* of tabanids and fleas, or the herpetomonads of *Musca, Pyrellia,* etc. As these invertebrates become infected and reinfected by the ingestion of infected feces, it is possible for them in the act of biting or of sucking wounds, to deposit the gregarine or other infecting forms of some of the flagellates with which they may be infected.

I have described[12] a fatal disease of this region caused by a minute microorganism, *Histoplasma capsulatum,* resembling *Leishmania* somewhat, and causing lesions very much like those of kala-azar, but apparently it is not closely related to the microorganism of Oriental sore described here.

## HISTOPATHOLOGY

Wright[9]: "The lesion consists essentially of a very extensive infiltration of the corium and papillæ by cells, accompanied by atrophy and disappearance of the epidermis of the part. The infiltrating cells are plasma cells, various kinds of lymphoid cells, and large cells with single vesicular nuclei, and a relatively large amount of cytoplasm, in which are large numbers of the microorganism. These large cells cover extensive areas, are very numerous and constitute the principal part of the infiltration. They are regarded as proliferated endothelial cells."

Manson[10]: "Section of a papule displays an infiltration of the derma by a mass of small, round granulation cells. These lie between the elements of the tissue, particularly about blood-vessels, lymphatics and sweat-glands; toward the center of the lesion they completely replace the normal structures."

Unna, from Scheube[5]: "There is an infiltration of the skin and subcutaneous tissue, with small, round oval cells, multigranulated and giant cells, and also a few leukocytes. In the center of the nodules over which the epithelium is attenuated the infiltration is so dense that the tissue elements are entirely disintegrated; while toward the periphery the cells form small centers, mostly situated in the vicinity of blood-vessels and lymphatics and sweat-glands. The lymphatic

---

12. Darling, S. T.: Histoplasmosis: A Fatal Infectious Disease Resembling Kala-Azar Found Among Natives of Tropical America, Arch. Int. Med., Chicago, 1908, ii, 107; The Morphology of the Parasite (*Histoplasma capsulatum*) and the Lesions of Histoplasmosis, A Fatal Disease of Tropical America, Jour. Exper. Med., 1909, xi, 515.

vessels and spaces are uncommonly wide and there is much edema. In the center of the infiltrated tissue small necrotic particles are inclosed and this, when the sections are stained, exhibits large fibrinous contents; the tissue, otherwise, also contains much fibrin."

Firth[13]: "The histology of these sores has been thoroughly worked out and if sections be made of the initial papule before ulceration, no difficulty is experienced in demonstrating that the whole thickness of the skin and subjacent tissue is infiltrated with lymphoid and epithelioid (mesoblastic) cells, accompanied by more or less complete disintegration of the normal tissue-elements thereby. In the center of the papule the infiltration by young, round cells is so complete that little can be seen of the sweat glands. Toward the edges of the diseased tissue the new cells occur in isolated clusters or groups, chiefly round blood-vessels or lymphatics. The infiltration does not seem primarily to involve either the hair follicles or the sebaceous glands. The individual cells of this infiltration vary from 7 to 9 microns; their nuclei from 5 to 6 microns; the nuclei are large, generally single, but in parts multiple. The anatomical structure of the papule and surrounding skin indicates that Oriental sore is the type of a granuloma; in fact, the most elementary microscopical examinations of the lesion show that it is a reaction of the skin against some virus of low virulenee which has produced granulomatous changes in the corium beneath and round the ulcer. So chronic are these changes which are sometimes met with that a close resemblance to tuberculosis may be occasioned. It is important to bear in mind because it has several times been suggested that certain of these lesions are tuberculous."

Thompson and Balfour[2]: "An increase in the rete Malpighii, long branching columns of which stretch down into the underlying tissues . . . In these respects the condition resembles a papilloma. There were typical cell nests. The papillary layer of the skin is hypertrophied, or at least appears to be so, invading and even cutting off and disintegrating portions of the rete, while itself invaded by infiltrating cells . . . examination with higher powers showed that the cytoplasm of numerous large cells with vesicular nuclei was full of Leishman bodies."

## MODE OF INFECTION

Most descriptions of this disease contain statements that the disease is transmitted through the bite of flies or other insects by their infecting a pre-existing wound or by the infection through the bite of a fly or other insect.

Its conveyance by flies was first claimed by Seriziat in 1875 and by Tscherepkin in 1876. The latter states that the people of Tashkent called the disease "pascha-churdj" which means "fly-bite" (Castellani and Chalmers).

Schulgin attributes its transmission to mosquitoes, and when one considers the location of many of the sores this is a very probable suggestion.

Laveran believes that flies transmit the virus mechanically. Nothing, however, of a positive nature is known. In the case reported here there is a very definite history of the sore following the bite of a tabanid.

The disease is directly inoculable from one individual to another, for the Jews of Bagdad were in the habit of inoculating their children, hoping to prevent a subsequent disfiguring scar. The disease is also autoinoculable.

---

13. Firth, R. H.: Allbutt's System of Medicine, ii, 490.

Dogs and camels have sores resembling Oriental sores and the sores of the dogs contain the "characteristic parasite" (Sambon).

The sores are frequently on exposed parts, easily accessible to flies or mosquitoes, and they are also not uncommonly located at hat and sleeve margins where friction would favor the introduction of an infecting agent into an abraded skin.

### PERIOD OF INCUBATION

Manson[10] saw "an unquestionable Oriental sore which did not appear until five months after the patient had been exposed to any possibility of infection." The period of incubation would seem to vary between the rather wide limits of a few days to several months.

### SYMPTOMATOLOGY

The first appearance is that of one or two small papules like those which follow insect-bites, and which may itch considerably. The papule increases in size by infiltration of the underlying derma and becomes hard and shotty. It has a hyperemic margin. When the papule becomes 10 to 15 mm. in diameter the sebaceous and sweat glands beneath have either been destroyed or have failed to secrete. The epithelium becomes dry and a film of gray epithelial scales forms on the surface. Later, the nutrition of this area has become so interfered with that necrosis and ulceration occurs. Accompanying the ulceration, there is some fluid exudation and desquamation which dries into a firm, hard, adherent crust overlying the ulcer. The margin of the ulcer is formed by normal skin, somewhat infiltrated, heaped up and pouting. Between the skin margin and the granulating surface of the ulcer is a depressed narrow fossa. The lymph-nodes draining the part may become tender, though they are said not to enlarge. This would be a diagnostic point, however, of doubtful value in a region such as this where there is so much general glandular enlargement among natives. The ulcer becomes smaller at length with each renewal of crust and finally heals, often leaving a depressed scar. The duration of the process may be from four or five to twelve or more months.

### DIAGNOSIS

Even in regions where the disease is common there is difficulty in some instances in establishing a diagnosis without the examination of films. The duration, location and appearance of the ulcer are usually suggestive. An isolated case was detected in Boston (Wright's case), and, though searching in vain for over five years for a case in this region, I felt confident when I saw the peculiar ulcer covered by the tough scab on the side of the patient's wrist that it was an Oriental sore. The presence of *L. tropica* is necessary to establish a diagnosis, though a prolonged and careful search may be necessary to detect the microorganism. James[14] found that surgeons whose experience with Delhi sore was considerable were unwilling to express a definite opinion as to whether a given sore was really Oriental sore. One of his cases seen at Delhi appeared superficially more like a ringworm than anything else.

## TREATMENT—PROPHYLAXIS

Those who have attempted to treat this type of ulceration are agreed that most methods are unsatisfactory. Surgical cleanliness and protection with antiseptic dressings are of paramount importance. The ulcers may be treated with bichlorid of mercury solution after removal of crusts, and then some antiseptic ointment should be applied. Castellani advocates the use of protargol by first washing the sores with a 5 per cent. solution, followed by the application of a 20 per cent. ointment. The protargol ointment cannot be used on Europeans when the *skin* of the face is affected, as the protargol after some time induces a discoloration of the skin.

The etiological factor, being a protozoon closely related to trypanosomes, the use of arsenic and its derivatives is suggested by the use of local applications or injections of *Trypanblau, Trypanroth,* salvarsan, etc. Other methods that have been used are the application of tincture of iodin 10 per cent., methylene blue 10 per cent., application of a thin piece of lead over the ulcer, *rausath,*[15] permanganate of potassium in powder and ointment, freezing the boil with ether, the application of a 10 per cent. solution of ferropyrin after cleansing the ulcer, and then an application of a 50 per cent. solution of bimuriate of quinin, daily.

In the case described here treatment consisted in free excision and closure beyond and below the area of involvement. The wound healed *per primam* and when patient was seen forty-two days later there had been no return of the sore.

The disease being contagious, the ulcer should after satisfactory disinfection be well protected from visits by flies, mosquitoes, etc. In an endemic region insect-bites should be treated surgically, particularly those becoming papular with marked infiltration and showing no tendency to resolve.

## THE ZOOLOGIC STATUS OF L. TROPICA

The zoological status of *L. tropica* has been investigated by the several workers mentioned below. Cultivation experiments have developed

14. James, S. P.: Oriental or Delhi Sore: Scientific Memoirs by the Officers of the Medical and Sanitary Departments of the Government of India, Calcutta, 1905, No. 13, New Series.

15. Aviss and Lincoln, C. S.: Treatment of Oriental Sore, Jour. Trop. Med. and Hyg., London, 1910, xiii, 206. *Rausath* is "a dark green fluid prepared from a gummy exudation of a native tree mixed with leaves."

the fact that the microorganism living in the bodies of endothelial cells in man in a gregarine phase becomes in cultures a monadine flagellate, having the characters of *Herpetomonas* or *Crithidia,* flagellates parasitic in the intestinal tracts of invertebrates.

*Herpetomonas muscæ domesticæ,* Burnett, 1851, and *Crithidia fasciculata,* Léger, 1902, are types of the genera. The dividing lines between them and the neighboring one, *Trypanosoma,* are not very sharply defined.

Representatives of the genus *Herpetomonas* are usually found in muscid flies, bugs, etc., while those of *Crithidia* are oftener found in such blood-sucking invertebrates as anophelines, tabanids, fleas, etc.

Flagellates having the morphology of trypanosomes are probably only found in their monadine phase in the blood-stream of vertebrates.

Now, while it is the monadine flagellated phase of these flagellates (trypanosomes) which chiefly excites our interest in trypanosomal disease, it is, on the other hand, the gregarine non-flagellated phase of *Herpetomonas* and *Crithidia* with which we are most familir in kala-azar, Oriental sore and kala-azar infantilis.

There are several gaps in our knowledge and a number of moot questions relative to the life cycle of these flagellates, but it will be of interest to give a brief summary of the life-cycle of one—*L. donovani.*

According to Captain Patton,[16] who has worked out the development of the parasite in *Cimex rotundatus,* the following changes take place when a bed-bug is fed on a patient suffering from kala-azar:

On the second day after being ingested by the bug the parasites begin to develop, their protoplasm increasing in volume; at the same time the macronuclei enlarge and show signs of commencing division. The parasites may now either pass on to flagellation, or further growth followed by the consecutive division of the macro- and micronuclei may result in the formation of rosettes. The single flagellates enlarge and begin to divide longitudinally to result in oval or spindle-shaped cells; while the rosettes, after flagellation, begin to divide up into separate elongated flagellates. The oval or spindle-shaped parasites divide repeatedly either by equal or unequal longitudinal division and result in smaller and more irregular forms. All these changes may be seen in the bug during the first three days. Still later longitudinal division of the oval and irregular flagellates progresses rapidly, so that by the fifth day the majority have become small or spirilla-like flagellates.

The exact mechanism of infection of man by bed-bugs is not known, nor is it known what phase of the life-cycle of *L. donovani* is the immediate antecedent of the gregarine form met with in man.

While it has not been definitely ascertained, it must be undoubtedly true that the bed-bug plays an important, if not the chief, rôle in the transmission of kala-azar.[17]

---

16. Patton, W. S.: A Critical Review of Our Present Knowledge of the Hemoflagellates and Allied Forms, Parasitology, Cambridge, 1909, ii, 91.

17. I have found in some of the native villages of Panama a tick *Ornithodoros talaje,* which has habits not unlike the bed-bug, and causes at times a peculiar pustular eruption in native children.

On account of its intimate relation to our subject, the following stages in the development of our knowledge in this department of medicine may be briefly outlined:

*The Discovery of Trypanosomal Diseases.*—This includes the many observations on trypanosomal infections in man, equines and other mammals, and the rapidly growing list of similar infections in other vertebrates.

*The Discovery of the Transmission of Trypanosomal Diseases by Biting Flies, Fleas, Lice, Etc.*

*The Cultivation of Trypanosomes on Artificial Media.*

*The Discovery of the Protozoal Nature of Kala-Azar, Oriental Sore and Leishmaniosis Infantum.*

Kala-Azar: Leishman,[18] in May, 1903, described certain small oval bodies from autopsy spleen smears in a case of chronic dysentery, cachexia and low fever. The patient had contracted the disease (kala-azar) in Dum-dum, near Calcutta, and died in London. Leishman had observed the bodies first in 1900. In his opinion they were residues of trypanosomes. Donovan, in 1903, reported finding similar bodies from three cases in Madras.

Marchand and Ledingham,[19] in 1904, published an account of a case of kala-azar in a German soldier, who had become infected while with his regiment in China. Leishman-Donovan bodies were detected in the tissue of this case in December, 1902, or in 1903.

Oriental Sore: Wright,[9] of Boston, in December, 1903, published a description of bodies found in the tissue of a case of "Delhi sore" in an Armenian girl. This established the protozoal nature of Oriental sore.

Kala-Azar Infantilis: Nicolle[20] observed eleven cases of this disease in Tunis occurring in young persons 8 months to 6 years old, associated with progressive anemia, irregular fever and gastro-intestinal disturbance. The etiological factor is *L. infantum.*

Cultivation of *L. Donovani:* Rogers'[21] cultivation experiments with splenic pulp from cases of kala-azar, using an acid sodium citrate medium

18. Leishman, W. B.: On the Possible Occurrence of Trypanosomiasis in India, Brit. Med. Jour., 1903, i, 1252; ibid., 1903, ii, 1376; Note on the Nature of the Parasites Found in Tropical Splenomegaly, ibid., i, 303.

19. Marchand, F., and Ledingham, J. C. G.: Ueber Infection mit "Leishman'schen Körperchen" (Kala-Azar?) und ihr Verhältniss zur Trypanosomen-Krankheit, Ztschr. f. Hyg. u. Infectionskr., Leipsic, 1904, xlvii, 1.

20. Nicolle, C. H.: Le kala-azar infantile, Ann. de. l'Inst. Pasteur, Paris, 1909, xxiii, 361; Culture du Parasite du Bouton d'Orient, Compt.-Rend. de l'Acad. de Sc., Paris, 1908, cxl, 482.

21. Rogers, L.: Preliminary Note on the Development of Trypanosoma in Cultures of the Cunningham-Leishman-Donovan Bodies of Cachexial Fever and Kala-Azar, Lancet, London, July 23, 1904, ii; The Development of Flagellated Organisms (Trypanosomes) from the Spleen Protozoic Parasites of Cachexial Fevers and Kala-Azar, Quart. Jour. Microsc. Sc., 1904, xlviii, pt. iii (Nov.).

in which he observed that at a temperature of 20 to 22 C. the Leishman-Donovan bodies became altered in morphology and assumed the characters of the monadine form of the genus *Herpetomonas.* This was a very important discovery.

*Captain Patton's Studies on the Development of L. Donovani in Cimex Rotundatus.*[22]

*The Discovery of L. Infantum in Pariah Dogs by Nicolle.*—On investigation Nicolle learned that in some of the cases of infantile kala-azar studied by him the patients had been in close contact with several dogs. He thereupon examined the cadavers of 222 dogs and found spontaneous kala-azar in four, or 1.8 per cent.

*Cultivation Experiments with L. Tropica by Row,*[23] *Nicolle and Carter.*—Carter gives the stages in the life-history of the parasite of Oriental sore as follows:

1. Monadine Crithidium. Very large, and several times the length of a red blood cell, staining blue, with a scarlet flagellum, carmin extranuclear centrosome and rosy violet nucleus.

2. Flagellated rosy-pink parasite; body oval or circular; apposed to the above at about the level of the nucleus of the monadine *Crithidium.* This presents a small, dark violet-staining nucleus, and an extranuclear centrosome, staining carmin, from which a long scarlet flagellum arises.

3. Gregariniform phase of clusters of small parasites circular, ovoid or bean-shape like enormous cocci. In these the nucleus stains violet. The extranuclear centrosome, when seen, stains rosy red, and the cytoplasm of the cell pale pink. A few are rose-colored throughout. These clusters are usually found surrounded by masses of bacteria and cocci, staining pale blue.

4. Early forms of the parasite showing pyriform, ovoid and torpedo-shaped elements as ordinarily seen in the infected tissues.

5. Larger pyriform cells.

6. Larger rosy bodies. The two latter frequently occur in the same group which may consist of 120 to 200 parasites.

*Observations on Insect Flagellates.*—These were first made by Ronald Ross[24] in 1898, in India, with the species described later, no doubt, by Léger as *Crithidia fasciculata.* Since then Durham, Chaterjee, Chris-

---

22. Patton, W. S.: Preliminary Report on the Development of the Leishman-Donovan Body in the Bed-Bug, Scient. Mem. by the Officers Med. and San. Departments of the Government of India, 1907, No. 27, New Series; The Development of the Leishman-Donovan Parasite in *Cimex Rotundatus,* Second Report; Scient. Mem. by the Officers Med. and San. Departments of the Government of India, 1907, No. 31, New Series.

23. Row, R.: Reported by Dr. Minchin, Brit. Med. Jour., 1909, i, 842.

24. Ross, R.: Notes on the Parasites of Mosquitoes Found in India Between 1895 and 1899, Jour. Hyg., Cambridge, 1906, vi, 101.

tophers, the Sergents, Patton, Novy and many others, by their researches, have added greatly to our knowledge of these groups of protozoa.

At the present time in these fields efforts are chiefly centered on determining exactly the mechanism of infection by trypanosomes and other pathogenic flagellates; the fate of these flagellates in the intestinal tracts of invertebrates, i. e., whether there is an exogenous life cycle; and the relationships between the genera *Trypanosoma, Crithidia* and *Herpetomonas.*

It is of the greatest importance that workers in these fields should recognize the fact emphasized by Patton, Nuttall and others, that though insects and acarids may ingest blood containing pathogenic flagellates, it is also true that of the species of invertebrates specially examined to date most, and probably all, are parasitized by non-pathogenic representatives of the genus *Crithidia* or *Herpetomonas* and that it is frequently impossible to differentiate between them at certain stages of their development.

The singularity of this isolated case in a man who had been living in the bush among native Panamans and Jamaicans suggests very strongly that the parasite in this case is a distinct species from those described from the Levant, India and South America. Morphologically, it resembles them very closely, but the gregarine stage of various crithidians and herpetomonads, while specifically distinct, are also morphologically identical. It is possible and very likely, then, that Oriental sore is caused by the development at the point of inoculation of the gregarine phase of various representatives of *Crithidia, Herpetomonas* or other flagellates. This could be accomplished by: (*a*) tabanids, mosquitoes, etc.; (*b*) fleas, ticks, bed-bugs, dermanyssids, etc.; (*c*) muscid flies, bugs, etc.

In the case of *a* and *b*, the host could be inoculated during the act of biting, or by rubbing or scratching infected feces into the wound by the patient. In *c* the infection of a sore could be accomplished by flies sucking the wound juices or by depositing feces containing the pathogenic agent.

Our knowledge of the number of hosts harboring flagellates which have a gregarine phase, resembling *Leishmania,* is increasing rapidly.

## TECHNIC

Smears were stained with Romanowski, Giemsa and Hastings' modification of Romanowski. I would like to urge the more general use of polychrome stains in the routine examination of autopsy smears and those from pathological tissue. Laboratory workers in the United States do not seem to be as familiar as they should be with the use of these beautiful and invaluable stains.

Hastings' stain is used first on nearly all smears, for it rapidly fixes and stains all the elements in the film. If, in selected slides, it is desired to intensify or improve the picture, this may be done by placing the stained slide in (a) Giemsa short method, (b) long method, or Romanowski. Overstaining may be corrected by differentiating in ethyl alcohol 95 per cent.

GIEMSA SHORT METHOD

| | |
|---|---|
| Azur II, eosin | 3 gm. |
| Azur II | 0.8 gm. |
| Glycerin (C. P.) | 250 gm. |
| Methyl alcohol (Kahlbaum) | 250 gm. |

One or more drops of this mixture to 1 c.c. of distilled water.

GIEMSA LONG METHOD

| | |
|---|---|
| Azur I, (1:1000 aqueous) | 3 parts |
| Azur II, (0.8:1000 aqueous) | 3 parts |
| Eosin solution (2.5 c.c. of 1 per cent. eosin aqueous in 500 of water) | 12 parts |

This mixture may be made up and placed in a staining pot and should be renewed every few days.

A cheaper modification of the Giemsa short method is to replace Azur II eosin by Hastings' stain in powder form.

The original Romanowski, when properly manipulated, gives excellent results; but time and careful adjustment of the proportions of eosin and methylene blue are necessary.

# THE USE OF BLOOD CHARCOAL AS A CLEARING AGENT FOR URINE CONTAINING GLUCOSE *

R. T. WOODYATT, M.D., AND H. F. HELMHOLZ, M.D.
EVANSTON CHICAGO

In the course of some experiments on the quantitative excretion of sugars after parenteral injection, we had occasion to use Bang's[1] method for the determination of glucose and experienced, as have others who have used this method, the difficulty of determining sharply the end point of the reaction when dealing with urines that were even moderately colored. This difficulty is obviated by clearing the urine before titration and, according to Bang and Bohmannsson,[2] this clearing is readily accomplished without the loss of any appreciable amount of glucose by shaking the urine with blood charcoal after having rendered the urine 5 per cent. acid by means of hydrochloric acid. The loss as indicated by Bang and Bohmannsson under these conditions is so small that it can be neglected. Our first control experiment, however, showed quite the contrary, and further determinations indicated losses that amounted to 61 per cent. as determined by the polariscope and 43 per cent. as determined by the Bang method. Such gross variations were impossible to overlook, and could scarcely have been encountered by Bang and Bohmannsson without mention. Further examinations were therefore made to ascertain the source of this discrepancy.

We selected six normal urines which were clear enough to permit accurate polariscopic readings. These samples were made saccharine by the addition of pure dry glucose. To eliminate the error due to any optical changes which might occur as a result of the action of the acid or clearing agents on other urinary constituents besides sugar, these normal specimens were examined with the polariscope before and after clearing prior to the addition of sugar. In some instances the change in the reading was negligible, in others considerable. One specimen, for example, having before clearing a rotation of minus 9 minutes in a 20 cm. tube, showed plus 3 minutes after acid clearing. Corrections for these variations were made in the readings which were obtained from the same urines after glucose had been added. Small losses of glucose might other-

*From the Medical Research Laboratory, Rush Medical College.

1. Bang, I.: Zur Methodik der Zuckerbestimmung, Biochem. Ztschr. 1906-1907, ii, 271.

2. Bang, I., and Bohmannsson, G.: Zur Methodik der Harnzuckerbestimmung, Ztschr. f. physiol. Chem., 1909, lxiii, 443.

EXPERIMENTS ON THE USE OF BLOOD CHARCOAL AS A CLEARING AGENT FOR URINE CONTAINING GLUCOSE

| | ROTATION | | | | | | | TITRATION | |
|---|---|---|---|---|---|---|---|---|---|
| Number of experiment | Normal urine | Normal urine cleared | Normal urine +glucose | Normal urine +glucose corrected | Normal urine +glucose cleared* | Normal urine +glucose cleared* corrected | Loss of glucose per cent. | Loss of glucose per cent. | Remarks |
| 1 | —0° 9′ | +0° 3′ | +1° 31′ | +1° 40′ | +1° 24′ | +1° 21′ | 16 | .. | .............. |
| 2 | —1° 6′ | +0° 4′ | +1° 38′ | +1° 40′ | +1° 22′ | 1° 18′ | 21 | .. | .............. |
| 3 | —0° 4′ | 0° 0′ | +1° 36′ | +1° 40′ | +1° 32′ | 1° 32′ | 8 | .. | .............. |
| 4 | —0° 6′ | +0° 1′ | +1° 38′ | +1° 38′ | +1° 37′ | 1° 36′ | 2 | .. | .............. |
| 5 | +0° 1′ | +0° 3′ | +1° 40′ | +1° 39′ | +1° 23′ | 1° 20′ | 20 | .. | .............. |
| 6 | +0° 1′ | +0° 3′ | +1° 40′ | +1° 39′ | +1° 18′ | 1° 15′ | 25 | .. | .............. |
| 7 | +0° 0′ | 0° 0′ | +0° 56′ | +0° 56′ | +0° 22′ | 0° 22′ | 61 | 43 | Bausch & Lomb, Blood cleared. |
| 8 | —0° 1′ | —0° 1′ | +0° 30′ | +0° 31′ | +0° 18′ | 0° 19′ | 39 | 40 | Bausch & Lomb. |
| 9 | —0° 1′ | —0° 1′ | +0° 30′ | +0° 31′ | +0° 28′ | 0° 29′ | 6 | 0 | Merck. |
| 10 | —0° 2′ | 0° 0′ | +1° 0′ | +1° 2′ | +1° 3′ | 1° 3′ | 0 | 0 | Merck. |
| 11 | —0° 2′ | 0° 0′ | +1° 0′ | +1° 2′ | +0° 39′ | 0° 39′ | 38 | .. | Bausch & Lomb. |
| 12 | —0° 4′ | 0° 0′ | +1° 4′ | +1° 8′ | +1° 7′ | 1° 7′ | 1 | .. | Merck |
| 13 | —0° 4′ | 0° 0′ | +1° 4′ | +1° 8′ | +0° 39′ | 0° 39′ | 43 | .. | Bausch & Lomb. |
| | | | Aqueous glucose sol. | | Aqueous glucose sol. cleared | | | | |
| 14 | .... | .... | +0° 48′ | ..... | +0° 20′ | ..... | 58.3 | 48.6 | Bausch & Lomb. |
| 15 | .... | .... | +1° 0′ | ..... | +0° 25′ | ..... | 58.3 | .. | .............. |
| 16 | .... | .... | +1° 0′ | ..... | +0° 25′ | ..... | 58.3 | .. | .............. |
| 17 | .... | .... | +1° 1′ | ..... | +0° 26′ | ..... | 58.7 | .. | .............. |
| 18 | .... | .... | +1° 1′ | ..... | +1° 6′ | ..... | 0 | 0 | Merck. |
| | | | Diabetic urine | | Diabetic urine cleared | | | | |
| 20 | .... | .... | +6° 35′ | ..... | +5° 55′ | ..... | .. | .. | Bausch & Lomb. |
| 21 | .... | .... | +6° 35′ | ..... | +6° 38′ | ..... | .. | .. | Merck. |

* Clearing always carried out with blood charcoal, 1 part to 10, in presence of 5 per cent. HCl.

wise pass unobserved. In this series, for special reasons, the urines were rendered only 2 per cent. acid, instead of 5 per cent. as according to Bang and Bohmannsson, and the weight of charcoal employed was smaller than these authors recommend. The glucose losses varied from a minimum of 2 per cent. to a maximum of 25 per cent., with an average of 15 per cent. The losses were not constant even in the same urines, but varied widely with the weight of charcoal used, the amount of shaking and the duration of contact. In Experiments 5 and 6, which represent two consecutive determinations on the same specimen of urine, the losses were 20 and 25 per cent. respectively. Occasionally two consecutive determinations gave the same figures, but not consistently.

Inasmuch as the statements of Bang and Bohmannsson are for the most part based on experiment with aqueous glucose solutions made 5 per cent. acid with hydrochloric acid, controls with such solutions were next made in exact accordance with the directions of these authors. In this series even higher percentage losses were encountered. Three determinations showed an average loss of 58 per cent. by polariscopic reading, and 48.6 per cent. by titration. Since the optical activity of the sugar solutions always fell more than their reducing power, we suspected the presence in the charcoal of an impurity that was either levorotatory, or of such a nature that it combined with the sugar to give reducing compounds having lower specific rotations than glucose. The possibility that the fall in rotation was merely a multirotational effect was eliminated by suitable precautions.

Since by extracting our charcoal with 5 per cent. aqueous hydrochloric acid we were unable to observe any optically active substance in the acid filtrate, and since charcoal so treated still exerted the same effect on glucose solutions as did the untreated charcoal, it seemed probable that we had to do with a substance in the blood charcoal that in some way combined with or metamorphosed the glucose.

With these considerations in view the experiments were continued with charcoal obtained from other sources. The original article was obtained from Bausch and Lomb; it was finely powdered and labeled "Charcoal from Blood." We made a second series of observations with Merck's "Blood Charcoal." This article had after pulverization a much coarser grain than the former. When used in the same proportion, the clearing was much less perfect than with the Bausch and Lomb product. Working with Merck's blood charcoal, however, we were able to confirm the findings of Bang and Bohmannsson and could demonstrate no significant loss of glucose from urinous or aqueous solutions, when these were cleared in the presence of a 5 per cent. hydrochloric acid.

Although it is naturally expected that pure chemicals be employed in the carrying out of any quantitative procedure, it is impossible in this connection to know beforehand, except by control experimentation, whether or not a given charcoal from blood will behave in the manner described by Bang and Bohmannsson, or otherwise, as in the present instance. Bang and Bohmannsson make no special mention as to what sort of *Blutkohle* shall be used. Different samples, however, acting in divergently opposite ways, make it necessary that, before any conclusions be drawn from measurements made by the Bang and Bohmannsson method, the individual sample of charcoal which is used shall be thoroughly tested in control experiments.

231 Dempster Street, Evanston—1449 Dearborn Avenue, Chicago.

# CHLORID AND WATER TOLERANCE IN NEPHRITIS *

KARL M. VOGEL, M.D.
NEW YORK

Widal, Achard, and Strauss some years ago called attention to the bearing of sodium chlorid retention on the still unsettled question of nephritic edema, and since then regulation of the chorid intake has been found of value, not only in nephritis, but also in the treatment of fluid accumulations of other origins. The measure has been applied with more or less success in cases of cardiac disease, inflammatory exudates, such, for example, as tuberculous peritonitis, and diabetes insipidus, and in conditions in which it is desirable to restrict the amount of fluid ingested. It is chiefly in nephritis, however, that resort to a salt-poor diet has been found useful, and it is becoming evident that while the therapeutic results are not invariably so brilliant as Widal predicted, investigation of the chlorid tolerance can furnish valuable diagnostic and prognostic indications. According to Widal, two clinical types of nephritis may be recognized, one in which nitrogen retention predominates, and another in which the permeability of the kidney for sodium chlorid has become impaired. Edema, he contends, depends solely on the retention of chlorids, and is largely a physical phenomenon, dominated by the body's intolerance of non-isotonic solutions. By determining, therefore, the fluid intake and output, the sodium chlorid intake and output, and the fluctuations of the patient's weight, it should be possible, provided the functional capacity of the kidneys has not been too seriously impaired, to manage the patient's dietary so as to dissipate existing fluid accumulations and guard against their recurrence. In general, these theoretical considerations of Widal's have received abundant clinical confirmation, but unfortunately experience shows that the problem of nephritic edema cannot be reduced to quite such simple terms, and instances are not infrequently encountered in which the condition proves refractory even to persistent reduction of the salt intake. Blooker,[1] indeed, who very carefully investigated the question of chlorid retention in a series of selected cases, comes to the conclusions that nephritic edema is only rarely the result of primary chlorid retention, and that resort to an extremely salt-poor diet is not often necessary.

---

* From the service of Dr. T. C. Janeway, St. Luke's Hospital, New York.

1 Blooker, J. W.: Deutsch. Arch. f. klin. Med., 1909, xcvi, 80.

The elaborate studies of Schlayer and Takayasu,[2] however, on the artificially induced nephritis of rabbits, furnish a very substantial experimental basis for further clinical work in this direction, and leave no doubt as to the interest of the chlorin balance in nephritis from the standpoint of diagnosis and prognosis, as well as of treatment.

These observers found that it was necessary to distinguish clearly between the effects of tubular and vascular lesions. Injury to the tubular epithelium invariably caused great reduction in the capacity for the excretion of sodium chlorid, the retention being directly proportional

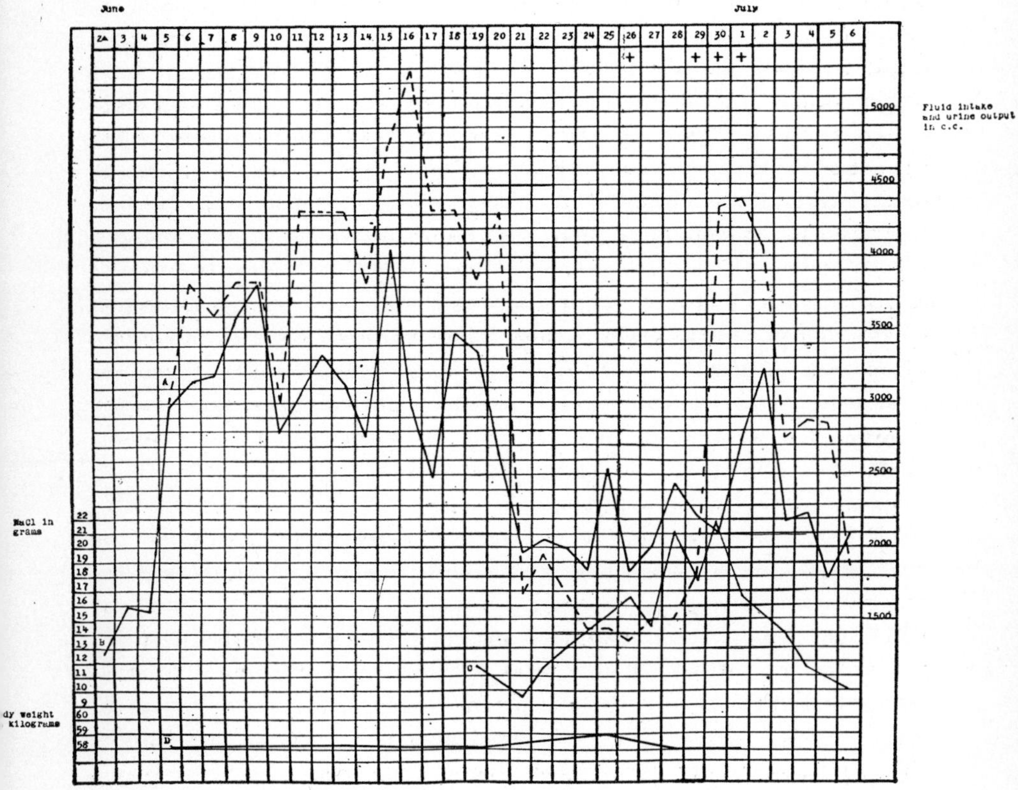


Chart 1.—Chlorid determinations in nephritis (Case 1). A, fluid intake; B, urine output; C, urinary chlorids; D, body weight; +, days on which 10 gm. of NaCl were added to diet.

to the intensity of the lesion. Vascular changes, on the other hand, were without influence on the elimination of the salt, and it was found that a low specific gravity urine might be the result of overirritability of the renal vessels, and in this case was not accompanied by any impairment of chlorid excretion; or it might be due to tubular lesions and then involved chlorid retention which might reach the highest grades.

2. Schlayer and Takayasu: Deutsch. Arch. f. klin. Med., 1910, xcviii, 17.

Clinically, there are, of course, many transitions between these two types, according as the tubular or the vascular lesion predominates, but some insight into the underlying conditions may certainly be gained by watching the sodium chlorid excretion, and particularly the manner in which known amounts of salt added to the diet are disposed of. In other words, just as it is essential to determine the carbohydrate tolerance of a diabetic, or the purin tolerance of a gouty patient as a preliminary to proper treatment, the ability of the nephritic to eliminate sodium chlorid and water must be investigated in order to secure a basis for the intelligent management of his disease. According to the information so elicited, a diet with no restriction as to salt content, or one that is salt-poor, or, in extreme cases, one that is as nearly as possible salt free, is employed, and the patient is subjected to no more hardship in the matter of salt abstention than the necessities of his case demand. At the same time, the manner in which the kidney deals with known amounts of sodium chlorid and water furnishes, at least in some measure, an index of its functional capacity in general and aids in establishing the anatomical diagnosis. It is, therefore, apparent that whatever may be thought of the salt-poor diet as a routine mode of treatment, the indications to be gained from a study of the chlorid and water intake and output are sufficiently valuable to render it advisable to make such determinations in beginning the treatment of every case of nephritis that is at all severe. The following three cases are cited briefly as an example of the behavior of the chlorid balance in different types of the disease.

CASE 1.—*Patient.*—T. L. (No. 81,341), an American carpenter, aged 27, admitted to the service of Dr. Norrie in St. Luke's Hospital, on June 2, 1910. The patient's family and previous history are negative. He takes two cups of tea and one of coffee a day. He uses no alcohol and is a moderate smoker.

*Present Illness.*—One month before admission he caught cold, had a sore throat, a chill, and some fever. His doctor said he had grip. Two weeks before admission his legs became swollen, remained so for a week, and then the swelling disappeared. His face was puffed at the same time. He urinates very frequently, especially during the night. The urine is very dark-colored, rather reddish sometimes. No visual disturbances. He has slight headache. The chief complaint is swelling of the legs, and frequent micturition.

*Physical Examination.*—The patient was a well-nourished young man without dyspnea, cyanosis, or edema. He was moderately prostrated; his skin was pale and the tongue coated. The heart was not enlarged; there were no murmurs, and the action was regular and forcible. The second aortic sound was slightly accentuated. Pulse: slight increase in tension; the vessel walls were palpable but soft. No edema. On admission, the blood-pressure was 160; it fell in four days to 130; and after that varied between 110 and 130. On admission, the patient's urine contained 10 per cent. of albumin by volume. A few hyaline and granular casts, a few leukocytes, and also some epithelial casts were found. The specific gravity varied between 1.008 and 1.020. After May 26, no more than a very faint trace of albumin was found.

The patient received no drugs and was on regular diet. During the period from June 5 to June 20 he was given very large amounts of water which, as the chart shows, were well excreted. From June 21 to June 29 he was told to follow his inclinations in regard to the amount of water taken, and from June 30 to July 2 his fluids were again increased. On June 26, 29 and 30, and July 1 he was given an additional amount of 10 gm. of sodium chlorid daily. This was followed by no increase in weight, and during the days following the administration of the extra salt the excess was completely excreted. During four days on regular diet the average excretion[3] of sodium chlorid was 11.4 gm. During eleven days in the course of which 40 extra gm. of salt were given, the total excretion of sodium chlorid was 188 gm. Deducting the 40 extra grams the average excretion for this period would be 13.4 gm., showing that the kidneys were able to excrete quantitatively all the excess, though its elimination was somewhat delayed.

Case 2.—*Patient.*—C. H. (No 82,055), a German butcher, aged 44, who was admitted to the service of Dr. Janeway on July 9, 1910. The patient's family history was irrelevant. He had had measles in childhood, Neisser infection twice

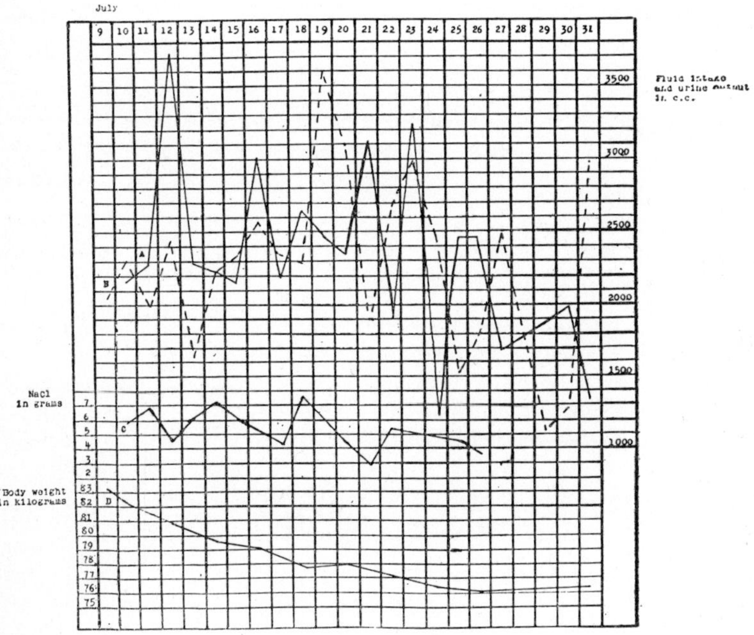


Chart 2.—Chlorid determinations in nephritis (Case 2). A, B, C and D as in Chart 1.

in early youth, and lues ten years ago. He takes six glasses of beer a day and some whiskey, and smokes six cigars. His general health has always been good.

*Present Illness.*—Six or seven weeks ago he noticed that his feet and legs were getting swollen, and later on his thighs, abdomen, and scrotum developed the same condition. At times there was puffiness about the eyes. He continued to work until three weeks ago, when he went to bed and has remained there most of the time ever since. His physician examined the urine frequently and told

3. Chlorid determinations by Mr. George M. Goodwin, Columbia University, 1911.

him he had kidney disease. The chief complaint was swelling of the abdomen and legs.

*Physical Examination.*—The patient was a large, well-nourished man. He did not appear prostrated, showed very slight dyspnea, and no cyanosis. The pupils were equal and reacted to light and accommodation. The tongue was coated; the teeth were in good condition. The apex impulse was not seen, but was faintly felt in the fifth space, five inches from the midline. The right border appeared to be 1 inch to the right, the left border 5 inches to the left of the midline. The sounds were of good quality; no murmurs or accentuations were made out. The heart action was regular. The pulse was of fair force, the tension 125 mm. Vessel wall not felt. Lungs: At the right base posteriorly there was dulness from the angle of the scapula down, with diminished breath sounds and voice. Fremitus came through. The abdomen was soft; the liver and spleen were not felt. There was marked edema of both legs, extending slightly up as far as the thighs.

On admission, the patient's urine contained 30 per cent. of albumin by volume, with a few hyaline casts. On July 12, it contained 60 per cent. of albumin, and after that date the amount steadily decreased until at the time of discharge there was only a trace. The specific gravity was 1.020 to 1.024. There was no sugar. Hyaline casts were always present. The diet was the hospital salt-poor diet (containing 3.25 gm. of sodium chlorid[4] per day) with no restrictions as to the amount of water taken. No drugs were given, except an occasional cathartic. The edema steadily decreased, at first rapidly, later more slowly, but on August 1, when the patient was allowed to leave his bed, there was very slight edema left over both tibiæ.

In this instance, in which no treatment was resorted to except the diet and the rest in bed, in a little over three weeks the patient's weight fell from 83 to 76 kilograms; the edema disappeared, and the chlorid output was greater than the intake. The kidneys are apparently still fairly permeable to sodium chlorid, and there is a strong likelihood that careful management of the patient's chlorid metabolism would do much to prevent further exacerbations.

Case 3.—*Patient.*—A. J. (No. 81,447), an Irish laborer, aged 50, sent into St. Luke's Hospital by Dr. A. W. Hollis, and admitted on May 16, 1910, to the service of Dr. Norrie. The family history is irrelevant to the present condition. For the past fifteen years he has had "rheumatism" every winter. Formerly the attacks were accompanied by pain, but of late there has been only swelling and impairment of function. There was a luetic infection about thirty years ago, treated and said to have been cured; Neisser infection denied. There was an infection of a finger twelve years ago. The patient's general hygiene is good. He takes tea twice a day; no coffee, and until the beginning of present illness eight to nine glasses of beer daily. For the last two years his appetite has been poor, but otherwise the patient has felt well.

*Present Illness.*—About one month before admission, the patient began to suffer from anorexia, nausea, and morning vomiting, which he relieved by taking a glass or two of whisky. Three weeks before admission his legs began to swell, there was puffiness of the left cheek and eyelids, and edema of the scrotum. No pain or urinary symptoms. Ten days before admission a severe headache lasting three days compelled him to stop work for two days. Some days before admission he "caught cold," had two chills, coughed with slight expectoration, and suffered from shortness of breath. During the past month he has been able to work only at intervals. The chief complaint is swelling of legs, shortness of breath, and morning vomiting.

---

4. Chlorid determinations by Mr. Harbeck Halsted, Columbia University, 1911.

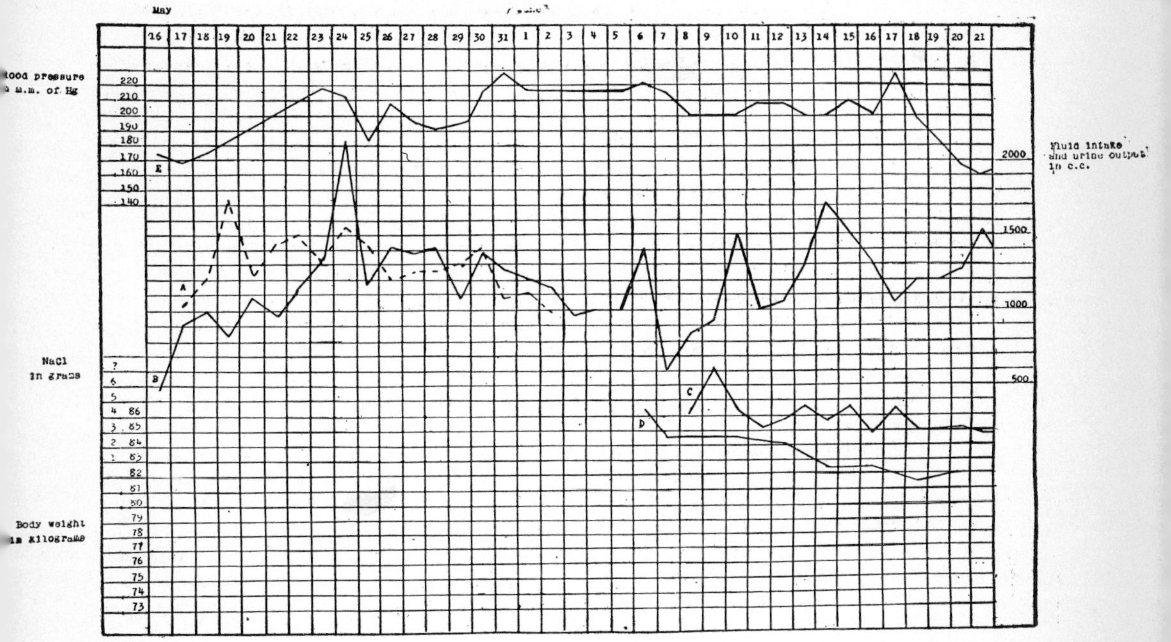


Chart 3.—Chlorid determinations in Case 3, nephritis. A, B, C and D as in Chart 1.

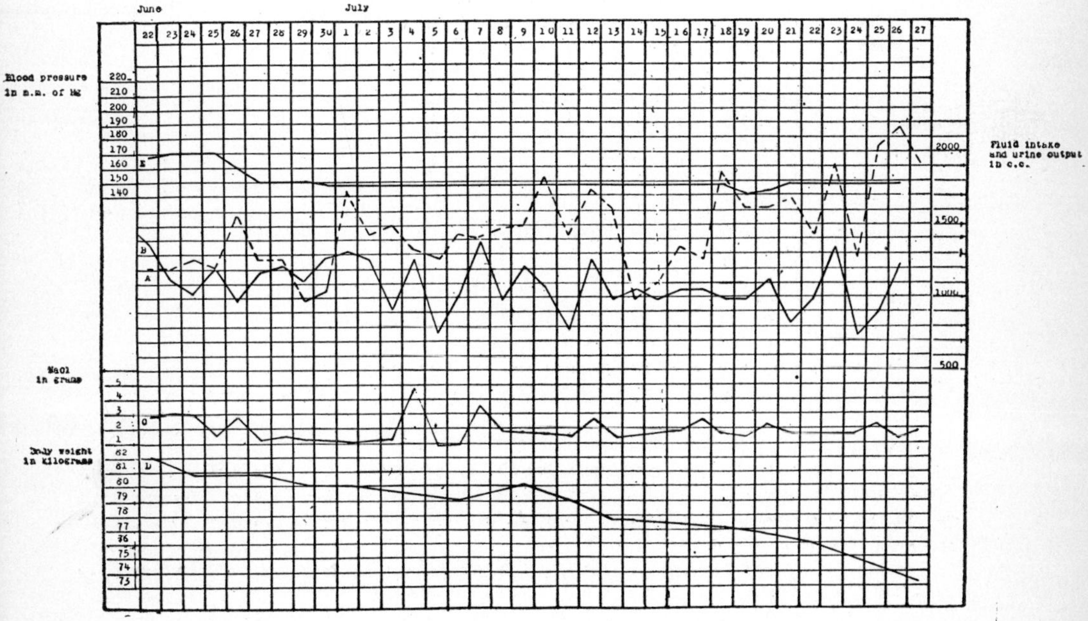


Chart 4.—Chlorid determinations in nephritis (Case 3). A, B, C and D as in Charts 1 and 2; E, blood-pressure.

*Physical Examination.*—The patient presented moderate edema of the lower extremities and about the trunk. There was slight cyanosis of the finger-tips, but no dyspnea. The apex-beat was in the fifth interspace, 6 inches from the midsternal line; no superficial impulse except in the epigastrium. The sounds at the apex were distant, but of good quality; second pulmonic sound faint; second aortic sound accentuated. The action was regular and forcible; pulse regular, of good force; the vessel wall was markedly thickened; blood-pressure, 176. At the apex of the left lung there was dulness, and many subcrepitant râles were heard immediately below the clavicle. Over both sides in front, sonorous and wheezing expiration; sibilant and sonorous breathing over the posterior chest. At both bases marked dulness, on the left side extending almost to the angle of the scapula. Fremitus, voice, and breathing were diminished. Coin sound was heard on both sides. The liver percussed slightly large, but its edge could not be felt. The spleen was not felt.

During the patient's stay in the hospital his urine usually showed a specific gravity of 1.020 and an albumin content of from 10 to 80 per cent. by volume. There was no sugar. Many hyaline and granular and a few waxy casts were found. On June 24, the left chest was tapped, and 1,560 c.c. of fluid removed. On July 11, the aspiration was repeated, and 1,740 c.c. of fluid, containing 19.1 gm. of sodium chlorid[5] were removed. At a third aspiration on July 26, 2,040 c.c. of fluid with 14.3 gm. of sodium chlorid were removed.

The treatment comprised the administration of digitalis, short periods on glonoin and diuretin, and hot packs, given from June 21 to July 11. On June 6 the hospital salt-poor diet was begun. On August 1, the patient came under the charge of Dr. Hollis, and a week of regular diet, begun on August 31, was accompanied by a gain in weight of 4 kilograms with the appearance of edema in the legs. A return to the salt-poor diet caused a prompt fall in weight, and on September 29, the patient was discharged weighing 73 kilograms, with slight edema of the legs and signs of fluid in the left chest.

The changes in the patient's condition observed while under the salt-poor régime may be summarized as follows, without of course attempting to ascribe them to this particular factor of the treatment: The blood-pressure dropped from the neighborhood of 200 mm. to the neighborhood of 140 mm., and remained there. The weight fell from 86 kilograms to 73 kilograms, the weight of the chest fluid removed at three tappings amounting to about 5 kilograms. The urine quantity remained fairly constant between 1,200 and 1,500 c.c. The urinary chlorids fell from about 5 gm. to about 2 gm., showing a retention of something over 1 gm. daily. This amount was probably accounted for by the amount stored up in the pleural effusion, as the fluid removed in the two instances in which the chlorin content was determined represented about 33 gm. of sodium chlorid. In the case of this patient, therefore, while a considerable reduction in edema was effected, still it was slow and not sufficient, as shown by the recurrence of the pleural effusion; and there was evidently pronounced impairment of the excretory capacity of the tubular epithelium.

In the accompanying table the sodium chlorid content of some of the commoner foodstuffs is given. The figures are from Strauss,[6] and apply to the substance in its raw, unprepared state.

---

5. Chlorid determinations by Mr. John A. Vietor, Columbia University, 1911.

6. Strauss, H.: Praktische Winke für die chlorarme Ernährung. Berlin, 1910, S. Karger. This contains very complete tables of analyses as well as many useful directions for the preparation of salt-poor diets. The most recent exposition of Widal's views, as well as a good bibliography, is to be found in Widal and Lemierre: Die diätetische Behandlung der Nierenentzündungen, Ergebn. d. inn. Med. u. Kinderh., 1909, iv, 523.

TABLE OF SODIUM CHLORID CONTENT OF COMMONER FOODSTUFFS

| Food | Per cent. | Food | Per cent. |
|---|---|---|---|
| Mutton | 0.17 | Gelatin | 0.75 |
| Veal | 0.13 | Eggs, whole without shell | 0.21 |
| Veal kidney | 0.32 | Milk | 0.16 |
| Calves' liver | 0.14 | Cream | 0.13 |
| Beef, lean | 0.11 | Butter, salted | 1.0 -3.0 |
| Pork, lean | 0.10 | Butter, unsalted | 0.02-0.21 |
| Trout | 0.12 | Swiss cheese | 2.0 |
| Codfish | 0.16 | Edam cheese | 3.30 |
| Salmon | 0.061 | Bread, wheat | 0.18 |
| Sole | 0.41 | Bread, rye | 0.18-0.59 |
| Halibut | 0.30 | Oatmeal | 0.29 |
| Mackerel | 0.28 | Celery | 0.25-0.49 |
| Duck | 0.14 | Cauliflower | 0.05-0.15 |
| Goose | 0.20 | Tomatoes | 0.11 |
| Chicken | 0.14 | Cabbage | 0.11-0.44 |
| Turkey | 0.17 | Lettuce | 0.12 |
| Oysters, washed in fresh water | 0.52 | Most other cereals, vegetables, fruits and nuts, less than 0.1. | |

680 Madison Avenue.

# STUDIES ON WATER-DRINKING:

## V. INTESTINAL PUTREFACTION DURING COPIOUS AND MODERATE WATER-DRINKING WITH MEALS *[1]

W. M. HATTREM AND P. B. HAWK, PH.D.
URBANA

In a previous paper from this laboratory (by Fowler and Hawk) data were presented indicating that copious water-drinking with meals was accompanied and followed by a decrease in the bacterial content of the feces. It was there shown that during a preliminary period in which a uniform diet was supplemented by a small water ration, that 5.3 gm. of dry bacteria was excreted per day, a value which was decreased to 4.6 gm. per day during an interval of five days in which the water ingestion was increased 1,000 c.c. per meal. Furthermore, data were presented which showed a further decrease in the daily output of bacteria during a post-water period of low water ingestion, the daily value for this period being 3.3 gm. In keeping with the figures for the excretion of bacterial substance in the feces were the results secured for bacterial nitrogen. These data showed a daily excretion of 0.48 gm. of bacterial nitrogen during the water period as against the higher excretion of 0.58 gm. for the preliminary period and the lower excretion of 0.38 gm. for the final period. Later experiments on other subjects[2] have verified these findings.

From the data above outlined it was evident that copious water-drinking with meals had brought about a decreased excretion of fecal bacterial substance. The logical explanation for this decreased output of bacterial substance during the days of increased water ingestion seemed to us to rest on the fact that the presence of the large volume of fluid in the intestine rendered a more rapid absorption of the digestive products possible. This being true, the microorganisms present in the intestine would be in contact with the nutritive matter of the intestinal contents for an interval of time shorter than normal. Therefore these bacteria would be more poorly nourished during the water period, thus decreasing the amount of bacterial substance and producing a lowered

*From the Laboratory of Physiological Chemistry of the University of Illinois.

1. The earlier members of this series were published as follows:

I. Hawk: Univ. Penn. Med. Bull., 1905, xviii, 7.

II. Fowler and Hawk: Jour. Exper. Med., 1910, xii, 388.

III. Rulon and Hawk: Jour. Am. Chem. Soc., 1910, xxxii, 1686.

IV. Rulon and Hawk: The Excretion of Chlorids Following Copious Water-Drinking with Meals, THE ARCHIVES INT. MED., 1911, vii, 536.

2. Mattill and Hawk: Reported before the American Physiological Society, 1909.

output of total bacterial nitrogen. Whether or not there was an accompanying decrease in the actual number of fecal bacteria during the water-drinking interval was not determined. It is entirely possible that the water caused not only a lessening of bacterial substance but an actual decrease in the number of bacteria excreted per day.[3]

After verifying with other subjects the finding of a lowered output of bacterial substance under the influence of copious water-drinking with meals, we next turned our attention to the question of a possible relation existing between this lowered bacterial output and the course of intestinal putrefaction. In other words, if water taken in large quantity at meal-time brought about an inhibition of the growth or activity of the intestinal flora, was this inhibitory influence exerted on the indol-forming organisms such, for example, as *B. coli* and *Bacterium welchii,* thus initiating a lowered intestinal putrefaction or was the principal force of the influence exerted on the non-indol-forming organisms? In keeping with the suggestion of Folin[5] and others, we were willing to accept the extent of the absorbed intestinal indol, measured by the indican content of the urine, as representative of the course of intestinal putrefaction.

### EXPERIMENTAL DATA AND COMMENTS

Experiments of three kinds were conducted. The influence of copious water-drinking with meals was first investigated. This was followed by a study of the influence of moderate water-drinking, and finally copious water-drinking by a man accustomed to drink large volumes of water at meal-time was investigated.

The urine was collected in twenty-four-hour samples. The feces were also passed regularly once a day. This latter feature is of prime importance in experiments in which determinations of urinary indican are to be made, inasmuch as retention of feces would naturally be followed by the absorption of added quantities of indol and a consequent increased output of indican. The urine was examined for indican according to the quantitative method of Ellinger,[6] and for ethereal sulphates according to the method of Folin.

*Ellinger's Method for Indican.*—There is at present no method for the quantitative determination of indican which can be said to be absolutely reliable. Ellinger's method as used in these experiments is accepted to-day as the most accurate, but even this method has its sources of error. The method employed is as follows:

Fifty c.c. of urine are placed in a small beaker and if neutral or alkaline in reaction is made faintly acid with acetic acid. Five c.c. of basic

3. This problem is to be investigated.
5. Folin: Am. Jour. Physiol., 1905, xiii, 99.
6. Ellinger: Ztschr. f. Physiol. Chem., 1903, xxxviii, 192.

lead acetate[7] is then added to precipitate the inorganic matter and pigment, after which the solution is mixed well and filtered. Forty c.c. of the clear filtrate are transferred to a separatory funnel, an equal volume of Obermayer's reagent (from 2 to 3 gm. ferric chlorid per liter concentrated hydrochloric acid) is added and the indigo thus formed extracted with chloroform. This extraction with chloroform should be repeated until the chloroform solution remains colorless. The chloroform extracts are filtered through a dry filter-paper into a dry Erlenmeyer flask. The chloroform is distilled off, the residue heated on a boiling water-bath for five minutes in the open flask, and the dried residue washed with hot water until the water is no longer colored. Concentrated sulphuric acid (10 c.c.) is added to the washed residue, which is then heated on the water-bath for from five to ten minutes, diluted with 100 c.c. of water and the blue solution titrated with a very dilute solution of potassium permanganate. The end-point is indicated by the dissipation of all the blue color from the solution and the formation of a pale yellow color.[8]

In making up the permanganate for titration an approximate 0.3 per cent. solution was first prepared. This stock solution was then diluted with forty volumes of water, as suggested by Wang.[9] The dilute solution was then standardized and employed in the titration.[10] One c.c. equalled 0.176 mg. indigo.

In starting these experiments, 50 c.c. of urine were used. The chloroform extract appeared thick and seemed full of small globules, which were so persistent that the solution would not filter. Some of these small globules were examined under the microscope and were found to contain beautiful blue crystals which were identified as indigo crystals. The solution, when evaporated without filtering, left a heavy brownish residue in the flask which could not be washed out without loss of indigo. This residue was due to small amounts of the supernatant liquid being entrapped between the globules of the chloroform extract and drawn off with it. This difficulty was finally overcome by using only 25 c.c. of urine and diluting it to 50 c.c. When urine from moderate water-drinking experiments was employed, 50 c.c. could be used without any difficulty. On the other hand, urines from the copious water periods were concentrated in order to insure the presence of enough indigo to make a satisfactory determination. Another difficulty we experienced was in getting a good blue solution in the chloroform. It was noticed in the first experiments that the chloroform solution was a bluish-red color. The residue, after the chloroform was distilled off, was reddish-

7. U. S. Pharmacopeia.

8. Hawk: Practical Physiological Chemistry, third edition, p. 387.

9. Wang: Ztschr. f. physiol. Chem., 1898, xxv, 409.

10. We are grateful to Dr. F. P. Underhill of Yale University for his courtesy in furnishing the pure indigo used by us in this standardization.

brown, and on being dissolved in sulphuric acid and diluted with water, gave a red solution which could not be titrated with potassium permanganate with any degree of accuracy. On investigation it was found that the source of the trouble was the thymol which was used as a urine preservative.

Making the determinations on fresh urine before the preservative was used resulted in a clear blue chloroform solution which on evaporation left the indigo in fine concentric circles on the bottom of the flask. It was very easy now to wash this residue without the danger of loss of indigo. Failure to wash the residue properly left some of the red coloring-matter, probably isatin,[11] which gave the solution which was to be titrated either a greenish or turbid blue appearance. This somewhat hindered the determination of the delicate end-point.

Methods for the determination of indican have been reported by various investigators, including Bouma, Folin and Imabuchi.[12] Bouma boiled the urine with hydrochloric acid containing isatin, thereby changing all the indoxyl of the urine into indigo red. Much of the other detail was the same as Ellinger's method. He finally titrated a red solution against permanganate, which certainly is anything but satisfactory as regards the securing of a visible end-point. He reports the formation of crystals of indigo red in the examination of urines of high indican content.

Folin used practically all of Ellinger's method except the final dissolving in sulphuric acid, dilution and titrating. He extracted the indigo with 5 c.c. of chloroform and then determined the amount colorimetrically by a comparison with Fehling's solution which he gave an arbitrary value of 100. The comparisons were made by means of a Duboscq colorimeter. In our experience this procedure does not yield as satisfactory results as the method of Ellinger. The procedure of Folin has not yet been placed on a strict quantitative basis.

Imabuchi conducted his method in much the same manner as did Ellinger, except that he used a few cubic centimeters of a 10 per cent. solution of copper sulphate with 40 c.c. of concentrated hydrochloric acid to oxidize the indican to indigo blue, whereas Ellinger used Obermayer's reagent. By an exhaustive series of experiments, he showed that with copper sulphate it was possible to obtain more indigo, and that it was not necessary to extract immediately with chloroform as was the case when Obermayer's reagent was used. His results varied only slightly after the solution had stood for a period of ten minutes, whereas longer standing caused lower results. He also determined that the best amount of copper sulphate solution (10 per cent.) to use was between 1

11. Ellinger: Ztschr. f. physiol. Chem., 1903, xxxviii, 192.

12. Bouma: Ztschr. f. physiol. Chem., 1901, xxxii, 82. Folin: Am. Jour. of Physiol., 1905, xiii, 53. Imabuchi: Ztschr. f. physiol. Chem., 1909, lx, 502.

and 3 c.c., 0.5 c.c. being insufficient to oxidize all of the indican to indigo and 5 c.c. causing superoxidation. He asserts that excess of reagent is less harmful in the case of copper sulphate than with Obermayer's reagent.

A few parallel determinations were made in connection with our experiments, in which the efficiency of Obermayer's reagent was compared with that of copper sulphate. The results obtained by us were practically the same in each instance.

TABLE 1.—INDICAN OUTPUT AS AFFECTED BY COPIOUS WATER-DRINKING WITH MEALS

(Subject W)

| No. of Day | Urine c.c. | Indican (Mg.) | Ethereal $SO_3$ (gm.) |
|---|---|---|---|
| PRELIMINARY PERIOD | | | |
| 1. | 888 | 38.0 | 0.1409 |
| 2. | 945 | 40.1 | 0.1273 |
| Av. | ... | 39.1 | 0.1341 |
| COPIOUS WATER PERIOD | | | |
| 3. | 3110 | 26.9 | 0.1500 |
| 4. | 4570 | 25.3 | 0.1618 |
| 5. | 4230 | 28.5 | 0.1257 |
| 6. | 3810 | 40.9 | 0.1446 |
| 7. | 3300 | 45.5 | 0.1497 |
| Av. | .... | 33.4 | 0.1460 |
| FINAL PERIOD | | | |
| 8. | 1100 | 33.6 | 0.1580 |
| 9. | 930 | 22.6 | 0.1489 |
| 10. | 965 | 24.8 | 0.1545 |
| Av. | .... | 27.0 | 0.1538 |
| THREE MONTHS LATER | | | |
| 1. | 578 | 36.9 | ...... |
| 2. | 710 | 31.7 | ...... |
| 3. | 825 | 30.2 | ...... |
| 4. | 715 | 43.6 | ...... |
| 5. | 828 | 40.7 | ...... |
| 6. | 785 | 44.6 | ...... |
| 7. | 772 | 32.1 | ...... |
| Av. | ... | 37.1 | ...... |

TABLE 2.—INDICAN OUTPUT AS AFFECTED BY MODERATE WATER-DRINKING WITH MEALS

(Subject W)

| No. of Day | Urine c.c. | Indican (Mg.) |
|---|---|---|
| PRELIMINARY PERIOD | | |
| 1. | 740 | 54.2 |
| 2. | 807 | 41.4 |
| 3. | 777 | 40.3 |
| Av. | ... | 45.3 |
| MODERATE WATER PERIOD | | |
| 4. | 2086 | 40.2 |
| 5. | 2412 | 44.4 |
| 6. | 2415 | 46.0 |
| 7. | 2560 | 44.5 |
| 8. | 1485 | 46.9 |
| 9. | 1660 | 39.5 |
| 10. | 1800 | 42.6 |
| 11. | 2336 | 41.5 |
| 12. | 2242 | 44.8 |
| 13. | 1720 | 34.7 |
| Av. | .... | 42.5 |
| FINAL PERIOD | | |
| 14. | 1370 | 68.8 |
| 15. | 760 | 46.5 |
| 16. | 781 | 47.6 |
| 17. | 700 | 42.4 |
| 18. | 783 | 40.8 |
| 19. | 650 | 40.6 |
| 20. | 760 | 55.8 |
| 21. | 793 | 60.9 |
| 22. | 690 | 45.6 |
| 23. | 757 | 35.1 |
| 24. | 677 | 42.1 |
| 25. | 757 | 49.2 |
| Av. | .... | 47.9 |

### 1. INFLUENCE OF COPIOUS WATER-DRINKING

The subject of this experiment (W) was a man 26 years of age. Nitrogen equilibrium was secured through the feeding of a uniform diet, the menu for each of the three meals of the day being as follows:

| | |
|---|---|
| Graham crackers | 150 gm. |
| Peanut butter | 20 gm. |
| Butter | 25 gm. |
| Milk | 450 c.c. |
| Water | 100 c.c. |

Three additional volumes of water of 200 c.c. each were taken at 10 a. m., 3 p. m., and 8:30 p. m., respectively. The experiment covered a period of ten days, consisting of a preliminary period of two days, a water period of five days and a final period of three days. During the water period an additional 1000 c.c. of water was taken at each of the three meals of the day.

It may be seen from Table 1 that the amount of indican in the urine was nearly the same for each of the two days preceding the copious water-drinking with meals. On the first day of the five-day water period, there was a decided drop in the output of indican, the lower daily excretion

TABLE 3.—INDICAN OUTPUT AS AFFECTED BY MODERATE WATER-DRINKING WITH MEALS

(Subject E)

| No. of Day | Urine c.c. | Indican (Mg.) |
|---|---|---|
| PRELIMINARY PERIOD | | |
| 1. | 1065 | 42.1 |
| 2. | 937 | 62.0 |
| 3. | 1047 | 77.9 |
| 4. | 1031 | 75.0 |
| 5. | 1062 | 38.6 |
| 6 | 1143 | 94.5 |
| 7. | 1301 | 105.3 |
| 8. | 1250 | 58.2 |
| Av. | .... | 69.2 |
| MODERATE WATER PERIOD | | |
| 9. | 2192 | 51.4 |
| 10. | 2465 | 45.5 |
| 11. | 2395 | 57.6 |
| 12. | 2110 | 60.6 |
| 13. | 2220 | 26.9 |
| 14. | 2760 | 37.7 |
| 15. | 1745 | 50.8 |
| 16. | 2277 | 46.6 |
| 17. | 2078 | 49.9 |
| 18. | 1090 | 52.1 |
| Av. | .... | 47.9 |
| FINAL PERIOD | | |
| 19. | 870 | 57.5 |
| 20. | 885 | 53.8 |
| 21. | 945 | 61.1 |
| 22. | 998 | 69.8 |
| Av. | .... | 60.5 |

TABLE 4.—INDICAN OUTPUT AS AFFECTED BY COPIOUS WATER-DRINKING WITH MEALS

(Subject E)

| No. of Day | Urine c.c. | Indican (Mg.) |
|---|---|---|
| PRELIMINARY PERIOD | | |
| 1. | 992 | 72.3 |
| 2. | 940 | 71.8 |
| 3. | 920 | 71.9 |
| 4. | 858 | 63.3 |
| 5. | 980 | 57.4 |
| Av. | .... | 67.3 |
| COPIOUS WATER PERIOD | | |
| 6. | 4550 | 30.9 |
| 7. | 4785 | 53.1 |
| 8. | 5220 | 86.0 |
| 9. | 4530 | 48.0 |
| 10. | 4850 | 52.6 |
| Av. | .... | 54.1 |
| FINAL PERIOD | | |
| 11. | 970 | 60.6 |
| 12. | 1009 | 68.3 |
| 13. | 880 | 75.8 |
| Av. | .... | 68.2 |

continuing with but slight variation for three days. The last two days of the period show, on the other hand, marked increases which, however, did not continue into the final period. The results for the final period agree fairly well with those of the first three days of the copious water period, showing that the effect of the copious water must have been carried over into this period. The effect is better observed by noting the average values for each period. The average for the copious water period, 33.4 mg., was lower than that of the preliminary period, 39.1 mg., thus indicating that copious water-drinking with meals decreased intestinal putrefaction. The average for the final period (27.0 mg.) was lower than that of the copious water period, showing that the effects of the increased water ingestion persisted even after the water quota had been reduced to the preliminary level.

This point is shown very nicely by an examination of Table 1. After the completion of the experiment on copious water-drinking, Subject W, on his return to the usual mixed diet, drank rather larger quantities of water at meal-time than had been his custom previous to the time he served as a subject in our tests. Three months later, as we wished to learn the exact reaction of his organism as regarded intestinal putrefaction when he was ingesting a diet of the same character as that employed in our water study, this individual was placed on such a diet and the urine examined. The data show that the daily average value for this seven-day period was 37.1 mg. as against 39.1 mg. for the period under the same conditions three months previous. There was, therefore, slightly less intestinal putrefaction. It is of interest to note also that the value as obtained was considerably higher than the daily average for the final period of the copious water-drinking study, i. e., 27 mg. This might be interpreted as indicating that the markedly inhibited putrefactive processes had been augmented by degrees above this final value during the period since the copious water ingestion, but that the conditions surrounding these processes had been so altered through this excessive intake of water as to require the lapse of a period of three months before they were enabled to assume their former activity.

Now if, as Baumann and others have claimed, the total ethereal sulphate excretion is an index of intestinal putrefaction, we should obtain a decreased output of this form of sulphur during the period of copious water-drinking. Table 1 shows the total daily output of ethereal sulphates for the interval during which indican determinations were made.[13] The average value for the preliminary period was found to be 0.1341 gm. On the first day of the copious water period there was an increase in the output to 0.1500 gm. while the average daily value for the entire period was considerably higher than that of the preliminary period, i. e., 0.146 gm. The first day of the final period showed an increase from 0.1479 gm. to 0.1580 gm., while the general average for the period, 0.1538 gm., was higher than that of the copious water period.

A comparison of the ethereal sulphate data with the indican values for the same urine fails to reveal any uniformity in the rate of excretion in the two instances. The indican values *decrease* during the water period and are still further depressed in the post-water interval, two observations which have been interpreted as indicating a progressively decreasing putrefaction. On the other hand, the output of total ethereal sulphates

13. These determinations were made by Mr. M. J. Eames.

is *increased* during the water period and still further increased during the period following the water. In other words, the course of the ethereal sulphate excretion is directly opposite to that of the indican.[14] It is logical to conclude, therefore, that they cannot correctly be considered as indexes of the intensity of the same metabolic process. This point is all the more significant when we consider that indican is itself an ethereal sulphate and therefore forms a part of the total output of this form of sulphur; hence the increase in the other forms of ethereal sulphates, except indican, was greater than the data show, inasmuch as the increase occurred during an interval in which the indican was considerably lessened in amount. These results lead us to believe that the statement that the ethereal sulphates may be taken as an index of intestinal putrefaction is incorrect.

### II. INFLUENCE OF MODERATE WATER-DRINKING

Following the investigation of the course of intestinal putrefaction as influenced by copious water-drinking with meals, a second experiment was undertaken, in which the topic of moderate water-drinking was under consideration. The added volume of water daily ingested with meals was only one-half that ingested per day during the study of copious water drinking, *i. e.*, 500 c.c. This volume was deemed representative of so-called moderate water-drinking. Two subjects were employed, one of whom, W, had already served as a subject in the copious water-drinking experiment. The other subject, E, was accustomed to drinking rather large amounts of water with meals. In fact, throughout the course of the investigation he frequently said that he was ingesting less water than he customarily ingested when living on an ordinary mixed diet. The experiment on this subject, E, may, therefore, be considered as embracing the study of the influence of moderate water-drinking with meals on a confirmed water-drinker. The daily program of the experiment was similar to that of the experiment on copious water-drinking.

Subject W ingested the following diet three times daily:

| | |
|---|---|
| Graham crackers | 125 gm. |
| Butter | 25 gm. |
| Peanut butter | 20 gm. |
| Milk | 400 c.c. |
| Water | 100 c.c. |

An additional volume of 200 c.c. of water was taken at 10 a. m., 3 p. m., and 8 p. m., respectively. His experiment was divided into a preliminary period of three days, a ten-day period of moderate water-drinking, and a final period of twelve days during which the same conditions were in force as during the preliminary period.

Subject E used a similar diet to that already mentioned in connection with W, with the exception that E's menu contained twenty-five grams of graham crackers additional per meal. He also drank an additional 200 c.c. of water at 10 a. m., 3 p. m. and 8 p. m. The experiment covered the same number of days as the experiment on W, but the periods were divided somewhat differently. It consisted of a preliminary period of eight days, a moderate water period of ten days, and a final period of four days.

14. Salant and Hinkel (Jour. Pharmacol. and Exper. Therap., 1910, i, 493) have recently made a similar observation in connection with a study of the influence of alcohol.

It may be seen from Tables 2 and 3 that there was a decrease in the average daily output of indican from the preliminary periods to the moderate water periods of both subjects. Also in both cases there was a noticeable increase as soon as the original low water ingestion was resumed. In the case of W, for instance, the average preliminary output was 45.3 mg. per day, a value which was lowered to 42.5 mg. under the influence of the moderate water-drinking. When the low water ingestion was again instituted, on the first day of the final period, there was an increase in the indican output for three days, followed by three days in which the output was below the level even of the water period. Taking the entire final period into consideration, we obtain a daily average of 47.9 mg. as compared with one of 45.3 mg. for the preliminary period. However, if we calculate on the basis of the last four days of the final period, we secure an average of 43.0 mg., which is lower than the preliminary level and practically the same as the daily output for the water period.

The data from Subject W indicate that moderate water-drinking exerted an inhibitory influence on intestinal putrefaction. However, on the withdrawal of the added water from the diet, the inhibitory factor being thus removed, there was no check to intestinal putrefaction and this process, which had been held in inhibition by the water, evidently again had full sway. This was noted during the first part of the final period. As the period progressed, however, conditions surrounding the putrefaction reactions became altered to such an extent as to yield an average daily value of practically the same magnitude as that secured during the water period.

From a comparison of Tables 1 and 2, it will be seen that on the same subject, W, the effect of moderate amounts of water with meals was not as pronounced as with the copious water-drinking. In the copious water experiment, there was a gradual decrease in the total daily output of indican which did not increase during the final period. In the moderate water experiment the amount of indican excreted daily decreased slightly during the water period. There was then an increased output during the first part of the final period which was not shown in the copious water experiment. These facts seem to indicate that there was less intestinal putrefaction during the copious ingestion of water with meals than when using only a moderate amount of water. Although there was a noticeable decrease during the moderate water period, the average daily output varied only slightly from that of the preliminary period, showing that the moderate amount of water did not have the pronounced effect which was in evidence during the experiment on the copious water ingestion.

Subject E (Table 3), showed a more pronounced effect with moderate water ingestion than did Subject W. From an average daily excretion of 69.2 mg., the value for the first day of the water period fell to 51.4 mg., with a general average of 47.9 mg. for the entire period. The output for the first day of the final period rose to 57.5 mg. with a general average of 60.5 mg. for the entire period.

Now Subject E, it will be remembered, was the subject accustomed to ingesting ordinarily larger amounts of water than he was receiving during the preliminary period of this experiment. In the face of this fact, it would seem that the additional 500 c.c. of water taken during the moderate water period acted in a manner similar to that in which the copious amounts of water acted on Subject W. Or we may suppose the lower water ingestion during the preliminary period of this subject to have increased the intestinal putrefaction, and that later during the moderate water-drinking the normal level for this individual was reached. This may be the true explanation, inasmuch as the subject frequently remarked that the added 500 c.c., ingested with each meal during the water period, was no more than he was accustomed to take. In the final period the increase during the four days may be interpreted as was the high value for the preliminary period, i. e., as due to the fact that the subject was not receiving as much water as he needed to keep his putrefaction processes properly regulated. That the value for these days is not as high as the preliminary level is probably due to the after-effects of the inhibitory influence of moderate water-drinking.

The average daily output of indican for Subject E is seen to be greater than that of Subject W throughout the experiments. This may be due to the factor of individuality, inasmuch as it has been pointed out by Herter[15] that the number of indol-producing bacteria in the intestinal tract varies with different subjects. It is doubtless true also that the percentage absorption of the indol formed would vary in different individuals.

INFLUENCE OF COPIOUS WATER-DRINKING ON A CONFIRMED WATER-DRINKER

Subject E, as has already been mentioned, was accustomed to drinking fairly large volumes of water at meal time. For this reason it seemed that the data secured from copious water ingestion by him might yield interesting findings, particularly when taken into comparison with similar data obtained from Subject W. At the close of the final period of the moderate water experiment he was, therefore, given a five-day preliminary period on the same diet. This was followed by a five-day copious water period, during which he ingested an additional 4,000 c.c. of water per day. Then followed a three-day final period with the regular low water ingestion. An inspection of Table 4 will show the results of this study.

The average amount of indican excreted daily in the urine during the preliminary period was 67.3 mg. During the first two days of the copious water ingestion, there was a large decrease in the daily excretion with an exceedingly large output on the third day. The remainder of

15. Herter: Bacterial Infections of the Digestive Tract, p. 263.

the period decreased again with an average for the period of 54.1 mg., showing a rather pronounced diminution of intestinal putrefaction during the ingestion of large amounts of water. The output of indican during the final period increased with an average daily excretion of 68.2 mg., a value slightly higher than the preliminary value.

Again, it is shown that the ingestion of large amounts of water with meals decreases the putrefaction in the intestinal tract. Here, as in the case of moderate water-drinking, the putrefactive processes were much more active in the case of Subject E than in the case of Subject W. In fact, this variation in the reaction of the two organisms in this respect was not limited to the water period, but was markedly in evidence throughout the various portions of the investigation. An interesting fact is brought out when the percentage decreases in the output of indican during copious water-drinking are calculated for Subjects E and W. Notwithstanding the actual output per day was greater in the case of E, the percentage decrease brought about in the indican excretion through the ingestion of the large volume of water was greater in his case. The values were 19.6 per cent. decrease for Subject E against a decrease of 14.6 per cent. for Subject W. It will be remembered that the diet was practically the same for the two subjects, the only variable factor being the water, of which W ingested 3,000 c.c. additional per day during the water period, whereas E's added intake was 4,000 c.c. The latter subject also ingested 150 c.c. less of milk per day than did W. It may be that this extra liter of water ingested by E over that taken by W may have been the efficient factor in causing a more marked lessening of intestinal putrefaction in the case of that individual. We would not expect, *a priori,* however, that the ingested water would prove as efficient in this regard in E's organism as in that of W, inasmuch as the former was an habitual water-drinker.

The pronounced increase in the output of indican on the third day of copious water-drinking by Subject E has already been mentioned. When this value was first obtained it was deemed incorrect, and the urine was again analyzed. Repeated analyses yielded similar values. An explanation was finally found when the feces data[16] were examined. These data showed that the average daily output for this subject had been about 135 gm. of moist feces per day for a long period previous to this time. On the first day of water-drinking the output was only 90.3 gm., whereas on the second day the output was only 37.2 gm. There was, therefore, evidently a retention of feces in the intestine, for on the next day, the third of water-drinking, a stool weighing 249.4 gm. was dropped. On the dry basis, conditions were similar to the above, as the data indicate

16. The feces data were taken from some unpublished results of Mathies and Hawk.

that the average normal output of dry feces per day had been about 32 gm. for some time. Under the influence of water this value was decreased progressively to 18.2 gm. and 10.2 gm. on the first two days of water-drinking, values which were followed by an output of 58.8 gm. of dry matter on the third day. Inasmuch as the urine sample tabulated as the urine of the third day of water-drinking was the urine collected between 7:15 a. m. on the third day and 7:15 a. m. on the fourth day, and further, inasmuch as the third stool of the water period which we have mentioned as weighing 249.4 gm. and having a dry matter content of 58.8 gm. was also passed on the morning of the fourth day of water-drinking, it is evident that this large mass of feces was in the intestine during the interval in which the urine of the high indican content was being passed into the bladder. The undue retention of this fecal mass gave more opportunity for the indol-forming bacteria to complete their task, thus causing the ultimate passage of an extra quota of indican into the urine.

A case very similar to this occurred during the moderate water-drinking experiment on Subject E (see Table 3). On the fifth day of the preliminary period there was an extremely low output of indican, far lower, in fact, than for several days preceding and following. An examination of the feces data showed that on the fourth day of the period a stool weighing 193.9 gm. was passed, whereas the stool for the fifth day weighed only 76.9 gm. and was followed on the sixth day by a stool weighing 207.7 gm. The dry weights of the stools for these days were 47.8, 20.1 and 47.3 gm. respectively. Thus, from the same reasoning as that advanced above, it is seen that the lower output of indican on this fifth day must have been due to the fact that on the fourth day of the period the intestine was more completely evacuated than usual, as shown by the defecation of a stool weighing 193.9 gm. as against an average of 135 gm. for the period. This unusually large output of feces, therefore, left but a comparatively small amount of residual matter within the intestine. The indol-forming microorganisms, consequently, were not able to produce the customary daily quota of indol and the low value for urinary indican was the result.

The last stool passed during the moderate water-drinking period of Subject W and the stool passed on the third day of the copious water-drinking period of Subject E were both acid in reaction to litmus. W's stool weighed 152.7 gm. against an average output of 105.3 gm. The stool was thus about 50 per cent. larger than the average daily output. Notwithstanding this fact, however, the indican output for the corresponding urine was only 34.7 mg., the lowest daily output for the period. The acid reaction of the intestinal contents during the time the *B. coli, Bacterium welchii* and other indol formers were producing the indol output evidently lowered the efficiency of the microorganisms in this respect. Hence less indol was available for subsequent detoxication, conjugation and final elimination as the indoxyl potassium sulphate.

In the case of the acid stool in E's water period, the conditions were somewhat similar. This stool was passed about fifteen hours sooner than it should have been in the usual course of events. On the morning of the day in question, a stool weighing 74.7 gm. was passed and in the afternoon a stool weighing 258 gm. and possessing an acid reaction was dropped. There were, therefore, 332.7 gm. of feces passed during the day as against a daily average of 152.5 gm., yet the urine corresponding to this fecal output showed an indican value of but 48.0 mg., which was nearly 50 per cent. lower than that of the previous day. Two factors evidently were instrumental in bringing about this result. In the first place, the stool was defecated fifteen hours sooner than usual, thus leaving a shorter interval for the microorganisms to accomplish the putrefaction of the protein residues; and, in the second place, the acid reaction of this stool would tend to lessen the efficiency of these bacteria even during the shortened time at their disposal. These two factors easily account for the markedly lessened indican output. In this connection, we would call attention to the fact that during the water periods of these experiments excessive amounts of hydrochloric acid were poured into the intestine through the influence of the water in stimulating gastric secretion.[17] This factor might further diminish the efficiency of the indol-forming bacteria.

The relation existing between the character of the ingested diet and the character, growth and development of the intestinal bacteria on the one hand, and the variation in the reaction of the intestinal contents on the other, coupled with the further relation which these factors bear to the course of intestinal putrefaction, combine to form an interesting and important problem.[18] Herter[19] reports important findings closely allied to this question. Bacteria of various sorts were injected directly into the small intestines of dogs and the course of intestinal putrefaction observed. It was found that *B. coli* and *B. proteus* brought about increased putrefactive changes whereas the injection of lactic acid bacteria caused a lessening of these processes. This furnished a very nice demonstration of the inhibitory influence of acid on the rate of intestinal putrefaction. Very recently Herter and Kendall[20] have reported some interesting findings on the influence of dietary alterations on the intestinal flora. They found in certain experiments on monkeys and cats that a change from a protein diet (meat and eggs) to one in which carbohydrate predominated

17. Wills and Hawk: Am. Soc. Biol. Chem., New Haven, 1910.

18. This problem will be investigated in connection with our water-drinking studies.

19. Herter: Brit. Med. Jour., 1897, p. 1898.

20. Herter and Kendall: Jour. Biol. Chem., 1910, vii, 203.

(sugar and milk) was followed by a change in the nature of the intestinal flora, a decreased putrefaction and a marked improvement in the "bodily and psychical well being" of the subjects.

## CONCLUSIONS

1. The drinking of copious (1,000 c.c.) or moderate (500 c.c.) volumes of water with meals *decreased* intestinal putrefaction as measured by the urinary indican output.

2. Copious water-drinking caused a more pronounced lessening of the putrefactive processes than did the moderate water-drinking.

3. In copious water-drinking the total ethereal sulphate output was increased coincidently with the decrease in the indican output. This observation furnishes strong evidence in favor of the view that indican has an origin different from that of the other ethereal sulphates, and that they cannot correctly be considered as indexes of the same metabolic process.

4. When Ellinger's method is employed, the determination of indican should be made on fresh urine before any preservative has been introduced. Especially is this true when thymol is used as the preservative.

5. The decreased intestinal putrefaction brought about through the ingestion of moderate or copious quantities of water at meal time is probably due to a diminution of the activity of indol-forming bacteria following the accelerated absorption of the products of protein digestion, and the passage of excessive amounts of strongly acid chyme into the intestine.

# THE DETERMINATION OF THE CATALYTIC ACTIVITY OF THE BLOOD AS A CLINICAL DIAGNOSTIC METHOD *

M. C. WINTERNITZ, M.D., G. R. HENRY, M.D., AND F. McPHEDRAN, M.D.
BALTIMORE

## *INTRODUCTION*

The examination of the blood as a diagnostic method has been confined until the present time almost entirely to the study of its cell content from a morphological point of view. This has included the enumeration of the various types of white cells and the red cells with the determination of the hemoglobin content. The importance of the results of these studies need not be emphasized here. It is, however, quite natural that the study of the morphology of the blood, no matter how complete, should only pave the way for further work which must be approached from physiological and chemical aspects. Just as a kidney may show great anatomical variations and still be functionally normal and *vice versa,* so the cells of the blood may vary, and no matter how complete our knowledge concerning the anatomy of the blood may be, the results to be derived must be limited. It seems, therefore, that with the trend of medical thought toward function as opposed to structure the time is propitious for closer observation concerning some of the functions of the blood from a chemical point of view.

### OXYGEN-CARRYING POWER OF THE BLOOD

The one function ascribed to the blood of most importance, is its oxygen-carrying power. All of the oxygen-carriers of the blood, of whatever nature, are contained in the formed elements and not in the plasma or serum. The oxygen catalysts of the blood include oxidases such as aldehydase, peroxidase, catalase and hemoglobin.

"To the oxidases we owe the oxidation of guaiacum, phenolphthalein, etc., as shown by aqueous solutions of the leukocytes. To the peroxidases we owe those oxidations which take place only in the presence of hydrogen peroxid or similar compounds. To the catalase we owe the active decomposition of hydrogen peroxid into water and molecular oxygen. These properties are all lost on boiling. On the other hand certain oxidations by means of hydrogen peroxid are induced by hemoglobin and its iron-

*From the Pathological and Medical Clinical Laboratories of the Johns Hopkins Hospital.

containing derivatives (which are not lost on boiling) and hence we find that the blood can still induce certain oxidations by means of hydrogen peroxid even after it has been boiled."[1]

It would lead us too far to enter into a discussion of these various oxygen-carriers here. Before proceeding further, however, the work of Kastle and Amoss[2] should be noted on the peroxidase activity of the blood in health and disease. These authors showed that the amount of phenolphthalein oxidized by the blood was decreased in many diseases and that in the majority at least this peroxidase activity or oxygen-carrying power is proportional to the hemoglobin.

## THE CATALASE OF THE BLOOD

Catalase is an enzyme of universal occurrence characterized by its power of decomposing hydrogen peroxid into water and molecular oxygen. The literature on this subject both prior to the discovery of the specificity of the ferment by Oscar Loew[3] in 1901 and the more recent literature, have been so thoroughly collected and correlated by Batelli and Stern,[4] and Kastle that it will be unnecessary to dwell on it here. It will suffice to recall the specific activity of the blood in this regard.

Bergengrün[5] demonstrated the catalase of the blood to be in the cellular elements, and while the white cells had a slight activity the red cells were most active. He was further able to show that the activity of the red cells was entirely independent of the hemoglobin, and that this latter substance had no activity after repeated crystallization. Following this Senter[6] prepared a catalase from the blood which he called "hemase." This was very active in decomposing hydrogen peroxid, but had no peroxidase activity.

## THE FUNCTION OF CATALASE

The only property of catalase of which we have any definite knowledge is its power of decomposing hydrogen peroxid. Loew was impressed with the wide distribution of the ferment and thought that it must have a specific function. He considered it possible that the catalase protected the cell from hydrogen peroxid which might be produced in the living cell as a result of the respiratory process, etc. Herlitzka has found that within certain limits the greater the concentration of catalase the greater was the concentration of peroxidase required to produce oxidation. This

1. Kastle, J. H.: This author has recently made an exhaustive review of the oxidases and other oxygen catalysts concerned in biological oxidation (Hyg. Lab. Bull. No. 59, p. 122, December, 1909).
2. Kastle and Amoss: Hyg. Lab. Bull. 31, Washington, 1906.
3. Loew: Report 68 U. S. Dept. Agric.; Washington, 1907.
4. Batelli and Stern: Arch. di fisiol., 1905, ii, 470.
5. Bergengrün: Inaug. Diss., Dorpat, 1888.
6. Senter: Ztschr. f. Physikal. Chem., 1903, xlix, 257.

would point to a protective action on the part of catalase against the peroxidase of the organisms.

Schaffer, and Battelli and Stern have brought forth experimental evidence in favor of this view. Bach and Chodat, on the other hand, have pointed out that catalase cannot decompose various substituted organic peroxids, etc., which are more powerful oxidizing agents than hydrogen peroxid and unless there exist specific substances which protect the organisms against these oxidizing substances, it would be necessary to modify the theory that the function of catalase is to protect the organism from excessive oxidation. The essential difference between catalase and other catalizers, as platinum black, is in the nature of the oxygen liberated. Catalase liberates relatively inactive molecular oxygen which is incapable of blueing guaiac, while other catalizers liberate active molecular oxygen, which has the power of turning guaiac blue (oxidizing it). Kastle has attempted to explain this discrepancy between the ferment catalase and other catalizers.

"Thus it is readily conceivable that the catalases like the peroxidases combine with hydrogen peroxid to form an unstable holoxid derivative, $K + H_2O_2 = H_2KO_2$. This might prove to be so unstable, however, that it would decompose in the sense of the equation $H_2KO_2 = K + H_2O + O$. Before it would have a chance to effect the oxidation of any oxidizable substance at hand; or in the event that oxidation occurred, it is conceivable that the catalase, itself potassium, might be more readily oxidizable than guaiac or any of the peroxidase reagents, in which event we would have $H_2KO_2 = H_2O + KO$. This would explain the fact that, while powerful catalysts, the catalases are not unlimited in their power to effect the decomposition of hydrogen peroxid. It is easier, however, and more in harmony with what we know regarding the conduct of other catalysts to suppose that both of these changes would occur simultaneously: viz., $H_2KO_2 = K + H_2O + O$ and $H_2KO_2$ + guaiac = $K + H_2O$ + guaiacum blue, in which event the given substance would exhibit the properties of both a catalase and a peroxidase, and it may be after all that when examined more closely, the catalases will show peroxidase reactions. As it is, the two sets of substances (catalases and peroxidases), if they are really distinct, are certainly found in the closest and most intimate association in both plant and animal tissues."[7]

## *THE DETERMINATION OF THE CATALYTIC ACTIVITY OF THE BLOOD AS A CLINICAL DIAGNOSTIC METHOD*

### I. LITERATURE

As early as 1893 Gottstein[8] observed that the power of the blood to split hydrogen peroxid was not affected in acute diseases like severe

7. Kastle: The Oxidases, Hygienic Lab. Bull. No. 59, p. 140.
8. Gottstein: Virchow's Arch. f. path. Anat., 1893, cxxxiii, 300.

anemias, diabetes and nephritis in man, and in anthrax and tuberculosis in rabbits and guinea-pigs. Gottstein simply makes the above statement without further detail.

A series of more important observations were made by Jolles and Oppenheim.[9] These authors first determined the catalytic activity of the blood of normal individuals and found that, while the vast majority were fairly constant, there were still occasional marked variations. They examined the blood of more than 100 individuals in this series and it is greatly to be regretted that they have omitted entirely any reference to the condition of the patients except that they were from Professor Finger's clinic. Naturally the results must lose significance without more precise knowledge concerning the individuals. They then examined the blood of twenty-seven hospital patients. They do not consider their series large enough to draw any general deductions especially since observations on the number of red blood cells and hemoglobin were not obtained. That, however, there may occur a marked fall in the power of the blood to split hydrogen peroxid is evident. This occurred in five of seven cases of tuberculosis, three of five cases of cancer, three of four cases of chronic nephritis (the lowest reading being obtained from an uremic patient). Three cases of diabetes were normal, as were also three cardiac cases; there was a marked fall in one case of catarrhal jaundice and one of leukemia and none in one case of sarcoma.

More recently Dalmady and Torday[10] have interested themselves in this work. They found the activity most often normal in anemias, but after severe anemias and large losses of blood there was a decrease, even though there was no constant relation between the grade of anemia and the catalytic activity. In nephritis there was a decrease, though this was marked only in very severe forms. In diseases of the respiratory tract there was no variation excepting in those cases of tuberculosis which had already led to severe anemia. Likewise with disease of the alimentary tract, there was no decline except in cancer or ulcer of the stomach which had caused severe anemia. But with diseases accompanied by high fever, pus and important disturbances of metabolism, there was always a decline.

Dalmady and Torday do not give any detailed information of their cases.

The above results are in themselves of sufficient significance to warrant further work on the catalytic activity of the blood in clinical conditions. It is, however, only fair to state that the following work was approached from an entirely different standpoint. It is perfectly evident that in dealing with such an unknown factor as the catalytic activity of the blood where the function of the enzyme is shrouded in obscurity the

9. Jolles and Oppenheim: Virchow's Arch. f. path. Anat., 1905, clxxx, 185.
10. Dalmady and Torday: Wien. klin. Wchnschr., 1907, xx, 457.

results must be empirical. We have attempted to place our work on as rational a basis as possible and have therefore preceded this article by a series of papers dealing with the catalytic activity of human tissues in health and disease and with various animal experiments. It will possibly be of value to summarize briefly our results.

The determination of the catalytic activity of pathological human tissues led us (Winternitz and Meloy)[11] to the conclusion that all of the tissues of the body were reduced in their power to split hydrogen peroxid in chronic nephritis, and that this reduction varied directly with the severity of the condition, the lowest activity being obtained in uremia. In no other disease was this universal decrease in the activity of the enzyme found. This seemed doubly important since the catalytic activity of the blood was reduced in uremia and was normal in two cases of eclampsia. It was perfectly natural that such an observation should be followed by experimental work, since here lesions can be produced at will and the conditions of the experiment governed. It was shown (Winternitz[12]) that the catalytic activity of a single rabbit's blood was constant from day to day over long periods of time; that following ligation of ureters, bilateral nephrectomy, or uremia following uranium nitrate nephritis there was a fall in the catalytic activity of the blood which became more and more marked as death was approached and that this tissue taken post mortem also had a decreased power to split hydrogen peroxid. We then attempted (Winternitz and Rogers[13]) to study the effect of salts on the catalytic activity of the blood, thinking that the retention of salt in nephritis might be responsible for the decrease in the activity, since it is well known that the power of the blood to split hydrogen peroxid is greatly influenced by the addition of salts of various kinds *in vitro*. The results were conclusive; acids, alkalies and salts all reduced the activity of the blood when injected intravenously.

During these experiments it was found that following an acute peritonitis there is an acute rise in the catalytic activity of the blood (Winternitz). This is entirely independent of the temperature and white blood-count (Winternitz and Pratt[14]), but varies directly with the red blood-count (Winternitz).

Further studies (Winternitz and Pratt[15]) on the relation of various organs to the catalytic activity of the blood were made with the following result: Following the extirpation of many organs there is a transient fall in the catalytic activity of the blood. The fall is permanent after extirpation of the thyroid, but is compensated if thyroid extract be fed.

11. Winternitz and Meloy: Jour. Exper. Med., 1908, x, 759.
12. Winternitz: Jour. Exper. Med., 1909, xi, 200.
13. Winternitz and Rogers: Not yet published.
14. Winternitz and Pratt: Jour. Exper. Med., 1910, xii, 1.
15. Winternitz and Pratt: Jour. Exper. Med., 1910, xii, 115.

From this work several important factors determining the activity of the blood in splitting hydrogen peroxid became evident. First, that there was a direct relation between the catalytic activity of the blood and the number of red blood cells; but that this was not the only factor determining the power of the blood to decompose hydrogen peroxid, since salts had a marked influence on the activity as did also the function of the thyroid gland and kidneys. It was also evident that there was an attempt on the part of the other tissues to keep the activity of the blood constant.

With this preliminary work as a basis we feel that the study of the catalytic activity of the human blood can be undertaken to a better advantage.

## II. METHOD

It is at once evident that if the test is to be at all practical a simple method must be adopted. We have modified the method of Kastle and Loevenhart,[16] described in detail in a previous paper (Winternitz and Meloy). The required amount of blood is obtained from an ear-prick, with a pipette (graduated to contain 0.025 c.c.). This is immediately diluted with 10 c.c. of distilled water, making 10 c.c. of a 1 to 400 dilution of blood in distilled water. This is divided, 5 c.c. being placed in each of two 100 c.c. salt-mouth bottles. One of these is retained as a check in case of emergency. In the other a small phial containing 5 c.c. of neutralized commercial hydrogen peroxid (Mallinckrodt's 3 per cent.) is placed and the large bottle is connected with a gas burette. This bottle is agitated for a period of one minute, readings of the amount of gas liberated being taken every fifteen seconds. The method has proved sufficiently accurate. The readings should be made as soon as possible (within several hours) after the blood is obtained. Under these conditions we have found it unnecessary to take any other precautions as, for instance, the temperature, etc.

## III. THE CATALYTIC ACTIVITY OF THE BLOOD OF NORMAL INDIVIDUALS

The first work to be reported consisted of a series of readings from normal individuals, including students, doctors, and patients suffering from hernia, fracture, etc. In each case the age and other particulars are recorded together with the red blood-count and in some instances the hemoglobin percentage.

During the first few days of life there is notoriously a marked variation in the number of red blood-cells and this is also true of the catalytic activity of the blood. These two curves bear no relation to each other. The number of cases in infants is too small to draw any conclusions and further discussion of them will therefore be omitted from the work.

16. Kastle and Loevenhart: Am. Chem. Jour., 1903, xxix, 397.

TABLE 1.—CATALYTIC ACTIVITY IN NORMAL INDIVIDUALS

INFANTS

| Age Days | Sex | Race | R.B.C. | Hg. % | Catalase—c.c. of Oxygen Liberated in 15″ | 30″ | 45″ | 60″ |
|---|---|---|---|---|---|---|---|---|
| 1 .... | .. | Bl. | 5728000 | ..... | 22. | 29. | 34. | 37.6 |
| 4 .... | F. | W. | 6368000 | ..... | 15.2 | 19. | 22. | 25. |
| 6 .... | M. | W. | 6176000 | ..... | 19. | 24. | 27. | 31. |
| 6 .... | M. | W. | 5120000 | ..... | 12.5 | 16. | 19.5 | 24. |
| 2 .... | M. | W. | 5248000 | ..... | 16.6 | 20.8 | 25. | 28. |

FIRST DECADE

| Age Yrs. | Sex | Race | R.B.C | Hg. % | Catalase—c.c. of Oxygen Liberated in 15″ | 30″ | 45″ | 60″ |
|---|---|---|---|---|---|---|---|---|
| 2½ .. | M. | W. | 3904000 | ..... | 14.6 | 18. | 21. | 25. |
| 9 .... | M. | W. | 4256000 | ..... | 14. | 16. | 17. | 18. |

SECOND DECADE

| Age Yrs. | Sex | Race | R.B.C | Hg. % | Catalase—c.c. of Oxygen Liberated in 15″ | 30″ | 45″ | 60″ |
|---|---|---|---|---|---|---|---|---|
| 19 .... | M. | W. | 5568000 | ..... | 14.6 | 18.8 | 24. | 28. |
| 18 .... | M. | W. | 4948000 | ..... | 13. | 16. | 19. | 22. |
| 17 .... | M. | W. | 4640000 | ..... | 14.4 | 18.6 | 22. | 25.2 |
| 11 .... | M. | W. | 4304000 | ..... | 12. | 14.8 | 17. | 19. |
| .. .... | M. | W. | 5040000 | ..... | 15. | 20. | 25. | 28. |
| 12 .... | M. | W. | 4240000 | ..... | 12. | 15. | 18. | 20. |

THIRD DECADE

| Age Yrs. | Race | Sex | R.B.C. | Hg. % | Catalase—c.c. of Oxygen Liberated in 15″ | 30″ | 45″ | 60″ |
|---|---|---|---|---|---|---|---|---|
| 28 .... | W. | M. | 4856000 | ..... | 14. | 18. | 21. | 25. |
| 25 .... | W. | M. | 5646000 | ..... | 14.3 | 19.6 | 24.6 | 23.6 |
| .. .... | W. | M. | 5221000 | ..... | 14.6 | 19.6 | 24. | 29.8 |
| 24 .... | W. | M. | 5200000 | ..... | 14.6 | 19.6 | 24. | 28. |
| 27 .... | W. | M. | 5488000 | ..... | 14.6 | 19.4 | 24. | 28. |
| 27 .... | W. | M. | 5072000 | ..... | 14. | 18.3 | 22.6 | 26.2 |
| 22 .... | W. | M. | 5248000 | ..... | 14.6 | 18.2 | 25. | 29.2 |
| 28 .... | W. | M. | 6080000 | ..... | 14.8 | 19.6 | 24.8 | 28. |
| 26 .... | W. | M. | 5160000 | 88. | 14.8 | 19.6 | 23.8 | 27. |
| .. .... | W. | M. | 4456000 | ..... | 14.3 | 19.2 | 23. | 27. |
| 29 .... | W. | M. | 5192000 | ..... | 15.2 | 19.2 | 24. | 27. |
| .. .... | W. | M. | 5112000 | ..... | 16.6 | 22. | 25. | 28. |
| 28 .... | W. | M. | 5496000 | ..... | 14.6 | 18. | 21.4 | 24.3 |
| 28 .... | W. | M. | 5528000 | ..... | 14. | 18. | 21. | 24. |
| .. .... | W. | M. | 5096000 | 99. | 18. | 22. | 25. | 28. |
| .. .... | W. | M. | 4516000 | 97. | 18. | 23. | 27. | 30.4 |
| 29 .... | W. | M. | 4448000 | 99.8 | 18. | 22. | 26. | 30.4 |
| 26 .... | B. | M. | 4336000 | ..... | 15. | 19. | 23. | 26.4 |
| .. .... | W. | M. | 5136000 | 100. | 18.4 | 24. | 29. | 34. |
| .. .... | W. | M. | 4664000 | ..... | 15.2 | 19. | 24. | 23. |
| .. .... | W. | M. | 5483000 | ..... | 15. | 19. | 21.6 | 25. |
| 25 .... | W. | F. | ....... | ..... | 14.2 | 18.6 | 22.5 | 26.3 |
| 25 .... | W. | M. | ....... | ..... | 16.4 | 21.9 | 28.4 | 29.2 |
| 26 .... | W. | F. | ....... | ..... | 14.2 | 18.8 | 21.8 | 24.6 |

FOURTH DECADE

| Age Yrs. | Race | Sex | R.B.C. | Hg. % | Catalase—c.c. of Oxygen Liberated in 15″ | 30″ | 45″ | 60″ |
|---|---|---|---|---|---|---|---|---|
| 34 .... | W. | M. | 4912000 | 87. | 13.2 | 17. | 20. | 23.8 |
| 37 .... | W. | M. | 4656000 | 80. | 17.6 | 22. | 25. | 29. |

| Age Yrs. | Race | Sex | R.B.C. | Hg. % | Catalase—c.c. of Oxygen Liberated in 15″ | 30″ | 45″ | 60″ |
|---|---|---|---|---|---|---|---|---|
| 36 .... | W. | M. | 4464000 | 103. | 15. | 18.8 | 21. | 24. |
| 37 .... | W. | M. | 5096000 | ..... | 14. | 18.2 | 22.3 | 27. |
| 31 .... | W. | M. | 5344000 | ..... | 14.8 | 19.6 | 24. | 27. |
| 34 .... | W. | M. | 5312000 | ..... | 14.6 | 19.6 | 24. | 27.6 |
| 30 .... | W. | M. | 4756000 | ..... | 14.6 | 19.8 | 24.2 | 27.8 |
| .. .... | W. | M. | 5216000 | ..... | 14.6 | 18.8 | 23.8 | 27.2 |
| 36 .... | W. | M. | 4624000 | ..... | 14.8 | 19. | 24. | 27.6 |
| 38 .... | W. | M. | 5113000 | ..... | 15. | 19. | 24. | 27.6 |
| 36 .... | W. | M. | 5860000 | ..... | 13.2 | 15.8 | 18. | 19. |
| 37 .... | W. | M. | 4168000 | ..... | 14.6 | 18. | 22. | 26. |
| 36 .... | W. | M. | 4840000 | ..... | 14.4 | 15. | 21. | 24.3 |
| 35 .... | W. | M. | 4736000 | ..... | 16.6 | 21. | 24.8 | 29. |
| 35 .... | W. | F. | 5152000 | 104. | 16.2 | 20.4 | 23.6 | 27.1 |

FIFTH DECADE

| Age Yrs. | Race | Sex | R.B.C. | Hg. % | Catalase—c.c. of Oxygen Liberated in 15″ | 30″ | 45″ | 60″ |
|---|---|---|---|---|---|---|---|---|
| 40 .... | W. | M. | 5880000 | 107. | 18. | 23. | 28. | 32. |
| 44 .... | W. | F. | 5156000 | ..... | 14. | 19.2 | 24. | 28. |
| .. .... | W. | M. | 5328000 | ..... | 14.6 | 19. | 23.8 | 28.2 |
| 46 .... | W. | M. | 5440000 | ..... | 14.6 | 19. | 23.8 | 28. |
| .. .... | B. | M. | 4736000 | ..... | 14.8 | 19. | 25.6 | 27.4 |
| 47 .... | W. | M. | 4928000 | ..... | 14.8 | 19. | 23.8 | 27.6 |
| .. .... | W. | M. | 5014000 | ..... | 14.8 | 19. | 23. | 26.8 |
| 44 .... | W. | M. | 5616000 | ..... | 14.6 | 19. | 22. | 26. |
| 41 .... | W. | M. | 5648000 | 97. | 18. | 22. | 26. | 28. |
| 47 .... | W. | M. | 4728000 | ..... | 16. | 22. | 26. | 29. |
| 47 .... | W. | M. | 4288000 | ..... | 16. | 22. | 26. | 30. |
| 41 .... | W. | M. | 5322000 | ..... | 14.6 | 19. | 22. | 26. |

SIXTH DECADE

| Age Yrs. | Race | Sex | R.B.C. | Hg. % | Catalase—c.c. of Oxygen Liberated in 15″ | 30″ | 45″ | 60″ |
|---|---|---|---|---|---|---|---|---|
| 50 .... | W. | M. | 4168000 | ..... | 14.8 | 19. | 23. | 27. |
| 57 .... | W. | M. | 4608000 | ..... | 14.8 | 18. | 21.6 | 24. |
| 53 .... | W. | M. | 5187000 | ..... | 14.8 | 18.6 | 44.6 | 27.8 |
| 57 .... | W. | M. | 4792000 | ..... | 12. | 16. | 20. | 25.6 |
| 57 .... | W. | M. | 5528000 | ..... | 12.4 | 15.6 | 19.6 | 24. |
| 52 .... | W. | F. | 4680000 | 82. | 14.8 | 18.8 | 21. | 23.8 |

SEVENTH DECADE

| Age Yrs. | Race | Sex | R.B.C. | Hg. % | Catalase—c.c. of Oxygen Liberated in 15″ | 30″ | 45″ | 60″ |
|---|---|---|---|---|---|---|---|---|
| 60 .... | B. | F. | 5056000 | ..... | 14.4 | 18. | 21. | 24.6 |
| 64 .... | W. | M. | 4944000 | ..... | 12. | 14. | 16. | 17.5 |
| 64 .... | W. | M. | 5328000 | 98. | 17. | 21. | 25. | 28. |
| 65 .... | W. | M. | 4000000 | ..... | 12.6 | 14.8 | 16.6 | 19. |
| 68 .... | W. | M. | 4080000 | ..... | 14.6 | 19. | 22. | 25. |
| 63 .... | W. | M. | 4960000 | ..... | 14. | 18. | 22. | 26. |

EIGHTH DECADE

| Age Yrs. | Race | Sex | R.B.C. | Hg. % | Catalase—c.c. of Oxygen Liberated in 15″ | 30″ | 45″ | 60″ |
|---|---|---|---|---|---|---|---|---|
| 70 .... | W. | M. | 5408000 | ..... | 21. | 24. | 28. | 31. |
| .. .... | W. | M. | 3520000 | ..... | 15. | 19. | 33. | 26. |

Table 1 can be summarized briefly as follows:

Total No. of cases, 74.

| Oxygen Liberated in First 15 Seconds c.c. | Cases No. | Cases % |
|---|---|---|
| 12-13 | 6 | 8.1 |
| 13-14 | 3 | 4.05 |
| 14-15 | 42 | 56.7 |
| 15-16 | 8 | 10.8 |
| 16-17 | 6 | 8.1 |
| 17-18 | 2 | 2.7 |
| 18-19 | 6 | 8.1 |
| 21-22 | 1 | 1.35 |

The vast majority of cases give a reading of from 14 to 15 c.c. of oxygen liberated within the first fifteen seconds. On the other hand the limit of error in any test of this nature could hardly be less than from 1 to 2 c.c. of oxygen liberated in the first fifteen seconds. We have therefore considered any reading between 13 and 17 to be within normal limits and with this as a premise 80 per cent. of the cases must be considered to fall within a physiological variation.

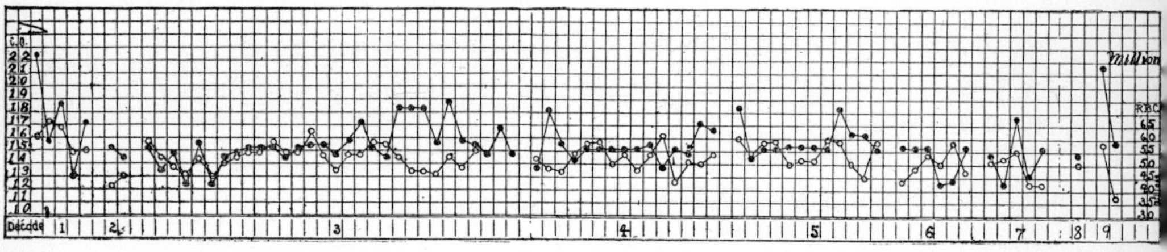

Chart 1.—Catalytic activity of blood compared with red blood count. Line determined by solid black dots represents cubic centimeters of oxygen liberated in first fifteen seconds. Line determined by hollow dots represents the number of red blood-cells.

It is of interest to compare the curve of the catalytic activity of the blood with the red blood-count (Chart 1).

Two facts at once become evident from this chart. First, the curve of the catalytic activity of the blood of a series of individuals is in many respects as constant as that of the red blood-count in those same individuals, and secondly, there is no absolute relation between the number of red blood-cells and the catalytic activity of the blood in different individuals. The second fact has been previously illustrated in rabbits (Winternitz and Pratt). It will be remembered that while in healthy rabbits a high blood-count is accompanied by a high catalytic activity in most instances, the number of red blood-cells is by no means the only factor determining the power of the blood to split hydrogen peroxid. Glands like the thyroid (Winternitz and Pratt) and salts (Winternitz and Rogers) likewise exert an influence on this activity. In a few instances in which there was a marked variation in the catalytic activity of the blood the hemoglobin content was determined. A glance at Table 1 will suffice to show that this is no more intimately connected with the power of the blood to split hydrogen peroxid than is the number of red blood-cells.

It is not our present aim to discuss in detail the variations found in supposedly normal individuals. This must form the basis for future work. It seems more logical, however, to consider the small percentage of marked variations to be based on physiological or pathological phenomena and that individuals with such variations must be considered abnormal rather than have it taken for granted on *a priori* evidence that the power of the blood to split hydrogen peroxid could vary to any marked extent in absolutely normal individuals.

The fact remains, however, that marked variations occur in 20 per cent. of normal individuals. This is of importance, and must be remembered in the interpretation of change in the catalytic activity of the blood in diseased conditions. Wherever possible, readings should be repeatedly taken, for the significance of the results must depend on variations from day to day as a result of the disease. When this is not possible, the significance of the results must suffer. In each case to be reported several readings were taken even though, for the sake of brevity, only one observation is recorded in many instances.

## IV. THE CATALYTIC ACTIVITY OF THE BLOOD OF A SINGLE NORMAL INDIVIDUAL OVER A LONG PERIOD OF TIME

TABLE 2.—CATALYTIC ACTIVITY OF BLOOD IN A SINGLE NORMAL INDIVIDUAL

| | Oxygen (c.c.) Liberated in | | | |
|---|---|---|---|---|
| Date | 15″ | 30″ | 45″ | 60″ |
| 10/16/08 | 14.6 | 19.2 | 23.4 | 27.4 |
| 10/17/08 | 14.2 | 18.8 | 23. | 27. |
| 10/18/08 | 13.9 | 18. | 21.9 | 25.6 |
| 10/19/08 | 14.9 | 18.8 | 23.1 | 26.8 |
| 10/21/08 | 14. | 18.5 | 22.6 | 26.2 |
| 10/24/08 | 14.7 | 19.6 | 23.8 | 27.3 |
| 11/ 2/08 | 15.2 | 19.5 | 22.6 | 25.6 |
| 11/ 4/08 | 15.2 | 20.4 | 23.7 | 27. |
| 12/10/08 | 14. | 18.5 | 22.6 | 26.2 |
| 1/20/09 | 14.9 | 18.8 | 23.1 | 26.8 |
| 3/10/09 | 16.2 | 20.4 | 23.7 | 27. |
| 5/ 5/09 | 15.2 | 19.6 | 22.4 | 26.6 |
| 7/10/09 | 14.8 | 18.2 | 22.6 | 26.4 |
| 12/17/09 | 14.8 | 19.6 | 24.6 | 28.6 |
| 3/10/10 | 14.6 | 19.4 | 24. | 26.8 |

The greatest variation (as illustrated in Chart 2) in the catalytic activity of a single individual's blood over a period of several months is 1.3 c.c. of oxygen liberated in the first fifteen seconds. This is remarkably constant and is what should have been expected from the animal experimentation where the same results were obtained with normal rabbits.

Briefly, we see that the blood in 80 per cent. of normal individuals has a very constant catalytic power—liberates 14 to 17 c.c. of oxygen in fifteen seconds, and that the activity of a single normal individual's blood may not vary within more than 1.3 c.c. of oxygen liberated in fifteen seconds over a period of seventeen months. On the other hand, 20 per cent. of normal individuals show such wide variations in the power of their blood to split hydrogen peroxid that, unless this is realized, the significance of the change in diseased conditions must suffer. The importance, therefore, of the determination of the catalytic activity of the blood rests, as will be seen, in variations in the activity from day to day or in any change from the normal activity of the *individual's* blood.

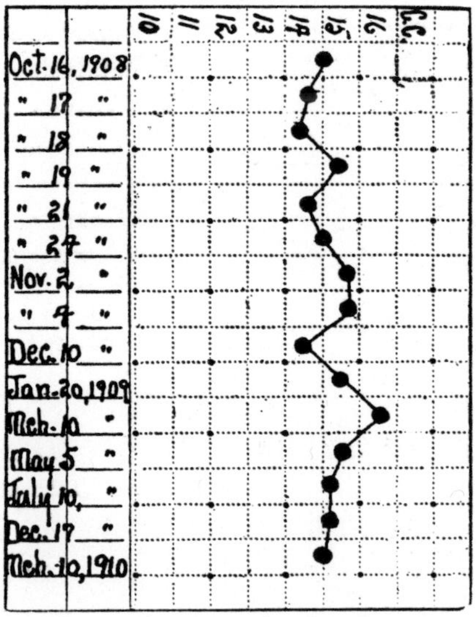


**Chart 2.—Curve of Table 2, representing cubic centimeters of oxygen liberated in first fifteen seconds.**

It should be emphasized that in these experiments no precautions as to temperature, etc., were used. Ordinary room temperature sufficed and thus modifies the method considerably.

## V. THE CATALYTIC ACTIVITY OF THE BLOOD IN DISEASED CONDITIONS

### *A. Acute Infectious Diseases*

A study of Table 3 shows that the catalytic activity of the blood varies within wide limits in typhoid fever. On further analysis, however, the variations are in part at least explainable. For this reason the table has been arranged according to day of disease, as has also the curve in

TABLE 3.—CATALYTIC ACTIVITY OF THE BLOOD IN TYPHOID FEVER PATIENTS

| No. | Med. No. | R.B.C. | W.B.C. | Hb. % | Catalase 15″ | Catalase 30″ | Catalase 45″ | Catalase 60″ | Day of Disease | Age | Sex | Race | Results | Complications |
|---|---|---|---|---|---|---|---|---|---|---|---|---|---|---|
| 1. | 23281 | 5100000 | 5400 | 80 | 17. | 22. | 26.6 | 30.6 | 1 | 38 | M. | W. | Recovery | Relapse |
| 2. | 23274 | 4202000 | 3600 | 58 | 14.5 | 19. | 23.4 | 27. | 1 | 17 | M. | W. | Recovery | Relapse |
| 3. | 23244 | 5360000 | 9600 | 92 | 14.1 | 18.6 | 22.5 | 26.6 | 1 | 23 | M. | W. | Recovery | Relapse |
| 4. | 23069 | 4844000 | 6200 | 68 | 14.5 | 19. | 23. | 26.7 | 3 | 31 | M. | B. | Death | Hemorrhages |
| 5. | 24460 | ? | 5800 | ? | 18.4 | 26.2 | 31.5 | 37.4 | 8 | 21 | M. | W. | Recovery | Hemorrhages |
| 6. | 24470 | ? | 4300 | 105 | 15.5 | 20.4 | 25.4 | 29. | 12 | 33 | M. | W. | Recovery | Hemorrhages |
| 7. | 24447 | ? | 3500 | ? | 13.6 | 18.2 | 22.8 | 27. | 14 | 9 | M. | W. | Recovery | Hemorrhages |
| 8. | 23145 | 3780000 | 5600 | 62 | 12.2 | 14.8 | 16.7 | 18.8 | 14 | 38 | M. | B. | Recovery | Pulmonary infarct |
| 9. | 23244 | 2624000 | 7000 | ? | 8.6 | 11.5 | 13.5 | 16.2 | 15 | 23 | M. | W. | Recovery | Albumin; epithelial casts in urine |
| 10. | ..... | ? | 5700 | 78 | 9.8 | 13.8 | 15.5 | 18. | 15 | 22 | M. | B. | Recovery | Albumin; epithelial and granular casts |
| 11. | 23194 | 3572000 | 5200 | 55 | 11.4 | 14. | 16.2 | 18.4 | 20 | 18 | F. | B. | Recovery | Parotitis; Bartholini gland abscess |
| 12. | 23193 | 300000 | 4680 | 62 | 10.9 | 13. | 14.4 | 16.2 | 25 | 26 | F. | W. | Recovery | Hemorrhages; mitral insufficiency; exophthalmic goiter; granular casts and albumin |
| 13. | 23116 | 3846000 | 5400 | 80 | 13.5 | 16.6 | 19. | 21.6 | 27 | 23 | F. | W. | Recovery | Acute thyroiditis |
| 14. | 24470 | 4784000 | 5000 | 65 | 14. | 17. | 19.6 | 21.5 | 40 | 33 | M. | W. | Recovery | Acute thyroiditis |
| 15. | 24399 | ? | ? | ? | 18. | 24.2 | 29.6 | 34.4 | 48 | 25 | M. | W. | Recovery | Relapse fifth day |

Chart 3, which represents the catalytic activity of the blood in terms of oxygen liberated in the first fifteen seconds (solid dots) and the number of red blood-cells (hollow dots).

The activity of the blood is normal during the early days of the illness, but declines during the later course, again rising to normal at the time of convalescence. This was confirmed in several cases when the activity was repeatedly determined during the illness. The curve is in part explainable by the anemia which accompanies the disease, as illustrated by the line of hollow dots in Chart 3. Whether the urinary findings and the low catalytic activity in Cases 9 and 10 are of significance

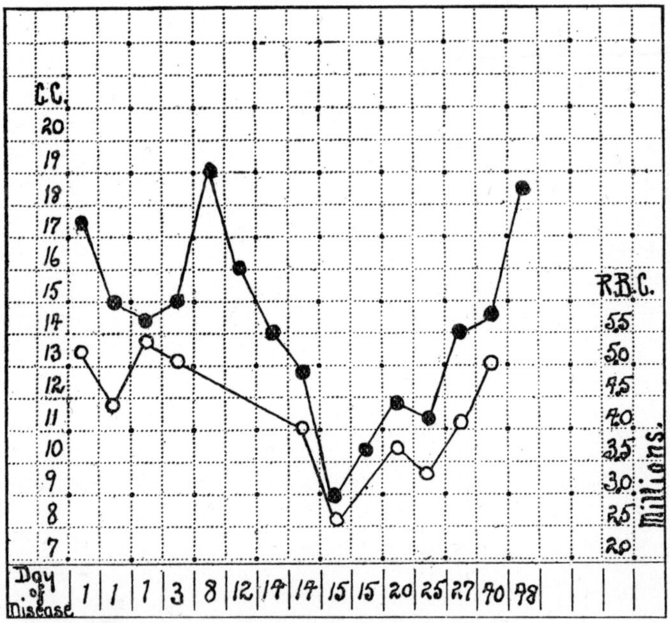


Chart 3.—Curve of Table 3, representing the catalytic activity of the blood in terms of oxygen liberated in the first fifteen seconds (line determined by solid dots), and the number of red blood-cells (line determined by hollow dots).

in relation to the function of the kidney can only be conjectured. This will be discussed in detail later.

DISEASES OF THE RESPIRATORY TRACT, INCLUDING LOBAR PNEUMONIA, TUBERCULOSIS AND EMPYEMA

CASE 1.—*Patient.*—J. S., colored man, aged 24. Medical No. 23570.

*Clinical Diagnosis.*—Lobar pneumonia, left upper and lower and lower right lobe.

Urine: Albumin in traces, few granular and epithelial casts.

Recovery.

CASE 2.—*Patient.*—C. S., colored girl aged 1. Medical No. 23572.

*Clinical Diagnosis.*—Lobar pneumonia; acute mastoiditis (bilateral), pneumococcus meningitis; cerebral hemorrhage.

Death.

*Anatomical Diagnosis.*—Lobar pneumonia with abscess formation (both upper lobes); acute pleuritis; bilateral acute otitis media; acute cerebrospinal meningitis with hemorrhage; cloudy swelling of viscera and acute splenic tumor.

Case 3.—*Patient.*—H. B. R., colored man aged 27. Medical No. 23268.

*Clinical Diagnosis.*—Lobar pneumonia (right lower).

Urine: Negative. Recovery.

Case 4.—*Patient.*—H. B. R., colored man aged 20. Medical No. 23490.

*Clinical Diagnosis.*—Lobar pneumonia (lower left).

Urine: Trace of albumin.

Recovery.

Case 5.—*Patient.*—W. M. B., colored man, aged 27. Medical No. 23506.

*Clinical Diagnosis.*—Lobar pneumonia (lower left).

Urine: Albumin in traces, casts throughout illness. Recovery.

Case 6.—*Patient.*—W. J. M., colored man, aged 23. Medical No. 23576.

*Clinical Diagnosis.*—Acute tuberculous bronchopneumonia.

Death.

*Anatomical Diagnosis.*—Chronic ulcerative pulmonary tuberculosis with cavity formation (left apex); caseous and gelatinous bronchopneumonia (left lung), etc.

Case 7.—*Patient.*—M. A. K., white woman, aged 32. Medical No. 23321.

*Clinical Diagnosis.*—Lobar pneumonia; empyema.

Operation; recovery.

Urine: Albumin in traces.

Case 8.—*Patient.*—W. B. B., colored man, aged 32. Medical No. 23577.

*Clinical Diagnosis.*—Acute pleurisy with effusion; probably tuberculous.

Table 4.—Catalytic Activity of the Blood in Eight Cases of Disease of the Respiratory Tract

| Case No. | Date | Catalase c.c. of Oxygen Liberated in | | | | Blood | | |
|---|---|---|---|---|---|---|---|---|
| .... | ..... | 15″ | 30″ | 45″ | 60″ | R.B.C. | W.B.C. | Hb. % |
| 1. | 1/14 | 16. | 20.5 | 26.4 | 36.8 | 4652000 | 18400 | 95 |
| 2. | 1/14 | 9.8 | 11.5 | 13.4 | 15.2 | 4840000 | 21160 | 55 |
| 3. | ..... | 15. | 18.5 | 23.2 | 26.8 | 5272000 | 32000 | 68 |
| 4. | 1/18 | 11.6 | 13.7 | 15.2 | 16.9 | 4120000 | 11000 | 65 |
| 5. | 1/14 | 14.9 | 18.8 | 22.2 | 25.5 | 4720000 | 10920 | 85 |
| 6. | 1/14 | 16.4 | 20.4 | 23.5 | 27. | 5152000 | 5840 | 63 |
| 7. | 11/ 6 | 16. | 19.9 | 23.4 | 26.5 | 4640000 | 39360 | 100 |
| 8. | 1/14 | 16.6 | 23.4 | 27.2 | 31.4 | 5255000 | 6800 | 90 |

Table 4 shows that in six of the eight cases the power of the blood to split hydrogen peroxid varies within normal limits in diseases of the lung. In the other two, Cases 2 and 4, there was a marked secondary anemia with a low hemoglobin percentage, but this could only in part explain the low activity, since No. 3, for example, has a low hemoglobin percentage and a normal activity. That there is a slight decline in the catalytic activity of the blood during the course of a lobar pneumonia is illustrated by Table 5.

Briefly, in four of six cases of lobar pneumonia, the catalytic activity of the blood is normal. In one of the other two the disease was so complicated by meningitis, etc., that any result must be considered from many standpoints. In the other no cause could be ascribed to the decreased activity. In the single case of acute pulmonary tuberculosis the activity was normal and this is what would be expected from Dalmady and Torday's report since there was no anemia. In the one case of acute pleurisy the activity was on the upper limits of normal. Whether the activity was influenced, raised, by the pleurisy can only be conjectured (see next section, on acute peritonitis).

Table 5.—Course of the Catalytic Activity in Pneumonia (Case 3)

| Date | C.c. of Oxygen Liberated in— | | | | Day of |
|---|---|---|---|---|---|
| ..... | 15″ | 30″ | 45″ | 60″ | Disease |
| 10/24 | 15. | 18.7 | 22.8 | 27. | 5 |
| 10/26 | 14.7 | 19.5 | 23.2 | 26.4 | 7 |
| 10/28 | 13.2 | 16.4 | 19.8 | 22.3 | 9 |

ACUTE PERITONITIS

Case 9.—*Patient*.—O. L., colored female, age unknown. Surgical No. 24320.
*Clinical Diagnosis*.—Acute appendicitis with rupture and general peritonitis.
Operation: Appendectomy with drainage.
Recovery.

Table 6.—Catalytic Activity in Acute Appendicitis (Case 9)

| | Catalase | | | | |
|---|---|---|---|---|---|
| Date | 15″ | 30″ | 45″ | 60″ | Remarks |
| 6/24 | 15.6 | 23. | 28.8 | 34.6 | 24 hrs. after operation. Peritoneum clear |
| 7/27 | 19.2 | 25.6 | 21.6 | 37.7 | Symptoms of acute peritonitis |

It is to be regretted that this case was not more thoroughly studied.

Case 10.—*Patient*.—M. K., white man, aged 29. Surgical No. 24957.
*Clinical Diagnosis*.—Appendicitis with acute spreading peritonitis.
Operation: Appendectomy with drainage.
Recovery.

Table 7.—Catalytic Activity in Acute Peritonitis (Case 10)

| | Catalase | | | | |
|---|---|---|---|---|---|
| Date | 15″ | 30″ | 45″ | 60″ | Remarks |
| 11/ 9 | 18. | 22.5 | 27. | 30.6 | Two hours before operation |
| 11/10 | 16. | 20. | 24.6 | 27.8 | Twelve hours after operation |
| 11/ 4 | 14.8 | 18.6 | 22.2 | 26. | Patient's condition excellent |

Case 11.—*Patient*.—A. S., colored man, aged 21. Surgical No. 25150.
*Clinical Diagnosis*.—General peritonitis; origin unknown.
Operation: Appendectomy and drainage.
Recovery.

Table 8.—Catalytic Activity in Acute Peritonitis (Case 11)

| | Catalase. | | | | | |
|---|---|---|---|---|---|---|
| Date. | 15″ | 30″ | 45″ | 60″ | R.B.C. | Remarks. |
| 12/17, 7:30 p.m. | 17. | 21.8 | 27. | 32. | 5480000 | Half hour before operation |
| 12/18, 10 a.m. | 12.6 | 15.4 | 19.2 | 22.8 | 4872000 | 14 hours after operation |
| 12/18, 3:30 p.m. | 12.6 | 16. | 19.8 | 23. | ........ | ........ |
| 12/19, | 8.8 | 11.8 | 14.4 | 17.2 | ........ | ........ |
| 12/20, | 8.8 | 15. | 17.6 | 20. | ........ | ........ |
| 12/21, | 8.8 | 15. | 17.8 | 20.8 | ........ | ........ |

CASE 12.—*Patient.*—C. M. J., colored man, aged 23. Medical No. 24,441.
*Clinical Diagnosis.*—Typhoid fever—perforation.
Operation: Closure of perforation—result recovery.
Urine: Albumin in traces and a few finely granular casts.

TABLE 9.—CATALYTIC ACTIVITY IN ACUTE PERITONITIS (CASE 12)

| | Catalase. | | | | |
|---|---|---|---|---|---|
| Date. | 15″ | 30″ | 45″ | 60″ | Remarks. |
| 7/19, 3:30 p. m.. | 19.8 | 26.8 | 32.4 | 37.2 | Patient seized with acute abdominal pain about 2:30 p. m. |
| 7/19, 6: p. m.. | 16.8 | 22.2 | 27. | 32.2 | Operation 4 p. m. |
| 7/23, ........... | 14. | 19. | 22.8 | 26. | ........................... |

CASE 13.—*Patient.*—M. S., colored woman, aged 23. Surgical No. 24,350. Illness of twenty-four hours' duration; acute onset.
*Clinical Diagnosis.*—Acute salpingitis; acute peritonitis.
Operation: Salpingo-oophorectomy; drainage.
Recovery.

| | Catalase. | | | | |
|---|---|---|---|---|---|
| Date. | 15″ | 30″ | 45″ | 60″ | Remarks. |
| 6/29, 9 a. m........ | 14.6 | 20.2 | 24.6 | 29.2 | Operation June 28, a. m. |

In the five cases of acute peritonitis above reported four show a characteristic rise in the power of the blood to split hydrogen peroxid. In the first there was a spreading peritonitis following operation. This was accompanied by an increased catalytic power of the blood, i. e., a rise of 3.6 c.c. oxygen liberated in the first fifteen seconds. In the other cases readings were obtained at the time of operation and then for several days afterward. In all of these cases the increase in the activity was not determinable, since the patient came under observation only after the peritonitis was suspected. In the fifth case the activity was normal, but here it must be remembered that the reading of the catalytic activity of the blood was not made until twenty hours after the operation.

These results on human beings correspond in every detail with the animal experiments (Winternitz). Here, it will be remembered, there was a marked rise in the catalytic activity of the blood within a few hours after an experimental peritonitis was produced, and this rise continued for a variable period, from six to thirty-six hours. It was later shown (Winternitz and Pratt) that the variation in the catalytic activity of the blood was entirely independent of the number of white blood-cells and the body temperature. On the other hand it has been shown (Winternitz) that following experimental peritonitis there is a rise in the number of red blood-cells which corresponds to the rise in the catalytic action. The nature of this change will be reported on in a subsequent article.

That some practical value might be acquired from the determination of the catalytic activity of the blood is emphasized in the two following cases. The second one (Case 15), in particular, is of interest. This patient was a child with high fever, leukocytosis, and obscure abdominal signs. Careful examination left the impression of an abdominal inflammation, and it was considered probable that this patient was suffering from a peritonitis either arising from a ruptured appendix or a typhoid perforation. The catalytic activity of the blood was normal. The peritoneum was clean. The next day a localized infection of the spine revealed itself.

SUSPECTED PERITONITIS

Case 14.—*Patient.*—M. G., white female, age unknown. Surgical No. 23,106.

*Clinical Diagnosis.*—Strangulated right femoral hernia; fecal fistula.

Operation: Incision and drainage abscess of groin about strangulated hernia; closure fecal fistula by lateral anastomosis of bowel.

Result unknown.

| Date. | Catalase. 15″ | 30″ | 45″ | 60″ | W. B. C. | Remarks. |
|---|---|---|---|---|---|---|
| 10/24 .......... | 14. | 18.6 | 22.4 | 28.5 | 20,300 | Operation Oct. 22. |

Case 15.—*Patient.*—C. M., white girl, aged 12.

*Clinical Diagnosis.*—Osteomyelitis of spine; general septicemia; metastatic abscesses.

On September 5 the child was first seen; history indefinite; temperature 103 F.; pulse 110; W. B. C. 32,000.

Operation: Exploratory laparotomy for peritonitis (probably either rupture of appendix or typhoid perforation. The peritoneum was found clean at operation.

On September 6 the back was found edematous. An incision was made; pus and dead bone were found in the lumbar spine.

Death. No autopsy.

| Date. | Catalase. 15″ | 30″ | 45″ | 60″ |
|---|---|---|---|---|
| 9/5 .......... | 14.8 | 18.2 | 23. | 27.2 |

While the above results are only suggestive, it seems that so simple a test as the one employed to determine the catalytic activity of the blood might be of value in the diagnosis of peritonitis whether from appendix rupture or typhoid perforation, etc., and further in the differentiation of these cases from obscure general infections which have not localized themselves in a serous cavity.

### *B. Diabetes Mellitus*

Case 16.—*Patient.*—F., white woman, aged 48. Medical No. 24,239.

Clinical Diagnosis: Diabetes mellitus; ulcer of toe.

Improvement.

Urine: Amount 490 to 1,528 c.c. Albumin trace. Sugar 1.6 to 2.4 per cent.

No coma.

Case 17.—*Patient.*—T., white man, aged 33. Medical No. 22,987.

*Clinical Diagnosis.*—Diabetes mellitus.

Improvement.

Urine: Albumin trace. Sugar 2, 6 and 6.1 per cent.

No coma.

Case 18.—*Patient.*—D., white man, aged 17. Medical No. 23,645.

*Clinical Diagnosis.*—Diabetes mellitus. Result improved.

Urine: Albumin, negative. Sugar 8 per cent. to none; on discharge 2 per cent. Diacetic acid and acetone constantly present.

TABLE 10.—CATALYTIC ACTIVITY IN DIABETES MELLITUS

| No. | Date. | Catalase. 15″ | 30″ | 45″ | 60″ | R. B. C. | Hb. % | |
|---|---|---|---|---|---|---|---|---|
| 1 | 10/18 .... | 16.7 | 23.5 | 28. | 32. | 4,886,000 | 83 | Sahli. |
| 2 | 1/16 .... | 15.8 | 20.6 | 25.2 | 29.8 | 3,832,000 | 79 | Sahli. |
| 3 | 1/25 .... | 14.4 | 17.8 | 20. | 22.2 | 5,764,000 | 90 | Urine sugar-free. Acetone plus. |

These three cases of diabetes suffice to show that it exerts no influence on the catalytic activity of the blood. This is in harmony with the results of the determination of the catalytic activity of the organs in a fatal case of diabetes (Winternitz and Meloy). It must be remembered, however, that none of these patients were in coma and that possibly the acidosis accompanying diabetic coma might affect the power of the blood to split hydrogen peroxid.

### C. *Catarrhal Jaundice*

CASE 19.—*Patient.*—J. T., white man, aged 41. Medical No. 65,924.

*Clinical Diagnosis.*—Catarrhal jaundice.

Patient had been jaundiced so long that operation was advised. He died from hemorrhage after operation. At autopsy only catarrhal inflammation of bile-ducts and extensive jaundice were found.

| Catalase. 15″ | 30″ | 45″ | 60″ |
|---|---|---|---|
| 14.8 | 18.2 | 23. | 27.2 |

The above case of catarrhal jaundice needs no further comment. Suffice it to say with severe jaundice and bile in the urine, etc., there was in this case no change in the catalase of the blood. This confirms the previous observation where there was no reduction in jaundiced tissues obtained from a fatal case of obstructive jaundice (Winternitz and Meloy).

### D. *Exophthalmic Goiter*

CASE 20.—*Patient.*—C., white woman, aged 26. Medical No. 23179.

*Clinical Diagnosis.*—Exophthalmic goiter; hypertrophy of thymus.

Improvement.

Urine negative.

TABLE 11.—CATALYTIC ACTIVITY IN EXOPHTHALMIC GOITER (CASE 10)

| Date. | Catalase. 15″ | 30″ | 45″ | 60″ | R. B. C. | Hb. % |
|---|---|---|---|---|---|---|
| 10/ 7 ........ | 19. | 25.2 | 31.4 | 37.2 | ........ | 85 |
| 10/18 ........ | 16.2 | 21.2 | 26.4 | 31.4 | ........ | .. |
| 10/19 ........ | 17.1 | 22.4 | 28. | 33.1 | ........ | .. |
| 10/21 ........ | 16.5 | 21.1 | 26.8 | 31.6 | 4640000 | 87 |
| 10/26 ........ | 18.6 | 22.4 | 27.7 | 31.6 | ........ | .. |

CASE 21.—*Patient.*—A. M. A., white woman, aged 41. Medical No. 23798.

*Clinical Diagnosis.*—Exophthalmic goiter. Tuberculosis of thyroid; myocarditis.

Urine: Specific gravity 1.004 to 1.022. Amount from 800 to 1,620 c.c. Albumin, trace; casts few. Slight edema of ankles. Blood-pressure from 82 to 130.

*Operation.*—January 9, ligation of right superior thyroid artery. January 23, partial thyroidectomy. Left lobe and isthmus.

Death.

*Pathologic Report.*—Advanced hypertrophy with disappearance of colloid. The epithelium of the alveoli is high and shows many invaginations. Diffuse increase in interstitial tissue containing nests of lymphoid cells. In another section a number of tubercles are found.

TABLE 12.—CATALYTIC ACTIVITY IN EXOPHTHALMIC GOITER (CASE 21)

| | Catalase | | | | | | |
|---|---|---|---|---|---|---|---|
| Date. | 15″ | 30″ | 45″ | 60″ | R.B.C. | Hb. % | |
| 1/12 ............ | 14. | 17. | 19.4 | 21.9 | ....... | .. | .... |
| 1/14 ............ | 18.8 | 23.8 | 27.6 | 31. | ....... | .. | .... |
| 1/18 ............ | 17.4 | 20.8 | 23.3 | 25.7 | ....... | .. | .... |
| 3/ 5 ............ | 16.4 | 20.4 | 23.6 | 26.4 | 5424000 | 94 | Sahli |
| 3/ 9 ............ | 18.6 | 23. | 26. | 29.4 | ....... | .. | .... |
| 3/15 ............ | 16.4 | 20.4 | 23.4 | 26.4 | ....... | .. | .... |

CASE 22.—*Patient.*—L. S., white woman, aged 36. Medical No. 24059.

*Clinical Diagnosis.*—Exophthalmic goiter.

*Operation.*—Partial thyroidectomy (right lobe removed).

Improvement.

*Pathological Report.*—Alveoli irregular, lined by invaginated columnar epithelium. Diminution in colloid. Increase in stroma.

| | Catalase | | | | | | |
|---|---|---|---|---|---|---|---|
| Date | 15″ | 30″ | 45″ | 60″ | R.B.C. | Hb. % | Remarks |
| 1/16 .... | 15.7 | 21.2 | 25.8 | 30.4 | 4840000 | 76 | Operation Jan. 5 (11 days before) |

CASE 23.—*Patient.*—W., white woman, aged 30. Medical No. 23227.

*Clinical Diagnosis.*—Exophthalmic goiter; dysthyreosis; pregnancy.

Patient treated with Rogers and Beebe's serum.

Urine: Acetone and diacetic acid present.

Improvement.

TABLE 13.—CATALYTIC ACTIVITY IN EXOPHTHALMIC GOITER (CASE 22)

| | Catalase | | | | | | |
|---|---|---|---|---|---|---|---|
| Date | 15″ | 30″ | 45″ | 60″ | R.B.C. | Hb. % | Remarks |
| 10/16 .. | 11.9 | 15.5 | 18.8 | 21.9 | 3304000 | 64 | Patient vomiting $NH_3$ in urine 14.6 per cent. of N. |
| 10/17 .. | 13. | 17.8 | 21.4 | 25. | ....... | .. | $NH_3$ in urine 10% of N. Sodium bicarbonate 45 gr. by mouth. Calcium lactate 10 gr. by mouth. |
| 10/18 .. | 12.4 | 16.5 | 20.1 | 23.6 | ....... | .. | Calcium lactate discontinued. Urine neutral to litmus. No acetone or diacetic in urine. |
| 10/19 .. | 12.8 | 17.5 | 20.6 | 24. | ....... | .. | ............ |
| 10/21 .. | 10.2 | 13.7 | 16.8 | 19.2 | ....... | .. | Urine alkaline to litmus. |
| 10/22 .. | 11.6 | 15.2 | 18.4 | 21. | ....... | .. | Urine alkaline to litmus. |
| 10/24 .. | 12. | 15.3 | 18.2 | 21.6 | ....... | .. | Urine neutral. |
| 10/25 .. | 11. | 14. | 17. | 19.7 | ....... | .. | ............ |
| 10/27 .. | 12.4 | 15.2 | 18. | 20.8 | 4720000 | 76 | (Dec. 12.) |

The above cases of thyroid disease are of interest. It will be remembered that in determining the catalytic activity of a single normal individual's blood over a long period of time practically no variation was found from day to day. In the above cases this is certainly not true. The variations are very marked. In several cases (1 and 2) the activity tends toward a high level while in Case 4 it is low. In the first two cases there were definite symptoms of hyperthyreosis while the fourth case was more obscure, being accompanied by symptoms of hypo- as well as hyperthyreosis. These findings can be readily interpreted from the experiments previously reported (Winternitz and Pratt). There it was shown that a permanent decline in the catalytic activity of the blood followed the extirpation of the thyroid gland in rabbits and that this fall could be compensated by feeding thyroid extract. With excessive function of the gland, therefore, an increased action on the part of the blood to split hydrogen peroxid can naturally be expected. And with a decreased function, a decreased catalytic activity of the blood should be expected. Case 4, therefore, would fall in the group of hypothyreosis.

### *E. Renal, Cardiac and Cardiorenal Diseases*

In this group several types of cases will be considered; first the cases of pure nephritis, then the pure cardiac cases, and finally a number of cases in which both the heart and kidneys are clinically insufficient and in which it is more difficult to determine which is the primary cause of the disease.

The cases of chronic nephritis will be arbitrarily divided. In the first division are included a number of chronic nephritics in whom, although the disease was evident, there were no clinical symptoms pointing to uremia.

CHRONIC NEPHRITIS

CASE 23.—*Patient.*—D., white man, aged 21. Medical No. 24219.

*Clinical Diagnosis.*—Chronic nephritis. Improved.

Urine: Total amount, 940-1000 c.c.; specific gravity 1007-1015; albumin, trace to 0.5 gm. per liter. Casts very few, hyaline and granular.

No edema, coma or convulsions. Blood-pressure 230-120.

| | Catalase | | | | | | |
|---|---|---|---|---|---|---|---|
| Date | 15″ | 30″ | 45″ | 60″ | R.B.C. | Hb. % | Remarks |
| 1/10 .. | 16.4 | 21.2 | 25. | 28.6 | 5800000 | 81 | Headache and vomiting on Jan. 8. Patient feels well at present. |

CASE 24.—*Patient.*—F., white girl, aged 18. Medical No. 24411.

*Clinical Diagnosis.*—Chronic nephritis.

Urine: Total amount 460-1130 c.c.; specific gravity from 1009-1027; albumin faint trace; casts, hyaline, granular and cellular.

Edema of feet for two years. Face puffy.

Eye-grounds negative. Blood-pressure from 112 to 115. No coma, convulsions in October, 1908.

Improvement.

| Date | Catalase 15″ | 30″ | 45″ | 60″ | R.B.C. | Hb. % |
|---|---|---|---|---|---|---|
| 7/29 | 15. | 20. | 25.4 | 29.8 | 5744000 | 100 |

Case 25.—*Patient.*—B., white man, aged 48. Medical No. 23582. Patient drowsy on admission. No coma or convulsions.

*Clinical Diagnosis.*—Chronic nephritis.

Urine: Total amount from 300 to 1780 c.c. Specific gravity from 1012 to 1032. Albumin trace. Casts few, hyaline and finely granular.

Improvement.

| Date | Catalase 15″ | 30″ | 45″ | 60″ | R.B.C. | Hb. % |
|---|---|---|---|---|---|---|
| 1/18 | 18.8 | 22.8 | 25.6 | 28.6 | 5100000 | 85 |

Case 26.—*Patient.*—S., colored woman, aged 45. Medical No. 23292.

*Clinical Diagnosis.*—Chronic nephritis. Tertiary syphilis.

Urine: Total amount 480-1450 c.c.; specific gravity from 1009 to 1019; albumin trace; casts occasional, granular.

No coma or convulsions. Blood-pressure from 204 to 110.

Improvement.

| Date | Catalase 15″ | 30″ | 45″ | 60″ | R.B.C. |
|---|---|---|---|---|---|
| 11/7 | 14.1 | 17.4 | 19. | 22.7 | 5220000 |

A glance at the above four cases suffices to show that here, even with outspoken nephritis, there may be no change in the catalytic activity of the blood.

The next group includes still more severe cases in which there were symptoms of uremia with edema, nausea, vomiting and more severe exacerbations which, however, never developed coma.

### CHRONIC NEPHRITIS WITH SLIGHT SYMPTOMS OF RENAL INSUFFICIENCY

Case 27.—*Patient.*—K., white woman, aged 42. Medical No. 23263.

*Clinical Diagnosis.*—Chronic nephritis; acute exacerbation.

Urine: Total amount 600-3300 c.c.; specific gravity 1005-1022; albumin from 1.5 to 4 gm. per liter. Casts hyaline, granular and cellular.

Edema and headache, vomiting. No coma. Blood-pressure from 157 to 172 mm. Hg.

Table 14.—Catalytic Activity in Chronic Nephritis (Case 27)

| Date | Catalase 15″ | 30″ | 45″ | 60″ | R.B.C. | Hg. % | Remarks |
|---|---|---|---|---|---|---|---|
| 10/22 | 13. | 16.5 | 19.8 | 23. | 4600000 | 90 | ............ |
| 10/24 | 12.4 | 16. | 19.5 | 22.8 | ....... | .. | ............ |
| 10/26 | 15.8 | 19.8 | 23.4 | 26.8 | ....... | .. | Patient much improved. |
| 10/27 | 16. | 20. | 24. | 27. | ....... | .. | ............ |
| 10/29 | 16.6 | 20.6 | 21.7 | 28.8 | 4136000 | 92 | ............ |

Case 28.—*Patient.*—G., white man, aged 57. Medical No. 23230.

*Clinical Diagnosis.*—Chronic nephritis; ascites.

Urine: Total amount 500-1600 c.c., specific gravity 1006-1015; albumin, trace to 1.5 gm. per liter. Casts few hyaline and granular. Edema and ascites present. Blood-pressure from 160 to 184.

No coma or convulsions.

Heart enlarged with systolic murmur and slight presystolic. Considered clinically to be a case of primary renal disease with secondary cardiac change, i. e., dilatation and hypertrophy.

Improvement.

TABLE 15.—CATALYTIC ACTIVITY IN CHRONIC NEPHRITIS (CASE 28)

| | Catalase | | | | | | |
|---|---|---|---|---|---|---|---|
| Date | 15″ | 30″ | 45″ | 60″ | R.B.C. | Hb. % | |
| 10/ 6 .. | 12.7 | 17. | 20.8 | 24.5 | 4472000 | 66 | ........ |
| 10/18 .. | 13.8 | 18.2 | 22.6 | 26.4 | ....... | .. | ........ |
| 10/19 .. | 14.5 | 19.6 | 24. | 28.8 | ....... | .. | ........ |
| 10/24 .. | 12.5 | 15.3 | 19.6 | 22.8 | 4128000 | 66 | (Oct. 26) |
| 10/29 .. | 14.5 | 18.3 | 21.1 | 23.2 | ....... | .. | ........ |
| 11/ 8 .. | 13. | 16. | 18.6 | 23.2 | 4280000 | 70 | ........ |

CASE 29.—*Patient.*—R., white man, aged 64. Medical No. 23316.

*Clinical Diagnosis.*—Chronic nephritis; myocarditis; dilatation of aortic arch.

Urine: Total amount 550-2000 c.c.; specific gravity 1013-1017; albumin trace; casts hyaline.

Edema of feet. Hydrothorax. Dyspnea; polyuria. No coma, vomiting, headache or convulsions. Blood-pressure from 213 to 244.

Improvement.

TABLE 16.—CATALYTIC ACTIVITY IN CHRONIC NEPHRITIS (CASE 29)

| | Catalase | | | | | | |
|---|---|---|---|---|---|---|---|
| Date | 15″ | 30″ | 45″ | 60″ | R.B.C. | Hb. % | |
| 11/ 6 .. | 9.9 | 12. | 13.7 | 15.4 | 3496000 | 64 | .................. |
| 11/ 8 .. | 9.9 | 12.2 | 14. | 15.8 | 3620000 | 62 | Blood pressure 244 mm. Hg. |

CASE 30.—*Patient.*—S., white man, aged 35. Medical No. 23108.

*Clinical Diagnosis.*—Chronic nephritis; pleurisy and pericarditis (acute).

Urine: Total amount 125-2550 c.c.; specific gravity 1010-1022; albumin from 5.5 to 15 gm. per liter; casts granular and hyaline.

Marked edema of dependent parts and ascites, headache and vomiting. No coma or convulsions.

Death. No autopsy.

TABLE 17.—CATALYTIC ACTIVITY IN CHRONIC NEPHRITIS (CASE 30)

| | | Catalase | | | | | | | |
|---|---|---|---|---|---|---|---|---|---|
| Date | Hr. | 15″ | 30″ | 45″ | 60″ | R.B.C. | Hb. % | W.B.C. | Remarks |
| 10/12 | ...... | .... | .... | .... | .... | 5336000 | 75 | 19400 | .................. |
| 10/16 | ...... | 12.6 | 17. | 20.6 | 25. | ....... | .. | ..... | .................. |
| 10/17 | ...... | 12. | 16. | 19.6 | 23. | ....... | .. | ..... | Urine alb. 6 gm. per liter. R.B.C., etc. Pericarditis. |
| 10/18 | ...... | 12. | 15.5 | 19. | 22. | ....... | .. | ..... | .................. |
| 10/19 | 4 p.m. | 13. | 18.4 | 22.2 | 24.9 | ....... | .. | ..... | .................. |
| 10/19 | 10 p.m. | 11.5 | 15.4 | 18.6 | 21.8 | 4088000 | .. | 31760 | Headache and vomiting. |
| 10/20 | ...... | 11.4 | 15. | 19.4 | 21.4 | ....... | .. | ..... | .................. |

CASE 31.—*Patient.*—C., white woman,[17] aged 22. Medical No. 23539.

*Clinical Diagnosis.*—Chronic nephritis (uremia) acute fibrinous pleurisy; exophthalmos.

Urine: Total amount 150-3200 c.c.; specific gravity 1005-1027; albumin from 1 to 8 gm.; casts.

Edema of face. Coma, several attacks, convulsions.

Blood-pressure 244-152 mm. Hg.

Patient had several attacks of uremia, coma while in hospital with gradual increasing blindness. Unimproved on discharge.

TABLE 18.—CATALYTIC ACTIVITY IN CHRONIC NEPHRITIS (CASE 31)

| | Catalase | | | | | | | |
|---|---|---|---|---|---|---|---|---|
| Date | 15″ | 30″ | 45″ | 60″ | W.B.C. | R.B.C. | Hb.% | Remarks |
| 1/12 .. | 12.1 | 14.3 | 16.4 | 18. | 13300 | 5400000 | 90 | (Jan. 2) |
| 1/14 .. | 11.5 | 13.8 | 15.4 | 16.8 | ..... | ....... | .. | ...... |
| 1/18 .. | 10.5 | 12.1 | 13.5 | 14.8 | ..... | ....... | .. | ...... |
| 2/10 .. | 12.4 | 15. | 17.3 | 19. | 35760 | 4176000 | 76 | ...... |
| | Condition improved. Headache, vomiting, coma. | | | | | | | |
| 3/ 5 .. | 11.4 | 13.6 | 16.4 | 18. | 8040 | 5336000 | 73 | ...... |
| 3/15 .. | 11.2 | 13.4 | 15.2 | 16.8 | 12880 | 5160000 | 80 | ...... |
| | Headache, convulsions. | | | | | | | |
| 3/20 .. | 10.8 | 13.4 | 15.5 | 17.2 | 7400 | 3976000 | 70 | ...... |

This group of five cases illustrates several facts. First, the curve of the catalytic activity of the blood is not constant from day to day; secondly, the activity is definitely decreased and tends to assume a lower level; and thirdly, the lowest activity is always obtained when the symptoms of renal insufficiency, headache, nausea, vomiting, etc., are most manifest. These findings correspond in every respect to the results obtained by producing chronic nephritis in rabbits with uranium nitrate (Winternitz). The power of the blood to split hydrogen peroxid becomes inconstant from day to day, but gradually assumes a lower level so that it may be only half as great as normal. With the decline in the catalase there is a fatal termination of the disease, even though the urinary picture and blood-pressure may be unchanged.

The next group of five cases illustrates the most severe type of disturbed renal function accompanied by definite uremic coma.

### CHRONIC NEPHRITIS WITH UREMIA

CASE 32.—*Patient.*—Y., white woman, aged 58. Medical No. 23633.

*Clinical Diagnosis.*—Acute mercurial poisoning.

Patient took bichlorid tablets with suicidal intent. Did not disclose fact till just before death. Mercury recovered from organs at autopsy.

Urine: Complete anuria.

Blood-pressure 132 mm. Hg.

---

17. This case should not be included in this group strictly, since the patient had been comatose during her stay in the ward. Unfortunately no reading was obtained during the time of coma and therefore the report is given with this group.

*Anatomic Diagnosis.*—Acute diphtheritic and ulcerative esophagitis, etc. Swelling and extensive necrosis of renal epithelium; edema of lungs; early bronchopneumonia.

| | Catalase | | | | | |
|---|---|---|---|---|---|---|
| Date | 15″ | 30″ | 45″ | 60″ | R.B.C. | Hb. % |
| 1/25 ........ | 10. | 13. | 16.2 | 18.8 | 4884000 | 92 |

This case represents the prototype of renal insufficiency in animals following a single injection of uranium nitrate (Winternitz). In both instances the disease is acute, ending fatally within a few days. The lesions in the kidney are identical, extreme necrosis of renal epithelium, causing complete anuria. The decline in the catalase is marked and needs no further comment.

CASE 33.—*Patient.*—McK., white man, aged 49. General No. 69412.

*Clinical Diagnosis.*—Chronic nephritis (uremia).

Urine: Total amount not learned. Specific gravity 1015-1020; albumin 3.5 gm. per liter; casts, many hyaline and granular.

Edema and coma. Headache, nausea, vomiting. Eyes, disks hazy. Heart enlarged but sounds clear. Blood-pressure 190 mm. Hg.

Patient improved.

TABLE 19.—CATALYTIC ACTIVITY IN CHRONIC NEPHRITIS WITH UREMIA (CASE 33)

| | Catalase | | | | | | |
|---|---|---|---|---|---|---|---|
| Date | 15″ | 30″ | 45″ | 60″ | R.B.C. | B.-P. | Remarks |
| 8/21 .. | 12.6 | 17. | 21. | 24.4 | ....... | 215-232 | Headache, nausea, vomiting, irrational. |
| 8/22 .. | 11.6 | 14.8 | 17.4 | 20. | 440000 | 190 | Comatose (venesection). |
| 8/23 .. | 10.4 | 13. | 15.8 | 18. | 3808000 | ... | Kidneys and skin reacting. |
| 8/24 .. | 10.2 | 13. | 16. | 18.6 | 3384000 | ... | Voiding, rational, still nauseated. |
| 8/26 .. | 12.4 | 15.2 | 18.4 | 21. | 4456000 | 170 | Much improved. |
| 8/29 .. | 13.6 | 17.2 | 21.4 | 25. | 4256000 | ... | Left hospital. |

Here again we find the same curve in the catalytic activity of the blood obtained in animal experiments. Accompanying the uremic coma there is a marked fall in the catalytic activity of the blood which, however, is not permanent but rises again with the improvement of the renal function.

CASE 34.—*Patient.*—M., white woman, aged 32. Medical No. 25160.

*Clinical Diagnosis.*—Chronic nephritis; uremia.

Urine: Total amount from 1600 to 20 c.c. Specific gravity from 1008 to 1012. Albumin trace to 225 gm. per liter. Casts few, granular.

Blood-pressure from 170 to 235 mm. Hg. Headache, nausea, vomiting. Dyspnea present. Eyes, disks swollen and edematous. Hemorrhages in fundi—exudation. Marked sclerosis of vessels of retina. Heart enlarged. Systolic blow follows sharp first sound. Coma. Edema of extremities and face.

Death. No autopsy.

TABLE 20.—CATALYTIC ACTIVITY IN CHRONIC NEPHRITIS WITH UREMIA (CASE 34)

| Date | Catalase 15″ | 30″ | 45″ | 60″ | R.B.C. | Hb. % | Remarks |
|---|---|---|---|---|---|---|---|
| 1/12 .. | 11. | 14.2 | 16.4 | 18. | 3752000 | 85 | Condition fair. |
| 2/ 3 .. | 10. | 13. | 15. | 17. | 3752000 | 88 | Nauseated, drowsy. |
| 2/11 .. | 9.6 | 12. | 14. | 15. | 3984000 | 92 | Coma, convulsions. |
| 2/13 .. | 8.2 | 10. | 11.6 | 13. | ? | ? | Coma, convulsions. |

CASE 36.—*Patient.*—Y., colored woman, aged 43.

*Clinical Diagnosis.*—Chronic nephritis; uremia.

Urine: Total amount and specific gravity not ascertained. Albumin; casts many hyaline and granular.

Edema, ascites, headache, exophthalmos, coma, etc., present.

*Anatomic Diagnosis.*—Acute and chronic diffuse nephritis; concentric hypertrophy of heart; general anasarca; bronchopneumonia (slight), etc.

TABLE 21.—CATALYTIC ACTIVITY IN CHRONIC NEPHRITIS WITH UREMIA (CASE 35)

| Date | Hr. | Catalase 15″ | 30″ | 45″ | 60″ | R.B.C. | Remarks |
|---|---|---|---|---|---|---|---|
| 8/26 | 17 m. .. | 9.6 | 13.4 | 16.6 | 19.4 | 4888000 | Comatose, Venesection 1 p. m. |
| 8/26 | 3 p. m. .. | 10.2 | 13.4 | 16.4 | 19.4 | 4344000 | ............... |

These two cases need no comment. The low activity corresponds in every respect to the low activity in the other cases of uremic coma.

CASE 36.—*Patient.*—K., white woman, aged 18. Medical No. 23039.

*Clinical Diagnosis.*—Chronic nephritis; purpura; pericarditis with effusion.

Urine: Total amount from 350 to 2440 c.c. Specific gravity from 1008 to 1026. Albumin 2.5 gm. per liter. Casts finely and coarsely granular.

Coma and edema, ascites, dyspnea; blood-pressure 80-144 mm. Hg.

Death November 14.

*Anatomic Diagnosis.*—Acute and chronic diffuse nephritis. Pleural and pericardial effusion; anemia with enlargement of spleen and liver; bronchopneumonia, etc.

TABLE 22.—CATALYTIC ACTIVITY IN CHRONIC NEPHRITIS WITH UREMIA (CASE 36)

| Date | Catalase 15″ | 30″ | 45″ | 60″ | R.B.C. | Hb. % | Remarks |
|---|---|---|---|---|---|---|---|
| 10/16 .. | 8.2 | 10.6 | 13. | 15.1 | 2632000 | 44 | .................. |
| 10/17 .. | 14.4 | 19. | 23.4 | 27. | ....... | .. | .................. |
| 10/18 .. | 15.2 | 20. | 24. | 28.6 | ....... | .. | .................. |
| 10/19 .. | 6.8 | 8.8 | 10.8 | 12.6 | ....... | .. | .................. |
| 10/24 .. | 7.6 | 9.7 | 13.6 | .... | 2888000 | 50 | Died Nov. 14. |

The marked rise in the activity in this case on the 17th and 18th deserves special comment. It was at this time that signs of pericarditis were most evident and possibly this could account for the increased catalytic activity of the blood (see under "Peritonitis").

CASE 37.—*Patient.*—N., white man, aged 45. Medical No. 23262.

*Clinical Diagnosis.*—Carcinoma of bladder; stricture of rectum; hydronephrosis; chronic nephritis.

Urine: Catheterized specimens. Albumin, heavy trace. Cellular casts.

Coma on admission continuing till death. Edema of ankles. Blood-pressure 106-186.

*Anatomic Diagnosis.*—Carcinoma of prostate with extension into rectum with stricture, into trigonum and near-by pelvic tissues; dilatation and hypertrophy of bladder; acute hemorrhagic cystitis; bilateral hydro-ureter and hydronephrosis. Chronic and acute diffuse nephritis (small white granular kidneys); cardiac dilatation and hypertrophy; edema of lungs and subcutaneous tissues; bronchopneumonia, not extensive, etc.

TABLE 23.—CATALYTIC ACTIVITY IN CHRONIC NEPHRITIS WITH UREMIA (CASE 37)

| | Catalase | | | | | | |
|---|---|---|---|---|---|---|---|
| Date | 15″ | 30″ | 45″ | 60″ | R.B.C. | Hb. % | Remarks |
| 10/22 .. | 5.8 | 8.2 | 10.3 | 13. | 2570000 | 45 | .................. |
| 10/23 .. | 4.8 | 6.6 | 8.2 | 9.8 | ....... | .. | .................. |
| .. | 4.8 | 7. | 8.4 | 9.8 | | | |
| 10/23 .. | 4.8 | 7. | 8.4 | 9.8 | ....... | .. | .................. |

Ten per cent. cloudy extract of kidney obtained at autopsy; 1 to 40 dilution.

It is with some hesitancy that this case is added to the series. As will be seen later, cancer in itself and the marked anemia are factors in reducing the power of the blood to split hydrogen peroxid. On the other hand, several observations were made on the patient during the last few days of life and a progressive decline in the catalytic activity of the blood was found. This, with the presence of a marked acute and chronic nephritis, has led us to include the case in this series.

OBSTRUCTION TO THE URINARY CANAL WITH SUPPRESSION OF URINE

CASE 38.—*Patient.*—B., white man, aged 74. Surgical No. 24325.

*Clinical Diagnosis.*—Cancer of bladder.

*Operation.*—Suprapubic cystostomy. Removal of right lateral wall of bladder. Transplantation of ureter.

Urine: No report. Coma.

Death. No autopsy.

TABLE 24.—CATALYTIC ACTIVITY IN URINARY OBSTRUCTION (CASE 38)

| | Catalase | | | | | | |
|---|---|---|---|---|---|---|---|
| Date | 15″ | 30″ | 45″ | 60″ | R.B.C. | Hb. % | Remarks |
| 7/ 3 .. | 6.2 | 7.5 | 9.4 | 11. | 2500000 | 40 | .................. |
| 7/ 6 .. | 5.6 | 7. | 8.4 | 9.5 | ....... | .. | Dull, almost comatose. |
| 7/20 .. | 6.6 | 8.5 | 10.6 | 12.2 | ....... | .. | Improved enough to be taken home. Died several days later. |

CASE 39.—*Patient.*—F., white man, aged 42. Surgical No. 24447.

*Clinical Diagnosis.*—Carcinoma of bladder.

Urine: Not reported. Loss of weight, retention of urine and coma, +.

Death.

Operation: Drainage of right kidney.

*Anatomic Diagnosis.*—Squamous-celled cancer of bladder; occlusion of ureteral orifices; bilateral pyonephrosis.

Metastases to left kidney, etc.

TABLE 25.—CATALYTIC ACTIVITY IN URINARY OBSTRUCTION (CASE 39)

| | Catalase | | | | | |
|---|---|---|---|---|---|---|
| Date | 15″ | 30″ | 45″ | 60″ | R.B.C. | Hb. % |
| 8/3 .......... | 7.8 | 10.8 | 13.7 | 15.8 | ....... | .. |
| 8/5 .......... | 6.8 | 10.2 | 12.4 | 14.6 | 1505000 | 30 |

These two cases illustrate how markedly the catalytic activity of the blood may be reduced over a long period of time. That the cancer and anemia took part in reducing this activity is without doubt and that these could not be the only factors becomes evident from the following cases:

Case 40.—*Patient.*—T., colored man, aged 66. Surgical No. 24471.

*Clinical Diagnosis.*—Prostatic hypertrophy.

Operation: Partial prostatectomy.

Death.

*Anatomic Diagnosis.*—Infection of perineal wound; encapsulated abscess in interior vesical space, acute purulent cystitis; bronchitis with edema and congestion of lungs; bronchopneumonia; chronic diffuse nephritis, etc.

Edema, coma present.

Urine: Specific gravity 1021. Albumin trace; casts hyaline and granular.

| | Catalase | | | | |
|---|---|---|---|---|---|
| Date | 15″ | 30″ | 45″ | 60″ | Remarks |
| 8/5 ..... | 6.2 | 8.4 | 10.8 | 12.6 | Operation in August |

Case 41.—*Patient.*—S., colored man, aged 52. Surgical No. 24342.

*Clinical Diagnosis.*—Gangrenous cystitis; pyonephrosis.

Operation: Urethrostomy for relief of impermeable stricture. Suprapubic drainage of bladder. Coma.

Urine: Pus, blood-cells, albumin in large quantities (++); casts granular and cellular.

Death.

*Anatomical Diagnosis.*—Acute and chronic cystitis with abscesses in bladder wall; purulent ureteritis; pyonephrosis extreme. Rupture of bladder with general purulent peritonitis, etc.

Table 26.—Catalytic Activity in Urinary Obstruction (Case 41)

| | Catalase | | | | | |
|---|---|---|---|---|---|---|
| Date | 15″ | 30″ | 45″ | 60″ | R.B.C. | Remarks |
| 6/26 .. | 9.4 | 12.6 | 15. | 17.6 | 2500000 | Operation, over a quart of pus evacuated from ureteral opening. |
| 6/27 .. | 10.6 | 14.8 | 17.4 | 20.4 | ....... | ......................... |
| 6/29 .. | 14.3 | 18. | 20.7 | 23.5 | ....... | Patient's condition excellent. Later developed perivesical abscess which was drained at a second operation. This led to peritonitis and a fatal termination. |

The last case is of particular interest. The patient entered the hospital comatose. The catalytic activity of his blood was low. Following drainage of the bladder and pyonephrotic kidneys the activity again assumed normal despite the anemia. There was therefore sufficient renal parenchyma left in the shell of tissue about the pyonephrotic sacs to maintain renal function, and a fatal termination was brought about later by an entirely different cause—rupture of prevesical abscess.

To summarize the changes in the catalytic activity of the blood accompanying disease of the kidney, it may be said that:

1. Despite the presence of a marked nephritis provided there are no symptoms of renal insufficiency, i. e., uremia, there will be no marked change in the catalytic activity of the blood.

2. Where there is a chronic nephritis accompanied by indefinite symptoms of renal insufficiency the catalytic activity of the blood will be irregular from day to day and will tend to assume a level lower than normal.

3. In acute mercurial nephritis there is a fall in the catalytic activity of the blood.

4. With uremic coma there is a marked fall in the catalytic activity of the blood, which is permanent if the coma ends fatally but which recovers should the coma disappear.

5. With retention of urine due to obstruction of the lower urinary tract there is a marked decline in the catalytic activity of the blood. This decline may persist for some time but, should the obstruction be removed, the catalase will again rise.

The changes in the red blood-cell count have not been followed sufficiently carefully in this series to make them of much value. Suffice it to say that there is as a rule some decrease in the number of red cells accompanying the fall in the catalase in uremic coma, but to what extent this will account for the decrease in the action of the enzyme cannot be stated. The retention of salts has been considered elsewhere (Winternitz and Rogers). Their importance depends on the following facts. Both in the test-tube and in the animal body they have the power not only of decreasing the catalytic activity of the blood temporarily, but if injected intravenously under the proper conditions can exhaust the compensating power of the tissues (which tend to keep the catalytic activity of the blood at a normal level). With the loss of the compensating action of the tissue, the power of the blood falls, the animal sinks into coma and dies.

The next group of cases will be considered preliminary to the group to follow, in which not only the cardiovascular system but the kidneys likewise are affected.

CASE 42.—*Patient.*—N., white woman, aged 22. Medical No. 24348 (24088).

*Clinical Diagnosis.*—Mitral and aortic insufficiency.

Urine: Amount 600-2200 c.c.; specific gravity 1009; albumin; casts, granular and cellular.

Edema of face and dependent parts. No coma or convulsions. Blood-pressure from 145 to 125 mm. Hg.

Improvement.

| | Catalase | | | | | |
|---|---|---|---|---|---|---|
| Date | 15″ | 30″ | 45″ | 60″ | R.B.C. | Hb. % |
| 7/10 ......... | 16.2 | 21.6 | 25.5 | 29.5 | 4960000 | 91 |

CASE 43.—*Patient.*—J. L. H., white man, aged 67. Medical No. 24428, etc.

*Clinical Diagnosis.*—Arteriosclerosis; myocarditis.

Urine: Specific gravity 1012-1025. Amount from 300 to 1390 c.c. Albumin; casts few granular.

Edema marked. Blood-pressure from 120 to 150. Delirium. No coma. Death.

*Anatomical Diagnosis.*—(Autopsy No. 3256.) Arteriosclerosis involving particularly the ascending aorta; hypertrophy and acute cardiac dilatation; chronic fibrous myocarditis; chronic passive congestion of the viscera; anasarca.

| | Catalase | | | | | |
|---|---|---|---|---|---|---|
| Date | 15″ | 30″ | 45″ | 60″ | R.B.C. | Hb. % |
| 6/10 ......... | 18.8 | 26.2 | 38. | 38. | ? | 87 |

CASE 44.—*Patient.*—J. A., white man, aged 43. Medical No. 24380.

*Clinical Diagnosis.*—Myocarditis.

Urine: Amount from 380 to 1210 c.c. Specific gravity 1011-1022. Albumin trace. Casts, hyaline and finely granular.

Edema of legs marked. Ascites; no coma; dyspnea marked. Blood-pressure 132 mm. Hg. Heart enlarged, etc.

Improvement.

| | Catalase | | | |
|---|---|---|---|---|
| Date | 15″ | 30″ | 45″ | 60″ |
| 7/20 .............. | 17.2 | .... | 28.8 | 34.2 |

CASE 45.—*Patient.*—K., colored girl, aged 15. Medical No. 24191.

*Clinical Diagnosis.*—Mitral stenosis and insufficiency; aortic insufficiency.

Urine: Amount 300-980 c.c.; specific gravity 1010-1015; albumin trace; casts coarsely granular.

Edema of legs, ascites. No coma.

Improvement.

| | Catalase | | | | | | |
|---|---|---|---|---|---|---|---|
| Date | 15″ | 30″ | 45″ | 60″ | R.B.C. | Hb. % | Remarks |
| 6/29 .. | 13. | 18.4 | 22.8 | 26.7 | 4756000 | 70 | (May 31) |

CASE 46.—*Patient.*—H., white man, aged 47. Medical No. 24262.

*Clinical Diagnosis.*—Mitral insufficiency; myocarditis; chronic nephritis; relative tricuspid insufficiency.

Urine: Total amount 2420 c.c. per day. Specific gravity 1015. Albumin trace, casts hyaline and granular.

Edema of feet, ascites. Dyspnea; vomiting. No coma. Heart enlarged. Gallop rhythm. Systolic murmur. Blood-pressure 130 mm. Hg.

Improvement.

| Catalase | | | |
|---|---|---|---|
| 15″ | 30″ | 45″ | 60″ |
| 13.2 | 18.2 | 22.8 | 26.1 |

CASE 47.—*Patient.*—B., colored man, aged 36. Medical No. 24354.

*Clinical Diagnosis.*—Myocarditis; mitral insufficiency; chronic nephritis.

Urine: Total amount 420-1660 c.c.; specific gravity 1005-1015; albumin, trace; casts, finely granular.

Edema, ascites, hydrothorax (left). No coma. Blood-pressure 32 mm. Hg.

Improvement.

| | Catalase | | | | | |
|---|---|---|---|---|---|---|
| Date | 15″ | 30″ | 45″ | 60″ | R.B.C. | Hb. % |
| 7/10 ......... | 15.5 | 21. | 24.6 | 28.5 | ? | 84 |

CASE 48.—*Patient.*—R., white woman, aged 56. Medical No. 24266.

*Clinical Diagnosis.*—Chronic nephritis; myocarditis.

Urine: Total amount from 690 to 3740 c.c. Specific gravity 1009-1025. Albumin.

Edema of legs, ascites and headache. No coma, convulsions or vomiting.
Blood-pressure 185-262 mm. Hg.
Improvement.

| Date | Catalase 15″ | 30″ | 45″ | 60″ | R.B.C. | Hb. % (June 19) | Remarks |
|---|---|---|---|---|---|---|---|
| 6/24 .. | 20.5 | 28. | 34. | 39.6 | 5150000 | 89 | Edema gone. |

This group can be dismissed rapidly. In severe cardiac disease there is no appreciable change in the catalytic activity of the blood and while the activity is slightly decreased in some this would hardly be sufficient even to suggest renal insufficiency when compared with the low readings in the group of renal diseases.

The next series, that of cases of cardiorenal disease, is of particular interest when compared with the following group. In all of these the kidney was considered clinically to be the seat of primary disease and the heart secondary. In all there were marked urinary changes, high blood-pressure and coma. In two of these, autopsies were obtained and the heart found to be primarily diseased with only secondary chronic congestive changes in the kidneys.

### CARDIORENAL DISEASE

CASE 49.—*Patient.*—D., white man, aged 53. Medical No. 24039.

*Clinical Diagnosis.*—Chronic nephritis; arteriosclerosis; myocarditis.

Urine: Total amount 470 to 2140 c.c. Specific gravity 1007-1026; albumin, trace; casts, numerous hyaline and granular with cells adherent.

Edema of ankles. No convulsions. Delirium and partial coma at times.

Blood-pressure from 205 to 145 mm. Hg. Cyanosis, dyspnea. Marked retinitis; choked disk, etc. Heart enlarged. Hydrothorax. Liver enlarged.

No improvement.

TABLE 27.—CATALYTIC ACTIVITY IN CARDIOVASCULAR DISEASE

| Date | Catalase 15″ | 30″ | 45″ | 60″ | Hb. % |
|---|---|---|---|---|---|
| 7/20 ............ | 16.6 | 22.7 | 27.7 | 32. | 75 |
| 8/21 ............ | 16.6 | 23. | 27.6 | 33. | .. |

CASE 50.—*Patient.*—T., colored woman, aged 50. Medical No. 23578.

*Clinical Diagnosis.*—Chronic nephritis (uremia); arteriosclerosis.

Urine: Amount 240-790 c.c.; specific gravity 1005-1023; albumin 0.25 gm.; casts, many hyaline and granular; red and white blood-cells.

General marked edema; ascites; coma; drowsy; vomiting. Blood-pressure 220-260 mm. Hg.

Death.

*Anatomic Diagnosis.*—Arteriosclerosis; chronic fibrous myocarditis; cardiac hypertrophy and dilatation (especially right ventricle). Chronic passive congestion of viscera; chronic diffuse nephritis (slight); obesity.

TABLE 28.—CATALYTIC ACTIVITY IN CARDIOVASCULAR DISEASE

| Date | Catalase 15″ | 30″ | 45″ | 60″ | R.B.C. | Hb. % |
|---|---|---|---|---|---|---|
| 6/14 ......... | 14. | 16.5 | 19.5 | 21.3 | 5192000 | 83 |
| 6/19 ......... | 13.4 | 16. | 17.1 | 20. | 4688000 | 80 |

CASE 51.—*Patient.*—D., white man, aged 69. Medical No. 24279.

*Clinical Diagnosis.*—Arteriosclerosis; myocarditis; mitral insufficiency.

Urine: Total amount 300-1780 c.c. Specific gravity 1015-1020; albumin; casts many hyaline and granular.

Edema of face and extremities, lungs. Coma? Patient drowsy but could be roused. Blood-pressure 180 mm. Hg. Heart enlarged. Gallop rhythm, loud systolic murmur.

Death.

Partial autopsy. Kidneys show typical chronic passive congestion.

| | Catalase | | | | | |
|---|---|---|---|---|---|---|
| Date | 15″ | 30″ | 45″ | 60″ | R.B.C. | Hb. % |
| 6/22 ......... | 16.6 | 22. | 25.2 | 28. | 4784000 | 95 |

These cases have been of particular interest since the constant normal activity of the catalase of the blood did not warrant a diagnosis of renal insufficiency despite the urinary findings, blood-pressure, and coma. The autopsy findings confirmed the results of the test during life.

One of the other conditions which sometimes may be difficult to differentiate from uremic coma is apoplexy. Two cases of coma complicating cerebral hemorrhage follow:

CASE 52.—*Patient.*—P., white man, aged 70. Medical No. 24489.

*Clinical Diagnosis.*—Cerebral hemorrhage; paralysis.

Urine: Albumin; casts hyaline, cells, pus.

Coma and Cheyne-Stokes respiration present. Blood-pressure 185 mm. Hg.

Improvement.

CASE 53.—R., colored man, aged 52. Medical No. 24237.

*Clinical Diagnosis.*—Arteriosclerosis; myocarditis; chronic nephritis. Apoplexy. Hemiplegia.

Urine: Total amount 660-1690 c.c.; specific gravity 1010-1025; albumin trace; casts, hyaline and granular; polyuria.

Heart enlarged, gallop rhythm. Blood-pressure 132-192 mm. Hg. Dyspnea.

Improvement.

TABLE 29.—CATALYTIC ACTIVITY IN CEREBRAL HEMORRHAGE

| No. | | Catalase | | | | | | |
|---|---|---|---|---|---|---|---|---|
| Case | Date | 15″ | 30″ | 45″ | 60″ | R.B.C. | Hb. % | Remarks |
| 52 .. | 6/16 | 17. | 23.2 | 29. | 34. | 6216000 | .. | Patient in coma. |
| 53 .. | 6/18 | 20. | 26.8 | 32.2 | 36. | ....... | 95 | Hemiplegia, coma |

In both of these cases of cerebral hemorrhage the catalytic activity of the blood is high, while the results are far too small to say there is an increased catalytic activity of the blood in apoplectic coma. One thing is clear: that there is no decrease and that in this respect a ready means offers itself for the differential diagnosis of the two conditions.

## *Toxemias of Pregnancy*

It will be remembered that in a previous paper (Winternitz and Meloy) the catalytic activity of the blood in cases of eclampsia was found to be normal. A number of cases of toxemia of pregnancy were studied in this series, but before the results of these observations were recorded

TABLE 30.—CATALYTIC ACTIVITY IN PREGNANCY

| Case | Obstetrical No. | Catalase 15″ | Catalase 30″ | Catalase 45″ | Catalase 60″ | R. B. C. | Age | Pregnancy | Time of Observation | Puerperium |
|---|---|---|---|---|---|---|---|---|---|---|
| 1 | 4211 | 14.6 | 18 | 20.6 | 23.2 | 4220000 | 22 | Second. | 1 day before delivery... | Normal. |
| 2 | 4280 | 16.2 | 19.8 | 22.6 | 24.8 | 4720000 | 18 | First. | 1 day before delivery... | Normal. |
| 3 | 4315 | 16 | 19 | 21.6 | 24 | 5240000 | 24 | Third. | 3 days before delivery.. | Normal. |
| 4 | 4320 | 14.6 | 17.8 | 20 | 22 | 4260000 | 16 | First. | 10 days before delivery. | Normal. |
| 5 | 4332 | 17 | 21 | 23.4 | 25.6 | 5040000 | 19 | First. | In labor, second stage.. | Normal. |
| 6 | 4281 | 14 | 17 | 19 | 21 | 4000000 | 21 | Second. | 20 days before delivery. | Normal. |
| 7 | 4307 | 16.6 | 21 | 23.4 | 25.8 | 4840000 | 15 | First. | 22 days before delivery. | Normal. |
| 8 | 4171 | 14.4 | 18.8 | 22.6 | 25.6 | 4280000 | 20 | First | 10 days before delivery. | Bartholinitis; conjunctivitis. |
| 9 | 4304 | 13.8 | 16.6 | 20.4 | 22.8 | 4200000 | 42 | Seventh | Just after delivery..... | Negative. |
| 10 | 4328 | 14.6 | 17.8 | 20 | 22 | 4560000 | 18 | First. | 2 hours after delivery.. | Negative. |

it seemed necessary to determine first whether there is any change in the catalytic power of the blood in pregnant women and, secondly, whether this power is influenced during labor.

The cases recorded in Table 30 will suffice to show that pregnancy has no appreciable effect on the power of the blood to split hydrogen peroxid. These cases were taken at varying intervals before, during and after labor, and it seemed of interest to determine whether the activity of the blood of a single individual was influenced by the course of pregnancy.

TABLE 31.—THE INFLUENCE OF LABOR AND CHILDBIRTH ON THE CATALYTIC ACTIVITY OF THE BLOOD OF A SINGLE INDIVIDUAL

| | | Catalase | | | | | |
|---|---|---|---|---|---|---|---|
| Date | Hr. | 15″ | 30″ | 45″ | 60″ | R.B.C. | Remarks |
| 2/ 9 | ..... .. | 14.6 | 18. | 20.6 | 23.2 | 4200000 | Patient walking about in perfect health. |
| 3/ 4 | ..... .. | 14.8 | 18. | 21. | 24. | 4358000 | Patient delivered March 5, 9:30 p. m. |
| 3/ 5 | 10:30 .. | 13.4 | 16.4 | 19. | 21.2 | 4184000 | Condition good. |
| 3/ 7 | ..... .. | 14.4 | 18.2 | 20.4 | 23.4 | 4096000 | Condition good |
| 3/17 | ..... .. | 14.6 | 18.4 | 21. | 23.6 | 4260000 | Discharged. |

Table 31 shows that there is a slight temporary decline in the catalytic activity of the blood just after delivery. This was confirmed repeatedly, though in some cases there was a slight rise in the activity of the blood after childbirth. These changes, however, are so small that they are negligible.

The consideration of the various toxemias of pregnancy and their relation to the catalytic activity of the blood will not be entered upon in detail. The cases to be reported are divided into two groups: first, those in which there was no change in the catalytic activity of the blood; secondly, those in which there was a decreased catalytic activity of the blood.

TOXEMIAS OF PREGNANCY IN WHICH THE FUNCTION OF THE KIDNEY IS NOT SUFFICIENTLY IMPAIRED TO INFLUENCE THE CATALYTIC ACTIVITY OF THE BLOOD

CASE 54.—*Patient.*—E. S., white woman, aged 32. Obstetrical No. 3879.

*Clinical Diagnosis.*—Eclampsia.

Delivery.

Urine: Total amount 6995-320 c.c.; specific gravity 1015; albumin 2 per cent; numerous hyaline and granular casts.

Blood-pressure 225 mm. Hg. Maximum coming down to normal. Convulsions, eight before delivery, five after. Coma present.

Recovery.

CASE 55.—*Patient.*—M. E. W., white woman, aged 32. Obstetrical No. 3876. This was the patient's fourth pregnancy. The last pregnancy normal though previously, following the second pregnancy, the patient had had a period of coma and convulsions lasting a number of days.

*Clinical Diagnosis.*—Chronic nephritis; uremia.

Urine: Total amount 4090-100 c.c.; specific gravity not ascertained; albumin 3 per cent. to 0.5 per cent.; numerous granular and hyaline casts; did not clear up completely.

The patient had ten convulsions during seven days after admission; then became normal. Coma for twenty-four hours. Blood-pressure 160 mm. Hg.

Improvement.

CASE 56.—*Patient.*—S., white woman, aged 21. Obstetrical No. 4173. This was the patient's second pregnancy. The first pregnancy had been normal.

*Clinical Diagnosis.*—Post-partum eclampsia.

Urine: Total amount 2700-1400 c.c.; specific gravity from 1015 to 1010; albumin 25 gm. per liter for first two weeks then disappeared; casts?

Convulsions, two following delivery. The patient was semi-comatose with headaches. Blood-pressure 170-100 mm. Hg.

Recovery.

CASE 57.—*Patient.*—J., white woman, aged 18. Obstetrical No. 4214. This was the patient's first labor.

*Clinical Diagnosis.*—Ante-partum eclampsia.

Convulsions began about seven hours before delivery, three in number, before delivery; but condition improved after delivery. Blood-pressure 190 mm. Hg, remaining high for nearly two weeks.

Urine: Amount 8500-2400 c.c.; specific gravity 1010-1012; albumin, trace; casts, numerous hyaline and granular casts on admission.

Recovery.

CASE 58.—*Patient.*—H., colored woman, aged 18. Obstetrical No. 4272. This was the patient's second pregnancy. The first was normal. The patient had edema of feet and headache for two weeks before admission; numerous general convulsions after delivery; nausea and vomiting; no coma.

*Clinical Diagnosis.*—Post-partum eclampsia.

Blood-pressure 165 mm. Hg at delivery, reaching 125 in four days.

Urine: Amount 3600-5250 c.c.; specific gravity 1012; albumin 2 per cent., disappearing in few days; casts negative.

Recovery.

CASE 59.—*Patient.*—D., white woman, aged 21. Obstetrical No. 4155. This was the patient's first pregnancy.

*Clinical Diagnosis.*—Intra-partum eclampsia.

The first convulsion occurred in the second stage of labor. Numerous general convulsions followed during operative delivery and until death. The patient was comatose. Blood-pressure 130 mm. Hg.

Urine: Amount 3730 c.c. ? c.c.; specific gravity 1018; albumin 1.5 gm. per liter; casts numerous, granular and hyaline.

Death.

*Anatomical Diagnosis.*—Peripheral necrosis of liver; cloudy swelling of viscera; acute splenic tumor; bronchopneumonia; edema of lungs, etc.

After death aqueous extracts were made of the liver, kidney and spleen in this case, and their power to split hydrogen peroxid was high. This is of interest compared with the low activity of organs from individuals dead of uremic coma (Winternitz and Meloy) and would of itself suggest that eclampsia may occur without any marked change in renal function.

TABLE 32.—CATALYTIC ACTIVITY OF ORGAN EXTRACTS FROM PATIENT DEAD OF ECLAMPSIA (CASE 59)

| | Catalase | | | | |
|---|---|---|---|---|---|
| No. | 15″ | 30″ | 45″ | 60″ | R.B.C. |
| 1. | 13. | 16. | 18.5 | 21.2 | ....... |
| 2. | 17.8 | 21.6 | 25.8 | 29.5 | ....... |
| 3. | 13.6 | 17.6 | 20.4 | 24. | ....... |
| 4. | 13.4 | 17.6 | 20.6 | 24. | 3832000 |
| 5. | 15. | 20. | 24. | 28. | 4320000 |
| 6. | 13. | 16. | 19. | 22. | ....... |

In all of these cases except the second (Case 55) a clinical diagnosis of eclampsia was made. In the sixth (Case 59) the post-mortem findings confirmed this clinical diagnosis. Case 55 deserves a moment's consideration. It concerned a woman in her fourth pregnancy. The second pregnancy was complicated by a period of toxemic coma, but the third pregnancy was normal. This fact alone would be of strong presumptive evidence in excluding a chronic nephritis for, with insufficient renal functions at one pregnancy, it would naturally be supposed that a succeeding pregnancy would bring about a similar condition. This was not true in this case, and only in the fourth pregnancy did a toxemia manifest itself. Had there been a renal insufficiency it is fair to assume that there would have been a marked fall in the catalytic activity of the blood such as is found in other types of renal insufficiency and in the following group of toxemias of pregnancy.

### TOXEMIAS OF PREGNANCY IN WHICH THE RENAL FUNCTION IS IMPAIRED SUFFICIENTLY TO CAUSE A FALL IN THE CATALYTIC ACTIVITY OF THE BLOOD

CASE 60.—*Patient.*—H., white woman, aged 29. Obstetrical No. 4225. This was the patient's first pregnancy. Albuminuria had been present during her early pregnancy, with marked increase in the seventh month, swelling of feet and face, and vomiting.

*Clinical Diagnosis.*—Toxemia.

Operative delivery, convulsions during labor. Blood-pressure (max. 240 mm. Hg) remained high for several days and only reached 160 mm. Hg one month later. Still later it again rose to 190 mm. Hg.

Urine: Total amount 150 c.c. on admission, later, large amounts; specific gravity 1045-1012. Albumin 35 gm. per liter on admission, decreasing to 4 gm. per liter. Casts, hyaline and granular.

TABLE 33.—CATALYTIC ACTIVITY IN TOXEMIA OF PREGNANCY (CASE 60)

| Date | Catalase 15″ | 30″ | 45″ | 60″ | |
|---|---|---|---|---|---|
| 12/16 ....... | 9.6 | 13. | 16. | 19. | On admission. |
| 12/20 ....... | 10.6 | 13.6 | 15.6 | 18. | .. .......... |
| 1/15 ....... | 12.2 | 15.4 | 17.8 | 20.2 | On discharge. |

CASE 61.—*Patient.*—C., white woman, aged 33. Obstetrical No. 4197. This was the fourth pregnancy, the first operative, the second and third normal. The patient had had two miscarriages. There had been continuous vomiting through present pregnancy; swelling of feet for several weeks, then general edema, dyspnea, frontal headache.

*Clinical Diagnosis.*—Pregnancy complicated by nephritis, toxemia.

The condition improved somewhat during the first week of residence in hospital when the pregnancy was terminated, Dec. 3.

Urine: Total amount 1600-4500 c.c.; specific gravity from 1010-1012; albumin, 1 gm. per liter; few hyaline and granular casts.

TABLE 34.—CATALYTIC ACTIVITY IN TOXEMIA OF PREGNANCY (CASE 61)

| Date | Catalase 15″ | 30″ | 45″ | 60″ | Remarks |
|---|---|---|---|---|---|
| 12/ 2 .. | 9.6 | 12.4 | 14.8 | 16.6 | Day before delivery |
| 12/17 .. | 12.8 | 16. | 18.4 | 20.2 | Condition improved |

CASE 62.—*Patient.*—S., white woman, aged 24. Obstetrical No. 4182. This was the patient's first pregnancy. Four days before admission the first convulsion occurred; before this headache, nausea and dimness of vision. General convulsions followed before delivery. Following delivery condition gradually improved.

*Clinical Diagnosis.*—Intrapartum eclampsia.

Urine: On admission 670 c.c.; specific gravity 1032; albumin 18 gm. per liter; many casts. Total amount, 5,000-6,000 c.c.; specific gravity 1010; albumin 0.2 gm. per liter. Occasional granular cast.

TABLE 35.—CATALYTIC ACTIVITY IN TOXEMIA OF PREGNANCY (CASE 62)

| | | Catalase | | | | | |
|---|---|---|---|---|---|---|---|
| Date | Hr. | 15″ | 30″ | 45″ | 60″ | R.B.C. | Remarks |
| 11/12 | ....... | 9. | 12. | 15. | 17.4 | 3120000 | Delivered at noon |
| 11/12 | 2 p.m. | 9.4 | 12.6 | 15. | 17.5 | ....... | Blood-pressure 160 mm. Hg. |
| 11/13 | ....... | 11. | 14.2 | 16.6 | 18.4 | ....... | Condition improved. |
| 11/14 | ....... | 10.4 | 13.4 | 16. | 16. | 3180000 | Condition improved. |
| 11/16 | ....... | 9.6 | 12. | 14.8 | 16. | ....... | Condition improved. |
| 11/18 | ....... | 10. | 12.4 | 15. | 16.4 | 3200000 | ....... ....... |
| 11/22 | ....... | 10.8 | 13.8 | 16. | 18. | 2984000 | Blood-pressure 130. Patient in bed. |
| 12/ 1 | ....... | 10.4 | 13.6 | 15.8 | 17.2 | ....... | Urine still contains albumin and casts. |

These three cases are distinct from the previous groups, inasmuch as they show a marked decrease in the catalytic activity of the blood. In two the activity became greater after delivery, while in the third the activity was still low on discharge. The urinary findings and blood-pressure likewise indicated marked renal disturbance.

It seems, therefore, that the toxemias of pregnancy can be differentiated into two groups by the determination of the catalytic activity of the blood.

1. Cases in which there is no change in the catalytic activity. These will include eclampsia without renal involvement.

2. Cases with decreased catalytic activity. These will include (a) chronic nephritis in which the excessive work thrown on the kidneys by the fetus will bring about renal insufficiency; and (b) eclampsia, etc., with marked renal involvement. The significance of this differentiation in the prognosis for future pregnancies is clear. In the first group future pregnancy may be normal. In the second it will most likely be complicated by a toxemia, the result of renal insufficiency.

### *Malignant Disease*

CASE 63.—*Patient.*—G., white man, aged 50. Medical No. 23524.

*Clinical Diagnosis.*—Sarcoma of liver.

Urine: Negative. Edema of extremities; slight jaundice.

Death.

*Anatomical Diagnosis.*—Alveolar sarcoma of liver with extensive metastases.

CASE 64.—*Patient.*—A. E., white man, aged 65. Surgical No. 29313.

*Clinical Diagnosis.*—Carcinoma of stomach confirmed by exploratory laparotomy.

Urine: Albumin, 0.75 gm. per liter.

Case 65.—*Patient.*—B. G., white man, aged 57. Medical No. 25329.

*Clinical Diagnosis.*—Carcinoma of stomach confirmed by exploratory laparotomy. Urine negative.

Table 36.—Catalytic Activity in Gastric Carcinoma (Cases 63, 64 and 65)

| No. | Catalase 15″ | 30″ | 45″ | 60″ | R.B.C. | Hb. % |
|---|---|---|---|---|---|---|
| 63 .......... | 9.8 | 11.4 | 14.6 | 15.5 | 4824000 | 77 |
| 64 .......... | 10. | 13. | 15. | 17. | 3688000 | 62 |
| 65 .......... | 10. | 14. | 17. | 20. | 4080000 | 70 |

In all three of these cases the disease was extensive though the anemia was moderate. In all three there was a decline in the catalytic activity of the blood which is apparently not in direct proportion to either the red blood-count or hemoglobin. It is evident therefore that with advanced malignant disease the power of the blood to split hydrogen peroxid is decreased. This is of importance in interpreting the two very low readings in cases of carcinoma of the bladder with retention of urine by partial occlusion of the ureters.

## *Diseases of the Hematopoietic System*

### SECONDARY ANEMIA

Case 66.—*Patient.*—J. L., white woman, aged 21. Medical No. 23736.

*Clinical Diagnosis.*—Gastric ulcer; hematemesis; melena.

Urine negative.

Recovery.

| Catalase 15″ | 30″ | 45″ | 60″ | R.B.C. | Hb. % |
|---|---|---|---|---|---|
| 8. | 9.6 | 10.6 | 11.7 | 1960000 | 35 |

### PERNICIOUS ANEMIA

Case 67.—*Patient.*—J., white man, aged 52. Medical No. 65564.

*Clinical Diagnosis.*—Pernicious anemia.

Urine negative. Blood-pressure 90-100 mm. Hg.

Improvement.

Table 37.—Catalytic Activity in Pernicious Anemia (Case 67)

| Date | Catalase 15″ | 30″ | 45″ | 60″ | R.B.C. | Hb.% |
|---|---|---|---|---|---|---|
| 10/17 ........ | 16. | 21. | 25. | 30. | 3200000 | 65 |
| 10/19 ........ | 14.6 | 19.2 | 23.4 | 27.6 | 3000000 | .. |
| 10/22 ........ | 13.2 | 17.2 | 20. | 22.7 | 3300000 | 66 |

### LEUKEMIA

Case 68.—*Patient.*—M. F., white man, aged 46. Medical No. 25142.

*Clinical Diagnosis.*—Lymphatic leukemia. Urine negative.

Case 69.—*Patient.*—S., white man, aged 31. Medical No. 24935.

*Clinical Diagnosis.*—Myeloid leukemia.

Urine negative.

Case 70.—*Patient.*—R., white man, aged 50. Medical No. 25430.

*Clinical Diagnosis.*—Myeloid leukemia.

Urine: Hyaline casts.

TABLE 38.—CATALYTIC ACTIVITY IN LEUKEMIA

| Case | Catalase 15″ | 30″ | 45″ | 60″ | R.B.C. | Hb. % | W.B.C. |
|---|---|---|---|---|---|---|---|
| 68 .... | 7. | 9. | 10.5 | 12. | 2041000 | 58 | 536000 |
| 69 .... | 3. | 3.5 | 4. | 4.8 | 840000 | 20 | 13200 |
| 70 .... | 11. | 14.4 | 17. | 22. | 2644000 | 48 | 600000 |

Differential Count:

| Case | P.M.N. % | L. M. % | L. Lym. % | S. Lym. % | Myel. % |
|---|---|---|---|---|---|
| 68 ........ | 2.6 | .6 | 4. | 92.6 | 0.6 |
| 69 ........ | 10. | 3. | 12. | 12. | 75. |
| 70 ........ | 57. | 2. | 4. | 4. | 38. |

These cases in themselves are too few to allow of any serious consideration. They only show that marked changes in the number of red blood-cells influence the catalytic activity of the blood while similar variations in the white blood-count are of no significance (compare leukemia Cases 1 and 6).

## *SUMMARY AND CONCLUSIONS*

### I. THE OXYGEN-CARRYING POWER OF THE BLOOD AND THE CATALASE OF THE BLOOD

The enumeration of the cellular elements of the blood and their hemoglobin content can be of only limited value in determining the oxygen-carrying power of the blood. The oxygen catalysts of the blood include oxidases, peroxidase, catalase and hemoglobin. Of these hemoglobin is the one which up to the present has received the widest attention. But it is needless to say that the time must come when the other oxygen-carriers will be investigated in relation to their changes in disease.

Aside from the fact that catalase has the power of decomposing hydrogen peroxid, little is known concerning the function of this enzyme. Its wide distribution throughout animal and plant kingdoms is responsible for its importance, and its intimate association with peroxidase seems to indicate that these two enzymes have a related function.

### II. THE CATALYTIC ACTIVITY AS A MEANS OF DIAGNOSIS

1. The literature on the diagnostic value of the determination of the catalase of the blood, while limited, is nevertheless suggestive. The complicated method of determination described by most authors possibly is responsible to some extent for its restricted application.

The study of the catalase of the blood in experimentally produced diseases of animals is confined to a few isolated observations. For this reason we have first interested ourselves in this direction. The results of this work are recorded elsewhere. Suffice it to say that these results form the nucleus of the clinical application of the test and they may be briefly summarized as follows:

**A.** The catalytic activity of human tissues is decreased in chronic nephritis and this reduction becomes more marked with the severity of the condition, the lowest readings being obtained from the tissues of individuals dead of uremia. In no other disease was a similar universal decrease in the power of the tissues to decompose hydrogen peroxid observed.

**B.** The catalytic activity of the blood of different rabbits varies within wide limits. This variation is not dependent on the red blood-count. On the other hand the catalytic activity of a single normal rabbit is constant from day to day over long periods of time.

**C.** The catalytic activity of rabbit's blood is reduced (1) after ligation of ureters; (2) after bilateral nephrectomy; (3) in uremic coma following uranium nitrate nephritis, etc. The tissues of these animals after death show a like reduction.

**D.** The catalytic activity of rabbit's blood is increased in early peritonitis, as is also the red blood-count. This change is, however, independent of the body temperature and white blood count.

**E.** The removal of the thyroid gland causes a drop in the catalytic activity of the blood which is compensated, however, if thyroid be fed.

**F.** Salts, acids, and alkalies inhibit the catalase of the blood when injected intravenously.

From the experiments outlined above it is evident that the power of the blood to split hydrogen peroxid is influenced by several factors: (1) the number of red blood-cells; (2) the thyroid gland; (3) the function of the kidney; and (4) the action of salts, acids, and alkalies.

2. The method adopted is as follows: Blood (0.025 c.c.) is removed from the lobe of the ear in a pipette. This is diluted in 10 c.c. of water. Five c.c. of this dilution suffices for a test. It is placed in a 100 c.c. bottle in which there is also a vial with 5 c.c. of neutral hydrogen peroxid. The large bottle is connected with a gas burette and the amount of oxygen liberated measured over a given period of time (fifteen seconds). The procedure requires only a few minutes, the error is slight and no precautions beyond ordinary room temperature and clean apparatus are necessary.

3. The catalytic activity of the blood of a series of normal individuals varies within physiological limits in 80 per cent. of the cases examined. In the other 20 per cent. the amount of oxygen liberated varied within wide limits. These variations are entirely independent of the number of red blood-cells and the hemoglobin. The nature of this variation is obscure. It is, however, of the utmost importance to bear this variation in mind when interpreting the activity of the blood in diseased conditions.

4. On the other hand, the catalytic activity of the blood of a single normal individual is constant from day to day over long periods of time and in this way a base-line can be obtained from which the significance of any change in the activity can be readily interpreted.

5. The catalytic activity of the blood in disease is a diagnostic factor to the extent indicated below:

A. Acute infectious diseases, including (1) typhoid fever, (2) diseases of the respiratory tract and (3) acute peritonitis presented the following variations:

1. In typhoid fever during the early days of illness there is no change in the catalytic activity of the blood, but toward the third week there is a gradual fall accompanying the anemia. During convalescence this activity as well as the red blood-count again becomes normal.

2. In diseases of the respiratory tract there is a slight decline in the catalytic activity of the blood during the course of lobar pneumonia. There is no marked variation in the power of the blood to split hydrogen peroxid except where the disease is accompanied by a severe anemia.

3. In four or five cases of acute peritonitis examined there was a characteristic rise in the catalytic activity of the blood. In one a reading had been made before the peritonitis occurred, while in the other three the increased activity was confirmed by the decline to normal following operation. In the one instance in which no rise was obtained the reading was only made twenty hours after operation. In two cases of suspected peritonitis with high fever and leukocytosis the catalytic activity of the blood was normal. In these cases the peritoneum was clean at operation.

B. Diabetes mellitus exerts no influence on the catalytic activity of the blood. The patients, however, were not in coma, and possibly the acidosis accompanying the coma might influence the catalase of the blood.

C. Catarrhal jaundice is likewise without effect.

D. In diseases of the thyroid gland, both hypothyreosis and hyperthyreosis, the catalytic activity of a single patient's blood is not constant from day to day. In hyperthyreosis the activity tends to increase, while in hypothyreosis the activity assumes a level lower than normal. This may be of significance in interpreting the condition of the thyroid gland where the signs and symptoms are atypical.

E. The group of renal cardiac and cardiorenal cases, like the group of acute infectious diseases, presents variations.

In the subgroup of renal disease there are also variations, as follows:

1. Despite the presence of a marked nephritis, provided there are no symptoms of renal insufficiency, i. e., uremia, there will be no marked change in the catalytic activity of the blood.

2. Where there is a chronic nephritis accompanied by indefinite symptoms of renal insufficiency the catalytic activity of the blood will be irregular from day to day and will tend to assume a level lower than normal.

3. In acute mercurial nephritis there is a fall in the catalytic activity of the blood.

4. With uremic coma there is a marked fall in the catalytic activity of the blood, which is permanent if the coma ends fatally but which recovers should the coma disappear.

5. With retention of urine due to obstruction of the lower urinary tract there is a marked decline in the catalytic activity of the blood. This decline may persist for some time, but should the obstruction be removed the catalase will again rise.

Even in severe cardiac disease there is no significant change in the catalytic activity of the blood. In some cases it is high. This may be normal for these individuals, as it will be remembered that some normal individuals have a high activity. In no single case was the activity sufficiently decreased, after many readings had been made, to suggest renal insufficiency.

In three cases of cardiorenal disease in which the clinical findings suggested a renal insufficiency, the catalytic activity of the blood was normal. At autopsy only a chronic passive congestion of the kidneys, the result of a decompensated heart was found.[18]

In two cases of cerebral hemorrhage the catalytic activity of the blood was high. Whether this is an increase over normal is not known but it is clear that the high reading would differentiate apoplectic coma from uremic coma.

F. Neither pregnancy nor labor as such has any appreciable effect on the catalytic activity of the blood. The toxemias of pregnancies accompanied by coma and convulsions can be differentiated into two groups by the determination of the catalytic activity of the blood.

1. Cases in which there is no change in the catalytic activity. These will include eclampsia without renal involvement.

2. Cases with decreased catalytic activity. These will include (a) chronic nephritis in which the excessive work thrown on the kidneys by the fetus will bring about renal insufficiency; and (b) eclampsia, etc., with marked renal involvement. The significance of this differentiation in the prognosis for future pregnancies is clear. In the first group future pregnancy may be normal. In the second it will most likely be complicated by a toxemia, the result of renal insufficiency.

G. In malignant disease (two cases of extensive carcinoma and one of sarcoma accompanied by a slight anemia) there was a decline in the catalytic activity of the blood. This did not vary with the anemia.

H. The cases of diseases of the hematopoietic system are too few to permit the drawing of any general conclusions. With marked anemia there is usually a fall in the catalytic activity though in the cases examined there is no direct relation between these two factors. Great variations in the white blood-cells in leukemias have no appreciable effect on the power of the blood to split hydrogen peroxid.

The interpretation of the above results has been almost entirely dependent on the preceding experimental work. Where this interpretation is unsatisfactory we can only suggest that it is from the incompleteness of the experimental studies.

In conclusion we wish to thank Drs. Barker, Thayer, Williams, Halsted and Kelly, who so kindly allowed us the privilege of the ward cases, and the members of the various staffs who have constantly informed us concerning the patients on whom it was desirable to have observations.

116 South Broadway.

---

18. Recently a fourth case has come under observation in which, though there were clinical signs of renal and cardiac insufficiency, it was difficult to decide which organ was causing the present symptoms. The catalase at first was high, 22 c.c. of oxygen being liberated in fifteen seconds. It was irregular from day to day, however, and toward the latter days of the patient's life fell so that three days before death only 16 c.c. of oxygen were liberated in the first fifteen seconds. At autopsy an acute hemorrhagic nephritis superimposed on a slight chronic nephritis was found. The heart was tremendously enlarged (weight 850 gm.) showed a chronic fibrous myocarditis and there was an extensive chronic passive congestion of the viscera. This case is particularly significant since, had the base-line not been obtained before the acute process with the renal insufficiency occurred, a reading of 16 c.c. might have been considered normal. As it was, the autopsy findings corroborate the clinical findings and the test. The patient probably suffered mostly from the cardiac condition at the time of the high reading, while with the onset of the acute nephritis there was a fall in the catalase of the blood.

# A STUDY OF THE INTERNAL FUNCTION OF THE PANCREAS IN CARBOHYDRATE METABOLISM *

JOSEPH H. PRATT, M.D., AND LESLEY H. SPOONER, M.D.
BOSTON

A recent study[1] showed that rapid atrophy and sclerosis of the entire pancreas was produced by tying the ducts and separating the pancreas from the duodenum. In a dog killed two months after the operation the gland was reduced to a small mass of dense fibrous tissue. On microscopic examination small areas of pancreatic acini were seen surrounded by connective tissue. Dr. Ordway, who made a careful histological study, failed to find any remains of the islands of Langerhans in the atrophied gland.

According to the theory most generally accepted the islands of Langerhans furnish an internal secretion to the blood that enables the organism to destroy sugar. The association of lesions of the islands and diabetes was observed by Opie[2] and Ssobolew[3] in 1900. Since that time many investigators have studied the nature and frequency of the pathological changes of these structures in diabetes, and definite lesions of the islands have been found in a large proportion of the cases. It is held that if the islands cease to furnish the internal secretion the sugar in the blood will not be consumed and diabetes will result.

In the observation cited above the dog did not develop diabetes in spite of the fact that the atrophy of the pancreas was extreme and the islands were destroyed. As our finding could not be explained by the island theory of diabetes, it was deemed important to inquire further into the effect of atrophy of the pancreas on carbohydrate metabolism. The limit of assimilation was determined in normal dogs and in animals in which atrophy of the pancreas had been produced.

---

*From the Laboratory of the Theory and Practice of Physic, Harvard University.

*Investigation made with the aid of a grant from the Proctor Fund for the Study of Chronic Diseases.

1. Pratt, Lamson, and Marks, Tr. Assn. Am. Phys., 1909, xxiv, 266.
2. Opie: Jour. Boston Soc. Med. Sc., 1900, iv, 251; Jour. Exper. Med., 1901, v, 397.
3. Ssobolew: Zentralbl. f. allg. Path. u. path. Anat., 1900, xi, 202.

## I. LIMIT OF ASSIMILATION FOR GLUCOSE IN NORMAL DOGS

F. Hoppe[4] fed dogs with large amounts of cane sugar up to 200 gm., but never detected a trace of sugar in the urine. Claude Bernard,[5] on the other hand, observed glycosuria after feeding dogs with smaller amounts of cane sugar (from 40 to 80 gm. per dog).

The first exact determinations of the limit of assimilation for carbohydrates in normal dogs were made by F. Hofmeister.[6] His figures are surprisingly low.

TABLE 1.—HOFMEISTER'S EXPERIMENTS

| Dog | Weight | Amt. Glucose which Produced Glycosuria | Limit of Assimilation | Per Kilo |
|---|---|---|---|---|
| ... | Gm. | Gm. | Gm. | Gm. |
| A | 2750 | 7.0 | 6 | 2.2 |
| B | 3400 | 10.0 | 8 | 2.4 |
| C | 1900 | 10.0 | 8 | 4.2 |
| F | 5400 | 16.2 | .. | less than 3.0 |
| G | 3850 | 5.0 | .. | less than 1.3 |

W. Schlesinger[7] found the limit of tolerance for glucose to be 10 to 11 gm. per kilogram of body weight. Boeri and De Andries[8] gave the limit as 4 to 6 gm. per kilo when the glucose was given to a fasting animal. There was a rise to 10 to 13 gm. when the sugar was fed with other food.

Quarta[9] asserts that the limit is much lower for male than female dogs. Tests made on four male dogs showed the average limit of tolerance to be 4.06 gm. per kilo while the average obtained in experiments on three female dogs was 10.28 gm. per kilo.

De Filippi[10] gave two dogs, each weighing 12,250 gm., after they had been fasting eighteen hours, 100 gm. of pure glucose dissolved in 500 gm. of water without other food. Neither dog developed glycosuria. When the dose was increased to 125 gm. the urine of one of the dogs remained free from sugar while the other showed within two hours a slight glycosuria. The limit of tolerance was more than 8.2 gm. per kilo for one dog, and more than 12.0 gm. for the other. De Filippi states that in an earlier investigation he gave to each of four normal dogs 100 gm. of glucose in the morning on a fasting stomach. None of the animals developed glycosuria.

4. Hoppe: Virchow's Arch. f. path. Anat., 1856, x, 144.
5. Bernard: Leçons sur le diabète, Paris, 1877, pp. 270, 320.
6. Hofmeister: Arch. f. exper. Path. u. Pharmacol., 1889, xxv, 240; xxvi, 355.
7. Schlesinger, W.: Wien klin. Wchnschr., 1902, xv, 768.
8. Boeri and De Andries: Policlinico, Medical Section, 1898, v, 477.
9. Quarta: Unpublished work quoted by De Filippi.
10. De Filippi: Ztschr. f. Biol., 1907, xlix, 511.

In Table 2 are given the results obtained by Pflüger.[11]

TABLE 2.—PFLÜGER'S EXPERIMENT

| Dog No. | Weight, Gm. | Amt. Glucose which Produced Glycosuria, Gm. | Limit of Assimilation, Gm. | Per Kilo Gm. |
|---|---|---|---|---|
| I | 11,900 | ... | more than 200 | more than 16.8 |
| II | 9,000 | ... | more than 100 | more than 11.1 |
| III | 11,700 | 225 | 200 | 17.1 |
| IV | 7,900 | ... | more than 100 | more than 12.6 |
| V | 13,000 | ... | more than 150 | more than 11.5 |

The first three dogs (I, II, III) in this series were animals from which the duodenum had been removed; the remaining two (IV, V) were normal. Pflüger was struck with the great variation between his results and those of Hofmeister. The latter investigator added the glucose to a thin meat soup, which was more rapidly absorbed when fed in this form than when given with chopped meat, which was the mode of administration adopted by Pflüger. In tests made on one animal Pflüger found that the limit of assimilation was lowered from "more than 11.5 gm." to "less than 8.0 gm." per kilo of dog weight when the sugar was given in soup instead of with hashed meat. It will be seen that Hofmeister's figures are much lower than those obtained by other investigators. No satisfactory explanation of this has been brought forward. It was certainly not due entirely to the fact that the sugar was given under conditions that favored rapid absorption, for De Filippi, who gave it in water without other food, obtained higher limits of assimilation, as did Pflüger in his single experiment with thin meat soup.

*Methods.*—We added the glucose to weighed amounts of finely chopped beef heart and after adding about 100 c.c. of water, the sugar and meat were thoroughly mixed together. Commercial glucose was used. This was tested and found to contain 95 per cent. pure glucose. Except during the early part of the investigation a standard diet was given composed of 300 gm. of meat and 300 c.cm. of milk on the day preceding the experiment. The animals were kept in metabolism cages, and the temperature of the room was noted. The amount of sugar in the urine was determined by the polariscope. The limit of assimilation was calculated for pure glucose.

The details of the tests on four normal dogs are given in Tables 3, 4, 5 and 6.

---

11. Pflüger: Arch. f. d. ges. Physiol., 1908, cxxiv, 1.

TABLE 3.—LIMIT OF GLUCOSE ASSIMILATION IN DOG 6*

| Date<br>....<br>1909 | Weight of Dog<br>Gm. | Food<br>....<br>.... | Amount<br>....<br>Gm. | Sugar<br>... | Amt. of Urine in c.c. | Amt. of Sugar Gm. | Notes<br>....<br>.... |
|---|---|---|---|---|---|---|---|
| 3/18.... | 5,300 | meat plus | | .. | 530 | .... | ............ |
| | | glucose | 10 | .. | ... | .... | ............ |
| 3/19.... | ... | meat | 250 | — | 560 | .... | ............ |
| | | lard | 10 | .. | ... | .... | ............ |
| | | glucose | 25 | .. | ... | .... | ............ |
| 3/20.... | ... | meat | 250 | — | 420 | .... | ............ |
| | | lard | 10 | .. | ... | .... | ............ |
| | | glucose | 30 | .. | ... | .... | ............ |
| 3/21.... | ... | meat | 250 | — | 440 | .... | ............ |
| | | lard | 10 | .. | ... | .... | ............ |
| | | glucose | 35 | .. | ... | .... | ............ |
| 3/22.... | ... | meat | 500 | — | 475 | .... | Fehling's solution turned green. |
| | | lard | 10 | | | | |
| | | glucose | 45 | .. | ... | .... | ............ |
| 3/23.... | ... | meat | 250 | .. | ... | .... | ............ |
| | | lard | 10 | .. | ... | .... | ............ |
| | | glucose | 45 | .. | ... | .... | ............ |
| | | Morning— | | — | ... | .... | ............ |
| 3/24.... | ... | meat | small amt. | — | ... | .... | Urine voided during the day free from sugar. |
| | | glucose | 55 | | | | |
| | | Evening— | | | | | |
| | | meat | 250 | + | 425 | 0.64 | Polariscope .15% |
| | | milk | 100 | .. | ... | .... | ............ |
| | | glucose | 75 | .. | ... | .... | ............ |

*The limit of assimilation was more than 9.8 gm. per kilo of body weight.

TABLE 4.—LIMIT OF GLUCOSE ASSIMILATION IN DOG 7 (FEMALE)*

| Date<br>....<br>1910 | Weight of Dog<br>...... | Food<br>....<br>.... | Amount<br>......<br>Gm. | Sugar<br>... | Specific Gravity<br>....... | Amt. of Urine c.c. | Amt. of Sugar Gm. | Room Temperature |
|---|---|---|---|---|---|---|---|---|
| 1/24...... | 6400 | meat | 200 | .. | .... | ... | ... | ..... |
| | | milk | 200 | .. | .... | ... | ... | ..... |
| 1/25...... | .... | meat | 300 | — | 1025 | 460 | ... | 20 C. |
| | | glucose | 75 | .. | .... | ... | ... | ..... |
| 1/31...... | .... | meat | 200 | .. | .... | ... | ... | ..... |
| | | milk | 200 | .. | .... | ... | ... | ..... |
| 2/1 ...... | .... | meat | 300 | + | 1055 | 212 | 0.6 | ..... |
| | | glucose | 90 | .. | .... | ... | ... | ..... |

*The limit of assimilation was more than 11.1 gm. per kilo of body weight.

TABLE 5.—LIMIT OF GLUCOSE ASSIMILATION IN DOG 8 (MALE)*

| Date<br>....<br>1910 | Weight of Dog<br>Gm. | Food<br>.....<br>..... | Amt.<br>....<br>Gm. | Sugar<br>.. | Specific Gravity<br>...... | Amt. of Urine c.c. | Amt. of Sugar<br>..... | Room Temperature |
|---|---|---|---|---|---|---|---|---|
| 2/25.... | 13,300 | meat | 300 | — | 1019 | 535 | ...... | 19.4 C. |
| | | glucose | 75 | .. | .... | ... | ...... | ...... |
| 3/1 .... | ...... | meat | 300 | — | 1022 | 575 | ...... | ...... |
| | | glucose | 100 | .. | .... | ... | ...... | ...... |
| 3/5 .... | ...... | meat | 300 | + | 1025 | 840 | Trace | 20 C. |
| | | glucose | 125 | .. | .... | ... | ...... | ...... |
| 3/9 .... | ...... | meat | 300 | — | 1029 | 375 | ...... | ...... |
| | | glucose | 115 | .. | .... | ... | ...... | ...... |
| 3/11.... | ..... | meat | 300 | — | 1025 | 905 | ...... | 14.4 C. |
| | | glucose | 120 | .. | .... | ... | ...... | ...... |
| 3/15.... | 11,900 | ...... | ... | .. | .... | ... | ...... | ...... |

*The limit of assimilation was 9.5 gm. per kilo.

TABLE 6.—LIMIT OF GLUCOSE ASSIMILATION IN DOG 9 (FEMALE)*

| Date .... 1910 | Weight of Dog Gm. | Food .... .... | Amt. gm. or c.c. ........ | Sugar ... | Specific Gravity ....... | Amt. of Urine in c.c. | Amt. of Sugar Gm. | Room Temperature |
|---|---|---|---|---|---|---|---|---|
| 3/8 ...... | 7,600 | meat | 300 | .. | .... | ... | .... | ...... |
| | | milk | 300 | .. | .... | ... | .... | ...... |
| 3/9 ...... | .... | meat | 300 | — | 1049 | 200 | .... | 15 C. |
| | | glucose | 85 | .. | .... | ... | .... | ...... |
| 3/14...... | .... | meat | 300 | .. | .... | ... | .... | ...... |
| | | milk | 300 | .. | .... | ... | .... | ...... |
| 3/15...... | .... | meat | 300 | — | 1029 | 300 | .... | 19.4 C. |
| | | glucose | 95 | .. | .... | ... | .... | ...... |
| 3/16...... | .... | meat | 300 | .. | .... | ... | .... | ...... |
| | | milk | 300 | .. | .... | ... | .... | ...... |
| 3/17...... | .... | meat | 300 | — | 1049 | 195 | .... | 17.3 C. |
| | | glucose | 110 | .. | .... | ... | .... | ...... |
| 3/31...... | .... | meat | 300 | .. | .... | ... | .... | ...... |
| | | milk | 300 | .. | .... | ... | .... | ...... |
| 4/1 ...... | .... | meat | 300 | + | 1054 | 155 | 4.75 | 22.2 C. |
| | | glucose | 125 | .. | .... | ... | .... | ...... |
| 4/3 ...... | .... | meat | 300 | .. | .... | ... | .... | ...... |
| | | milk | 300 | .. | .... | ... | .... | ...... |
| 4/4 ...... | .... | meat | 300 | — | 1060 | 148 | .... | 21.1 C. |
| | | glucose | 125 | .. | .... | ... | .... | ...... |
| 4/5 ...... | .... | meat | 300 | .. | .... | ... | .... | ...... |
| | | milk | 300 | .. | .... | ... | .... | ...... |
| 4/6 ...... | .... | meat | 300 | — | 1052 | 175 | .... | 23.8 C. |
| | | glucose | 125 | .. | .... | ... | .... | ...... |
| 4/11...... | .... | meat | 300 | .. | .... | ... | .... | ...... |
| | | milk | 300 | .. | .... | ... | .... | ...... |
| 4/12...... | .... | meat | 300 | + | 1032 | 290 | 0.14 | 21.1 C. |
| | | glucose | 135 | .. | .... | ... | .... | ...... |
| 4/13...... | .... | meat | 300 | .. | .... | ... | .... | ...... |
| | | milk | 300 | .. | .... | ... | .... | ...... |
| 4/14...... | .... | meat | 300 | — | 1060 | 140 | .... | ...... |
| | | glucose | 135 | .. | .... | ... | .... | ...... |

*The limit of assimilation was more than 15.6 gm. per kilo of dog weight.

It will be seen by consulting Table 5 that Dog 9 developed glycosuria on April 1 when 125 gm. of glucose were fed, but in two subsequent tests the urine remained free from sugar when this amount of glucose was given. This is probably explained by the fact that the dog was allowed to run about in a yard on the days preceding the feeding of sugar, April 3, and April 5. In March the dog was kept in her cage most of the time. From April 6 to April 10 considerable exercise was given. On April 11 she was confined in a cage and the following day was fed 135 gm. of glucose. Slight glycosuria developed. On April 13 she was allowed the freedom of the "run" and the usual preliminary diet given. Although 135 gm. of glucose were given on April 14 the urine remained free from sugar. These observations suggest that exercise prior to the day of the feeding experiment may alter the limit of assimilation.

Our results on normal dogs, which are summarized in Table 7, accord with those reported by Boeri and De Andries, Schlesinger, and Pflüger.

TABLE 7.—LIMIT OF ASSIMILATION FOR GLUCOSE PER KILO OF BODY WEIGHT IN NORMAL DOGS

| | | |
|---|---|---|
| Dog 6 | more than | 9.8 grams |
| Dog 7 | more than | 11.1 grams |
| Dog 8 | | 9.5 grams |
| Dog 9 | more than | 15.6 grams |
| Average | more than | 11.5 grams |

## II. LIMIT OF ASSIMILATION FOR GLUCOSE IN DOGS WITH ATROPHY OF THE PANCREAS

As stated in the beginning of this paper, Pratt, Lamson and Marks[12] have shown that if all the pancreatic ducts are occluded extreme atrophy of the gland occurs. The absorption of fats and proteins is so seriously affected that the animals lose weight rapidly.

DOG 5.—Young female. Weight 5,700 gm. On Nov. 19, 1908, Dr. Murphy under ether anesthesia separated the pancreas from the duodenum, cutting all the tissues that unite the two except the main branches of the pancreaticoduodenal artery and vein, the preservation of which was necessary in order to prevent the necrosis of the duodenum. Two pancreatic ducts were recognized and these were cut between double ligatures. The omentum was inserted between the duodenum and the corpus pancreatis, thus interposing a barrier of living tissue through which pancreatic juice escaping from open ducts would have to pass before it could enter the intestine.

As soon as the dog began to eat meat the bulky stools contained a large amount of undigested muscle tissue. A metabolism experiment showed that only 31.0 per cent of fat and 32.1 per cent. of nitrogen were absorbed. There was a steady loss of weight in spite of an abundant diet. On January 12 it had fallen to 4,700 gm. The urine was repeatedly examined, but it always was free from sugar.

Feb. 13, 1909: Weight 5,100 gm.

February 23: Ten gm. of *glucose* were added to the food, which consisted of meat and milk. The urine gave no reduction with Fehling's solution.

February 24: Urine contains no sugar.

February 26: Thirty-five gm. of *glucose* given with the regular food. Urine, amount 650 c.c. Fehling's test positive.

February 28: Urine, 350 c.c., specific gravity 1027, slight trace of albumin; sugar present.

March 1: Urine is free from sugar.

March 2: Weight 5,900 gm. Fed 30 gm. of *glucose*. Two hours later voided 25 c.c. of urine with 1.6 per cent. = 0.4 gm. of sugar. (Quantity estimated with Fehling's solution.) During the following twenty-four hours 610 c.c. of urine collected. This was free from sugar.

March 3: Urine, 975 c.c.; specific gravity 1024; no sugar; slight trace of albumin.

March 4: No glucose given. Urine, 1700 c.c.; sugar present; 1.5 per cent. = 25.5 gm. (Fehling's method).

March 5: Urine, 1000 c.c.; no sugar.

March 6: Urine, 575 c.c.; no sugar.

March 8: Weight 6000 gm.

March 9 to March 29: Urine examined daily and found free from sugar.

12. Pratt, Lamson and Marks: Tr. Assn. Am. Phys., 1909, xxiv, 277.

April 24: Fed 30 gm. of *glucose* with 200 gm. of meat and 225 c.c. of milk. Four hours later found 65 c.c. of urine which contained 3.7 per cent. of sugar, amount 2.4 gm. The urine passed later in the day was free from sugar.

April 28: Weight 6400 gm.

May 12: Given 20 gm. of *glucose* with 500 gm. of meat and 250 c.c. of milk. In the evening 200 c.c. of urine had been collected, which contained 0.6 gm. of sugar.

May 29: Given 15 gm. of *glucose* with a meal consisting of 250 gm. of meat and 250 c.c. of milk. During the day voided 440 c.c. of urine which reduced Fehling's solution. Amount of sugar 1.8 gm.

May 30: Urine, 460 c.c.; no sugar.

June 2: Weight 6,800 gm.

June 3: Food, 10 gm. of *glucose;* 250 gm. meat. Urine free from sugar.

June 4: No glycosuria.

June 9: Food, 10 gm. *glucose;* 250 gm. meat. Urine passed later in the day contained no sugar.

June 11: Weight 7000 gm.

July 1: Weight 7000 gm.

July 6: Food, 15 gm. *glucose;* 250 gm. meat; 250 c.c. milk. Urine, 265 c.c.; specific gravity, 1028. No reduction of Fehling's solution at time test was performed, but after one hour fluid had a greenish color; the following day a yellow precipitate had formed and settled to the bottom of the tube.

July 14: Weight 6,900 gm.

July 28: Weight 6,300 gm.

September 24: Food, 300 gm. meat, 15 gm. *glucose.* Urine, 210 c.c.; specific gravity, 1039, no sugar.

September 27: Food, 1000 gm. meat, 30 gm. *glucose.* Urine, 700 c.c.; specific gravity; 1023, no sugar. Limit of assimilation more than 4.7 gm. per kilo.

October 17: Weight, 6,500 gm.

November 10: No food for twenty-four hours.

November 11: Food, 500 gm. meat, 35 gm. *glucose.* Urine 260 c.c.; specific gravity, 1045, no albumin, trace of sugar.

November 12: Urine free from sugar.

December 1: Weight 6,300 gm.

December 6: Weight 6,100 gm.

December 13: Weight 5,800 gm.

January 5, 1910: Weight 5.306 gm.

January 11: Weight 5,100 gm.

January 12: Food: 300 gm. meat, 30 gm. *glucose.* Urine, 215 c.c.; 0.89 gm. sugar. Limit of assimilation less than 5.9 gm. per kilo.

January 24: Weight 5000 gm.

January 25: Food, 300 gm. meat, 15 gm. *glucose.* Urine, 265 c.c.; no albumin, no sugar.

January 31: The dog is very thin and weak. She cannot go up more than one flight of stairs without resting, and is unable to jump from the floor into her cage, as she could formerly.

February 1: Weight, 4,700 gm. Food, 300 gm. meat, 25 gm. *glucose.* Urine: 230 c.c.; specific gravity 1038, no sugar. Limit of assimilation more than 5.3 gm. per kilo.

February 3: To-day the fresh pancreas of the sheep was added to the diet. (The dog was given two or three glands a day.)

February 9: The dog is now very lively and apparently stronger than she has been for two months. The stools are now small and firm, and do not contain any excess of fat. On microscopic examination only a few muscle fibers, and no starch granules are seen. A metabolism experiment conducted over four days

—February 8 to February 11—showed that 88.7 per cent. of the fat contained in the food was absorbed and 82.2 per cent. of the nitrogen.

February 14: Weight 5,300 gm.

February 18: Weight 5,800 gm. Food, 300 gm. meat, 300 c.c. milk, two sheep's pancreas.

February 19: Food, 40 gm. *glucose;* 300 gm. meat; two sheep's pancreas. The dog appears ravenously hungry; she eats the pancreas first, picking the glands out from the mixture of pancreas and chopped beef-heart. Urine, 275 c.c.; specific gravity 1041; no sugar. Room temperature 16.2 C.

February 21: Weight, 5,900 gm.

February 23: Weight, 6,000 gm. Food, preliminary diet with three pancreatic glands.

February 24: Food, 50 gm. *glucose,* 300 gm. meat, three pancreatic glands. Urine 240 c.c.; specific gravity, 1049; no sugar.

February 28: Weight, 6,400 gm. The dog has never been in better condition.

March 3: Weight, 6,400 gm.

March 8: Weight, 6,600 gm. Preliminary diet of 300 gm. of meat and 300 c.c. of milk with three fresh pancreas.

March 9: Sixty-five gm. of *glucose* with 300 gm. of meat and three pancreas. Urine, 320 c.c.; specific gravity 1040; no sugar. Room temperature 15 C.

March 15: Weight 6,900 gm. The dog was fed to-day 80 gm. of *glucose* with 300 gm. of meat and three pancreatic glands. Urine, 350 c.c.; specific gravity 1039; no sugar. Room temperature 19.5 C.

March 16: Food, 300 gm. of meat, 300 c.c. of milk and three fresh pancreas.

March 17: Food, 100 gm. of *glucose* with 300 gm. of meat and three pancreas. Urine, 240 c.c.; specific gravity 1039. Sugar present; amount 0.81 gm. Temperature 17.3 C.

March 18: Weight, 6900 gm. The feeding of the fresh pancreas was stopped to-day.

March 21: Food, 300 gm. of meat and 300 c.c. of milk.

March 22: Weight 6600 gm.

March 23: Food, 80 gm. of *glucose* with 300 gm. of meat. Urine, 225 c.c.; specific gravity 1040. No sugar. Room temperature 18.9 C.

March 30: Weight 6500 gm.

March 31: Preliminary diet of 300 gm. meat and 300 c.c. milk.

April 1: Given 80 gm. of *glucose* with 300 gm. of meat. Urine, 230 c.c.; specific gravity 1031. No sugar. Temperature 22.2 C.

April 3: Preliminary diet of 300 gm. of meat and 300 c.c. of milk.

April 4: One hundred gm. of *glucose* with 300 gm. of meat. Urine, 230 c.c.; specific gravity 1036; no sugar. Room temperature 21.1 C.

April 5: Regular preliminary diet.

April 6: Weight 6000 gm. Fed 100 gm. of *glucose* and 300 gm. of meat. Urine, 170 c.c.; specific gravity 1054; no sugar. Room temperature 23.9 C.

April 11: Preliminary diet.

April 12: Weight, 5,800 gm. Fed 100 gm. of *glucose* with 300 gm. of meat. Urine, 285 c.c.; specific gravity 1031; sugar 1.45 gm. Temperature 21.1 C.

April 21: Preliminary diet.

April 22: Weight 5,600 gm. Given 100 gm. of *glucose* with 300 gm. of meat. Urine, 265 c.c.; specific gravity 1034; no sugar.

April 26: Weight 6,200 gm.

April 29: Preliminary diet.

April 30: Given 100 gm. of *glucose* with 300 gm. of meat. Urine, 300 c.c.; specific gravity 1032. Sugar 2.01 gm.

May 1: Urine, 475 c.c.; specific gravity 1020; no sugar.

This dog has lived without any pancreatic secretion entering the intestine from Nov. 19, 1908, until the present time. In one experiment 95.2 per cent. of the fat in the food was excreted in the feces.

TABLE 8.—LIMIT OF GLUCOSE ASSIMILATION IN DOG 5*

| Date | Weight Gm. | Sugar in Food | Gm. | Limit of Assimilation for Glucose† per kilo | Gm. | | Sugar in Urine Gm. |
|---|---|---|---|---|---|---|---|
| 3/2 /09.... | 5,900 | glucose | 30 | less than | 6.5 | + | 0.4 |
| | | lactose | 10 | ........ | ... | .. | ..... |
| | | | 40 | | | | |
| 5/12/09.... | 6,400 | glucose | 20 | ........ | ... | .. | ..... |
| | | lactose | 13 | ........ | ... | .. | ..... |
| | | | 33 | less than | 4.9 | + | 0.6 |
| 5/29/09.... | 6,800 | glucose | 15 | ........ | ... | .. | ..... |
| | | lactose | 13 | ........ | ... | .. | ..... |
| | | | 28 | less than | 3.9 | + | 1.8 |
| 6/3 /09.... | 6,800 | glucose | 10 | more than | 1.6 | 0 | ..... |
| 6/9 /09.... | 7,000 | glucose | 10 | more than | 1.2 | 0 | ..... |
| 7/6 /09.... | 7,000 | glucose | 15 | ........ | ... | .. | ..... |
| | | lactose | 13 | ........ | ... | .. | ..... |
| | | | 28 | less than | 3.8 | + | Trace |
| 9/27/09.... | .... | glucose | 30 | more than | 4.4 | 0 | ..... |
| 11/11/09... | 6,500 | glucose | 35 | less than | 5.1 | + | Trace |
| 1/12/10.... | 5,100 | glucose | 30 | less than | 5.6 | + | 0.89 |
| 1/25/10.... | 5,000 | glucose | 45 | more than | 2.9 | 0 | ..... |
| 2/1 /10.... | 4,700 | glucose | 25 | more than | 5.0 | 0 | ..... |
| 2/19/10.... | 5,800 | glucose | 40 | more than | 6.6 | 0 | ‡ |
| 2/24/10.... | 6,000 | glucose | 50 | more than | 7.9 | 0 | ‡ |
| 3/9 /10.... | 6,600 | glucose | 65 | more than | 9.3 | 0 | ‡ |
| 3/15/10.... | 6,900 | glucose | 85 | more than | 11.7 | 0 | ‡ |
| 3/17/10.... | 6,900 | glucose | 100 | more than | 13.8 | 0 | ‡ |
| 4/4 /10.... | 6,000 | glucose | 100 | more than | 15.8 | 0 | ..... |
| 4/12/10.... | 5,800 | glucose | 100 | less than | 16.3 | + | 1.45 |
| 4/22/10.... | 5,600 | glucose | 100 | more than | 16.9 | 0 | ..... |
| 4/30/10.... | 6,200 | glucose | 100 | more than | 15.3 | 0 | ..... |

*Young female, weight 5700 gm.; pancreas separated from duodenum Nov. 19, 1908.

‡Fresh pancreas fed from February 3 to March 18.

†Calculated for pure glucose.

Atrophy of the pancreas takes place with rapidity after all the ducts are occluded and Hess found sclerosis of the pancreas of high degree one month after the operation, and Pratt, Lamson and Marks observed extensive atrophy and sclerosis in two months. As all the dogs have shown atrophy of the pancreas, varying in extent with the length of time after operation, there is every reason to believe that in Dog 5 there has been extreme atrophy of the pancreas for many months.

In spite of the progressive atrophy of the epithelial structure of the pancreas, the dog has not developed diabetes. A summary of the results in the glucose assimilation tests is given in Table 8. The tolerance for carbohydrates was not determined previous to the operation on Nov. 19, 1908. The first experiment on March 2, 1909, about three and a half months after occlusion of the ducts, showed that the limit of assimilation was less than 6.5 gm. per kilo, while the average assimilation in our normal dogs was more than 11.5 gm. This observation furnishes additional evidence of the important part played by the pancreas in carbohydrate metabolism. From the seventh to the ninth month after the onset of atrophy of the organ the assimilation was less than 3.9 gm. per kilo. Then a slight increase occurred and in the eleventh month (test made September 27) more than 4.4 gm. per kilo were taken without producing glycosuria. The gain was slight and near the end of the twelfth month the assimilation was less than 5.1 gm. per kilo.

This study gives no definite support for the view that there is compensation by other organs when the internal function of the pancreas becomes impaired.

No direct relation can be traced between the general condition and the power to assimilate sugar. In July, 1909, when the dog weighed its maximum and was strong and active, the limit of assimilation was less than 3.8 gm. per kilo, while on Feb. 1, 1910, when the weight had dropped to the minimum, the limit was more than 5.0 gm. per kilo.

Dog 4.—Male, weight, Dec. 2, 1908, 11,100 gm. The operation of occluding the ducts and separating the pancreas from the duodenum was performed by Dr. Murphy on December 12.

Metabolism experiments on this dog have been reported.[1] There was severe disturbance in the absorption of fats and proteins after the exclusion of the pancreatic juice from the intestine and the dog lost weight rapidly. During January the urine occasionally caused a slight reduction of Fehling's solution.

February 22: Weight 7,800 gm.

February 23: Dog given 10 gm. of *glucose*. The urine remains free from sugar.

February 24: Dog given 20 gm. of *glucose*. No glycosuria.

February 26: Dog given 35 gm. of *glucose*. The urine reduces Fehling's solution. Limit of assimilation less than 4.5 gm. per kilo.

February 27 to March 2: The urine each day reduced Fehling's solution, although no more glucose was fed.

March 3: Urine did not reduce Fehling's solution.

April 20: Weight 7,600 gm.

April 24: Food, 30 gm. of *glucose*, 200 gm. of meat, 225 c.c. of milk. No glycosuria resulted.

April 25: Food, 35 gm. of *glucose*, 150 gm. of meat, 10 gm. of lard. Urine, 250 c.c.; 0.6 per cent. sugar, amount 1.5 gm.

May 11: Weight 7,800 gm.

May 16: Food, 300 gm. of *glucose*, 250 gm. of meat, 250 c.c. of milk. Urine free from sugar. Including in the estimation the lactose of the milk, the limit of assimilation is more than 5.4 gm. per kilo.

June 3: Weight 6,600 gm. The dog was given 30 gm. of *glucose* with meat. In the afternoon 150 c.c. of urine were found which contained 4.5 gm. of sugar. Limit of assimilation less than 4.3 gm. per kilo.

June 4: Weight 6,400 gm. Urine, slightly acid, specific gravity 1021, slight trace of albumin, no sugar. Sediment contained many red blood corpuscles, some leukocytes and a few hyaline and finely granular casts.

On June 4, Dr. Murphy removed the dense inflammatory tissue which occupied the side of the pancreas. The outlines of the organ were completely lost. The sclerotic mass was identified as the remains of the pancreas by the dilated duct passing through it. In breaking up dense adhesions the liver was torn.

June 5, the dog was found dead. He had passed 55 c.c. of urine. This was acid and had a specific gravity of 1012. Fehling's solution was turned green, and after standing a slight deposit of yellow cupric oxid formed at the bottom of the test-tube. The polariscopic examination showed about 0.1 per cent. of glucose.

*Autopsy.*—June 5, 1909, by Dr. Thomas Ordway.

Anatomical Diagnosis: Massive hemorrhage into the peritoneal cavity; sacculated periduodenal abscess with fistula into duodenum; chronic fibrous peritonitis (adhesion of omentum, duodenum, pancreas and liver); contusion of liver; distention of gall-bladder; acute and chronic pyelonephritis; atrophy of pancreas and dilation of pancreatic duct.

Body is that of a fairly well-developed and poorly nourished, somewhat emaciated, young male dog. Weight 6,170 gm. There is marked rigor mortis; no edema. Between the ensiform and umbilicus in the median line is a recent incised wound sutured with interrupted sutures of silk-worm gut. The edges are clean and agglutinated. Subcutaneous and thoracic abdominal fat very scant.

Peritoneal Cavity: Peritoneum is everywhere blood-stained and the pelvis is filled with fluid blood. Pelvis and flanks contain about 60 c.c. of fluid blood. The omentum, duodenum and liver are bound together by firm adhesions, forming a mass which is 6 by 5 cm. in size. On the outside this is blood-stained (apparently caused by attempt to break up adhesions at operation on June 4). No pancreatic tissue can be recognized. The lymph-nodes in the vicinity of this mass are considerably enlarged. On section they are of a dark red color. On the left hand and lower portion of the mass above referred to is a hemorrhagic stump with apparently dilated pancreatic duct in the center. Incision into the mass discloses an irregular, sacculated, abscess cavity surrounding the duodenum anteriorly and laterally, and communicating with the duodenum by the fistulous tract 2 cm. below the pylorus. For 10 cm. from this point the duodenum is markedly thickened, the wall varying from 0.3 to 1.2 cm. The mucosa is elevated, roughened, reddened and in places ulcerated. Serial sections through the thickened duodenal wall adjacent to the abscess and the mass of surrounding adhesions show no definite evidence of pancreatic tissue. Dilated ducts are found, about which is firm, fibrous tissue in which is an occasional small punctum, possibly the remains of glandular tissue.

Pleural and Pericardial Cavities: Normal.

Heart: The right auricle and ventricle are much distended by cruor clot. All cavities are apparently moderately dilated, particularly on the right side. The myocardium, endocardium and valves are normal.

Lungs: These are very pale, collapsed and normally crepitant throughout.

Spleen: Weight and size normal (estimation). On the outer border are three or four slightly elevated, yellowish nodules varying from 1 to 4 cm. in diameter. On section these are sharply circumscribed, circular areas without definite softening.

Gastro-Intestinal Tract: Stomach is empty; rugæ prominent; duodenum described above. The small intestine is collapsed and empty. The large intestine contains considerable slate-colored, pasty, fecal material.

Pancreas: See "Peritoneal Cavity."

Liver: The right lobe is adherent at the lower portion to the mass above described. At one portion the adhesions are somewhat separated, leaving a hemorrhagic surface. Three cm. from the area of adhesions in the substance of the right lobe is a large nodule 3 by 2 cm. in diameter, considerably firmer than the liver tissue elsewhere. On section this is of a general grayish yellow color and has a somewhat fibrous appearance, being in marked contrast to the normal chocolate-brown liver parenchyma. The gall-bladder is enormously distended, measuring 5 by 6 by 3 cm. The common duct runs through the mass of adhesions about the duodenum and is apparently pressed on by the periduodenal abscess. Pressure on the gall-bladder, however, causes thin, yellowish fluid to flow freely into the duodenum.

Kidneys: Weight, 90 gm. The capsule strips freely, leaving a smooth surface. On section the pyramids in their inner third have a distinctly vacuolated or finely fenestrated appearance. This increases as the pelvis is approached. The mucosa of the pelvis is roughened, reddish and has a granular appearance. The pelves contain 0.5 c.c. of slightly turbid fluid.

Adrenals, Bladder, Genital Organs and Aorta: Normal.

Organs of Neck: Thyroid Gland: Both lobes are easily found and the two are equal in size, measuring 3.5 by 1.4 by .8 cm.

*Microscopical Examination.*—Fragments of tissue removed by Dr. Murphy at operation consist of dense connective tissue with a few dilated ducts. No definite islands of Langerhans or acini are seen. Many sections from the stump of the pancreas, i. e., the proximal portion and the vicinity of the periduodenal abscess show acute and chronic inflammatory tissue.[13]

A search of the literature fails to reveal an instance of such extreme sclerosis of the pancreas as developed in this case. On naked-eye examination no pancreatic tissue could be found. Microscopic examination showed only a small nodule 0.6 cm. by 0.6 cm., made up of acini and islands of Langerhans imbedded in dense connective tissue. Although there was almost total destruction of the pancreas, not only did diabetes not develop but the dog was able to assimilate three weeks before its death more than 5.4 gm. of glucose per kilo. On the other hand, the profound effect of atrophy of the pancreas on carbohydrate metabolism was shown by the reduction of the limit of assimilation to less than 4.5 gm. per kilo within three months after the onset of the atrophy. Slight variation in the tolerance occurred. There was no definite increase with the passage of time, and the last test, made two days before the dog's death, showed the limit of assimilation to be as low as it had been three months previously. The significance of the glycosuria following the removal of the pancreas is not clear owing to the speedy death of the animal. Transitory glycosuria may follow severe operative procedures when the pancreas is healthy. So in this case it may have been the result of the operation, although the conclusion that it was due to the removal of a few areas of pancreatic tissue that remained is more probable. No dog has ever failed to develop diabetes when the entire pancreas has been extirpated. The hypothesis that the organism will compensate in some way if the internal function of the pancreas is gradually lost has as yet no clear evidence to support it.

Dog 8.—Male, weight March 15, 1910, 11,900 gm.

March 16: Operation under ether anesthesia by Dr. F. T. Murphy. The corpus pancreatis measured 11 cm. by 2.7 cm., the processus uncinatus 8 cm. by 2 cm., and the processus lienalis 8 cm. by 3 cm. A duct was found near the center of the

13. In one block of tissue examined since this paper was written, a small nodule of pancreatic tissue 0.6 by 0.6 cm. in size was found, and in this among the acini numerous islands of Langerhans can be clearly made out.

corpus pancreatis. A wedge-shaped mass of gland tissue, 1 cm. by 1 cm. in size, was left around this duct with its base in contact with the duodenum. At the distal end of this mass the duct was cut between double ligatures. The remainder of the pancreas was entirely separated from the duodenum, except for a few connecting blood-vessels, which were left intact. Only two pancreatic ducts were recognized. The omentum was placed between the cut surface of the pancreas and the duodenum. The dog made a rapid recovery.

March 20: Weight, 10,000 gm.

March 22: The abdominal wound is clean and dry. Food, 150 gm. of meat, 400 c.c. of milk. The urine is high-colored, specific gravity 1019. There is a large amount of albumin; no sugar. The sediment contains many fresh red-blood corpuscles, and a large number of spermatozoa.

March 23: Urine smoky. Albumin present. No sugar. The sediment contains a few fatty and brown granular casts, and many fresh and disintegrated red-blood corpuscles.

March 30: The dog is active and strong, although he looks emaciated. Weight, 8,200 grams. Food, 100 gm. of *glucose;* 300 gm. of meat. Urine, 320 c.c.; specific gravity, 1036; no albumin; sugar, 0.63 per cent.; amount, 2.02 gm. The feces are normal in appearance, but contain an excess of muscle fibers; no fat visible.

March 31: Preliminary diet, 300 gm. of meat and 300 c.c. of milk.

April 1: Food, 90 gm. of *glucose* and 300 gm. of meat. Urine, 295 c.c.; specific gravity, 1039; a slight trace of albumin; sugar, 0.61 per cent.; amount, 1.80 gm.; sediment contains very many blood cells and a few spermatozoa; no casts found. Room temperature 22.2 C.

April 3: Preliminary diet as before.

April 4: Food, 65 gm. of *glucose;* 300 gm. of meat. Urine, 265 c.c.; sugar, 0.14 per cent.; amount, 0.37 gm. Room temperature 21.1 C.

April 5: Preliminary diet. The dog had the freedom of the yard.

April 6: Weight, 8.400 gm. Food, 50 gm. of *glucose*; 300 gm. of meat. Urine 225 c.c.; no sugar. Room temperature 23.9 C.

April 11: Preliminary diet.

April 12: Food, 60 gm. of *glucose;* 300 gm. of meat. Urine, quantity not determined as some was lost; sugar, 2.9 per cent. Room temperature 21.1 C.

Table 9.—Summary of Glucose Feeding Experiments After Separating Pancreas from Duodenum (Dog 8)

| Date | Weight, Gm. | Amt. of Sugar (Glucose) in Food, Gm. | Limit of Assimilation for Glucose per Kilo* | Sugar in Urine, Gm. |
|---|---|---|---|---|
| 1910 | | | | |
| 3/30 ......... | 8,200 | 100 | less than 11.6 | 2.02 |
| 4/ 1 ......... | .... | 90 | less than 10.8 | 1.80 |
| 4/ 4 ......... | .... | 65 | less than 7.5 | 0.37 |
| 4/ 6 ......... | 8,400 | 50 | more than 5.6 | 0. |
| 4/12 ......... | .... | 60 | less than 6.8 | Amount not determined. |

*Calculated for pure glucose.

Before the operation it was necessary to feed the dog 125 gm. of glucose in order to produce glycosuria. Within three weeks after the onset of atrophy of the pancreas sugar appeared in the urine when 65 gm. of glucose were given. This represented a decrease in the limit of assimilation from 10 gm. per kilo to less than 7.9 gm.

Schulze,[14] Ssobolew[15] and De Witt[16] assert that after occlusion of the pancreatic ducts the islands of Langerhans remain intact. The statement that the acini degenerate, but the islands undergo no change has often been brought forward in support of the island theory of diabetes. If tying *all* the ducts produces no pathological alterations in the islands how can the rapid loss in the power of the pancreas to destroy sugar in the organism which was observed in this animal be explained? It would certainly be difficult for defenders of the island theories to reconcile the great reduction in the limit of assimilation with the observations of the investigators just cited. To shut off all the pancreatic secretion from the intestine is a difficult task, as was first recognized by Hess.[17] It has been often attempted, but rarely accomplished. In dogs and cats in which we have entirely prevented the entrance of pancreatic juice into the intestine there was a speedy and progressive destruction of the islands of Langerhans. At the same time, marked disintegration and destruction of the acini took place, so that our observations offer as much support for the acinar theory as for the island theory of the origin of diabetes. The view that alterations in the acini are the cause of diabetes is held by Hansemann,[18] Herxheimer,[19] Gutmann,[20] Schmidt,[21] and Karakascheff.[22]

### III. LIMIT OF ASSIMILATION INCREASED BY FEEDING FRESH PANCREAS

Pflüger[23] has shown in a careful critical study that the glycosuria in diabetes has never been diminished by the introduction into the body of pancreas or pancreatic preparations. Zuelzer[24] has recently stated that he has caused a temporary decrease in the amount of sugar in the urine of diabetic men and dogs by the intravenous injection of a pancreatic "hormone." It seems quite evident from the studies of Forschbach[25] that the decreased elimination of sugar was due to the toxic action of the material injected rather than to the presence of a specific substance in the preparation.

Hédon[26] has asserted that the existence of an internal secretion of the pancreas will not be demonstrated until it is possible to check diabetes in a depancreatized dog by the introduction of a pancreatic product.

---

14. Schulze: Arch. f. mikr. Anat. u. Entwcklngsgesch., 1900, lvi, 491.
15. Ssobolew: Virchows Arch. f. path. Anat., 1902, clxviii, 91.
16. De Witt: Jour. Exper. Med., 1906, viii, 193.
17. Hess: Arch. f. d. ges. Physiol., 1907, cxviii, 536.
18. Hansemann: Verhandl. d. deutsch. pathol. Gesellsch., 1901, iv, 187, Berlin.
19. Herxheimer: Virchows Arch. f. path. Anat., 1906, clxxxiii, 228.
20. Gutmann: Virchows Arch. f. path. Anat., 1903, clxxii, 493.
21. Schmidt: München. med. Wchnschr., 1902, xlix, 51.
22. Karakascheff: Deutsch. Arch. f. klin. Med., 1904, lxxxii, 60.
23. Pflüger: Archiv. f. d. ges. Physiol., 1907, cxviii, 267.
24. Zuelzer: Ztschr. f. exper. Path. u. Therap., 1908, v, 307.
25. Forschbach: Deutsch. med. Wchnschr., 1909, xxxv, 2053.
26. Hédon: Travaux de la Physiologie, 1898. Quoted by Pflüger.

The study of the effect of feeding fresh pancreas to animals with a lowered limit of assimilation for glucose was undertaken with the hope of gaining some information in regard to the internal secretion of the pancreas.

The limit of assimilation in Dog 5 was tested at frequent intervals over a period of fourteen months following the separation of the pancreas from the duodenum. As has already been stated, the tolerance for glucose varied during this time from less than 4 gm. per kilo of body weight to more than 5.3 gm. per kilo. On Jan. 12, 1910, nearly fourteen months after the operation, the feeding of 30 gm. of glucose produced glycosuria. From February 3 to March 18 the dog was fed two to three raw pancreas a day. The limit of assimilation rose rapidly and steadily as is shown in Table 8. On March 17, the day the administration of pancreas was discontinued, the limit of assimilation was more than 14.5 gm. per kilo, which represented an increase of more than 100 per cent. in the dog's power to destroy glucose. While the pancreas was fed the absorption of fat and protein was almost normal and the dog gained more than 2 kilos. As soon as the feeding of the gland was discontinued there was a loss of weight. The limit of assimilation did not fall for more than a month afterward. This is a remarkable fact. The test made on April 30, six weeks after the last fresh pancreas had been given, showed that this dog with an atrophied and sclerotic pancreas had a greater power to assimilate sugar per kilo of body weight than any normal animal in our series. It would be futile to speculate on the cause of this increase until more experimental data have been accumulated.

## IV. SUMMARY

There is a rapid decrease in the power to assimilate glucose after the onset of atrophy of the pancreas.

The persistence of a low limit of assimilation for more than a year shows that the other organs of the body compensated imperfectly if at all for the pancreatic insufficiency. Diabetes did not develop in any animal, although in two the atrophy and sclerosis of the pancreas were extreme. It cannot be denied that the retained ability to consume sugar in animals with the pancreas almost totally sclerosed was possibly due to some compensating action elsewhere in the organism.

The limit of assimilation in a dog with atrophy of the pancreas which had been under observation fourteen months was increased more than 100 per cent. by feeding fresh pancreas.

313 Beacon Street.

# TUBERCULOUS RETROPERITONEAL ADENITIS CONNECTING BY A SINUS WITH THE DUODENUM

## REPORT OF A CASE WITH AUTOPSY

MERRICK LINCOLN, M.D.
WORCESTER, MASS.

Tuberculous mesenteric retroperitoneal glands are so common and so much has been written about them that only a special research or some unusual peculiarity warrants one in broaching the subject. It is the latter reason that leads me to offer this report.

Involvement of a few of the glands is very commonly found at operation or autopsy; general involvement occurs frequently. Localized in the appendix region tuberculous adenitis forms a well-known surgical and clinical picture. Localized in the region of the duodenum, as in the case here reported, producing certain clinical aspects, it may occur more often than we know, but a search of the literature of the past thirty years has brought to light only one similar case coming to autopsy.

This is described by Moynihan[1] in his recent work on duodenal ulcer and is included in his list of cases of tuberculous ulceration of the duodenum. It was first reported by Trier in 1863. The patient had pain for seven years a little above and to the right of the umbilicus, coming on within three or four hours after eating. He had one attack of severe hematemesis, was jaundiced and had a tender tumor in the epigastrium. Necropsy revealed in the duodenum close to the pylorus a circular opening leading into a cavity containing in its lumen a thrombus. There were obsolete tubercles in the apices of both lungs.

Only one other case was found with similar clinical symptoms, and in this no statement was made localizing the processes beyond stating it was one of intestinal tuberculosis. In 1899 Drs. D. R. Brower and C. J. Habheggar[2] reported a case of intestinal tuberculosis in which there were glands palpable in the neck, axillæ and groins, tenderness and pain in the epigastrium, a subicteric tinge to the skin and vomiting of blood. The patient reacted to an injection of tuberculin. There was no autopsy.

The subject of tuberculous ulcerations of the pylorus and adjacent glands was thoroughly covered in 1905 by Ricard and Chevrier,[3] and since it is a closely

1. Moynihan, B. G. A.: Duodenal Ulcer, Philadelphia and London, 1910, p. 81, quoting F. Trier, Ulcus corrosivum duodeni, Copenhagen, 1863.
2. Brower, D. R., and Habhegger, C. J.: Further Observations on the Chlorid of Gold and Sodium, Jour. Am. Med. Assn., 1899, xxxiii, 1337.
3. Ricard and Chevrier: Rev. de Chir., Paris, 1905, xxxi, 557, 736; 1905, xxxii, 74.

related condition a few words in that connection may be of interest. Out of eighty-five cases of gastric tuberculosis the pylorus was involved in thirty cases, with stenosis in sixteen cases. In four of these sixteen the duodenum was also involved. Among the eighty-five cases the duodenum was involved in ten. The ulcers at the pylorus were surrounded by a circle of caseous glands, into some of which fistulous openings led. Some of these leading from the stomach to the duodenum under the ulcer are referred to as *fistules gastro-duodénales.* The perigastric glands were involved in 32.7 per cent. Among the cases with pyloric stenosis the number of tuberculous glands amounted to 56.25 per cent. In some cases there was glandular enlargement involving the pylorus, but without any ulceration. Ricard and Chevrier state that tuberculosis of the perigastric glands occurs in 2.1 per cent. of all cases of primary tuberculous adenitis. Beside the suprapyloric and retropyloric glands, glands were often noted at the hilum of the liver, that is, subpyloric. These tuberculous glands are always multiple and may form very large tumors in the pyloric and pancreoduodenal region. Ricard and Chevrier conclude that the bacillus of Koch gains entrance through the lymphatic system in the cases of stenosing adenitis, and through the mucous membrane in the non-stenosing local and most of the mixed cases.

The following case, then, is worthy of reporting on account of its rarity:

## REPORT OF CASE

*History.*—An Irish widow aged 52, occupation housework, previously a laundress, entered the Worcester City Hospital Oct. 9, 1909. Her father died of consumption; otherwise there is nothing of importance in the family history. The patient remembered nothing about the diseases of childhood, but thought, on account of deafness which she had had for many years, that she had had scarlet fever. The menopause occurred six years before admission. After March, 1907, she had abscesses on both sides of her neck, some of which ruptured spontaneously; others were operated on at various times, the first time being May 10, 1907. Most of these had not healed but had continued to discharge. For these the patient was treated by the ordinary surgical methods, also with Tuberculin R. and a *Staphylococcus pyogenes albus* vaccine; later with Tuberculin B. E. for about six months with no apparent effect. She had been given potassium iodid in good-sized doses at two or three different times without result. There had been some cough for a few months, but she did not complain of it, and her lungs were found normal in October, 1907. In March, 1908, there were found a few moist râles at the apex of the left lung in front, with diminished resonance and fremitus. On March 20, 1909, she was sent to the Worcester City Hospital for an attack of jaundice. She had pain over the region of the gall-bladder, and at McBurney's point for three days, and was markedly jaundiced for several days, with bile in the urine. Her lungs showed a few crackling râles at the left lower back. Her breath sounds were harsh. A few tubercle bacilli were found in her sputum. The liver was felt almost down to the umbilicus with a tender mass in the right lower quadrant just below the edge of the liver. Five days after entrance the urine was free from bile; the bowels were free and the stools of normal color three days later. The blood showed: hemoglobin 85 per cent., white count 7,400; differential count of white cells: polymorphonuclear neutrophils 52 per cent., small lymphocytes 31 per cent., large lymphocytes 16 per cent., eosinophils 1 per cent. Convalescence was soon established. The patient left the hospital April 18, with no abdominal symptoms; the diagnosis was acute catarrhal jaundice, no gall-stones having been found. The patient was given large doses of potassium iodid with no effect on the adenitis. On Oct. 5, 1909, four days before readmission to Worcester City Hospital, the patient had three small hemorrhages from the stomach, severe pain about the lower right costal region and considerable diarrhea. She had been slightly jaundiced for several months, but more so of late. She had noticed that the urine was highly colored, but the stools had not been observed. The patient's head ached a little, and she had no appetite.

*Physical Examination.*—The patient was a fairly developed and poorly nourished woman with yellow pigmentation of the skin and sclera. There were a dozen or so scars, crusts and discharging sinuses about the neck and the upper part of the chest. The heart sounds were of fair intensity but somewhat intermittent. There was a loud blowing systolic murmur at the apex transmitted to the axilla. The apex was in the fifth costal interspace, exactly in the nipple line. The left border of cardiac dulness extended just outside of the nipple line; the right border was at the right edge of the sternum. The pulse was of fair tension, 90 per minute. The radial arteries were firm but did not show arteriosclerotic beading. The lungs showed prolonged expiration at the left apex, both in front and in back, and also slight dulness. There were no râles; and no dulness or abnormal respiration was found elsewhere.

The abdomen was soft and tympanitic, except in the right hypochondriac region. Here there was a firm mass, the smooth, dull edge of which could be palpated about two fingers' breadth below the right costal margin but could not be palpated across the epigastrium. The dulness was increased on full inspiration. There was a suggestion of a rounded mass at the edge of the liver, corresponding to the gall-bladder, but it could not be definitely made out. Above, the relative dulness of the liver extended to the fourth interspace, the absolute dulness to the sixth interspace. There was tenderness over the right upper quadrant of the abdomen, more marked in the region of the gall-bladder.

The knee-jerk, plantar, wrist and triceps reflexes were present and active. There was no Babinski reflex or ankle-clonus. The extremities showed no edema. Temperature was 101 and respirations 20. The blood examination was as follows:

Hemoglobin 70 per cent. White cells 7,000. Red cells 3,344,000.

Differential count of white cells:

| | % |
|---|---|
| Polymorphonuclear neutrophils | 75 |
| Large mononuclear lymphocytes | 22 |
| Small mononuclear lymphocytes | 2 |
| Eosinophils | 1 |

The red cells showed no abnormal forms.

The urine showed an acid reaction, specific gravity 1.024, albumin absent, sugar absent, bile present.

The temperature was normal for twenty-four hours on October 11. The patient had two movements of the bowels in the night. The stool was of dark brown color, containing blood (guaiac test). Fat was not present by microscopical examination and nothing otherwise abnormal was found.

On October 12 the patient had had no more hemorrhages. She had been on a semisolid diet, and the pain in the right costal region had subsided considerably. This morning the side of the left ear and the skin below the chin were inflamed and angry, the area of this being well circumscribed. The temperature rose to 101.3 and the count of white blood corpuscles was 8,000. A diagnosis of erysipelas was made.

The patient was not very sick, but on October 13 the erysipelas spread to the right side of her face. A vaccine made of streptococci of thirty-eight strains was obtained and 25,000,000 given every eight hours.

The erysipelas gradually subsided, and by October 16 had wholly disappeared. At times the patient became more jaundiced, and complained of an uncomfortable feeling in the region of the liver, but on the whole she seemed to have had fewer symptoms referable to her abdomen during the course of the erysipelas. During the afternoon of the 16th the patient complained of some epigastric pain, and shortly afterward vomited about two ounces of dark blood. There were no more hemorrhages for several days.

On October 19, the examination of the stool, which was watery and black, showed blood by the guaiac test.

On October 22, the patient seemed as comfortable as she had previously been but still complained of indefinite pains about the liver area. At 3 p. m. she vomited half a pint of fairly bright blood, containing many thick clots. She was given morphin, gr. ¼, and cracked ice, and an ice-bag was applied to her epigastrium. A surgeon advised no operative interference. Between 3 and 6 p. m. the patient had five small hemorrhages of the same character as before, amounting in all to about a pint. At 5 p. m. morphin, gr. ¼, was repeated. Examination of the abdomen showed nothing new except slight dulness just below the left costal margin near the median line, which, later developments showed, probably was due to blood in the stomach. The patient became very anemic, but her pulse remained good. At 7 p. m. 10 c.c. of rabbit serum were given. At 9 p. m. the patient began to show signs of failing circulation. Strychnin, gr. 1/30 was given, and the pulse improved markedly. The patient complained of epigastric pain, and morphin, gr. ¼, was given again. At 11 p. m. her general condition was the same, but her pulse was good, and she had vomited no more blood. At 2:25 a. m., October 23, she died, being conscious and uncomplaining up to the last.

AUTOPSY

This was performed Oct. 23, 1909, at 11:45 a. m., by Dr. F. H. Baker, about nine hours after death.

The body was that of a middle-aged woman, fairly well developed and poorly nourished, body length 5 feet 3 inches, skin and conjunctivæ of a very faint yellow color, mucous membranes of the lips of extreme pallor, left pupil normal, the right slightly contracted with a small internal and a small inferior coloboma. The usual suggillations were present on the posterior aspect of the body. On both sides of the neck, anterior and posterior to the sternocleidomastoid and also below the clavicle, were multiple openings one-quarter to one-half inch in length, surrounded by a narrow zone of pink tissue, some healed, some incrusted, some discharging pus. These were openings of cavities formed by broken down and caseating lymph-glands. Incision showed about half an inch thickness of deep yellow subcutaneous fat.

*Heart.*—The muscle was pale and somewhat friable. The weight was 300 gm. The thickness of the wall of the right ventricle was about one-eighth of an inch, and of the left seven-sixteenths of an inch, with a layer of fatty tissue between it and the epicardium about three thirty-seconds of an inch thick. The valves were normal, except that the mitral had a slight thickening of the cusps along the edge, while the aortic orifice showed a slender cartilaginous ridge just above two of the cusps at the junction of the heart-wall and aorta. Microscopically, the heart muscle showed nothing of interest.

*Pleural Cavities.*—The right showed old adhesions of the pleura, readily broken at the apex and on the lateral wall. The right lung weighed 330 gm. and showed thickening with fibrous structure at the apex and with a few scattered tubercles the size of a pin-head. The middle lobe was small and atelectatic, adherent throughout to the upper and lower lobes. The left pleural cavity showed old adhesions at the apex, lateral wall and posterior wall, being readily broken. There was at the apex of the left lung an area about 2 inches in diameter, of thickened fibrous tissue, and scattered throughout it were small tubercles and an occasional small purulent caseating area. This lung weighed 330 gm. Both lungs showed a small amount of edema. Throughout there were a few small black nodules of black pigment about the size of peas. Microscopically, the left lung showed many small areas of tuberculosis. The right lung showed similar but less marked changes especially in the middle lobe.

*Abdominal Cavity.*—There were various areas of old adhesions. In the pelvic region were many old adhesions. The uterus was bound down in front to the bladder, and behind to the rectum. A loop of the sigmoid flexure was bound down in the cul-de-sac of Douglas. The appendix was atrophied like an old fibrous cord adherent throughout. The cecum was likewise bound down by similar dense adhesions. From the lesser curvature of the stomach to the under surface of the right lobe of the liver ran eight to a dozen moderately firm fibrous bands.

*Liver.*—The weight was 1,390 gm. The peritoneal covering was smooth; when this was stripped off the surface appeared finely granular. A cut section was pale yellow brown, mottled as of fatty degeneration. The right lobe was slightly lengthened downward. Microscopically, the liver cells showed marked cloudy swelling. The acini were considerably separated by spaces in which was an exudation with leukocytes, red blood cells and lymphocytes. The portal spaces were frequently considerably dilated. The interlobular hepatic veins, arteries and ducts were often surrounded with a moderate excess of connective tissue containing leukocytes, lymphocytes, a few red blood corpuscles and an occasional eosinophil.

*Gall-Bladder.*—This was firmly adherent to the lower surface of the liver, its walls being considerably thickened. It contained two brown gall-stones each one-half inch in diameter, with two or three mulberry-like surfaces and four or five smooth facets. These consisted chiefly of cholesterin. The common duct was patent.

*Pancreas.*—The organ was pale, firm and hard, and slightly enlarged. At its head was a firm, hard mass of enlarged glands, half or three-quarters of an inch in length each, adherent and caseating, surrounded by thickened tissue. Dissection revealed a cavity an inch and a half in diameter just to the right of the head of the pancreas, and behind the first portion of the duodenum, lined with an inflamed tissue in places showing small areas of granulation tissue with newly formed blood-vessels. This cavity contained a little blood-stained fluid and a few small clots. This cavity communicated with a smaller pocket below, three-quarters of an inch in diameter containing some thick, dark red, grumous, bloody fluid. There was no connection between the abscess cavity and the bile-ducts.

*Duodenum.*—The first cavity mentioned above also communicated by means of a small sinus with the surface of the duodenum, the mucous membrane of which was slightly drawn out into a funnel, like a traction-diverticulum. The edges of the opening were thickened. This communicating sinus was about half an inch long. The duodenum showed no other changes. There were no ulcers elsewhere. The duodenum was filled with bloody material and clots as were the intestines for some distance below. The pylorus showed nothing but the normal thickening.

*Stomach.*—This was filled with a blood-clot in the form of a cast of the stomach weighing 180 gm. and showing a slight constriction at the junction of the upper and middle third. The mucous membrane was pale and smooth. No ulcerations or abrasions of any kind could be found.

Microscopically, the pancreas showed a considerable interlobular as well as interacinous connective tissue. It was especially marked around the blood-vessels and ducts. There was infiltration with lymphocytes, polymorphonuclear lymphocytes and eosinophils, and occasionally a large eosinophilic mononuclear cell and red blood corpuscle, altogether showing an acute process in addition to a chronic one. A few polymorphonuclear leukocytes had wandered into the interacinous structure, as well as an occasional lymphocyte and mononuclear eosinophil. The epithelium of the acini showed some cloudy swelling and a slight amount of vacuolization.

The mass around the sinus showed one tubercle with a caseating center, not quite filling the low-power field, surrounded by a zone of spindle-cells, leukocytes, lymphocytes, a dozen giant cells and a few plasma cells with an irregular zone of lymphocytes outside containing occasionally the above-mentioned cells. There was scarcely anything left of the normal gland tissues. It was represented in isolated spots by a few lymphatic cells. The rest of the mass was taken up with connective tissue, some young, with frequent nuclei, and the fibers close together staining purple, some much older with a few nuclei, and a considerable separation of fibers staining pink. Scattered throughout were many lymphocytes, a few leukocytes and an occasional epithelioid cell. In many places were round oval or longitudinal bundles of nerve-fibers of a diameter up to one-half the width of

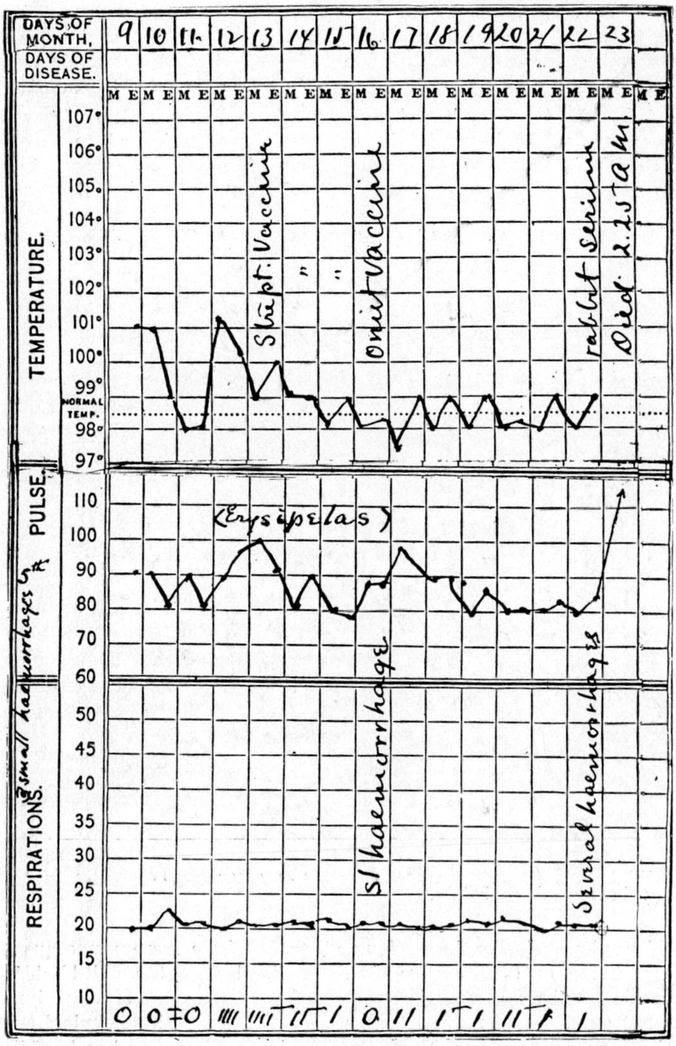


Fig. 1.—Chart of temperature, pulse and respiration in case of tuberculous retroperitoneal adenitis.

the low-power field, surrounded by a thin capsule formed by a few layers of connective tissue cells. These often were subdivided by sub-bundles of tissue separated by spaces. The histologic picture of the mass around the sinus was that of the remains of a tuberculous lymph-gland for the most part replaced by connective tissue, which had caught up and included some of the nerve-fibers in the neighborhood. No tubercle bacilli were found.

A section along the sinus showed the mucous membrane of the duodenum extending up to it, where it ended curled up and folded on itself. In between the villi were many leukocytes and lymphocytes. The wall of the sinus was formed by connective tissue rather loose, infiltrated with lymphocytes and leukocytes, and resting in places on circular and then on longitudinal muscle fibers from the duodenal wall, and then on the connective tissue of the gland itself. The connective tissue of the duodenum merged slowly into that of the gland, there being no definite line of demarcation except that the blood-vessels were larger and more numerous where the glandular element apparently began.

*Various Lymphatic Glands.*—There was tuberculous adenitis of several other lymphatic glands. The bronchial lymph-glands were enlarged to three-quarters of an inch or so in length, usually black from pigment, and caseous in part. A gland near the pancreas showed normal gland tissue in one small area; the rest

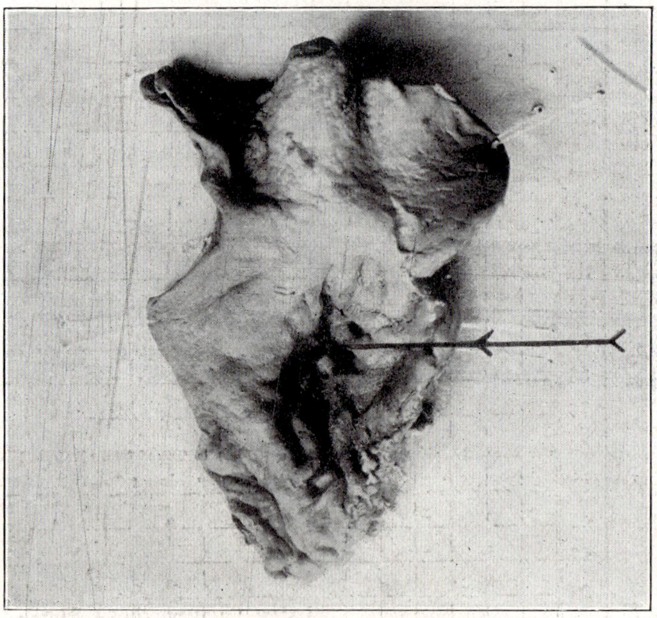

Fig. 2.—Portion of duodenum opened up, showing pylorus and opening of sinus about half an inch below.

showed tuberculous disease in various stages. There were numerous scattered areas of caseation of considerable size. A gland near the gall-bladder showed a considerable number of good-sized areas of caseation. A cervical lymph-gland showed about one-third of its area taken up with two or three typical tuberculous areas. There were no other enlarged lymph-glands except as has been previously stated.

*Spleen.*—This weighed 240 gm. It was slightly pale and flabby. A cut surface showed a mottled appearance with an excessive marking of the trabeculæ. The pulp was moderately soft. Microscopically, there was nothing markedly abnormal.

*Kidneys.*—The weight of each was 110 gm. The capsules stripped easily and the surfaces were smooth. Cut sections showed the cortices and pyramids of normal size, but the markings were pale yellowish streaks very noticeable in both. The section resembled that of a chronic toxemia. Microscopically, the right kidney showed considerable swelling of the convoluted tubules and occasional necrosis. The Malpighian corpuscles showed some hyperemia and some indentations with some loss in places of cellular elements. Bowman's capsule was in places thickened. The ascending and descending loops of Henle showed an increase in the intercanalicular tissue. The left kidney showed a similar condition, but more variable, the cloudy swelling and Malpighian degeneration

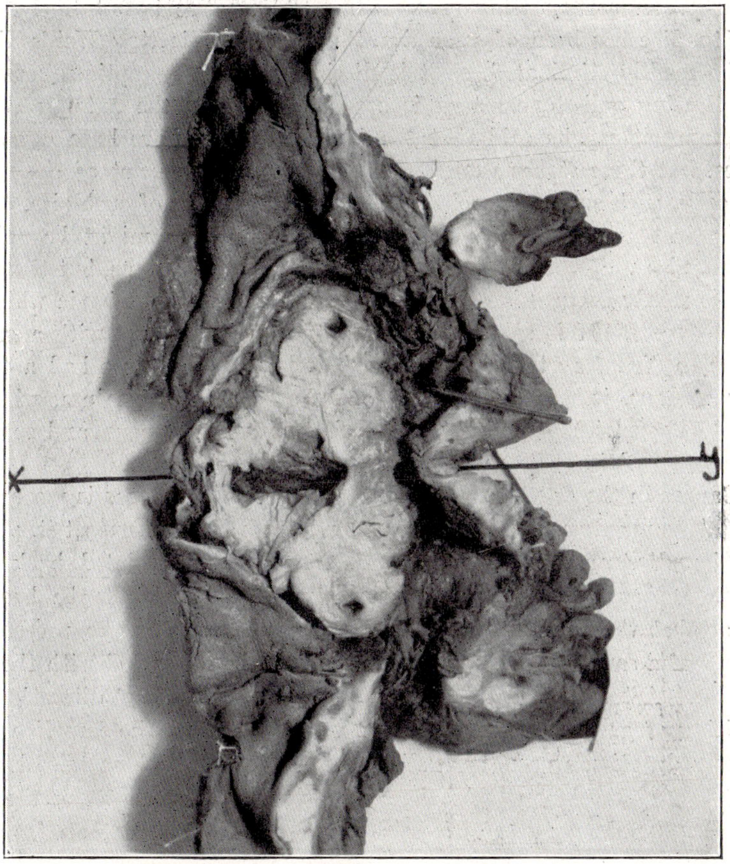


Fig. 3.—Duodenum, split open through sinus, lymph-gland and inflammatory mass, front portion turned down on *x-y* as axis; sinus leading from duodenum into abscess cavity above gland and inflammatory mass; probe entering abscess cavity from a second connecting cavity posterior.

being more marked in some places, and less marked in others. There was very little hyperemia.

The adrenal glands were normal.

A point of interest in this case is the differential diagnosis, which is of considerable complexity. Limiting ourselves to a consideration of gross conditions characterized by gastric hemorrhage, the diseases under consideration before autopsy should have been gastric ulcer, duodenal ulcer, gastric cancer, duodenal or pancreatic cancer, with gall-stones or acute catarrhal jaundice complicating any of these. We were not able to obtain the gastric contents on account of the hemorrhages.

Against gastric ulcer, there is nothing to be said except that it does not complete the picture. The pain usually comes on soon after eating or two or three hours afterward. But peptic ulcer does not explain the jaundice. A complicating acute catarrhal jaundice is not likely, since the jaundice has been of some duration. A complicating Weil's disease can be readily eliminated, as it is distinctly an acute septic process. A complicating gall-stone attack is a possibility. As the autopsy showed gall-stones it can be said that the jaundice might have been caused by stones, but these stones were large, and the pain was not of the nature of a colic, such as would probably be caused by stones of such size.

Against cancer of the stomach much the same might be said as against ulcer. The trouble was of some duration, it is true, but there was not the steady progressive emaciation or the picture of cachexia which we would expect. It is also an unusual thing for a patient with a gastric cancer to die of acute hemorrhage. Further, although we had a tumor mass present, it was located to the right of the epigastrium, where it would (if gastric) be connected probably with the pylorus, and so cause dilatation and its concomitant symptoms (absent here).

Cancer in the duodenum or in the head of the pancreas is more probable. The mass was felt approximately where we would expect it. There was jaundice and hematemesis and the disturbance dated back some months. Against this, there is nothing very effective to be brought, except that the character of the tumor was not such as to present the feeling of a cancer here, but seemed rather to be connected with the gall-bladder. After such a duration we expect symptoms of dilatation and vomiting of gastric residue. We must also note that the jaundice while of long duration was not steadily increasing, but had remained slight until toward the last attack. There was no steady progress of the local disturbance; simply an attack in the spring, and then freedom from epigastric distress until shortly before her last entrance to the hospital. Lastly there was no typical cachexia.

The most natural diagnosis was ulcer of the duodenum. There were hematemesis and melena. There was tenderness to the right of the epigastrium. There was a palpable mass which could be due to inflammatory thickening. There was jaundice, which might be caused by pressure from the mass or by a catarrh extending up the duct. Yet jaundice is not to be expected with the ordinary duodenal ulcer. The pain of ulcer is usually two hours or so after meals, while here it was constant while it lasted, and came irrespective of meals.

Gall-stones *per se* are a possibility. Jaundice, tenderness in the right epigastrium, a palpable mass, all are consistent with gall-stones in the gall-bladder and ducts. The hemorrhage, however, cannot be accounted for by this unless we can conceive of a stone rupturing a vessel in close communication with the duodenum, or when rupturing into the duodenum at the same time tearing a blood-vessel. But in this process we would expect colic, or at least a more severe pain than was present, and the possibility seems remote.

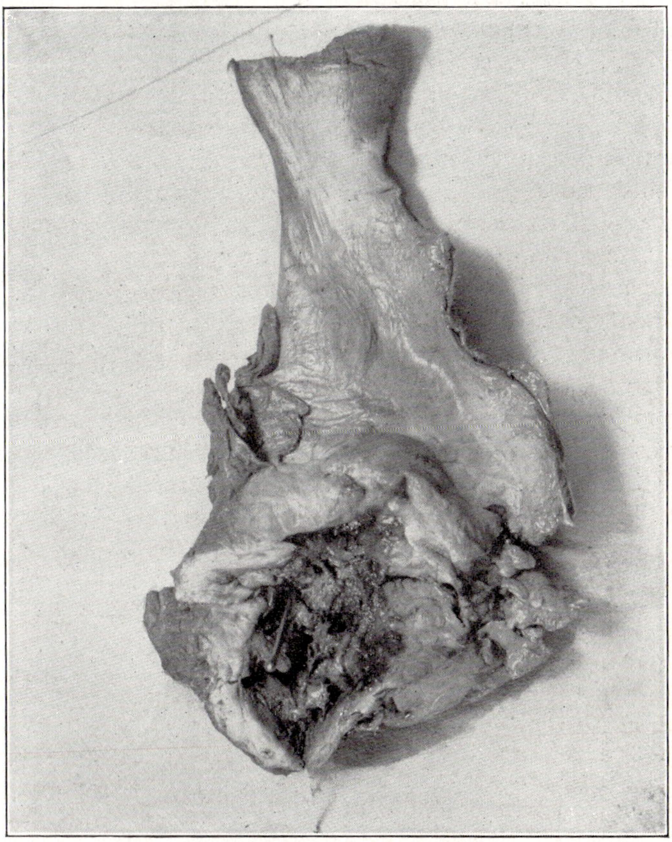

Fig. 4.—Posterior view of duodenum and inflammatory mass showing second abscess cavity laid open with probe entering from the first cavity.

A pure tuberculous ulcer in the duodenum needs not to be considered, as references in the literature to such cases are extremely rare. A tuberculous ulcer of the stomach would be ruled out for the same reasons as a simple ulcer, as well as on account of its rarity.

Chronic pancreatitis needs hardly to be considered. Jaundice and tumefaction are consistent with it, but the tumor should be more toward the center, and not distinct, and hemorrhage from the stomach is not a symptom of pancreatitis.

A consideration of these possibilities left us more or less undecided, but against rather than for any of them. Hemorrhage from the duodenum from some undetermined cause was our diagnosis.

Taking all the knowledge gained by autopsy, we can explain the case as follows: A tuberculous gland became necrosed and formed an abscess cavity; connective tissue formation took place, with considerable induration round about. The abscess gradually formed a fistulous communication with the duodenum. Later, some one of the larger blood-vessels on the wall of the abscess cavity gave way with the resulting hemorrhage.

The essential factors on which we might in the future establish a diagnosis would be:

1. A tuberculous person.

2. Tenderness in or to the right of the epigastrium.

3. A mass felt in or to the right of the epigastrium.

4. Jaundice from compression or swelling of the mucous membrane by extension of the inflammation.

5. Hematemesis or melena.

I have reported this case from an academic point of view rather than from a practical one. It is of interest only as adding one more possibility in making our differential diagnosis. It would hardly be expected that anything radical could be done by way of a cure by surgery. The extensive inflammatory condition and the inaccessibility and friability of the parts would lead us to expect no help in this direction. It is, therefore, chiefly as a rarity that I have reported this case, and with the hope that other similar cases may come to light.

In conclusion, I wish to thank Dr. F. H. Baker for pathological suggestions, and Miss Ora M. Mills for cutting and staining sections.

2 Linden Street.

# SYNCHRONOUS CARDIAC AND RESPIRATORY RATE

## REPORT OF A CASE

GEORGE WILLIAM NORRIS, M.D.
PHILADELPHIA

The patient from whom the accompanying tracings were made was admitted to the Pennsylvania Hospital in March, 1910, suffering with an attack of broken cardiac compensation. He was an Italian laborer, aged 19. A moderate user of alcohol and tobacco, he denied all previous disease except an attack of scarlatina twelve years previously. He presented the usual picture of an individual suffering from dilatation of the heart following disease of the aortic and mitral valves (insufficiency). Further examination disclosed the absence of leukocytosis with a marked diminution of the number of erythrocytes, and some depression of the percentage of hemoglobin, as well as an irregular fever, which sometimes reached 102. Blood-cultures were sterile on a number of occasions. Two months after admission well-marked signs of an acute pericarditis were noted, which gradually disappeared.

I saw the patient for the first time during August, while in charge of Dr. Tyson's service. At this time he still suffered from orthopnea, anemia and occasional fever. The following diagnosis was made: subacute endocarditis, aortic, mitral and tricuspid insufficiency; hypertrophy and dilatation of the heart, passive congestion of the lungs, the kidneys and of the portal system. Blood-pressure 110-85, hemoglobin 66 per cent., erythrocytes 3,160,000, leukocytes 8,400.

On August 23 he became very much worse, the heart dulness increased greatly in size, and the heart-sounds became muffled and distant. In the belief that he had developed a pericardial effusion, paracentesis pericardii was performed with negative results. The respirations were very rapid, but the pulse-rate very slow. At this time Tracing 1 was made, which shows that the pulse-rate and the respiratory rate were absolutely synchronous, 72 per minute. The jugular tracing was of the positive or systolic type, and the cardiogram definitely excludes the possibility of a non-conducted bigeminus. The brachial tracing shows an extrasystole. This condition persisted for about twenty-four hours, during which time the cardiac and respiratory rate remained absolutely synchronous. For twelve days preceding, the patient had been taking 10 minims of the tincture of strophanthus thrice daily. A right-sided hydrothorax of small size was also present.

Gradual improvement occurred. The cardiac dulness receded, and when last seen on October 28, the patient was very much more comfortable although still bedfast. Tracing 2, which was made at this time, shows a pulse and respiratory ratio of about four to one.

In so far as a brief search of the literature disclosed, this case is unique. The fact that the pulse and respiration remained accurately synchronous for such a long time, under careful observation, indicates that there must have been a definite cause and that the condition could not have been due to mere coincidence. There were of course reasons enough in the pulmonary congestion, hydrothorax, ascites, etc., to account for the rapidity of the respirations, but all these factors should, according to physiological laws, as we know them, have increased the pulse-rate

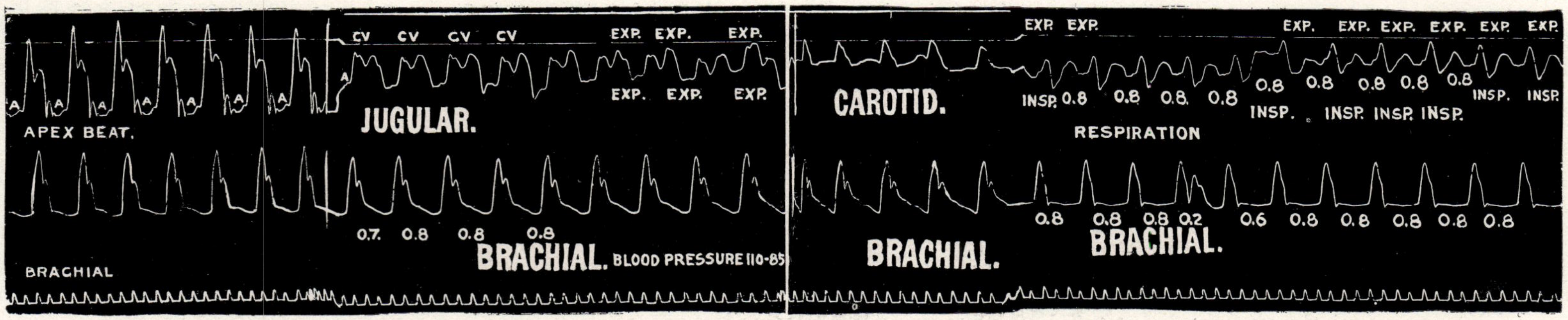


Tracing 1.—Synchronous cardiac and respiratory rate: a, the apex-beat in coordination with the brachial; b, a positive venous pulse, with a large, early "v" wave; c, the carotid in coordination with the brachial; d, the respiration exactly synchronous with the brachial, except after the fourth beat, following which an extrasystole is seen.

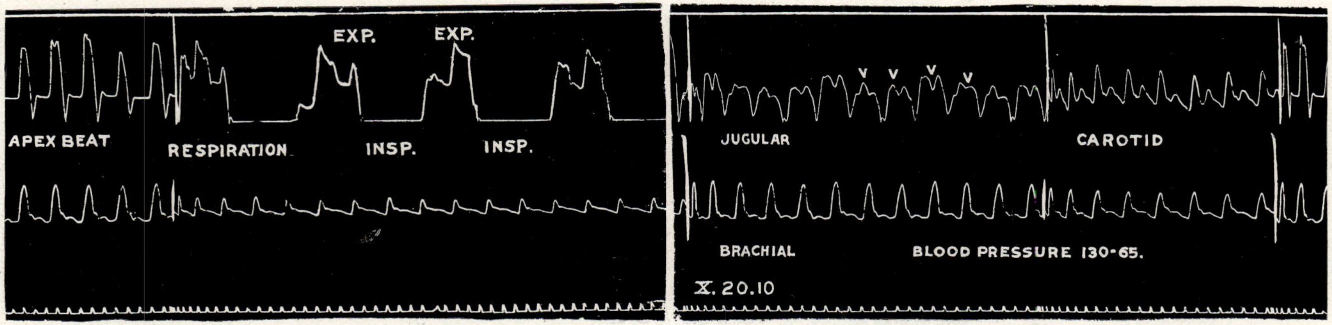


Tracing 2.—Tracing from same patient: a, a positive venous pulse with a large, early "v" wave; b, the carotid and brachial tracings in coordination; c, the apex-beat and the brachial in coordination; d, fairly normal pulse-respiration ratio.

also. The tracings from the jugular pulse and the apex-beat definitely eliminate the possibility of either heart-block or a pseudobradycardia resulting from extrasystoles.

The only explanation which I have to offer is as follows: It is a well-established fact that inspiration, by increasing the negative pressure in the thorax, favors diastolic filling of the heart, and in a similar manner expiration assists in systolic emptying. Now a glance at the last part of Tracing 1 shows that the expiration did correspond with systole and inspiration with the diastole of the heart. The patient had suffered from an acute dilatation of the heart, associated with great circulatory embarrassment, and it seems not improbable that this polypnea was automatically adopted by the organism in an effort at compensation. This hypothesis does not, of course, explain the relative bradycardia, to account for which we must assume that either as the result of medicinal action or as the effect of pathologic alteration there was sufficient overstimulation of the vagus, or depression of the chronotropic function of the heart-muscle to prevent an increase of the rate.

**In conclusion I wish to express my indebtedness to Dr. James Tyson for his courtesy in allowing me to report the case.**

**1530 Locust Street.**

# THE UTILIZATION OF FATS AND OILS GIVEN SUBCUTANEOUSLY *

LLOYD H. MILLS, M.D.
WITH THE ASSISTANCE OF ERNEST A. CONGDON, CHEMIST
NEW YORK

## HISTORICAL REVIEW

Attention was called to the possible value in nutrition of oils and fats given subcutaneously, by von Leube[1] in 1895. He remarked the rapid disappearance of very large injections of camphorated oil which he was giving for stimulation and sought to find whether oils remained in the tissue spaces or were utilized in nutrition.

An emaciated dog, previously brought into nitrogenous equilibrium at a very low level, was given daily subcutaneous injections of butter-fat for over six weeks in an amount which equaled about 1,400 gm. The weight rose from 4.4 kilos to 5.4 kilos. A laparotomy performed at the end of the injection period showed large masses of extraperitoneal fat, two-thirds of which was butter-fat. The omental fat consisted wholly of dog-fat. On a very low ration of fat-free meat at the end of a further three and one-half months, the same dog weighed 4.1 kilos, which was assumed to be an indication of the complete use of the foreign fat. Dissection showed but 3 to 4 gm. of subcutaneous fat and barely 2 gm. from the internal fat depots, 0.5 gm. of the former being butter-fat. From this and similar work von Leube believed that fats given hypodermically were of distinct benefit in nutrition.

In commenting on this experiment, Winternitz[2] and Henderson and Crofutt,[3] who oppose von Leube's interpretation, both conclude that this furnishes evidence that the absorption of fat is too slow to be practical.

Butter contains about 80.8 per cent. pure fat. So in Leube's experiment 1,131 gm. of fat were used in 135 days or 8.4 gm. daily. Placing the requirement of this dog at 70 calories per kilogram, a liberal figure, and using Stohmann's figures for the caloric value of butter fat, this fat must have furnished 78 calories per day or 18 calories per kilo,

---

* From the Laboratory of Physiology, Cornell University Medical School, New York City.

* This research has been aided by a grant from Prof. John Hays Hammond.

1. von Leube, W.: Sitzungsb. d. physik.-med. Gesellsch. zu Würzburg, 1895, p. 5.

2. Winternitz, H.: Ztschr. f. klin. med., 1903, l, 80.

3. Henderson, Yandell, and Crofutt, E.: Am. Jour. Physiol., 1905, xiv, 193.

one-quarter of the full requirement.[4] Further evidence of the value of this fat is given by the fact that the animal could endure five months on a minimal protein ration.

In 1898, Du Mesnil de Rochemont[5] in a series of clinical reports covering twenty-eight cases, gives tables to show that daily injections of from 60 to 200 gm. of olive oil produced a retention of nitrogen or a reduction in the amount excreted, which, however, did not become apparent until after the fourth or fifth days of injection. He believed that the subcutaneous use of oils was a rational mode of feeding, but remarked the slowness of absorption. His patients were nearly all very ill with wasting diseases and the poor absorption in these practically starving and sometimes moribund patients gave point to the severe criticism of Winternitz, who was led to condemn the entire method. Winternitz,[2] working with olive and sesame oils to which iodin had been added, took the amount of potassium iodid appearing in the urine as quantitative evidence of the destruction of iodized oils given subcutaneously. His conclusion, drawn largely from work on starving animals or patients ill with such wasting diseases as cancer, are that oils are absorbed from the subcutaneous tissue at the rate of from 2 to 3 gm. a day, and that if time enough elapses, all of the injected fat is utilized, a fact on which all observers are agreed.

Henderson and Crofutt[3] worked with cotton-seed oil because of its easy recognition in the tissues. In common with Winternitz, they noticed the wonderfully rapid diffusion of oil in the direction of gravity, and observed the accumulations of non-absorbed oil, which formed in the dependent parts of the abdomen, and in the groins. They found emulsions made with sodium hydroxid and with acacia to be difficult of absorption, the soluble part of the emulsion being taken up, leaving free oil in the tissue. They concluded that "oil injections in any moderate amounts are practically without nutritive value." Some of their own work can, however, be adduced against their view. In their most careful experiment, a well-nourished dog, weighing 7.8 kilos, was fed with 200 gm. of lean beef daily for two weeks, after which daily injections of 165 gm. of cottonseed oil were superimposed on this diet for ten days. At the end of this time the animal had become so weak that its ration of beef was doubled. As this was not enough to produce nitrogenous equilibrium, a need apparently not recognized by the investigators, normal vitality was never recovered and the dog was killed at the end of a month. The method of recovering oil left in the tissue was to squeeze the subcutaneous tissue in a small hand press and rinse the fibrous residue twice

4. From the present writer's experience, it is highly probable that had the animal been killed earlier, a much higher daily utilization would have been obtained.

5. Du Mesnil de Rochemont: Deutsch. Arch. f. klin. Med., 1898, lx, 474.

with naphtha. This gave an absorption figure of about 13 gm. daily. No mention is made of attempted extraction of skin and hair or of the outer layers of the abdominal or thoracic muscles, which always contain such considerable amounts of oil as to make conclusions regarding absorption valueless unless their extraction and analysis for foreign fat is accomplished. A dog weighing 7.8 kilos would require about 65 calories per kilo per day, a total of 500 calories. In the 200 gm. of lean beef, the animal received during the preliminary period about 250 calories daily. The daily injection of 165 gm. of cottonseed oil had a caloric value of 1,548, or from fat alone over three times the total requirement. The introduction of such excessive quantities of oil, to the absorption of which there were definite mechanical deterrents, and possibly also the inability of the body, from its low protein condition at the time, to furnish the comparatively large quantity of lipase or other enzymes necessary for the hydrolysis and metabolism of such food, inevitably produced accumulation in the tissue spaces.

The mistake of all previous investigators has been that they have attempted to show that plain oils given subcutaneously in starvation or on a very low protein diet, will give the same metabolic results as when fats, carbohydrates and proteins combined are administered. In reality, however, there are no grounds for assuming that fats given subcutaneously are differently oxidized than when fed by mouth. The work of Voit, Rubner and Schulz[6] has long since proved that fat fed alone has no influence on protein waste, save possibly slightly to increase it, and that under such conditions protein waste continues until some vital organ can no longer functionate and death ensues. Accordingly, granting the absorbability of injected fats, no successful application can be made of such injections which does not recognize the necessity of a sufficient protein supply.

As most of the previous experimental work was done on starving animals or in diseased conditions in man which closely simulated starvation, the faulty interpretation of such investigations has gone far toward discrediting the positive facts which the work of von Leube and du Mesnil exhibited and toward discouraging further investigation.

### OBJECTS OF THIS RESEARCH

The immediate objects of this work were to determine:

1. The absorbability of injected oil from the subcutaneous spaces.[7]

6. Quoted by Lusk in The Science of Nutrition, 1909, 72-75 and 165.

7. In a preliminary paper Mills and Murlin, using the respiratory apparatus of Pettenkoffer and Voit, have shown that oil in emulsion given subcutaneously to starving animals influences the respiratory metabolism to practically the same extent as identical amounts of similar oil fed by mouth. Mills, Lloyd H., and Murlin, John R.: Proc. Soc. Exper. Biol. and Med., 1910, vii, 166.

2. The conditions, if any, which favor absorption.
3. The method of utilization of fat so absorbed.
4. The organic effects of such utilization.

The ultimate object of this demonstration was the application of fat injections in wasting diseases as tuberculosis, and certain of the marasmic or cachectic states resulting from imperfect metabolic processes. Tuberculosis[8] was, however, the especial aim, for in this disease aversion and intolerance to fats is so universal as to be almost symptomatic, and any arrest of the progressive and extreme exhaustion of body fat would, if successful, mean at least an increase in general resistance.

## PLAN OF PRESENT RESEARCH

The general plan of this work was as follows:

1. Selection of unirritating fats and fixed oils for injection.
2. Development of absorbable emulsions of such oils and fats.
3. Injection of plain and emulsified oils into animals during (a) starvation, (b) low protein diet, (c) full mixed diet.

At the end of sufficiently long periods the animals were killed by ether and subjected to

4. Complete extraction of the various tissues of the body for fats.[9]
5. Determination of the amount of oil absorbed by comparing the iodin values (a) of the extracts of the skin and hair, subcutaneous tissues, skeleton and muscles with (b) the iodin indices of similar tissues from normal or starved cats, according to the type of experiment, and also with (c) the iodin index of the injected oil. Thus determined, any loss in the amount of oil from the amount injected could be considered as utilized oil, for examination of the ether extract of a large number of the internal and visceral fats gave no reactions such as were characteristic of the unchanged oils before injection.
6. Determination of the influence of injected oils on the visceral and internal adipose tissue fats by examination of the iodin values, weights and percentage of their ether extracts.

Cats were used throughout this work, for the reason that they were obtainable without difficulty, were not so large as to make a long series of complete extractions unduly difficult, and, being carnivorous, were capable of metabolizing fat in quantities. Gray male cats with tiger markings were used almost exclusively, for experience indicated that

8. Further work, to be published shortly, bears on the effect of oils given subcutaneously on the nitrogen balance in tuberculosis of man.

9. The brain and skull were not considered in this work except to make the gross observations that the meningeal lymph-spaces contained no macroscopic oil.

cats of this type were more than commonly resistant to tissue insult of all kinds.

## SELECTION OF OILS

All the fixed oils used were furnished by Fairchild Brothers & Foster, whose many courtesies I wish to acknowledge here. The purity of these oils was corroborated by their iodin values and by their characteristic reactions whenever obtainable.

J. F., a man affected with pulmonary tuberculosis, willingly offered himself as a test subject for irritant properties. Oil of lard, cocoanut oil, peanut, cotton-seed, olive and sesame oils produced no irritation and proved to be diffusible in about the order given. In addition to these, lard, butter-fat and human oils were used in animals. Corn oil and cod-liver oil produced intense and long-continued inflammation.

Investigation of the oils used gave the figures in Table 1.

Table 1.—Iodin Index and Specific Gravity of Various Oils

| Oil. | Iodin Index. | Specific Gravity. |
|---|---|---|
| Olive | 88.0 | 9.2 |
| Cotton-seed | 111.0 | 9.24 |
| Sesame | 105.0 | 9.23 |
| Peanut | 87.0 | 9.20 |
| Corn | 123.0 | 9.26 |
| Lard | 57.0 | 9.36 |
| Human | 54.8 | .... |

## EXPERIENCE WITH EMULSIONS

Emulsions made with acacia and with sodium hydroxid were unsatisfactory.

Casein produced a perfect permanent emulsion, but after ten to fourteen days the solution became cheesy and incapable of injection.

Theoretically, casein should produce the ideal emulsion and work is under way to prevent caseation in such emulsions if possible. Egg lecithin (Fairchild) in from 3 to 5 per cent. solution gave satisfactory emulsions, the oils usually taking up about 4 per cent. of lecithin at room temperature. An alcoholic solution of egg lecithin of value known to equal 5 gm. of dry lecithin, was added to 70 gm. of oil and the alcohol dissipated by distillation *in vacuo* at a temperature not exceeding 50 C., the lecithin going into solution in the oil as the alcohol distilled off. The emulsion was produced by the addition of 25 gm. of sterile water and shaking.[10]

10. The addition of pigs' bile salts was made to some of these emulsions, but either the bile had not been freed of electrolytic salts and these precipitated the lecithin out of its mixture with oil, or the well-known affinity of lecithin for bile was greater than for oil, and the solution was broken up. Physiological salt solution was also used to replace sterile water, but, in common with many other electrolytes, it precipitates the colloidal lecithin from its solution, thus exposing a fallacy in the hypodermic administration of lecithin in salt solution.

I would suggest, from the perfect emulsification produced by mixtures of lecithin, oil and water, that the rôle which the lecithin content of the bile plays in the absorption of fat from the intestine, is not so much that of an activator of pancreo-lipase, as suggested by Hewlett, as it is of a simple colloid, for lecithin swells like tragacanth on the addition of water.

Injections of 10 per cent. lecithin in oil produced no inflammatory reaction, but the emulsions above 8 per cent. were made so viscid by the lecithin that it interfered with absorption.

To discover the effect of living tissue on these emulsions 35 c.c. of 67.5 per cent. sesame oil with 3.5 per cent. lecithin was injected into the subcutaneous tissue of a cat and the same quantity into the peritoneal cavity of another. Both cats were killed by ether at the end of twenty-four hours. In the peritoneum only unemulsified oil was found from which no lecithin could be precipitated by acetone alone or combined with a few drops of a saturated solution of magnesium chlorid in alcohol. There was no peritoneal inflammation. From the subcutaneous tissue of the other cat about 3 gm. of free oil were recovered and this gave no lecithin precipitate. Nearly all the oil remaining in the tissue was in the form of emulsion.

### METHOD OF INJECTION

An all-glass syringe which could be carefully cleaned and sterilized was used. This gave an accurate gauge of the rapidity of injection. Comparatively fine needles were found to allow the passage of oil at sufficient speed. The skin was prepared for injection, both in cats and man, by placing a drop of 10 per cent. tincture of iodin on the desired spot. In animals under long experimentation all injections were given into the dorsal region, which was arbitrarily divided into eight injection places, in order to develop the absorbing capacity of the subcutaneous tissues to the largest possible extent.

The needle-point was inserted between the subcutaneous fat and the muscular aponeurosis below and when correctly placed could be moved about without obstruction. When beginning injection the development of a tiny globe of oil about the needle-point was carefully watched for, as indicating that the needle was not placed in the lumen of some blood-vessel.[11]

Injection was performed very slowly in order to avoid distention and consequent pain. About 20 gm. of plain oil or its equivalent in emulsion was the average quantity given, and when it was correctely administered the animal needed no restraint beyond having its head stroked. In man single slow injections of about 60 gm. could be tolerated without discom-

11. The work of Graham (Jour. Med. Research, 1907, xvi, 459), shows that plain oil injected into the ear vein of rabbits causes death by cerebral or pulmonary embolism after doses of 1 c.c. of plain oil for every 1,100 gm. weight.

fort. Beyond that point, however, the distention caused pain and when the experiment called for larger dosage multiple injections were given.

After withdrawal of the needle the oil was gently massaged away until no evidences of injection remained. So rapid is the diffusion of oil through the tissue spaces that gentle massage accomplished this result usually within a minute.

### DIFFUSION OF OILS THROUGH THE TISSUE SPACES

In all cases in which daily injections of over 30 c.c. of oil were given, careful palpation of the lowest part of the abdomen and of the groins soon showed the tissue to be thickened by accumulations of oil which could be transferred by massage in the direction toward which pressure was exerted. If very large injections were given the accumulations of oil produced elephantoid legs and thighs, from which the oil could be temporarily massaged. This seepage through the tissue is not peculiar to oil, for in anasarca the greatest collections of fluid lie in the dependent parts and autopsies after hypodermoclyses show a similar gravitation. The difference is merely one of degree, in that movement of oil along the fascial planes is much more rapid. Careful palpation also disclosed the fact that a gradual hypertrophy of the inguinal lymph-nodes occurred. This was most rapid and pronounced in injected cats that were well fed, and unusually marked in those cases in which peanut oil was used. Hypertrophy did not occur to any noticeable extent in starving animals in which plain oils were used, a difference possibly ascribable to the lack of protein material for constructive processes in the latter animals.

### METHOD OF TISSUE SEPARATION: AUTOPSY FINDINGS

At the end of the injection period each animal was killed by etherization and a complete separation of the different tissues made, in a dissection which seldom took less than five hours. The subcutaneous fat with its content of oil was dissected from muscle and skin, and preserved separately. The first case showed that muscular action, gravity and lymphatic absorption had carried a large amount of oil deep into and between the muscular layers of the abdomen and lower thorax, and made obvious the need for complete separate extraction of the skeletal muscles, the entire subcutaneous tissue and the skin and hair. Included in the group of skeleton and skeletal muscles were the cord, genitalia, bladder, the diaphragm, the contents of the posterior mediastinum, and the entire deep lymphatic system. The superficial lymph-glands were included with the subcutaneous fat.

When the thorax was opened—and this was always done with clean instruments—in nearly every case following the prolonged use of oil, each lower intercostal space was seen to carry a lymphatic vessel dilated with very fluid oil. On removal of the heart and lungs, these tributaries were found to unite with a dilated tortuous trunk having a wall like tissue-paper. This occupied the position of the thoracic duct. Osmic acid and the microscope showed that its content was thin plain oil in which occasional fat-filled leukocytes were seen.

In all such cases the bronchial lymphatic glands in the posterior mediastinal space were hypertrophied and yielded thin plain oil on section. The pericardium was separated and saved for extraction and comparison with the rest of the internal fats of the body, these being mesentery, omentum, the perirenal and pelvic fats, and the fat which fills in the point of muscular deficiency in the diaphragm and which is designated as diaphragmatic. This last fat is frequently absent after starvation.

The abdomen was opened through the diaphragm to prevent any possible contamination with oil. Whenever instruments were soiled with oil they were replaced at once. The omentum was dissected absolutely clear from the stomach and duodenum, the mesentery carefully freed from the intestine down to the anus and each preserved separately. In this separation the spleen was removed and with much difficulty the pancreas, usually in one large and several smaller accessory portions. Lying behind, on, and sometimes in the pancreatic tissue, an enlarged oil-carrying lymphatic gland was frequently found. Its enucleation required much care to prevent the pancreas from becoming contaminated. This gland apparently connected with the pelvic glands via the vena cava inferior, and seemed to empty directly into the receptaculum chyli. The gullet, stomach and intestine were removed together, the contents carefully pressed out, weighed, and this weight deducted from the body weight taken immediately after death. The intestine was then split and washed out carefully. The pelvic lymph-nodes were usually much hypertrophied and colored with oil which exuded on section. The kidneys were decapsulated and their capsules added to the perirenal and pelvic fat, which were removed together, as they have physical continuity, are identical on inspection, and give identical iodin reactions.

In the smaller animals the perirenal fat is separated by a very thin musculo-aponeurotic layer from a layer of fat lying in Petit's triangle, here a very long, narrow affair. This latter fat is invariably mixed with oil and without careful separation may easily be included with the perirenal fat and give incorrect extraction results. None of the previous observers has stated what precautions were used to prevent contamination of visceral and natural fat tissue; the most scrupulous care has to be taken throughout the entire dissection, else admixture with oil is reasonably sure. All of the viscera were immediately placed in 95 per cent. alcohol.

In a number of similar dissections the most noteworthy point was the general hypertrophy and complete saturation with oil of all the glands of the lymphatic system. In the use of peanut oil the superficial inguinal nodes reached diameters of 2 by 3 cm. and their lymph-courses were dilated by oil carriage to channels of 0.1 to 0.4 cm. diameter.

In several cats the connection of the lymphatics of the anterior intercostal spaces and the so-called suspensory ligament of the diaphragm was well shown, the former, where it joins diaphragm and thoracic wall, receiving oil from the latter and distinctly transmitting it to the upper mediastinal glands. The presence of oil in the lung tissue was noticed several times. In one case in which lard had been given, the lung was cut twenty-four hours after death, and lard was squeezed from the cut surface. This was verified by the greasiness, solubility in ether and microscopic examination. No evidences of infarction were found.

In some cats the oil in the subcutaneous tissue seemed almost on the point of being built into the fat cells. These are enlarged and suggest the cells of a grape-fruit with their thick spindle shape. Whether this is preliminary to absorption, or merely a soaking through fibrous tissue wall, there is no present means of knowing, but the latter seems more probable.

The tissues under separate investigation were:

I. Subcutaneous fat
II. Skin and hair
III. Skeleton and skeletal muscles
IV. Viscera
  1. Liver
  2. Kidneys
  3. Heart
  4. Lungs
  5. Spleen
  6. Pancreas
  7. Stomach and Intestines
V. Natural Fats
  1. Omentum
  2. Mesentery
  3. Pericardial fat
  4. Perirenal and pelvic fat
  5. Diaphragmatic fat
VI. Blood
VII. Feces

METHOD OF EXTRACTION

The method of extraction best adapted to our purposes was the alcohol-ether method of Otto Frank.[12] The saponification method of Libermann and Székely[13] and of Kumagawa and Suto[14] gives closer results where the more complex fats are sought. Residues left after ether extraction were treated by the saponification method and negative or negligible results obtained. In the method used there is no doubt of the completeness of the extraction of all of the foreign fats, all of which are easily soluble in ether. Again the results are strictly comparable, as they were

12. Frank, Otto: Ztschr. f. Biol., 1897, xxxv, 549. Voit, E., ibid., 1897, xxxv, 549.

13. Liebermann and Székely: Arch. f. d. gesamte Physiol., lxii, 360.

14. Kumagawa and Suto: Muneo Kumagawa and Kenzo Suto: Biochem. Ztschr., 1907-1908, viii, 212-347.

obtained in the same manner and under the same conditions. All results are given as "ether extract," for, as is well known, in addition to the triglycerids of the fatty acids, such bodies as the cholesterins, the lecithins and other phosphatids are extracted with the true fats. The fragmented tissue was covered with 95 per cent. alcohol and evaporated to dryness three times in a steam bath. As the point of dryness was approached the heat was turned off so that the temperature, kept considerably below 100 C., did not volatilize any possible volatile acid present. The final drying was done on a hot plate at 96 C. to 98 C.[15]

For ether extraction the whole of each viscus, natural fat and subcutaneous fat was used. A 20-gm. sample of the skin and hair, and 40 gm. of the powdered skeleton and muscle were taken and the total ether extract calculated from the result. All specimens, placed in Schleicher and Scholl fat-free capsules, were extracted for twenty-four hours in Soxhlet extractors, and the ether was then boiled from the flasks in a steam bath. Finally the flasks were placed in a hot air chamber for eight hours at 98 C. They were weighed when cool.

### METHOD OF DETERMINATION OF AMOUNT OF OIL ABSORBED

The iodin values of the extract of the skin and hair,[16] subcutaneous fat and oil, and of skeleton and muscle were obtained, and by plotting a chart the proportions of foreign oil to normal cat fat were easily determined. Subtraction of the amount of foreign oil thus calculated, from the amount of oil given, may fairly be said to give the amount of oil utilized. After repeated examinations of natural fat and visceral extracts by the Halphen or furfurol tests, I have been unable to find any evidence of deposit in these tissues of unchanged cotton-seed or sesame oils, and therefore consider the assumption of utilization (meaning by this either combustion or conversion to body fat) to be logical.

Iodin indices were obtained from the ether extracts of the separate organs and tissues of three normal cats and of one starved cat which lived thirty-seven days. These indices were used as the basis of calculation in superposition and starvation experiments respectively, for in starving

15. Without complete dehydration the water remaining will dissolve mineral salts from the tissue during ether extraction and this will produce high weight and low iodin values.

16. Hanus' modification of Hübl's method (Bulletin No. 107. Revised. U. S. Dept. of Agriculture, Bureau of Chemistry, 1908) was used. The iodin value of a fat is the weight of iodin which 100 parts of the fat will absorb, or it may be the parts by weight of either of the other halogens, chlorin and bromin, expressed in chemically equivalent terms of iodin. There is a direct addition of the halogen to the molecule which takes place only with unsaturated compounds and is due mainly to the two unsaturated valencies of the oleic acid radicle of the fat.

injected cats, the indices approached more nearly to those of the starvation content than of the normal well-nourished controls.

The results of extraction and the iodin values of the tissues of the control animals used as a basis for calculation are shown in Table 2.

TABLE 2.—ETHER EXTRACT AND IODIN IN NORMAL AND STARVED CATS

| | Ether Extract in Grams | | | | | Iodin Indices | | | | |
|---|---|---|---|---|---|---|---|---|---|---|
| | Normal cats | | | | Starvation | Normal cats | | | | Starvation |
| Tissue | Cat 27 | Cat 41 | Cat 64 | Normal Av. | Cat 13 | Cat 27 | Cat 41 | Cat 64 | Normal Av. | Cat 13 |
| Subcutaneous fat | 15.41 | 78.75 | 78.91 | 51.7 | 0.234 | 64.0 | 58.2 | 67.3 | 63.1 | 78.7 |
| Skin and hair | 15.67 | 13.36 | 23.69 | 17.6 | 6.680 | 54.1 | 50.0 | 55.0 | 53.0 | 50.0 |
| Skeleton and muscle | 84.63 | 125.83 | 130.57 | 113.7 | 12.620 | 65.4 | 64.3 | 65.1 | 64.9 | 71.0 |
| Total | 115.71 | 217.94 | 233.17 | 184.0 | 19.53 | .... | .... | .... | .... | .... |

The total amount of ether extract of the entire body amounted to 1.42 per cent. of the end weight in the starved cat and to 4.83 per cent. in Cat 27, 7.55 per cent. in Cat 41, and 9.05 per cent. in Cat 64, a very fat animal.

Any method in which average figures are applied to individual instances is likely to be misleading, but that the error here is slight the following calculations will show.

The extraction results of the tissues containing unchanged oil in an animal which had been injected with 469 gm. of cotton-seed oil during twenty-three days of starvation were as given in Table 3.

TABLE 3.—EXTRACTION RESULTS OF TISSUES IN ANIMAL INJECTED WITH 469 GM. OF COTTON-SEED OIL DURING TWENTY-THREE DAYS OF STARVATION

| Tissue. | Ether Extract. gm. | Iodin Index. |
|---|---|---|
| Subcutaneous oil and fat | 70.027 | 110 |
| Subcutaneous fat | 43.480 | 109 |
| Skin and hair | 41.850 | 101.8 |
| Skeleton and muscle | 65.270 | 97.5 |
| Total | 220.63 | ..... |

To calculate the amount of foreign oil in the subcutaneous tissue, a chart was plotted with the index of normal subcutaneous fat extract, 63.1, and of the cotton-seed oil used, 111. On this line the iodin indices, 110 and 109, show 98 per cent. and 95.7 per cent. respectively of the ether extract to be cotton-seed oil. Replacing the figure of normal subcutaneous tissue by that of the starvation animal the percentages become 97 and 94 respectively. Similar comparison of the other tissues leads to the results given in Table 4.

TABLE 4.—CALCULATED OIL RECOVERED, USING NORMAL AND STARVATION FIGURES

| Tissue. | Normal. | Starvation. |
|---|---|---|
| | gm. | gm. |
| Subcutaneous fat........ | 110.24 | 108.80 |
| Skin and hair........... | 34.65 | 35.07 |
| Skeleton and muscle..... | 46.01 | 43.08 |
| Total............. | 190.90 | 186.95 |
| Oil given............... | 469 | 469 |
| Oil recovered............ | 191 | 187 |
| Oil utilized............. | 278 | 282 |
| Grams per day.......... | 12.08 | 12.26 |
| Calories per day......... | 112.4 | 114.0 |

From these results it seems reasonable to assume that the error in such calculation is very slight.

## INJECTION OF PLAIN OIL IN STARVATION

Sesame, peanut, olive, cotton-seed and human oils were used in this work, and while it is unfortunate that complete extraction was made of but one animal, the clinical pictures and autopsy findings were so constant for the entire group that at the time of experiment but one typical extraction was considered necessary.

Cat 4, a very fat cat weighing 3.91 kilos, was given 347 gm. of plain cotton-seed oil subcutaneously over a period of fourteen days, no other food being administered. Rapidly progressive accumulation and weakness were apparent after the ninth day, and the animal was found dead in its cage on the morning of the fifteenth day. Its appearance was characteristic, in that the upper part of the body was much wasted, while the legs, root of tail and the abdomen were those of a very large, robust animal. The loss in weight was 27.6 per cent. in fourteen days.

Autopsy showed that protein starvation was the fundamental cause of death, for the muscles were remarkably wasted and flabby for an animal so shortly in good health, and microscopically were characteristic of starvation. The duration of life was too short to dissipate the large internal masses of normal cat-fat to any great extent. Their somewhat high iodin indices, which appear below, indicate that enough combustion of fat of low iodin value had occurred to make appreciable the alteration in the normal proportions of the ordinary triglycerids and of the lecithins. The total true tissue extract was 8.8 per cent. of the true body weight at the close of the experiment, the true weight in all cases being the end weight less oil recovered. "True tissue extract" may be considered as "cat-fat" characteristic of the animal. Of 347 gm. of oil injected, 317, as shown in Table 5, were recovered, a utilization of 2.14 gm. or 20 calories a day.

TABLE 5.—TISSUE EXTRACT IN CAT 4

| Structure. | Ether Extract. gm. | Iodin Index. | Cotton-Seed Oil. gm. | True Tissue Extract. gm. |
|---|---|---|---|---|
| Subcutaneous fat and oil... | 171.82 | 95.2 | 87.63 | 84.2 |
| Skin and hair ............ | 74.07 | 82.3 | 39.4 | 34.7 |
| Skeleton and muscle....... | 224.03 | 105.0 | 109.4 | 33.6 |
| Total................. | 469.92 | ..... | 317.4 | 1525. |

These figures are perhaps emphasized by the partial extraction results of a similarly treated cat, No. 57, into which 369 gm. of sesame oil were injected during twenty days. This cat lost 25 per cent. of its weight, the end weight including the unabsorbed fat still in the tissue, against a loss of 19 per cent. in the previous animal weighed under similar conditions. From the subcutaneous tissue alone 121 gm. of sesame oil were recovered. The furfurol test for sesame oil applied to the ether extracts of the lung, omentum, perirenal and pericardial fats, was negative in each case. These figures suggest corroboration of the results obtained with Cat 4, but when combined with the clinical and autopsy findings, they lead to the conclusion that except for the slight differences in the *specific absorbability* of the various fixed oils, the amount of utilization of these fixed oils in absolute starvation is negligible.[17]

The sharp attack on the protein tissue of the body in starvation is accompanied by a diminution of all the visceral functions. The digestive juices are no longer secreted, and since some lipase or other similar enzyme must be used for the transference of outlying fat to the liver, further production of these enzymes must take place at the expense of still further protein destruction. On the other hand, the need for enzymes with emulsified oils is minimized, for the oil is in a physical state which makes entrance to the small-calibered lymphatics easier.[18] It was further noticed that oils thrown out of emulsion by tissue action seemed much more fluid and lighter-colored than before emulsification, which was possibly the result of an intimate mixture with tissue fluid. Such oil dried in the hot-air chamber lost about 5 per cent. of its weight by evaporation in eight hours.

## INJECTION OF EMULSIFIED OILS AND FATS IN STARVATION

Cat 5, weighing 3 kilos, received daily injections of 20 gm. of cottonseed oil in 66.5 per cent. emulsion containing 5 per cent. lecithin during a starvation period of twenty-three days. On account of protein loss there was a steady reduction in weight, progressive emaciation and, after

17. By "specific absorbability of oils" is meant the characteristics of oils which make them more diffusible through the tissue spaces and consequently more easily absorbable, as well as to characteristics such as the stimulation to vigorous lymph-node hypertrophy which peanut oil seems to produce.

18. The lymphocytes may take part in this.

the nineteenth day, great muscular weakness. Accumulation of oil was first noticed on the fifteenth day. In twenty-three days 1.39 kilos were lost by the animal, 44 per cent. of its original weight. The results of extraction were as given in Table 6.

TABLE 6.—RESULTS OF EXTRACTION IN CAT 5

| Tissue. | Ether Extract. | Iodin Index. | Cotton-Seed Oil. | True Tissue Extract. |
|---|---|---|---|---|
| | gm. | | gm. | gm. |
| Subcutaneous oil (and fat)* | 70.03 | 110.0 | 108.8 | 4.7 |
| Subcutaneous fat | 43.48 | 109.0 | | |
| Skin and hair | 41.85 | 101.8 | 35.1 | 6.7 |
| Skeleton and muscle | 65.27 | 97.5 | 43.1 | 22.2 |
| Total | 220.62 | ..... | 187.0 | 33.6 |

* As directly withdrawn on autopsy.

Of 469 gm. injected, 187 were recovered and 282 were utilized, giving a daily absorption figure of 12.26 gm. or 114 calories, about half of the energy requirement of this animal. The total true tissue extract was 3 per cent. of the true end weight.

This experiment was repeated, using an emulsion of lard as a contrast to the vegetable oils, with the idea that more closely related animal fats might be more easily taken up by animal tissue. The omenta of several freshly slaughtered hogs were tried out by continuous jets of steam and 446 gm. of the resultant lard were injected in the form of a 72 per cent. emulsion during sixteen days. The animal was starved and lost weight steadily, as in all similar experiments, but no accumulation could be ascertained until the injection was increased from 35 to 70 c.c. a day. Following the appearance of marked accumulation the animal's weakness increased and the experiment was closed under anesthesia at the end of the sixteenth day. The index of the lard used was 57, which made it impossible to employ the ordinary method of calculation. Accordingly the extraction figures of four cats, similarly starved and injected with vegetable oils during a similar period were averaged for each group of the tissues and the average figure used, the results being given in Table 7.

TABLE 7.—RESULTS OF EXTRACTION IN CAT 26

| Structure. | Ether Extract. | Iodin Index. | Average Tissue Ether Extract. | Calculated Weight of Lard Recovered. |
|---|---|---|---|---|
| | gm. | | gm. | gm. |
| Subcutaneous fat and oil | 93.11 | 59 | 17.32 | 75.79 |
| Skin and hair | 42.35 | 50 | 12.30 | 30.09 |
| Skeleton and muscle | 77.36 | 56.3 | 12.70 | 64.63 |
| Total | 212.82 | .... | 42.32 | 170.50 |

By this calculation we find 170 gm. recovered, giving a daily utilization of over 17 gm. or over 160 calories. This corresponds with what the dissection promised. Should this be considered an excessively high result, it will be found on estimating the entire ether extract as unabsorbed lard that 233 gm. of lard must have been utilized in sixteen days, 14.5 gm. per day or 135 calories, a large amount in an animal whose total requirement was not greater than 210 calories a day.

The results obtained from the use of lard and from brief, but to me, equally conclusive experiments with human oil and to a lesser extent with butter, suggest that the fats whose chemical characteristics are similar to those of man may be much more readily absorbable than other fats, and that specific absorbability may be found to depend in a measure on the closeness of chemical resemblance which an injected fat bears to the fat of the host.[19]

## INJECTION OF PLAIN OIL IN CONDITIONS OF PROTEIN INGESTION

The cats of this entire series were fed with about 70 gm. of lean beef heart daily, or about a third of the average energy requirement, with the object of preventing part of the protein waste while forcing the animal to live mainly on its own and the foreign fat.

The series is unfortunately incomplete, for no complete extractions were made of cats injected with plain oils under such conditions of nutrition. Clinically and at autopsy the absorption results seemed slightly better than those following the use of plain oils in absolute starvation, but not sufficiently better to warrant the laborious separation and extraction.

## INJECTION OF EMULSIFIED OILS IN CONDITIONS OF PROTEIN INGESTION

Cat 14, weighing 2.8 kilos, received 627 gm. of cotton-seed oil in 66.5 per cent. emulsion with 5 per cent. lecithin over a period of thirty-four days. Up to the twenty-fourth day the cat remained fairly vigorous, but weakness and accumulation of oil in the tissues had become moderately marked when the animal was killed at the close of the thirty-fourth day.

Autopsy disclosed moderate amounts of fat in the natural adipose tissues. The subcutaneous and structural extracts gave a brilliant Halphen reaction,[20] denoting the presence of cotton-seed oil which, however, was given by none of the visceral or internal adipose fat extracts. The results of extraction were as given in Table 8.

19. In this connection R. L. Sutton (Brit. Med. Jour., May 23, 1908, p. 1225), reports experiments tending to show that animal fats, and especially lard, are much better absorbed through the unbroken skin than vegetable oils.

20. Bull. 107, Revised, Bureau of Chemistry, U. S. Dept. Agric.

TABLE 8.—RESULTS OF EXTRACTION IN CAT 14*

| Structure. | Ether Extract. | Iodin Index. | Cotton-Seed Oil. | True Tissue Extract. |
|---|---|---|---|---|
| | gm. | | gm. | gm. |
| Subcutaneous fat and oil | 229.50 | 110 | 222.50 | 7.00 |
| Skin and hair | 50.30 | 90.6 | 33.45 | 16.85 |
| Skeleton and muscle | 64.54 | 63.0 | 2.00 | 62.54 |
| Total | 344.34 | ..... | 257.95 | 86.39 |

* In this and in several other cases the muscles had been washed practically free of cotton-seed oil by rinsing with ether. This, of course, lowers the iodin index to a figure so approximately normal as to make the small content of oil remaining incalculable by this method. In each of such cases 2 gm. would probably be an excessive allowance and this is the amount arbitrarily chosen.

Of the 627 gm. of oil given, 369 were utilized, or 10.85 gm. per day, the equivalent of 100 calories. The weight at the end of the experiment, less recovered oil, was 2,016 kilos, a loss of 0.784 kilos, or 28 per cent. The true tissue ether extract made 7.4 per cent. of the true end weight.

A similar result, under the same food conditions, was shown by Cat 10, which was given 560 gm. of olive oil in a 71.5 per cent. emulsion containing 3.5 per cent. lecithin during thirty-two days. It was killed with ether while still moderately active.

TABLE 9.—RESULTS OF EXTRACTION IN CAT 10

| Structure. | Ether Extract. | Iodin Index. | Olive Oil. | True Tissue Extract. |
|---|---|---|---|---|
| | gm. | | gm. | gm. |
| Subcutaneous fat and oil | 110.870 | 83.5 | 62.090 | 47.780 |
| Skin and hair | 55.097 | 78.4 | 41.322 | 13.775 |
| Skeleton and muscle | 47.610 | 76.8 | 16.664 | 30.946 |
| Total | 213.57 | .... | 120.07 | 93.50 |

Five hundred and sixty-six grams of oil were given and 120 gm. recovered (Table 9), a daily utilization of 13.97 gm. or 131 calories; but here, as in the previous experiment, not enough protein was given to check the protein waste, and the weight fell from 3.53 kilos to 2.83 kilos, a loss of 20 per cent. The total true tissue extract was 3.6 per cent. of the end weights, less the oil recovered.

These experiments are interpreted to mean that the comparatively large amount of fat absorbed was directly burned for heat and energy with a corresponding sparing of normal tissue fat, or that the foreign fat was broken down in the liver and resynthesized into cat-fat, which was transferred to the tissue and used as needed.[21]

21. The work of J. B. Leathes (Lancet, London, 1909, i, 593), of J. Rosenfeld (Ergebn. d. Physiol., 1902, p. 673) and of A. Lebedeff (Arch. f. d. ges. Physiol., 1883, xxxi, 11) on this point in normal digestive processes and in pathological conditions is of great interest.

### SUBCUTANEOUS INJECTION OF PLAIN OIL SUPERIMPOSED ON A NORMAL MIXED DIET

Cat 45, weighing 3.2 kilos, was fed a rich mixed diet and was injected with 369 gm. of plain cotton-seed oil during twenty days. The cat remained perfectly well and gained 18 per cent. in weight, excluding the weight of the oil recovered.

Table 10.—Results of Extraction in Cat 45

| Structure. | Ether Extract. gm. | Iodin Index. | Cotton-Seed Oil. gm. | True Tissue Extract. gm. |
|---|---|---|---|---|
| Subcutaneous fat and oil .... | 252.80 | 95. | 167.4 | 83.4 |
| Skin and hair.............. | 37.62 | 73. | 13.0 | 24.6 |
| Skeleton and muscle......... | 116.09 | 68. | 8.1 | 108.0 |
| Total.................. | 406.50 | ... | 190.5 | 216.0 |

One hundred and ninety grams were recovered (Table 10) of the 369 gm. of oil injected, giving a daily utilization of 8.95 gm. or 83 calories. No Halphen reaction was obtainable from the extracts of the internal fats.

A similar although more marked result followed the injection of 669 gm. of plain peanut oil similarly superimposed on a rich mixed diet. The animal weighed 3.2 kilos and gained 27 per cent. in thirty-six days. The inguinal lymph-nodes were remarkably hypertrophied and the lymphatics and thoracic duct contained considerable amounts of free oil in process of transference from the subcutaneous spaces. The extraction results were as given in Table 11.

Table 11.—Results of Extraction in Cat 63

| Structure. | Ether Extract. gm. | Iodin Index. | Peanut Oil. gm. | True Tissue Extract. gm. |
|---|---|---|---|---|
| Subcutaneous fat and oil..... | 285.00 | 78.3 | 182.4 | 102.6 |
| Skin and hair............. | 37.77 | 71.0 | 20.4 | 17.4 |
| Skeleton and muscle......... | 146.50 | 71.4 | 35.2 | 111.3 |
| Total.................. | 469.27 | .... | 238.0 | 231.3 |

Of 662 gm. injected, 238 were recovered, giving a daily utilization amount of 11.77 gm. or 109 calories.

At the start of this experiment the animal was an average-sized, well-nourished cat. At autopsy its fat depots were found to be extraordinarily well filled with normal cat-fat, the amount of omental fat extract being twice as great as the largest normal extraction figure, and the subcutaneous, perirenal and diaphragmatic weights appreciably above the highest normal results.

This case presents additional evidence of the utilization of oil so administered and undoubtedly means that most of the fat entering the system after intestinal absorption was deposited as cat-fat, the foreign oil supplying the heat and energy necessary.[22]

The quite different results which follow the injection of plain oils superimposed on a rich mixed diet, results seen both in starvation and in very low protein feeding, bear out the supposition that the slight absorption of plain oils in starvation is due to lessened or absent enzyme formation and action, for with the lymphatic apparatus equally open to absorption in both instances, absorption of plain oils occurs in practically utilizable amounts only where there is a sufficient protein supply or sufficient glandular activity to furnish enzymes to act on the oil.

### SUBCUTANEOUS INJECTION OF EMULSIONS SUPERIMPOSED ON A NORMAL MIXED DIET

Cat 39, weighing 2.48 kilos, was fed with more than its requirement in fat, meat and milk, covering a period of twenty-three days, during which it received 270 gm. of cotton-seed oil in the form of a 66.5 per cent. emulsion containing 5 per cent. lecithin. During the experiment the animal became ill with a nasopharyngitis and was unable to eat or to drink for four days, during which time it lost 0.38 kilos.[23] This was more than regained, the final weight being 2.86 kilos, a gain of 15.4 per cent. of the original weight and 30 per cent. of the weight after illness. At the close of the experiment the cat was very active, ate well and gave every evidence of excellent health.

Table 12.—Results of Extraction in Cat 39

| Structure. | Ether Extract. gm. | Iodin Index. | Cotton-Seed Oil. gm. | True Tissue Extract. gm. |
|---|---|---|---|---|
| Subcutaneous fat and oil.... | 121.200 | 96.5 | 83.63 | 37.57 |
| Skin and hair.............. | 49.775 | 70.0 | 14.44 | 35.34 |
| Skeleton and muscle........ | 80.627 | 64.3 | 2.00 | 78.63 |
| Total................... | 251.602 | .... | 100.07 | 151.54 |

One hundred of the 270 gm. of oil given were recovered from the cat's body, which indicated a daily utilization of 7.4 gm. or 68 calories (Table 12). No Halphen reaction could be obtained from the visceral or internal fats. The total true tissue extract was 6.7 per cent. of the true body weight.

22. It might be highly significant to repeat this experiment under conditions of accurate calorimetry in order to contrast the amount of carbon excreted with the carbon content of the foreign oil used, the latter being determined by complete extraction of the animal.

23. All our animals under experiment at the time were ill with epidemic rhinitis and pharyngitis, which affected cats receiving oil with the same intensity as control untreated cats.

The smaller utilization of foreign fat was probably due to the smaller demand for fat as food. The foreign absorbed fat was apparently burned to spare the normal fat.

To determine the influence of the intercurrent illness and enforced starvation on the absorption, the experiment was repeated using the same diet.

Three hundred and thirty-one grams of peanut oil in a 67.5 per cent. emulsion containing 3.5 per cent. lecithin were injected into Cat 36, weighing 2.68 kilos, during twenty-six days. The cat remained perfectly well but gained only 0.1 kilo. Autopsy showed well-filled fat depots, but the total true tissue extract was only 4.5 per cent. of the end weight, although the utilization figure was practically identical with that of the previous experiment.

Table 13.—Results of Extraction in Cat 36

| Structure. | Ether Extract. gm. | Iodin Index. | Peanut Oil. gm. | True Tissue Extract. gm. |
|---|---|---|---|---|
| Subcutaneous fat and oil..... | 125.300 | 82.5 | 102.1 | 23.2 |
| Skin and hair.............. | 39.263 | 71.2 | 20.8 | 18.5 |
| Skeleton and muscle......... | 79.210 | 69.6 | 16.5 | 62.7 |
| Total.................. | 243.773 | .... | 139.4 | 104.4 |

One hundred and forty grams of the 331 gm. injected were recovered, giving a daily utilization of 7.35 gm. or 69 calories (Table 13). The absorbability of oils is still further demonstrated by these experiments in superimposition and the fact elicited that under such conditions plain oils are somewhat more absorbable than emulsified oils.

## INJECTION OF EMULSIONS SUBJECTED TO LIPOLYSIS

An emulsion of 70 per cent. cotton-seed oil with 4 per cent. lecithin was subjected to digestion by a very active lipase for half an hour, after which the lipase action was inhibited by heating to 60 C. In amounts above 0.1 per cent. the emulsion was broken up by digestion, but from 0.1 per cent. to 0.05 per cent. the emulsion remained perfect, although microscopically the fat globules showed considerable digestive fragmentation.

Emulsions treated with lipase in proportions from 0.05 per cent. to 1 per cent., in which after sufficient digestion the lipase was destroyed by heat, were injected into several cats. The object was to ascertain whether the chemical products of lipolysis of oils given subcutaneously were irritating and to what extent, if any, they were absorbable. The following experiment is typical of the result.

Cat 15, weighing 3.77 kilos, was given 23 gm. of cotton-seed oil daily for seven days, in the form of an emulsion subjected to the action of

0.2 per cent. lipase for two hours. The intention had been to superimpose this injection on normal feeding, but from the first injection the animal refused food, soon became careless of habit and showed such evidences of toxic effect that it was killed at the end of the seventh day. The weight had fallen 20 per cent. Complete extraction showed that 8.3 gm. of oil had been utilized daily. As there was no great evidence of local irritation it was at first supposed that the lipase had split the lecithin and that cholin poisoning had resulted. Analogous results were given, however, by plain oil similarly lipolyzed, and hence the constitutional and local effects may have been due in both forms of injection to the production and action of free oleic acid, possibly with the formation of minute quantities of toxic soaps. No evidences of hemolysis were seen.

From the experience with oils subjected to lipolysis it is obvious therefore that their practical utilization is prevented by the production of toxic substances formed during their preparation. Table 14 shows the utilization of foreign fats administered subcutaneously to cats, including only those animals which were completely extracted

TABLE 14.—UTILIZATION OF FOREIGN FATS ADMINISTERED SUBCUTANEOUSLY TO CATS WHICH WERE COMPLETELY EXTRACTED

| Cat. | Oil Used. | Days of Injection. | Fat Injected. gm. | Fat Utilized. Total. gm. | Fat Utilized. Per Day. gm. |
|---|---|---|---|---|---|
| | STARVATION | | | | |
| 4 | Plain cotton-seed | 14 | 347.0 | 30.0 | 2.1 |
| 5 | Cotton-seed emulsion | 23 | 469.0 | 282.0 | 12.3 |
| 9 | Olive oil emulsion | 16 | 332.0 | 94.0 | 5.9 |
| 11 | Olive oil emulsion | 5 | 117.0 | 54.5 | 10.9 |
| 16 | Olive oil emulsion | 10 | 214.0 | 84.0 | 8.4 |
| 23 | Cotton-seed emulsion | 14 | 274.0 | 101.0 | 7.2 |
| 26 | Lard emulsion | 16 | 446.0 | 276.0 | 17.3 |
| 32 | Human oil emulsion | 11 | 212.0 | 56.0 | 5.1 |
| 15 | Lipolyzed cotton-seed emulsion | 7 | 164.0 | 58.0 | 8.3 |
| | LOW PROTEIN DIET | | | | |
| 10 | Olive oil emulsion | 32 | 566.0 | 46.0 | 13.97 |
| 12 | Olive oil emulsion | 17 | 311.0 | 136.0 | 8.00 |
| 14 | Cotton-seed emulsion | 34 | 627.0 | 369.0 | 10.85 |
| 30 | Sesame emulsion | 13 | 187.0 | 120.0 | 9.66 |
| 34 | Corn oil emulsion | 13 | 139.0 | 85.0 | 6.50 |
| 44 | Liquid petrolatum emulsion | 15 | 172.0 | 44.0 | 3.00 |
| | FULL MIXED DIET | | | | |
| 35 | Sesame emulsion | 26 | 289.0 | 148.0 | 5.70 |
| 36 | Peanut oil emulsion | 26 | 331.0 | 191.0 | 7.35 |
| 39 | Cotton-seed emulsion | 23 | 270.0 | 170.0 | 7.40 |
| 43 | Peanut oil emulsion | 17 | 211.0 | 95.0 | 5.60 |
| 45 | Plain cotton-seed | 20 | 369.0 | 179.0 | 8.95 |
| 63 | Plain peanut oil | 36 | 662.0 | 424.0 | 11.77 |

## INFLUENCE OF INJECTED OILS ON THE VISCERAL FATS AND THE INTERNAL ADIPOSE TISSUE FATS

The influence on the internal fats of oils absorbed after injection was first sought by an experiment on two animals of approximately the same weight and given the same normal mixed diet over the same period, one receiving injections of plain peanut oil.

Cat 63, an animal in good nutrition, was given 662 gm. of plain peanut oil in thirty-six days, during which time, as extraction proved, 424 gm. of this oil were utilized. The animal's weight rose from 3.203 kilos to a final weight of 4.32 kilos. The recovered oil weighed 238 gm. Hence the true weight was 4.08 kilos, a gain of 27 per cent. during the period.

Cat 64, an animal in good condition, and weighing 3.556 kilos, was given the same full mixed diet over the same period. This cat ate quite as heartily as its fellow and gained 0.324 kilo or 8.3 per cent. The two animals were killed at the same time, dissected on the same day and extracted simultaneously. The results are given in Table 15.

TABLE 15.—RESULTS OF EXTRACTION

| Organ or Tissue | Fresh Weight Cat 63 | Fresh Weight Cat 64 | Dry Weight Cat 63 | Dry Weight Cat 64 | Weight o[f] Ether Extra[ct] Cat 63 | Weight o[f] Ether Extra[ct] Cat |
|---|---|---|---|---|---|---|
| Liver | 159.5 | 113.0 | 53.0 | 43.0 | 5.35 | 4 |
| Kidneys | 48.3 | 44.7 | 15.0 | 16.4 | 1.60 | 1 |
| Heart | 20.2 | 18.7 | 6.0 | 6.2 | 1.79 | 2 |
| Lungs | 51.2 | 21.0 | 12.2 | 6.3 | 1.44 | [illegible] |
| Spleen | 11.0 | 9.0 | 2.7 | 2.3 | 0.25 | 0 |
| Pancreas | 10.0 | 6.2 | 3.0 | 2.7 | 0.66 | 1 |
| Stomach and intestines | 142.0 | 157.5 | 31.5 | 40.5 | 3.71 | 5 |
| Omentum | 97.5 | 52.5 | 89.2 | 48.7 | 86.32 | 45 |
| Mesentery | 26.7 | 29.5 | 18.5 | 20.2 | 16.60 | 17 |
| Pericardial fat | 10.0 | 10.5 | 5.5 | 6.0 | 3.90 | 4 |
| Perirenal fat | 67.0 | 36.0 | 52.5 | 31.5 | 46.64 | 27 |
| Diaphragmatic fat | 10.0 | 8.1 | 8.0 | 7.6 | 7.62 | 7 |
| Subcutaneous fat and oil | 481.0 | 130.5 | 354.0 | 110.5 | 284.90 | 78 |
| Skin and hair | 373.0 | 481.0 | 193.0 | 230.0 | 37.70 | 23 |
| Skeleton and muscle | 2038.0 | 2390.0 | 701.0 | 805.0 | 146.50 | 130 |
| Total | 3544.0 | 3508.0 | 1545.1 | 1376.9 | 644.98 | 351 |

*10 c.c. blood from Cat 63 gives 0.027 gm. of ether extract; 10 c.c. blood from Cat 64 giv

From this table it is seen that the total fresh weight is about the same in each animal, but that the amount of ether extract is much larger in the animal which had received oil. Deducting the amount of peanut oil recovered from the tissues, or 238 gm., the true fresh weight of the tissues under extraction is 3,306 gm. Also it must be considered that the cat receiving oil was over 200 gm. lighter than the control cat at the start of the experiment. Hence in the injected cat whenever there is any increase or even equalization of the weight of a viscus or in the amount of natural fats, or of the ether extracts as compared with similar tissue in the control, it may reasonably be ascribed to some factor invoked during the period of increase in weight. The single factor in the entire experiment not common to the two animals is that the smaller received injections of oil. Comparison of the weights shows the following points.

1. The originally smaller animal contained over 17 per cent. more ether extract after the amount of oil recovered from the tissue had been deducted. This increase is seen to be greatest in the adipose tissue ether extracts and may therefore be considered as true fat increase.

2. The weights of the liver and of its ether extracts are greater than in the control. This organ[21] is the one most actively engaged in the chemical transformation of fat and the fact that this is the only viscus and the only visceral fat extract which shows an increase over the control is extremely significant.[24]

3. The great internal depositories for fat, the omentum and perirenal, with the pelvic adipose tissues, are nearly twice as full of true fat as in the control. The true subcutaneous tissue extract, 102 gm., is also greater than that of the control.

AT 63 (TREATED) AND CAT 64 (CONTROL)*

| Per Cent. of Ether Extract of Fresh Weight | | Per Cent. of Ether Extract of Dry Weight | | Per Cent. of Ether Extract of Total Tissue Extract | | Per Cent. Ether Extract of Total Fresh Body Weight | | Iodin Index of Ether Extract | |
|---|---|---|---|---|---|---|---|---|---|
| Cat 63 | Cat 64 | Cat 63 | Cat 64 | Cat 63 | Cat 64 | Cat 63 | Cat 64 | Cat 63 | Cat 64 |
| 3.37 | 4.11 | 10.09 | 10.78 | 1.31 | 1.31 | 0.13 | 0.12 | 95 + | 95 + |
| 3.31 | 4.18 | 10.66 | 11.33 | 0.39 | 0.52 | 0.04 | 0.05 | 48.6 | 48.0 |
| 8.88 | 12.24 | 29.75 | 36.93 | 0.44 | 0.65 | 0.04 | 0.06 | 65.0 | 64.0 |
| 2.85 | 7.64 | 11.84 | 25.50 | 0.35 | 0.45 | 0.035 | 0.044 | 89.1 | 69.2 |
| 2.31 | 2.74 | 9.41 | 10.74 | 0.06 | 0.07 | 0.006 | 0.007 | 85.0 | 66.0 |
| 6.63 | 19.51 | 22.10 | 44.81 | 0.16 | 0.34 | 0.016 | 0.034 | 60.0 | 66.0 |
| 2.62 | 3.19 | 11.77 | 12.42 | 0.91 | 1.44 | 0.09 | 0.13 | 73.1 | 68.6 |
| 88.54 | 86.45 | 96.77 | 97.33 | 21.20 | 2.12 | 2.12 | 1.17 | 65.0 | 66.0 |
| 62.17 | 58.38 | 90.00 | 84.25 | 4.10 | 4.86 | 0.41 | 0.47 | 64.6 | 66.0 |
| 39.00 | 39.30 | 70.90 | 68.78 | 0.95 | 1.17 | 0.095 | 0.106 | 65.0 | 60.0 |
| 69.61 | 75.58 | 88.84 | 86.06 | 11.64 | 7.74 | 1.16 | 0.72 | 67.3 | 65.1 |
| 76.20 | 92.40 | 95.25 | 97.43 | 1.89 | 2.10 | 0.19 | 0.19 | 63.5 | 62.0 |
| 59.23 | 66.46 | 80.48 | 91.40 | 25.33 | 22.47 | 2.53 | 2.03 | 78.3 | 67.3 |
| 10.14 | 4.42 | 79.57 | 10.30 | 4.26 | 6.74 | 0.42 | 0.64 | 71.0 | 65.0 |
| 7.13 | 5.46 | 20.90 | 16.22 | 27.60 | 37.19 | 2.76 | 3.65 | 71.4 | 65.1 |

*25 gm. of ether extract.

Comparison of the iodin indices gives further corroboration of the presence of fat of a higher iodin value than that usually found in the fatty tissues after ordinary food fats have been absorbed from the intestine, for the average index of the visceral and internal adipose fats in the injected cat is 67.8 and in the control 60.1. The indices of the spleen and pancreas are much above our highest normal figures, and while this may be due to an uncommonly large proportion of some phosphatid-lipoid, it is more probably due to the same cause which has generally raised the indices.

24. In estimating the iodin indices of ether extracts of the liver it is often very difficult to obtain the exact end reaction point owing to the deep brown color of liver fat. The iodin indices placed at or about 95 are not exact readings and indicate simply that the iodin value was not lower than that figure.

It has long been known and recently been emphasized by Williams and Forsyth[25] that the nature of the fat in the body is determined by the nature of the fat eaten and stored. As a considerable absorption of oil with a high iodin index has been demonstrated in the case of the treated cat under consideration, and as all other experimental conditions were identical, it is but logical, therefore, to conclude that this oil has had a direct influence in generally raising the iodin values of the visceral and adipose tissue fats of the injected animal.

The ether extracts of the blood are not significant. The fat in the rapidly circulating blood-stream under ordinary conditions of health is soon stored and as each specimen was taken from the external jugular vein, the likelihood of a distinct increase in the fat content of blood taken from a point so remote from the place of entry of fat, is slight. No examination of the fat content of the feces was made in these animals. Previous examination of feces from starving and fed cats under treatment and from the controls had shown that the normal fat content of these excreta from each animal was about 16 per cent. and was unaffected by the subcutaneous injections of oils.

The influence on the internal fats of oils given subcutaneously was further demonstrated by comparison of the weights of visceral and adipose tissue, and their ether extracts; also by the iodin indices of the fat of animals which had absorbed enough oil over sufficiently long periods to allow the possibility of an influence. In general this influence was demonstrated for the average index of an organ to be higher in treated animals than in the controls under the same nutritive conditions.

The liver, the most important of the viscera as regards fat storage, distinctly shows the influence of oil injection.

TABLE 16.—RESULTS OF EXTRACTION OF LIVER

| Cat | | Oil Utilized gm. | Days of Treatment | Ether Extract gm. | Iodin Index | Per Cent. of Ether Extract | Per Cent. Total True Fresh Body Weight |
|---|---|---|---|---|---|---|---|
| | STARVATION | | | | | | |
| 13 | Untreated | ... | 37 | 1.79+ | 95. | 7.27 | 0.10 |
| 5 | Cotton-seed emulsion | 282 | 23 | 1.81 | 100. | 4.40 | 0.13 |
| 26 | Lard emulsion | 276 | 16 | 4.72 | 96. | 7.90 | 0.21 |
| | LOW PROTEIN DIET | | | | | | |
| 10 | Olive emulsion | 446 | 32 | 2.82 | 90. | 2.74 | 0.10 |
| 14 | Cotton-seed emulsion | 269 | 34 | 2.93 | 111. | 1.58 | 0.15 |
| | NORMAL MIXED DIET | | | | | | |
| 63 | Plain peanut | 424 | 36 | 5.35 | 95.+ | 1.31 | 0.13 |
| 30 | Cotton-seed emulsion | 170 | 23 | 5.92 | 110. | 3.01 | 0.20 |
| 35 | Sesame emulsion | 148 | 26 | 2.73 | 92. | 7.67 | 0.24 |
| 41 | Control | ... | .. | 7.25 | 97. | 2.18 | 0.16 |
| 64 | Control | ... | .. | 4.64 | 95.+ | 1.32 | 0.12 |

25. Williams, Owen T., and Forsyth, Charles: Brit. Med. Jour., 1909, ii, 1120.

In the starved cat, No. 26, the large weight of fat after sixteen days of starvation is significant. This cat showed the largest absorption result of all the animals under experiment, 17 gm. of lard a day, and these extraction figures are indicative of an active mobilization of fat from the subcutaneous spaces to the liver where as Leathes[21] and Hartley have shown, modification of the saturated fatty acids occurs with the production of acids having higher halogen absorption values. The influence of the type of oil is shown by the iodin indices of the three cotton-seed oil cats used for illustration, and the comparatively low figure in the animal given olive oil.

The lung, the first organ to exercise any possible filtration effect on oil reaching the systemic circulation through the thoracic duct, was, in several cases, found to contain oil in macroscopic form but in no case was infarction or pneumonitis observed.

TABLE 17.—RESULTS OF EXTRACTION OF LUNGS

| Cat | | Oil Utilized gm. | Days of Treatment | Ether Extract gm. | Iodin Index | Per Cent. Total Ether Extract | Per Cent. of True Fresh Body Weight |
|---|---|---|---|---|---|---|---|
| | STARVATION | | | | | | |
| 13 | Control | ... | 37 | 0.407 | 69.5 | 1.61 | 0.002 |
| 5 | Cotton-seed emulsion | 282 | 23 | 0.528 | 72.0 | 1.20 | 0.038 |
| 26 | Lard emulsion | 276 | 16 | 0.854 | 61.0 | 1.44 | 0.039 |
| | LOW PROTEIN DIET | | | | | | |
| 10 | Olive emulsion | 446 | 32 | 0.553 | 62.8 | 0.54 | 0.019 |
| 14 | Cotton-seed emulsion | 369 | 34 | 2.250 | 80.5 | 1.98 | 0.111 |
| | NORMAL MIXED DIET | | | | | | |
| 63 | Plain peanut | 424 | 36 | 1.445 | 89.1 | 0.35 | 0.035 |
| 41 | Control | ... | .. | 1.243 | 75.1 | 0.37 | 0.028 |
| 64 | Control | ... | .. | 1.606 | 69.2 | 0.45 | 0.044 |

In all the treated animals cited in this table, except Cat 10, oil or fat was observed macroscopically. This accounts directly for the increased weights and percentages and for the variation in the iodin indices, that of the cat given lard being unusually low, while the cats given cotton-seed and peanut oils show an increase.

The general effect of injected oil on the iodin index of the kidney is to raise it. The average renal ether extract has an iodin value of about 50. The average index of the cats given normal food and injected is 60.8 and of the starved animals similarly injected 58.1.

The average splenic and pancreatic indices in starvation and normal health are approximately 70. In the treated starvation animals the average of splenic indices is 73.6 and on a full diet 76.9. Average pancreatic indices for similar groups of animals are 67 and 69.7 respectively, indicating practically no influence on the pancreas and but slight effect on the spleen.

The indices for the stomach and intestine are practically unaffected in the starving animals under treatment. In the fat-treated animals on a full diet the average is 78, as opposed to 70 for the controls.

All averages of the indices of the internal adipose tissue extracts in the starvation and in the full diet experiments (both with superimposed subcutaneous fat injections) show very little, if any, increase over the normal figures. This fact indicates that the foreign oils are not found in the functionally active viscera unless these exist there in a changed form. If any of the foreign oil absorbed is not immediately consumed for the production of heat and energy it may possibly be converted into normal cat-fat before it is stored.

The average amount of ether extract obtained from the 10 c.c. sample of jugular vein blood was 0.035 for the normal cats, 0.037 for treated and normally fed animals, 0.222 for the starvation control, and 0.088 for the treated and starved animals. The index of the starvation control specimen was 57.2. The only extract of sufficient size to be treated, 0.124 gm. from the blood of Cat 10, which utilized 446 gm. of olive oil in thirty-two days of low protein diet, gave the index of 77.3. A group of treated and superimposed cats gave the index of 63.5. Not enough work has been done as yet to allow interpretation of these figures, although the relatively high index given by the blood of Cat 10 is suggestive. It will be seen therefore that injections of oil, acting over a sufficient period, will influence the character and amount of the fatty tissue of the body to an appreciable extent.

## SUMMARY AND CONCLUSIONS

1. Olive, peanut, cocoanut, sesame, cotton-seed, lard oils, unsalted butter-fat and lard may be given hypodermically and over a considerable period without local irritation, provided aseptic care is used, and no constitutional disturbance occurs provided precautions are used to prevent injection into the blood-stream.

2. Emulsions of these oils made with 3 to 5 per cent. of egg lecithin and water are permanent, and cause no irritation if given subcutaneously.

3. Oils and fats given subcutaneously are absorbed by means of the lymphatic system and eventually reach the thoracic duct.

4. Lymphatic vessels and glands in contact with and transmitting oil for any length of time become hypertrophied and are thus better able to carry oil.

5. The amount of absorption of plain oil from the subcutaneous tissues after injection during starvation is so small as to be negligible. Emulsified oils and fats injected during starvation are absorbed in amounts sufficient to furnish from one-half to two-thirds of the full calorific requirement of the animals injected.

6. Oils and fats so injected and absorbed have no more influence on the destruction of protein in starvation than has fat given alone by mouth.

7. Plain oils injected subcutaneously under conditions of low protein ingestion are little, if any, better absorbed than when similarly given during starvation. Emulsified oils injected under these conditions are absorbed quite as well as similar oils given to starving animals.

8. Plain and emulsified oils are absorbed about equally well when the animals injected are given a plentiful supply of protein in their food. This probably furnishes the large quantity of lipolytic enzymes necessary for body action on plain oil.

9. The injection of oils subjected to lipolysis causes death, which is due apparently to the production of oleic or other acids with the possible formation of toxic quantities of soaps.

10. Oil absorbed from the tissues after subcutaneous injection is (a) burned in the body for the production of heat and energy, thus sparing the body fat; (b) retained as such within the organism; or (c) possibly converted into body fat by reconstruction in the liver from which it may be sent for storage to the various fat depositories, after which it is drawn on as needed. Proof of this last proposition is lacking.

11. It seems likely, from comparative examination of the iodin indices of the ether extracts of visceral and adipose tissue that the actively functioning viscera use oil and fat absorbed after subcutaneous injection for the direct performance of their functions, and that the storage of the foreign fat given in excess of the nutritive requirement takes place principally in the subcutaneous tissue, liver and lungs, to a small extent in the kidneys and spleen, while the pancreas and stomach and intestines are practically uninfluenced.

12. This demonstration that after injection under suitable conditions oils can be absorbed to an amount capable of covering so large a proportion of the calorific requirement suggests the application of such injections to the treatment of wasting diseases, to the cachectic conditions associated with imperfect metabolic processes and especially to tuberculosis, in which the intolerance to fats is almost symptomatic.

In conclusion I wish to express my obligations to Professor Graham Lusk for the courtesies of the laboratory and to both Professor Lusk and Assistant Professor Murlin for many valuable suggestions.

## CORRECTION OF AN IMPORTANT ERROR IN DR. HART'S PAPER ON THE ACIDOSIS INDEX

*To the Editor:* By an error, "ethyl acetate" appears in place of the correct name, "ethyl aceto-acetate" in my paper on "The Acidosis Index," which appeared in THE ARCHIVES OF INTERNAL MEDICINE (March, 1911, p. 369). This unfortunate mistake, which escaped my attention both in the typewritten manuscript and in the proofs, invalidates the whole paper. The sentence should read as follows:

The "standard solution" consists of ethyl aceto-acetate, 1 c.c.; alcohol 25 c.c.; and distilled water to 1,000 c.c.

T. STUART HART, M.D., New York.

The Archives of Internal Medicine

Vol. VII JUNE, 1911 No. 6

# CALCIFICATION AND OSSIFICATION *

H. GIDEON WELLS, M.D.
CHICAGO

It is the merit of Jacques Loeb to have shown us the necessity of simplifying our methods of attacking biologic problems. Instead of investigating the effects of complex substances on still more complex living organisms, he took up the simplest things imaginable, the familiar inorganic salts, and for his living subject the least complex complete organism possible—the single cell, *sans* blood, *sans* nerves, *sans* soul, *sans* everything. We pathologists cannot so readily reduce our subjects of investigation to such simple terms, but are forced too often, by the nature of our problems, to the opposite extreme, with such unsatisfactory results as might be expected. The situation of a pathologist, trying to investigate the action of a bacterial toxin of absolutely unknown composition on the equally unknown compounds of a complex mammalian organism, reminds us pathetically of the grotesque figure in "Confessio Medici," of the blind man searching in a dark room for a black hat which is not in the room. To be sure, in our gropings we have occasionally blundered into some great truth, but I fear that when our eyes are opened and the daylight comes, we shall be shocked at the wreckage our blind efforts have caused. For example, is it not possible that, stumbling about in the darkness, we have buried the simple key to the mystery of immunity beneath a mass of false data and distorted facts?

Calcification, dry and unpromising a problem as it may seem to be, possesses at least one of the cardinal virtues on which Loeb has insisted: The participants at one end of our reactions are of known and simple nature. Calcium salts we can isolate, estimate, and investigate to our hearts' content, and with all the accuracy which modern chemical methods afford us. And indeed the other end of the reaction seems to be somewhat simpler than the biological reactions of living cells, for in pathological calcification the organic structures are commonly dead, inert, chemically inactive; and even in ossification a relative chemical inactivity seems to characterize the calcifying structure. A pathologist working along chemical lines, therefore, has the right to feel that in the field of calcification he has a favorable place in which to try his feeble flights with the best hope of success.

---

*Harvey Lecture, Delivered March 25, 1911.

The accumulation and deposition of insoluble calcium salts by living organisms is so universal a process, exhibited by even the simplest protozoa, that in the investigation of the problems of calcification and ossification one is carried far afield into the territory of the zoologist, the biologist, and the plant physiologist. On the chemical side we find the newer developments of colloid chemistry coming to our assistance with many suggestive disclosures, and so our problem, which at first may seem somewhat limited, broadens out into a most interesting one. Furthermore, the existence of such diseases as rickets, osteomalacia, and osteoporosis, and questions concerning repair and regeneration of bone, make the discussion of more than merely academic interest.

Calcification, as observed in the formation of shells by mollusks and crustacea, seems to be a comparatively simple matter, and if the commonly accepted interpretation of the chemical processes is correct, we can find here little to help us in our study of physiological and pathological calcification in the mammals. The essential discrepancy is that with the latter the calcium salts are brought to the place of deposition in the blood of the animal, while with the marine invertebrates the calcium is apparently provided by the surrounding fluid. The hypothesis of Murray and Irvine,[1] which von Fürth[2] seems to consider the most adequate explanation of the facts, is that the calcium of the molluscan shells and of coral reefs is provided by the sea-water, in which it exists dissolved in the form of the relatively soluble sulphate, and that it is precipitated as calcium carbonate by the ammonium carbonate which is formed in the metabolism of the animals. This carbonate is excreted through the integument, where the deposition takes place according to the following equation:

$$CaSO_4 + (NH_4)_2CO_3 = CaCO_3 + (NH_4)_2SO_4$$

Another important difference is that in all these lower forms the calcium deposits consist chiefly of carbonate, with but little phosphate, whereas in the mammals and in most other vertebrates the calcium deposits are chiefly phosphate with relatively little carbonate. An important exception to this last statement is furnished by the shells of birds' eggs, the calcium in these being almost all carbonate,[3] and this in spite of the fact that the bones of birds closely resemble the bones of mammals

1. Murray and Irvine: Coral Reefs and Other Carbonate of Lime Formations in Modern Seas, Proc. Royal Soc., Edinburgh, 1889, xvii, 79.

2. Von Fürth: Vergleichende chemische Physiologie der niederen Tiere, Jena, 1903, p. 578.

3. Shells of hens' eggs contain approximately 97 per cent. $CaCO_3$, 1 per cent. $Ca_3(PO_4)_2$, including some small quantities of magnesium phosphate and carbonate, and also 2 per cent. of organic matter. (Bronn: Klassen und Ordnung des Thierreiches, 1891, $vi_4$, 875). This carbonate probably exists in the form of calcit. (Kelly, Agnes: Beiträge zur mineralogischer Kentniss der Kalkausscheidung im Tierreiche, Jenaische Ztschr. f. Naturwissensch., 1901, new series, xxviii, 439.)

in composition, and consist chiefly of phosphate with about one-sixth as much carbonate of calcium (Hiller,[4] Weiske[5]). A particularly remarkable feature of the formation of egg-shells is the constancy of composition, for if a hen is deprived of calcium until she begins to lay eggs with very little inorganic matter in the shell membranes, on the addition of silicate, phosphate, nitrate, or sulphate of calcium to the food, she will begin, in a few days, to lay eggs with shells of the usual thickness and containing calcium carbonate in normal proportion (Murray and Irvine). Concerning the manner and means by which the egg-shells are formed, we know very little, beyond that in the hen the egg usually remains about twenty hours in that part of the generative tract where the shell is formed. The interesting experiments of Pearl and Surface[6] show that the shell-glands secrete the calcium in response to mechanical stimulation, for when they anastomosed the intestine to the oviduct the feces which passed over the "shell-glands" were covered with a calcareous shell. This observation recalls Leo Loeb's demonstration that the formation of the maternal placenta in guinea-pigs takes place when a mechanical stimulus acts upon a uterine mucosa which has been sensitized by a hormone from the corpus luteum.

How the daily deposition of 4 or 5 gm. of calcium carbonate is accomplished by laying hens has not been explained. As hen's blood contains but 0.007 to 0.020 per cent. of calcium oxid, all the calcium of about 15,000 to 30,000 c.c. of blood must be secreted by the shell-glands to form an average shell, which contains 2 or 3 gm. of calcium oxid. One may imagine that the calcium is carried through the walls of the shell-glands in the form of the soluble bicarbonate, the carbonate being precipitated either by a neutralization process, or by simple escape of the excessive carbon dioxid. The chemistry of shell formation by birds seems to have received little investigation, as yet, although it is an interesting problem; but its solution probably will give us little information as to how calcium phosphate is deposited in mammalian tissues.

### THE RELATION OF CALCIFICATION AND OSSIFICATION

With the double topic of calcification and ossification before us, we may properly begin by ascertaining whether we are here concerned with two separate processes, or with two manifestations of a single process. The essential differences between ossification and calcification seem to be chiefly morphological. In calcification we have deposited in dead tissues,

4. Hiller: Vergleichende Knochenuntersuchungen am Skelett eines Vogels, Landwirthschaftliche Versuchsstationen, 1885, xxxi, 319.

5. Weiske: Untersuchungen über Qualität und Quantität der Vogel-Knochen und Federn in verschiedenen Altersstadien, Landwirtschaftliche Versuchsstationen, 1889, xxxvi, 81.

6. Pearl and Surface: The Nature of the Stimulus which Causes a Shell to be Formed on a Bird's Egg, Science, 1909, xxix, 428.

or in tissues of low vitality, a considerable quantity of inorganic calcium salts, which appear at first in granular form, although later there may be more or less fusion and resulting areas of homogeneity. Within such deposits there are usually no living cells, and, so far as we know, no further change takes place in the calcified area unless it be absorption or addition of more calcium salts. We have no information as to whether resorption of this calcium can take place to supply a deficit in the diet or the unusual demands of lactation and pregnancy, but we do know that it is not necessarily permanent, for the experimentally produced deposits of calcium in the kidney of the rabbit may be reabsorbed (von Werra[7]) within a few weeks, and even if such deposits have undergone secondary ossification they may disappear within a year (Maximow[8]). In normal ossification, however, the homogeneous calcium deposits are closely related to living cells, which not only determine the form of the deposits, but which also are able to dissolve the insoluble salts or to cause their deposition as may be needed, thus rendering the inorganic salts of bone the reserve supply of a tissue of active metabolism, entirely comparable to deposits of glycogen or of fat, and perhaps quite as important in view of the necessity of maintaining strict neutrality of the blood, a vitally important process in which the bone salts are of the utmost value.

Beyond this, however, there seem to be no differences between normal ossification and pathological calcification. Even morphologically there are many points of resemblance. In each case the insoluble salts are laid down in a matrix especially prepared to receive them; in bone formation the homogeneous acellular matrix of the cartilage; in calcification some acellular necrotic tissue, or, more especially, homogeneous elastic fibers or hyaline degenerated connective tissue, each of these latter bearing marked structural resemblance to the hyaline matrix of the cartilage or osteoid tissue. If we dissolve out the salts with acids we find remaining alike in bone and calcified areas an insoluble ground substance of homogeneous organic material, usually showing an affinity for basic dyes; however, the proportion of salts and stroma is less constant in pathological calcification than it is in adult bone. Finally when the inorganic salts are first deposited in normal ossification they are in a finely granular form (Pacchioni[9]) even although they later appear to be homogeneous, so that even this distinction between calcification and ossification is not absolute. Chemically the resemblance is even more close, for with few exceptions the proportion of the different inorganic salts in all sorts of

---

7. Werra, von: Ueber die Folgen des vorübergehenden und dauernden Verschlusses der Nierenarterie, Virchows Arch. f. path. Anat., 1882, lxxxviii, 197.

8. Maximow: Ueber experimentelle Erzeugung von Knochenmarkgewebe, Anat. Anz., 1906, xxviii, 609.

9. Pacchioni: Untersuchungen über die normale Ossification des Knorpels, Jahrb. f. Kinderh., 1902, lvi, 327.

areas of pathological calcific deposits has been found quite the same as that characteristic of normal bone. I grant that in the literature there may be found a few analyses of pathological materials indicating that the calcium salts present were not in a proportion similar to that of the inorganic substance of normal bone, which in the mammals is invariably from 85 to 90 per cent. of calcium phosphate and from 10 to 15 per cent. calcium carbonate, but there is every reason to believe that these atypical results are to be ascribed to improper methods of analysis. Nothing can be more misleading than to analyze an ash for bases and acids, and then to give the resulting figures as indicating the composition of the inorganic elements present in the tissues during life. In the case of bone-ash the results for the carbonate will inevitably be incorrect, for during the burning there develops a great quantity of carbon dioxid, more or less of which will unite with the bases present; with subsequent heating, however, all the carbon dioxid can be driven off, leaving only the oxids of the metals. In a test experiment, 2 gm. of pure gelatin and 2 gm. calcium phosphate [$(Ca_3(PO_4)_2$] were mixed by means of a little hot water, dried, and fused over a Bunsen burner until only a little carbon was left, as shown by the gray color of the ash. Analysis showed the presence in this ash of 0.0356 gm. carbon dioxid, which indicates the presence of 0.080 gm. calcium carbonate; therefore, about 4 per cent. of the calcium of the phosphate had become united as carbonate. A repetition of this experiment, carrying the fusion until there was practically no free carbon left, yielded 0.026 gm. carbon dioxid, or 0.059 gm. calcium carbonate.

The danger of error from addition or loss of carbon dioxid in ashing, although generally recognized in bone analyses, seems to have been overlooked in several of the reports of analyses of pathological calcific deposits which speak of the amount of carbon dioxid in the ash. That the phosphoric acid determinations in ash are also unreliable, seems not to have been considered, even in most of the recorded analyses of bone. We have, however, in bone tissue, a greater or less proportion of nucleo-proteins and lecithin, especially when the marrow is included, from which phosphoric acid is freed on heating, and which will unite with the bases, especially the carbonates.[10] For example, in a test analysis, a mixture containing (1) 2 gm. of $CaCO_3$, (2) 2 gm. of dog spleen from which all phosphorus soluble in water, ether, or boiling alcohol had been extracted; and (3) 0.5 gm. lecithin, was fused until white, washed thoroughly with water to remove soluble phosphates, and analyzed. No less than 0.0635 gm. of

10. The method used by Gabriel, decomposing the bone with an alkaline solution of glycerin, offers the same opportunity of converting organic phosphorus compounds into calcium phosphate, and in fact gives the same proportion of calcium phosphate as the ashing method. It is an interesting fact, emphasized by Aron (Stutzgewebe und Integumente der Wirbeltiere, Handbuch der Biochemie, 1908, ii, 178), that both methods indicate the presence of sodium and potassium held in the bone ash in an insoluble form.

insoluble $P_2O_5$ was found, corresponding to 0.1344 gm. of $Ca_3 (PO_4)_2$, which had undoubtedly been formed from the organically bound $P_2O_5$ during the fusion, changing 6.6 per cent. of the calcium of the carbonate into phosphate.

There have been made in my laboratory by R. L. Benson, Conrad Jacobson, and myself, many analyses of normal and pathological calcified materials, both natural and experimental, by a method devised to exclude these sources of error, and without exception, whether the material was early or late calcification, large or small in amount, natural or experimental, human, bovine, or rabbit, we have always obtained results showing that in pathological deposits the calcium salts are always present in the ratio of phosphate and carbonate which is, within certain limits, characteristic of normal bone. Of the analyses in the literature, a large proportion show a similar ratio of carbonate and phosphate. Where the results are different from this they usually can be explained by the use of the ashing method in the presence of a large amount of organic material.

## PATHOLOGICAL CALCIFICATION

Perhaps the most striking evidence of the relation of calcification to ossification is the frequency with which we find an area of pathological calcification of some dead tissue undergoing a metamorphosis into true bone. Surely nothing can be more remarkable, more spectacular, indeed, than that a human eye may come to be lined with a shell of true living bone, perhaps containing marrow, as a sequel to the deposition of calcium salts in dead material left unabsorbed after a suppuration within the eye. Neither is this an unusual, isolated observation, for we find it to be a rule that when areas of calcified pathological tissues remain long enough in the body, ossification will take place in a certain proportion of cases, irrespective of any proximity or relation to bone tissue. This is particularly true of the eye, the ophthalmologists having reported many cases of ossification of calcific deposits within the eye-ball; and Poscharissky[11] found that of twenty-nine such calcified areas which he examined, true bone could be found in all but four. Calcified nodules from the lungs of twenty-eight persons were examined by the same author, and in seventeen of the bodies (60 per cent.) bone was found. Bone-marrow, or a tissue resembling it, was found in three of fourteen calcified nodules from heart-valves, and bone was present in four of thirty-one calcified aortic plaques. Calcified nodules in the liver and in the mesenteric glands are also often ossified, and in fact there is hardly a tissue in the animal body in which transformation of calcified into ossified tissue has not been observed (Harvey[12]).

11. Poscharissky: Ueber heteroplastische Knochenbildung, Beitr. z. path. Anat. u. z. allg. Path. (Ziegler's), 1905, xxxviii, 135.

12. Harvey: Experimental Bone Formation in Arteries, Jour. Med. Research, 1907, xvii, 25.

The process by which these inert dead calcified areas are converted into living bone tissue is entirely analogous to the normal formation of bone in endochondral ossification. The calcified material simply takes the place of the primordial cartilage, vascular granulation tissue eroding it, the cells of the granulation tissue undergoing a differentiation into osteoblasts which constitute an osteogenetic layer and form the new bone. When there is no preliminary calcification of a necrotic tissue we get no subsequent ossification, and it seems that the *calcium salts exert a specific influence on the connective tissue cells which causes them to take on active growth, and to undergo a metaplasia, not only into osteoblasts and bone corpuscles, but apparently even into marrow cells with hematogenetic function,* since, according to Bunting[13] and others, the evidence indicates that the marrow tissue which so commonly accompanies pathological ossification[14] is derived from the proliferated connective tissue cells.[15] According to Poscharissky a further point of resemblance between normal and pathological ossification is that in senile cartilage which is undergoing or is about to undergo ossification, the characteristic microchemical tests for amyloid can be obtained, and the same reactions are given by the decalcified ground substance of ossifying calcified areas.[16] It is nothing less than remarkable how rapidly ossification can occur in areas of pathological calcification, for Liek[17] was able to obtain bone formation constantly in the pelvis of the rabbit's kidney within sixteen or twenty days after ligating the renal artery, provided that he wrapped the kidney with omentum to secure a free collateral circulation; without this collateral circulation it requires about three months for ossification to appear. These and other experiments by the same author show that the amount of blood-supply is an important factor in determining pathological ossification; with too free a circulation there is no calcification and no ossification, with too little circulation necrosis is followed by slow calcification and either late or no ossification.

---

13. Bunting: Formation of True Bone with Cellular, Red Marrow in a Sclerotic Aorta, Jour. Exper. Med., 1908, viii, 365.

14. Poscharissky (see Note 11) states that marrow tissue is *always* present when bone is formed in calcified tissues, and that in 10 per cent. of his cases there was marrow without true bone, but it is possible that he is too liberal in his interpretation of the histological criteria of marrow.

15. Maximow (see Note 8) ascribes the marrow formation to metaplasia of lymphocytes from the blood.

16. The only attempt with which I am familiar, to corroborate this interesting observation was made by Buerger and Oppenheimer (Bone Formation in Sclerotic Arteries, Jour. Exper. Med., 1908, x, 354) with negative results in the one specimen of ossifying arteries which they examined. It may be recalled that Wichmann [Die Amyloiderkrankung, Beitr. z. path. Anat. u. z. allg. Path. (Ziegler's), 1893, xiii, 487] also throws doubt on many of the earlier statements concerning the presence of amyloid in cartilage and bone.

17. Liek: Heteroplastische Knochenbildung in Nieren, Arch. f. klin. Chir., 1908, lxxxv, 118.

The essential part played by the calcium salts in stimulating osteogenesis is further demonstrated by Barth's[18] experiments on the healing of bone defects by implantation of dead and living bone. He found that living bone thus implanted always dies, and then the dead bone is replaced by a process of substitution, new layers of osteoid tissue invading and replacing layer by layer the dead bone. If the bone is dead and sterile when implanted, or if ashed bone is used, the results are quite the same. Calcium sulphate placed in bone cavities also favors rapid ossification.[19] If, however, decalcified bone is similarly implanted it is quickly absorbed, and is replaced by fibrous tissue, without ossification except such growth of bone as may invade the scar tissue from the living bone tissue about the margins. Stoeltzner[20] has also indicated the importance of calcium in natural ossification, not only as forming a part of the bone, but also in stimulating osteogenetic tissue to form bone.

The observations cited above indicate to us the specific osteogenetic influence exerted by deposits of calcium salts, alike whether in dead tissue or in cartilage which is to be ossified. But how is this influence exerted? It is hard to imagine that it is chemical, since the calcium salts concerned are most insoluble, and it does not seem probable that the fluids bathing them will contain appreciably more calcium than the normal body fluids, which seem to be pretty nearly saturated with calcium salts. Possibly it is a tactile stimulus—if so we might have ossification induced by rough mineral deposits other than calcium, but such a thing has never been described. In any case, in order to have ossification of calcific deposits, certain conditions of relationship between calcium salts, fibrous tissues and blood-supply evidently must be very exactly met, as shown by Liek's experiments with the rabbit's kidney, and by his failure to produce ossification by the implantation of pieces of decalcified bone and masses of calcium phosphate or carbonate into the peritoneal cavity and soft tissues of rabbits.[21] Morpurgo and Martini[22] also obtained negative results in similar experiments. On the other hand, even in extreme old age the senile connective tissues are still able, under suitable conditions, to undergo active osteogenetic metamorphosis (Bunting).

18. Barth: Histologische Untersuchungen über Knochenimplantationen, Beitr. z. path. Anat. u. z. allg. Path. (Ziegler's), 1895, xvii, 65.

19. Barth: Ueber künstliche Erzeugung von Knochengewebe und über die Ziele der Osteoplastik, Berl. klin. Wchnschr., 1896, xxxiii, 8.

20. Stoeltzner, W.: Die zweifache Bedeutung des Calciums für das Knochenwachstum, Arch. f. d. ges. Physiol. (Pflüger's), 1908, cxxii, 599.

21. Barth (see Note 18) states that he found some isolated islands of young bone in a piece of bone ash implanted into the peritoneal cavity of a cat six weeks previously, which Liek believes due to a misinterpretation of the histological findings.

22. Morpurgo and Martini: Atti d. R. Accad. d. fisiocrit. di Siena, 1898, x, quoted by Sacardotti and Frattin: Virchows Arch. f. path. Anat., 1902, clxviii, 431.

THE PROBLEMS OF CALCIFICATION

All the above facts, when taken together, leave little ground for the belief that there is any essential dissimilarity between the processes of ossification and calcification. In either case histological elements of similar structure are infiltrated with inorganic salts of identical composition, and even if at first the calcific area is dead, inert, and of pathological origin, it may later by gradual change be transformed into true living bone. Therefore it is permissible for us to consider both processes together, and the evidence afforded by either can be applied to the other with but slight modification and few reservations. We may summarize the problems awaiting solution under the following heads:

1. Why is calcium deposited in the tissues at all?
2. Why is it deposited in some tissues and not in others?
3. How is the calcium carried in the blood?
4. How is it held in the tissues where deposited?
5. Why is the composition of calcified deposits so constant qualitatively and quantitatively?
6. What are the causes of rickets and osteomalacia?

In the first problem we must consider in the beginning that in mammals only one normal tissue is the site of calcific infiltration, the developing bone, while *any* tissue may become calcified provided that its vitality is reduced sufficiently and that it remains long unabsorbed. Even such highly specialized structures as the ganglion cells of the brain may become calcified so completely that there results a perfect cast of the original cell, dendrites, axis cylinder and all. Furthermore, not all cartilages calcify, and indeed only certain portions of those cartilages which are eventually to become entirely ossified are calcified at first. Why is it that the ribs calcify up to a certain definite line, leaving the costal cartilage uncalcified for a long space of years, only eventually to undergo in old age a final senile calcification and ossification? Why do only certain particular spots in the great mass of fetal cartilage become calcified, one by one and in a definite order, until finally only a narrow margin of cartilage is left about each to form the joint surfaces? In all these cases the process seems to follow a definite order, with an early deposition of calcium salts; this is followed by an increased vascularity at these places, the newly formed vessels and the cells which accompany them forcing their way into and partly absorbing the calcified cartilage; a new structure is now laid down in place of the resorbed cartilage, containing the invading cells in the form of osteoblasts and bone corpuscles; this new tissue is then infiltrated with calcium salts and we have true bone. This series of processes, it will be seen, is exactly the same as occurs in the ossification of pathological calcified areas, and in each case it is the deposition of calcium which is the primary step. Therefore the problem of ossification is, after all, the problem of calcification of tissues, normal or pathological.

### THE CHEMICAL FIXATION THEORY

To account for the primary deposition of calcium salts (for the magnesium and other bases are relatively so insignificant in amount that we can disregard them for the present) many hypotheses have been advanced, and none is simpler or older than the idea of a precipitation of insoluble salts of calcium because of a chemical reaction, certain acid radicals formed within the tissues combining with and precipitating the calcium contained in the blood and tissue fluids. To this idea no better name can be given than that used by the Germans, the *Kalkfänger* hypothesis.

As most of the calcium of bones is phosphate, the first idea that occurs is that phosphoric acid is the *Kalkfänger,* and we have no difficulty in finding possible sources of phosphoric acid. In ossification it might come from autolysis of the nuclei of the cartilage cells (Grandis and Mainini[23]), or these cells might secrete soluble phosphates; in calcification $P_2O_5$ might come from the autolysis of the nucleoproteins and lecithin of the dead tissues. Such an explanation, however, has failed of proof. In calcified necrotic areas there is far more inorganic phosphoric acid than could possibly be derived from the phosphorus which was originally held there in organic combination; so, too, in ossification, the amount of nuclein phosphorus present in cartilage is much too small to account for the phosphates present in the bone, and the traces of soluble inorganic phosphorus present in ossifying cartilage are not greater in amount than in other, non-calcifying tissues.[24] Furthermore, I have found by experiment that dead sterile pieces of tissue rich in nucleo-protein (thymus and spleen) do not take up calcium more rapidly than do similar pieces of tissue poor in phosphorus compounds (muscle[25]). One might, of course, imagine an active secretory formation of phosphoric acid by the osteoblasts, but such a process has not been demonstrated, and we shall later give evidence which apparently excludes this possibility.

Another way in which we might account for the phosphate in the event phosphoric acid is not the true *Kalkfänger,* is by double decomposition; any precipitated calcium salts of whatever sort present in the tissues being converted into the phosphate, because this is one of the most insoluble of calcium salts, and, according to the law of double decomposition, the least soluble salt is formed when solutions of two salts are mixed. It is unquestionably true that other calcium salts within the tissues do become replaced to at least some extent by phos-

23. Grandis and Mainini: Arch. ital. de biol., 1900, i, 73.

24. Wells and Benson: Studies on Calcification and Ossification, II, Jour. Med. Research, 1907, xii, 15.

25. Wells: Pathological Calcification, Jour. Med. Research, 1906, xiv, 491.

phate, as we have found true for calcium sulphate[26] implanted into the tissues of rabbits. In view of the fact that calcium sulphate is a salt of calcium which is only slightly soluble, and that cartilage is characterized by containing a compound of sulphuric acid with chondrosin (chondroitin-sulphuric acid) this source of a possible *Kalkfänger* is at once evident. But since the calcium salt of chondroitin sulphuric acid is very soluble, this compound itself cannot precipitate calcium, and the total amount of $SO_4$ present in cartilage is far too small to account for any appreciable precipitate of calcium sulphate—indeed it would require quite a considerable quantity of calcium and $SO_4$ present together at one time in the tissues to produce a precipitate, in view of the relatively considerable solubility of $CaSO_4$ (2.73 gm. per liter in water at 18° C., Kohlrausch and Rosa[27]), and numerous analyses have failed to show the presence of an appreciable amount of $CaSO_4$ in calcifying tissues at any stage of the process.[25]

Carbonic acid certainly cannot be looked on as a precipitant, since the more $CO_2$ present the more soluble are the calcium salts, which readily form the soluble bicarbonate; indeed it is probable that solution of bone takes place through this reaction.

### CALCIUM SOAPS

The available inorganic acids being exhausted by the foregoing list, we must fall back on a possible organic *Kalkfänger,* and here several well-known facts at once call our attention to the fatty acids. In the first place, we know that calcium soaps do at times form in pathological processes, as seen especially in areas of fat necrosis where the formation of calcium soaps is an almost constant process. Indeed, necrotic areas in fat tissue commonly form calcium soaps, calcification of a lipoma with the presence of calcium soaps having been described as long ago as 1851 by Fürstenberg,[28] while Jaeckle[29] found 29.5 per cent. of the calcium in a calcified lipoma combined with fatty acids. Secondly, areas of pathological tissues which calcify are commonly areas in which fatty degeneration has taken place, e. g., caseous tubercles, atheromatous vessels, old infarcts, etc.

It is easy to imagine calcium soaps formed in this way becoming slowly transformed *in situ* into calcium phosphate and carbonate, by double decomposition in the presence of soluble phosphates and carbonate

---

26. Wells and Mitchell: Studies in Calcification and Ossification, III, Jour. Med. Research, 1906, xxii, 501.

27. Kohlrausch and Rosa: Ztschr. f. physik. Chem., 1893, xii, 234.

28. Fürstenberg: Magazin f. Tierheilk., 1851, xvii, 1; quoted by Hofmeister: See Note 30.

29. Jaeckle: Ueber die Zusammensetzung des menschlichen Fettes, Ztschr. f. physiol. Chem., 1902, xxxvi, 53.

formed in the degenerating tissues or brought from the blood, and the hypothesis is most plausible. We must, indeed, admit that calcification by soap formation does occur, as witness the calcification of foci of fat necrosis and lipomas. Hofmeister[30] also states that Tanaka has found that when various tissues are acted on by calcium solutions, either *in vitro* or *in vivo,* only the fat tissue takes up calcium in appreciable amounts, and when solutions of calcium salts are injected into the peritoneal cavity there is formed a certain amount of calcium soaps in the subserous fat tissue. But that calcium soaps are formed in areas of necrotic fat is one thing, and that their formation is the usual first step in pathological calcification, is quite another.

This calcium soap hypothesis is certainly a most attractive one, and one that has long interested me greatly, especially as I supposed for some years that it was a discovery of my own, until I made a thorough search of the older literature. If true it settles all questions concerning pathological calcification, and leaves us with a closed chapter on this subject, certainly a condition most to be desired, and so for some nine years I have been endeavoring to prove that it is true, but without success.

The first point of attack naturally consists in seeking for calcium soaps in areas of calcification, especially during the early stages. There are technical difficulties involved which make the task almost impossible, except in cases in which the amount of calcium soaps is large, and on which I need not expatiate. It is sufficient here to state that I have never obtained convincing evidence of the presence of calcium soaps in areas of calcification of many kinds and at all stages, including some specimens, both experimental and natural, in which the process was known to be very early. A similar negative result was obtained by Baldauf[31] who analyzed atheromatous aortas, in which all stages of the process are occurring side by side in the numerous lesions. On the other hand, to prevent our case from being conclusively and finally settled, I have commonly found most minute traces of calcium in solutions obtained by prolonged extraction of calcified tissues with ether, ethyl alcohol and amyl alcohol at near the boiling point of each solvent. The amounts so obtained, however, were so extremely minute (usually 1 or 2 mg., sometimes less, from quantities of calcified tissues containing as much as 5 or 6 gm. of calcium and 3 to 4 gm. of fat) that it is very doubtful if this finding is of any significance. Experiments show that mixtures of calcium phosphate, calcium carbonate, fats and pure proteins, when submitted to a correspondingly vigorous extraction with the same solvents, may give off to the solvents corresponding minute quantities of calcium,

---

30. Hofmeister: Ueber Ablagerung und Resorption von Kalksalzen in den Geweben, Ergebn. d. Physiol., 1910, ix, 429.

31. Baldauf: The Chemistry of Atheroma and Calcification, Jour. Med. Research, 1906, xv, 355.

since inorganic calcium salts are only relatively and not absolutely insoluble.

Therefore we are obliged to conclude that no appreciable amount of calcium exists in the form of soaps in any calcified areas that we have examined. To be sure, the objection at once presents itself that the amount of calcium soaps that is present at any one time during calcification may be too small to detect by chemical means, since according to the hypothesis the calcium is only transitorily in the form of soaps before going over to the inorganic form. This argument is, of course, unanswerable, if one wishes to insist on the sufficiency of infinitesimally minute quantities of calcium soap; and it is just this possibility alone that prevents us from saying positively that the calcium soap hypothesis of calcification is untenable. But we add to the improbability when we consider the very large size of the calcium soap molecule; in calcium stearate, for example, the calcium represents by weight but about one-fifteenth of the molecule; hence in an area of calcification containing 1 gm. of calcium, the soap hypothesis demands that 15 gm. of calcium soap shall have been formed during the process of calcification. On this basis the amount present at any one time in an area of rapid calcification should be easily detected unless the rate of change of soap into phosphate and carbonate is much more rapid than we have any right to believe it can be. To take a specific example, I have analyzed a crumbling chalky calcified thrombus, which was formed as a result of an occlusion of the jugular vein by pressure from rapidly growing cancerous lymph-glands. From the history of the case it is improbable that this thrombus was over two months old, but to be liberal let us assume that it was 100 days old and that calcification had begun as soon as the thrombus was formed, instead of some days or weeks later, as is more probably the case. In this thrombus was found 0.730 gm. of calcium. If this was laid down by first passing through a stage of soap formation there must have been all told about 11 gm. of calcium soaps formed. Now if we assume that only the amount of calcium soap formed on a single day was present at any one time (which certainly represents a very rapid rate for this sort of chemical transformation to take place in so avascular an area as a large thrombus), there would be present 0.110 gm. of calcium soaps, containing about 7 mg. of calcium. Nevertheless analysis of this thrombus yielded in the fat and soap fraction a mere trace of calcium, too small to be weighed, but probably less than 1 mg.; and even this trace presumably is to be ascribed to the solubility of inorganic calcium salts in the solvents used. Many other analyses of equally early stages of calcification give a similar lack of evidence of calcium soaps, and also show that the calcium is always present as phosphate and carbonate in the same proportions as in normal bone.

But even if calcium soaps are formed in a calcifying tissue, is it certain that the calcium so precipitated in the dead area would remain and be changed to phosphate and carbonate? In favor of this view we may refer to Jaeckle's calcifying lipoma, which contained, besides the 29.5 per cent. of calcium as soaps, much carbonate (28.61 per cent.) and phosphate (41.80 per cent.) of calcium, according to his analysis; this we may interpret as an illustration of incomplete transformation of calcium soap into carbonate and phosphate.[32] I have performed a number of experiments (elsewhere described[24, 26]) to determine whether sodium soaps can become transformed within the body into calcium soaps and, if so, whether the calcium soaps are then replaced by calcium phosphate and carbonate. To simulate as closely as possible the conditions existing in calcifying tissues, in which the salts concerned are contained in an avascular mass of colloids, the soaps were imbedded in solidified agar jelly and implanted in the peritoneal cavity of rabbits. It was found that under these conditions a considerable proportion (30 to 40 per cent.) of the soap does become combined with calcium, and that a very small amount of inorganic salts of calcium (from 1 to 2 per cent.) appears. A strange feature of this process is that the same proportion of inorganic calcium is obtained whether the soaps have been implanted but a few days or several months, suggesting that possibly an equilibrium is here established. When calcium soaps are implanted the end results are much the same, the greater part of the soaps disappearing and a very small amount (from 1 to 2 per cent.) of carbonate and phosphate remaining, the two latter being always in the same ratio to each other as in normal bone.

From these results it may be considered as established that implanted sodium soaps do to some extent become changed into calcium soaps, but we are unable to consider the evidence clear as to whether the new-formed calcium soaps do or do not become changed into phosphate and carbonate. While these two inorganic salts are always found present in such implanted materials, yet the amount is so small that its presence might as well be explained as the result of simple infiltration of the implanted mass of soap and agar by calcium from the blood, irrespective of any reaction with the soaps. Speaking most strongly against the soap hypothesis, however, is the finding that most of the calcium which is introduced as soaps is absorbed, instead of being replaced by inorganic salts. This agrees entirely with my experiments on fat necrosis[33] in which it was

32. Possibly one may consider as examples of a similar process the *Fettgewebesteine* described by O. M. Chiari (Ueber die herdweise Verkalkung und Verknocherung des subkutänen Fettgewebessteine, Ztschr. f. Heilk., 1908, xxviii Suppl. 1), which are found in the subcutaneous tissue of the lower extremities following arterial occlusion, but unfortunately chemical studies of this material have not been made.

33. Wells: Experimental Fat Necrosis, Jour. Med. Research, 1903, ix, 70.

found that in spite of early formation of calcium soaps in areas of experimental fat necrosis, complete healing and reabsorption may again take place in a few days or weeks. In other words, although fatty acids may cause calcium to be precipitated, yet they do not hold the calcium permanently in the tissues either as soaps or as inorganic compounds of calcium. This is presumably to be explained by the observation of Hofmeister[30] that the colloids of blood-serum enable it to keep large quantities of calcium soaps in solution. Also, as Hofmeister points out, pathological calcification is not always preceded by fatty degeneration, and, furthermore, if calcium soaps act catalytically, as has been maintained, calcification should be a most common, if not universal occurrence since it is as soaps that fatty acids are transported, and soaps are often if not always present in the tissues without calcification taking place.

The affirmative side of the question has been most strongly supported by Klotz,[35] largely on a basis of microscopical evidence. This consisted chiefly in finding in calcifying areas granules staining "pinkish yellow" with Sudan III, which Klotz states distinguishes them as soaps because neutral fat stains golden red. By staining with von Kossa's silver nitrate stain for calcium salts, granules staining black were found in the same location as the granules which stain "yellowish pink" with Sudan III, and hence Klotz considered that this "suggests strongly that we are dealing with a deposit of calcium soap." Unfortunately for this doctrine, calcium soaps have been shown by Baldauf[36] not to stain at all with Sudan III,[37] and in the second place in von Kossa's silver nitrate method, the silver reacts with phosphoric acid and not with calcium; hence the results of these observations merely show that insoluble phosphates are present in the earliest stages of calcification, and do not give any evidence whatever that calcium soaps or any other kinds of soaps are present and demonstrable by microchemical measures. We can, indeed, scarcely hope to obtain microchemical evidence of calcification if chemical procedures are unavailing; my analyses show that if calcium soaps are present at all in calcifying tissues, they can represent not over one-thousandth of

35. Klotz: Studies on Calcareous Degeneration, Jour. Exper. Med., 1905, vii, 633.

36. Baldauf, Leon K.: An Investigation of the Nature of Proteid-Soap Compounds and of the Staining of Pure Fats and Lipoids by Scharlach R and Sudan III, Jour. Am. Med. Assn., 1907, xlix, 642.

37. To quote from Baldauf, "Neither calcium nor sodium soaps, palmitic nor stearic acids, will at room temperature take the stain with Sudan III or Scharlach R, hence the material staining by these substances, which Klotz described as occurring at certain stages of calcareous degeneration, cannot be any of these compounds. In all probability it is a mixture of oleic acid, triolein and lecithin." Aschoff [Zur Morphologie der lipoiden Substanzen, Zeitr. z. path. Anat. u. z. allg. Path. (Ziegler's), 1909, xlvii, 1] also takes exception to the supposed differentiation of soaps by Sudan III.

the total calcium, and to distinguish by the microscope such minute quantities of a calcium soap from all the remaining 999 parts of inorganic calcium with which it is mingled, is evidently impossible. Other features of this work, which time does not permit me to take up at length, are also open to criticism, and in the final analysis I can find in it no satisfactory support for the calcium soap hypothesis. Hofmeister,[30] in a recent review of the literature of calcification, also refuses to accept this work as establishing the calcium soap theory of calcification.

A point that should be especially mentioned is that there is no reason whatever to believe that the formation of normal bone from cartilage takes place through a stage of soap formation, hence the acceptance of the soap theory would compel us to separate sharply ossification and calcification, whereas most of the evidence indicates the unity of these two processes.

To recapitulate, then, we can say that while there is some reason from a theoretical standpoint to support the idea that fatty acids formed in necrotic areas may combine calcium from the blood and precipitate it in the tissues where it may later undergo transformation into carbonate and phosphate, yet that this is the ordinary process by which calcification occurs, is unproved. Other considerations, to be expressed later, make it seem improbable.

Besides fatty acids, few other organic *Kalkfänger* have been suggested. Special proteins with a specific affinity for calcium, or products of protein hydrolysis, such as albumoses, have been thought of, but no proof of their existence has been brought forward, nor has their existence been made probable.

Another possible method of precipitation of calcium salts would be by an *increased alkalinization* of the degenerating tissues, which might cause mono- and dicalcium phosphates and bicarbonate of calcium to be converted into the less soluble basic salts and precipitate from the blood. That a change in reaction can be a sufficient cause for precipitation of calcium salts from the blood into normal tissues, is made probable by that unusual type of calcification which was first described by Virchow under the title of "metastatic calcification."

## METASTATIC CALCIFICATION

Here we find calcium salts deposited throughout the body in what seem to be perfectly normal tissues, but especially in the lungs, the kidneys and the gastric mucosa. Of the twenty-nine cases recorded in the literature[38] in all but four there was demonstrated some extensive

38. Askanazy (Beiträge zur Knochenpathologie, Festschr. f. Jaffe, Brunswick, 1901; quoted by Hofmeister; see Note 30) in 1901 collected reports of twenty-one cases, to which Hofmeister (see Note 30) added two more. In addition to these

destructive disease of the bones,[39] supporting the assumption made by Virchow that the primary cause of the disease is an overloading of the blood with calcium salts. Recent experimental work by Hofmeister and Tanaka leaves no question that this assumption is correct, for they found it possible to cause extensive and typical metastatic calcification by intraperitoneal injection of soluble calcium salts into rabbits.[40] The fact that the deposition of calcium takes place most often in these three tissues (lungs, stomach and kidneys), where otherwise calcification is not commonly seen independent of local lesions, such as tubercles, thrombi, etc., is of special significance, for as has been pointed out elsewhere (Askanazy,[38] Wells[25]) in these three tissues we have the three chief places in the body where acids are excreted. In the lungs we have bicarbonates giving up $CO_2$ and passing on in the blood as carbonates; in the stomach HCl is excreted, and in the kidneys acid phosphates are excreted by a reaction which leaves basic phosphates and carbonates in the blood and tissues. We therefore believe that the coincidence of the location of the calcium deposits and the acid-excretion function of the tissues leaves little or no room for doubt that the precipitation of calcium occurs in this condition of metastatic calcification because calcium salts are

---

I have noted cases reported by Hedinger (Ueber Verkalkung der Leber, Corrsbl. f. Schweiz. Aerzte, 1909, xxxix, 833), Pari (Ueber einen Fall von Kalkinkrustation der Lungen mit Fragmentation der elastischen Fasern, Virchows Arch. f. path. Anat., 1910, cc, 199), Versé (Ueber ausgedehnte Verkalkungen der Lungen, Verhandl. d. Deutsch. path. Gesellsch., 1910, xiv, 281), Jadassohn (Ueber Kalkmetastasen in der Haut, Arch. f. Dermat., 1910, c, 317), Lazarus and Davidsohn (Hirnhautsarkom mit zahlreichen Kalkmetastasen im Herzen, Ztschr. f. klin. Med., 1906, lx, 314), and Tschistowitsch and Kolessnikoff (Multiples diffuses Myeloma mit reichlichen Metastasen in die Lungen und andere Organe, Virchows Arch. f. path. Anat., 1904, cxcvii, 112). This does not include the remarkable cases of generalized subcutaneous calcification of unknown etiology, recently discussed by Lhermitte (La calcinose généralisée et ses formes anatomiques interstitielle et sous-cutanée, Sem. méd., 1910, xxx, 553).

39. In many cases nephritis also exists, which Hedinger (see Note 38) believes may be a factor by interfering with calcium excretion. However, since normally most of the calcium excretion takes place through the bowel, it seems improbable that disease of the kidney can have much influence on the calcium content of the blood, although Erben (Ueber die chemische Zusammensetzung des Blutes, Ztschr. f. klin. Med., 1903, l, 441) did find an increased amount of calcium in the blood in nephritis.

40. A human case quite comparable to these experimental calcifications has been reported by Thayer and Hazen (Calcification of the Breast Following a Typhoid Abscess, Jour. Exper. Med., 1907, ix, 1). A typhoid patient was given during eleven days, on account of hemorrhages, 132 gm. calcium lactate by mouth, and 5 gm. calcium chlorid as a subcutaneous injection. At the site of the latter there developed an abscess, in the margins of which some days afterwards a deposition of calcium salts took place, later becoming absorbed under a diet free from carbohydrates. The form in which the calcium was held was not determined, beyond noting that it dissolved in HCl without effervescence.

slightly less soluble in the more alkaline fluids present in these tissues.[41] The histological findings in the calcified areas of the stomach are remarkably conclusive as to this point for, as Hofmeister points out, the calcium deposits are limited to the interglandular tissue about the upper portion of the glands of the fundus—in other words, exactly corresponding to the location of the parietal cells which are (as the observations of Mabel Fitzgerald[42] show finally) the cells which secrete the hydrochloric acid. In some cases of bone absorption we also find wide-spread calcium deposits in the walls of the heart, arteries and capillaries, independent of degenerative changes in the tissues of these vessels; thus Lazarus and Davidsohn[38] described extensive internal calcification of the left auricle, which is expressly noted to have come from the blood within the auricle, and not from the vessels of the heart wall; Versé[38] found, in a case of leukemia, deposits in the lungs, pulmonary veins, and most extensively beneath the endocardium of the left side of the heart; Jadassohn[38] observed deposits in the left auricle in a case of myocarditis, and Küttner[43] in a case of rarefying osteitis noted generalized arterial deposits in and on the intima, without deposits present in the media or in the vein walls. In these cases the explanation is somewhat similar to that given above for the visceral deposits, for here, it will be noted, the calcification has taken place in the walls of those vessels whose contents have the smallest amount of $CO_2$. In other words, the carrying of calcium salts by the blood is, at least in the cases of excessive bone absorption, largely dependent on the carbon dioxid of the blood. Whether this is the normal condition or not will be considered later. In this place we are concerned with the question of whether a similar process of alkalinization takes place in calcifying and ossifying tissues, to cause precipitation in them of calcium salts brought in the tissue fluids. One can readily imagine that ammonia set free during autolysis in necrotic areas might cause such an alkaline reaction, but the evidence which we have speaks rather for the development of an excess of acids in such areas. Not only are acids

---

41. There seem to have been no quantitative analyses made of the deposits in metastatic calcification. Pari (see Note 38) could find no $P_2O_5$ by microchemical methods. Jadassohn (see Note 38) found both carbonate and phosphate in the skin metastases of his case. Hofmeister in experimental metastatic calcification found calcium phosphate and a little carbonate, no matter what salt had been injected. Hedinger (see Note 38) in calcified areas in the liver found $P_2O_5$, but observed no effervescence on addition of acid. Versé (see Note 38) found in his case both carbonate and phosphate. Tschistowitsch and Kolessnikoff (see Note 38) found the ash of the lungs, kidneys and aorta in their case to contain greatly increased amounts of Ca and $P_2O_5$, but no analysis of isolated calcific material was made.

42. Fitzgerald, Mabel: The Origin of Hydrochloric Acid in Gastric Tubules, Proc. Roy. Soc. London, 1910, lxxxii, 346.

43. Küttner: Ein Fall von Kalkmetastase, Virchows Arch. f. path. Anat., 1872, lv, 521.

supposed to be formed during autolysis of tissues *in vitro*,[44] but certain histological evidence is in favor of the view that calcification takes place in acid tissues. In the first place cartilage, which is the favorite site of calcium deposition, takes on a basic stain, implying that it is of an acid reaction which probably is caused by the chondroitin-sulphuric acid. It is also said that in rickets osteoid tissue which is not capable of calcification fails to assume this basophilic character. In areas of calcification after removal of the calcium salts we also find that the ground substance shows the same basophilic (therefore presumably acid) character. Finally, Schmidt[45] has noted that iron pigment present in splenic infarcts is rapidly removed; he does not explain this, but as iron salts are uniformly insoluble in alkalies and soluble in very weak acids, we may consider this fact to be a natural experiment indicating the development of acids in necrotic infarcted areas, which are so prone to calcify. The well-known tendency of muscle fibers to calcify in the vicinity of recent wounds may perhaps also be placed in this category, since there is much evidence of an accumulation of lactic acid in injured muscle fibers[46] and this might be neutralized in part by calcium from the blood; in any case we here again find calcification taking place in acid rather than in alkaline tissues.

We must conclude, therefore, that while in conditions of oversaturation of the blood with calcium salts, either from bone absorption or experimental injection, the presence of a local alkalinity or, perhaps more accurately stated, a decreased amount of $CO_2$ in the fluids and tissues, may determine the deposition of calcium in otherwise normal structures, yet it is not probable that any such reaction is responsible for the ordinary deposition of calcium in ossifying cartilage or in necrotic tissues. We must admit, however, that in this case also the negative evidence is not absolutely conclusive, and we cannot leave out of our considerations the possibility that local changes in tissue reaction may determine calcium deposit. Especially is this reservation necessary since we have abundant evidence that the occurrence of both normal and pathological calcification depends in large measure on the amount of calcium present in the blood. Animals starved of calcium develop, if adult, an osteoporosis, and if young a pseudo-rickets. Experimental calcification in the kidneys is favored by a calcium-rich diet or injections of calcium

---

44. The investigations of Jackson, Wolbach, and Saiki (The Rate of Autolysis and the Appearance of Gases and Acids in the Autolysis of So-Called Sterile Livers of the Dog, Jour. Med. Research, 1909, xxi, 281) have opened the question as to how much of the acidity observed in so-called aseptic autolysis depends on hitherto unrecognized anaerobic bacteria, and how much upon the autolysis itself.

45. Schmidt, M. B.: Ueber Schwund des Eisens in der Milz, Verhandl. d. deutsch. path. Gesellsch., 1908, xii, 271.

46. Wells: The Pathogenesis of Waxy Degeneration of Striated Muscles, Jour. Exper. Med., 1909, xi, 1.

salts (von Kossa[47]). Rabbits are the most favorable animals for use in studies of experimental calcification because of the high calcium content of their blood, but if they are fed on a calcium-poor diet, calcification of the arteries will not follow epinephrin injections (Loeper and Boveri[48]), nor can experimental atheroma be produced in pregnant rabbits whose calcium supply is being utilized by the fetus. Therefore it is evident that both normal and pathological calcification are dependent at least to some extent on the amount of calcium in the blood, which brings us to the subject of the conditions of the solution of calcium by the blood.

### THE SOLUTION OF CALCIUM BY THE BLOOD

In the blood we have present the anomalous condition of calcium in solution in a fluid containing carbonates, phosphates, and sulphates, any one of which would throw it down in the test-tube. According to Abderhalden the red corpuscles contain no appreciable amount of calcium, which is all in the serum, the amount of CaO varying but little in mammals,[49] being from 0.0110 to 0.0131 per cent. Birds' blood contains similarly 0.007 to 0.02 per cent. of CaO (Hiller[4]). Water will hold in solution but about 0.0079 per cent. of tri-calcium phosphate, the form of calcium phosphate which is assumed to be present in the blood, because of the alkali carbonate it contains; therefore tri-calcium phosphate is normally contained in the blood of various mammals *in two to four times as large an amount as it can be held in solution in water.* To account for this phenomenon we have at least two possible agencies, the colloids and the $CO_2$. It is a well-known property of colloids to keep otherwise insoluble substances in solution or in suspension, and the property varies definitely with different colloids, which fact is taken advantage of in the study of the characteristics of colloids by determination of their *Goldzahl.* This *Goldzahl* refers to the number of milligrams of an emulsion colloid (such as the proteins) which is required to prevent precipitation of a characteristic suspension colloid (colloidal gold) by a standard quantity of sodium chlorid.

Colloids maintain the solution of crystalloids in the following manner: in a solution containing crystalloids, which are in solution, and colloids which are in suspension, we have really a solution with two phases, colloid and water. In such two-phase systems part of the crystalloid is concentrated at the surfaces of the colloid particles where the two phases meet, and held here in higher concentration than elsewhere. Consequently the water phase is relieved of part of its load of crystalloid,

47. Von Kossa: Ueber die im Organismus künstlich-erzeugbaren Verkalkungen, Beitr. z. path. Anat. u. z. allg. Path. (Ziegler's), 1901, xxix, 163.

48. Loeper and Boveri: La chaux et les artères, Presse Méd., 1907, xv, 401.

49. Von Kossa gives for rabbits' serum the incredibly high figure of 0.150 per cent. while Abderhalden found in the same animal but 0.0116 per cent.

and is able to take up still more before becoming saturated, so that the total amount of crystalloid dissolved by an aqueous colloidal solution is greater than the amount that can be dissolved by the same quantity of water.

Another possibility is the presence of soluble ion-protein compounds in the blood, but the fact that all the calcium can be readily precipitated from the blood by ammonium oxalate is, according to Hofmeister, conclusive evidence that the calcium is not carried dissolved as such ion-protein compounds. Furthermore, Michaelis and Rona have shown that in milk the calcium is in true solution and not in colloidal solution or suspension, and the same is probably equally true of the blood.

Since the solution and precipitation of calcium by blood-serum is a typical case of colloidal solution of crystalloids, we must carry the above facts into all our considerations of calcification, as Schade[50] has done with such success in the related field of concrement formation.

Pauli and Samac[51] have studied the solubility of calcium salts in dialyzed serum, and contrast the results with their solubility in water and in gelatin, as shown in Table 1.

Table 1.—Solubility of Calcium Salts

| | Percent. Soluble in— | | |
|---|---|---|---|
| | Water | Serum | 1.5 Per Cent. Gelatin |
| $CaSO_4$ | 0.223 | 0.226 | 0.295 |
| $Ca_3(PO_4)_2$ | 0.011 | 0.021 | 0.018 |
| $CaCO_3$ | 0.004 | 0.023 | 0.015 |
| $SiO_2$ | 0.023 | 0.030 | 0.027 |
| Uric Acid | 0.040 | 0.057 | ..... |

Hofmeister[30] found that when calcium chlorid and disodium phosphate react in an alkaline horse-serum there is no precipitation until the concentration of newly-formed tri-calcium phosphate is 0.15 per cent., which is five to ten times greater than the amount of this salt which is present in normal horse-serum.

We may therefore assume that the colloids of the blood are adequate to account, at least in part, for the power of the blood to carry calcium salts in solution. If all the calcium of the blood, however, exists as phosphate and carbonate, the degree of solubility which Hofmeister and Pauli found for these salts in serum is not nearly so great as would be required to account for the amount of calcium (from 1 to 2 per cent. of dry weight or about 0.15 per cent. of entire blood) which von Kossa found in the blood of rabbits. The 0.014 per cent. of CaO found in dog's blood by

50. Schade: Beiträge zur Konkrementbildung, München. med. Wchnschr., 1909, lvi, 3; Zur Enstehung der Harnsteine, Kolloide Ztschr., 1909, iv, 175, and 261.

51. Pauli and Samac: Löslichkeitsbeeinflussung von Elektrolyten durch Eiweiskörper, Biochem. Ztschr., 1909, xvii, 235.

Boggs[52] would, if in the form of tri-calcium phosphate, amount to about 0.026 per cent., which is a little more than the amount of this salt (0.021 per cent.) which Pauli and Samec found soluble in dialyzed serum free from $CO_2$ and salts. We need, therefore, to consider the influence of $CO_2$, which is known to be capable of dissolving calcium, even as it exists in bone, converting it into the relatively soluble acid calcium carbonate and at the same time causing the formation of the mono- and di-calcium phosphates, both of which are more soluble than the tri-calcium phosphate. It is, indeed, probable that it is the $CO_2$ which accomplishes the resorption of dead bone in the living body, and perhaps also the normal resorption of bone in the various conditions in which this process takes place. It was long ago demonstrated by Maly and Donath that $CO_2$ in solution will dissolve calcium from pieces of bone and that $NaHCO_3$ will not dissolve it, and Hofmeister and Tanaka[30] have studied quantitatively this solubility *in vitro* and *in vivo,* finding that pieces of ivory are absorbed most rapidly in tissues whose metabolism is the most active and where, by inference, there is the most $CO_2$ production.[53] The influence of $CO_2$ on the solution of calcium salts has been studied most extensively by Barillé[54] who concludes that calcium is carried in the blood in the form of a definite compound, a carbon-phosphate of calcium. This author finds that 1 liter of water saturated with $CO_2$ at 10 kg. pressure can dissolve 0.923 gm. of tri-calcium phosphate, which forms a solution of an unstable compound, supposedly according to the following reaction:

$$Ca_3P_2O_8 + 4H_2CO_3 = H_2O + P_2O_8Ca_2H_2 : 2CO_2(CO_3H)_2Ca$$

(tri-basic calcium carbon-phosphate)

If this solution is evaporated to dryness the salt decomposes, yielding 0.975 gm. of precipitate, which consists of 0.709 gm. $CaHPO_4$ and of 0.260 gm. $CaCO_3$. Only those bases which form bicarbonates (namely K, Na, $NH_4$, Ca, Mg and Ba) can form carbon-phosphates, all of which are unstable and decompose to form a biphosphate and a bicarbonate. Phosphates of other bases form simple solutions in $CO_2$ and water. Barillé believes that these six bases, or rather the first five, which are normal constituents of the body, all exist in the blood in the form of the carbon-phosphates, and when the $CO_2$ is given off, or neutralized by other bases, the mixture of carbonate and phosphate is precipitated. If the precipitation takes place in an alkaline medium or in one with acid-neu-

52. Boggs: Variations in the Calcium Content of the Blood Following Therapeutic Measures, Johns Hopkins Hosp. Bull., 1908, xix, 201.

52. Bunge: Kochsalzgehalt des Knorpels und das biogenetische Grundsatz, Ztschr. f. physiol. Chem., 1899, xxviii, 452.

53. According to Morpurgo and Satta (Sur quelques particularités de l'autolyse, Arch. ital. de biol., 1908, xlix, 380) calcium may be dissolved from bone tissue during autolysis of bone, but by what process they do not determine.

54. Barillé: Carbonphosphates tricalcique, Jour. de pharm. et chim., Jan. 1 to March 16, 1904, series 6; 1910, series 7, i, 342, 377.

tralizing properties, such as the blood, the phosphate comes down as the tricalcium phosphate, as in bones, intestinal concretions, atheromatous vessels, etc.; if in an acid medium, as in normal urine, we have the dicalcic phosphate. Analyses of different sorts of calcific deposits give results agreeing with this. Now if we recur to Hofmeister's studies of the precipitation of calcium when dissolved to excess in the body fluids, or to the phenomena of metastatic calcification, especially such cases as those of Versé, Jadassohn and Küttner, where we have precipitation of calcium in and on the intima of the vessels containing the least $CO_2$, we find much support for this hypothesis of Barillé's. Furthermore, there is the well-known fact that, no matter how sclerotic the walls of the veins may become, they rarely, if ever, calcify so long as there is venous blood rich in $CO_2$ flowing through them. As soon as they are occluded, however, calcification occurs readily enough (e. g., phleboliths). We may consider that the solution of calcium in the blood is as the carbon-phosphate, in part or in whole, and that under ordinary conditions the precipitation of calcium is prevented by the colloids, no matter how completely the $CO_2$ is removed from the blood, for, as Hofmeister's experiments as well as general experience shows, a watery solution of colloids can maintain a much higher percentage of a crystalloid in solution in the presence of precipitants than it can dissolve from masses of the precipitated salt; e. g. Hofmeister found that when calcium phosphate was precipitated in serum there was no precipitate until the concentration reached 0.15 per cent., while Pauli and Samec had found that serum dissolves but 0.023 per cent., one-seventh as much, of solid tricalcium phosphate. Only in such extreme conditions of oversaturation of the blood with calcium as occurs after experimental injection of calcium salts, or rarely when great quantities of bone are being rapidly absorbed by tumors and other active disease processes, does it become impossible for the blood to hold in solution the carbon-phosphate, which is then precipitated, especially in those places where the $CO_2$ is given off (the lungs) or neutralized by acid excretion (stomach and kidneys) or where the $CO_2$-rich and colloid-poor lymph gives up its $CO_2$ to the arterial blood (the intima of the arteries). This hypothesis receives further support when we consider that tricalcium carbon-phosphate was found by Barillé to be decomposed on evaporation of its aqueous solution into seventy-seven parts of dicalcium phosphate and twenty-three parts of calcium carbonate; now in potentially alkaline solutions, such as the tissue fluids, the dicalcium phosphate would go over to the tricalcium phosphate, and from seventy-seven parts of dicalcium phosphate would be formed 87.7 parts of the tricalcium salt, or exactly the proportion of calcium phosphate which all my analyses have shown to prevail in bone and calcified tissues. It may also be mentioned that Hofmeister and Tanaka found that in experimental metastatic calcification, no matter what soluble salt of calcium they had injected, the deposits always consisted "aus Calciumphosphat mit wenig Calciumcarbonat."

## THE RELATION OF THE COMPOSITION OF CALCIUM SALTS IN BLOOD AND TISSUE

It is indeed unfortunate that erroneous methods of analysis have kept us so long from appreciating the constancy and identity of composition of both normal and pathological deposits of calcium within the tissues, for this is an important consideration in our problems. If we take into account, however, the conditions of circulation in the body, we at once find that it would not be possible for anything except a practically constant and identical composition of bone and calcified tissue deposits to exist for any length of time. The same blood which furnishes the calcium salts to the calcifying tissues is also passing and repassing through great areas of capillaries within the bone-tissue, where are present large quantities of calcium phosphate and carbonate that are in a proportion which is practically constant, not only for the bones of the same animal, but also for the bones of all mammals as far as they have yet been investigated. In both the normal and pathological tissue calcium is being given off to or taken up from the surrounding fluids according to the laws of solution tension and of chemical and osmotic equilibrium, and therefore no matter what the composition of the pathological deposit may have been originally, there can be no question that eventually it will become the same as that of the bone; and even more certainly if the calcium salts are deposited from the blood the resulting precipitate cannot from the beginning be very different from what it is in the calcium storehouse, the bones. Direct experiments made by J. H. Mitchell and myself[26] have shown that mixtures of calcium phosphate and sodium carbonate, and of sodium phosphate and calcium carbonate, when shaken together for some time come to an equilibrium which is quite the same in either case, the calcium carbonate and phosphate being present in the precipitate and in the solution according to their relative solubility.

Likewise when we implanted masses of calcium carbonate or of calcium phosphate into animals we found that in time phosphate is taken up by the carbonate, and carbonate by the phosphate (see Table 2) so that even in so unnatural and extreme a condition as this artificial implantation, in due time we should undoubtedly have present the salts in the same proportion as in the normal bones. Hofmeister and Tanaka[30] have independently obtained corroborative results.

In pathological calcification the deposit is from the first (except in the case of calcifying fat tissue), undoubtedly a mixture of carbonate and phosphate in nearly or quite the standard proportions. That the compo-

TABLE 2.—RESULTS OF IMPLANTATION OF CALCIUM SALTS

| Salt Implanted | Days Before Removal | $Ca_3(PO_4)_2$ in Inorganic Ca Salts Percent. | $CaCO_3$ in Inorganic Ca Salts Percent. |
|---|---|---|---|
| Calcium sulphate | 98 | 76.3 | 8.8 |
| | 160 | 92.6 | 4.6 |
| | 197 | 61.2 | 38.8 |
| Calcium carbonate | 90 | 1.15 | 98.85 |
| | 190 | 8.1 | 91.9 |
| | 200 | 9.8 | 90.2 |
| Calcium phosphate | 80 | 94.1 | 5.9 |
| | 190 | 91.8 | 8.2 |
| | 220 | 93 | 7 |

sition of the bone itself is constant we must ascribe, not to any special combination of ions of calcium, magnesium, $P_2O_5$ and $CO_2$ with the stroma, but to the relative solubility of these salts in the blood-stream. In support of this idea may be cited the experiments of Hofmeister and Tanaka, who found that if $Ca_3(PO_4)_2$ was acted on for twelve days at 37° C. by a solution composed, in imitation of the blood, of 0.9 per cent. NaCl, 0.1 per cent. $Na_2CO_3$, and 0.1 per cent. $NaHCO_3$, the precipitate contained 85.2 per cent. calcium phosphate and 12.75 per cent. calcium carbonate, i. e., the same composition as bone. If a different concentration of alkali was used the ratio of phosphate to carbonate could be changed, the more alkaline the solution the more calcium carbonate in the precipitate. Just as the blood is of nearly constant, yet incessantly varying composition, so too the bone salts may vary within very narrow limits, as they are laid down or taken up according to the relative amount present in the blood, not only of calcium salts, but also of $CO_2$, of colloids, and of other salts, each of which modifies to some extent the solubility of the calcium salts. For example, we may greatly modify the composition of the bone by feeding food poor in calcium and rich in magnesium and strontium,[55, 56] substituting the latter two bases for a considerable proportion of the calcium[57] and also, as is well known, calcium may be withdrawn to a large extent to neutralize acids in acidosis, experimental or pathological, or to meet drains on the bases from pancreatic and biliary fistulæ (Babkin,[58] Looser,[59] Seidel[60]). Conversely, excess

55. Stoeltzner, Helene: Ueber den Einfluss von Strontiumverfütterung auf die chemische Zusammensetzung des wachsenden Knochens, Biochem. Ztschr., 1908, xii, 119.

56. Lehnerdt: Zur Frage der Substitution des Kalziums im Knochensystem durch Strontium, Beitr. z. path. Anat. u. z. allg. Path. (Ziegler's), 1909, xlvi, 468; 1909, xlvii, 215.

57. However, hens are unable to substitute magnesium or strontium for calcium in their shells (See Note 1).

58. Babkin: Material zur experimentellen Pathologie und Therapie der Hunde, Zentralbl. f. Stoffwechsel, 1910, xi, 561.

59. Looser: Ueber Kochenveranderungen bei chronischen Fisteln der grossen Verdauungsdrüsen, Verhandl. d. deutsch. path. Gesellsch., 1907, xi, 291.

60. Seidel: Permanente Gallenfistel und Osteoporose beim Menschen, München. med. Wchnschr., 1910, lvii, 2034.

introduction of calcium can lead to a certain amount of deposition of calcium in the bones (Goitein[61]), although most of the excess is excreted in the urine and feces.

It has been found that there is a regular increase in the ratio of phosphate to carbonate in the bones with advancing years. Wildt[62] gives the figures of Table 3 for the ash of rabbits' bone at different ages.

TABLE 3.—ASH OF RABBITS' BONES AT DIFFERENT AGES

| | At Birth | 1 Mo. | 6 Mo. | 1 Yr. | 4 Yrs. |
|---|---|---|---|---|---|
| Ca phosphate ............ | 86.04 | 85.87 | 84.47 | 82.45 | 82.25 |
| Ca carbonate ........... | 8.30 | 9.09 | 11.23 | 12.98 | 12.86 |
| Mg phosphate ........... | 3.01 | 2.66 | 2.29 | 1.99 | 1.81 |

Similar results have been obtained by Graffenberger[63] and by Gabriel,[64] the latter of whom also notes slight constant differences in the ash (by the glycerin method) of bones of different vertebrates, as follows:

TABLE 4.—PHOSPHORUS PENTOXID AND CALCIUM DIOXID IN BONES OF MAN, THE OX AND THE GOOSE

| | Human | Ox | Goose |
|---|---|---|---|
| $P_2O_5$ ...................... | 36.65 | 37.46 | 38.19 |
| $CO_2$ ...................... | 5.86 | 5.06 | 4.11 |
| Total ................ | 42.51 | 42.52 | 42.30 |

These regular variations in the proportion of calcium carbonate and phosphate present in normal bones of different ages and species, dispose entirely of the hypothesis of Hoppe-Seyler that there is in bones a complex chemical compound of calcium phosphate-carbonate of definite composition.

It is probable that we shall find these variations in the salts of bone to be dependent on differences in the composition of the blood which affect its solvent power for calcium salts. In osteomalacia, the calcium is taken out of the bones in the same ratio of phosphate and carbonate as it there exists (Levy[65]), fully supporting the hypothesis that the salts exist in the bones according to the laws of solubility.

---

61. Goitein: Ueber den Einfluss verschiedener Ca- und Mg-Zufuhr auf den Umsatz und die Menge dieser Stoffe im tierischen Organismus, Arch. f. d. ges. Physiol. (Pflüger's), 1906, cxv, 118.

62. Wildt: Zusammensetzung des Knochen des Kaninchens in verschiedenen Altersstufen, Landwirtschaftliche Versuchsstationen, 1872, xv, 404.

63. Graffenberger: Ueber die Zusammensetzung der Kaninchenknochen im hohen Altersstufen, Landwirtschaftliche Versuchsstationen, 1891, xxxix, 115.

64. Gabriel: Chemische Untersuchungen über die Mineralstoffe der Knochen und Zähne, Ztschr. f. physiol. Chem., 1893, xviii, 257.

65. Levy: Chemische Untersuchungen über osteomalacische Knochen, Ztschr. f. physiol. Chem., 1894, xix, 239.

THE PHYSICAL CHEMISTRY OF CALCIFICATION

Granting that the work of Hofmeister, Pauli, Barillé and others has given us some rational understanding of how the calcium is carried in the blood and why the composition of the deposits of calcium is constantly what it is, yet we have been unable so far to explain why the deposition of calcium salts occurs in the places where it does occur. I have failed, as Pfaundler had before, to find any chemical substance in these places which will account for the deposition of calcium, and the evidence at hand indicates that the calcium is carried in and precipitated from the blood as a mixture of phosphate and carbonate, hence rendering unwarranted any hypothesis of a primary chemical combination of the calcium of the blood with any tissue element. Only in metastatic calcification have we secured evidence of chemical processes which can account for the calcium precipitation. Therefore, finding no clue on the chemical side we naturally turn to the physical aspects, and here we obtain some interesting evidence. The first systematically to consider this possibility seems to have been Pfaundler,[66] who based his work on the earlier observations of Hofmeister and Spiro, that disks of gelatin placed in solution containing various crystalloids are able to absorb some and not others; that is, colloids exert a specific absorption affinity for crystalloids. Pfaundler observed that cartilage immersed in solutions of calcium chlorid takes up more calcium than chlorin, suggesting to him the existence of a specific ion affinity. Other tissues were also found to exhibit a similar but less marked affinity for calcium. However, many of the results obtained by Pfaundler were based on a miscalculation,[67] and I have been unable to secure any positive evidence that there is any marked affinity of cartilage *in vitro* for calcium ions, although it is probable that cartilage does absorb calcium salts to some extent, just as it and many other colloids absorb many different crystalloids; *e. g.*, cartilage absorbs uric acid (Almagia,[68] Brugsch and Citron[69]). Pfaundler was unable to ascribe calcification to this absorption affinity, however, because crystalloids absorbed *in vitro* are washed out readily and not held firmly in the colloids; furthermore, adsorption of calcium seems to be a general colloidal property, not at all limited to the cartilage but exhibited by muscle

66. Pfaundler: Ueber die Elemente der Gewebsverkalkung und ihre Beziehung zur Rachitisfrage, Jahrb. f. Kinderh., 1904, lx, 123.

67. The results of Pfaundler's experiments with pseudo-rachitic limbs are even more doubtful, because the injection of calcium chlorid was preceded by injections of NaCl solution to wash out the blood, and apparently the author has not taken into account the NaCl which would be absorbed by the tissues from the wash water and then given back to the $CaCl_2$ solution.

68. Almagia: Ueber das Absorptionsvermögen der Knorpelsubstanz für Harnsäure, Beitr. z. chem. Physiol. u. Path. (Hofmeister's), 1905, vii, 466.

69. Brugsch and Citron: Ueber die Absorption der Harnsäure durch Knorpel, Ztschr. f. exper. Path. u. Pharm., 1908, v, 401.

and other tissues. Also, as Aron[10] has pointed out, these experiments concern adsorption of calcium ions, while in calcification we have to do with the accumulation of neutral salts. Hofmeister, however, comes to the rescue with an interesting suggestion, which may be stated as follows:

We may imagine the cartilage causing by its absorptive powers an accumulation within itself of calcium salts from the blood, up to or near the limit of saturation. Now the amount of these salts which the tissue fluids can hold in solution depends, as we have seen, partly on the amount of $CO_2$ which is present, and this is a variable quantity. If the amount of $CO_2$ is reduced there will result a precipitation of part of the calcium salts, thus restoring to the cartilage the power of adsorbing more calcium salts whenever the tissue fluids come to it with a higher degree of saturation with calcium salts and $CO_2$; this process can be imagined as going on until the cartilage is entirely incrusted with calcium deposits so that its adsorptive affinity is entirely lost. This hypothesis possesses one great advantage, in that it leaves out of consideration any activity on the part of the cartilage itself, for my own experiments have conclusively shown that calcium deposition takes place in cartilage more than in other tissues *independent of any "vital action"* on the part of the cartilage.[25] As the following table shows, when various tissues, sterilized and killed by heating to 100° for half an hour on each of two days, are left in the abdominal cavity of rabbits for some time, only the cartilage takes up any considerable amount of calcium, but the cartilage comes to contain so much calcium that this is visible to the naked eye as thin scales as large as from 1 to 2 mm. in width.

TABLE 5.—MILLIGRAMS OF CALCIUM OXID IN EACH GRAM OF DRY TISSUE

| | Control | 4 Weeks | 6 Weeks | 8 Weeks | 10 Weeks | 12 Weeks | 14 Wks. |
|---|---|---|---|---|---|---|---|
| Muscle .. | ±0.4 | .... | 4.7 | 6.4 | 11.3 | ..... | ..... |
| Fat ..... | trace | .... | 1.0 | ... | 3.3 | 4.7 | ..... |
| Spleen ... | ±0.3 | .... | 3.3 | ... | 8.4 | ..... | 12.0 |
| Thymus . | trace | .... | ... | 8.7 | ..... | ..... | 12.0 |
| Cartilage. | 3.3 | 15.5 | ... | ... | 124.6 | 162.0 | 154.0 |

Here there can be no question of any cellular activity on the part of the killed cartilage, and as the calcium was found to be combined with phosphoric acid in quite the same proportion as in bone, we may exclude such calcium-ion adsorption as Pfaundler considers. I know of no reason, however, why Hofmeister's theoretization cannot be applied here. The objection may be raised that in the normal body some sorts of cartilage ossify and some do not, which may be considered as evidence of a difference in physiological activity, since no structural difference can be found which accounts for the difference in behavior. I have found,[33] however, that if cartilages which normally do not ossify (tracheal and costal cartilages) be implanted in a similar way, they do not take up nearly so much calcium as the epiphyseal cartilages, as seen in Table 6.

TABLE 6.—MILLIGRAMS OF CALCIUM OXID PRESENT IN THE ENTIRE IMPLANTED MATERIAL

| Weeks | 2. | 4. | 6. | 8. | 10. | 12. | 14. | 16. | 18. |
|---|---|---|---|---|---|---|---|---|---|
| Costal | .. | 0.5 | .. | 1 | 6 | 15 | ... | absorbed | ... |
| | .. | ... | .. | 5 | 12 | absorbed | ... | ........ | ... |
| | .. | ... | .. | 4 | .. | ........ | ... | ........ | ... |
| Tracheal | 5 | ... | 10 | 1.8 | .. | 20 | 28 | 46 | ... |
| | .. | ... | 19 | .... | .. | ........ | ... | ........ | ... |
| | .. | ... | 3 | .... | .. | ........ | ... | ........ | ... |
| Epiphyseal | .. | 10 | 37 | 54 | 134 | 109 | 167 | ........ | 151 |
| | .. | ... | 37 | 88 | 117 | 128 | ... | ........ | ... |

Therefore we must admit that the characteristic difference which these cartilages exhibit in respect to their tendency to lay on calcium salts is not in any way dependent on any physiological or vital activity of their cells, for it is exhibited just as strikingly by the dead cartilage. We have been unable to detect any chemical differences in the three sorts of cartilage sufficient to account for this difference in behavior,[33] and we have not found any corresponding variation in their adsorptive affinity for calcium salts *in vitro*.[22] It must be borne in mind, however, that all forms of hyaline cartilage are prone to calcify—far more so than any other normal tissue in the body—so that in old age more or less calcification and ossification always takes place in tracheal, costal, laryngeal, and articular cartilages. That is to say, the difference between the different cartilages in respect to calcification is one of degree only, which may not be discernible under the unnatural conditions of an experiment *in vitro*.

Furthermore, if we not only consider the cartilages, but also take into account the nature of the tissues in which pathological calcification takes place, we find further support for the physical theory. What have these many and various sites of calcification in common? Certainly not a common chemical composition, for we find most widely differing sorts of materials the seat of calcium deposition; contrast, for example, the elastic coat of arteries, ganglion cells, necrotic epithelium, and hyaline cartilage; in fact every dead or dying tissue may calcify. What these various tissues do have in common are: (1) a poor blood-supply and slow lymph-stream, with conditions retarding the rate of exchange by osmosis; (2) a more or less homogeneous, usually hyaline, ground substance.

Even in metastatic calcification a hyaline ground substance seems to be the point of election for the deposition of the calcium salts, for Huebschmann[70] found that in the lungs in this condition the deposit is first and chiefly in the elastic fibers. Furthermore, that tissues which are to calcify have a high affinity for inorganic salts is shown by their well-

---

70. Huebschmann: Histologie der Kalkmetastase, Centralbl. d. allg. Path., 1908, xix, 737.

known tendency to lay on iron when this is available, e. g., in the vicinity of hemorrhages.[71]

Taking ossification and calcification by and large as the processes occur, we cannot fail to be impressed with these two factors of a homogeneous ground substance and a poor circulation; pathologists especially have been familiar with the coincidence and have repeatedly called attention to it (see Ricker,[72] Aschoff[73]). Therefore, all things considered, we are fairly driven back to the conception of a physical *Kalkfänger,* which serves as a point where condensation of the poorly soluble calcium salts takes place until, perhaps because of variation in $CO_2$ content in the solvent fluids, precipitation begins and continues rhythmically as Hofmeister has suggested. Precipitation is ordinarily in excess of re-solution because of the known slowness of solution of precipitates by a fluid in which the precipitated substance exists at all times nearly at the saturation point, although when for any length of time the amount of calcium in the blood is reduced resolution exceeds deposition, and absorption of calcium occurs.[74]

Taking all the evidence as it stands we find ourselves best satisfied with that which indicates that *calcification begins as a simple physical adsorption by hyaline substances,* which have a more or less specific adsorption affinity for calcium. That the substances which take up calcium have strong and specific absorption affinities is well established. For example, cartilage itself is the richest of all tissues in NaCl (Bunge[52]

71. S. Ehrlich (Eisen und Kalkimpragnation in menschlichen Geweben, Centralbl. f. allg. Path., 1906, xvii, 177) holds that the iron serves as a mordant for the calcium which is subsequently deposited.

72. Ricker: Verkalkung und Steinbildung, Ergebn. d. allg. Path. (Lubarsch-Ostertag's), 1896, iii, 643.

73. Aschoff: Verkalkung, Ergebn. d. allg. Pathol. (Lubarsch-Ostertag), 1902, viii, 561.

74. Lichtwitz (Ueber die Bedeutung der Kolloide für die Konkrementbildung und die Verkalkung, Deutsch. med. Wchnschr., 1910, xxxvi, 704) has suggested another hypothesis of calcification which can be applied to pathological calcification, perhaps, but not so well to ossification. He considers especially the part played by the colloids in keeping the calcium salts in solution, and notes that in areas where calcification occurs we have had a precipitation of these colloids; e. g., in caseous areas there has been precipitation of proteins, in atheroma the fatty changes represent a precipitation of lipoids. When in these areas the colloids are thus precipitated the calcium salts which they have kept in solution will then fall out. Of course the amount of dissolved calcium salts present in the area at any one time would not, when precipitated, cause any noticeable calcification, but because of the withdrawal of the calcium from the solution the osmotic equilibrium is disturbed, and there being now a relatively greater concentration of calcium salts in the surrounding fluids, these will continue to diffuse into this area and to be precipitated until the area is entirely filled up with precipitated calcium salts. This is an attractive hypothesis, but objections may be raised. In the first place, it does not seem possible to apply it to ossification, and in the second place it seems probable that under the conditions specified the invading calcium would be promptly precipitated on the inner surface, or even in the walls of the diffusion membrane, thus blocking further infiltration.

found that 70.7 per cent. of the ash of nasal cartilage from the pig is NaCl), yet contains very little potassium, although the circulating blood contains much potassium, and in most tissues the proportion of potassium is greater than of sodium. In the shark, indeed, so great is the affinity of the cartilaginous skeleton for NaCl that this easily soluble salt takes almost the same place as does calcium in the mammals, constituting 16.69 per cent. of the total fresh weight and 94.24 per cent. of the ash of the cartilage (Peterson and Soxhlet[75]). On the other hand, in rickets the cartilage seems unable to take up even the calcium which is present in the blood and tissues in normal amounts (Brubacker[76]). As before mentioned, cartilage also shows a decided adsorption affinity for uric acid and many other crystalloids.

The hyaline degenerated tissues in which calcification commonly occurs also show a strong adsorption affinity, especially for pigments, such as iron, and often for various dyes that stain by physical rather than by chemical union. May we not, indeed, liken the process of calcification to its analogues, the infiltration of foreign bodies in the bladder with urinary salts, or even the petrefaction of trees and similar objects? Schade[50] points out that in the former case the part played by the foreign body is not to be compared to the starting of crystallization, since in crystallization the substance initiating crystallization must be of the same nature as the crystals, and the solution must be saturated. Rather is it to be considered as a surface phenomenon, concentration at the surface of colloidal particles leading to saturation and precipitation, which is progressive as long as new supplies come in, and permanent when the stroma of the precipitated mass is a non-reversible colloid. After all, to what extent does a mass of calcifying dead tissue in the body, e. g., a thrombus, differ from the saturation of a fibrin clot in the urinary bladder with the salts of the urine? In each case the colloid is permeated by a fluid nearly saturated with certain salts, and when the process is completed we have alike in each a ground substance of irreversibly coagulated colloids in which the crystalloidal deposit is held. We do not question that the formation of the urinary concretion may be initiated by purely physical causes; then why not admit the same possibility for calcification in the tissues?

## RECAPITULATION

So far as the knowledge gained from the literature and personal investigation permits me to form opinions, my present understanding of the essentials of calcification and ossification may be summarized as

75. Petersen and Soxhlet: Ueber die Zusammensetzung des Knorpels vom Haifisch, Jour. f. prakt. Chem., 1841, vii, 179.

76. Brubacker: Ueber den Gehalt an anorganischen Stoffen, besonders an Kalk, in den Knochen und Organen normaler und rachitischer Kinder, Ztschr. f. Biol., 1890, xxvii, 517.

follows: Calcium is carried in the blood in amounts not far from the saturation point, held in solution by the colloids and the carbon dioxid, and existing probably in the form of an unstable double salt of calcium bicarbonate and dicalcium phosphate. In normal ossification, and in most instances of pathological calcification, the deposition is probably initiated by a process of colloidal adsorption causing a concentration of this double salt in the hyaline matrix which is to be calcified, and which has a strong affinity for calcium salts. Reduction in the amount of carbon dioxid in such areas, or some unknown agency, causes a precipitation of calcium salts in this colloid matrix, and permits of further infiltration of dissolved calcium salts whenever the concentration of $CO_2$ in the fluids may be greater (Hofmeister). The composition of bone and of most pathological deposits of calcium exhibits an almost constant ratio of phosphate (from 85 to 90 per cent.) and carbonate (from 10 to 15 per cent.) which constancy of composition is to be ascribed to the relative solubility of these calcium salts in the blood, and the approximately constant composition of this solvent. Slight variations in the composition of the blood may cause corresponding slight changes in the composition of the calcium deposits in the body. It is inconceivable that a mass of calcium salts anywhere in the body can for long possess a chemical composition essentially different from that of the bone, with which it is in constant exchange through the medium of the circulating blood.

There is no acceptable evidence that in ossification, or ordinarily in pathological calcification, the deposition of calcium is initiated as a chemical precipitation by some precipitating ion present in the tissues which are to be calcified. *From the beginning the calcium seems to be deposited as carbonate and phosphate in about the same ratio as in mature bone.*

Hyaline cartilage possesses an affinity for calcium which is not exhibited to an equal degree by other tissues, and this affinity is more marked in cartilage which normally ossifies than in cartilages which normally do not ossify. This specific affinity does not depend on any functional activity of the cells, for it is shown by dead cartilage. No difference in chemical composition can be found to explain this difference between ossifying and non-ossifying cartilage in regard to their absorption affinity for calcium salts. A homogeneous, hyaline structure is the usual characteristic of calcifying substances, which resemble each other much more in physical qualities than in chemical composition.

There seem to be no essential differences between the processes involved in normal ossification and in most instances of pathological calcification; any area of calcification may be changed to true bone in the course of time. Calcium salts seem to exert a specific influence on connective tissue cells, causing them to form bone; without this stimulus they cannot form bone, at least not readily and normally.

Exceptional cases of calcification occur in which other processes are involved than in ossification. One of these, "metastatic calcification," occurs whenever from any cause the proportion of calcium present in the blood is so great that it requires the effect of both the colloids and of the $CO_2$ in maximum concentration to keep it in solution; then the calcium salts are deposited in those points in the body where the $CO_2$ content of the fluids is least. Another exception is seen whenever there is a considerable splitting of fats, the new-formed fatty acids in some cases combining with calcium to form calcium soaps. These calcium soaps are ordinarily absorbed, but exceptionally, when in large amounts, e. g., calcifying lipoma, etc., the fatty acid radicals may be replaced by $P_2O_5$ and $CO_2$. There is no satisfactory evidence, however, that this is a common, much less a usual method of calcification, and there is much evidence that it is not. *Calcium deposition seems to depend, alike in normal and in most pathological conditions, rather on physico-chemical processes than on chemical reactions.*

University of Chicago.

# INTRA-ABDOMINAL PRESSURES

HAVEN EMERSON, M.D.
NEW YORK

## INTRODUCTION

The subject of intra-abdominal pressure falls naturally under four heads, namely:

1. Pressure on solid viscera (liver, kidney, spleen), which cannot be other than that existing in the free peritoneal cavity.

2. Pressures within hollow viscera; which have been fairly established under a variety of conditions, and may be wholly independent of the pressure in the abdominal cavity.

3. Pressures within blood and lymph spaces which have been accurately determined, and are modified by the pressure in the abdominal cavity.

4. Pressures within the peritoneal space proper.

Except in so far as the pressures within the hollow viscera and the blood-vessels affect or are affected by the intraperitoneal pressure proper, they will not be treated of in this study. The pressures on the viscera must be identical with the pressure conditions of the cavity within which they are exposed wholly or in part, except where there is some inflammatory or neoplastic process, which might cause a local variation of pressure within or without the capsule of an organ, or in its secretory spaces or its vessels. We come then to a discussion of previous statements concerning the normal pressure within the peritoneal cavity, which will be followed by experimental evidence directed toward settling some doubtful points, and leading attention to the application of our knowledge in this regard, to the work of the internist and the surgeon.

I shall use the term "intra-abdominal pressure" to indicate the pressure in the free peritoneal cavity.

While the conditions causing and modifying intra-thoracic pressures have been the subject of exact research, and the conclusions offered meet general acceptance, this is not the case with intra-abdominal pressures. Inasmuch as intrathoracic and intra-abdominal pressures are to a certain degree complementary and serve somewhat similar functions, it seems worth while to put intra-abdominal pressure on as exact a basis as intrathoracic. This seems especially desirable when the bearing of intra-abdominal pressure on circulation, respiration and absorption is considered. The relation of intra-abdominal pressures to some of the problems of internal medicine, obstetrics, gynecology and surgery warrants a more exact study of the question than has yet appeared.

HISTORICAL SKETCH

The standard text-books of obstetrics, gynecology and surgery treat of the matter so rarely, and when it is mentioned, so inaccurately, that no information is to be had from them. In medical writings the matter is oftenest found under discussions of splanchnoptosis, ascites and circulatory conditions, but nowhere is there anything approaching a full statement of the case. Most of the text-books of physiology fail to mention intra-abdominal pressure at all.[1]

A few of the more comprehensive physiologies do mention the matter, but treat it quite superficially. DuBois-Reymond (1908) merely states that there is a variation in intra-abdominal pressure due to the action of the diaphragm. Hall (1900) considers intra-abdominal pressure at zero when the abdominal muscles are at rest, but illustrates the rise above that on descent of diaphragm and contraction of the abdominal muscles. Although his tracings are probably correct, he gives neither base-line nor statement as to what fluid he used in his manometers to obtain the pressure records. He notes the effect of abdominal pressure on venous and lymphatic flow. Landois (1900) refers to Hamburger's work of 1895-96, and makes the curious statement that expiration causes a rise in intra-abdominal pressure in man and dogs, but that inspiration has this effect in guinea-pigs. A slight increase in abdominal pressure causes increased heart action and arterial pressure, but excessive pressure in the abdomen decreases both.

Luciani describes the use of rectal and esophageal bougies, and gives tracings of intrathoracic and intra-abdominal pressures, but no figures as to the facts observed in etherized dogs. The essential fallacy of testing such pressures through a contractile hollow organ he does not observe. He finds that the abdominal pressure varies with the descent of the diaphragm and contraction of the abdominal walls.

Schaefer (1900) after noting the effect of abdominal conditions on the circulation, points out the very important fact that the tone of the abdominal wall muscles is maintained by the respiratory center. The abdominal pressure as maintained by the abdominal walls is of the utmost importance, as it tonically maintains the caliber of the great veins and can compress them or allow them to expand.

Tigerstedt (1906) says, "By abdominal pressure we mean the pressure on abdominal viscera produced by the simultaneous contraction of

1. Brubaker, 1908; Bunge, 1905; Dalton, 1882; Foster, 1896; Halliburton, 1907; Nagel, 1907; Ott, 1907; Howells, 1907; Kirke, 1907; Starling, 1907; Stewart, 1905; Hermann, 1880; Hill, 1906.

the diaphragm and the abdominal muscles." He gives no figures or tracings, and considers the pressure of importance only in relation to defecation and in labor.

A review of the literature is very interesting aside from the many points of view from which the matter of intra-abdominal pressure has been approached by clinicians.

In 1851 Weber, and Donders, in 1854, called attention, the former to a condition in man, the latter to experimental conditions in animals, which tended to prove that extreme expiratory effort caused a diminution or disappearance of the arterial pulse at various points of the body, as in the radial at the wrist, and a marked diminution in cardiac sounds. They note that expiratory effort assists venous return from the abdominal to the thoracic cavity. They suggest that it would be interesting to know whether expiratory pressure is associated with strong pressure on the abdominal viscera.

Hammernik, in his publication of 1858, makes the first definite statement in the literature that the opposed surfaces of the abdominal viscera are held together by "horror vacui," or suction of surfaces, and he even states that opening of the abdomen allows entrance of air into the cavity just as is the case on opening the pleural space. He practically states that under normal conditions there is a constant negative pressure within the abdominal cavity; "the diaphragm being held down by negative pressure, ascending in a higher dome when this pressure is released on opening abdomen." This statement is quoted by Schatz and evidently had strong influence on the writers of the last half of the nineteenth century.

Marey in his "Physiologie médicale de la circulation du sang," Paris, 1863, says that the effects that respiration produces on the thorax are the inverse of those present in the abdomen. In other words, he seems to have recognized a fluctuating positive pressure in the abdomen, modified by the fluctuating negative pressure in the thorax, but he describes no tests and gives no records or figures.

In 1865 two writers, Braune in Germany and Duncan in Edinburgh, wrote on this subject, and they have been frequently quoted.

Braune tested abdominal pressure by the use of rectal bougies with human beings of different sizes and weights, and concluded that abdominal pressure depended on hydrostatic conditions in the abdomen; he says that it varies from 40 cm. water to 100 cm., according to the amount of voluntary abdominal contraction. He says that it is lowest in the horizontal, and highest in the vertical position. Positive pressure exists only when the abdominal muscles contract, or within hollow viscera.

Duncan, on the other hand, describes a retentive power of the abdomen as a moderate negative pressure which assists circulation, and the position of viscera, but which straining overcomes. In both reports the method of observation is altogether unreliable.

In 1870 Paul Bert published his admirable volume on the comparative physiology of respiration, in which he notes the errors necessarily arising from recording pressures within hollow organs and reasoning from such records as to intra-abdominal pressures. He therefore avoids offering figures to indicate absolute abdominal pressures, but draws some excellent conclusions from numerous tests on chloroformized mammals by tracheal and rectal tubes. If the descent of the diaphragm predominates, the abdominal pressure will rise in inspiration. If thoracic expansion predominates, abdominal pressure will fall in inspiration. He finds that the conditions of reciprocal muscular tone and contraction of diaphragm, abdominal and thoracic muscles vary infinitely.

In 1872 Schatz went into the subject in detail from the experimental and clinical standpoint. He used a Ludwig kymograph and a mercury manometer connected with a balloon and rigid tube, the balloon being placed within the uterus during labor. He concludes that the abdominal pressure itself is positive or negative. His other figures, relating as they do to intra-uterine and not intraperitoneal conditions, are not of immediate interest here. "Intra-abdominal pressure must be positive because, if it were not, the amniotic fluid would not flow out." Here again he reasons falsely, attributing to abdominal pressure conditions existing in the uterus.

Again, he says that intra-uterine pressure varies with abdominal pressure, having under certain conditions a negative pressure when pressure in the abdomen is positive. He reasons also from pressure conditions in the urinary bladder with equal error. He says that the pressure in the pelvis in pregnancy differs from abdominal pressure because of separation of the cavities by the uterus.

Schatz suggests that there is an adjustment of the abdominal muscles to meet distention by the pregnant uterus. He says pressure is from 4 to 5 mm. Hg lower in the dorsal than in the sitting or standing positions, and is negative in the knee-chest or knee-elbow positions, even — 2 to — 4 mm. Hg tested by gastric and rectal bougie balloons. He finds that pure thoracic respiration diminishes abdominal pressure. Pure diaphragmatic breathing raises abdominal pressure.

In the cadaver and in the puerperal state the abdominal pressure is negative because of relaxation of the abdominal muscles.

During pregnancy intra-abdominal pressure rises slightly though not in proportion to the increase in the size of the uterus, until the last month, when usually the abdominal muscles are stretched beyond their ability to respond, and there is then usually a fall of pressure below normal.

In other words, abdominal pressure depends on the muscular strength and support of the back muscles against the stretching of the abdominal and thoracic muscles. Schatz notes that the blood-pressure in the inferior cava must be at least as high as intra-abdominal pressure to avoid obliteration of its lumen, at least 20 cm. water. By the same reasoning the pressure in the liver capillaries must be higher than the caval pressure.

The capillaries in the soft tissues of the abdominal viscera are supported by a moderate abdominal pressure which assists them to withstand the blood-pressure, in somewhat the same way that the capillaries in compact tissues, such as muscle, are supported.

A moderate positive intra-abdominal pressure, slightly increased in the erect position, assists the return flow of blood, and the flow of chyle from the abdominal viscera.

Wendt (1873) followed Schatz with a further study of rectal pressures, and concludes that the higher the abdominal pressure the less the secretion of urine.

Emminghaus (1874) found negative pressure in human beings, but by unreliable methods in the cadaver.

Odebrecht (1875) concludes from testing pressure in the urinary bladder and in the rectum that the intra-abdominal pressure is normally positive. He found only two cases which showed a negative pressure, out of a large number tested. One was a case of localized peritonitis involving the fundus of the bladder and its lateral and posterior attachments during pregnancy, but after complete recovery and a readjustment of the organs after delivery, there was a return to normal positive pressures in the rectum and in the bladder. The other case was one of hydronephrosis, in which the bladder was found to show a negative pressure on catheterization.

Dubois (1876) notes the errors of Schatz' method and warns against drawing conclusions as to intraperitoneal pressure from pressures found in hollow viscera.

Luciani (1877) in a monograph on the oscillation of intrathoracic and intra-abdominal pressure, states that the contraction of the diaphragm is not properly accessory, but essential in causing an inspiratory rise of pressure in blood-vessels. The statement is distinct, but the curves before and after section of the phrenic nerves do not show it perfectly. Again in 1878 he made a full report and notes the necessity of observing whether the test animal is under deep narcosis or not. He did not use a cannula in the intact abdomen.

Wegner (1877) tested the rate of absorption of fluids from the peritoneal surface and in a very suggestive study concludes that one of the factors in the mechanics of absorption is the filtration which the normal positive intra-abdominal pressure accomplishes. He notes that one factor which interferes with absorption of fluid exudates or transudates, in cases in which large tumors or large accumulations of peritoneal fluids have been removed from the abdominal cavity, is the drop in abdominal pressure to zero or negative, which change affects directly the circulatory and absorptive functions. This disadvantage does not persist if there has been no severe injury to the abdominal muscles. The result of stretching the abdominal walls is a diminution, a slowed and perhaps wholly checked absorption.

Quincke in 1878 states that abdominal pressure is positive and increases with inspiration and decreases with expiration. He draws his conclusions from tests on patients with ascites. He notes the probably obstructive effect of high abdominal pressure on venous return from abdominal viscera.

Landau wrote, in 1881, on floating kidney, in the course of which study he remarks that intra-abdominal pressure falls below zero where the abdomen is pendulous with a resulting difficulty in expiration.

Schwenburg (1882) concluded from animal experiments that the respiratory change of blood-pressure was due chiefly to pressure increase in the abdomen on descent of the diaphragm in inspiration, but confessed to his inability to prove it in the case of human beings.

Mosso and Pellacani (1882) using a catheter in the bladder, decided that there was a positive abdominal pressure as well as an active pressure by the bladder walls.

Rosenthal (1882) by the use of a gastric bougie showed that abdominal pressure seemed to be positive and to rise on inspiration.

Schreiber (1883) concludes from tambour tracings with a stomach bougie that abdominal pressure is negative, — 5 to — 10 mm. water. All positive pressures are merely local in various visceral cavities, and are not caused by abdominal pressure which is normally negative. In a case of ascites he found inspiratory increase and expiratory decrease in positive abdominal pressure. Abdominal pressure is positive only under abnormal conditions, as ascites.

Kronecker and Meltzer (1883) in the course of studies on the mechanism of deglutition, found by the use of a gastric bougie that there was a fall in pressure on inspiration and a rise in expiration below the diaphragm.

Senator (1883) notes that abdominal pressure is much diminished by weakness of the abdominal walls. A common cause of floating kidney is stretching of the abdominal walls by repeated pregnancies.

Martin (1885) in discussing the causes of displacement of the uterus says that intra-abdominal pressure is the essential factor, and that failure of the pelvic floor allows diminution of this pressure, and a fall of the uterus. He notes that the abdominal pressure, if positive, must be very slight.

Hegar (1886) says that pelvic viscera are dislocated, not only by relaxed ligaments, but by diminution of intra-abdominal pressure. This lowered pressure causes dislocation of other viscera and allows congestion and dilatation of abdominal and crural vessels (veins especially). Large hernias always cause a fall of intra-abdominal pressure (1873). He concludes that negative pressure does not exist in the rectum or bladder normally, but may be created by relaxing the abdominal walls, and then making deep thoracic inspiratory efforts.

C. Hasse (1886) gives the following as proofs that abdominal pressure is positive and fluctuating: (1) tonus of abdominal walls; (2) pressure of intestinal contents; (3) prolapse of intestines on opening the abdomen; (4) issue of fluid on puncture; (5) non-entrance of air on opening crural vein below Poupart's ligament. He says that abdominal pressure rises in inspiration and falls in expiration, and at no time is negative.

Schroeder (1886) notes but slight increase of intra-abdominal pressure in pregnancy, and supposes that there must be some adaptation of abdominal tension to the increasing size of the uterus. He also notes a negative pressure in the abdomen in the knee-chest and other similar positions.

Verstraeten (1887) thinks that pressure rises in expiration and falls in inspiration.

Weisker (1888) made a summary of the facts as understood at that time, and says: "Pressures in hollow viscera vary within wide limits and are independent of intra-abdominal pressure." "Pressure in any cavity depends on its content (its character, bulk and compressibility) and its wall (elasticity of various parts, its ability to contract, support or change its shape)." He finds inspiratory and expiratory changes of pressure in the abdomen to be constant within from 1 to 2 cm. of water. Inspiratory increase in pressure is minimized by the yielding of the abdominal walls. In the same way there is rarely high pressure in ascites. From tests he made himself in the rectum and in the stomach he concludes that if proper precautions are taken the gastric pressure is never negative, and usually only slightly above zero. Positive abdominal pressure can be brought into play only when the abdominal muscles contract.

Timofeevsky in 1888 concluded in a study on the pressure in the inferior vena cava that the normal pressure varied but slightly from zero, and that it was not constant, varying with different positions of the body, the weight and fulness of abdominal viscera, and with the contraction and development of the abdominal wall and exterior pressure.

Hasse in 1890 notes that intra-abdominal pressure increases with the descent of the diaphragm in inspiration, and that this variation in pressure plays a large part in assisting the flow of blood in the portal vein.

Heinricius (1890) made exact observations by carotid cannula, tracheal cannula and abdominal cannula, but did not record absolute pressures graphically. He found that pressures of from 27 to 46 cm. water, in cats and guinea-pigs were fatal owing to prevention of respiration and a steadily diminishing amount of inspired air. Any interference with thoracic expansion allows pressure of lungs against heart, a diminution of diastolic distention and a low blood-pressure.

Under curare and artificial respiration he found that increased abdominal pressure caused a vagus effect on the heart, a marked slowing with rise in arterial blood-pressure. A pressure of 32 mm. Hg in the abdomen caused the pulse-rate to fall from 226 to forty per minute, and pressure in carotid to fall from 134 to 130 mm. Hg. Rapid distention at low pressure is of much harm, while high pressure gradually established may be well borne for some time. A pressure of even 60 mm. Hg, he says, may be borne within the abdomen. That this does not close the veins is proved by the absence of a prompt fall in arterial pressure, which such obstruction always causes. If pressure is extreme and prolonged collateral paths may be developed.

Reprieff (1890) found intra-abdominal pressure zero in living and dead dogs, and often negative when they were put in horizontal dorsal position.

Schatz (1891) still denies that there is a positive abdominal pressure.

Hogge (1892) after noting the futility of pretending to get absolute intra-abdominal pressure by recording appliances, inserted in hollow viscera, gives a number of good theoretical reasons for expecting to have an increase of abdominal pressure when inspiration causes a drop in thoracic pressure. He also follows the work of Heinricius closely, and points out that pathological conditions which cause excessive pressure or absence of normal support in the abdomen, result in interference with the circulation. He considers a positive pressure fluctuating with respiration, rising on inspiration, normal and useful in assisting secretion and excretion.

Kelling (1892) agrees with Schrieber (1883) after testing gastric pressures with bougie and water manometer, that normally, abdominal pressure is negative, and that this is more marked in inspiration because at that moment the costal arch is increased and enlarges the abdominal volume more than the descending diaphragm decreases it. In expiration there is no rule, the pressure rising or falling. He asserts that gastric pressure is negative except when the gastric musculature is either distended by contents or irritated and contracted. His conclusions as to abdominal pressure are all based on observations on intragastric pressures.

Moritz in 1895 tested pressures by a bougie balloon in the stomach connected with a recording water manometer. He notes that accurate intra-abdominal pressure can be determined only by a cannula in the peritoneal cavity. He finds stomach pressure but little affected by external pressure of the abdominal walls.

Hamburger (1896) is the first writer to state definitely that he thinks pressures are different at different levels in the abdomen, a fallacy which occurs even in more recent writings.

His tests of abdominal pressure were incidental to experiments on the absorption of fluids from the peritoneal space from the intestines. Excessive abdominal pressure, 45 cm. water, causes failure of respiration by fatigue of the diaphragm in rabbits. Moderate pressure increases blood-pressure, and if persisted in causes cardiac weakness from fatigue due to overcoming unnecessary resistance applied to the surface of the abdominal vessels. This is more marked the higher the pressure. Absorption of fluids from the normal intestine is increased in rate by increase of intra-abdominal pressure, within moderate limits, from 8 to 14 cm. water. If intestinal pressure falls to zero absorption ceases, and if as low as 0.5 cm. it is very slow. On inspiration, the diaphragm, and on expiration, the abdominal muscles, compress the abdominal contents, but pressure rises on inspiration and falls on expiration. It takes a pressure of from 20 to 40 cm. water in the abdomen to obliterate the effect of respiration on abdominal pressures. The intra-intestinal pressure at which the absorption stream ceases, must lie under the capillary pressure. How much lower it is depends on the power of cellular imbibition and the accompanying suction of the blood-stream.

Schwerdt (1896), in an able article on enteroptosis, notes that intra-abdominal pressure is probably positive under normal conditions, but sinks with relaxed abdominal walls. Usually pressure is the same throughout the abdominal cavity, and the hollow viscera are but little affected in shape or volume. His conclusions are based on the use of a water manometer and bougie in the rectum and stomach. Normal pressure probably varies from zero to + 3 cm. water.

Kelling (1896), as a result of tests in the stomach and the rectum, denies the existence of a positive intra-abdominal pressure. He makes no direct tests in the abdominal cavity, but tests stomach pressure and volumes in etherized dogs and in cat and rabbit cadavers.

Hasse (1901) considers a fluctuating positive intra-abdominal pressure as the result of coincident contraction of the diaphragm and abdominal muscles in inspiration, but he reports no tests.

Quirin (1901) used narcotized dogs, cats, guinea-pigs and rabbits and a glass cannula tied in the opened abdomen. He reports positive pressures, greater in inspiration than in expiration, except during active movements, when the reverse is the case. He notes diminished tone as a cause of low pressure in anesthetized animals, and cautions against the error of drawing conclusions from visceral records. His records give no abscissa, but show fairly constant results. The errors in his method are opening the abdomen before testing, and the absence of a base-line in his tracings.

Meyer (1902) denies the presence of a positive intra-abdominal pressure, and says it must vary in different parts of the abdomen, and at different times. His ideas show a total lack of understanding of physics and are based on no direct observations.

Jurgensen (1899) notes the effect of abdominal pressure which when increased in inspiration raises aortic pressure.

Hagentorn (1902) considers abdominal pressure positive, except when the diaphragm or abdominal muscles are paralyzed or have lost their tone. All bodily movement is accompanied by increased intra-abdominal pressure. No experimental evidence is reported.

Hormann (1905) points out the defects in the reports of earlier writers, and declares that he will determine pressure in the intact abdomen. His observations on a recently killed dog, and on a dog killed by chloroform, cannot be taken as correct, as the maintenance of muscular tone is necessary for accurate tests. He concludes from these tests that pressure is different in different parts of the abdomen, an error that even careless technic should not allow any one to perpetuate. Using an abdominal trochar he found negative pressure in the upper part of the peritoneal cavity and positive pressure in the lower part, in animals held vertically and recently killed by chloroform.

One animal tested during life showed negative pressure rising in inspiration. Hormann illustrates his ideas by models which have rigid and not tonically contracted walls, and the conclusions are not at all justified. He denies a constant abdominal pressure. In complete repose abdominal muscles exert no pressure. He notes that animals used in his tests were either dead or under deepest narcosis, and the four living dogs under narcosis he notes as being emaciated and with sunken abdominal walls, conditions which explain his failure to obtain correct results.

Mathes (1906) makes an excellent statement to the effect that "the greater is the traction effected by the lungs (i. e., negative thoracic pressure), the less is the portion of the pressure on the viscera which the abdominal and pelvic walls have to support." He agrees in general with Kelling and considers pressure in the abdomen to be positive and to increase in inspiration.

Smith (1908) in a summary of the subject, presents no new data and is misled by some of the earlier writers. He notes, however, that when abdominal pressure is raised by contraction of the abdominal muscles, the pressure is transmitted undiminished in all directions. Negative pressure he considers as common beneath the diaphragm, if the abdominal walls are rigid at that spot, a statement that seems impossible since a fall in pressure is likely to be distributed just as much as a rise to all parts of the abdomen, and undiminished.

Barrett (1908) adds no further proof to the subject, and moreover says that "because of constant disturbance of body equilibrium, and because of the sluggishness of contents to respond to fluid pressure, this pressure varies in different localities at different times."

Weitz, in 1909, working in Quincke's clinic, made a number of tests of intra-abdominal pressure by a manometer in connection with a trocar used in abdominal paracentesis for the removal of ascitic fluid. He found positive pressure in the fluid and noted that it was due to a combination of the forces of hydrostatic pressure and tension of the abdominal wall. If the fluid is of long standing and the walls are relaxed the pressure is lower than under the reverse conditions. He finds that the pressure rises in inspiration and falls in expiration.

He evidently considers pressure in the normal abdomen to be less in the upper than in the lower portions. "As pressure after the removal of part of the ascitic fluid is but slightly above atmospheric pressure at the level of the trocar, the pressure in the upper abdomen must be often negative." "This must be beneficial as it lightens the work of the abdomen." Finding pressure in the urinary bladder in ascites higher than pressure in the free peritoneal cavity, he notes that the contraction of the walls of hollow viscera may make any such records quite misleading.

Undoubtedly his observations as regards the presence of positive pressure in the fluid accumulation in an ascitic abdomen, and the negative pressure in the space left in such a distended and pendulous abdomen above the fluid, are correct, but that is far from saying that in the normal abdomen with no fluid and with a gaseous medium to distribute pressures among the movable intestines, there may be different or opposite kinds of pressure in different parts of the abdomen at the same time.

Herrick (1910) notes the probable existence of negative pressure in the uppermost portions of the abdomen of dogs in the dorsal position when they are deeply narcotized by morphin and ether, and mentions the demonstration of negative pressure in the bladder in human beings in the knee-chest position, as supporting this theory. In reply to this it may be said that it is of course true that with deeply narcotized animals in a condition of absolute muscular relaxation, in the dorsal position, and with women with enteroptosis, or relaxed abdominal walls after repeated pregnancies, in the knee-chest position, negative pressure may be demonstrable, but be it clearly understood that this is abnormal and unusual in each instance, and furthermore the negative pressure has nothing to do with which part of the abdominal cavity is uppermost, for the negative pressure will be created by the thoracic expansion and the failure of the tone of the abdominal walls to serve their usual function of support. Differences of pressure will be found only between different closed cavities, and certainly not in different parts of the same cavity, where a gaseous medium is the distributer of the pressures.

## THE OBJECTS OF EXPERIMENTAL STUDY

From this summary, which I believe gives a correct idea of the previous results of study of intra-abdominal pressure, I found it difficult to construct any intelligible statement, and it was this dilemma which prompted me to make the following tests, which I think must settle at least a few of the questions at issue.

I think it only fair to state that it is quite inconceivable to me that under normal conditions there can be different pressures in different parts of the peritoneal cavity. The space is but a single compartment from diaphragm to pelvic floor, and from the vertebral column to the abdominal walls. I have tested this repeatedly, and whenever I found a difference in pressure the error has been due to obstruction of one of the cannulas from which I was reading my pressures. When we speak of zero pressure we mean atmospheric pressure, negative and positive pressures being read below and above the zero thus taken.

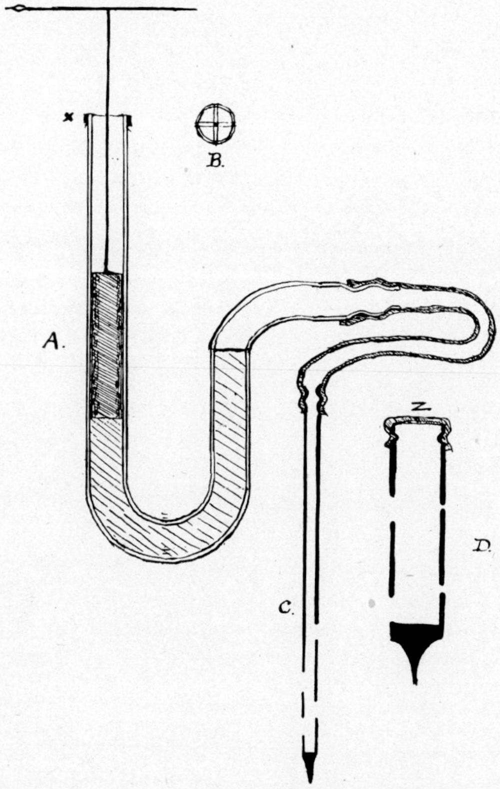


**Fig. 1.—Apparatus for ascertaining abdominal pressure. A, water manometer with aluminum float carrying writing-point guided at x by system of crossed hairs as shown in B. C, the small fenestrated trocar shown attached to manometer by rubber tubing. D, the large fenestrated trocar through the heavy rubber head of which at z the small trocar is plunged after D is forced through the abdominal wall.**

The primary objects of the study were to determine the pressure conditions in the peritoneal space, and if possible to discover the causes of the pressure, the function of such pressures as were found, and the disturbances resulting from variations from the normal pressures.

The method was of the simplest. Rabbits, cats, dogs and calves, under the influence of local or general anesthesia, were used. A straight fenestrated trocar was plunged through one or another part of the abdominal wall and so arranged as to prevent the entrance into or exit from the abdominal cavity of air. This trocar was connected with a recording water manometer, as described in 1904 in an earlier publication. The tracings were written from a base-line on a smoked drum. In some instances synchronous records were taken of the pleural pressure and of the carotid blood-pressure.

PROTOCOLS AND GRAPHIC RECORDS OF EXPERIMENTS

*Experiment* 1.—May 19, 1904: Male fox terrier, under ether anesthesia. Trocar inserted at level of umbilicus three-fourths of an inch to right of mid-line; again in left hypochondriac region and two inches below and to left of umbilicus. In all positions the water manometer registered negative pressures varying from 40 to 90 mm. This fluctuated, increasing with inspiration and decreasing with expiration. The explanation for this unexpected phenomenon was found on opening the abdomen, each trocar being left in place and clamped to prevent change of pressure conditions. Each trocar had failed to penetrate the internal aponeurosis, thus making an artificial space between the more superficial layer of muscle and the deep aponeurosis. Result: Failure of technic and false records.

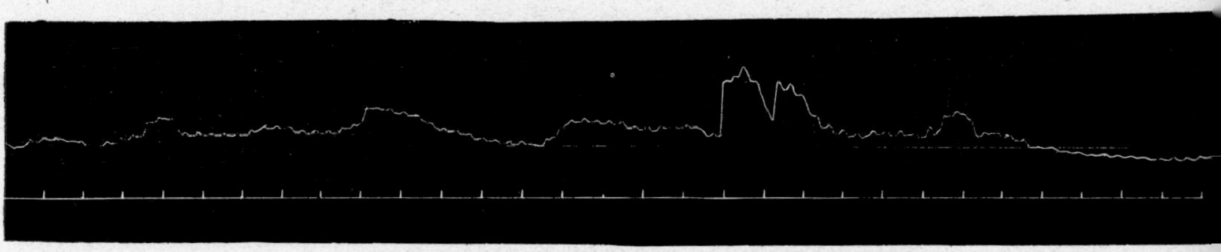

Fig. 2.—Record of intra-abdominal pressure in a decerebrated cat (Experiment 3, May 26, 1904). No anesthetic for past two hours. Tracing during slight asphyxia. Time marks 2 seconds and time line is used for abscissa. The small fluctuations in the tracing are due to respirations, the large ones to general bodily movements. Reduced to three-fourths size of the original tracing.

*Experiment* 2.—May 26, 1904: Rabbit under ether anesthesia. A much sharper and smaller fenestrated trocar was inserted just below the ribs in the right side in front. The pressure was from 20 to 25 mm. aq. rising in inspiration and falling in expiration. The trocar was withdrawn and the opening closed by clamp. The trocar inserted in left side, half-way between ribs and pelvis, registered from 10 to 15 mm. aq.; again withdrawn and reinserted in mid-line an inch and a half above pubic arch, it registered from 10 to 12 mm. aq. This fall, as will be explained later, was due partly to the failure to close the first two holes perfectly, but more to the gradually failing muscular tone during anesthesia. The trachea was clamped. Asphyctic convulsions resulted, forcing the pressure again up to 22 mm. aq., which, as the stage of exhaustion ensued, fell gradually to 8 mm. and remained there, as I found after opening the abdomen, because of obstruction to the trocar by omentum. If this obstruction had not occurred there would probably have been a fall to zero pressure, such as occurred in later tests.

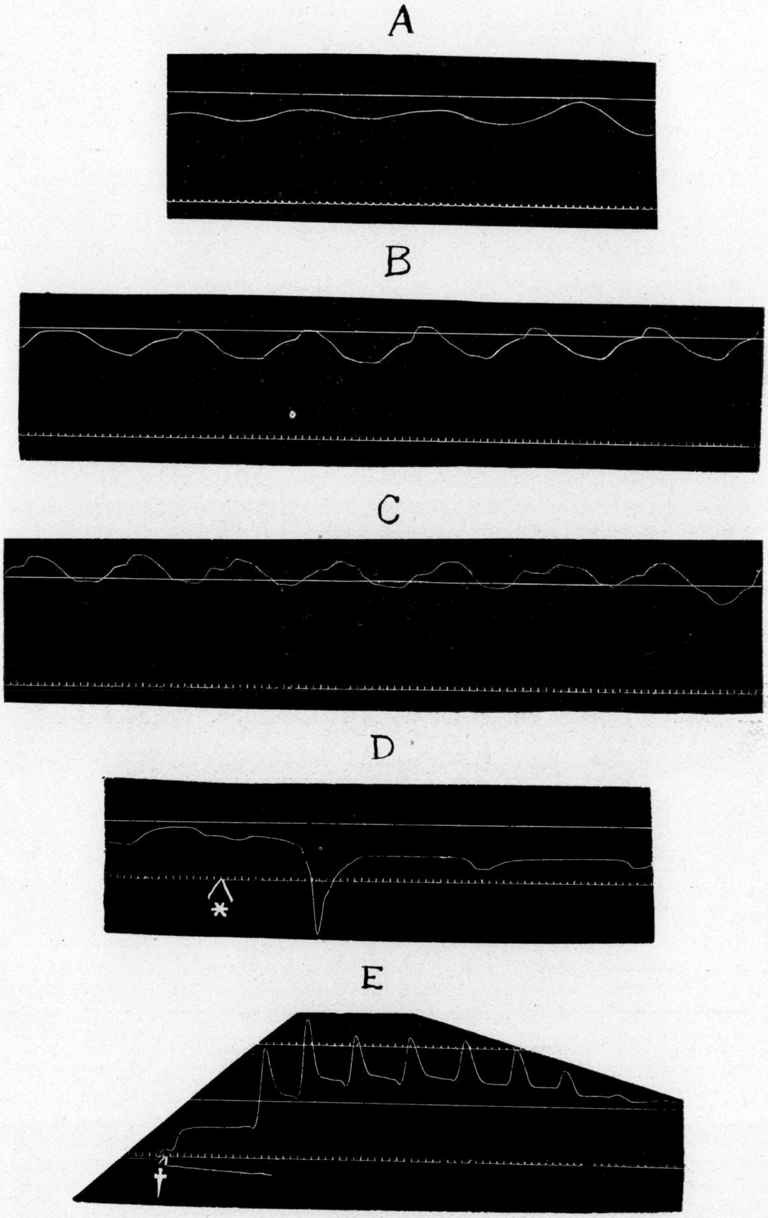


Fig. 3.—Cat under ether anesthesia (Experiment 4, Nov. 25, 1904). The lower straight line represents time in fifths of a second; the upper is the abscissa; the wavy line is the intra-abdominal pressure tracing. Up stroke represents inspiration except in D. A, deep narcosis; B, moderate narcosis; C, light narcosis; D, beginning asphyxia; E, release from asphyxia. Star (*) trachea clamped; dagger (†) trachea released. Reduced to three-fourths.

*Experiment* 3.—Nov. 22, 1904: A decerebrated cat that had been used for demonstration purposes was tested without an anesthetic. The trocar was inserted in the right flank. Pressure fluctuated above and below the zero mark. On eliciting vigorous muscular movements or during temporary closure of the trachea, the pressure rose to 10 to 15 mm. water (Fig. 2).

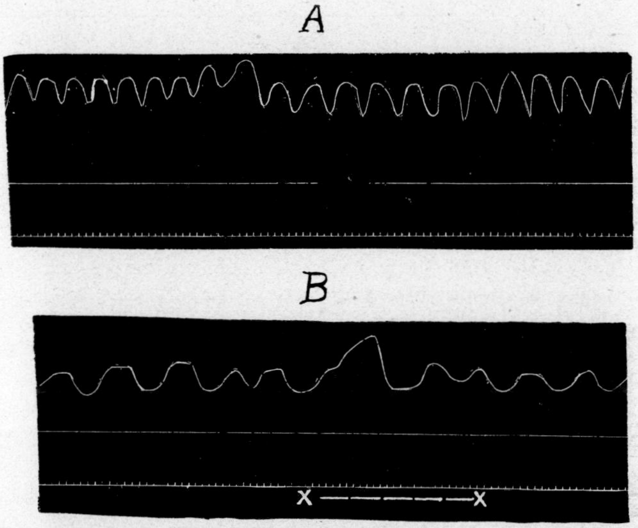


Fig. 4.—Continuous record of positive intra-abdominal pressure (Experiment 5, Nov. 26, 1909) in a cat under light ether narcosis. Prolonged inspiration, x....x. Rising pressure during inspiration. Reduced to three-fourths.

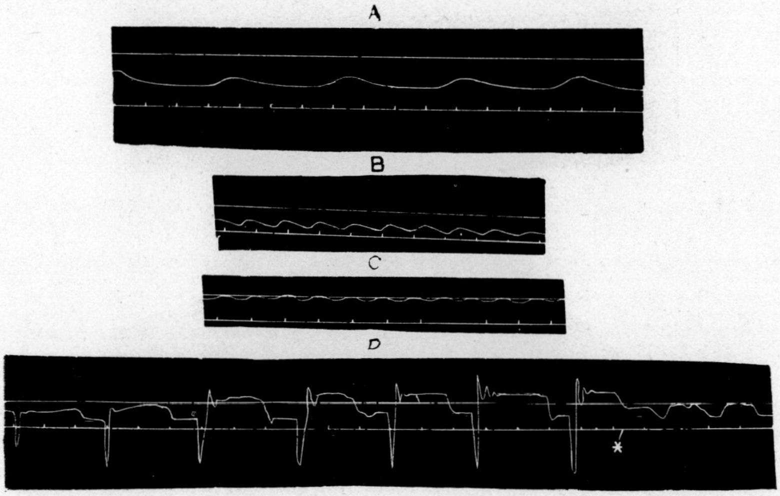


Fig. 5.—Small fox terrier (Experiment 6, Nov. 29, 1909). Uppermost line, abscissa; middle line, abdominal pressure; bottom line, time. Up stroke represents inspiration. A, deep narcosis. B, moderate narcosis. C, light narcosis. D, effect of obstruction of trachea and sudden release. Star (*) trachea released, Reduced one-half.

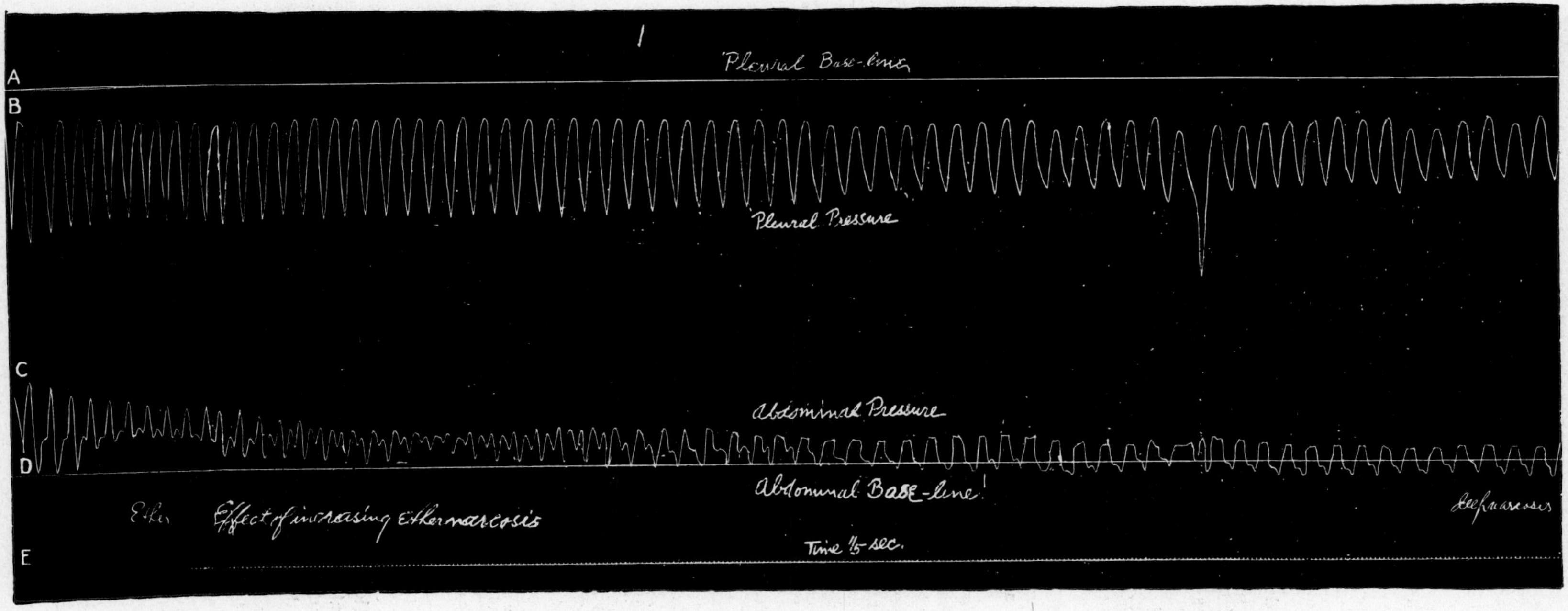


Fig. 6.—Effect of increasing ether narcosis (Experiment 8, Jan. 3, 1905); deep narcosis at end. A, pleural base-line. B, pleural pressure. C, abdominal pressure. D, abdominal base-line. E, time in fifths of a second. Reduced to two-thirds.

*Experiment* 4.—Nov. 25, 1904: Cat under ether anesthesia. It is to be especially noted that this cat was an unusually emaciated and feeble specimen, as a result of a paralyzed right hind leg from an earlier injury. The trocar was inserted in the left loin and negative pressure, i. e., less than atmospheric, was recorded under deep narcosis. As narcosis was diminished in intensity the pressure gradually rose and at the height of inspiration the pressure was positive to a slight degree. In this animal it was noticeable that the up-stroke (during inspiration) of the pressure curve was made of two elements, the first long and gradual and the second abrupt and short. The second part occurred when full costal expansion had been reached and appeared to be due to a contraction of the diaphragm. During a slight struggling that occurred when the anesthesia was light, the pressure even at its lowest point (i. e., during expiration), kept above zero. Apparently the returning tone of the abdominal muscles allowed positive pressure to prevail even against the negative pull of the thorax. On obstructing the trachea the first long inspiratory effort resulted in a great drop in pressure, the pressure remaining well below zero until the following great expiratory movement caused a rise, and then on releasing the trachea a still further rise in pressure occurred as the inrush of air into the lungs satisfied the negative pressure which had been operative in causing unnatural low pressure in the abdomen (Fig. 3).

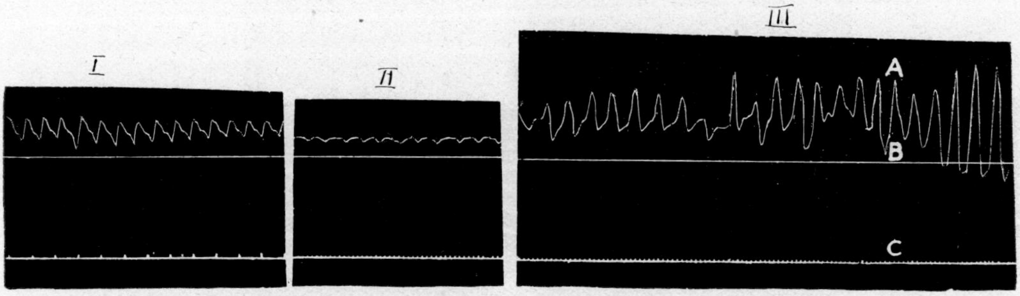


Fig. 7.—Experiment 8, continued. I, effect of moderate narcosis. II, deep narcosis. III, recovery from ether narcosis. Upper line intra-abdominal pressure; middle line abscissa; lowest line, time in fifths of a second. Reduced to two-thirds.

*Experiment* 5.—Nov. 26, 1904: A large powerful cat of unusual muscular development was used. Ether anesthesia. When inserted through four different places in the abdominal wall the trocar registered positive pressure at each point (Fig. 4). The urinary bladder was finally entered by mistake and further observations were unreliable.

*Experiment* 6.—Nov. 29, 1904: Small fox terrier which had been anesthetized by ether at 2:15 p. m. and had been operated on for demonstration of localization of brain function and was kept continuously under ether until 3:45 p. m., when these observations were made. There was, as is apt to be the case after severe cerebral operations have been performed, extreme muscular relaxation. The animal was put in ventral horizontal position and the trocar inserted at various points and only at deep inspiration did the pressure rise to zero or slightly above it (Fig. 5).

*Experiment* 7.—Dec. 24, 1904: Having failed occasionally to get reliable graphic records with the recording manometer in the previous experiments because of obstruction of the fenestræ of the cannula by omentum or mesentery, I used in this and the following experiments a double trocar. A large trocar half an inch in diameter, with four large holes directly above the steel lance-shaped tip, was closed at its upper end by a heavy piece of rubber tied so as to be quite air-tight.

This was inserted where desired, and then the smaller trocar, previously connected with the manometer but with the connecting tube clamped, was quickly forced through the rubber cap, making an air-tight joint. The chances of obstruction of the large openings in the large trocar are much less than was the case with the smaller one, and the smaller one thus protected and yet subject to the pressure changes proved a reliable recording instrument for long periods in the abdominal cavity, without the errors and risks attendant on changing the position or point of insertion. A heavy pug dog was used. The stomach was full of a large meal of meat and dog biscuit (a pint). Ether anesthesia. In the dorsal position. Trocar in mid-line above umbilicus showed a positive pressure. On clamping the trachea a rise still further above zero occurred with the violent movements. A pleural cannula was also applied to test coincidently intrapleural pressures.

*Experiment* 8.—Jan. 3, 1905: Medium-sized cat. Ether; dorsal position. Trocar as described in previous protocol in mid-line above umbilicus. Pleural

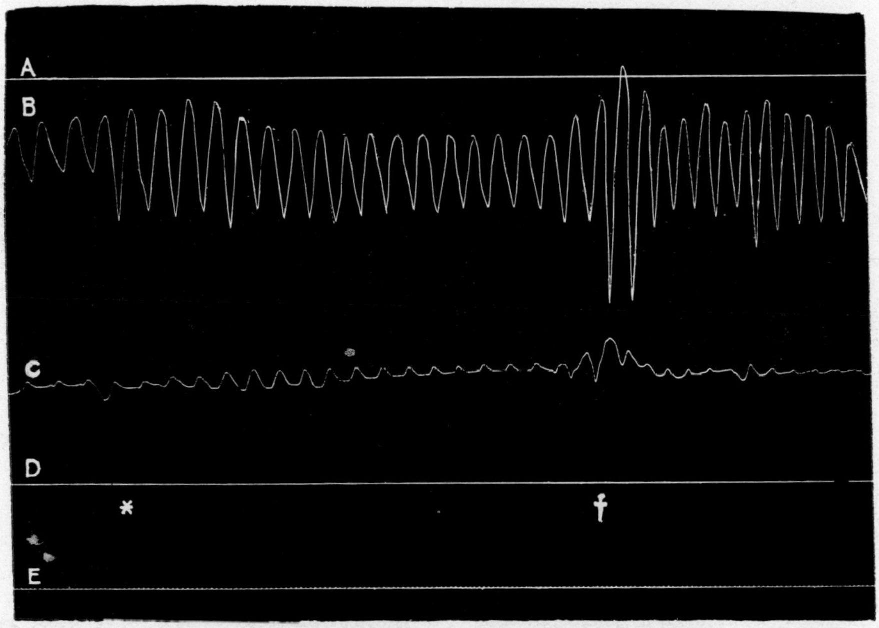


Fig. 8.—Effect of recovery from light narcosis (Experiment 8 continued). A, B, C, D and E as in Figure 6; star (*) light narcosis; dagger (†) struggle. Reduced to two-thirds.

cannula connected with recording manometer (equal parts aqua destil. and glycerin C. P.). The pleural trocar recorded persistent but fluctuating negative pressure, while the abdominal pressure was positive, except when deep narcosis abolished the muscular tone of the abdominal muscles, and allowed of zero or negative pressures.

For details of tracings see Figures 6, 7 and 8.

It will be seen that the abdominal pressure becomes positive, zero or negative according to the amount of anesthesia produced by the ether. Deep asphyxia causes the well-recognized increase in negative pleural pressure, and at the same time almost obliterates the abdominal positive pressure, so much more powerful is the expansion of the rigid thorax than is the downward descent of the diaphragm. The effect of 300 c.c. of 7 per cent. salt solution was to raise abdominal pressure to a considerable height, and cause a persistence of this relatively high positive pressure even when the animal was under deep narcosis. This pressure was evidently harmful, as artificial respiration had to be resorted to because of the limited respiratory excursion permitted.

*Experiment* 9.—Jan. 5, 1905: Large male rabbit. Ether narcosis, tracheotomy. Right phrenic nerve exposed in the neck, and esophagus cut and tube passed to stomach and tied in place. Abdominal and pleural cannulas. Dorsal position. The usual record of low positive or negative abdominal pressure was obtained during deep narcosis and a fluctuating positive pressure during light narcosis was obtained. Cutting the right phrenic nerve caused a marked diminution in the inspiratory rise in abdominal pressure (Fig. 9). Ammonia inhaled failed to cause any change in the pressures. Curare (2 cg.) was given by subcutaneous injection and in ten minutes a gradually increasing muscular paralysis resulted in death with both pleural and abdominal pressures registering zero.

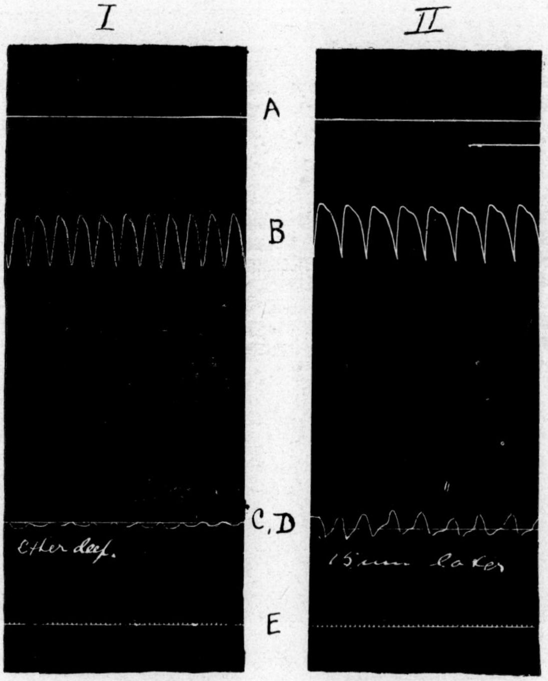


Fig. 9.—Effect on rabbit of deep and light ether narcosis (Experiment 9, Jan. 5, 1905). A, pleural base; B, pleural pressure; C, abdominal pressure; D, abdominal base; E, time in fifths of a second. I, deep narcosis; II, fifteen minutes later. Reduced to two-thirds.

*Experiment* 10.—Jan. 12, 1905: Black and tan dog, 5.5 kilo. Ether, tracheotomy; both phrenic nerves exposed above the subclavian artery. Bougie tube tied into the esophagus. The effects of quiet respiration, the distention of the stomach with salt solution and cutting the phrenic nerves were observed. The usual records were obtained in quiet respiration. Thoracic excursion was hindered and abdominal pressure rose on distending stomach with 400 c.c. of salt solution. Cutting phrenic nerves at the high level indicated did not materially affect abdominal pressure (Fig. 10).

*Experiment* 11.—Jan. 14, 1905: White rabbit. Cocain used for local anesthesia to right of mid-line just below umbilicus. Trocar inserted and pressure recorded with water manometer. Positive pressure persisted throughout the observations, and was doubled on slight exertion or any sudden bodily movement. The trocar was withdrawn and the abdominal wound closed. Recovery from puncture uneventful.

*Experiment* 12.—Jan. 24, 1905: A large brown male rabbit had been under ether for two hours for a demonstration on the functions of the cervical sympathetic nerves, both of which had been cut. At the end of this prolonged narcosis the abdominal pressure was found to be persistently below zero, to the extent of from 2 to 4 mm. aq.

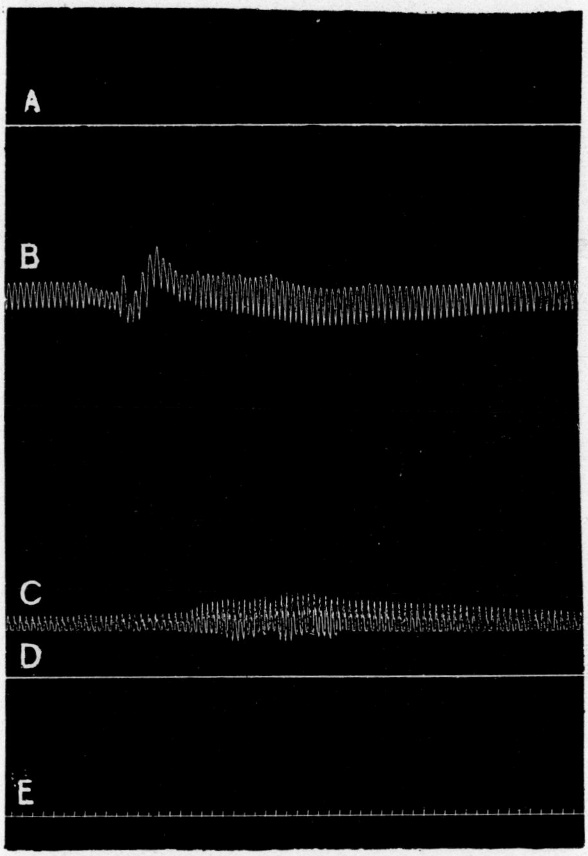


Fig. 10.—Moderate ether narcosis in dog (Experiment 10, Jan. 12, 1905). A, pleural base; B, pleural pressure; C, abdominal pressure; D, abdominal base; E, time in single seconds. Reduced to two-thirds.

*Experiment* 13.—Feb. 8-9, 1905: Two cats used for demonstration purposes and under very light ether narcosis for a brief period, were tested and positive intra-abdominal pressure recorded.

*Experiment* 14.—March 6, 7, 8, 1905; Three calves, each of which had been under ether narcosis for an hour and a half, were tested and only one showed a positive pressure within the abdomen, from 2 to 6 mm. The other two exhibited extreme muscular relaxation, and the dorsal position allowed of collapse of the normal abdominal shape, causing a slight negative pressure.

*Experiment* 15.—April 18, 1905: Rabbit under deep ether narcosis. Recording manometer with equal parts glycerin and water showed abdominal pressure from — 1 to 3 mm. aq.

*Experiment* 16.—April 20, 1905: Powerful male cat. Ether. Tracheotomy. Dorsal position. Carotid cannula to mercury manometer. Trocar in left pleural space to water-and-glycerin manometer. Trocar in mid-abdomen to recording water manometer. Effect of raising foot of board was a rise of abdominal pressure. Raising head gave sometimes rise and sometimes fall; a rise if under light narcosis and a fall if under deep narcosis. Effect of manual pressure on abdomen noted. A fatal dose of strychnin nitrate killed the animal by gradually increasing muscular spasm and with a steadily rising intra-abdominal pressure. The pressure in the abdomen was positive throughout the experiment and the

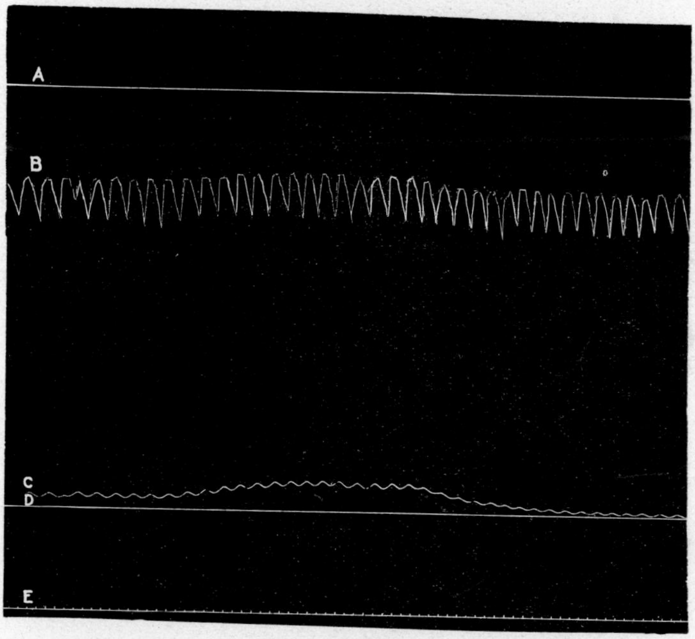


Fig. 11.—Effect of raising foot of dog-board 6 inches (Experiment 16, April 20, 1905). A, pleural base; B, pleural pressure; C, abdominal pressure; D, abdominal base; E, time in fifths of a second. Reduced to two-thirds.

thoracic pressure was negative. The carotid pressure fluctuated slightly, coincident with the rise and fall in abdominal pressure (Fig. 11).

*Experiment* 17.—April 21, 1905: Test of abdominal pressure on an etherized cat showed a fluctuation between 2 and 5 mm., by a glycerin-and-water manometer (sp. gr. 1120).

*Experiment* 18.—April 22, 1905: Dog, 5.5 kilos ether, tracheotomy, carotid cannula. Abdominal pressure positive except on deep narcosis. Raising hind end of the animal always caused rise of abdominal and carotid pressure. Raising of head end caused fall of both pressures. The recording abdominal trocar was in the costal angle just below the free edge of the liver. Another cannula connected with a mercury manometer and an air-pressure bottle was then inserted in the

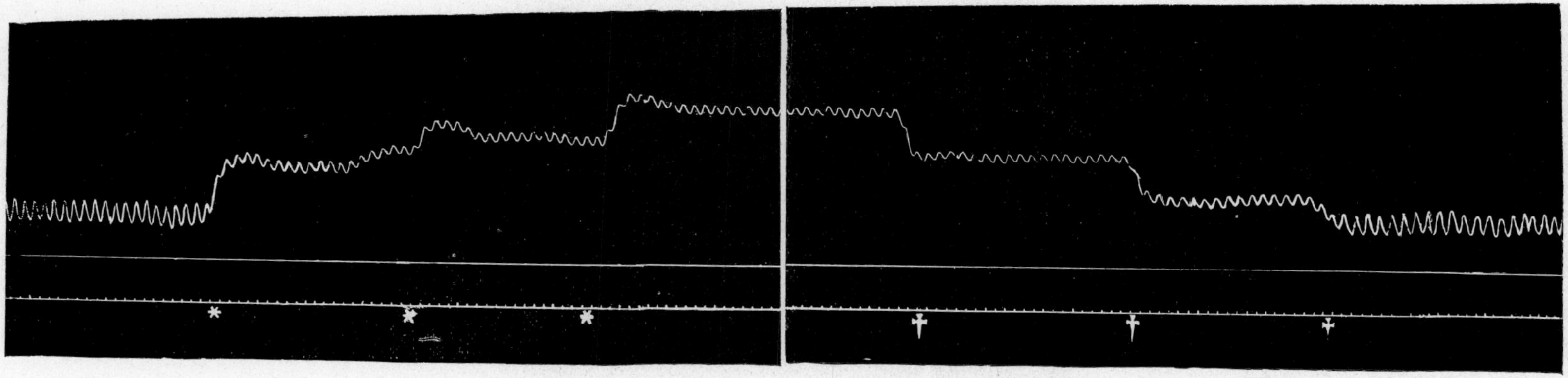

Fig. 12.—Effect on intra-abdominal pressure of distending abdomen with 150 c.c. of saline and withdrawal of same amount (Experiment 18, April 22, 1905). Star (*) injection of 50 c.c.; dagger (†) withdrawal of same amount. Reduced to two-thirds.

mid-line as near the bladder as possible. Air was blown into the abdomen through the second cannula on three occasions, and the change in abdominal pressure was instantly recorded through the upper cannula. Each rise of abdominal pressure was accompanied by a rise in the carotid pressure. The slightest increase or alteration in the abdominal pressure was recorded equally by the two manometers in the abdominal cavity. The abdomen was then distended until 40 mm. water was recorded. Curare (4 cg. Eimer and Amend) was injected subcutaneously, and in sixteen minutes death occurred with a gradual fall of both carotid and abdominal pressures (Fig. 12).

*Experiment* 19.—March 5, 6, 7, 1907: In the course of three class demonstrations on the musculature of respiration, it was noted in the case of three etherized dogs that on section of the spinal cord at the level of the sixth cervical vertebra, the abdominal pressure suddenly rose. This was due to the sudden cessation of the negative thoracic pressure owing to paralysis of all the intercostal muscles, and to the increased contraction of the diaphragm on spinal irritation.

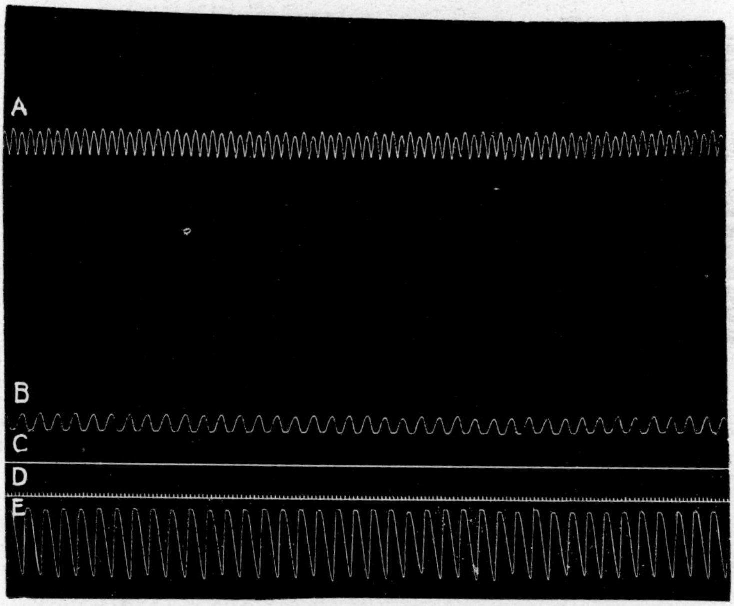


Fig. 13.—Pressures under normal conditions in moderate ether anesthesia (Experiment 22, May 20, 1907). A, carotid pressure; B, abdominal (intraperitoneal) pressure; C, abscissa; D, time in fifths of a second; E, in intrapleural pressure. Reduced to two-thirds.

That this increase in abdominal pressure is due to diaphragm action, and not to the increase of blood content in the abdomen as a result of abdominal vasoparesis, is proved by its sudden onset and its persistence at the same level. On cutting the cord at the level of the second cervical vertebra, the abdominal pressure dropped at once to zero, and did not vary at all thereafter, although the cardiac contractions continued to register slight fluctuations in the thoracic pressure.

*Experiment* 20.—April 2, 3, 4, 1907: Three calves were tested as in March, 1905, and by the use of light anesthesia it was found that the abdominal pressure in each instance varied between 3 mm. and 10 mm. of water-pressure.

*Experiment* 21.—April 10, 11, 1907: Two dogs under ether, registered from 2 to 10 mm. water pressure in the abdomen. After the skeletal muscles had been paralyzed by the use of curare, the pressure fell to zero and thereafter even the pressure necessary to distend the lungs by artificial positive pressure respiration failed to cause a rise in the abdominal pressure, since the paralysis of the abdominal wall muscles was as complete as the paralysis of the diaphragm, thus allowing flaccid distention and retraction of the abdomen with each respiratory cycle.

In light narcosis abdominal pressure, +2 to +10 mm. aq.
In deep narcosis abdominal pressure, +2 to +4 mm. aq.
After curare (10 mm.) abdominal pressure, 0 to 1 mm. aq.
Artificial respiration, 0 to 0
One hour after death, 0

*Experiment* 22.—May 20, 1907: Male dog, 9 kilos. Ether; tracheotomy; carotid cannula to mercury manometer. Intra-abdominal cannula to water manometer. Intrapleural cannula to water manometer. Base line and time record in half seconds. All three manometers were arranged to write from the same base-line, and from the same perpendicular on the drum, and when the experiment was

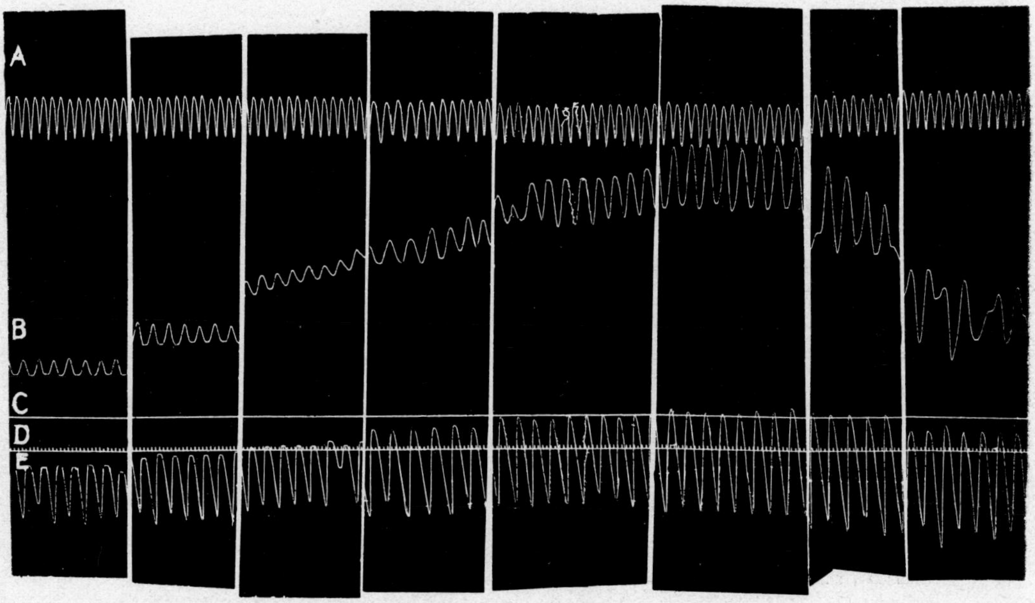


Fig. 14.—Effect of inflation of abdomen with air, on carotid, intra-abdominal and pleural pressures (Experiment 22, continued). A, carotid; B, abdominal; C, abscissa; D, time in fifths of a second; E, pleural. Reduced to two-thirds.

finished all three recording needles returned to the same point on the abscissa, except the one on carotid manometer, which was 1 mm. out of line. Records were made of normal conditions and variations due to inflation of the abdomen and during artificial respiration (Figs. 13 and 14).

*Experiment* 23.—May 21, 1907: Three vigorous well-developed cats were put under ether. Their weights and respirations were as follows:

| | Weights | Respirations |
|---|---|---|
| A | 3300 gm. | 34 to the minute |
| B | 4300 gm. | 34 to the minute |
| C | 3640 gm. | 34 to the minute |

Into the abdominal cavity of each, 100 c.c. of 0.7 per cent. sodium chlorid solution was put by trocar. This amount increased the diameter of the abdomen 1 cm.

and did not increase abdominal pressure. In B the abdomen was opened by a 10 cm. incision in the mid-line. In C sufficient air was blown into the abdominal cavity to distend it 5 cm. in diameter. The three cats were kept under the lightest possible narcosis for an hour and as no manipulations were under way, they lay motionless. At the end of that time the abdominal cavity of each was opened from pubis to ensiform, and all the fluid from the abdominal cavity was collected in a basin over which the animal was inverted. It was found that A (under normal conditions) had absorbed 0.01066 of its weight of saline solution in the hour, B 0.00581, and C 0.00684.

The object of this test was to illustrate the importance of maintaining as nearly as possible normal conditions of pressure within an abdomen, for the sake of assisting in the return flow of lymph and chyle from the abdomen to the thorax. Whether normal pressure is exceeded as in the rigid abdomen of acute peritonitis or in ascites, or whether there is a loss of normal pressure as in enteroptosis or after abdominal operations or abdominal paracentesis, there is a delay in absorption.

*Experiment* 24.—May 23, 1907: Dog, 6 kilos. Ether, tracheotomy. Carotid pressure recorded by mercury manometer. Abdominal pressure recorded by water

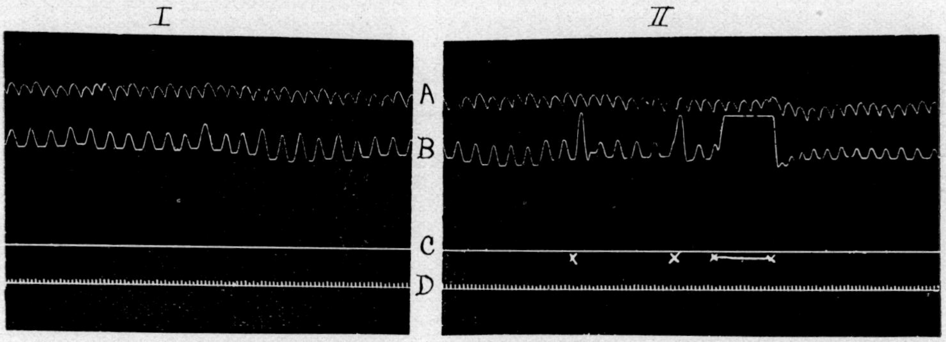


Fig. 15.—May 23, Experiment 24. I. Normal record before section of phrenics; II, effect of faradization of both phrenics in continuity. A, carotid; B, abdominal; C, abscissa; D, time in fifths of a second. Reduced to two-thirds.

manometer. Phrenic nerves isolated deep in neck. Normal record taken and then phrenic nerves stimulated, showing rise of intra-abdominal pressure and fall in carotid pressure. The phrenic nerves were cut as far down as possible, and a low pressure recorded. Under deep narcosis after section of the phrenic nerves, the respiratory variation in abdominal pressure caused by the thoracic expansion was almost *nil*, while during light narcosis the tone of the abdominal wall muscles was sufficient to develop some resistance, and the fluctuations of abdominal pressure became distinct and prominent in spite of the paralysis of the diaphragm (Figs. 15-18).

*Experiment* 25.—May 24, 1907: Dog, 7 kilos. Local cocain anesthesia in mid-abdominal line just above the umbilicus. Trocar inserted and pressure read at 5 mm. by a water-and-glycerin (sp. gr. 1160) manometer. After I had assured myself by a number of readings that this was a normal pressure for this animal, i. e., 5 mm. in expiration and 10 mm. in inspiration, 2 c.c. of dilute hydrochloric acid were injected directly into the abdominal cavity. Instant and marked rigidity of the abdominal muscles resulted. The pressure fluctuated between 15 and 20

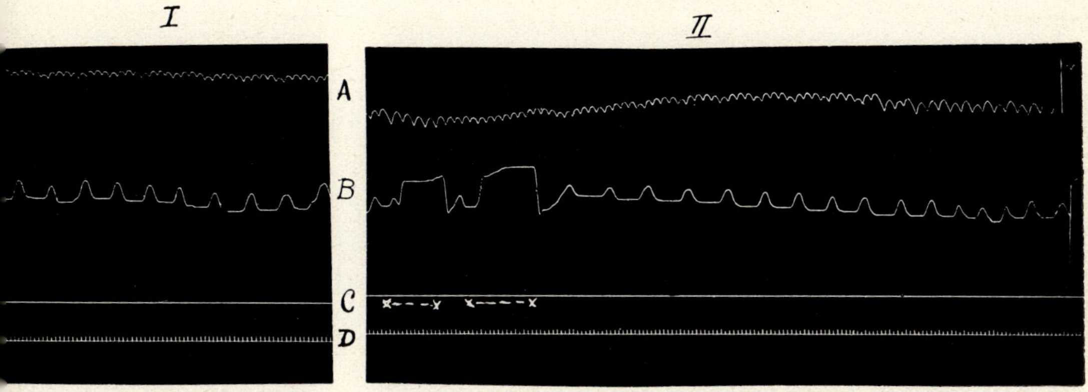


Fig. 16.—Experiment 24, continued. I, normal before section of phrenics; II, effect of faradization of both phrenics in continuity. Note slowing of respiration between crosses after fatigue of diaphragm. A, B, C, and D as in Figure 15. Reduced to two-thirds.

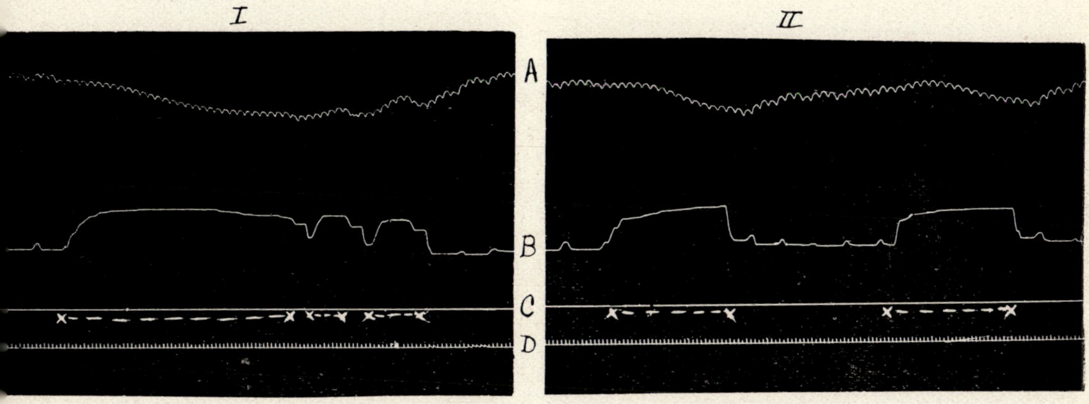


Fig. 17.—Experiment 24, continued. Effect of prolonged faradization of both phrenics immediately after section of both phrenics. Electrodes on distal stumps. A, B, C, and D as in Figures 15 and 16. Reduced to two-thirds.

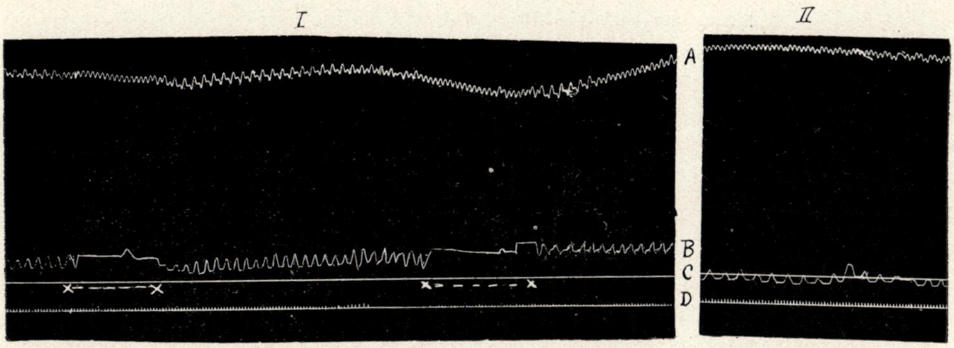


Fig. 18.—Experiment 24, concluded. I, fifteen minutes after section of phrenics; between crosses, faradization of right phrenic distal end. II, thirty minutes after section of phrenics. A, B, C, and D as in preceding figures. Reduced to one-half.

mm. The dog was then chloroformed, and during the narcosis the body was immersed in water and an opening 10 cm. long was made in the abdomen under an inverted bell jar full of water. Only a few bubbles of air that were retained in the clamped tube connected with the cannula escaped, and no gas appeared in spite of complete evisceration into the bell jar. The animal was killed by chloroform.

## CONCLUSIONS

It was apparent that under normal conditions the viscera completely fill the abdominal cavity.

The contraction of the diaphragm is the chief, if not the only factor in the normal rise in pressure during quiet inspiration.

Debilitated states show a low pressure.

Ether anesthesia causes a gradual drop in pressure, until with complete loss of muscular tone, the pressure reaches zero.

Curare likewise causes a progressive fall to zero pressure.

Asphyxia develops great rises in pressure during inspiration until muscular relaxation allows a drop to zero just before death.

Excessive pressure artificially produced within the peritoneal cavity, causes death from cardiac failure before the obstruction to respiratory excursion has developed a marked asphyxia.

Summing up the results of the foregoing experiments it will be granted, I think, that it is normal in the animals tested to exhibit a pressure within the free abdominal cavity which is above atmospheric pressure. This true positive intra-abdominal pressure is seen to fluctuate with the respiratory excursion of the thorax and diaphragm. This pressure is seen to depend on the contraction of the diaphragm, and the tone or the active contraction of the abdominal wall muscles, including the pelvic floor, acting from relatively fixed points of the thorax, pelvis and vertebral column. Whatever diminishes or abolishes the tone of the diaphragm and abdominal muscles, causes a fall in the positive abdominal pressure. If at the same time the thoracic expansion is active, there will be a fall of abdominal pressure below atmospheric pressure. If at any time the tone or activity of the diaphragm and abdominal muscles is increased, whether the thoracic expansion is diminished or normal, the abdominal pressure will rise above its usual positive points.

The tone or contractility of the abdominal muscles must persist or the pressure will fall to atmospheric or below. Distention of the abdomen, by fluid or gas, raises abdominal pressure.

The pressure recorded at any point in the abdominal cavity is equivalent to the pressure at the same moment at any other point in the cavity.

The normal moderate positive pressure is better for absorption of fluid from the peritoneal space than atmospheric pressure, and *a fortiori,* a pressure below this, or than a pressure much above atmospheric pressure. Pressure much above the normal intra-abdominal pressure causes a fall in general arterial blood-pressure, due apparently to diminished venous inflow through the inferior cava, and a resultant diminution of systolic output from the left ventricle.

The questions at once come to mind as to the neuromuscular mechanism that maintains this pressure, and as to what useful purpose this positive or supra-atmospheric pressure within the abdominal space serves, for it would be contrary to all experience that any force should be found to be exerted by an animal organism that did not serve some good end. Is this pressure a waste or by-product of necessary muscular activity serving other purposes, or is it of itself helpful in the body economy? Paralysis of the abdominal muscles and of the diaphragm experimentally, abolishes the positive abdominal pressure. The action of the diaphragm is under the direct control of the respiratory center, and to a lesser degree the same center controls the abdominal wall muscles. Schaefer states that the tone of the abdominal muscles is maintained by the respiratory center.

The descent of the diaphragm meets for its main resistance the tone of the abdominal muscles. If, as seems probable, the respiratory center allows of a diminished tone of the abdominal muscles during inspiration, and maintains a greater tonicity during expiration, then the expansion of the lungs would be accomplished by the minimum of effort, and their collapse ensured by prompt recoil on the part of the elastic and slightly stretched abdominal walls. Whether this can be definitely proved by animal experiment or not, the clinical facts are abundant to show that a relaxed or paralytic condition of the abdominal walls, as in transverse laceration of the spinal cord (Hogge), or after pregnancy, removal of tumor mass, or ascitic fluid, or in extreme splanchnoptosis, or in a milder degree after removal of corsets in one who is habituated to their support, or in cases of pleural exudate, will cause a more or less severe objective and subjective dyspnea. In spite of the fact that the diaphragm has less resistance to contract against in these conditions, there is really a diminished respiratory excursion, for expiration is only partially accomplished owing to the failure of the abdominal recoil.

If, on the other hand, there is excessive intra-abdominal pressure, the difficulty in breathing is even more marked, and this often plays an important rôle in the circulatory emergencies in infectious diseases where meteorism, abdominal distention and interference with the descent of the diaphragm may determine cardiac failure. The function of intra-abdominal pressure as regards respiration is then to offer but slight resistance to the descent of the diaphragm during the inspiratory phase, and assist promptly in the ascent of the diaphragm when it is relaxed, thereby assisting in the rapid and complete emptying of the lungs during the expiratory phase. Pressure as high as 45 cm. aq. in the abdomen will usually kill a small animal, cat or rabbit, by fatiguing the diaphragm, as well as by diminishing venous return to the heart (allowing of asphyxia). The maintenance of a slight positive pressure in the abdomen assists the circulation by aiding the return of venous blood to the thorax. Abdominal pressure is below the pressure in the femoral veins (5.4 mm. Hg according to Opitz), even at the height of inspiration, and the highest abdominal pressure is not as high as the pressure in the portal vein (8.9 mm. Hg according to Opitz). The normal conditions of pressure within the abdomen do not hinder the return of venous blood, and it is to be noted that at the time when the abdominal pressure is highest and might tend to hinder venous flow, the suction exerted by the thoracic expansion is at its maximum.

Any marked loss of abdominal tone is recognized clinically as a contributing cause of venous stagnation in the abdominal viscera, and this means a delayed or insufficient venous return to the right heart, a diminished output and a fall in arterial pressure, or a pressure maintained only at the expense of greater cardiac action. In general it may be stated that a lack of normal abdominal pressure is a contributing cause of general arterial low pressure. On the other hand increase in abdominal pressure will usually serve as an increased peripheral resistance, and cause a rise in blood-pressure as long as the heart is competent, but this higher pressure which is necessitated by the obstruction to the arterial and venous flow will, if persistent, cause cardiac fatigue and serve as a direct cause of overloading the heart muscle, with more or less serious results. The palpitation, the precipitation of incompetence in a previously competent heart, the onset of irregularity of force and frequency in heart action as a result of distention of the abdomen with gas or fluid, as in typhoid fever, ascites, or peritonitis, are evidences of the interference with the heart action by overloading the resistance in the splanchnic area. Relief of the laboring heart is constantly seen after removal of ascitic fluid. It is well to note, however, that withdrawal of the fluid although it relieves the obstruction in the circulation, also removes a certain support which the veins had, and unless some artificial support is provided, as by a binder, the sudden drop from a high abdominal pressure to atmospheric pressure or below, may cause further disturbance in both respiratory and circulatory functions.

The flow of chyle from the abdomen to the thorax is largely determined by the suction exerted by thoracic expansion, and this is materially assisted by the coincident rising pressure in the abdomen, the same muscular movement of the diaphragm which sucks the chyle to the thorax, pressing it out of the abdomen. Insufficient or abnormally low abdominal pressure allows of a less advantageous condition of lymph flow. Increased pressure will tend to collapse the tender walls of the lacteals and the receptaculum chyli, exposed as they are without the support of surrounding tissue.

The inefficient absorption in relaxed abdominal conditions, as after abdominal operations, if sufficient support is not given by artificial means, and the improved absorption after a portion of ascitic fluid is removed, parallel clinically the experiment in absorption as described above.

120 East Sixty-Second Street.

BIBLIOGRAPHY

Bert: Physiologie comparée de la respiration, 1870, Paris, p. 339.

Barrett: Surg., Gynec. and Obst., 1908, viii, 369.

Braune: Centralbl. f. d. med. Wissensch., 1865, iii, 913.

Capps, J. A.: Some Observations on the Effect on the Blood-Pressure of the Withdrawal of Fluid from the Thorax and Abdomen, Jour. Am. Med. Assn., 1907, xlviii, 22.

Depage, Rouffart and Mayer: Jour. méd. de Bruxelles, 1904, ix, 425, 527.

Donders: Ztschr. f. rat. Med., 1854, new series, iv, 230.

Dubois: Deutsch. Arch. f. klin. Med., 1876, xvii, 148.

DuBois-Reymond: Physiologie des Menschen und der Säugethiere, 1904, Berlin, p. 554.

Duncan: Edinburgh Med. Jour., 1865, xl, 516.

Edgar: Obstetrics, 1904, Philadelphia, Chap. xl, 357.

Emerson: Proc. Soc. Exper. Med. and Biol., 1904-05, xi, 38.

Emminghaus: Deutsch. Arch. f. klin. Med., 1874, xiii, 446.

Foster: Physiology, 1888-90, London. Vol. 1, Book iii, 434.

Hall: Text-Book of Physiology, 1900, London, 206.

Hasse: Arch. f. Anat. u. Entwicklungsgesch. Anat. Abtheil., 1886, 185; Die Formen des menschlichen Körpers, Jena, 1890, Abtheil. 11, 53; Arch. f. Anat. u. Physiol. Anat. Abtheil., 1901, 273.

Hormann: Arch. f. Gynäk., 1905, lxxv, 527.

Hagentorn: Centralbl. f. Gynäk., 1902, xxxiv, 891.

Hammernik: Das Herz und seine Bewegung, Prague, 1858.

Herrick, W. W.: A Study of Pneumoperitoneum, with a Means for Its Diagnosis, The Archives Int. Med., 1910, v, 246.

Hegar: Arch. f. Gynäk., 1872, iv, 531; Deutsch. med. Wchnschr., 1886, xii, 582.

Heinricius: Ztschr. f. Biol., 1890, new series, viii, 113.

Hamburger: Arch. f. Anat. u. Physiol., Phys. Abtheil. (Du Bois-Reymond), 1896, p. 36.

Hogge: Arch. d. Biol. d. Gand., 1892, xii, 573.

Jurgensen: Nothnagel's specielle Pathologie und Therapie, Bd. xv, Theil 1, 47.

Kelling: Deutsch. med. Wchnschr., 1892, xviii, 1160, 1191; Samml. klin. Vortr. (Volkmann's), new series, Inn. Med., 1896, No. 44, 487.

Kronecker and Meltzer: Arch. f. Anat. u. Physiol. Phys. Abtheil., 1883, p. 328. (DuBois-Reymond's Festschrift.)

Landau: Wanderniere, Berlin, 1881, p. 29; Wanderleber und Hängebauch, Berlin, 1883.

Landois: Lehrbuch der Physiologie des Menschen, Berlin, 1899, 1st Halfte, p. 218.

Lesshaft: Anatom. Anzeig, 1888 iii, 823, 838.

Lenbuscher: Jenaische Ztsch. f. Naturw., 1888, xvi, 424, 818.

Leyden: Charité Ann. (1876), Berlin, 1878, iii, 264. Pub. 1878.

Luciani: Delle oscillazione delle pressione intratoracico e intraabdominale, 1877, Turin; Arch. p. scienz. med., 1878, ii, 177; Physiologie des Menschen, 1905, Berlin, I, 347.

Marey: Physiologie médicale de la circulation du sang, Paris, 1863.

Martin: Frauenkrankheiten, Vienna, 1885.

Meinert: Samml. klin. Vortr. (Volkmann's), 1896, new series, Inn. Med., No. 35, p. 207.

Mathes: Arch. f. Gynak., 1906, lxxvii, 357.

Meyer: Centralbl. f. Gynäk., 1902, xxvi, 579.

Moritz: Ztschr. f. Biol., 1895, n. s. xiv (old series xxxii), 313; Berhandl. d. Gesellsch. Deutsch. Naturf. u. Aerzte, 1896, lxv, 18.

Mosso and Pellacani: Arch. ital. d. biol., 1882, i, 97.

Odebrecht: Berl. klin. Wchnschr., 1875, xii, 175.

Quincke: Deutsch. Arch. f. klin. Med., 1878, xxi, 453.

Quirin: Deutsch. Arch. f. klin. Med., 1901, lxxi, 79.

Reprieff: Russk. Vrach., 1890, xi, 405, 460, 505.

Rosenthal: Sitzungsb. d. phys. med. Soc. zu Erlang., 1881, xiii, 19-23.

Roth: Beitr. d. Klin. d. Tuberk., 1905, iv, 437.

Rovsing: Hospitalstidende, 1905, xiii, 1213.

Schaefer: Physiology, London, 1900, ii, 44, 162.

Schatz: Jubelfestgrusse z. Gynäk., 45 Versammlung Deutsch. Naturforsch. u. Aerzte, Leipsic, 1872.

Schroeder: Handbuch der weiblichen Geschlechtsorgane, 1886, Leipsic, p. 151.

Schulein: Deutsch. med. Wchnschr., 1906, xxxii, 1198.

Schwenburg: Arch. f. Anat. u. Physiol., 1882, Phys. Abth., p. 540.

Schwerdt: Deutsch. med. Wchnschr., 1896, xxii,, 53.

Senator: Charité-Ann., 1883, viii, 307.

Smith: Am. Jour. Obst., 1908, lviii, 288.

Tigerstedt: Text-Book of Physiology (Murlin), New York, 1906, p. 299.

Timofeefsky: Inaug. Diss., Moscow, 1888.

Veit: Zentralbl. f. Gynäk., 1906, xxx, 201.

Verstraeten: Ann. de la Soc. de Méd. de Gand., 1887, lxvi, 11.

Wagner: Russk. Vrach, 1888, ix, 223, 247, 264.

Weber: Arch. f. Anat. Phys. u. wissensch. Med. (Müller's), 1851, p. 88.

Weitz: Deutsch. Arch. f. klin. Med., 1909, xcv, 257.

Wegner: Arch. f. klin. Chir., 1877, xx, 51.

Weisker: Schmidt's Jahrb. d. Med., 1888, ccxix, 277.

Wendt: Arch. d. Heilk., 1876, xvii, 527.

# THE EFFECTS ON BLOOD-PRESSURE OF INTRAVENOUS INJECTIONS OF EXTRACTS OF THE VARIOUS ANATOMICAL COMPONENTS OF THE HYPOPHYSIS

DEAN LEWIS, M.D., JOSEPH L. MILLER, M.D., AND S. A. MATTHEWS, M.D.
CHICAGO

This work was undertaken with the hope of determining the origin of the pressor substance in the hypophysis and its mode of secretion, and of reconciling, if possible, the divergent views concerning the depressor substance in the anterior lobe.

The ox hypophysis was used in making the extracts because the pars intermedia is sharply demarcated from the pars nervosa and can be cut away from the latter without taking nervous tissue with it (Fig. 1). In preparing the extracts an attempt was made to isolate the different portions of the gland in as pure a condition as possible. The anterior and posterior lobes were separated in the usual way by inserting scissor points in the depression anteriorly which indicates the position of the hypophysial cleft and by then cutting along the margins of the cleft until the separation was completed. The cleft is frequently filled with a rather thick colloid. The colloid appears in the form of thin platelets and but a small amount is obtained from a relatively large number of glands. There is almost constantly found within the cleft a small amount of thick yellow fluid which adheres to the surface of the knife or scissors and can be scraped off from the epithelial surfaces bounding the cleft. This fluid has the same physical properties as that obtained by curetting the epithelial covering of the posterior lobe. It is probably secreted by the cells of the pars intermedia. Whether the colloid found in the cleft is a thickened, hard stage of the fluid just mentioned, we are not prepared to say.

We have never been able to find any evidence of an antecedent secretion in the cells of the pars intermedia which resembles the colloid occurring in the cleft or the hyaline bodies described by Herring. Cysts which can be seen with the naked eye are rare. We have examined over 1,200 glands in making extracts and have found but two large cysts. A colloid-like material is frequently found in the lumen of the gland-like tubules of the pars intermedia.

At the margins of the hypophysial cleft, the cells of the pars intermedia are grouped so that a distinct mass of gland-like tubules is formed (Fig. 2). The transition between the pars intermedia and the anterior lobe at the margin of the cleft is quite abrupt but the anatomical relations are such that tissue with the histologic characteristics of the pars intermedia remains attached to the anterior lobe in the process of separation usually employed. The cells of the anterior lobe adjacent to the cleft have many of the histologic characteristics of those of the epithelium covering the posterior lobe, and we believe that the form and staining properties of these cells suggest that they may belong to the pars intermedia and that the hypophysial cleft lies within the pars intermedia, rather than between it and the anterior lobe.

In the method usually employed in separating the two lobes of the hypophysis masses of cells belonging to the pars intermedia remain attached to the anterior lobe at the margins of the cleft and a fringe of tissue with all the physical properties of the pars intermedia can often be

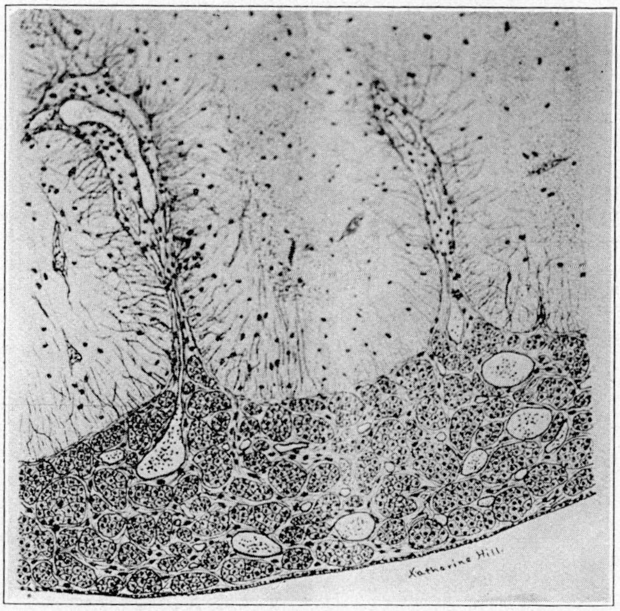


Fig. 1.—Section through the posterior lobe showing relation of the pars intermedia to pars nervosa. The pars intermedia at this level—middle of infundibular lobe—has a glandular structure. In the ox it is sharply separated from the subjacent nervous tissue. In man, cat, and some other animals the cells of the pars intermedia are scattered throughout the pars nervosa, some of the cells extending almost to the infundibular canal.

removed from the margins of the lobe. This tissue contains none of the elements of the pars nervosa and therefore represents the pars intermedia in its purest form.

We have examined the effects of intravenous injections of the following extracts with the view of determining the origin and mode of secretion of the different substances acting on blood-pressure.

1. Extracts of the entire anterior lobe.

2. Extracts of the part of the anterior lobe away from the hypophysial cleft.

3. Extracts of the part of the anterior lobe immediately adjacent to the cleft.

4. Extracts of the entire posterior lobe.

5. Extracts of the pars intermedia.

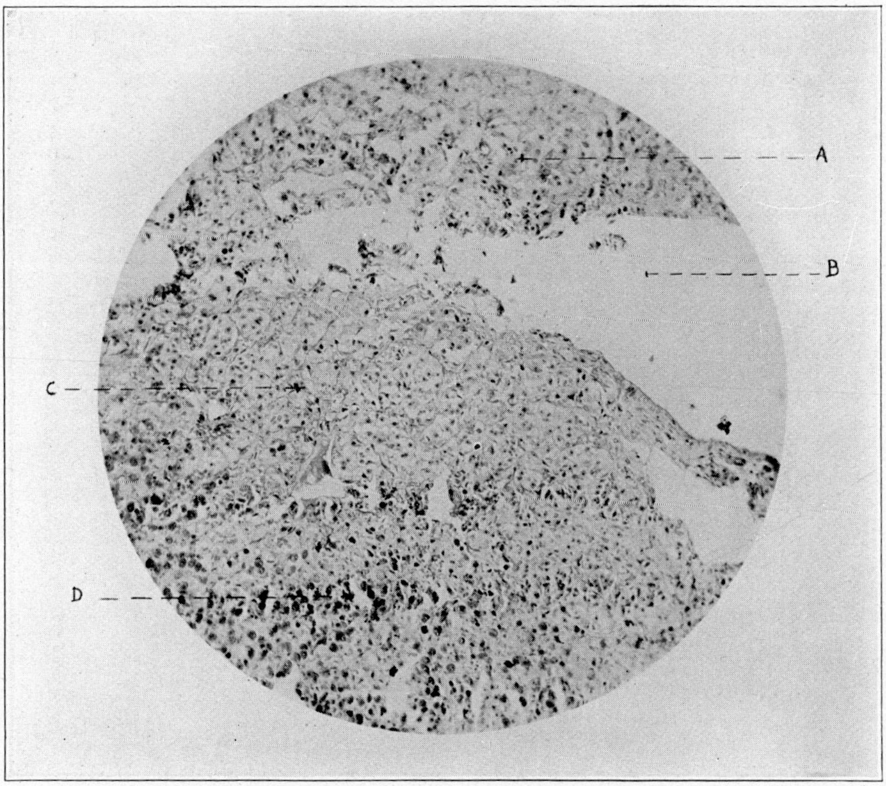


Fig. 2.—Section through the hypophysis at margin of the cleft, showing the pars intermedia and zone of transition between it and the anterior lobe. The cleft is bounded at the sides and to the front by the pars intermedia. The entire anterior boundary of the cleft is formed by cells which resemble more closely histologically those of the pars intermedia than those of the anterior lobe. Groups of cells belonging to the pars intermedia remain attached to the anterior lobe at the margin of the cleft after separation of the posterior lobe. A, pars intermedia. B, cleft. C, group of cells belonging to pars intermedia at margin of the cleft. D, anterior lobe containing a few dark granule cells. Magnification 110 diameters.

6. Extracts of the fringe of the pars intermedia, which frequently remains attached to the anterior lobe at the margins of the cleft after separation of the lobes.

7. Extracts of the pars nervosa entirely freed of the pars intermedia.

8. Extracts of the stalk uniting the infundibulum to the floor of the third ventricle.

9. Contents of cysts in the pars intermedia and the thick colloid removed from the cleft.

The material with which we worked was obtained fresh from Armour & Co. The cattle were killed in the forenoon and the hypophyses were removed, packed in ice and taken immediately to the laboratory. This was done to avoid the possibility of error due to putrefactive changes, for

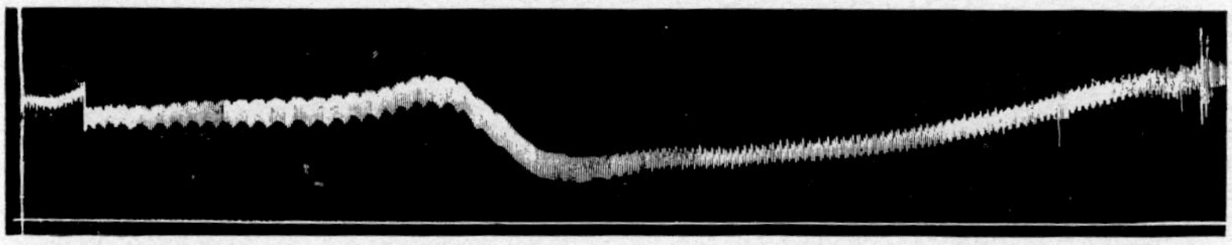

Fig. 3.—Effect of intravenous injections of 0.17 gm. fresh anterior lobe in a dog weighing 3 kilos.

Schäfer and Herring state that any active properties in the anterior lobe are due to post-mortem changes.

The amount of fresh gland substance to be used was weighed and then cut into small pieces which were mixed with white sand and thoroughly ground into a fine pulp in a mortar. Normal salt was then added to the mixture to make the solution. The sand and tissue particles were removed by sedimentation or filtration. In some instances the glands were extracted with acidulated water, the solution being neutralized. In many cases the extracts were made from glands cut into fine pieces which were dried in a hot-air blast or a thermostat. The glands were dried to

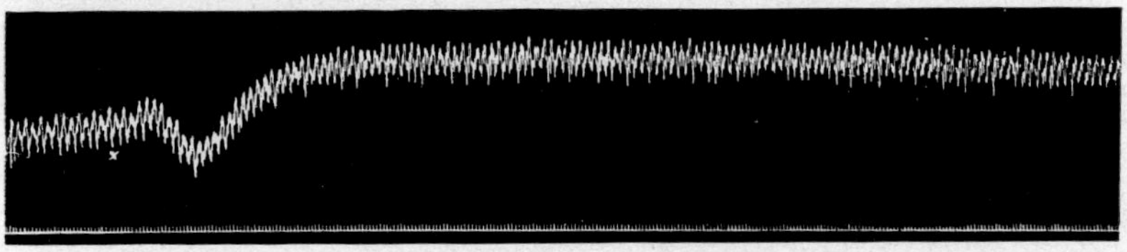

Fig. 4.—Injection of extract made from 2 gm. of the anterior lobe. In most instances the primary fall in pressure was greater than shown here.

avoid putrefactive changes. The dried material was extracted either with normal salt solution or with alcohol to remove the depressor substance; and the residue, from which the alcohol had been removed by evaporation, was then extracted with normal salt solution.

Dogs weighing 6 to 10 kilos were used. The injections were made into the femoral vein, the blood-pressure tracings being taken with a mercury manometer connected with a carotid cannula. In all about sixty dogs were injected. The animals were thoroughly etherized. Any changes in blood-pressure which might possibly be due to anesthesia were carefully excluded. While many animals received several injections only the results of the primary injection were recorded, as Howell has shown that when two injections are made with but a short interval between, the effect of the second is much less intense. The amount of gland substance used and the exact changes in pressure are recorded in the tables.

### EFFECTS OF EXTRACTS OF THE ENTIRE ANTERIOR LOBE

Saline extracts of the fresh anterior lobe, boiled extracts and extracts from dried portions of the gland were employed. Following the injection there was usually an immediate fall in pressure. This fall in many cases was followed by a rise. Two readings were taken, one immediately after the injection and one at the time of the maximum rise, usually within two minutes after the injection.

Nine animals received injections of fresh unboiled preparations of the entire anterior lobe. In two of these animals the blood-pressure after

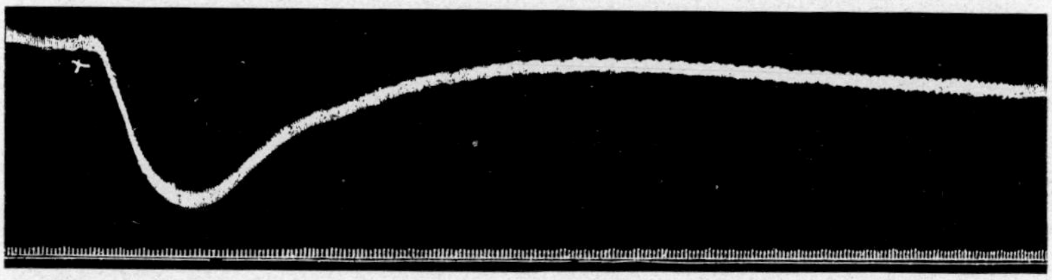

Fig. 5.—Blood-pressure curve after injecting a saline extract made from 0.5 gm. of fresh ox brain.

the fall did not return to the level existing before it. In three of the animals the pressure mounted considerably above the level existing before the primary fall—15, 32 and 58 mm. respectively. This increase continued for several minutes, the pressure gradually returning to the primary level. In some instances considerable bradycardia was noted during the rise. This rise was not, however, necessarily associated with slowing of the pulse. In the animal that succumbed to the injection, there was marked slowing of the pulse, the heart finally stopping while the respirations continued quite normally for more than a minute. When injections were repeated at intervals of two or three minutes, the succeeding falls in pressure grew less after each injection, the results resembling in this way those following injections of the depressor substance of the posterior lobe. Characteristic pressure curves are shown in Figures 3 and 4.

Two animals received injections of 0.68 and 1 gm. respectively of a boiled extract of the anterior lobe. As in the preceding experiments there was a temporary fall in pressure succeeded by a rise above the previous level of 12 and 14 mm. respectively.

Three animals received injections of extracts made from dried pieces of the anterior lobe. In two of the animals there was a primary fall followed by a rise of from 10 to 18 mm. of mercury. In one animal the rise occurred without a primary fall.

In 57 per cent. of the cases—fourteen animals being used—there was an ultimate rise in blood-pressure of 10 mm. or more. In thirteen of the animals there was a primary fall. A rise of 10 mm. is very slight, but after injections of extracts of brain (Fig. 5) the rise following the primary fall is at most to the previous level. In a few of the animals the rise in pressure was so decided as to leave little doubt that extracts of the entire anterior lobe may give a pressor reaction. The depressor substance, however, is so powerful that its effect predominates in most cases. When an animal received repeated injections at short intervals each succeeding injection caused less rise and less fall in pressure, until finally a dose, which if administered at the beginning would have killed the animal, could be given without modifying the pressure curve. Howell first called attention to the lessened effect of repeated injections, referring especially to the pressor substance. Subsequent investigators have reported that the effect of the depressor substance is not lessened by repeated injections. All of our results indicate that both the pressor and the depressor substances behave alike in this respect. The results obtained by us correspond very closely with those noted by Hamburger.

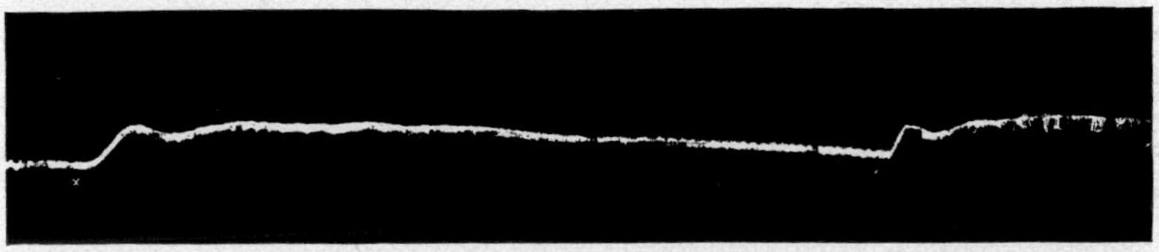

Fig. 6.—Dog weighing 7 kilos received at first x mark 0.5 c.c. = 0.21 gm. of dried anterior lobe with depressor substance removed. The second x shows the effect of injecting 0.63 gm. of the same.

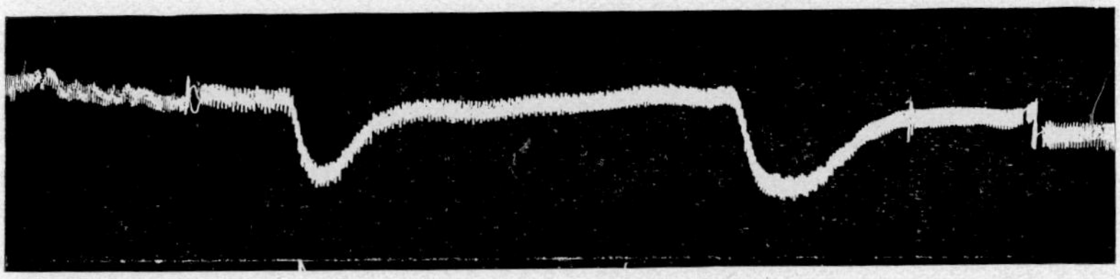

Fig. 7.—The first x indicates an injection of 1 c.c. = 4 gm. of alcoholic extract of posterior lobe, representing the depressor substance; the second x, 4 c.c. of same.

The presence of a depressor substance, the existence of which is denied by Schäfer and Herring, can be demonstrated almost constantly in fresh glands extracted with salt solution. It has the characteristics of the depressor substance which is found in other tissues.

It was thought that if this depressor substance, which is soluble in alcohol—the pressor substance is not—could be removed, a more marked and constant effect might be elicited by extracts of the anterior lobe. With this in view, the fresh anterior lobe, thoroughly washed to free it from any adherent secretion from the posterior lobe, was dried by exposure to the hot-air blast. The dried gland was thoroughly powdered and extracted with alcohol, the insoluble residue then dried and extracted with normal salt. The normal salt extract thus obtained should be free of the depressor substance. A solution containing the extract from 0.2 gm. of the dried anterior lobe prepared in this way gave a sharp rise in pressure without a preliminary fall, the rise being maintained for several minutes as indicated in Figure 6. A second injection after the lapse of

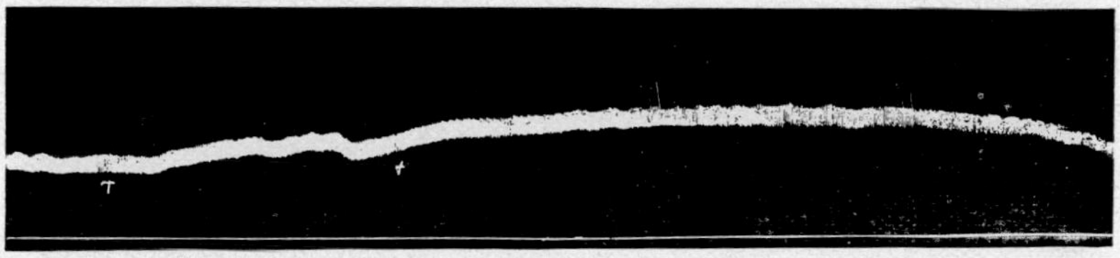

**Fig. 8.—Injection of 2 c.c.=0.8 gm. of anterior portion of anterior lobe with** depressor substance removed. Injection given slowly, the crosses marking time **consumed in making the injection.**

six minutes gave a characteristic rise. The curve corresponds quite closely to curves from extracts of the pars intermedia which will be given later. The alcoholic extract after evaporation—the residue being dissolved in salt solution and injected—gave uniformly a fall in pressure without a subsequent rise (Fig. 7).

As that portion of the anterior lobe adjacent to the cleft resembles histologically the pars intermedia to which Herring ascribes on histological grounds the secretion of the pressor substance, the narrow strip of tissue immediately bounding the cleft was cut away from the large part of the lobe distal to the cleft.

Extracts were made from both of these divisions of the lobe, the depressor substance having been previously removed by alcohol. Extracts of the portion of the lobe adjacent to the cleft gave a decided rise in blood-pressure. Extracts of the portion distal to the cleft either gave no rise at all or a slight rather continuous rise but not the sharp decided rise which is caused by the pressor substance (Figs. 8 and 9).

During the process of separation of the anterior from the posterior lobe a fringe of tissue with all the physical properties of the pars intermedia frequently remains attached to the anterior lobe at the margins of the cleft. An extract of this fringe previously extracted with alcohol gave a decided pressor reaction (Fig. 10). This demonstration of a pressor substance in the anterior lobe confirms the work of Hamburger concerning the secondary rise after the primary fall caused by the injec-

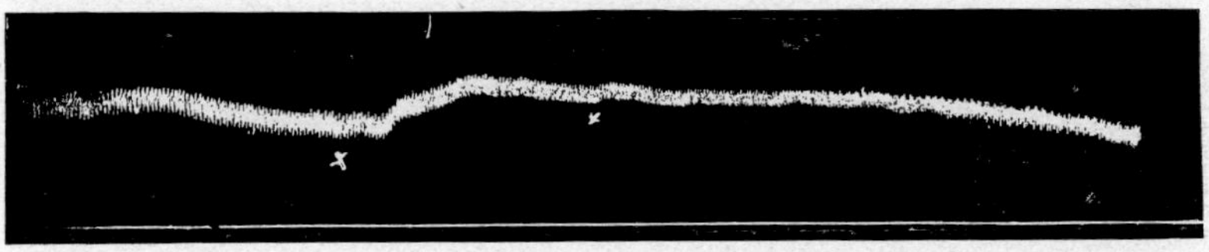

Fig. 9.—The first x indicates injection of 0.5 c.c.=0.2 gm. of dried posterior portion of anterior lobe with depressor substance removed; the second x, 1 c.c. of same.

tion of extracts of the anterior lobe and Franchini's results with Ehrmann's test. That these results have not been noted more frequently is due, we believe, to the existence of a depressor substance which counteracts the pressor. The pressor substance is evidently confined to the part of the anterior lobe adjacent to the cleft—in that part containing cells belonging to the pars intermedia.

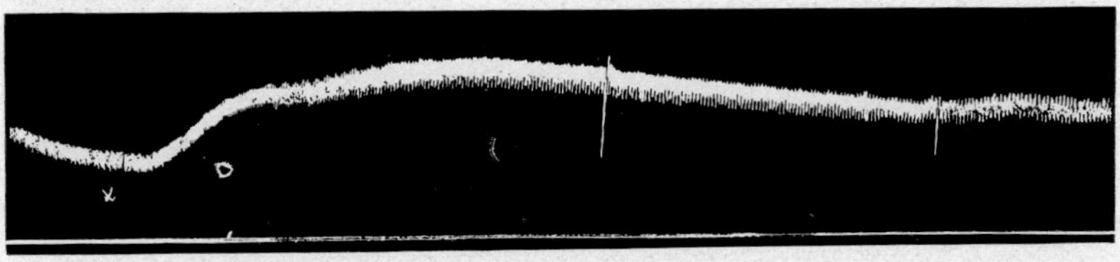

Fig. 10.—Injection of 2 c.c. extract from epithelial fringe on the anterior lobe which histologically is pars intermedia.

EFFECTS OF EXTRACTS OF THE ENTIRE POSTERIOR LOBE

Nine dogs received injections of extracts of the entire fresh posterior lobe. In almost every instance there was a marked fall in blood-pressure of about the same degree as has been noted after injections of the same amount of the anterior lobe. Following the fall in pressure there was a gradual rise, which in 55 per cent. of the cases exceeded the previous level. In 33 1/3 per cent. of the animals the blood-pressure did not return to the previous level. Very marked slowing and irregularity of the heart occurred in most cases. Rarely was there any disturbance of respiration, although decided slowing was noted in a few instances.

When we compare these results with those of corresponding preparations from the anterior lobe, we find that 33 1/3 per cent. of the animals receiving injections of the anterior lobe reacted by a mean rise in pressure of 32 mm., while 55 per cent. of the animals receiving extracts of the entire posterior lobe reacted by a mean rise in pressure of 29 mm. The failure of a constant pressor effect renders these results different from those of Howell and Schäfer. Two types of reaction are shown in Figures 11 and 12.

The majority of tracings from extracts of the posterior lobe show a sudden sharp rise in pressure immediately after the injection, followed by a sharp fall; the first effect is apparently due to the action of the pressor substance, but this is almost invariably overcome by the depressor substance. This primary rise was not observed after injections of the anterior lobe.

Three injections were made with extracts of the dried posterior lobe. The primary fall in pressure was much less, resembling in this respect

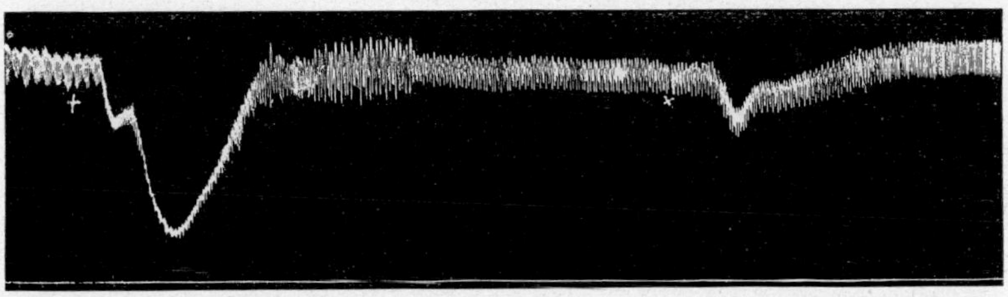

Fig. 11.—At the first x, an injection of 0.2 gm. fresh posterior lobe; at the second x, a second injection of 0.4 gm. During the primary fall a slight transitory rise is noted.

the effects of injections of dried preparations of the anterior lobe. Apparently the depressor substance is partially destroyed by drying.

Five animals received injections of a boiled extract made from the fresh posterior lobe. Only one gave evidence of a pressor substance.

### EFFECTS OF EXTRACTS OF THE PARS INTERMEDIA

The pars intermedia in the ox forms a distinct layer of tissue which may be cut away from the pars nervosa, if care is exercised. With manicure scissors thin pieces of yellowish tissue were cut away from the surface of the posterior lobe bounding the hypophysial cleft. Only the superficial layers were removed with the idea of keeping away from the subjacent pars nervosa, which can easily be recognized by its white or reddish-white color.

In some instances the surface of the pars intermedia was scraped with a small curette, the yellowish fluid filling the cup of the curette being dissolved in salt solution, to which it gives an opalescent appearance.

The thin pieces of tissue which were removed from the surface of the pars intermedia were dried and in the later experiments were extracted with alcohol before the saline extracts were made, because a depressor effect similar to that in the anterior lobe was observed after some injections of the saline extract without previous extraction with alcohol (Fig. 13). A mean rise of 22 mm. occurred in 43 per cent. of the animals after injection of the pars intermedia. The pressor effect caused by the injection of extracts of the purest form of the pars intermedia—the fringe adhering to the anterior lobe after separation of the two lobes of the gland—is not associated with slowing of the pulse.

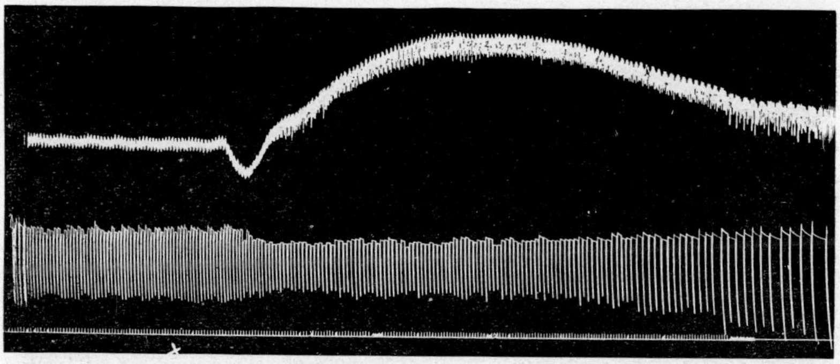

Fig. 12.—At x, injection of 0.5 gm. boiled posterior lobe. Upper curve carotid; lower curve shows slowing of respiration.

In the instances in which the surface of the pars intermedia was curetted and the material removed dissolved in relatively large amounts of salt solution no result except an increase in the amplitude of the pulse wave followed the injection. After evaporation of the salt solution and washing with alcohol, a more concentrated saline solution gave a typical pressor reaction.

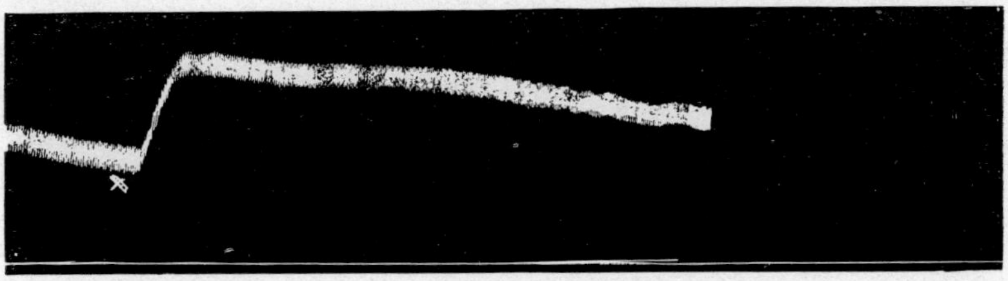

Fig. 13.—Injection of 0.018 gm. dried pars intermedia with depressor substance removed.

EFFECTS OF EXTRACTS OF THE PARS NERVOSA

In making extracts of the pars nervosa, the yellow, overlying pars intermedia was cut away and in order to be sure that none of it remained considerable portions of the pars nervosa were sacrificed. As some of the material covering the surface of the pars intermedia adhered to the scissors, these were frequently washed and the parts of the gland removed were hurriedly washed in salt solution with the idea of removing any of the secretion of the pars intermedia that might have adhered to the surface of the part to be used for injection.

Four animals received injections of extracts of the pars nervosa. One-half of these reacted by a mean rise in pressure of 30 mm. The rise in pressure was more marked than that following the injection of extracts of the pars intermedia (Fig. 14).

Several intravenous injections were made with an infundibular extract put on the market by Burroughs, Wellcome & Co. An amount equivalent to 0.2 gm. of the fresh gland produced the same effect as fresh posterior lobe, i. e., a marked fall in pressure with a gradual return to the previous level or somewhat higher (Fig. 15). Occasionally an animal reacted by a primary rise without a secondary fall.

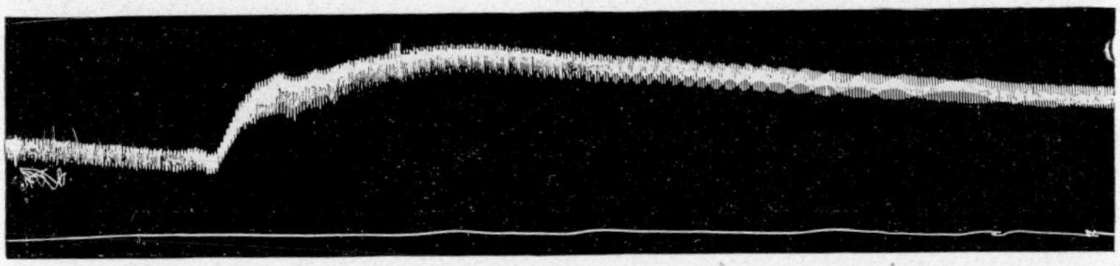

Fig. 14.—Dog 6 kilos received 0.9 gm. fresh pars nervosa of the posterior lobe. Except in this single instance there was a marked secondary fall after the primary rise.

## EFFECTS OF INJECTIONS OF EXTRACTS OF THE PARS NERVOSA AFTER EXTRACTION WITH ALCOHOL

An attempt was made to remove the depressor substance of the pars nervosa by first extracting it with alcohol. A small dose of a saline extract of the residue, equivalent to 0.2 gm. of the dried pars nervosa, gave a rise in pressure without a preliminary fall. If the dosage were increased in 0.6 gm., there was an abrupt, rapid rise with a secondary fall to the level at which the experiment was started and then a gradual rise to the same or a higher level, as previously noted by Howell. The secondary rise continued for some time.

The fall, after the primary rise, is not observed after the injection of extracts of the pars intermedia or of the anterior lobe. The fall in pressure is coincident with marked weakening of the heart, but not necessarily with slowing. Coincident with the secondary rise there is evidence of an increased systolic output with very decided slowing of the pulse which continues for several minutes. Atropin relieves the slowing. The substance producing this fall—after the primary rise—is insoluble in alcohol and thus differs from the depressor substance found in the pars intermedia and anterior lobe, and on account of its insolubility in alcohol may be considered specific in character, as the depressor substance normally present in nervous tissue can be removed by extracting with alcohol.

With the pressor substance obtained from the part of the anterior lobe adjacent to the cleft and from the pars intermedia we were never able to obtain such a powerful effect on the pulse-rate and it seems not improbable that the pars nervosa contains a specific substance which produces it.

It is evident from the results which have been given that both the pars intermedia and pars nervosa contain a pressor substance. It is highly improbable that tissues which differ so markedly histologically

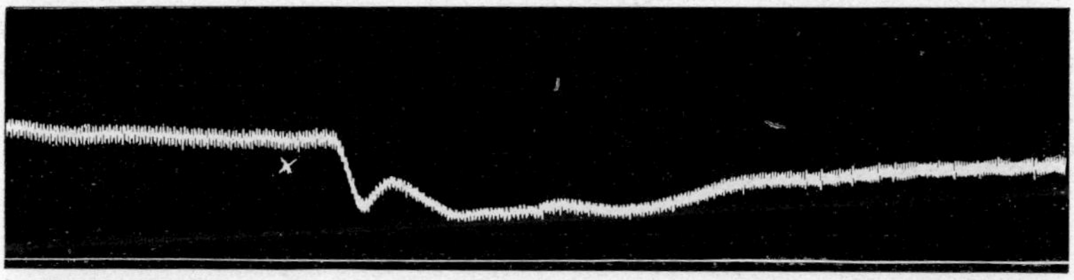

Fig. 15.—Injection of 1 c.c. Burroughs, Wellcome & Co.'s infundibular extract, equivalent to 0.2 gm. Dog 7 kilos.

should secrete the same pressor substance. We believe that the pressor substance is secreted by the pars intermedia. It exerts its effect, however, without coming into contact with the pars nervosa, and does not need to be activated as suggested by Cushing.

We do not believe that one can say whether the pressor substance passes into the pars nervosa by way of the blood-stream or the hyaline bodies. The latter do not form a striking picture in the histology of the

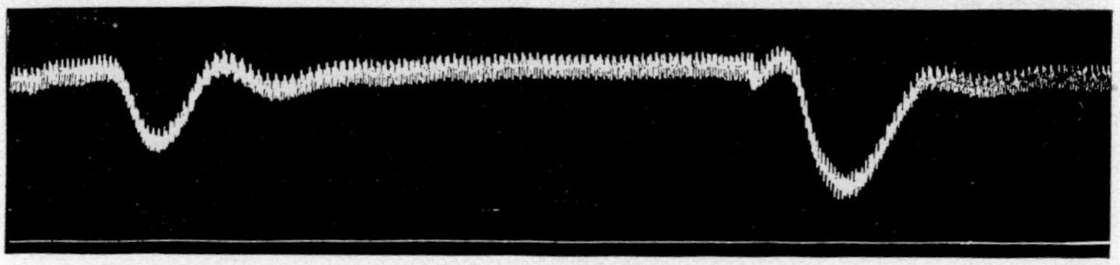

Fig. 16.—Injection of extract made from 0.3 gm. of the fresh stalk.

ox hypophysis, and besides we shall later adduce evidence which we believe will show that these pressor substances do not pass by way of the stalk into the third ventricle.

## EFFECTS OF INJECTIONS OF EXTRACTS OF THE STALK

If the hyaline bodies which Herring believes contain the pressor substance pass into the third ventricle where they become mixed with the cerebrospinal fluid, we believe that the pressor reaction should be obtained from extracts of the stalk through which these bodies must pass to reach the third ventricle. Cushing and Goettsch have recently called attention to the presence in the cerebrospinal fluid of a substance which gives the same pressor reaction as extracts of the posterior lobe, indicating that the active principle of the posterior lobe is actually secreted into the ventricular cavity.

Four dogs each received 0.3 gm. of the fresh stalk extracted in salt solution, the amount of solution injected varying from 4 to 10 c.c. In each instance there was an immediate fall in blood-pressure averaging 35 mm. This was followed by a gradual rise to the previous level but never

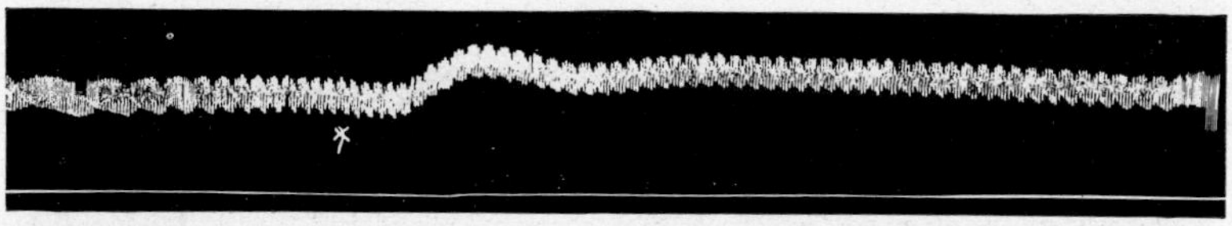

Fig. 17.—Injection of contents of a cyst of the pars intermedia 0.5 c.c.

above it. The pulse and respiration were unaffected (Fig. 16). The results resemble those obtained by injecting extracts of parenchymatous organs.

Several experiments were made with extracts of stalks which were dried and extracted in alcohol, the residue being dissolved in salt solution. When the depressor substance was removed, injections of the saline extract had no effect whatever.

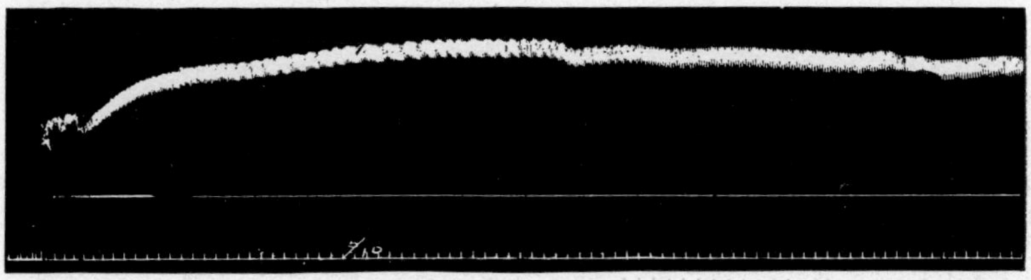

Fig. 18.—The effect on blood-pressure of injecting an extract from the colloid found in the cleft.

The results of these injections were carefully watched because of the importance which has recently been attached to the hyaline bodies described by Herring and to their peculiar mode of secretion. As previously stated, Cushing and Goettsch have attributed an hypophysial origin to the pressor substance in the cerebrospinal fluid and state that it is obvious from the distribution of the hyaline that the infundibular wall must be as active as the pars nervosa, for it often contains a large amount of hyaline.

In the ox, at least, there is a distinct break in the path of secretion of the pressor substance from the pars nervosa to the third ventricle and we believe this to be a strong argument against Herring's theory, which is based on histological findings.

Effects on Blood-Pressure of Injections of Extracts of Various Portions of the Hypophysis

| Part of Gland Used | Amount of Fresh Gland gm. | Quantity of Fluid c.c. | Blood Pressure: Before Injecting | Blood Pressure: Immediately After | Blood Pressure: After 1-2 Minutes |
|---|---|---|---|---|---|
| Entire anterior lobe | 0.30 | 10.0 | 110 | 98 | 110 |
| Entire anterior lobe | 0.40 | 10.0 | 140 | 36 | 88 |
| Entire anterior lobe | 0.40 | 10.0 | 175 | 20 | 0 |
| Entire anterior lobe | 0.17 | 2.0 | 72 | 42 | 70 |
| Entire anterior lobe | 1.50 | 1.5 | 142 | 130 | 200 |
| Entire anterior lobe | 1.00 | 1.0 | 110 | 110 | 110 |
| Entire anterior lobe | 1.00 | 2.0 | 116 | 96 | 148 |
| Entire anterior lobe | 0.50 | 1.5 | 100 | 92 | 116 |
| Entire anterior lobe | 0.30 | 2.0 | 140 | 140 | 140 |
| Entire posterior lobe, fresh | 0.30 | 10.0 | 110 | 60 | 100 |
| Entire posterior lobe, fresh | 0.30 | 7.0 | 90 | 44 | 74 |
| Entire posterior lobe, fresh | 0.40 | 10.0 | 128 | 38 | 138 |
| Entire posterior lobe, fresh | 0.30 | 1.0 | 130 | 90 | 180 |
| Entire posterior lobe, fresh | 0.30 | 1.0 | 70 | 58 | 100 |
| Entire posterior lobe, fresh | 1.00 | 2.0 | 134 | 76 | 160 |
| Entire posterior lobe, fresh | 0.60 | 2.0 | 144 | 50 | 100 |
| Entire posterior lobe, fresh | 0.20 | 2.0 | 104 | 46 | 134 |
| Entire posterior lobe, fresh | 0.20 | 2.0 | 140 | 46 | 140 |
| Dried posterior lobe | 0.50 | 1.0 | 142 | 138 | 142 |
| Dried posterior lobe | 0.50 | 1.0 | 60 | 50 | 100 |
| Dried posterior lobe | 0.20 | 1.0 | 140 | 120 | 160 |
| Boiled extract of post. lobe | 0.25 | 0.5 | 116 | 136 | 118 |
| Boiled extract of post. lobe | 0.15 | 2.0 | 120 | 50 | 120 |
| Boiled extract of post. lobe | 0.30 | 1.0 | 100 | 84 | 114 |
| Boiled extract of post. lobe | 0.45 | 1.5 | 134 | 40 | 0 |
| Boiled extract of post. lobe | 0.45 | 3.0 | 92 | 48 | 80 |
| Pars intermedia | 0.2 | 2.0 | 80 | 66 | 86 |
| Pars intermedia | 0.15 | 2.0 | 108 | 120 | 108 |
| Pars intermedia | 0.45 | 3.0 | 152 | 170 | 148 |
| Pars intermedia | 0.25 | 2.0 | 92 | 80 | 114 |
| Pars intermedia | 1.00 | 3.0 | 130 | 50 | 164 |
| Pars intermedia | 0.10 | 2.0 | 120 | 86 | 108 |
| Pars intermedia | 0.25 | 2.0 | 126 | 76 | 150 |
| Pars nervosa | 1.60 | 8.0 | 144 | 90 | 85 |
| Pars nervosa | 0.45 | 10.0 | 156 | 84 | 130 |
| Pars nervosa | 0.50 | 10.0 | 140 | 60 | 160 |
| Pars nervosa | 0.90 | 3.0 | 100 | 130 | 140 |
| Colloid | ? | 4.0 | 110 | 122 | ... |
| Colloid | ? | 0.5 | 118 | 148 | ... |
| Colloid | ? | 3.0 | 98 | 110 | ... |
| Colloid | ? | 2.0 | 160 | 168 | ... |

## EFFECT OF THE INJECTION OF THE CONTENTS OF A CYST OF THE PARS INTERMEDIA AND OF COLLOID

Considerable fluid of a light straw color was obtained from a cyst in the pars intermedia. We have encountered but two cysts in over 1,200 glands. The fluid obtained from these gave a decided pressor effect, as shown in Figure 17. In examining contents of cysts of the pars intermedia we should keep in mind the possibility of cysts developing from inclusions of craniopharyngeal duct epithelium, the contents of which should not be active. One of the most typical pressor effects that we have seen followed the injection of fluid removed from one of the two cysts which we have encountered. As we were dependent on small pieces of colloid, the amount available for injection in any single instance was small, never more than three pieces at a time, one-fourth the size and about the thickness of the little finger-nail. In all four dogs were injected with solutions of colloid. The effect on the blood-pressure is shown in Figure 18. The increase in pressure averaged 15.5 mm. and was maintained for some time. The respiration and pulse were unaffected.

## CONCLUSIONS

1. Extracts of the pars intermedia (*Korkschicht, Epithelsaum*) when injected intravenously cause a decided rise in blood-pressure. The extract does not need to come in contact with the pars nervosa to become active.

2. Extracts of the pars nervosa also give a pressor effect. The primary rise is followed by a fall, which is succeeded by a rise associated with a marked slowing of the pulse.

3. Extracts of the anterior lobe give a primary fall, which is followed in the majority of instances by a secondary rise in pressure above the level existing at the beginning of the experiment. These results confirm Hamburger's findings. The pressor substance is confined to that part of the anterior lobe bounding the cleft which contains groups of cells belonging to the pars intermedia. Ehrmann's test elicited by Franchini with extracts of the anterior lobe is explained in the same way.

4. The contents of a cyst of the pars intermedia gave a decided pressor effect.

5. A depressor substance, soluble in alcohol, is found in the anterior lobe, the pars intermedia and the pars nervosa.

6. It is not probable that two structures differing so much histologically as the pars intermedia and the pars nervosa would secrete a substance having the same effect on blood-pressure. We believe that the pressor substance is secreted by the pars intermedia and that it then passes into the pars nervosa. Whether it passes by way of the blood or the hyaline bodies we cannot say. The latter, however, do not form a striking feature in the histology of the ox hypophysis.

7. We have never been able to obtain any pressor effect from extracts of the hypophysial stalk. If the hyaline bodies pass through this and represent the pressor substance, we believe that we should be able to elicit a pressor reaction with extracts of the stalk. In the ox, at least, there

is a distinct break in the paths of secretion between the pars nervosa and the ventricular cavity.

122 South Michigan Boulevard—5221 Jefferson Avenue.

BIBLIOGRAPHY

1. Oliver, G., and Schaefer, E. A.: The Physiological Action of Extracts of Pituitary Body and Certain other Glandular Organs, Jour. Physiol., 1894, xvi, 1; 1895, xviii, 277.

2. Howell, W. H.: The Physiological Effects of Extracts of the Hypophysis Cerebri and Infundibular Body, Jour. Exper. Med., 1898, iii, 245.

3. Hamburger, W. W.: The Action of Intravenous Injections of Glandular Extracts and other Substances on the Blood-Pressure, Am. Jour. Physiol., 1904, xi, 282.

4. Franchini, G.: Die Funktion der Hypophyse und die Wirkungen der Injektion ihres Extraktes bei Thieren, Berl. klin. Wchnschr., 1910, xlvii, 722.

5. Cushing, H.: Experimental Hypophysectomy, Bull. Johns Hopkins Hosp., 1910, xxi, 151.

6. Schaefer, E. A., and Vincent, S.: Physiological Effect of Extracts of Pituitary, Jour. Physiol., 1900, xxv, 87.

7. Herring, P. T.: The Histological Appearance of the Mammalian Pituitary Body, Quart. Jour. Exper. Physiol., 1908, ii, 154.

8. Halliburton, W. D.: The Physiological Effects of Extracts of Nervous Tissues, Jour. Physiol., 1900-1901, xxvi, 229.

9. Cleborne and Vincent: A Contribution to the Study of the Pituitary Body, Brit. Med. Jour., 1900, i, 502.

10. Cushing and Goettsch: Concerning the Secretion of the Infundibular Lobe of the Hypophysis and Its Presence in the Cerebrospinal Fluid, Am. Jour. Physiol., 1910, xxvii, 60.

# THE VALUE OF TROPHIC BONE CHANGES IN THE DIAGNOSIS OF LEPROSY *

A. B. HERRICK, M.D., AND T. W. EARHART, M.D.
ANCON HOSPITAL, CANAL ZONE

The diagnosis of anesthetic leprosy is often very difficult, as the bacillus of Hansen is obtained in only a small proportion of the early cases and consequently the diagnosis usually rests on the symptoms and signs of the neuritis and the gross trophic changes arising from it. These trophoneurotic changes are usually most marked in the extremities and may affect any or all of the tissues of the extremity.

The changes which take place in the nerves, muscles, subcutaneous tissue and skin have been emphasized by the writers on this disease and are well known to all. But the corresponding changes occurring in the bone, although of equal if not of greater diagnostic significance, have been simply mentioned in the descriptions of this disease. This is readily understood when we consider the difficulty of determining these changes early in the disease, before it has advanced to such a stage that these lesions become curious and interesting features of the process, rather than aids in diagnosis.

These bone lesions have been described by several writers. In 1886, Heiberg[1] called attention to peculiar atrophies of bone occurring in this disease. In 1898, Miura[2] described the pathological changes and also followed these changes with the aid of the *x*-ray. Hansen and Looft[3] also described the various processes. More recently Hirschberg and Bichler[4] have shown that a true leprous osteomyelitis and periostitis often occurs. In 1905, Deycke[5] traced the sequence of certain of these changes by means of the *x*-ray, and in 1909, Harbitz,[6] from a study of pathological speci-

---

* Read at the meeting of the Canal Zone Medical Association, Nov. 9, 1910.

1. Heiberg, H.: Om lepra mutilans og trofoneurotiske forandringer ved spedalskhed, klin. Aarb., 1886, iii.

2. Miura, K.: Ueber die Veränderungen der Knochen an den Händen und Füssen bei Lepra mutilans, Mitt. a. d. med. Fac. d. Kais. jap. Univ. zu Tokio, 1898, iv, 107.

3. Hansen and Looft: Die Lepra vom klinischen und pathologisch-anatomischen Standpunkte, Biblioth. med. int., 1894, ii, 2.

4. Hirschberg and Bichler: Lepra der Knochen, Dermat. Ztschr., 1909, xvi, 415.

5. Deycke: Knochenveränderungen bei Lepra nervorum in Roentgengraph, Fortschr. a. d. Geb. d. Roentgenstrahlen, 1905-6, ix, 9.

6. Harbitz: Trophoneurotic Changes in Bones and Joints in Leprosy, THE ARCHIVES INT. MED., 1910, vi, 147.

mens, called attention to a peculiar atrophy in this disease which he describes as concentric bone atrophy.

The pathological changes in the bones in leprosy occur in three different ways:

1. The true trophic disturbance due to the altered innervation, in which there takes place a simple atrophy or gradual absorption of the bone.

2. An osteomyelitis or periostitis caused by the lepra bacillus.

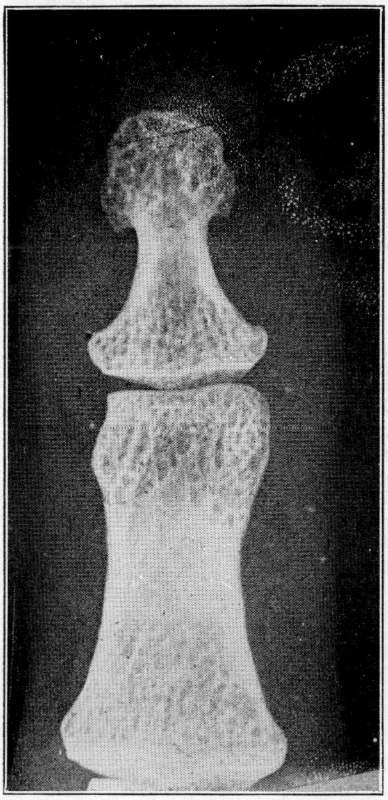

Figure 1.

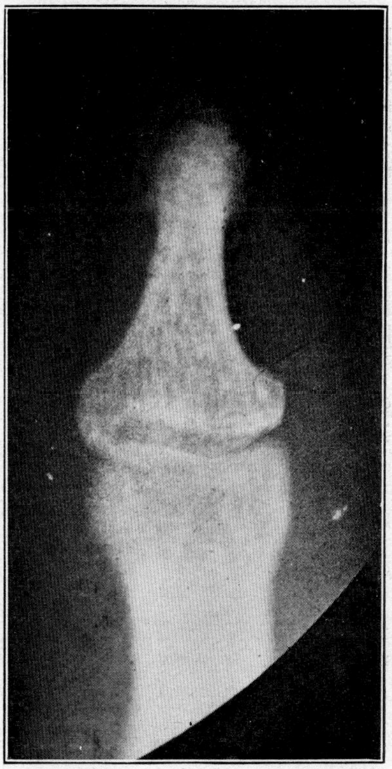

Figure 2.

Fig. 1.—Middle and distal phalanges of a normal index-finger.

Fig. 2.—Beginning absorption of the bulbous tip of the distal phalanx of the thumb, and an associated narrowing of the shaft. Both the shaft and the distal end are involved.

3. A necrosis or inflammation of either of the above arising from secondary involvement by pyogenic organisms.

These processes occur mainly in the fingers and toes and lead to a loss of the digits, from which this form of the disease gets its name of lepra mutilans.

Clinically the process in which a finger or toe is cast off or disappears presents two entirely different forms. The one shows simple atrophy and absorption of the digit without gross disturbance. The other presents an associated inflammatory process of various types. The former would represent a pure trophic type, and the latter a tropho-inflammatory method of the mutilating process.

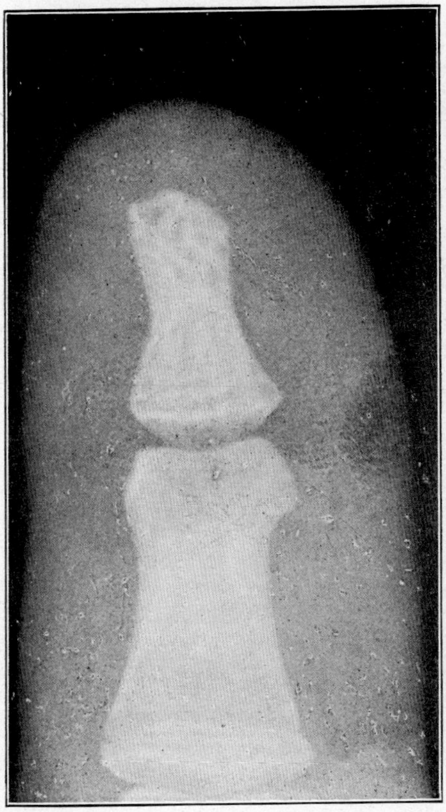

Figure 3.

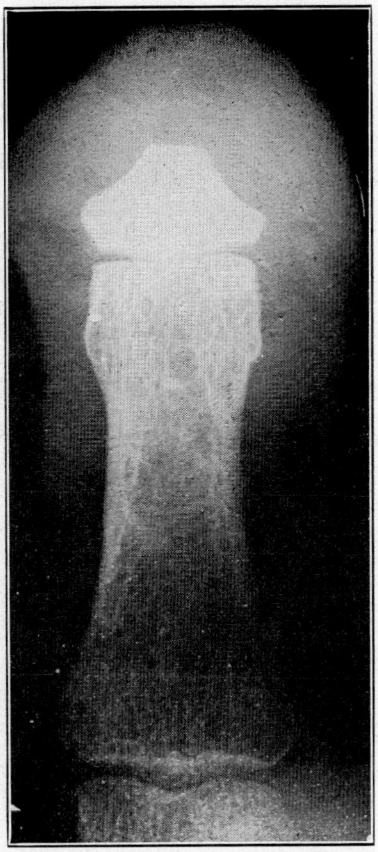

Figure 4

Fig. 3.—Absorption of the greater part of the bulbous tip of the distal phalanx of the index-finger. No change in the shaft.

Fig. 4.—Absorption and disappearance of the tip and shaft of the distal phalanx of the finger, only the base remaining.

In the tropho-inflammatory type there occurs a casting off of the digits in various ways, but in all the ways there is the underlying trophic change to which is added a secondary infection arising by different methods and thus causing the clinical variations. A perforating ulcer may form, which gradually extends to the shaft of a bone or to a joint and thus through a chronic suppurative process results in a casting off of the bone or that portion of the member distal to the ulcer. An abscess close to the bone may destroy the periosteum and lead to necrosis of the bone, or a necrosis of the bone of the atrophic type might become secondarily infected and thus lead to loss of the bone with later shrinking of the soft parts. A gangrene-like process might occur through involvement

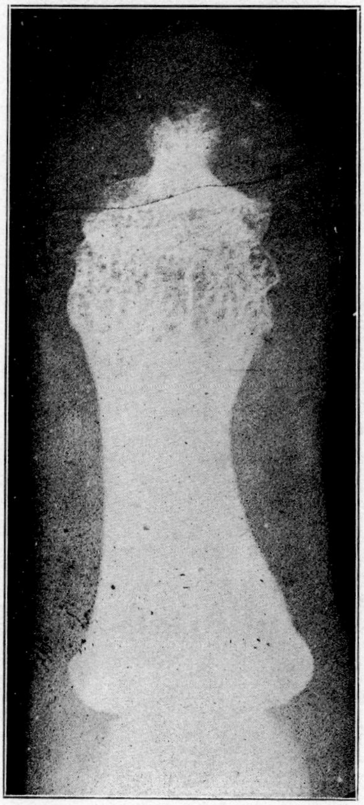

Figure 5.

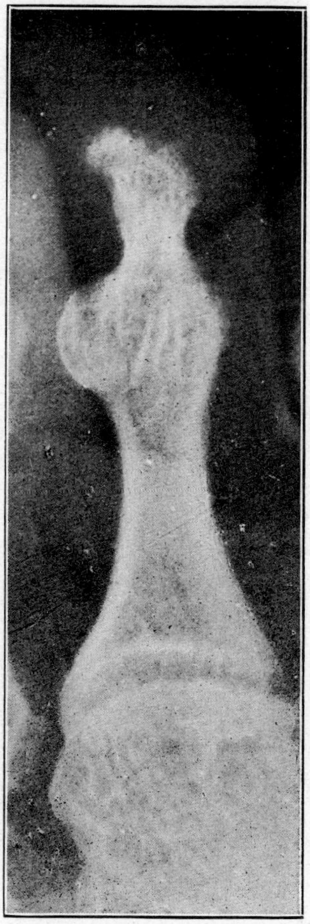

Figure 6.

Fig. 5.—Typical concentric atrophy with absorption and shrinking of the distal phalanx of the middle finger, the process affecting both tip and shaft but more marked in the shaft. It also involves the shaft of the middle phalanx.

Fig. 6.—Typical concentric atrophy of all the phalanges of the third toe; the distal phalanx almost absorbed; the middle phalanx markedly shrunken; the proximal phalanx showing incipient atrophy.

of the vessels by the leprous formations and thus cause the loss of a finger or toe. All of these forms depend on the secondary inflammatory process and consequently show no lesions characteristic of the disease.

The pure trophic type has been variously described. Scheube[7] speaks of it as "simple absorption of the tissues." Manson[8] describes it as "a curious interstitial absorption of one or more phalanges, the shaft of the phalanx wasting more rapidly than either of the articular surfaces." Harbitz speaks of it as "atrophy of the bone of characteristic appearance. The atrophy is concentric and chiefly involves the most peripheral parts of the phalanx."

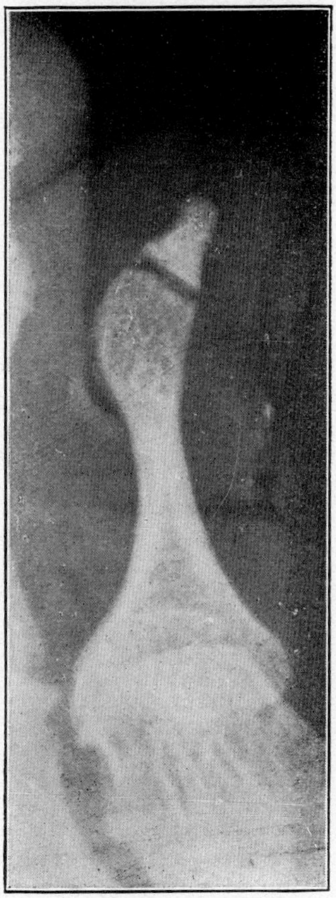

Figure 7.

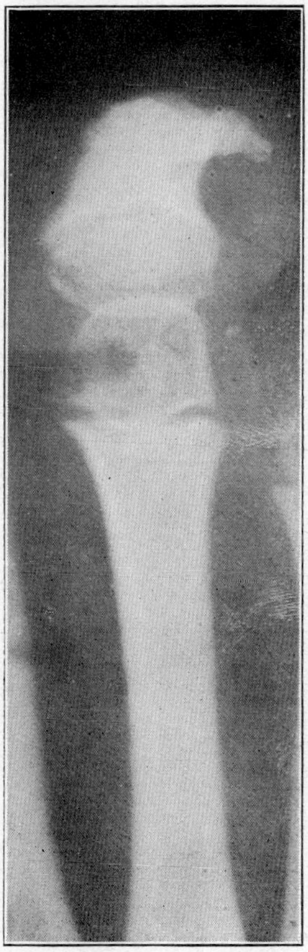

Figure 8.

Fig. 7.—Advanced concentric atrophy of all phalanges of fourth toe. The distal and middle phalanges are almost entirely absorbed. The proximal phalanx shows marked shrinking and narrowing of the shaft.

Fig. 8.—Very advanced concentric atrophy of all the phalanges of the ring finger.

In addition to this simple atrophy of the bone there is described an ainhum-like process which leads to the loss of a toe but which cannot

7. Scheube: Diseases of Warm Countries, 1904, Edition 2, p. 255.
8. Manson: Tropical Diseases, 1909, Edition 4, p. 546.

be distinguished from true ainhum except that other manifestations of leprosy are present.

The relative frequency of these two processes in the causation of mutilation is stated differently by writers. Harbitz says that "many, perhaps the majority, are dependent on ulcerative necrosis and chronic suppurative inflammation." Van Bergman and Guill say that "the

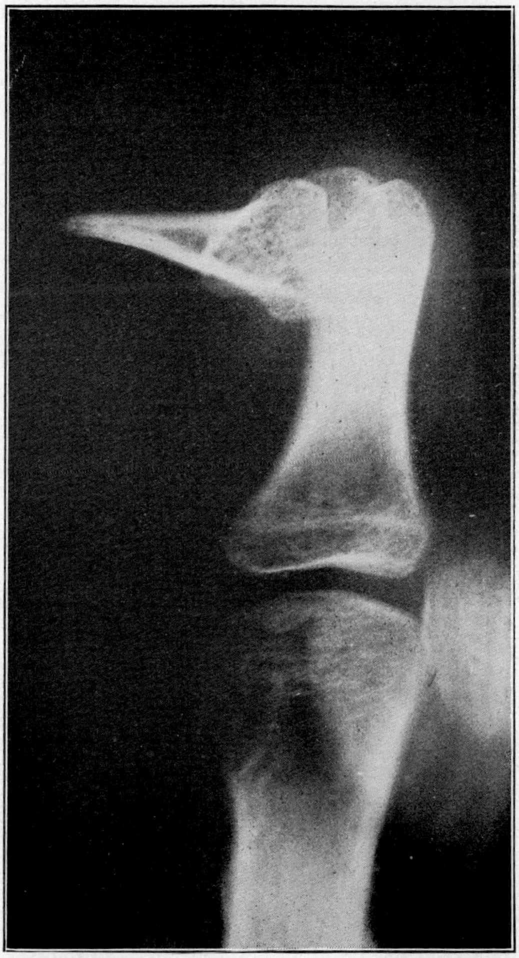

Fig. 9.—E. L., leprosy suspect. Typical concentric atrophy of distal phalanx of right thumb.

phalanges become necrotic and are cast off through suppuration. This is the case as a rule." Balz describes simple absorption of the tissue as the usual cause of the mutilation. From a study of the cases accessible here, I believe that mutilations arise in almost equal numbers by the two methods, but that if we could examine the case before the secondary infective processes took place, we would find that the great majority of these would show trophic changes in the bone. Most of the mutilating processes, at present in the course of development in the cases here, are taking place by the trophic method. In the course of years a certain number of these will undoubtedly fall into the other class, secondary infections arising in them from trauma or other causes. This is shown in the case of a boy at Palo Seco who has lost all the fingers and thumbs of both hands. Of

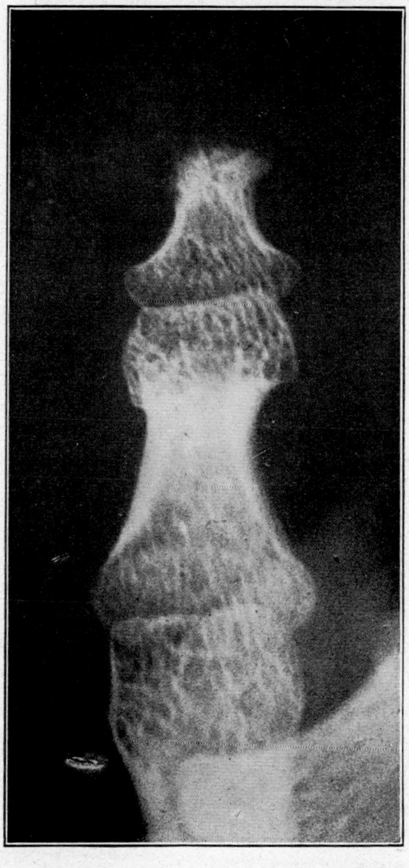

Fig. 10.—E. L., leprosy suspect. Typical distal atrophy of distal phalanx of index-finger of right hand.

the ten digits lost, four were removed on account of suppurative processes, and in the other six there was simply a gradual atrophy and shrinking of the fingers.

The pure trophic type presents bone lesions which are characteristic of the disease. This has been shown by Harbitz in his work on pathological specimens showing characteristic trophic changes late in the disease. These trophic changes in many cases begin early and present definite pictures which give important additional aid in the diagnosis. This trophic disturbance usually begins in the tip of the distal phalanx and may involve one or more fingers. As the process advances in the distal phalanx, changes are found in the middle and later in the proximal phalanx, and may even extend to the metacarpal or metatarsal bones. This same trophic change extends to other bones, but we are interested only in the earliest changes when the diagnosis of the case might be doubtful. These early changes are easily observed by means of the $x$-ray.

During the past two years we have been giving special attention to the bone changes in the cases of leprosy which have been brought before the medical examining board of this hospital. The study of the $x$-ray plates taken in these cases and also in several others from Palo Seco has revealed bone changes varying greatly in degree. These changes we have arranged according to the character and extent of the bone involvement so as to illustrate the development and progress of the trophic bone lesions of this disease. In order to understand these, especially the earlier lesions, the appearance of the distal phalanx with its cellular bulbous tip must be recalled (Fig. 1).

The earliest change noticed is in the bulbous tip of the terminal phalanx. This becomes smaller and shrinks, generally with some associated narrowing of the shaft (Fig. 2), or the process may affect the bulbous tip mainly, in which case there appears to be a definite absorption starting at the most distal point, and progressing almost transversely toward the base (Fig. 3). As this process progresses, the tip disappears and then the shaft becomes gradually absorbed, and a stage is reached in which only the base of the distal phalanx remains (Fig. 4). So far the process shows a distal type of atrophy in which the absorption is mainly in the distal extremity of the bone. In the true concentric type, when the process becomes more advanced, the distal phalanx shows marked shrinking and shortening in both the shaft and the distal extremity, and there is also a shrinking in the shaft of the middle phalanx as is shown by the increase of the concave outline of its borders (Fig. 5). In this form the process involves the shaft more than the distal extremity. In a later stage the terminal phalanx almost entirely disappears, being represented by a very slight shadow on the $x$-ray plate. The middle phalanx becomes greatly shrunken and smaller, and the proximal phalanx shows the incipient changes in the narrowing and shrinking of the shaft (Fig. 6). The interphalangeal joint spaces disappear, the joints becoming partially or totally ankylosed. In a more advanced stage the distal and middle phalanges are reduced to very small fragments, and the proximal phalanx shows a very marked concentric atrophy, almost obliterating the shaft of the bone, with marked absorption of the distal extremity (Figs. 7 and 8).

The same changes may progress farther and involve the metatarsal and metacarpal bones, but by this time the disease is usually so far advanced that the diagnosis is comparatively easy from the gross signs. These later changes are well shown in the pathological specimens radiographed by Harbitz, and also in some of the cases reported by Deycke.

The successive changes shown in these enlargements have been taken from positive leprosy cases and represent the gradually increasing lesions in the progress of the disease. The earliest changes occur in the distal extremity of the terminal phalanx and on account of its small size in the ordinary *x*-ray plate, it is readily overlooked. Also radiographs from suspected cases usually reveal only one or two of these lesions at the most.

In the usual case of anesthetic leprosy, the simple trophic lesion alone is not always found, for frequently secondary inflammatory changes have taken place, as would be expected when we consider that a perforating ulcer is one of the earliest and most common signs of this form of the disease. Accordingly in many cases there occurs a combination of the concentric bone atrophy with ulcerative bone necrosis. This combination occurs in the majority of the cases of anesthetic leprosy, but even with this additional bone necrosis, the true trophic lesion can be readily made out.

These trophic bone changes may appear early and are of great aid in the diagnosis of the disease, as they furnish an additional sign and one quite characteristic. This is shown in the case of a recent leprosy suspect under examination here. The case was that of a little Jamaican girl, 18 years old, presenting an anesthetic type of the disease. She has marked analgesia of both hands and feet. The hands show the beginning contractures of the claw-hand. In the left hand there is beginning ankylosis of the joints of the little and ring fingers with simple atrophy of the tip of the index-finger. The right hand shows a later stage of the claw-hand involving all four fingers. There is marked atrophy of the tip of the thumb and partial atrophy of the tip of the index-finger. In both feet the second toe is swollen and discolored and presents an ulcer at the tip. There is a neuritis of both peroneal nerves, the child walking with a partial foot-drop.

Examinations of the mucous membrane of the nose and of all lesions were negative for the bacillus of Hansen four months ago, and remain negative at this time.

Radiographs of the hands show typical concentric atrophy of the distal phalanx of the right thumb and of the distal and middle phalanges of the left little finger. They also show typical distal atrophy of the terminal phalanges of the index-fingers; slight distal atrophy of the end phalanx of the left middle finger; and very marked in the right middle finger, the entire distal phalanx having been absorbed. The last represents the most advanced lesion of distal atrophy we have found in the cases here (Figs. 9 and 10).

In any consideration of the value of these trophic changes it is necessary to determine under what conditions more or less similar bone changes might occur. There are some conditions which produce bone lesions somewhat resembling these, but as a rule they can be readily differentiated by a proper history and examination of the case. Similar changes could arise as a result of previous injuries; in the atrophy of disuse as might occur in paralysis or in nerve lesions; in Morvan's disease, and in ainhum. Also the race and occupation of the individual must be taken into consideration in the interpretation of the radiograph.

In a study of the early lesions occurring in the feet, a knowledge of the race and occupation of the individual becomes necessary, for in the barefoot native the phalanges of the toes are broader, larger, and far better developed than in the members of the races wearing shoes. This is well shown in the radiographs of the feet of Americans when compared with those of the islanders or natives.

In the case of injuries involving the bones of the phalanges changes more or less similar to progressing distal atrophy may occur, but the history of the case would serve to differentiate this condition.

Similar lesions might occur following injuries to nerves or in the atrophy of disuse, but in these cases the lesions would be limited to a certain definite area and all the bones in this area would be similarly involved. Also an extra point of differentiation could be obtained from the history of the case.

In syringomyelia, more especially that variety known as Morvan's disease, a mutilating process takes place which in great part resembles the same process in anesthetic leprosy. The description of this process as detailed in the literature would point to its occurrence by means of an ulcerative-necrotic method rather than by true concentric atrophy, as the descriptions of Morvan's disease speak of this mutilation as occurring through an inflammatory process.

In ainhum there is a peculiar trophic disturbance which shows bone changes very similar to those occurring in leprosy. The process involves the proximal phalanx primarily and there is a lengthening with narrowing and absorption of the shaft rather than a shortening and absorption as occurs in the concentric atrophy of leprosy. But what the bone change would be in a case of leprosy in which the loss of the toe was taking place by an ainhum-like process we are unable to say, as we have seen no such case.

In a study of the radiographs taken from the various cases of leprosy accessible here, there are two main methods by which the atrophy of the bone takes place. The one could be called progressive distal atrophy. It starts at the distal extremity of the terminal phalanx and progresses almost transversely toward the base. We have not been able to follow this process beyond the distal phalanx. It appears to be the more rapid method of mutilation and occurs more often in cases of a mixed type of the disease. It also bears a close resemblance to the bone changes following injuries, or to amputation stumps. The other method presents the true concentric atrophy well described by Harbitz. In this there is a general shrinking and absorption of the distal portion and shaft of a phalanx simultaneously. This process is very characteristic of the disease, but a similar process might occur in the atrophy of disuse or in a severe injury or lesion of the innervating nerve.

These trophic bone lesions, while not absolutely pathognomonic of the disease, are very characteristic of it. Any condition which might present a similar bone lesion could be readily differentiated by the previous history of injury or disease taken in connection with the examination of the case. Of all the trophic lesions of leprosy these are the most characteristic, and while not occurring in all cases they are found in the majority and very often sufficiently early to be of great aid in the diagnosis. It is in the anesthetic form of leprosy especially that these two forms of bone changes—the progressive distal atrophy and the concentric atrophy—furnish an additional diagnostic sign and one very characteristic of the disease.

# AN EXPERIMENTAL STUDY OF THE CAUSES WHICH PRODUCE THE GROWTH OF THE MAMMARY GLAND *

ROBERT T. FRANK, M.D., AND A. UNGER, B.S.
NEW YORK

Hyperplasia of the breasts is regularly noted in pregnancy. This change in the breasts, for a time passively accepted as a fact, has in late years been made the subject of intensive study, which aimed to discover the primary cause of the tissue growth, and to analyze the nature of the stimulus which gave rise to it. The subject is not only of great interest to biologists, but to investigators in all branches of medicine. The sweeping analogies, drawn from some of the theories which have been based on experimental work, are so far-reaching that confirmation is imperatively needed; otherwise there is danger of basing future research, some in allied, others in entirely separate fields, on an insecure or even false foundation.

The breast hyperplasia of pregnancy can best be studied in animals, and as a matter of laboratory convenience, small animals are preferred. Most workers have employed rabbits in their study. To some extent, however, clinical observations made by physicians on the human subject, or by veterinarians on the domestic animals, have been so striking that they have been used to fill gaps in our knowledge, or as confirmation of the results obtained by experiment.

### CLAYPON AND STARLING'S EXPERIMENTS

Although not the first in chronological order, Starling's theory of breast hypertrophy will first be considered, and as our investigation concerns itself chiefly with his work, a somewhat detailed description of his experiments must be given.

In 1906 Claypon and Starling[1] published an article entitled "An Experimental Enquiry Into the Factors Which Determine the Growth and the Activity of the Mammary Gland," in which they asserted that the breast hyperplasia of pregnancy was due to the formation of chemical substances in the embryo. These substances reached the blood-stream of the mother by way of the placenta, and

*From the Department of Pathology, College of Physicians and Surgeons, Columbia University (The George Crocker Special Research Fund). Presented at the meeting of the Alumni Association of the College of Physicians and Surgeons, Jan. 30, 1911. Received for publication Feb. 21, 1911.

1. Lane-Claypon and Starling: Proc. Roy. Soc., 1906, Series B, lxxvii, 520.

activated the growth of the breast. They designated this activator as the breast hormone (from ὁρμάω) and throughout we shall adhere to this term. The methods employed by Claypon and Starling were as follows. They first determined the size and appearance of the breast in young virginal rabbits which had reached adult age. To do this the breasts were exposed by reflecting the skin, and fixed in continuity with the surrounding connective tissue and fat. After fixation the tissues were stained with dilute hematoxylin in bulk, and then partly decolorized with acid alcohol. The ducts with all their ramifications became visible against their less deeply stained surroundings. The tissue was then dehydrated, cleared and permanently mounted in balsam between glass slides. Thus with little trouble clear and permanent records of results are obtained. Similar studies of breasts at various stages of pregnancy were likewise made. Claypon and Starling's illustrations are here reproduced (Figs. 1 to 7). It was found that by the fourth or fifth day after impregnation the breasts had considerably increased in size (Fig. 2) chiefly by the extension and the branching of the ducts. By the ninth day the margin of adjacent breasts were almost contiguous, the ducts longer and more branching, and at the periphery the breast tissue was raised and, in the fresh state, of pinkish color (Fig. 3). Under the microscope the beginning of acini with several layers of epithelium lining their lumen, could be recognized. More advanced stages of pregnancy manifest themselves chiefly by a still greater increase in the number of acini, and by the presence of secretion, at first of colostrum, later of true milk, within the lumina of acini and ducts.

With few exceptions virgin rabbits, born and raised in their laboratory, were employed in the experiments. As at the outset of the experiments it was not known which of the many possible tissues involved, gave rise to the hormone, they were all tried alone or in combination. The following tissues were employed—ovaries, uterine wall or mucous membrane, placenta, placenta and uterus combined, fetus together with placenta and membranes, fetus alone.

Perusal of Table 1 will show that four rabbits were injected with the extract of ovaries, obtained from pregnant rabbits. The longest experiment lasted fifteen days and in it twenty-six ovaries were used. The results were negative.

The mucous membrane of pregnant uteri was injected into two animals, likewise with negative results.

Rabbit's placentas (respectively press juice, boiled and unboiled extract) were injected into three animals without producing breast changes.

Extracts of fetuses were injected into ten rabbits. Press juice, unboiled extract passed through a Berkefeld filter, and boiled extracts were employed. Two animals proved to be multiparous, so that in their cases no definite conclusions could be drawn. Two animals showed no increased growth. The six remaining animals showed a varying degree of hypertrophy of the breasts. The best results were obtained in Experiment 10 (Fig. 4), in which during the course of forty-one days twenty-two injections of the press juice of 154 fetuses, placentas and uterine mucous membrane were given intraperitoneally. The breasts were greatly hypertrophied, almost contiguous and the margins raised and pink, corresponding to the breasts of the ninth or tenth day of pregnancy. On microscopic section marked proliferation of the ducts, with mitoses in their lining epithelium were found. In the thickened borders the formation of alveoli was just commencing. In five other rabbits in whom the injections were given intraperitoneally for lesser periods of time, similar but not as marked proliferation was noted.

A control experiment, in which normal rabbit's serum from non-pregnant animals was injected subcutaneously during three weeks showed little or no enlargement of the breasts. The ducts, however, showed a certain amount of proliferation with some mitoses in their epithelium.

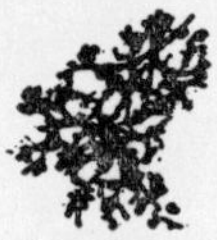

FIG. 1.

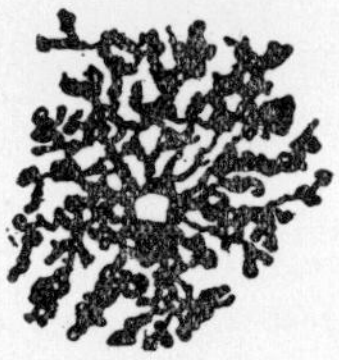

FIG 2.

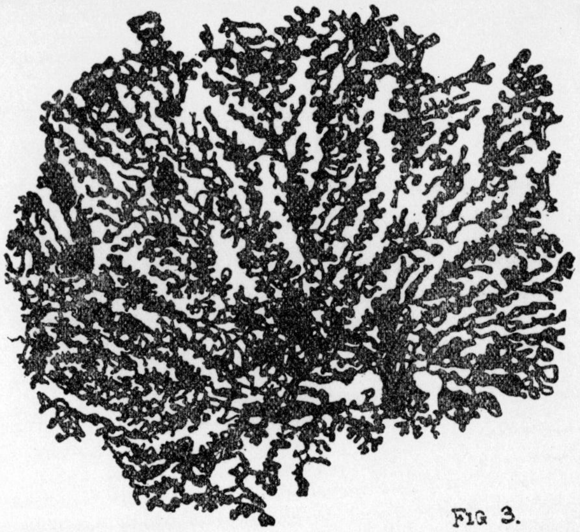

FIG 3.

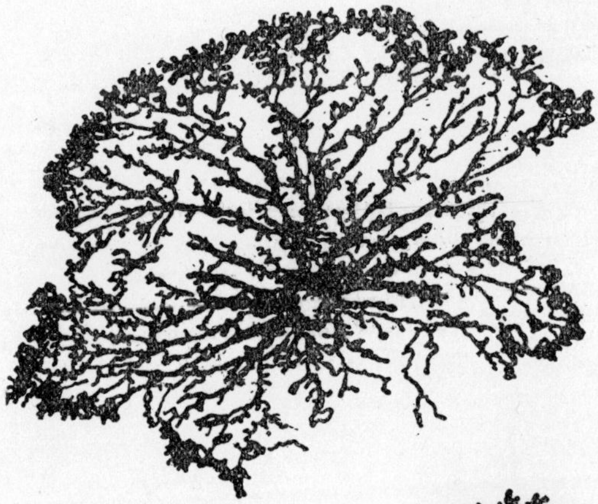

FIG. 4.

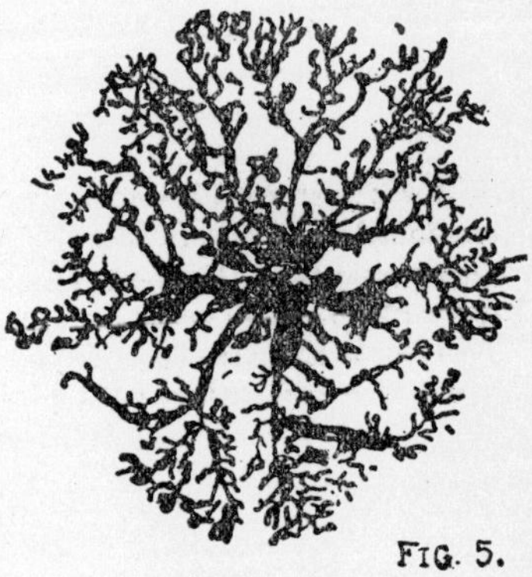

FIG. 5.

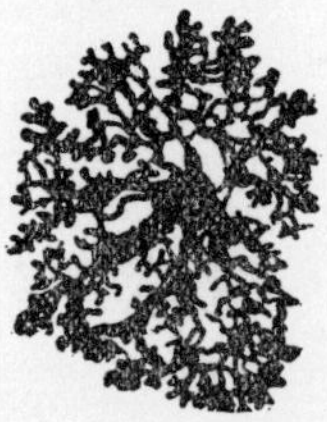

FIG. 6.

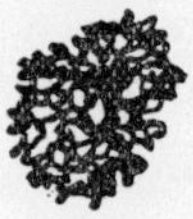

FIG. 7.

Figures 1 to 7 inclusive are natural size.

Figures 1-7 inclusive are reproduced from Starling's plates. As will readily be noticed by comparing Figures 1 and 22 (both figures of the virgin rabbits' breast) *our illustrations* (Figures 8-27) *are drawn somewhat more lightly and are reduced slightly below the natural size* (4/5 of normal size).

Fig. 1.—Gland from virgin rabbit.

Fig. 2.—Mammary gland from primiparous rabbit, five days after impregnation.

Fig. 3.—Mammary gland from primiparous rabbit, nine days after impregnation.

Fig. 4.—Mammary gland from virgin rabbit which had received injections of extracts of fetuses, uterus, and placentas during five weeks (Exp. 10).

Fig. 5.—Mammary gland of virgin rabbit, showing growth produced by injection of extracts of fetal viscera during a period of seventeen days.

Fig. 6.—Mammary gland of virgin rabbit, showing growth produced by injection of extracts of fetal bodies and placentas over seventeen days.

Fig. 7.—Mammary gland of virgin rabbit, showing slight growth induced by daily subcutaneous injection of rabbit's serum (from non-pregnant rabbits) during a period of three weeks.

CONCLUSIONS OF CLAYPON AND STARLING

From these experiments Claypon and Starling conclude[2] that the hormone is produced in the growing embryo, but not stored there to any large amount. Consequently injections will introduce only small quantities of the hormone into the experimental animal. The exact site of production of the hormone within the fetus was not determined. The wide-spread distribution within the fetal body points to a highly diffusible substance, which from the fact that it probably withstands boiling, and passes through a Berkefeld filter is of non-proteid nature. For the same reasons it is diffusible, not of large molecular structure and not a colloid. The fetus is probably not the only source of the hormone; at puberty the ovaries exert their influence. Possibly at an early stage of pregnancy the chorionic villi elaborate the hormone, a function later taken up by the fetus.

In multiparous rabbits milk is secreted during the course of the injections, probably because the hormone is exhausted after a few hours, with the result that the already present glands (acini) are first inhibited (by the presence) and then stimulated (by the absence) of the hormone—alternatingly an inhibitory and assimilative impulse.

Claypon and Starling also fed a kitten with rabbit's embryos for three weeks, with no increase in the mammary glands. In conclusion they propounded two questions, the first of which they had not determined to their complete satisfaction, the second of which they had not really attempted to prove. Does boiling not destroy the hormone? Is the active substance specific to animals of a given species?

Starling's results appeared to offer a definite solution of the mechanism of the breast hyperplasia of pregnancy. The result assuredly invited corroboration and extension of the researches along the lines indicated by himself. For several years, however, his conclusions, which seem to have been accepted, with more or less reserve, have been widely quoted in many different connections, but have given rise rather to speculation than to further continuance of experimental work.

Since we undertook the research which we shall now report, several recent publications dealing with the same subject have come to our attention, though unknown to us at the time we began our experiments. From what is to follow, however, it will be seen that the question of priority does not arise. Two of the articles dealing with the pregnancy hyperplasia confirm Starling's findings and represent continuations of his work. The others deal with different theories, and will therefore be discussed further on.

---

2. See also Starling, E. H.: Chemical Correlations of the Functions of the Body, Croonian Lectures. Lecture IV, Lancet, 1905, ii, 579.

Table 1.—Summary of Claypon and Starling's Experiments*

| Tissue Extract | Animal | No. of Inj. and Method of Preparation | Site of Injection | Duration of Experiment, days | Result |
|---|---|---|---|---|---|
| 1. 2 Ov. preg. rab. 15 d. | Rab. Non-Preg. | 1 implantation | Implanted intra-perit. | 11 | Breasts neg.; graft vascularized. In heat. |
| 2. Ov. preg. rab. 15 d. | Rabbit | 3 inj. chloroform water extr. 6 ov. | Injection site ? | 17 | Breasts and ut. neg. |
| 3. Ov. preg. rab. 11-14 d. | Virgin Rabbit | 6 inj. emulsion 10 ovaries | Injection site ? | 19 | Breasts invisible; ut. enlarged, congested; mucosa proliferating. |
| 4. Ov. preg. rabbits | Virgin Rabbit | 13 inj. saline extract of 26 ovaries | Injection site ? | 15 | Breasts unaffected; ut. congested. |
| 5. Muc. membrane 4 preg. ut. | Virgin Rabbit | 4 inj. chloroform water extract | Injection site ? | 20 | Breasts unaffected; ut. unaffected. |
| 6. Muc. membrane 7 preg. ut. | 2 Virgin Rabbits | (A) Boiled saline extr.; (B) Unboiled | Injection site ? | 19 | (A) Breasts unaffected (in heat); (B) ditto; ut. congested. |
| Two other experiments. | No details | | | | Results Negative. |
| 7. Press juice, mucous membr. 14 ut. 123 placenta | Virgin Rabbit | 14 inj., press juice | Injection site ? | 17 | Breast unaltered; uterus congested |
| 8. Boiled ext. of 55 plac. | Virgin Rabbit | 8 inj., boiled extract | Injection site ? | 19 | Breast unaltered; uterus neg. |
| Unboiled ext. of 55 placenta | Virgin Rabbit | 8 inj. unboiled extract | Injection site ? | 21 | Breast unaltered; uterus sl. congested. |

| Extracts of Fetuses | | 5-7 injections | No details | | Results Negative |
|---|---|---|---|---|---|
| 9. Saline ext. 57 fetuses and placentæ | Virgin Rabbit | 15 inj. saline extr. Berkefeld | Subcutaneous | 17 | Marked hypertrophy of breasts; ovaries large; ut. congested, vulva showed signs of heat. |
| 10. Press juice of 154 fetuses, plac. and uterine mucosa | Virgin Rabbit | 22 inj., press juice | Intraperitoneal | 41 | Breasts nearly contiguous, raised pinkish margin; beginning of alveoli; ov. not mentioned. |
| 11. I Part of 182 fetuses | Not virgin | ? Press juice viscera | Intraperitoneal | 29 | Milky fluid after 17 inj. Multipara, many alveoli; ducts with milk, only one layer epith. |
| II Pt. of 182 fetuses | Virgin | ? Filtered boiled extract viscera | Intraperitoneal | 29 | Water, fluid after 17 inj., Macroscopic not much enlarged. Microscopic branching ducts with two layer of cells. |
| III Pt. of 182 fetuses | Virgin | ? Unboiled press juice of bodies | Intraperitoneal | 29 | Watery fluid (trace) after 12 inj., glands large, hypertrophied, watery fluid. Alveoli present; ducts proliferating. |
| IV Pt. of 182 fetuses | Multiparous | ? Boiled extr. of bodies | Intraperitoneal | 29 | Milky fluid after 17 inj. Glands fully marked, distended with milky fluid. Hypertrophy (?) |
| Viscera of fetuses 138 | Virgin (?) Immature | 16 inj. Press juice (Kieselguhr) | Intraperitoneal (?) | ? | Breasts negative. |
| 12. Saline extr. viscera fetuses | Virgin | 15 inj. | Intraperitoneal | 17 | Distinct growth of mammary glands with duct proliferation (Fig. 5). |
| 13. Saline extr. bodies & placentæ | Virgin | 15 inj. | Intraperitoneal | 17 | Marked growth of mammary glands with plentiful mitotic figures (Fig. 6). |
| Normal rabbit's serum | Virgin | ? | Subcutaneous | 21 | Glands little if any enlarged. Microscopic mitoses in epithelium of ducts & certain amt. of proliferation of ducts. |

*Abbreviations: epith.=epithelium; inj.=injection; preg.=pregnant; ov.=ovaries; extr.=extract; muc. membrane=mucous membrane; ut.=uterus.

Foa[3] reported in 1908 that he had been able to obtain proliferation of the breasts in rabbits by injecting extracts, prepared from cows' fetuses with unboiled extracts only. He therefore concluded that he had proved that heterologous extracts were able to produce hyperplasia.

Quite recently Biedl and Königstein[4] have repeated, extended and varied Starling's experiments, *also using rabbits,* arriving at the same conclusions. In a small number of their experiments, they excised portions of breasts before and after they had performed the injections, but apparently examined these specimens only microscopically. In order to accentuate the effect of the injections, in a few animals, they first seared the surface of the ovaries, as they believe that ovarian activity has an inhibiting action on breast hyperplasia (on milk secretion ?). In two instances animals castrated three weeks previously were used. In almost all of the fetus injections they report breast hyperplasia, including castrated animals; while placental injections produced no result. The amount of hyperplasia, according to Biedl and Koenigstein, depends not on the duration of the injections but on the amount of fetal tissue injected.

## AIMS OF OUR RESEARCH

Starling had asked whether or not the breast hormone is specific to the animal of a given species.[5] This question is interesting and important from a twofold point of view: first, from a strictly biological standpoint; second, if fetus extracts of cows, sheep or swine could be made to produce hyperplasia in the breasts of small laboratory animals a method would be at our disposal to use enormous quantities of extracts, in order to determine what effect exaggerated doses of the hormone exert. By summation of stimuli it might prove possible to transform physiological into pathological effects!

As hypertrophy of the breasts occurs in all mammals, we felt at liberty to choose almost any species. Partly for the sake of employing a small inexpensive animal, partly because we hoped to extend our work into the effect of local hyperplasia on growing tumors, we chose white rats, which are extensively employed in tumor research.

## WHITE RATS INJECTED WITH SOWS' FETUSES

*Technic and Experiments.*—Fresh sows' fetuses were obtained daily at a slaughter house. Fetuses not larger than 3 or 6 inches in length were used. They were passed through a meat machine, thoroughly ground up with sand, and, after adding normal salt solution, were kept for two hours at 0 C. The thick extract was squeezed through thin toweling by means of a meat press, and then centrifuged. Part was passed through a Berkefeld filter, part slightly acidified with acetic acid, boiled for three minutes, and filtered through a sterile paper filter. Eight female white rats raised to maturity in the laboratory were used in the series.

---

3. Foa, C.: Arch. di fisiol., 1908, v, 520.

4. Biedl and Koenigstein: Ztschr. f. exper. Pathol. u. Therap., 1910, vii, 358.

5. As previously stated, Foa's paper was not known to us when we began our work. Biedl and Königstein's article appeared after completion of our experiments.

TABLE 2.—WHITE RATS INJECTED INTRAPERITONEALLY WITH FETUSES OF SOWS

| Extract | Daily Amount c.c. | No. of Inject. | Duration of Exper. Days | Result |
|---|---|---|---|---|
| 1. Berkefeld | 1.5 | 29 | 33 | Negative |
| 2. Berkefeld | 1.0 | 23 | 26 | Negative |
| 3. Berkefeld | 0.5 | 29 | 33 | Negative |
| 4. Boiled | 1.5 | 30 | 33 | Negative |
| 5. Boiled | 1.0 | 27 | 31 | Negative |
| 6. Boiled | 0.5 | 30 | 34 | Negative |
| 7. Berkefeld, 1 week old | 1.0 | 22 | 25 | Negative |
| 8. Boiled, 1 week old | 1.0 | 22 | 25 | Negative |

In rats 7 and 8 one cubic centimeter of Berkefeld and of boiled extract was each day put aside and kept for one week at 0 C., and then daily injected, in order to test with the same material whether the hormone lost its activity on standing.

*Results.*—After killing the animal, its hair was removed with sodium sulphid. Two strips, which consisted of the entire abdominal wall, including the peritoneum, were then removed at an ample distance from the nipples. Similar strips were taken from the thorax, in order to preserve all of the ten to fourteen breasts (in liquor formaldehydi). Three to five breast areas from each animal were then studied in serial section (paraffin, hematoxylin-eosin). Starling's technic of staining and clearing the breasts, as in the rabbit, could not be employed in the rats. Numerous normal animals had been previously prepared and studied as controls.

In all the eight injected rats no breast hyperplasia was noted. It therefore seemed justified to conclude that heterologous hormones did not produce breast hyperplasia, unless Starling's theory did not have a general applicability; or that, as might happen with a certain species, the white rat was refractory.

## WHITE RATS INJECTED WITH FETUSES OF WHITE RATS

In order to determine these two points, we injected white rats with fetuses of white rats.

As a matter of interest we extended these experiments to include also placenta and serum of pregnant rats, in addition to the fetus extracts. Pregnant rats were obtained from a breeder. The exact ages of the fetuses were not known, but the number and combined weight of the fetuses are recorded in the protocols. As a matter of convenience passage of the unboiled extract through a Berkefeld filter was omitted. To avoid the possibility of infection the entire process of obtaining and preparing the extracts were performed with all aseptic precautions. The extract called by us "centrifuge extract" could contain quantitatively only more, certainly not less of the active substance than Starling's "Berkefeld extract." Injection of these extracts was well borne. The boiled extracts were not well tolerated by the rats. We finally gained the impression that the amount of acetic acid used to precipitate the proteid during the boiling, might be at fault.

With the exception of the centrifuge extract just referred to, the material was prepared as in the preceding series, divided into approximately equal parts, of which one was used as centrifuged, the other as boiled extract. Each animal therefore, received about one-quarter to one-third of the entire extract obtained each day, depending on how many animals were being injected on a given day (see protocols).

TABLE 3.—WHITE RATS INJECTED INTRAPERITONEALLY WITH EXTRACTS OF FETUSES, ETC., OF RATS*

| Extract | Daily Amount c.c. | No. of Inject. | Duration of Exp. Days | Result |
|---|---|---|---|---|
| 1. Centrifuged Fetuses, 130 used | 2.0 | 19 | 19 | Negative |
| 2. Centrifuged Fetuses, 65 used | 2.0 | 9 | 9 | Negative (died) |
| 3. Centrifuged Fetuses, 165 used | 2.0 | 23 | 28 | Negative |
| 4. Boiled Fetuses, 89 used | 0.5-3.0 | 11 | 17 | Negative (died) |
| 5. Placental extr.; placentæ, 177 used. | 2.0 | 25 | 27 | Negative |
| 6. Placental extr.; placentæ, 105 used. | 1.5-2.0 | 16 | 24 | Negative |
| 7. Blood serum preg. rats | 0.5-3.0 | 24 | 31 | Negative |

*Rats 3 and 6 were castrated twenty-six and twenty-one days before injections were begun. The "centrifuged" fetal extract corresponded to Starling's "Berkefeld extract." The placental extract was prepared in a manner similar to the centrifuged extract.

In none of the injected animals was any increase in size of the breasts noted. Therefore our negative results with heterologous extract were of no significance, as apparently white rats were refractory to fetal extracts of both homologous and heterologous origin. Some further experiments on white rats made at this time will be referred to later.

### RABBITS INJECTED WITH RABBITS' FETUSES

Before attempting to use heterologous extracts in rabbits, we determined to repeat Starling's experiments of injecting rabbits with rabbits' fetuses. The technic employed was that of Starling, except that we did not pass the unboiled extract through a Berkefeld filter. Instead, we used aseptic precautions in the preparation as in the preceding series.

In addition to the boiled and unboiled fetal extract, we prepared and injected intraperitoneally also the extract of placentæ, the extract of ovaries of pregnant rabbits and the extract obtained from the hypophysis. Hypophyseal extract was used because this gland undergoes marked changes during pregnancy, and because considerable evidence obtains that it has important relations to the genital organs.[6] The rabbits used for the injections had been obtained young and kept segregated for two months. They were approximately seven or eight months old.

---

6. The literature will be found in Frank, R. T.: Has Ovotherapy, as Now Practiced, an Experimental Basis, THE ARCHIVES INT. MED., 1910, vi, 314.

TABLE 4.—RABBITS (SERIES 1) INJECTED WITH RABBITS' FETUSES

| Rabbit | Source of Extract | No. of Inj. | Days | Result. |
|---|---|---|---|---|
| 1. Virgin | Unboiled extr. of fetuses (111 used) | 21 | 28 | Little hypertrophy (Fig. 8) |
| 2. Virgin (?) | Boiled extr. of fetuses (88 used) | 15 | 36 | Much enlarged breasts—multipara (?) |
| 3. Virgin | Unboiled extr. of ovaries (49 used) | 22 | 30 | Breasts considerably enlarged, ducts fine, margin raised, epithelium proliferating (Fig. 9) |
| 4. Virgin | Unboiled placental extr. (120 used) | 22 | 30 | No hypertrophy |
| 5. Virgin | Unboiled hypophyseal extr. (11 used) | 11 | 15 | Increase in size; marks of activity even greater than in No. 3 (Fig. 10) |

TABLE 5.—RABBITS (SERIES 2) INJECTED WITH RABBITS' FETUSES

| Rabbit | Source of Extract | No. of Inj. | Days | Result |
|---|---|---|---|---|
| 1. Virgin | Unboiled fetus extr. (76 used) | 11 | 11 | Slight increase (Fig. 11) ducts narrow with many fine branches |
| 2. Virgin | Boiled fetus extr. (59 used) | 8 | 10 | Breasts slightly larger than No. 1. Many branches, no terminal buds (Fig. 12) |
| 3. Virgin | Unboiled ovarian and (22) hypophysis extr. (11 used) | 11 | 11 | Ducts narrow, few branches. A breast was removed before beginning the exp. (Fig. 13). The corresponding breast after was larger (Fig. 14) |
| 4. Virgin | Unboiled placental extr. (76 used) | 11 | 11 | Breast not much enlarged, but many terminal buds, broad and active-looking ducts (Fig. 15) |

TABLE 6.—RABBITS (SERIES 3, CASTRATES) INJECTED WITH RABBITS' FETUSES*

| Rabbit | Control of Breast Removed | Source of Extract | No. of Inject. | Days | Result |
|---|---|---|---|---|---|
| 1. Virgin | 24 days before castration | Rabbits' fetuses, 101 used | 17 | 17 | Slight increase (Figs. 16 and 17) |
| 2. Virgin | 20 days before castration | Preg. rabbits' ov., 34 used | 17 | 17 | Size of breast enormously increased; ducts thin; no acini (Figs. 18 and 19) |
| 3. Virgin | 18 days before castration | Preg. rabbits' hypophyses 17 used. | 17 | 17 | Size of breast double that of control, not as large as No. 2, but of same type (Figs. 20 and 21). |

*Rabbit 1 was castrated eleven days, the other two ten days before beginning the injections. The fact that eighteen or twenty-four days intervened between the time of removing the control breast and castration, in the light of our subsequent results, deprives the injection effects of their significance.

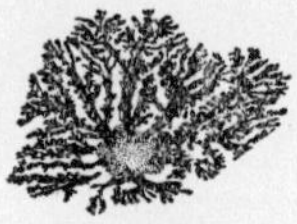
Fig. 8

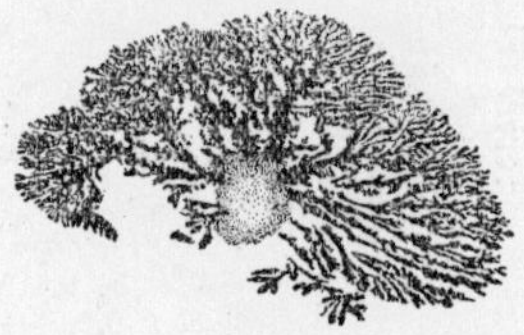
Fig. 9

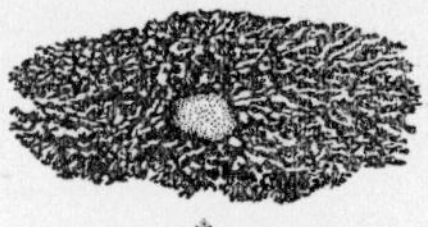
Fig. 10

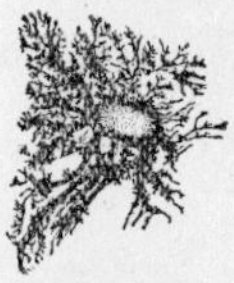
Fig. 11

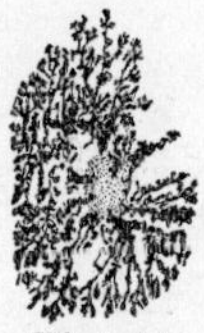
Fig. 12

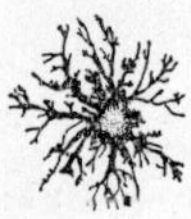
Fig. 13

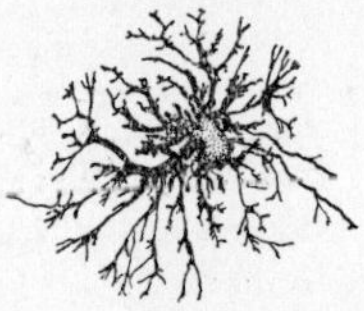
Fig. 14

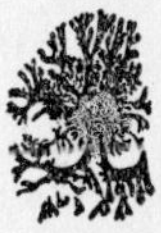
Fig. 15

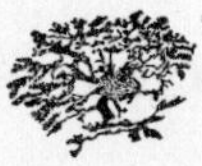
Fig. 16

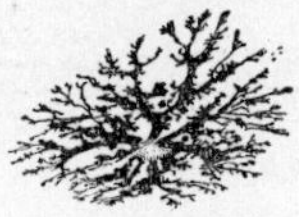
Fig. 17

Figures 8 to 27, inclusive, are four-fifths natural size.

Fig. 8.—Breast of rabbit 1, series 1, which was injected with unboiled extract of rabbit fetuses. In this and the following illustrations, the breasts, stained, cleared and mounted exactly as Starling has directed, have been projected by means of an Edinger projection apparatus directly on the paper. In order to facilitate the drawing of details a magnification of three diameters was employed. The reproductions are reduced slightly below natural size. A careful outline of each breast was drawn, the ducts, though sometimes, when of large caliber, apparently hollow, are shown as solid cords.

Fig. 9.—Breast of rabbit 3, series 1, which was injected with unboiled extract of rabbit ovaries.

Fig. 10.—Breast of rabbit 5, series 1, which was injected with unboiled extract of rabbit hypophyses.

Fig. 11.—Breast of rabbit 1, series 2, which was injected with unboiled extract of rabbit fetuses.

Fig. 12.—Breast of rabbit 2, series 2, which was injected with boiled extract of rabbit fetuses.

Fig. 13.—Rabbit 3, series 2; breast removed before starting experiment.

Fig. 14.—Rabbit 3, series 2; breast removed after injection of rabbits' hypophyses and ovaries.

Fig. 15.—Rabbit 4, series 2; breast removed after injection of rabbits' placentæ.

Fig. 16.—Rabbit 1, series 3; breast removed before castration and injection.

Fig. 17.—Rabbit 1, series 3; breast removed after injection of rabbits' fetuses.

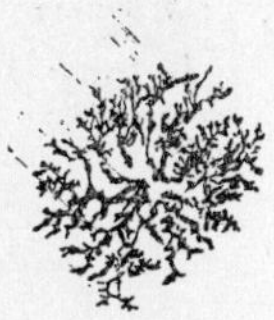

Fig. 18

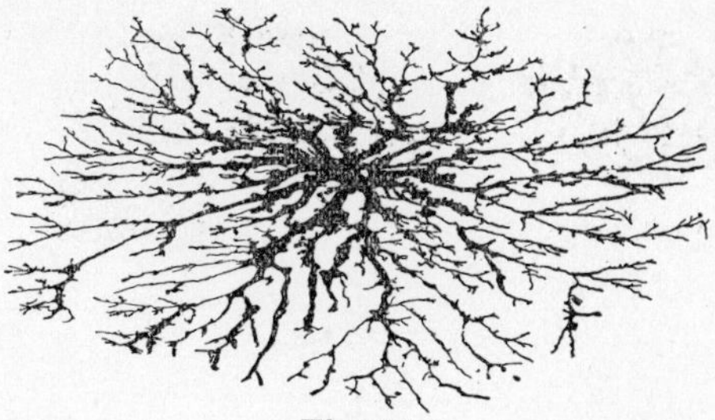

Fig. 19

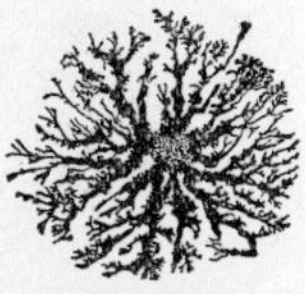

Fig. 20

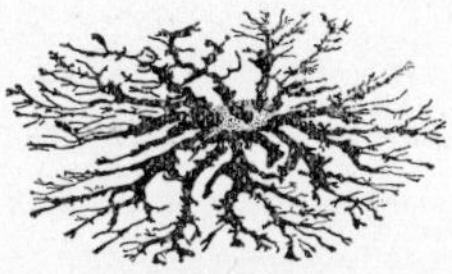

Fig. 21

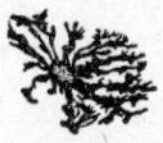

Fig. 22

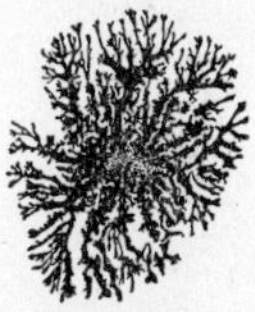

Fig. 23

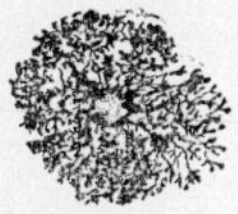

Fig. 24

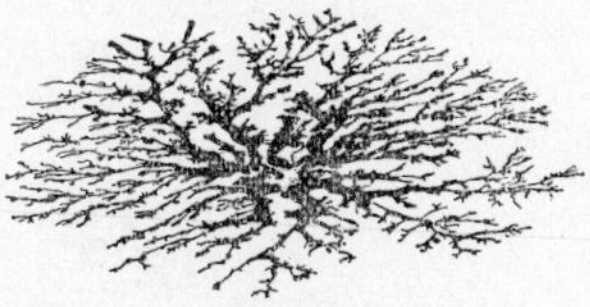

Fig. 25

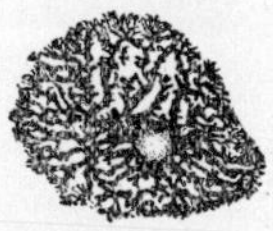

Fig. 26

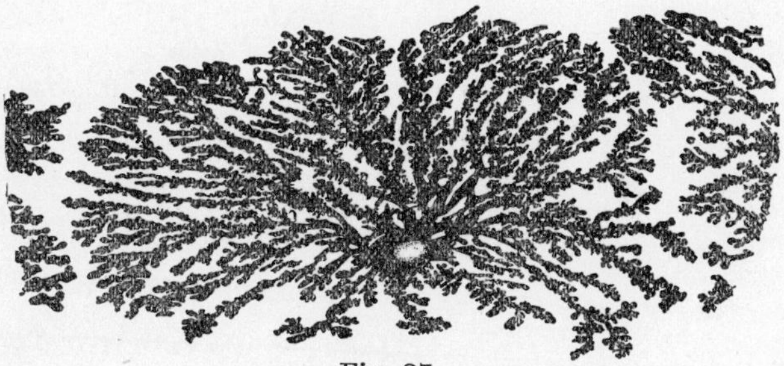

Fig. 27

Fig. 18.—Rabbit 2, series 3; breast removed before castration and injection.

Fig. 19.—Rabbit 2, series 3; breast removed after injection of rabbits' ovaries.

Fig. 20.—Rabbit 3, series 3; breast removed before castration and injection.

Fig. 21.—Rabbit 3, series 3: breast removed after injection with rabbits' hypophyses.

Fig. 22.—Normal virgin rabbit's breast before first estrum (Rabbit 24).

Fig. 23.—Corresponding breast removed nine days later (Rabbit 24).

Fig. 24.—Normal virgin rabbit's breast, already showing slight growth (Rabbit 15).

Fig. 25.—Corresponding breast removed twenty-six days later (Rabbit 15).

Fig. 26.—Normal virgin rabbit's breast, showing slight growth (Rabbit 14).

Fig. 27.—Corresponding breast removed twenty-four days later (Rabbit 14).

This series showed startling results. The unboiled fetal extract had produced only slight hyperplasia. In the boiled, no definite conclusion as to increase could be determined, as the breasts appeared to belong to a multiparous animal. The placental animal showed negative results. The ovarian and hypophysial injections apparently produced very active hyperplasia.

In view of these differences we determined to repeat the experiments, using the same technic, except that we injected both ovarian and hypophysis extract into the same animal with the hope of thus still further increasing the degree of hyperplasia.

In the second series the animals treated with extract of fetuses again showed the least proliferation. Rabbit 3, which received combined ovarian and hypophysis extract, had a breast removed nine days before the injections were begun. On completion of the experiment the corresponding breast of the other side was found nearly double in size but no subdivision of ducts had occurred. The placental animal, however, showed a breast nearly as large and with more active proliferation.

We determined to obtain another series, using castrated rabbits, in order to exclude any direct effect of the extracts on the ovaries, or any indirect action independently exerted by these glands.

A number of nulliparous rabbits were castrated through lumbar incisions and of these we selected three of about equal age for the injections. We had previously removed from each a single breast, partly for control and partly to assure ourselves that the glands were virgin in type.

Of the three castrated rabbits, that injected with fetal extract again showed the least growth of the breast. The ovarian experiment was followed (?) by an enormous hyperplasia; the hypophysis injections were intermediate.

*Summary of Rabbit Experiments.*—Three rabbits had been injected with unboiled extract with but little result. Of two injected with boiled fetal extract one had large breasts, possibly multiparous, though the nipples were minute; the other showed hardly any change. Two injected with ovarian extract showed much hyperplasia; one with combined ovarian and hypophysis extract very slight increase. Of the two placental rabbits one showed some breast activity, the other none. The two animals which received the hypophysis injections both showed considerable increase.

It seemed advisable to study the anatomy and the physiology of the rabbits' breast more closely because our results not only differed from those of Starling, but also because our series did not correspond sufficiently. Some disturbing factor remained to be accounted for.

## FURTHER STUDY OF THE RABBIT'S BREASTS

We selected a number of apparently virgin adult female rabbits, which had been segregated for a month or more, and under anesthesia and aseptic precautions removed a breast. The operation is simple and primary union is usually obtained. The loose subcutaneous layer down to the external oblique fascia is removed in one sheet, stretched on cork, and prepared as described by Starling. Whenever we obtained breasts which corresponded to Starling's description of the virginal type, the animal was used for further study. At various intervals of time other breasts from the same animal were removed.

Using this method we then noted that in some animals, sometimes within a period of three to five days, a marked increase in size of the breast, accompanied by a striking change in the width of the ducts, number of side branches and terminal buds, occurred. Further study convinced us that at a given period of time all the breasts of any one animal were the same in size and in general structure, although corresponding breasts (as for instance the third right and left) removed at different periods, differed greatly in size. At first we used only animals in which the first breast removed corresponded in size to the virginal type described by Starling (Fig. 22), but it soon became apparent that this distinction does not apply, as a comparison of Figures 22 and 23 will show. These two figures illustrate breasts removed from a rabbit which had been previously isolated for several months, only nine days intervening between the removal of the two breasts. The breasts of multiparous animals apparently do not return to smaller size, although the ducts may grow thin in caliber and resemble a leafless tree.

Figures 24 and 25 show two breasts of a virgin rabbit, a period of twenty-six days intervening between the removal of the breasts. Figure 27 pictures the breast of a rabbit which closely resembles the mammary development seen about the tenth or twelfth day of pregnancy. The breast margins were raised and pinkish, adjoining breasts were nearly contiguous, and both ducts and acini were well developed as microscopic sections proved. Figure 26, however, which is taken from the corresponding breast of the same rabbit (removed twenty-four days before) abundantly proves that the rabbit was virgin. This rabbit had been purchased quite young and had been kept isolated for two months before the first breast was removed. The uterus, also, was subjected to careful microscopical examination. It showed the changes noted when the corpus luteum is active. The ovaries of this animal were found to contain numerous flourishing corpora lutea. Thus in a virgin animal we were able to demonstrate changes which were indistinguishable from those seen at the end of the first third of pregnancy.

In searching the literature we finally discovered an article of Bouin and Ancel[7] which describes variations in the size and appearance of the rabbit's breast corresponding to the development of the corpus luteum. According to these authors after the corpus luteum begins to regress, the breasts, which have previously grown to large proportions, rapidly involute and diminish in size. This involution has not yet been fully corroborated by us. Various other points mentioned by these authors also require further study which is now being pursued. These investigations will be published separately.

In this connection it will suffice to note that virgin rabbits, without injections, can have breasts which are more developed than those described by Starling as corresponding to the ninth or tenth day of pregnancy. As will be seen in Figure 27 adjacent breasts are nearly contiguous; the ducts are wide and show many branchings. The edges in this breast were raised and pinkish. Microscopical sections through this raised portion showed ducts surrounded by smaller ducts and alveoli. Intermediate stages are readily found, and this increase in size can be followed from day to day. That the operation *per se* does not stimulate the growth of the breasts is abundantly proved by the fact that in several animals, breasts removed at the usual intervals showed no increase in size or change in type. It may be added that in the winter months (during which most of these experiments were performed) some rabbits apparently do not ovulate.[8]

The facts brought out by the above experiments fully explain why our results and those of Starling do not correspond. They also account for the discrepancies noted in our three series. In view of our results it will not prove necessary to consider the papers of Starling, Foa, and Biedl and Koenigstein separately. The experiments of all these authors were performed on rabbits. Apparently Foa (who even reproduces Starling's illustration of the virgin breast) and Biedl and Koenigstein accepted Starling's controls without personal study of the virgin breast.

Both Claypon and Starling, and Biedl and Koenigstein report that injections of placental extract produced no change. In one of our own experiments (Series 2, Rabbit 4) the breasts were at least as large and active as those of corresponding animals injected with fetal extract. The

7. Bouin and Ancel: Compt. rend. Soc. d. biol., 1909, lxvii, 466. Since our article has been received for publication, Bouin and Ancel (Jour. de physiol. exper., Jan. 16, 1911) have reported further on the growth of the heart in the rabbit. They believe that the mammary growth is due to the action of the corpus luteum (resulting from "sterile coitus"). They no longer assert that regression of the ducts takes place. The proof offered is. however, not conclusive.

8. Bouin and Ancel (Compt. rend. Soc. d. biol., 1909, lxvii, 464) assert that in rabbits, and in all other animals which have an interstitial gland in the ovary, a corpus luteum does not form except after coitus. This observation also requires corroboration. W. Heape (Proc. Roy. Soc., 1905, lxxvi, 260) found that ovulation did not take place except after coitus in the rabbit. He further says that the doe will not accept the male except during estrum. Our experience does not agree with this finding, as even pregnant rabbits (the existence of pregnancy was not suspected) submitted to vigorous males, abortion subsequently resulting.

question is raised because it might be objected that, even if Starling's views are not entirely correct, the fetal extracts might stimulate the ovary and thus inaugurate the hyperplasia.

Basch[9] has announced a theory, based on experiments, in which such an interrelation is supposed to bring about hyperplasia of the breast and secretion of milk. Only instead of a fetal-ovarian complex, he favors an ovarian-placental activation.

Basch's experiments may be divided into two groups. In the first he injected multiparous animals in which the milk secretion had ceased (apparently subcutaneously, though no experimental details are given) with heterologous and homologous placental extracts. Various degrees of milk secretion were noted, the breast nearest the site of injection always producing most milk. Placental fragments, implanted subcutaneously, likewise gave rise to secretion. Of the second group of experiments he describes one in greater detail. In a virgin bitch he subcutaneously implanted two ovaries removed from a pregnant one, using the back of the animal for the site of the implantation. After fourteen days all the breasts showed distinct increase in size. Six weeks later the glands corresponded in size to those of a pregnant animal, although the implanted ovaries had shrunken to very small size. When, eight weeks after the beginning of the experiment (a time which corresponds approximately to the duration of pregnancy in the bitch), he gave placental extract injections, milk secretion set in and the animal was able to nurse puppies. Breasts excised at intervals during the experiment showed a gradual change from the virginal to the fully secreting breast.

## EXPERIMENTS DEALING WITH BASCH'S THEORY

In this connection we shall recur to some of our own experiments, previously referred to, performed on rats. In one adult virgin rat we transplanted the ovaries of a pregnant rat subcutaneously into two pockets on the back. The ovaries contained numerous fresh corpora lutea. Seven days later we began injections of rat's placental extract, giving sixteen injections in eighteen days. No increase in the breasts either macroscopically or microscopically was noted. In another rat the ovaries of five pregnant rats were similarly implanted at intervals of a few days during the course of twelve days, the animal being killed four days after the last implantation. Here also no change occurred. The implanted ovaries had all healed aseptically. Microscopically the corpora lutea showed various degrees of necrobiosis, depending on the time since which they had been transplanted.

*Discussion of Basch's Results.*—In criticizing Basch's first experiments we concur entirely with the objections offered by Biedl and Koenigstein. Multiparous animals are unfit for studying breast hyperplasia. Ducts and acini after parturition remain present for an indefinite period. Our study of multiparous rabbits convinced us that this period extends over several months. Basch, therefore, stimulated already present breast tissue by his subcutaneous injections. That this stimulus was in no sense specific is shown by the fact that the breast nearest to the site of

9. Basch, K.: Monatschr. f. Kinderh., 1909, viii, 513.

injection reacted first and most strongly. Furthermore, just as Biedl and Koenigstein report, we also were able to observe renewed milk secretion, occurring in the breasts of multiparous rabbits in which abscesses developing near the breast had caused increased congestion. That the secretion consisted of milk was shown by microscopical examination. No direct comparison of Basch's placental extract and that of other investigators is possible, as Basch carefully refrains from mentioning his mode of preparation. He states, moreover, that he has entered into negotiation with a commercial chemical laboratory ("which as may be well understood, reserves for itself every right in the manufacture") to supply him with larger quantities of material!

The one successful experiment in a virgin bitch, reported by Basch and previously mentioned, does not appear convincing. That ovaries which were transplanted from a pregnant animal, and which evidently underwent rapid regression, should have caused growth of the breasts, appears unlikely. If the corpus luteum is to be considered the activator, it is well known that this delicate gland does not permit of transplantation, although the remainder of the ovary may do so, and L. Loeb,[10] in another connection, has found it impossible to produce uterine changes due to the action of the corpus luteum of an homologous animal, by daily subcutaneous injection. Our own unsuccessful injections with ovarian extract, containing fresh rabbit's corpus luteum, have already been mentioned. Possibly further study may show that in the bitch rut changes of the breast similar to those observed by us in the rabbit occur.[11] Basch's paper, moreover, both from the fact that neither the site of injections is more than hinted at, nor the method of preparation of the extract mentioned, hardly deserves serious consideration. Furthermore, Basch does not distinguish with sufficient clearness between milk secretion and growth of the breasts.

### HYPERPLASIA VERSUS SECRETION

While it probably is correct to assume that as soon as breast acini have reached a certain stage of development, milk secretion can and perhaps does set in, the amount of milk secreted is no index or guide of the amount of hyperplasia which has occurred. Therefore, in studying the growth of the breast attention should be focused on the increase in development of the acini and ducts, not on their catabolic activity.

Foa[3] in the paper previously referred to, has shown that the secretory activity of the breast is not inhibited by the presence of fetal products, as was assumed by Starling. Foa also showed that the blood of pregnant

10. Loeb, L.: Med. Rec., 1910, lxxvii, 1083.

11. Starling (see note 1) quotes Heape and Kehrer who recorded cases of bitches which had not been impregnated at the normal time, and who after two months not only made a bed for their young, but had swelling of their mammary glands, with, in some cases, actual secretion of milk.

goats does not contain a substance which increases the secretory activity of the breasts. Lederer and Pribram[12] injected placental extract intravenously into goats, and assert that after from two to ten minutes an enormous increase in the quantity of milk secreted was noted for a short period (one and one-half to three minutes). As was pointed out to us by Dr. H. Auchincloss, an anatomical observation already mentioned by Sir Astley Cooper[13] might account for this effect in a different way. The terminal ducts in the cow, goat, etc., form a reservoir which can contain a large amount of milk. Lederer and Pribram inserted a catheter into the nipple and recorded the quantity of milk which entered a calibrated glass tube within a given period. If, for instance, injection of placental extract should produce an increased muscular contraction or tonus of the chest muscles,[14] this elevation of pressure would naturally serve to empty the breast reservoir more rapidly without necessarily indicating an increased secretion. The question, however, does not concern us further in this connection.

Halban's theory,[15] based largely on clinical observations, hardly comes within the scope of this paper. He believes that the ovary exerts its trophic influence on the breast, except in pregnancy. During gestation, according to this author, the ovary is quiescent (many facts strongly controvert this assumption) and the placenta, its temporary antagonist, inaugurates the breast's growth. No experimental proof corroborates Halban's views, while all the facts he mentions are equally well accounted for in other ways.

Our experiments, which showed that the rabbit's breast, without the artificial stimulus of injections, may reach a size corresponding closely to that observed in the tenth day of pregnancy, prove that the results of Starling, Foa, and Biedl and Koenigstein are accounted for by accidental and purely physiological variations. It does seem strange, however, that Starling never encountered hyperplasia of the breast in the ten animals injected with ovarian, placental and mucous membrane extracts, particularly as he states that in several the uterus was congested and the animal was in heat. No exact study of the ovaries appears to have been made, nor is the presence or absence of corpora lutea mentioned. Biedl and

---

12. Lederer and Pribram: Arch. f. ges. Physiol., 1910, cxxxiv, p. 531.

13. Cooper, Sir Astley: The Anatomy and Diseases of the Breast, Philadelphia, Lea & Blanchard, 1845, p. 49.

14. Dixon and Taylor (Brit. Med. Jour., 1907, ii, 1150), asserted that the placenta contained pressor principles. O. Rosenheim (Jour. Physiol., 1909, xxxviii, 337) in his studies found that the so-called pressor principles of the placenta were due to bacterial putrefaction, and that the resulting pressor bases were identical with those found in putrefying meat. Whether these findings could be applied to the work of Lederer and Pribram appears doubtful, as in most experiments they employed fresh extracts.

15. Halban, J.: Arch. f. Gynäk., 1905, lxxv, 353.

Koenigstein in four animals injected with placenta also report negative results.

We, in all our injected animals (also in those in which breasts were excised at intervals, and in the case of the castrated rabbits), examined both ovaries in serial section, and studied numerous sections, removed from different levels of the uterus. Two rabbits, whose breasts showed very active hyperplasia (Figs. 10 and 27) had numerous large corpora lutea in their ovaries, and the uterine mucosa was thrown into numerous folds. There were, however, in many cases, no corpora lutea, although the breast showed increase in size.[16]

CONCLUSIONS

It is not our intention in this paper to discuss in detail certain observations we have made relating to the sexual cycle of the rabbit. We have, however, shown that a breast hormone, elaborated by the fetus, has not been demonstrated, and must be considered purely hypothetical. Basch's theory of an ovarian placental interaction, likewise, lacks all proof. Halban's conception of a cessation of ovarian activity during pregnancy is made most unlikely not only by the persistence, but also by the hypertrophic state of the corpus luteum, which is now definitely known to be an actively functionating gland. Our own views, many of which yet require proof, can be summarized in the following. These views not only harmonize with all facts now known to us, but also regard the breast changes of pregnancy merely as an exaggeration of the cyclical changes of the sexual cycle, similar to the uterine changes, which occur at regular intervals, in preparation for the function of reproduction.

1. Intra-uterine, prepuberty and puberty growth of the breasts is directly dependent on ovarian function (Tandler[17]), Foges.[18]

2. A cyclical change in the virgin breast occurs under the influence of the ovary.

3. Castration does not cause rapid regression of the cyclical breast hyperplasia.

4. No proof has been offered to show that the fetus or placenta directly produces growth of the breast in pregnancy.

5. Evidence points to the fact that the persistent corpus luteum of pregnancy may produce this breast growth.

6. The factors which favor or cause the persistence of the corpus luteum are unknown.

7. Certain evidence (increase of the breast produced by hydrated mole without fetus, chorio-epithelioma) makes it unlikely that the fetus is at any time the controlling factor.

---

16. In studying the rabbit's ovary not only the corpus luteum but also the state of development of the interstitial gland may have to be considered.

17. Tandler, J.: Wien. klin. Wchnschr., 1910, xxiii, 459.

18. Foges, A.: Wien. klin. Wchnschr., 1908, xxi, 137.

8. Nature's process is more complicated than the simple chemical stimulus assumed by Starling. As yet hyperplasia of the breasts has not been experimentally produced except by parabiosis, which does not explain the stimulus. Possibly the influence of other glands of internal secretion complicates the problem.

9. Milk secretion is no index of quantitative increase in breast tissue.

10. Under physiological conditions milk secretion sets in when the ovarian influence is removed—in the new-born after birth; in the puerpera as the corpus luteum of pregnancy regresses; sometimes postoperatively after castration in the virgin (if the breast has been activated by the corpus luteum of menstruation?).

Further study may show that some of these conclusions require modification. Our present aim has been to emphasize the fact that the fetus does not directly cause hyperplasia of the breast in pregnancy—fascinating and simple as this theory appears. The fact that breast changes in the rabbit are noted as early as the fourth day, although nidation does not occur until the ninth, confirms the view that neither fetus nor placenta is the causative factor.

The ovary, on the other hand, inaugurates cyclical changes in the uterus, and similar but more exaggerated changes during pregnancy. The mammary changes under consideration are analogous in their relation to the reproductive function, and likewise manifest themselves by tissue hyperplasia.

The results of our research make it evident that the primary end for which we undertook the work—to study physiological hyperplasia of breast tissue under controllable conditions, and to study transplantable animal tumors when under the influence of artificially stimulated environment—cannot be attained by this method.

The results should also influence the conclusions drawn by several authors, who have sought to correlate Starling's findings in the study of tumor growth—notably P. Ehrlich, E. F. Bashford and M. Askanazy.[19] Ehrlich and Bashford apparently experienced some difficulty in harmonizing their own findings with Starling's experiments. Askanazy considered

19. Ehrlich, P. (Beiträge zur experimentellen Pathologie und Chemotherapie, Leipsic, 1909) says that Starling's experiments show that the growth-substances are quite specific, and by their stimulation of certain definite cells likewise enable them to become more resistant to athreptic influences. Bashford, Murray, and Haaland (Resistance and Susceptibility to Inoculated Cancer, The Imperial Cancer Research Fund, Third Sc. Report, London, 1908, p. 356) believe that Starling's experiments may show a fundamental difference between normal cells of the mamma and those of an adenocarcinoma of the same organ. M. Askanazy (Ztschr. f. Krebsforsch., 1910, xi, 393) considers the possibility that certain progressive hyperplastic developments, especially those of the genital organs seen with tumors of the pineal gland, kidney, ovary, and testis, bear evidence to the fact that the embryonal tissue of the tumor induces the hyperplasia. He regards Starling's experiments as confirmatory.

the breast changes corroborative evidence in substantiating his hypothesis, which in substance is, that embryonal tissues in tumors exert a hormone action leading to hyperplastic development. And finally, our results force us to admit that, though we may in rare instances succeed in producing a very limited tissue hyperplasia by artificial means (such as epithelial proliferation due to injection of Scharlach R, oils, etc.), the subtler processes of Nature cannot at the present time, or with our present methods, be imitated.

983 Park Avenue—437 West Fifty-Ninth Street.

RAT SERIES 1.—WHITE RATS INJECTED INTRAPERITONEALLY WITH FETUSES OF SOWS

Rat 1.—Virgin Female

Weight 110 gm.; Berkefeld Extract

| Date | Amount of Extract, c.c. | Weight of Fetuses, gm. | Date | Amount of Extract, c.c. | Weight of Fetuses, gm. | Date | Amount of Extract, c.c. | Weight of Fetuses, gm. |
|---|---|---|---|---|---|---|---|---|
| 6/14 | 1.5 | 42.5 | 6/25 | 1.5 | 140.0 | 7/7 | 1.5 | 78.0 |
| 6/15 | 1.5 | 35.5 | 6/27 | 1.5 | 165.0 | 7/8 | 1.5 | 36.0 |
| 6/16 | 1.5 | 13.0 | 6/28 | 1.5 | 27.0 | 7/9 | 1.5 | 37.0 |
| 6/17 | 1.5 | 207.0 | 6/29 | 1.5 | 54.0 | 7/11 | 1.5 | 14.0 |
| 6/18 | 1.5 | 192.0 | 6/30 | 1.5 | 240.0 | 7/12 | 1.5 | 120.0 |
| 6/20 | 1.5 | 23.0 | 7/1 | 1.5 | 280.0 | 7/13 | 1.5 | 5.0 |
| 6/21 | 1.5 | 39.0 | 7/2 | 1.5 | 325.0 | 7/13 | 1.5 | 700.0 |
| 6/22 | 1.5 | 128.0 | 7/4 | 1.5 | 100.0 | 7/14 | 1.5 | 128.0 |
| 6/23 | 1.5 | 135.0 | 7/5 | 1.5 | 290.0 | 7/15 | 1.5 | 74.0 |
| 6/24 | 1.5 | 0.5 | 7/6 | 1.5 | 330.0 | 7/16 | 1.5 | 74.0 |

Killed July 18, 1910.

Nipples barely visible; breasts not visible; uterus and ovaries small. Microscopical, breasts unchanged.

Rat 2.—Virgin Female

Weight 105 gm.; Berkefeld Extract

| Date | Amount of Extract, c.c. | Weight of Fetuses, gm. | Date | Amount of Extract, c.c. | Weight of Fetuses, gm. | Date | Amount of Extract, c.c. | Weight of Fetuses, gm. |
|---|---|---|---|---|---|---|---|---|
| 6/14 | 1 | 42.5 | 6/23 | 1 | 135.0 | 7/2 | 1 | 325.0 |
| 6/15 | 1 | 35.5 | 6/24 | 1 | 0.5 | 7/4 | 1 | 100.0 |
| 6/16 | 1 | 13.0 | 6/25 | 1 | 140.0 | 7/5 | 1 | 290.0 |
| 6/17 | 1 | 207.0 | 6/27 | 1 | 165.0 | 7/6 | 1 | 330.0 |
| 6/18 | 1 | 192.0 | 6/28 | 1 | 23.0 | 7/7 | 1 | 78.0 |
| 6/20 | 1 | 23.0 | 6/29 | 1 | 54.0 | 7/8 | 1 | 36.0 |
| 6/21 | 1 | 39.0 | 6/30 | 1 | 240.0 | 7/9 | 1 | 37.0 |
| 6/22 | 1 | 128.0 | 7/1 | 1 | 280.0 | | | |

Killed July 10, 1910.

Breasts unchanged; fresh corpus luteum, uterus vascular.

Rat 3.—Virgin Female

Weight 189 gm.; Berkefeld Extract

| Date | Amount of Extract, c.c. | Weight of Fetuses, gm. | Date | Amount of Extract, c.c. | Weight of Fetuses, gm. | Date | Amount of Extract, c.c. | Weight of Fetuses, gm. |
|---|---|---|---|---|---|---|---|---|
| 6/14 | 0.5 | 42.5 | 6/27 | 0.5 | 165.0 | 7/9 | 0.5 | 37.0 |
| 6/15 | 0.5 | 35.5 | 6/28 | 0.5 | 23.0 | 7/11 | 0.5 | 14.0 |
| 6/16 | 0.5 | 13.0 | 6/29 | 0.5 | 54.0 | 7/12 | 0.5 | 120.0 |
| 6/17 | 0.5 | 207.0 | 6/30 | 0.5 | 240.0 | 7/13 | 0.5 | 5.0 |
| 6/18 | 0.5 | 192.0 | 7/1 | 0.5 | 280.0 | .... | ... | 700.0 |
| 6/20 | 0.5 | 23.0 | 7/2 | 0.5 | 325.0 | 7/14 | 0.5 | 128.0 |
| 6/21 | 0.5 | 39.0 | 7/4 | 0.5 | 100.0 | 7/15 | 0.5 | 74.0 |
| 6/22 | 0.5 | 125.0 | 7/5 | 0.5 | 290.0 | 7/16 | 0.5 | 74.0 |
| 6/23 | 0.5 | 135.0 | 7/6 | 0.5 | 330.0 | | | |
| 6/24 | 0.5 | 0.5 | 7/7 | 0.5 | 71.0 | | | |
| 6/25 | 0.5 | 140.0 | 7/8 | 0.5 | 36.0 | | | |

Killed July 18, 1910.

Breasts unchanged; uterus and ovaries small.

RAT 4.—VIRGIN FEMALE

Weight 99 gm.; Boiled Extract

| Date | Amount of Extract, c.c. | Weight of Fetuses, gm. | Date | Amount of Extract, c.c. | Weight of Fetuses, gm. | Date | Amount of Extract, c.c. | Weight of Fetuses, gm. |
|---|---|---|---|---|---|---|---|---|
| 6/13 | 1.5 | 5.0 | 6/25 | 1.5 | 149.0 | 7/8 | 1.5 | 36.0 |
| 6/14 | 1.5 | 42.5 | 6/27 | 1.5 | 165.0 | 7/9 | 1.5 | 37.0 |
| 6/15 | 1.5 | 35.5 | 6/28 | 1.5 | 23.0 | 1/11 | 1.5 | 14.0 |
| 6/16 | 1.5 | 13.0 | 6/29 | 1.5 | 54.0 | 7/12 | 1.5 | 120.0 |
| 6/17 | 1.5 | 207.0 | 6/30 | 1.5 | 240.0 | 7/13 | 1.5 | 5.0 |
| 6/18 | 1.5 | 192.0 | 7/1 | 1.5 | 280.0 | .... | ... | 700.0 |
| 6/20 | 1.5 | 23.0 | 7/2 | 1.5 | 325.0 | 7/14 | 1.5 | 128.0 |
| 6/21 | 1.5 | 39.0 | 1/4 | 1.5 | 100.0 | 7/15 | 1.5 | 74.0 |
| 6/22 | 1.5 | 128.0 | 7/5 | 1.5 | 290.0 | 7/16 | 1.5 | 74.0 |
| 6/23 | 1.5 | 135.0 | 7/6 | 1.5 | 330.0 | | | |
| 6/24 | 1.5 | 140.0 | 7/7 | 1.5 | 78.0 | | | |

Killed July 16, 1910.

Breasts unchanged; uterus and ovaries small.

RAT 5.—VIRGIN FEMALE

Weight 78 gm.; Boiled Extract

| Date | Amount of Extract, c.c. | Weight of Fetuses, gm. | Date | Amount of Extract, c.c. | Weight of Fetuses, gm. | Date | Amount of Extract, c.c. | Weight of Fetuses, gm. |
|---|---|---|---|---|---|---|---|---|
| 6/13 | 1 | 5.0 | 6/24 | 1 | 140.0 | 7/6 | 1 | 330.0 |
| 6/14 | 1 | 42.5 | 6/25 | 1 | 140.0 | 7/7 | 1 | 78.0 |
| 6/15 | 1 | 35.5 | 6/27 | 1 | 165.0 | 7/8 | 1 | 36.0 |
| 6/16 | 1 | 13.0 | 6/28 | 1 | 23.0 | 7/9 | 1 | 37.0 |
| 6/17 | 1 | 207.0 | 6/29 | 1 | 54.0 | 7/11 | 1 | 14.0 |
| 6/18 | 1 | 192.0 | 6/30 | 1 | 240.0 | 7/12 | 1 | 120.0 |
| 6/20 | 1 | 23.0 | 7/1 | 1 | 280.0 | 7/13 | 1 | 500.0 |
| 6/21 | 1 | 39.0 | 7/2 | 1 | 325.0 | .... | . | 700.0 |
| 6/22 | 1 | 128.0 | 7/4 | 1 | 100.0 | | | |
| 6/23 | 1 | 132.0 | 7/5 | 1 | 290.0 | | | |

Killed July 14, 1910.

Breasts unchanged; uterus and ovaries small.

RAT 6.—VIRGIN FEMALE

Weight 88 gm.; Boiled Extract

| Date | Amount of Extract, c.c. | Weight of Fetuses, gm. | Date | Amount of Extract, c.c. | Weight of Fetuses, gm. | Date | Amount of Extract, c.c. | Weight of Fetuses, gm. |
|---|---|---|---|---|---|---|---|---|
| 6/13 | 0.5 | 5.0 | 6/25 | 0.5 | 149.0 | 7/8 | 0.5 | 36.0 |
| 6/14 | 0.5 | 42.5 | 6/27 | 0.5 | 165.0 | 7/9 | 0.5 | 37.0 |
| 6/15 | 0.5 | 35.5 | 6/28 | 0.5 | 23.0 | 7/11 | 0.5 | 14.0 |
| 6/16 | 0.5 | 13.0 | 6/29 | 0.5 | 54.0 | 7/12 | 0.5 | 120.0 |
| 6/17 | 0.5 | 207.0 | 6/30 | 0.5 | 240.0 | 7/13 | 0.5 | 500.0 |
| 6/18 | 0.5 | 192.0 | 7/1 | 0.5 | 280.0 | .... | ... | 700.0 |
| 6/20 | 0.5 | 23.0 | 7/2 | 0.5 | 325.0 | 7/14 | 0.5 | 128.0 |
| 6/21 | 0.5 | 39.0 | 7/4 | 0.5 | 100.0 | 7/15 | 0.5 | 74.0 |
| 6/22 | 0.5 | 128.0 | 7/5 | 0.5 | 290.0 | 7/16 | 0.5 | 74.0 |
| 6/23 | 0.5 | 135.0 | 7/6 | 0.5 | 330.0 | | | |
| 6/24 | 0.5 | 140.0 | 7/7 | 0.5 | 78.0 | | | |

Killed July 18, 1910.

Breasts unchanged; uterus vascular; fresh corpora lutea.

RAT 7.—VIRGIN FEMALE

Weight 103 gm.; Berkefeld Extract; 1 Week Old

One c.c. of extract given each day (except July 3 and 10) from June 29 to July 23.

Killed July 24, 1910.

Breasts not enlarged; uterus vascular; fresh corpora lutea.

RAT 8.—VIRGIN FEMALE

Weight 104 gm.; Boiled Extract; 1 Week Old

Killed July 24, 1910.

One c.c. of extract given each day (except July 3 and 10) from June 29 to July 23.

Breasts unchanged; hydrometra; large corpora lutea.

## RAT SERIES 2.—WHITE RATS INJECTED INTRAPERITONEALLY WITH FETUSES, ETC., OF RATS

### Rat 1.—Virgin Female

Centrifuged extract of rat fetuses; 19 injections; 130 fetuses.

| | Fetuses | | Amount of Extract Injected, c.c. | | Fetuses | | Amount of Extract Injected, c.c. |
|---|---|---|---|---|---|---|---|
| Date | No. | Weight, gm. | | Date | No. | Weight, gm. | |
| 7/20 | 9 | 26.0 | 3.0 | 7/30 | 5 | 26.0 | 2.0 |
| 7/21 | 11 | 32.0 | 2.5 | 7/31 | 7 | 24.0 | 2.0 |
| 7/22 | 7 | .... | 2.5 | 8/1 | 6 | 24.5 | 2.0 |
| 7/23 | 8 | 39.0 | 2.8 | 8/2 | 7 | 17.0 | 2.0 |
| 7/24 | 8 | 23.0 | 2.5 | 8/3 | 9 | 16.5 | 2.0 |
| 7/25 | 6 | 30.0 | 2.0 | 8/4 | 5 | 18.2 | 2.0 |
| 7/26 | 7 | 15.5 | 2.0 | 8/5 | 5 | 18.3 | 2.0 |
| 7/27 | 3 | 14.5 | 2.0 | 8/6 | 7 | 32.0 | 2.0 |
| 7/28 | 6 | 16.0 | 2.0 | 8/7 | 7 | 32.0 | 2.0 |
| 7/29 | 8 | 19.0 | 2.0 | | | | |

Killed Aug. 8, 1910.

Breasts unchanged; uterus and ovaries small.

### Rat 2.—Virgin Female

Centrifuged extract of rat fetuses; 9 injections; 65 fetuses.

| | Fetuses | | Amount of Extract Injected, c.c. | | Fetuses | | Amount of Extract Injected, c.c. |
|---|---|---|---|---|---|---|---|
| Date | No. | Weight, gm. | | Date | No. | Weight, gm. | |
| 6/8 | 8 | .... | 2.0 | 6/12 | 7 | 34.0 | 2.0 |
| 6/9 | 9 | 20.0 | 2.0 | 6/13 | 7 | 6.0 | 2.0 |
| 6/10 | 9 | .... | 1.2 | 6/14 | 8 | 7.0 | 2.5 |
| 6/11 | 10 | 40.0 | 2.0 | 6/15 | 8 | 26.0 | 2.0 |
| | | | | 6/15 | Died suddenly after injection. | | |

Breasts unchanged.

### Rat 3.—Virgin Female

Ovaries removed (?) June 15; centrifuged extract of rat fetuses; 23 injections; 165 fetuses.

| | Fetuses | | Amount of Extract Injected, c.c. | | Fetuses | | Amount of Extract Injected, c.c. |
|---|---|---|---|---|---|---|---|
| Date | No. | Weight, gm. | | Date | No. | Weight, gm. | |
| 7/11 | 10 | 40.0 | 2.0 | 7/28 | 6 | 16.0 | 2.0 |
| 7/12 | 7 | 34.0 | 2.0 | 7/29 | 8 | 19.0 | 2.0 |
| 7/15 | 8 | 26.0 | 2.0 | 7/30 | 5 | 26.0 | 2.0 |
| 7/19 | 9 | 13.0 | 3.5 | 7/31 | 7 | 24.0 | 2.0 |
| 7/20 | 9 | 26.0 | 2.0 | 8/1 | 6 | 24.5 | 2.0 |
| 7/21 | 11 | 32.0 | 2.0 | 8/2 | 7 | 17.0 | 2.0 |
| 7/22 | 7 | .... | 1.2 | 8/3 | 9 | 16.5 | 2.0 |
| 7/23 | 8 | 38.0 | 3.0 | 8/4 | 5 | 18.5 | 2.0 |
| 7/24 | 8 | 23.0 | 1.5 | 8/5 | 5 | 18.2 | 2.0 |
| 7/25 | 6 | 30.0 | 2.0 | 8/6 | 7 | 32.0 | 2.0 |
| 7/26 | 7 | 15.5 | 2.0 | 8/7 | 7 | 32.0 | 2.0 |
| 7/27 | 3 | 14.5 | 2.0 | | | | |

Killed Aug. 8, 1910.

Breasts unchanged; small remnant of right ovary had been left *in situ;* uterus not atrophic.

### Rat 4.—Virgin Female

Boiled extract of rat fetuses; 11 injections; 89 fetuses.

| | Fetuses | | Amount of Extract Injected, c.c. | | Fetuses | | Amount of Extract Injected, c.c. |
|---|---|---|---|---|---|---|---|
| Date | No. | Weight, gm. | | Date | No. | Weight, gm. | |
| 7/8 | 8 | .... | 1.5 | 7/15 | 8 | 26.0 | 3.0 |
| 7/9 | 9 | 20.0 | 2.0 | 7/19 | 9 | 13.0 | 1.5 |
| 7/10 | 9 | 20.0 | 3.0 | 7/20 | Sick; no injection. | | |
| 7/11 | 10 | 40.0 | 2.0 | 7/22 | Better. | | 1.2 |
| 7/12 | 7 | 34.0 | 2.0 | 7/23 | 8 | 39.0 | 2.0 |
| 7/13 | 7 | 6.0 | 0.5 | 7/24 | 8 | 23.0 | 2.0 |
| 7/14 | 8 | 7.0 | 2.0 | 7/25 | Found dead. | .... | |

Breasts unchanged.

RAT 5.—VIRGIN FEMALE

Centrifuged extract of rat placenta; 25 injections; 177 placentas.

| Date | Placentas, No. | Amount of Extract, c.c. | Fetuses, Weight, gm. | Date | Placentas, No. | Amount of Extract, c.c. | Fetuses, Weight, gm. |
|---|---|---|---|---|---|---|---|
| 7/9 | 9 | 2.0 | 6.0 | 7/26 | 7 | 1.5 | 3.0 |
| 7/10 | 9 | 2.0 | 6.0 | 7/27 | 3 | 2.0 | 2.0 |
| 7/11 | 10 | 2.0 | 4.0 | 7/28 | 6 | 2.0 | 4.0 |
| 7/12 | 7 | 2.0 | 4.0 | 7/29 | 8 | 1.0 | 4.0 |
| 7/13 | 7 | 2.0 | 3.0 | 7/30 | 5 | 2.0 | 2.5 |
| 7/14 | 8 | 3.5 | 3.0 | 7/31 | 7 | 2.0 | 3.0 |
| 7/15 | 8 | 2.0 | 4.0 | 8/1 | 6 | 2.0 | 3.0 |
| 7/19 | 9 | 2.0 | 4.0 | 8/2 | 7 | 2.0 | 4.5 |
| 7/20 | 9 | 2.0 | 4.0 | 8/3 | 9 | By mistake 2 c.c. centrifuged fetus extract. | 4.0 |
| 7/22 | 4 | 2.0 | ... | | | | |
| 7/23 | 8 | 2.0 | 4.0 | 8/4 | 5 | 2.0 | 2.2 |
| 7/24 | 8 | 2.0 | 5.5 | 5/5 | 5 | 2.0 | 4.2 |
| 7/25 | 6 | 2.0 | 3.0 | 8/6 | 7 | 2.0 | 4.0 |

Killed Aug. 7, 1910.
Breasts unchanged; uterus congested; recent corpus luteum.

RAT 6.—VIRGIN FEMALE

Castrated June 20; centrifuged extract of rat placenta; 16 injections; 105 placentas.

| Date | Placentas, No. | Amount of Extract, c.c. | Fetuses, Weight, gm. | Date | Placentas, No. | Amount of Extract, c.c. | Fetuses, Weight, gm. |
|---|---|---|---|---|---|---|---|
| 7/11 | 10 | 2.0 | 4.0 | 7/28 | 6 | 1.8 | 4.0 |
| 7/12 | 7 | 2.0 | 4.0 | 7/30 | 5 | 1.0 | 2.5 |
| 7/15 | 8 | 2.0 | 4.0 | 8/1 | 6 | 1.5 | 3.0 |
| 7/19 | 9 | 2.0 | 4.0 | 8/2 | 7 | 1.5 | 4.0 |
| 7/22 | 4 | 1.2 | ... | 8/3 | 9 | 2.0 | 4.0 |
| 7/23 | 8 | 1.0 | 4.5 | 8/4 | 5 | 2.0 | 2.2 |
| 7/25 | 6 | 2.0 | 3.0 | 8/5 | 5 | 2.0 | 2.3 |
| 7/27 | 3 | 1.5 | 2.0 | 8/6 | 7 | 2.0 | 4.0 |

Killed Aug. 7, 1910.
Breasts unchanged; uterus atrophic.

RAT 7.—VIRGIN FEMALE

Blood-serum of pregnant rats; 24 injections; serum from 24 rats.

| Date | Amount of Serum, c.c. | Date | Amount of Serum, c.c. | Date | Amount of Serum, c.c. |
|---|---|---|---|---|---|
| 7/8 | 2.0 | 7/20 | 1.0 | 7/30 | 1.2 |
| 7/9 | 1.1 | 7/21 | 3.0 | 7/31 | 1.5 |
| 7/11 | 1.0 | 7/22 | 1.8 | 8/1 | 1.5 |
| 7/13 | 2.0 | 7/23 | 3.0 | 8/2 | 2.0 |
| 7/14 | 2.0 | 7/25 | 1.0 | 8/3 | 2.0 |
| 7/15 | 0.5 | 7/26 | 2.0 | 8/4 | 2.0 |
| 7/16 | 0.5 | 7/27 | 0.8 | 8/5 | 2.0 |
| 7/19 | 1.5 | 7/28 | 2.0 | 8/6 | 2.0 |

Killed Aug. 7, 1910.
Breasts unchanged; uterus vascular; fresh corpus luteum.

## RABBIT SERIES 1. — RABBITS INJECTED INTRAPERITONEALLY WITH FETUSES, OVARIES, PLACENTAS AND HYPOPHYSES OF RABBITS

RABBIT 1.—VIRGIN; NIPPLES BARELY VISIBLE

Weight 1,830 gm.; 21 injections centrifuged extract; 111 rabbit fetuses used.

| Date | Fetuses No. | Fetuses Weight, gm. | Amount of Extract Injected, c.c. | Date | Fetuses No. | Fetuses Weight, gm. | Amount of Extract Injected, c.c. |
|---|---|---|---|---|---|---|---|
| 9/3 | 1/2 of 6 | 82.0 | 20.0 | 9/21 | 1/2 of 5 | 82.0 | 23.0 |
| 9/4 | 1 | 1.5 | 7.5 | 9/22 | 1/2 of 7 | 139.0 | 24.0 |
| 9/5 | 5 | 6.0 | 10.0 | 9/23 | 1/2 of 3 | 16.0 | 18.0 |
| 9/8 | 1/2 of 6 | 71.5 | 22.0 | 9/24 | 1/2 of 6 | 14.0 | 11.0 |
| 9/9 | 1/2 of 4 | 131.0 | 23.0 | 9/25 | 1/2 of 8 | 10.0 | 23.0 |
| 9/10 | 5 | 5.0 | 13.0 | 9/26 | 7 | 3.5 | 15.0 |
| 9/11 | 2 | 8.5 | 15.0 | 9/27 | 1/2 of 4 | 50.0 | 25.0 |
| 9/15 | 1/2 of 6 | 148.5 | 22.0 | 9/28 | 1/4 of 5 | 83.5 | 13.0 |
| 9/16 | 2/5 of 6 | 242.0 | 22.0 | 9/29 | 7 | 5.0 | 22.0 |
| 9/17 | 1/2 of 7 | 100.5 | 22.0 | 9/30 | 1/2 of 7 | 26.5 | 20.0 |
| 9/18 | 4 | 4.0 | 11.0 | | | | |

Killed Oct. 2, 1910.
Nipples not enlarged; slight amount of clear fluid expressed; stained breasts show considerable enlargement; ovaries small; uterus vascular but resting. Microscopically: no alveoli, no mitoses; smaller ducts have some wedge-shaped projections of epithelium (Fig. 8).

### Rabbit 2.—Multipara (?); Nipples Barely Visible

Weight 1,940 gm.; 15 injections boiled extract of fetuses; 88 fetuses used.

| Date | Fetuses No. | Fetuses Weight, gm. | Amount of Extract Injected, c.c. | Date | Fetuses No. | Fetuses Weight, gm. | Amount of Extract Injected, c.c. |
|---|---|---|---|---|---|---|---|
| 9/3 | 1/2 of 6 | 82.0 | 12.0 | 9/23 | 1/2 of 3 | 16.0 | 13.0 |
| 9/8 | 1/2 of 6 | 71.5 | 9.0 | 9/24 | 1/2 of 6 | 14.0 | 12.0 |
| 9/9 | 1/2 of 4 | 131.0 | 20.0 | 9/25 | 1/2 of 8 | 101.0 | 30.0 |
| 9/15 | 1/2 of 6 | 148.5 | 22.0 | 9/27 | 1/2 of 4 | 50.0 | 16.0 |
| 9/16 | 2/5 of 6 | 242.0 | 24.0 | 9/28 | 1/2 of 5 | 83.5 | 21.0 |
| 9/17 | 1/2 of 7 | 200.5 | 23.0 | 9/30 | 1/2 of 7 | 26.5 | 13.0 |
| 9/21 | 1/2 of 5 | 82.0 | 13.0 | 10/2 | 8 | 5.0 | 15.0 |
| 9/22 | 1/2 of 7 | 139.0 | 22.0 | | | | |

Killed Oct. 3, 1910.

Nipples not enlarged; stained breasts nearly contiguous; margins raised; uterus moderate in size; ovaries small. Microscopically the connective tissue is old and fibrous; the medium-sized ducts have one and two layers of epithelium. In a few sections acini were present. The size and microscopical picture closely resemble that of Rabbit 14 (Fig. 27), but no corpus luteum was present. Furthermore, the pericanalicular connective tissue in Rabbit 2 is more fibrous.

### Rabbit 3.—Virgin; Nipples Just Visible

Weight 2,150 gm.; 22 injections of saline extract of ovaries of pregnant rabbits; 49 ovaries used.

| Date | Ovaries No. | Ovaries Weight, gm. | Amount of Extract Injected, c.c. | Date | Ovaries No. | Ovaries Weight, gm. | Amount of Extract Injected, c.c. |
|---|---|---|---|---|---|---|---|
| 9/3 | 2 | 2.0 | 6 | 9/21 | 2 | 0.5 | 7 |
| 9/4 | 4 | 2.0 | 9 | 9/22 | 2 | 1.0 | 7 |
| 9/5 | 2 | 1.0 | 5 | 9/23 | 2 | 0.5 | 7 |
| 9/8 | 2 | 1.0 | 7 | 9/24 | 2 | 0.5 | 6 |
| 9/9 | 2 | ... | 7 | 9/25 | 2 | 0.7 | 6 |
| 9/10 | 4 | 1.5 | 9 | 9/26 | 2 | 0.5 | 6 |
| 9/11 | 2 | 0.5 | 6 | 9/27 | 1 | 0.3 | 6 |
| 9/15 | 2 | 1.0 | 7 | 9/28 | 2 | 1.0 | 7 |
| 9/16 | 2 | 0.5 | 7 | 9/29 | 2 | 5.0 | 6 |
| 9/17 | 2 | 1.5 | 6 | 9/30 | 2 | 1.0 | 6 |
| 9/18 | 2 | 1.0 | 7 | 10/2 | 4 | 1.5 | 15 |

Killed Oct. 3, 1910.

Stained breasts much enlarged, more than in Rabbit 1; margin slightly raised; uterus and ovaries small. Microscopically many medium-sized ducts, with proliferating epithelium. The connective tissue is embryonal in type (Fig. 9).

### Rabbit 4.—Virgin; Nipples Just Visible

Weight 2,140 gm.; 22 injections of centrifuged placental extract; 120 rabbits' placentas used.

| Date | Placentas No. | Placentas Weight, gm. | Amount of Extract Injected, c.c. | Date | Placentas No. | Placentas Weight, gm. | Amount of Extract Injected, c.c. |
|---|---|---|---|---|---|---|---|
| 9/3 | 6 | 23.5 | 20 | 9/21 | 5 | 16.0 | 20 |
| 9/4 | 1 | 1.5 | 10 | 9/22 | 7 | 18.0 | 22 |
| 9/5 | 6 | 6.5 | 20 | 9/23 | 3 | 10.5 | 22 |
| 9/8 | 6 | 20.5 | 17 | 9/24 | 6 | 8.0 | 21 |
| 9/9 | 4 | 13.5 | 17 | 9/25 | 8 | 25.0 | 22 |
| 9/10 | 5 | 4.5 | 12 | 9/26 | 7 | 7.0 | 14 |
| 9/11 | 2 | 4.5 | 16 | 9/27 | 4 | 10.0 | 26 |
| 9/15 | 6 | 23.0 | 22 | 9/28 | 5 | 20.0 | 26 |
| 9/16 | 6 | 28.0 | 23 | 9/29 | 7 | 5.5 | 25 |
| 9/17 | 7 | 27.0 | 23 | 9/30 | 7 | 13.0 | 23 |
| 9/18 | 4 | 5.0 | 12 | 10/2 | 8 | 7.0 | 15 |

Killed Oct. 3, 1910.

No enlargement of breasts; uterus small; also ovaries. Microscopically there were found only small, straight ducts with a single layer of epithelium.

### Rabbit 5.—Virgin; Nipples Just Palpable

Weight 1,980 gm.; 11 injections of saline extract of hypophyses of pregnant rabbits; 11 hypophyses used.

| Date | Amount of Extract, c.c. | Date | Amount of Extract, c.c. | Date | Amount of Extract, c.c. |
|---|---|---|---|---|---|
| 9/18 | 6 | 9/25 | 6 | 9/29 | 6 |
| 9/22 | 7 | 9/26 | 6 | 9/30 | 6 |
| 9/23 | 5 | 9/27 | 6 | 10/2 | 8 |
| 9/24 | 6 | 9/28 | 6 | | |

Killed Oct. 4, 1910.

Breasts much enlarged, rather elliptical in shape; margins raised and pink; uterus vascular; fresh corpora lutea. Microscopically looks very active; many small ducts disposed about main ones (Fig. 10).

## RABBIT SERIES 2.—RABBITS INJECTED INTRAPERITONEALLY WITH EXTRACTS OF RABBIT FETUSES, OVARIES AND HYPOPHYSES

### Rabbit 1.—Virgin; Nipples Very Small

Eleven injections of centrifuged extract of rabbits' fetuses; 76 fetuses used.

| Date | Fetuses No. | Fetuses Weight, gm. | Amount of Extract Injected, c.c. | Date | Fetuses No. | Fetuses Weight, gm. | Amount of Extract Injected, c.c. |
|---|---|---|---|---|---|---|---|
| 11/11 | 1/2 of 8 | 526.0 | 23.0 | 11/17 | 1/2 of 7 | 30.5 | 20.5 |
| 11/12 | 1/2 of 7 | 72.0 | 17.0 | 11/18 | 1/2 of 6 | 33.0 | .... |
| 11/13 | 1/2 of 12 | 64.0 | 22.0 | 11/19 | 3 | 4.0 | 21.0 |
| 11/14 | 1/2 of 6 | 22.0 | 24.0 | 11/20 | 1/2 of 7 | 85.0 | 20.0 |
| 11/15 | 1/2 of 6 | 26.0 | 23.0 | 11/21 | 7 | 5.0 | 24.0 |
| 11/16 | 7 | 9.0 | 20.5 | | | | |

Killed Nov. 22, 1910.

Breasts slightly enlarged with numerous buds; uterus small. Microscopical: moderate number of medium-sized and large ducts with single layer of epithelium (Fig. 11).

### Rabbit 2.—Virgin; Nipples Very Small

Eight injections of boiled extract of rabbits' fetuses; 59 fetuses used.

| Date | Fetuses No. | Fetuses Weight, gm. | Amount of Extract Injected, c.c. | Date | Fetuses No. | Fetuses Weight, gm. | Amount of Extract Injected, c.c. |
|---|---|---|---|---|---|---|---|
| 11/11 | 1/2 of 8 | 526.0 | 23.0 | 11/15 | 1/2 of 6 | 26.0 | 20.0 |
| 11/12 | 1/2 of 7 | 72.0 | 15.0 | 11/17 | 1/2 of 7 | 30.5 | 18.0 |
| 11/13 | 1/2 of 12 | 64.0 | 15.0 | 11/18 | 1/2 of 6 | 33.0 | 21.0 |
| 11/14 | 1/2 of 6 | 22.0 | 15.0 | 11/20 | 1/2 of 7 | 85.0 | 15.5 |

Killed Nov. 21, 1910.

Breasts slightly enlarged with fair amount of buds; uterus congested; ovaries small; no corpora lutea. Microscopical: large ducts with single layer of epithelium (Fig. 12)

### Rabbit 3.—Virgin

On November 2 a breast was removed for control (Fig. 13); 11 injections of the combined saline extract of two ovaries of pregnant rabbits and one hypophyses were given daily.

| Date | Hypophyses, No. | Ovaries, No. | Amount of Extract Injected, c.c. | Date | Hypophyses, No. | Ovaries, No. | Amount of Extract Injected, c.c. |
|---|---|---|---|---|---|---|---|
| 11/11 | 1 | 2 | 9.0 | 11/17 | 1 | 2 | 9.5 |
| 11/12 | 1 | 2 | 13.0 | 11/18 | 1 | 2 | 9.0 |
| 11/13 | 1 | 2 | 16.0 | 11/19 | 1 | 2 | 9.0 |
| 11/14 | 1 | 2 | 12.0 | 11/20 | 1 | 2 | 10.0 |
| 11/15 | 1 | 2 | 8.0 | 11/21 | 1 | 2 | 9.5 |
| 11/16 | 1 | 2 | 9.0 | | | | |

Killed Nov. 22, 1910.

Breasts small, consisting of a few main ducts only; uterus congested; ovaries small. Microscopical: few ducts with single layer of epithelium (Figs. 13 and 14).

### Rabbit 4.—Virgin; Nipples Very Small

Eleven injections of centrifuged extract of rabbits' placentas; 76 placentas used.

| Date | Placentas No. | Placentas Weight, gm. | Amount of Extract Injected, c.c. | Date | Placentas No. | Placentas Weight, gm. | Amount of Extract Injected, c.c. |
|---|---|---|---|---|---|---|---|
| 11/11 | 8 | 28.0 | 25 | 11/17 | 7 | 11.0 | 25 |
| 11/12 | 7 | 16.5 | 25 | 11/18 | 6 | 12.5 | 19 |
| 11/13 | 12 | 23.0 | 25 | 11/19 | 3 | 4.0 | 22 |
| 11/14 | 6 | 9.0 | 26 | 11/20 | 7 | 20.5 | 25 |
| 11/15 | 6 | 11.0 | 23 | 11/21 | 7 | 8.0 | 17 |
| 11/16 | 7 | 7.0 | 25 | | | | |

Killed Nov. 23, 1910.

Breasts only slightly enlarged, but with many buds; chiefly large ducts with several layers of epithelium; uterus not congested; ovaries negative (Fig. 15).

## RABBIT SERIES 3.—CASTRATED RABBITS INJECTED INTRAPERITONEALLY WITH EXTRACT OF RABBITS' FETUSES, OVARIES AND HYPOPHYSES

### Rabbit 1.—Virgin

Breast removed December 6 for control; castrated through two lumbar incisions December 30; 17 injections of centrifuged extract of rabbits' fetuses; 101 fetuses used.

| Date | Fetuses No. | Fetuses Weight, gm. | Amount of Extract Injected, c.c. | Date | Fetuses No. | Fetuses Weight, gm. | Amount of Extract Injected, c.c. |
|---|---|---|---|---|---|---|---|
| 1/10 | 6 | 5.0 | 15.0 | 1/19 | 6 | 121.0 | 25.0 |
| 1/11 | 3 | 1.0 | 15.0 | 1/20 | 6 | 119.0 | 24.0 |
| 1/12 | 6 | 7.5 | 15.0 | 1/21 | 6 | 13.5 | 15.0 |
| 1/13 | 5 | 17.0 | 24.0 | 1/22 | 6 | 7.0 | 14.0 |
| 1/14 | 6 | 2.0 | 15.0 | 1/23 | 5 | 132.0 | 25.0 |
| 1/15 | 6 | 11.5 | 14.5 | 1/24 | 10 | 30.0 | 22.0 |
| 1/16 | 5 | 9.0 | 17.0 | 1/25 | 3 | 9.0 | 15.0 |
| 1/17 | 6 | 29.0 | 20.0 | 1/26 | 4 | 17.0 | 15.0 |
| 1/18 | 12 | 294.0 | 23.0 | | | | |

Killed Jan. 27, 1911.

No great increase in size compared with control breast; fewer branchings, chiefly main ducts (Figs. 16 and 17).

### Rabbit 2.—Virgin

Breast removed December 12 for control; castrated through double lumbar incision January 1; 17 injections of saline extract of pregnant rabbit ovaries; 34 ovaries used.

| Date | No. of Ovaries | Amount of Extract Injected, c.c. | Date | No. of Ovaries | Amount of Extract Injected, c.c. | Date | No. of Ovaries | Amount of Extract Injected, c.c. |
|---|---|---|---|---|---|---|---|---|
| 1/10 | 2 | 8.0 | 1/16 | 2 | 9.5 | 1/22 | 2 | 9.0 |
| 1/11 | 2 | 10.0 | 1/17 | 2 | 10.0 | 1/23 | 2 | 8.5 |
| 1/12 | 2 | 9.0 | 1/18 | 2 | 10.0 | 1/24 | 2 | 8.5 |
| 1/13 | 2 | 10.0 | 1/19 | 2 | 9.0 | 1/25 | 2 | 9.0 |
| 1/14 | 2 | 10.0 | 1/20 | 2 | 9.0 | 1/26 | 2 | 9.0 |
| 1/15 | 2 | 10.0 | 1/21 | 2 | 9.0 | | | |

Killed Jan. 27, 1911.

Enormous increase in size of breasts compared with that of controls; only main branches; no finer ducts (Figs. 18 and 19).

### Rabbit 3.—Virgin

Breast removed December 14 for control; castrated through double lumbar incisions January 1; 17 injections of saline extract of hypophyses of pregnant rabbits; one injection a day from Jan. 10, 1911, to Jan. 26, 1911; 17 hypophyses used, 1 each day.

Amount of extract, 6 c.c. each day, except January 10 (5 c.c.) and January 13 (6.5 c.c.). Rabbit killed Jan. 27, 1911.

Moderate increase in size over control breast; again only large ducts found (Figs. 20 and 21).

## RATS WITH PLACENTAL INJECTION AND OVARIAN TRANSPLANTATION

### Rat 1.—Virgin

July 13, two ovaries from pregnant rat transplanted subcutaneously in back; 16 intraperitoneal injections of rat placentas; 103 placentas used.

| Date | Placentas No. | Placentas Weight, gm. | Amount of Extract Injected, c.c. | Date | Placentas No. | Placentas Weight, gm. | Amount of Extract Injected, c.c. |
|---|---|---|---|---|---|---|---|
| 7/20 | 9 | 4.0 | 2.0 | 7/30 | 5 | 2.5 | 0.5 |
| 7/22 | 4 | ... | 1.2 | 7/31 | 7 | 3.0 | 1.5 |
| 7/23 | 8 | 4.5 | 1.5 | 8/1 | 6 | 3.0 | 1.5 |
| 7/24 | 8 | 5.5 | 1.5 | 8/3 | 9 | 4.0 | 2.0 |
| 7/25 | 6 | 3.0 | 1.0 | 8/4 | 5 | 2.2 | 2.0 |
| 7/26 | 7 | 3.0 | 1.0 | 8/5 | 5 | 2.3 | 2.0 |
| 7/27 | 3 | 2.0 | 1.0 | 8/6 | 7 | 4.0 | 2.0 |
| 7/28 | 6 | 4.0 | 1.0 | | | | |
| 7/29 | 8 | 4.0 | 1.0 | | | | |

Killed Aug. 15, 1910.

Breasts show no increase; implanted ovaries healed in; corpora lutea show necrobiosis; uterus moderately congested; ovaries negative.

### Rat 2.—Virgin

On August 4 four ovaries of pregnant rats were implanted subcutaneously in back; on August 6, 11 and 16, six ovaries in all were implanted, two on each of the days mentioned.

Killed Aug. 20, 1910.

All implanted ovaries have healed firmly; their corpora lutea show varying degrees of necrobiosis; ovaries are all well vascularized; breasts unchanged; uterus congested; ovaries show corpora lutea large and regressing.

# INDEX TO VOLUME VII


PAGE

Abdomen, pressure within; H. Emerson .......... 754
Acidosis index; T. S. Hart .......... 367
Acidosis, retention of alkali by kidney with special reference to; H. M. Adler and G. Blake .......... 479
Adams-Stokes' syndrome with heart-block, two cases of; W. S. Thayer and F. W. Peabody .......... 289
Adenitis, tuberculous retroperitoneal, connecting by a sinus with the duodenum; M. Lincoln .......... 680
Adler, Herman M., and Blake, G.: Retention of alkali by the kidney with special reference to acidosis .......... 479
Alkali, retention of, by the kidney with special reference to acidosis; H. M. Adler and G. Blake .......... 479
Allergy; C. E. von Pirquet .......... 259, 383

Bacillus-carriers, diphtheria; H. Page .......... 16
Biedl's Innere Sekretion, review of .......... 437
Blackwater fever, nature of; a manifestation of malaria or a disease sui generis? C. F. Craig .......... 56
Blackwater fever, treatment of; W. Brem .......... 153
Blake, Gerald and Adler, H. M.: Retention of alkali by the kidney with special reference to acidosis .......... 479
Blood charcoal as a clearing agent for urine containing glucose; R. T. Woodyatt, and H. F. Helmholz .......... 598
Blood, determination of the catalytic activity of, as a clinical diagnostic method; M. C. Winternitz, G. R. Henry, and F. McPhedran .......... 624
Blood-pressure, effects of intravenous injections of extracts of the various anatomical components of the hypophysis on; D. Lewis, J. L. Miller and S. A. Matthews .......... 785
Blood-pressure in tuberculosis; H. Emerson .......... 441
Bone changes, trophic value of, in the diagnosis of leprosy. A. B. Herrick and T. W. Earhart .......... 801
Book Reviews—
Biedl's Innere Sekretion .......... 437
Flexner's Medical Education in the United States and Canada .......... 134
Lusk's Elements of the Science of Nutrition .......... 58
Boos, William F., Newburgh, L. H., and Marks, H. K.: Use of digipuratum in heart-disease .......... 551
Brem, Walter: Treatment of blackwater fever .......... 153
Briggs, LeRoy H.: A blood-crisis occurring with primary sarcoma of the stomach .......... 246
Bullock, F. D., Rohdenburg, G. L., and Johnston, P. J.: Effects of certain internal secretions on malignant tumors .......... 491
Bybee, Addison and Lorenz, W. F.: Report of fifty examinations of cerebrospinal fluid with special reference to the cell-count .......... 38

Calcification and ossification; H. G. Wells .......... 721
Cammidge reaction, technic of, and the substance giving rise to the so-called typical crystals; J. C. Roper and R. G. Stillman .......... 252
Carbohydrate metabolism, study of internal function of pancreas in; J. H. Pratt and L. H. Spooner .......... 665

PAGE

Cardiac disease, diagnostic value of the orthodiagram in; J. G. van Zwaluwenburg and L. F. Warren .... 137
Cardiac disease, use of digipuratum in; W. F. Boos, L. H. Newburgh and H. K. Marks .... 551
Cardiac rate synchronous with respiratory rate; G. W. Norris .... 691
Carpenter, Thorne M., and Murlin, J. R.: Energy metabolism of mother and child just before and just after birth .... 184
Catalytic activity of the blood, determination of, as a clinical diagnostic method; M. C. Winternitz, G. R. Henry, and F. McPhedran .... 624
Cell-count, a report of fifty examinations of cerebrospinal fluid with special reference to; A. Bybee and W. F. Lorenz .... 38
Cerebrospinal fluid, a report of fifty examinations of, with special reference to the cell-count; A. Bybee and W. F. Lorenz .... 38
Child and mother, energy metabolism of, just before and just after birth; T. M. Carpenter and J. R. Murlin .... 184
Chlorid and water tolerance in nephritis; K. M. Vogel .... 602
Chlorids, excretion of, following copious water-drinking between meals; S. A. Rulon, Jr., and P. B. Hawk .... 536
Christian, Henry A.: Observations on the spirilla of relapsing fever .... 1
*Cicuta maculata*, poisoning due to eating; A. Egdahl .... 348
Cohn, Alfred E., and Kessel, L.: Function of the sino-auricular node .... 226
Complement-fixation and conglutination reactions, a study of streptococci with; H. F. Swift and W. C. Thro .... 24
Corset, meralgia paresthetica due to pressure of; J. L. Miller .... 182
Craig, Charles F.: *Entamœba tetragena* as a cause of dysentery in the Philippine Islands .... 362
Craig, Charles F.: Is hemoglobinuric fever a manifestation of malaria or a disease *sui generis?* .... 56
Crowder, Thomas R.: The ventilation of sleeping-cars .... 85

Darling, S. T.: Oriental sore in Panama .... 581
Digipuratum in heart-disease; W. F. Boos, L. H. Newburgh and H. K. Marks. 551
Diphtheria bacillus-carriers; H. Page .... 16
Duodenum, tuberculous retroperitoneal adenitis connecting by a sinus with; M. Lincoln .... 680
Duval, Charles W., and Gurd, F. B.: Studies on the biology of and immunity against the bacillus of leprosy .... 230
Dysentery, *Entamœba tetragena* as a cause of, in Philippine Islands; C. F. Craig .... 362

Earhart, T. W., and Herrick, A. B.: Value of trophic bone changes in the diagnosis of leprosy .... 801
Egdahl, Anfin: Poisoning due to eating poison-hemlock (*Cicuta maculata*) ... 348
Emerson, Haven: Blood-pressure in tuberculosis .... 441
Emerson, Haven: Intra-abdominal pressures .... 754
Energy metabolism of mother and child just before and just after birth; T. M. Carpenter and J. R. Murlin .... 184
*Entamœba tetragena* as a cause of dysentery in the Philippine Islands; C. F. Craig .... 362

Fats and oils, given subcutaneously, utilization of; L. H. Mills .... 694
Fever, blackwater, treatment of; W. Brem .... 153
Fever, relapsing, observations on the spirilla of; H. A. Christian .... 1
Flexner's Medical Education in the United States and Canada, review of.. 134
Frank, Robert T., and Unger, A.: An experimental study of the causes which produce the growth of the mammary gland .... 812

PAGE

Gage, John G.: A case of *Strongyloides intestinales* with larvæ in the sputum 561
Gastric sarcoma, blood-crisis occurring with; L. H. Briggs ............... 246
Gestation period, energy metabolism of; T. M. Carpenter and J. R. Murlin .. 184
Glucose, urine containing, blood charcoal as a clearing agent for; R. T. Woodyatt and H. F. Helmholz ............ 598
Gurd, Fraser B., and Duval, C. W.: Studies on the biology of and immunity against the bacillus of leprosy ............ 230

Hart, T. Stuart: The acidosis index ............ 367
Hattrem, W. M., and Hawk, P. B.: Intestinal putrefaction during copious and moderate water-drinking with meals ............ 610
Hawk, P. B., and Hattrem, W. M.: Intestinal putrefaction during copious and moderate water-drinking with meals ............ 610
Hawk, P. B., and Rulon, Jr., S. A.: Excretion of chlorids following copious water-drinking between meals ............ 536
Heart-block, two cases of Adams-Stokes' syndrome with; W. S. Thayer and F. W. Peabody ............ 289
Heart-disease, diagnostic value of orthodiagram in; J. G. Van Zwaluwenburg and L. F. Warren ............ 137
Heart-disease, digipuratum in; W. F. Boos, L. H. Newburgh and H. K. Marks 551
Heart, function of sino-auricular node of; A. E. Cohn and L. Kessel ........ 226
Heart-rate synchronous with respiratory rate; G. W. Norris .............. 691
Helmholz, Henry F.: Pyrogenic action of salt solutions in rabbits ......... 468
Helmholz, H. F., and Woodyatt, R. T.: Use of blood charcoal as a clearing agent for urine containing glucose ............ 598
Hemoglobinuria, erythrolytic, pernicious anemia with; W. Brem .......... 153
Hemoglobinuric fever, nature of: a manifestation of malaria or a disease *sui generis?* C. F. Craig ............ 56
Henry, G. R., McPhedran, F., and Winternitz, M. C.: Determination of the catalytic activity of the blood as a clinical diagnostic method ......... 624
Herrick, A. B., and Earhart, T. W.: Value of trophic bone changes in the diagnosis of leprosy ............ 801
Hypophysis, effects on blood-pressure of intravenous injections of extracts of the various anatomical components of; D. Lewis, J. L. Miller and S. A. Matthews ............ 785

Intestinal putrefaction during copious and moderate water-drinking with meals; W. M. Hattrem and P. B. Hawk ............ 610

Johnston, P. J., Rohdenburg, G. L., and Bullock, F. D.: Effects of certain internal secretions on malignant tumors ............ 491

Kessel, Leo and Cohn, A. E.: Function of the sino-auricular node .......... 226
Kidney, retention of alkali by, with special reference to acidosis; H. M. Adler and G. Blake ............ 479

Leishmaniosis in Panama; S. T. Darling ............ 581
Lenhart, C. H., and Marine, D.: Pathological anatomy of the human thyroid gland ............ 506
Leprosy, studies on the biology of and immunity against the bacillus of; C. W. Duval and F. B. Gurd ............ 230
Leprosy, value of trophic bone changes in diagnosis of; A. B. Herrick and T. W. Earhart ............ 801
Lewis, Dean, Miller, J. L., and Matthews, S. A.: Effects on blood-pressure of intravenous injections of extracts of the various anatomical components of the hypophysis ............ 785
Lincoln, Merrick: Tuberculous retroperitoneal adenitis connecting by a sinus with the duodenum ............ 680

PAGE
Liver, acute yellow atrophy of; E. Novak and E. L. Whitney .............. 376
Lorenz, W. F., and Bybee, A.: Report of fifty examinations of cerebrospinal fluid with special reference to the cell-count ....................... 38
Lusk's Elements of the Science of Nutrition, review of .................. 580

Malaria, alleged relation of hemoglobinuric fever to; C. F. Craig ......... 56
Malaria, pernicious, with erythrolytic hemoglobinuria; W. Brem ........... 153
Mammary gland, an experimental study of the causes which produce the growth of; R. T. Frank and A. Unger ............................ 812
Marine, David, and Lenhart, C. H.: Pathological anatomy of the human thyroid gland ................................................ 506
Marks, Henry K., Boos, W. F., and Newburgh, L. H.: Use of digipuratum in heart-disease ............................................... 551
Matthews, S. A., Lewis, D., and Miller, J. L.: Effects on the blood-pressure of intravenous injections of extracts of the various anatomical components of the hypophysis ..................................... 785
McPhedran, F., Winternitz, M. C., and Henry, G. R.: Determination of the catalytic activity of the blood as a clinical diagnostic method ......... 624
Medical Education in the United States and Canada, by Abraham Flexner, review of ................................................ 134
Megaloblasts, ameboid activity of; W. S. Thayer ........................ 223
Meralgia paresthetica due to pressure of the corset; J. L. Miller .......... 182
Metabolism, carbohydrate, study of internal function of pancreas in; J. H. Pratt and L. H. Spooner ....................................... 665
Miller, Joseph L.: Meralgia paresthetica due to pressure of the corset ...... 182
Miller, Joseph L., Matthews, S. A., and Lewis, D.: Effects on blood-pressure of intravenous injections of extracts of the various anatomical components of the hypophysis ...................................... 785
Mills, Lloyd H.: Utilization of fats and oils given subcutaneously .......... 694
Mother and child, energy metabolism of, just before and just after birth; T. M. Carpenter and J. R. Murlin ................................ 184
Murlin, John R., and Carpenter, T. M.: Energy metabolism of mother and child just before and just after birth ............................. 184

Nephritis, chlorid and water tolerance in; K. M. Vogel .................. 602
Newburgh, L. H., Marks, H. K., and Boos, W. F.: Use of digipuratum in heart-disease ............................................... 551
Node, sino-auricular, function of; A. E. Cohn and L. Kessel .............. 226
Norris, George William: Synchronous cardiac and respiratory rate ........ 691
Novak, Emil and Whitney, E. L.: Acute yellow atrophy of the liver ........ 376
Nutrition, Elements of the Science of, by Graham Lusk, review of ......... 580

Oils and fats, given subcutaneously, utilization of; L. H. Mills ............ 694
Opsonic index in diagnosis of mixed infection in pulmonary tuberculosis; R. T. Pettit ................................................ 357
Oriental sore in Panama; S. T. Darling .................................. 581
Orthodiagram, diagnostic value of, in heart disease; J. G. Van Zwaluwenburg and L. F. Warren ........................................... 137
Ossification and calcification; H. G. Wells .............................. 721
Owen, Robert Goldsborough: Schürmann's color test for syphilis ........... 52

Page, Henry: Diphtheria bacillus-carriers ............................... 16
Panama, Oriental sore in; S. T. Darling .................................. 581
Pancreas, study of internal function of, in carbohydrate metabolism; J. H. Pratt and L. H. Spooner ....................................... 665
Peabody, F. W., and Thayer, W. S.: A study of two cases of Adams-Stokes' syndrome with heart-block ......................................... 289

PAGE

Pettit, Roswell T.: The opsonic index in the diagnosis of mixed infection in pulmonary tuberculosis ........ 357
Philippine Islands, dysentery in, *Entamœba tetragena* as a cause of; C. F. Craig ........ 362
Pirquet, C. E., von: Allergy ........ 259, 383
Poison-hemlock, poisoning due to eating; A. Egdahl ........ 348
Pratt, Joseph H., and Spooner, L. H.: The internal function of the pancreas in carbohydrate metabolism ........ 665
Pressures, intra-abdominal; H. Emerson ........ 754
Pyrogenic action of salt solutions in rabbits; H. F. Helmholz ........ 468

Rabbits, pyrogenic action of salt solutions in; H. F. Helmholz ........ 468
Reaction, Cammidge, technic of, and the substance giving rise to the so-called typical crystals; J. C. Roper and R. G. Stillman ........ 252
Reactions, complement-fixation and conglutination, a study of streptococci with; H. F. Swift and W. C. Thro ........ 24
Relapsing fever, observations on the spirilla of; H. A. Christian ........ 1
Respiratory rate synchronous with cardiac rate; G. W. Norris ........ 691
Rohdenburg, G. L., Bullock, F. D., and Johnston, P. J.: Effects of certain internal secretions on malignant tumors ........ 491
Roper, Joseph C., and Stillman, R. G.: Technic of the Cammidge reaction and the substance giving rise to the so-called typical crystals ........ 252
Rulon, Jr., S. A., and Hawk, P. B.: Excretion of chlorids following copious water-drinking between meals ........ 536

Salt solutions, pyrogenic action of, in rabbits; H. F. Helmholz ........ 468
Sarcoma, primary, of the stomach, blood-crisis occurring with: L. H. Briggs. 246
Schürmann's color test for syphilis; R. G. Owen ........ 52
Sekretion, innere, by Artur Biedl, review of ........ 437
Sino-auricular node, function of; A. E. Cohn and L. Kessel ........ 226
Sleeping-cars, ventilation of; T. R. Crowder ........ 85
Spooner, Lesley H., and Pratt, J. H.: Study of the internal function of the pancreas in carbohydrate metabolism ........ 665
Stillman, Ralph G., and Roper, J. C.: Technic of the Cammidge reaction and the substance giving rise to the so-called typical crystals ........ 252
Stomach, blood-crisis occurring with primary sarcoma of; L. H. Briggs ........ 246
Streptococci, a study of, with the complement-fixation and conglutination reactions; H. F. Swift and W. C. Thro ........ 24
*Strongyloides intestinalis*, case of, with larvæ in the sputum; J. G. Gage ........ 561
Swift, Homer F., and Thro, W. C.: A study of streptococci with the complement-fixation and conglutination reactions ........ 24
Syphilis, Schürmann's color test for; R. G. Owen ........ 52

Thayer, William Sydney: Ameboid activity of megaloblasts ........ 223
Thayer, W. S., and Peabody, F. W.: A study of two cases of Adams-Stokes' syndrome with heart-block ........ 289
Thro, W. C., and Swift, Homer F.: A study of streptococci with the complement-fixation and conglutination reactions ........ 24
Thyroid gland, human, pathological anatomy of; D. Marine and C. H. Lenhart ........ 506
Todd, John L.: Duration of trypanosome infections ........ 500
Trypanosome infections, duration of; J. L. Todd ........ 500
Tuberculosis, blood-pressure in; H. Emerson ........ 441
Tuberculosis, pulmonary, opsonic index in diagnosis of mixed infection in; R. T. Pettit ........ 357
Tumors, malignant, effects of certain internal secretions on; G. L. Rohdenburg, F. D. Bullock and P. J. Johnston ........ 491

PAGE

Unger, A., and Frank, R. T.: An experimental study of the causes which produce the growth of the mammary gland .......... 812
Urine containing glucose, blood charcoal as a clearing agent for; R. T. Woodyatt and H. F. Helmholz .......... 598

Van Zwaluwenburg, J. G., and Warren, L. F.: Diagnostic value of the orthodiagram in heart-disease .......... 137
Ventilation of sleeping-cars; T. R. Crowder .......... 85
Vogel, Karl M.: Chlorid and water tolerance in nephritis .......... 602
Von Pirquet, C. E.: Allergy .......... 259, 383

Warren, L. F., and Van Zwaluwenburg, J. G.: Diagnostic value of the orthodiagram in heart-disease .......... 137
Water and chlorid tolerance in nephritis; K. M. Vogel .......... 602
Water-drinking, studies on; S. A. Rulon, Jr., and P. B. Hawk .......... 536
Water-drinking, studies on; W. M. Hattrem and P. B. Hawk .......... 610
Wells, H. Gideon: Calcification and ossification .......... 721
Whitney, E. L., and Novak, E.: Acute yellow atrophy of the liver .......... 376
Winternitz, M. C., Henry, G. R., and McPhedran, F.: Determination of the catalytic activity of the blood as a clinical diagnostic method .......... 624
Woodyatt, R. T., and Helmholz, H. F.: Use of blood charcoal as a clearing agent for urine containing glucose .......... 598